EIGHTH EDITION   VOLUME ONE

TEXTBOOK OF
DIAGNOSTIC SONOGRAPHY

EIGHTH EDITION   VOLUME ONE

TEXTBOOK OF
DIAGNOSTIC
SONOGRAPHY

Sandra L. Hagen-Ansert, MS,
RDMS, RDCS, FASE, FSDMS

Cardiology Department
Manager, Echo Labs
Scripps Clinic & Hospitals—La Jolla, California

ELSEVIER

ELSEVIER

3251 Riverport Lane
St. Louis, MO 63043

TEXTBOOK OF DIAGNOSTIC SONOGRAPHY, EIGHTH EDITION   ISBN: 978-0-323-35375-5

Notices

Knowledge and best practice in this field are constantly changing. As new research and experience broaden our understanding, changes in research methods, professional practices, or medical treatment may become necessary.

Practitioners and researchers must always rely on their own experience and knowledge in evaluating and using any information, methods, compounds, or experiments described herein. In using such information or methods they should be mindful of their own safety and the safety of others, including parties for whom they have a professional responsibility.

With respect to any drug or pharmaceutical products identified, readers are advised to check the most current information provided (i) on procedures featured or (ii) by the manufacturer of each product to be administered, to verify the recommended dose or formula, the method and duration of administration, and contraindications. It is the responsibility of practitioners, relying on their own experience and knowledge of their patients, to make diagnoses, to determine dosages and the best treatment for each individual patient, and to take all appropriate safety precautions.

To the fullest extent of the law, neither the Publisher nor the authors, contributors, or editors, assume any liability for any injury and/or damage to persons or property as a matter of products liability, negligence or otherwise, or from any use or operation of any methods, products, instructions, or ideas contained in the material herein.

Previous editions copyrighted 2012, 2006, 2001, 1995, 1989, 1983, and 1978.

International Standard Book Number: 978-0-323-35375-5

Executive Content Strategist: Sonya Seigafuse
Content Development Manager: Lisa P. Newton
Content Development Specialist: Betsy McCormac
Publishing Services Manager: Julie Eddy
Senior Project Manager: Marquita Parker
Design Direction: Amy Buxton

Working together
to grow libraries in
developing countries

www.elsevier.com • www.bookaid.org

Printed in China
Last digit is the print number: 9 8 7 6 5 4 3

To my family,
Art, Becca and Eric, Aly, and Kati,
who mean the world to me

CONTRIBUTORS

Alicia Armour, MA, BS, RDCS
Cardiovascular Sonographer
Duke University Health System
Duke Cardiac Diagnostic Unit,
    Level III
Durham, North Carolina

Joan P. Baker
President, Sound Ergonomics
Kenmore, Washington

Carolyn Coffin
CEO, Sound Ergonomics
Kenmore, Washington

Marveen Craig, RDMS
Tucson, Arizona

M. Robert DeJong, RDMS, RVT, FAIUM, FSDMS
Radiology Technical Manager,
    Ultrasound
The Johns Hopkins Hospital
Baltimore, Maryland

Terry J. DuBose, MS, RDMS, FSDMS, FAIUM
Associate Professor Emeritus
Diagnostic Medical Sonography
University of Arkansas for Medical
    Sciences
Austin, Texas

Pamela M. Foy, MS, RDMS, FSDMS
Maternal Fetal Medicine
Imaging Manager
Clinical Associate Professor,
    Department of OB/GYN
Columbus, Ohio

Candace Goldstein, BS, RDMS
Sonographer Educator Scripps Clinics
Scripps Clinic–Carmel Valley
San Diego, California

Joy Guthrie, PhD, RDMS, RDCS, RVT, FSDMS
Advanced Practice Sonographer
Program Director Diagnostic Medical
    Sonography
Community Regional Medical Center
Fresno, California

Charlotte G. Henningsen, MS, RT(R), RDMS, RVT, FSDMS, FAIUM, ADU, RT(R)
Chair and Professor
Sonography Department
Adventist University of Health
    Sciences
Orlando, Florida

Talisha Hunt, BSRT, RDMS, RDCS, RVT
Clinical Sonographer
Mayo Clinic, Department of
    Sonography
Rochester, Minnesota

Mariana Kozirovsky, MS, RDMS, RDCS
Assistant Professor
Long Island University
Brooklyn, New York
Research Scientist
NYU School of Medicine
New York, New York

Fredrick W. Kremkau, PhD, RACR, FAIMBE, FAIUM, FASA
Professor of Radiologic Sciences
Director, Program for Medical
    Ultrasound
Center for Applied Learning
Wake Forest University School of
    Medicine
Winston-Salem, North Carolina

Daniel I. Lebovic, MD
Reproductive Endocrinologist/Fertility
    Specialist
Center for Reproductive Medicine
Minneapolis, Minnesota

Daniel A. Merton, BS, RDMS, FSDMS, FAIUM
ECRI Institute
Senior Project Officer
Health Devices Group
Plymouth Meeting, Pennsylvania

Carol Mitchell, PhD, RDMS, RDCS, RVT, RT(R), FASE, FSDMS
University of Wisconsin
    Atherosclerosis Imaging Research
    Program
Assistant Professor
Section of Cardiovascular Medicine
Madison, Wisconsin

Cindy A. Owen, RT, RDMS, RVT, FSDMS
Global Luminary and Research
    Manager
Radiology and Vascular Ultrasound
GE Healthcare
Milwaukee, Wisconsin

Susan Raatz Stephenson, MEd, BSRT-U, RDMS, RT(R)(C)
International Foundation for
    Sonography Education and
    Research
AIUMcommunities.org
Sandy, Utah

Deziree Rada, RDMS, RVT
Sonography Department
Adventist University of Health Sciences
Orlando, Florida

Mitzi Roberts, EdD, RDMS, RDCS, RT(R)
Director of Institutional Effectiveness
Baptist College of Health Science
Memphis, Tennessee

Jean Lea Spitz, MPH, RDMS
Nuchal Translucency Quality Review
    Program
Maternal Fetal Medicine Foundation
Oklahoma City, Oklahoma

Diana M. Strickland, BS, RDMS, RDCS
Clinical Assistant Professor and
    Co-Director
Ultrasound Program
Department of Obstetrics and
    Gynecology
Brody School of Medicine
East Carolina University
Greenville, North Carolina

Shpetim Telegrafi, MD
Assistant Professor
Director, Diagnostic Ultrasound
NYU School of Medicine, Department
    of Urology
New York City, New York

Barbara Trampe, RN, RDMS
Chief Sonographer
Meriter/University of Wisconsin
    Perinatal Ultrasound
Madison, Wisconsin

Kevin R. Volz, PhD, RVT
Research Lab Manager
Laboratory for Investigatory Imaging
Instructor/Vascular Technology
    Clinical Coordinator
School of Health and Rehabilitation
    Sciences
Division of Radiologic Sciences and
    Therapy
Ohio State University–College of
    Medicine
Columbus, Ohio

**Kerry Weinberg, PhD, RDMS, RDCS,
    RT(R), FSDMS**
Director and Associate Professor
Diagnostic Medical Sonography
    Program
Long Island University–Brooklyn Campus
Brooklyn, New York

Marquita Williams, BS, RDMS
Technical Site Manager
Ultrasound System Modality Manager
Florida Hospital Radiology Enterprise
Orlando, Florida

Janette Wybo, BAS, RDMS, RDCS, RVT
Diagnostic Medical Sonography
    Program Coordinator
Providence Hospital/Madonna
    University
Southfield, Michigan

**Kathryn E. Zale, MS, BA, RDMS,
    RVT**
Former Clinical Coordinator
    Sonography/Vascular Technology
Radiologic Sciences and Therapy
Ohio State University–College of
    Medicine
Columbus, Ohio

Sheena Bhimji-Hewitt, MAppSc, RVT, RDMS, CRGS
Professor
The Michener Institute for Applied Health Sciences
Toronto, Ontario, Canada

Scott Andrew Blanchard, RDMS
Sonography Instructor
Meridian College
Sarasota, Florida
Ultrasound Program Director
Gwinnett College
Lilburn, Georgia

Marcia J. Cooper
Clinical Coordinator
Diagnostic Medical Sonography Program
Morehead State University
Morehead, Kentucky

Theresa L. Moore, RT/RDMS
Adjunct Faculty
Delaware Technical Community College
Wilmington, Delaware

Catherine E. Rienzo, MS, RT(R), RDMS, FSDMS
Professor and Program Director
Diagnostic Medical Sonography Program
Northampton Community College
Bethlehem, Pennsylvania

INTRODUCING THE EIGHTH EDITION

The eighth edition of *Textbook of Diagnostic Sonography* continues the tradition of excellence that began when the first edition was published in 1978. Like other medical imaging fields, diagnostic sonography has seen dramatic changes and innovations since its first clinical experimental days. Phenomenal strides in transducer design, instrumentation, three-dimensional (3D) and four-dimensional (4D) imaging, image processing, tissue harmonics, and contrast agents continue to improve image resolution and the diagnostic clinical value of sonography. The eighth edition has kept abreast of advancements in the field by inviting new contributors currently working in different areas of medical sonography throughout the country. The critiques and suggestions from multiple reviewers have helped ensure that this edition includes the most complete and up-to-date information needed to meet the requirements of the modern student of sonography.

Distinctive Approach

This textbook can serve as an in-depth resource both for students of sonography and for practitioners in any number of clinical settings, including hospitals, clinics, and private practices. Care has been taken to cultivate readers' understanding of the patient's total clinical picture even as they study sonographic examination protocol and technique. To this end, each chapter covers the following:

- Key terminology
- Normal anatomy (including cross-sectional anatomy)
- Normal physiology
- Laboratory data and values
- Pathology
- Sonographic evaluation of an organ
- Sonographic findings
- Pitfalls in sonography
- Clinical findings
- Differential considerations
- "Key Pearls"

The full-color art program is of great value to the student of anatomy and pathology for sonography. Detailed line drawings illustrate the anatomic information a sonographer must know to successfully perform specific sonographic examinations. Multiple color photographs of gross pathology help the reader visualize some of the pathology presented, and color Doppler illustrations are included where relevant.

To make important information easy to find, key points are pulled out into numerous boxes; tables throughout the chapters summarize the pathology under discussion and break the information down into Clinical Findings, Sonographic Findings, and Differential Considerations.

Sonographic findings for particular pathologic conditions are always preceded in the text by the following special heading:

Sonographic Findings This icon makes it very easy for students and practicing sonographers to locate this clinical information quickly.

Study and Review Opportunities

Study and review are also essential to gaining a solid grasp of the concepts and information presented in this textbook. Learning objectives, chapter outlines, "Key Pearls" that summarize the chapter highlights, comprehensive glossaries of key terms, full references for cited material, and a list of common medical abbreviations printed on the inside back cover all help students learn the material in an organized and thorough manner.

Scope and Organization of Topics

The *Textbook of Diagnostic Sonography* is divided into eight parts:

Part I introduces the reader to the foundations of sonography and patient care and includes the following:
- Foundations of sonography, which includes the basic principles of ultrasound physics and medical sonography
- Terminology frequently encountered by the sonographer
- Patient care for the sonographer
- Ergonomics and musculoskeletal issues for practitioners
- Anatomic and physiologic relationships within the abdominopelvic cavity
- Comparative sectional anatomy of the abdominopelvic cavity
- Imaging and Doppler artifacts

Part II presents the abdomen in depth. The following topics are discussed:
- Anatomic relationships and physiology
- Abdominal scanning techniques and protocols
- Abdominal applications of ultrasound contrast agents
- Ultrasound-guided interventional techniques
- Emergent abdominal ultrasound procedures
- Sonographic techniques in the transplant patient
- Separate chapters for the vascular system, liver, gallbladder and biliary system, spleen, pancreas, gastrointestinal tract, urinary system, retroperitoneum, and peritoneal cavity and abdominal wall

Part III focuses on the superficial structures of the body, including the breast, thyroid and parathyroid glands, scrotum, and musculoskeletal system.

Part IV is completely new and explores sonographic examination of the neonate and pediatric patient.

Part **V** focuses on the thoracic cavity and includes the following topics:
- Anatomic and physiologic relationships within the thoracic cavity
- Hemodynamics
- Echocardiographic evaluation and techniques
- Introduction to clinical echocardiography
- Fetal echocardiography

Part **VI** comprises four chapters on extracranial and intracranial cerebrovascular imaging and peripheral arterial and venous sonographic evaluation.

Part **VII** is devoted to gynecology and includes the following topics:
- Normal anatomy and physiology of the female pelvis
- Sonographic and Doppler evaluation of the female pelvis
- Separate chapters on the pathologic conditions of the uterus, ovaries, and adnexa
- Updated chapter on the role of sonography in evaluating female infertility

Part **VIII** takes a thorough look at obstetric sonography. The following topics are discussed:
- The role of sonography in obstetrics
- Clinical ethics for obstetric sonography
- Normal first-trimester findings and first-trimester complications
- Sonography of the second and third trimesters
- Obstetric measurements and gestational age and fetal growth assessment
- Sonography in the high-risk pregnancy
- Prenatal diagnosis of congenital anomalies
- Chapters are devoted to the placenta, umbilical cord, amniotic fluid and fetal membranes, fetal face and neck, neural axis, thorax, anterior abdominal wall, abdomen, urogenital system, and skeleton

New to This Edition

Eight new contributors joined the eighth edition to update and expand existing content, bringing with them a fresh perspective and an impressive knowledge base. They also helped contribute the more than 1000 images new to this edition, including color Doppler, 3D and 4D, and contrast-enhanced images. More than 30 new line drawings complement the new chapters found in the eighth edition.

Essentials of Patient Care for the Sonographer (Chapter 2) covers all aspects of patient care the sonographer may encounter, including taking and understanding vital signs, handling patients on strict bed rest, patients with tubes and oxygen, patient transfer techniques, infection control, isolation techniques, emergency medical situations, assisting patients with special needs, and patient rights.

Ergonomics and Musculoskeletal Issues in Sonography (Chapter 3) outlines the importance of proper technique and positioning throughout the sonographic examination as a way to avoid long-term disability problems that may be acquired with repetitive scanning.

Anatomic and Physiologic Relationships within the Abdominopelvic Cavity (Chapter 4) introduces the reader to body systems and anatomic relationships, which include membranes and ligaments and potential spaces in the body.

Comparative Sectional Anatomy of the Abdominopelvic Cavity (Chapter 5) is an introduction to sectional anatomy incorporating gross anatomy with comparative ultrasound and computed tomography sectional images.

Basic Ultrasound Imaging: Techniques, Terminology, and Tips (Chapter 6) describes scanning techniques, terminology, abdominal ultrasound protocol, and abdominal Doppler technique.

Imaging and Doppler Artifacts (Chapter 7) is an outstanding review of all the artifacts commonly encountered by sonographers. There are numerous examples of the various artifacts and detailed explanations of how these artifacts are produced and how to avoid them.

Sonographic Techniques in the Transplant Patient (Chapter 20) is completely new to this edition and focuses on criteria required for organ transplantation, including liver transplant, renal transplant, and pancreatic transplant.

Thyroid and Parathyroid Glands (Chapter 22) is completely updated with beautiful illustrations.

The entire pediatrics section (Chapters 25 to 29) has been fully updated with exquisite new illustrations for each chapter.

Understanding Hemodynamics (Chapter 31) introduces the student to blood flow dynamics, intracardiac pressures and volumes, Doppler basics, and quantification of intracardiac pressures by ultrasound.

Introduction to Clinical Echocardiography: Left-Sided Valvular Heart Disease (Chapter 33) and *Introduction to Clinical Echocardiography: Pericardial Disease, Cardiomyopathies, and Tumors* (Chapter 34) have been added to this edition to provide understanding of significant cardiac findings that may be encountered by the general sonographer or clinician.

The entire cerebrovascular section (Chapters 37 to 40) has been updated with new images and current techniques for the sonographer.

Student Resources

Workbook. Available for separate purchase, *Workbook for Textbook of Diagnostic Sonography* has also been completely updated and expanded. This resource gives the learner ample opportunity to practice and apply the information presented in the textbook.
- Each workbook chapter covers all the material presented in the textbook.
- Each chapter includes exercises on image identification, anatomy identification, key term definitions, and sonographic technique.
- A set of 30 case studies using images from the textbook invites students to test their skills at identifying key anatomy and pathology and describing and interpreting sonographic findings.
- Students can also test their knowledge with the hundreds of multiple-choice questions found in the four

examinations covering different content areas: General Sonography, Pediatric, Cardiovascular Anatomy, and Obstetrics and Gynecology.

Evolve. On the Evolve site, students will find review questions for each chapter.

Instructor Resources

Resources for instructors are also provided on the Evolve site to assist in the preparation of classroom lectures and activities.

- PowerPoint lectures for each chapter that include illustrations
- Test bank of 1500 multiple-choice questions in Examview and Word
- Electronic image collection that includes all the images from the textbook both in PowerPoint and in jpeg format

Evolve Online Course Management. *Evolve* is an interactive learning environment designed to work in coordination with *Textbook of Diagnostic Sonography*. Instructors may use *Evolve* to include an Internet-based course component that reinforces and expands on the concepts delivered in class. *Evolve* may be used to do all of the following:

- Publish the class syllabus, outlines, and lecture notes
- Set up virtual office hours and email communication
- Share important dates and information on the online class calendar
- Encourage student participation with chat rooms and discussion boards
- Post examinations and manage grade books

For more information, visit http://www.evolve.elsevier.com/HagenAnsert/diagnostic/ or contact an Elsevier sales representative.

ACKNOWLEDGMENTS

I would like to express my gratitude and appreciation to a number of individuals who have served as mentors and guides throughout my years in sonography. Of course it all began with Dr. George Leopold at UCSD Medical Center. His quest for knowledge and his perseverance for excellence have been the mainstay of my career in sonography. I would also like to recognize Drs. Dolores Pretorius, Nancy Budorick, Wanda Miller-Hance, and David Sahn for their encouragement throughout the years at the UCSD Medical Center in both Radiology and Pediatric Cardiology.

I would also like to acknowledge Dr. Barry Goldberg for the opportunity he gave me to develop countless numbers of educational programs in sonography in an independent fashion and for his encouragement to pursue advancement. I would also like to thank Dr. Daniel Yellon for his early-hour anatomy dissection and instruction; Dr. Carson Schneck, for his excellent instruction in gross anatomy and sections of "Geraldine"; and Dr. Jacob Zutuchni, for his enthusiasm for the field of cardiology.

I am grateful to Dr. Harry Rakowski for his continued support in teaching fellows and students while I was at the Toronto Hospital. Dr. William Zwiebel encouraged me to continue writing and teaching while I was at the University of Wisconsin Medical Center, and I appreciate his knowledge, which found its way into the liver physiology section of this textbook.

My good fortune in learning about and understanding the *total patient* must be attributed to a very dedicated cardiologist, James Glenn, with whom I had the pleasure of working while I was at MUSC in Charleston, South Carolina. It was through his compassion and knowledge that I grew to appreciate the total patient beyond the transducer, and for this I am grateful.

For their continual support, feedback, and challenges, I would like to thank and recognize all the students I have taught in the various diagnostic medical sonography programs: Episcopal Hospital, Thomas Jefferson University Medical Center, University of Wisconsin-Madison Medical Center, UCSD Medical Center, and Baptist College of Health Science. These students continually work toward the development of quality sonography techniques and protocols and have given back to the sonography community tenfold.

The continual push toward excellence has been encouraged on a daily basis by our Medical Director of the Echo Lab, Dr. David Rubenson and outstanding staff of Scripps Clinic Cardiologists.

The Cardiac Sonographers at Scripps Clinic have been invaluable in their excellent image acquisition. Special thanks to Kristen Billick for her excellent echocardiographic images. The general sonographers at Scripps Clinic have been invaluable in providing the outstanding images for the obstetrics and gynecology chapters.

I would like to thank the very supportive and capable staff at Elsevier who have guided me though yet another edition of this textbook. Megan Chandler and Betsy McCormac and their staff are to be commended on their perseverance to make this an outstanding textbook.

I would like to thank my family, Art, Becca, Aly, and Kati, for their patience and understanding, as I thought this edition would never come to an end.

I think that you will find the 8th Edition of the *Textbook of Diagnostic Sonography* reflects the contribution of so many individuals with attention to detail and a dedication to excellence. I hope you will find this educational experience in sonography as rewarding as I have.

Sandra L. Hagen-Ansert
MS, RDMS, RDCS, FASE, FSDMS

CONTENTS

PART III Superficial Structures

PART IV Pediatrics

VOLUME TWO

PART V The Thoracic Cavity

Part VI Cerebrovascular

PART I

Foundations of Sonography

Foundations of Clinical Sonography

Sandra L. Hagen-Ansert

OBJECTIVES

On completion of this chapter, you should be able to:
- Describe the role of the sonographer and the career path
- Know the historical developments in medical ultrasound
- List the basic principles and terminology of medical ultrasound
- Identify the transducers necessary for specific ultrasound applications
- Explain the multiple display modes on ultrasound instrumentation
- State the Doppler effect

OUTLINE

The Role of the Sonographer
Historical Overview of Sound Theory and Medical Ultrasound
Introduction to Basic Ultrasound Principles
    Acoustics

Transducer Selection
Pulse-Echo Display Modes
Harmonic Imaging
Three-Dimensional and Four-Dimensional Ultrasound

System Controls for Image Optimization
Doppler Ultrasound

KEY TERMS

Absorption
Acoustic impedance
Aliasing
Amplitude
Angle of incidence
Angle of reflection
Attenuation
Axial resolution
Azimuthal resolution
Color flow Doppler
Compression
Continuous wave (CW) Doppler
Crystal
Cycle
Decibel (dB)
Doppler angle
Doppler shift
Dynamic range
Far field (Fraunhofer zone)

Focal zone
Frame rate
Frequency
Gain
Gate
Gray scale
Hertz (Hz)
Intensity
Interface
Kilohertz (kHz)
Laminar
Lateral resolution
Megahertz (MHz)
Near field (Fresnel zone)
Nyquist limit
Piezoelectric effect
Power
Pulse duration
Pulse repetition frequency (PRF)

Pulsed wave (PW) Doppler
Rarefaction
Real-time
Reflection
Refraction
Resistance
Resolution
Scattering
Slice thickness
Spectral analysis
Spectral broadening
Temporal resolution
Time gain compensation (TGC)
Transducer
Velocity
Wave
Wavelength

The primary purpose of this chapter is to introduce the sonographer to the fascinating field of diagnostic medical ultrasound. Historians will tell us that we cannot know where we are going until we know where we have been. Therefore a brief background into the historical development of ultrasound will be presented to enable the sonographer to understand the progress that has been made with technology in the medical application of ultrasound. It is important for sonographers to understand their role in the health care field, as well as to have a global concept of anatomic reconstruction. An introduction into the terminology of the basic principles of ultrasound is critical for the student to understand how and why an anatomic image appears as it does on the ultrasound monitor.

The terms *diagnostic medical ultrasound, ultrasound,* and *ultrasonography* have all been used to describe the instrumentation used in ultrasound. *Sonography* is the term used to describe a specialized imaging technique to visualize soft tissue structures in the body. The term *echocardiography,* or simple *"echo,"* refers to an ultrasound examination of only the cardiac structures.

A *sonographer* is a member of the allied health professions who has received specialized education in diagnostic medical sonography and has successfully completed the national boards given by the American Registry of Diagnostic Medical Sonography. A *sonologist* is a physician who has received specialized training in ultrasound and has successfully completed the national boards granted by their respective specialty (radiology, cardiology, obstetrics, etc.).

The field of diagnostic medical ultrasound has grown to become a well-respected and valuable addition to diagnostic imaging by providing pertinent clinical information to the physician and to the patient. The applications of ultrasound are extensive; they include, but are not limited to, the following areas:

1. General ultrasound (abdominal, renal, retroperitoneal, chest)
2. Superficial ultrasound (breast, thyroid, scrotum)
3. Neonatal and pediatric ultrasound (abdomen, renal, hips, brain, spine)
4. Echocardiography (adult, pediatric, neonatal, fetal)
5. Interventional and therapeutic-guided ultrasound
6. Obstetric and gynecologic ultrasound
7. Intraoperative ultrasound
8. Musculoskeletal ultrasound
9. Ophthalmologic ultrasound
10. Point-of-care ultrasound

Extensive research has verified the safety of ultrasound as a diagnostic procedure. No harmful effects of ultrasound have been demonstrated at power levels used for diagnostic studies when performed by qualified and nationally certified sonographers, under the direction of qualified and board-certified sonologists, using appropriate equipment and techniques.

Diagnostic ultrasound has developed into a valuable imaging technique for many reasons. First is the lack of ionizing radiation for the ultrasound procedure compared with the various other imaging modalities, such as computed tomography (CT) or nuclear medicine. The second reason is the portability of the ultrasound equipment. Even the high-end ultrasound equipment may be moved into the intensive care unit, emergency department, operating room, cardiac catheter laboratory, or small doctor's office. The low-end systems are now so portable, they can fit into the physician's laboratory coat to be used at the bedside as an *initial quick look* evaluation of the patient physical examination.

Ultrasound is unique in other ways as well. The ultrasound image is presented in a real-time cine clip format, which makes it possible to see the image transition from one cardiac structure to another, or from one organ system to another. The flexible multiplanar imaging capability allows the sonographer to "follow" the path of a tortuous vessel, a moving cardiac structure, or a moving fetus to capture the necessary images. Moreover, Doppler techniques allow the qualitative and quantitative evaluation of blood flow hemodynamics within a vessel. Finally, the cost analysis of an ultrasound system is superior compared with the other imaging diagnostic systems.

Today nearly every hospital and medical clinic has some form of ultrasound instrumentation to provide the clinician with an inside look at the soft tissue structures within the body. Ultrasound manufacturers continue their research to improve image acquisition, develop efficient transducer functionality and design, and create software to improve computer assessment of the acquired information. Two-dimensional (2D) ultrasound information can be recreated in a three-dimensional (3D) or four-dimensional (4D) (real-time) format to provide an "en face" surface rendering of the specific area. Color Doppler, harmonics, tissue characterization, and spectral analysis have greatly expanded the utility of ultrasound imaging. The development of specialized contrast agents for use with ultrasound has enabled clinicians to make specific diagnoses with greater precision.

To obtain even more information from the ultrasound image, various medical centers and manufacturers have been working toward the development of effective contrast agents that may be ingested or administered intravenously into the bloodstream to facilitate the detection and diagnosis of specific pathologies. Early attempts at producing a contrast effect with ultrasound imaging involved administration of aerated saline or carbon dioxide. Research today is focused on the development of gas microspheres, which are injected into the patient to provide visual contrast during the ultrasound study. Specific applications of ultrasound contrast are found in Chapter 17.

THE ROLE OF THE SONOGRAPHER

The sonographer is an allied health professional who has received specific training in diagnostic medical sonography (general applications) or cardiovascular technology (cardiac and vascular applications). The sonographer performs ultrasound procedures and gathers diagnostic data under the direct or indirect supervision of a physician. Sonographers are known as "image makers" who have the ability to create images of soft tissue structures and organs inside the body, such as the liver, pancreas, biliary system, kidneys, heart, vascular system, musculoskeletal system, uterus, and fetus. In addition, sonographers can record hemodynamic information with velocity measurements through the use of color Doppler and spectral analysis to determine whether a vessel or cardiac valve is patent (open) or restricted.

Sonographers work directly with physicians and patients as a team member in a medical facility. They also interact with nurses and other medical staff as part of the health care team. The sonographer must be able to review the patient's records to assess clinical history and clinical symptoms; to interpret laboratory values; and to understand other diagnostic examinations. The sonographer is required to understand and operate complex ultrasound instrumentation using the basic principles of ultrasound physics.

To produce the highest quality sonographic image for interpretation, the sonographer must possess an in-depth understanding of anatomy and pathophysiology and be able to evaluate a patient's problem specific to the examination ordered. Sonographers use their knowledge and skills to provide physicians with clinical information such as the rapid focused assessment with sonography for trauma (FAST) scan evaluation of a trauma victim's injury, visualization of detailed fetal anatomy, measurement and evaluation of fetal growth and progress, or even to evaluate the patient for cardiac abnormalities or injury. In addition to technical expertise and knowledge of anatomy and pathophysiology, several other qualities contribute to the sonographer's success.

What makes the sonographer distinct from the other health care professionals? The sonographer has the following responsibilities:

- Reviews the clinical chart and speaks directly with patients to identify symptoms that relate directly to the ultrasound examination
- Explains the procedure to the patient and performs the examination using the protocol established by the department
- Analyzes each image and correlates the information with patient information
- Uses independent judgment in recognizing the need to make adjustments with the sonographic protocol to answer the clinical question
- Reviews the previous sonograms and provides an oral or written summary of the technical findings to the physician for the medical diagnosis
- Alerts the physician if critical findings or new changes are found on the sonographic examination

The Sonography Career

Advantages. Sonographers with specialized education in ultrasound obtained from a nationally accredited diagnostic medical sonography or cardiovascular technology program have demonstrated their ability to analyze the clinical situation and to produce high-quality sonographic images, thereby earning the respect of other allied health professionals and clinicians. Every day, sonographers are faced with varied human interactions and opportunities to solve problems. These experiences give sonographers an outlet for their creativity by requiring them to come up with innovative ways to meet the challenges of performing quality sonographic examinations on difficult patients. Sonographers must have the creative ability to alter their normal protocol as difficult situations arise (e.g., trauma patient, immobile patient, postoperative surgical patient with multiple bandages). New applications in ultrasound and improvements in instrumentation create a continual challenge for the sonographer. Flexible schedules and variety in examinations and equipment, not to mention patient personalities, make each day interesting and unique. Certified sonographers find that employment opportunities are abundant, schedule flexibility is high, and salaries are attractive.

Disadvantages. On the other hand, some sonographers find their position to be stressful and demanding, with the constant changes in medical care and decreased staffing causing increased workloads. Hours of continual scanning may lead to tendinitis, arm and shoulder pain, and back strain.

Qualities of a Sonographer

The sonographer must possess the following qualities and talents:
Intellectual curiosity to keep abreast of developments in the field
Perseverance to obtain high-quality images and the ability to differentiate an artifact from structural anatomy
Ability to conceptualize two-dimensional images into a three-dimensional format; ability to reconstruct a 2D image into a 3D format to product an "en face" image
Quick and analytical mind to continually analyze image quality while keeping the clinical situation in mind
Technical aptitude to produce diagnostic-quality images
Good physical health because continuous scanning may cause strain on back, shoulder, or arm; equipment is mobile, thus the sonographer must be able to manipulate equipment weighing greater than 250 pounds; Doppler is audible, thus sonographers

must have adequate hearing to interpolate the returning Doppler audible sound
Independence and initiative to analyze the patient, the history, and the clinical findings and tailor the examination to answer the clinical question
Emotional stability to deal with patients in times of crisis; this means the ability to understand the patient's concerns without losing objectivity
Communication skills for interactions with peers, clinicians, and patients; this includes the ability to clearly communicate ultrasound findings to physicians and the ability *not* to disclose or speculate on findings to the patient during the examination
Dedication because a willingness to go beyond the "call of duty" is often required of the sonographer

(Chapter 3 focuses on ergonomics and musculoskeletal issues in sonography.)

Sonographers may become frustrated when dealing with terminally ill patients, which can lead to fatigue and depression.

Employment. The field of sonography continues to expand. The demand for certified sonographers exceeds the supply nationwide. Sonographers may find employment in the traditional setting of a hospital or medical clinic. Staffing positions within the hospital or medical setting may include the following: Director of Imaging, Technical Director, Supervisor, Chief Sonographer, Sonographer Educator, Clinical Staff Sonographer, Research Sonographer, or Clinical Instructor. Clinical research opportunities may be found in the major medical centers throughout the country. Sonographers with advanced degrees (i.e., BS, MS, or PhD) may serve as faculty in diagnostic medical sonography programs as Program Director, Department Head, or Dean of Allied Health. Many sonographers have entered the commercial world as Clinical Application Specialists or Director of Education/ Continuing Education Director, marketing specialist, product design/engineering, sales, service, or quality control. Other sonographers have become independent business partners in medicine by offering mobile ultrasound services to smaller community hospitals.

Resource Organizations. Specific organizations are devoted to developing standards and guidelines for ultrasound:

- American Institute of Ultrasound in Medicine (AIUM), www.aium.org. This organization represents all facets of ultrasound to include physicians, sonographers, biomedical engineers, scientists, and commercial researchers.
- American Society of Echocardiography (ASE), www.asecho. org. This very active organization represents physicians, sonographers, and scientists involved with cardiovascular applications of sonography.
- Society of Diagnostic Medical Sonography (SDMS), www. sdms.org. This is the principal organization for more than 25,000 sonographers. The website contains information regarding the SDMS position statement on the code of ethics for the profession of diagnostic medical ultrasound; the nondiagnostic use of ultrasound; the scope of practice for the diagnostic ultrasound professional; and diagnostic ultrasound clinical practice standards.
- Society for Vascular Ultrasound (SVU), www.svunet.org. This is the principal organization representing physicians, sonographers, and scientists in vascular sonography.

Certification. The National Certification Examination for Ultrasound is provided by the following organization:

- American Registry for Diagnostic Medical Sonography (ARDMS), www.ardms.org. This is the primary organization offering international credentials for sonographers once their training has been completed.

Joint Review Committee. The national review boards for educational programs in sonography are provided by two groups:

- Joint Review Committee on Education in Diagnostic Medical Sonography (includes general ultrasound, echocardiography, and vascular technology) (JRC-DMS), www.jrcdms.org
- Joint Review Committee on Education in Cardiovascular Technology (includes noninvasive cardiology [echocardiography], invasive cardiology [cardiac catheterization], and vascular technology) (JRC-CVT), www.jrccvt.org

HISTORICAL OVERVIEW OF SOUND THEORY AND MEDICAL ULTRASOUND

A complete history of sound theory and the development of medical ultrasound is beyond the scope of this textbook. The following is a brief overview, designed to provide readers a sense of the extensive history and exciting developments in this area of study. For a more detailed outline of historical data, the reader is referred to Dr. Joseph Woo's excellent online article titled "A Short History of the Development of Ultrasound in Obstetrics and Gynecology" and other resources listed in the Bibliography at the end of this chapter.

The story of acoustics began with the Greek philosopher **Pythagoras** (sixth century BC), whose experiments on the properties of vibrating strings led to the invention of the sonometer, an instrument used to study musical sounds. Two thousand years later, in 1500 AD, **Leonardo da Vinci** (1452–1519) discovered that sound traveled in waves and discovered that the **angle of reflection** is equal to the **angle of incidence. Galileo Galilei** (1564–1642) is said to have started modern studies of acoustics by elevating the study of vibrations to scientific standards. In 1638 he demonstrated that the frequency of sound waves determined the pitch. **Sir Isaac Newton** (1643–1727) studied the speed of sound in air and provided the first analytical determination of the speed of sound. **Robert Boyle** (1627–1691), an Irish natural philosopher, chemist, physicist, and inventor, demonstrated the physical characteristics of air, showing that it is necessary in combustion, respiration, and sound transmission. **Lazzaro Spallanzani** (1729–1799), an Italian biologist and physiologist, essentially discovered echolocation. Spallanzani is famous for extensive experiments on bat navigation, from which he concluded that bats use sound and their ears for navigation in total darkness. **Augustin Fresnel** (1788–1827) was a French physicist who contributed significantly to the establishment of the theory of wave optics, forming the theory of wave diffraction named after him. **Sir Francis Galton** (1822–1911) was an English Victorian scholar, explorer, and inventor. One of his numerous inventions was the Galton whistle used for testing differential hearing ability. This is an ultrasonic whistle, which is also known as a dog whistle or a silent whistle. **Christian Johann Doppler** (1803–1853) was an Austrian mathematician and physicist. He is most famous for what is now called the *Doppler effect,* which is the apparent change in frequency and wavelength of a wave as perceived by an observer moving relative to the wave's source. In 1880 **Paul-Jacques Curie** (1856–1941) and his brother **Pierre Curie** (1859–1906) discovered *piezoelectricity,* whereby physical pressure applied to a crystal resulted in the creation of an electric potential. **John William Strutt (Lord Rayleigh)** (1842–1919) wrote *The Theory of Sound.* The first volume, on the mechanics of a vibrating medium which produces sound, was published in 1877; the second volume on acoustic wave propagation was published the following year. **Paul Langevin** (1872–1946) was a French physicist noted for his work on paramagnetism and diamagnetism. He devised the modern interpretation of this phenomenon in terms of spins of electrons within atoms. His most famous work was on the use of ultrasound using Pierre and Jacques Curie's piezoelectric effect. During World War I, he began working on the use of these sounds to detect submarines through echolocation.

SONAR is an acronym for *SOund Navigation and Ranging.* Sonar is a technique that uses sound propagation, usually underwater, to navigate, communicate with other vessels, or detect other vessels. Sonar may be used as a means of acoustic location and measurement of the echo characteristics of "targets" in the water. The term *sonar* is also used for the equipment necessary to generate and receive the sound. The acoustic frequencies used in sonar systems vary from very low (infrasonic) to extremely high (ultrasonic). World War II brought sonar equipment to the forefront of military defense, and medical ultrasound was influenced by the advances in sonar instrumentation.

In the 1940s, **Dr. Karl Dussik** (1908–1968) made one of the earliest applications of ultrasound to medical diagnosis when he used two transducers positioned on opposite sides of the head to measure ultrasound transmission profiles. He discovered that tumors and other intracranial lesions could be detected by this technique. **Dr. William Fry,** an electrical engineer whose primary research was in the field of ultrasound, is credited with being the first to introduce the use of computers in diagnostic ultrasound. Around this same time, he and **Dr. Russell Meyers** performed craniotomies and used ultrasound to destroy parts of the basal ganglia in patients with parkinsonism.

Between 1948 and 1950, three investigators, Drs. **Douglass Howry,** a radiologist, **John Wild,** a clinician interested in tissue characterization, and **George Ludwig,** who was interested in reflections from gallstones, each demonstrated independently that when ultrasound waves generated by a piezoelectric crystal transducer are transmitted into the body, ultrasound waves of different acoustic impedances are returned to the transducer.

One of the pioneers in the clinical investigation and development of ultrasound was **Dr. Joseph Holmes** (1902–1982). A nephrologist by training, Dr. Holmes' initial interest in ultrasound involved its ability to detect bubbles in hemodialysis tubing. Holmes began work in ultrasound at the University of Colorado Medical Center in 1950, in collaboration with a group headed by **Douglass Howry.** In 1951, supported by Joseph H. Holmes, Douglass Howry, along with **William Roderic Bliss** and **Gerald J. Posakony,** both engineers, produced the "immersion tank ultrasound system," the first 2D B-mode (or plan position indicator [PPI] mode) linear compound scanner. Two-dimensional cross-sectional images, published in 1952, demonstrated that interpretable 2D images of internal organ structures and pathologies could be obtained with ultrasound. The *Pan Scanner,* put together by the Holmes, Howry, Posakony, and **Richard Cushman** team in 1957, was a landmark invention

in the history of B-mode ultrasonography. With the Pan Scanner, the patient sat on a modified dental chair strapped against a plastic window of a semicircular pan filled with saline solution, while the transducer rotated through the solution in a semicircular arc (Figure 1-1, *A*).

In 1954 echocardiographic ultrasound applications were developed in Sweden by Drs. **Hellmuth Hertz** and **Inge Edler,** who first described the M-mode (motion) display.

An early obstetric contact compound scanner was built by **Tom Brown** and **Dr. Ian Donald** (1910–1987) in Scotland in 1957. Dr. Donald went on to discover many fascinating image patterns in the obstetric patient; his work is still referred to today. Meanwhile, in the early 1960s in Philadelphia, **Dr. J Stauffer Lehman** designed a real-time obstetric ultrasound system (Figure 1-1, *B*).

In 1959 the Ultrasonic Institute (UI) was formed at the National Acoustic Laboratory in Sydney, Australia. **George Kossoff** and his team, including **Dr. William Garrett** and **David Robinson,** developed diagnostic B-scanners with the use of a water bath to improve resolution of the image (Figure 1-1, *C* and *D*). This group was also responsible for introducing gray-scale imaging in 1972. Kossoff and his colleagues were pioneers in the development of large-aperture, multitransducer technology in which the transducers were automatically programmed to operate independently or as a whole to provide high-quality images without operator intervention, as was required with the contact static scanner that had been developed in 1962 at the University of Colorado.

The advent of real-time scanners changed the face of ultrasound scanning. The first real-time scanner (initially known as a fast B-scanner) was developed by **Walter Krause** and **Richard Soldner.** It was manufactured as the Vidoscan by Siemens Medical Systems of Germany in 1965. The Vidoscan used three rotating transducers housed in front of a parabolic mirror in a water coupling system and produced 15 images per second. The image was made up of 120 lines with basic gray-scale imaging. The use of fixed-focus, large-face transducers produced a narrow beam to ensure good resolution and a good image. Fetal life and motions could be demonstrated clearly. In 1973 **James Griffith** and **Walter Henry** at the National Institutes of Health produced a mechanical oscillating real-time scanning device that could produce clear 30-degree sector real-time cardiac images with good resolution. The phased-array scanning mechanism was first described by **Jan Somer** at the University of Limberg in the Netherlands and was in use from 1968, several years before the appearance of linear-array systems.

Medical applications of ultrasonic Doppler techniques were first implemented by **Shigeo Satomura** and **Yasuhara Nimura** at the Institute of Scientific and Industrial Research in Osaka, Japan, in 1955 for the study of cardiac valve motion and pulsations of peripheral blood vessels. The Satomura team pioneered transcutaneous Doppler flow measurements in 1959. In 1966 **Kato** and **T. Izumi** pioneered the directional flow-meter using the local oscillation method whereby flow directions were detected and displayed. This was a breakthrough in Doppler instrumentation because reverse flow in blood vessels could

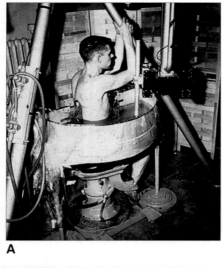

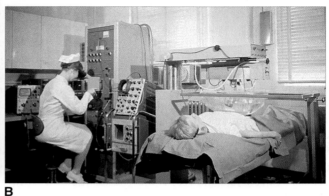

A

B

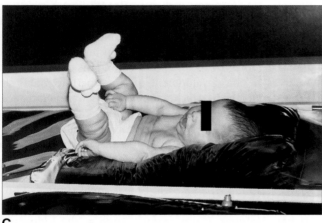

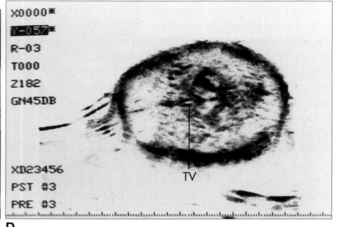

C

D

FIGURE 1-1 A, One of the early ultrasound scanning systems used a B-52 gun turret tank with the transducer carriage moved in a 360-degree path around the patient. **B,** Dr. Lehman used a water path system to scan his obstetric patients. **C,** The Octoson used eight transducers mounted in a 180-degree semicircle and completely covered with water. The patient would lie on top of the covered waterbed, and the transducers would automatically scan the patient. **D,** Real-time image of the neonatal head. *TV,* Third ventricle.

now be documented. In the United States **Robert Rushmer** and his team did groundbreaking work in Doppler instrumentation, beginning in 1958. They pioneered transcutaneous continuous-wave flow measurements and spectral analysis in 1963. **Donald Baker,** a member of Rushmer's team, introduced a pulsed-Doppler system in 1970. In 1974 Baker, along with **John Reid** and **Frank Barber** and others, developed the first duplex pulsed-Doppler scanner, which allowed 2D scale imaging to be used to guide placement of the ultrasound beam for Doppler signal acquisition. In 1985 a work titled "Real-Time Two-Dimensional Blood Flow Imaging Using an Autocorrelation Technique" by **Chihiro Kasai, Koroku Namekawa,** and **Ryozo Omoto** was published in English translation. The autocorrelation technique described in this publication could be applied to estimating blood velocity and turbulence in color flow imaging. The autocorrelation technique is a method for estimating the dominating frequency in a complex signal, as well as its variance. The algorithm is both computationally faster and

significantly more accurate compared with the Fourier transform, because the resolution is not limited by the number of samples used. This provided the rapid means of frequency estimation to be performed in real-time that is still used today.

In 1987 the Center for Emerging Cardiovascular Technologies at **Duke University** started a project to develop a real-time volumetric scanner for cardiac imaging. In 1991 they produced a matrix array scanner that could image cardiac structures in real-time and in 3D. By the second half of the 1990s, many other centers throughout the world were working on laboratory and clinical research into 3D ultrasound. Today 3D ultrasound has developed into a clinically effective diagnostic imaging technique.

INTRODUCTION TO BASIC ULTRASOUND PRINCIPLES

To produce high-quality images that are free of artifacts, the sonographer must have a firm understanding of the basic principles of ultrasound. This section introduces the basic principles of acoustics, measurement units, instrumentation, real-time sonography, 3D ultrasound, harmonic imaging, and optimization of gray-scale and Doppler ultrasound to reinforce the sonographer's understanding of scanning techniques. The student sonographer is introduced to a new language and terminology with ultrasound physics. This serves as a brief overview of the material that will be covered in depth in a dedicated ultrasound physics textbook.

Acoustics

Acoustics is the branch of physics that deals with sound and sound waves. It is the study of generating, propagating, and receiving sound waves. Within the field of acoustics, *ultrasound* is defined as sound frequencies that are beyond (ultra-) the range of normal human hearing. Most human hearing ranges between 20 **hertz (Hz)** and 20 **kilohertz (kHz).** Thus ultrasound refers to sound frequencies greater than 20 kHz.

Sound is the result of mechanical energy that produces alternating **compression** and **rarefaction** of the conducting medium as it travels as a wave (Figure 1-2). (A **wave** is a propagation of energy that moves back and forth or vibrates at a steady rate.) Diagnostic ultrasound uses short sound pulses at frequencies of 1 to 20 million **cycles**/sec (**megahertz [MHz]**) that are transmitted into the body to examine soft tissue anatomic structures (Table 1-1). In medical ultrasound, the piezoelectric vibrating source within the transducer is a ceramic element that vibrates in response to an electrical signal. The vibrating motion of the ceramic element in the transducer causes the particles in the surrounding tissue to vibrate. In this way the ultrasound transducer converts electrical energy into mechanical energy as the sonographic imaging is produced. As the sound beam is directed into the body by the transducer at various angles to the organs, reflection, absorption, and scatter cause the returning signal to be weaker than the initial impulse. Over a short period of time, multiple anatomic images are acquired in a real-time format.

The **velocity** of propagation is constant for a given tissue and is not affected by the frequency or wavelength of the pulse. In soft tissues, the assumed average propagation velocity is 1540 m/sec (Table 1-2). It is the stiffness and the density of a medium that determine how fast sound waves will travel through the structure. The more closely packed the molecules, the faster is the speed of sound.

The velocity of sound differs greatly among air, bone, and soft tissue, although the velocity of sound varies by only a little from one soft tissue to another. Sound waves travel slowly through gas (air), at intermediate speed through liquids, and quickly through solids (metal). Air-filled structures, such as the lungs and stomach, or gas-filled structures, such as the bowel, impede the sound transmission, whereas sound is attenuated through most bony structures. Small differences among fat, blood, and organ tissues that are seen on an ultrasound image may be better delineated with higher-frequency transducers that improve resolution, but lose the depth penetration.

Measurement of Sound. The decibel (dB) unit is used to measure the intensity (strength), amplitude, and power of an ultrasound wave. Decibels allow the sonographer to compare the intensity or **amplitude** of two signals. **Power** refers to the rate at which energy is transmitted. Power is the rate of energy flow over the entire beam of sound and is often measured in watts (W) or milliwatts (mW). **Intensity** is defined as power per unit area. It is the rate of energy flow across a defined area of the beam and can be measured in watts per square meter (W/m²) or milliwatts per square centimeter. Power and intensity are directly related: If you double the power, the intensity also doubles.

Frequency. Sound is characterized according to its frequency (Figure 1-3). Frequency may be explained by the following analogy: If a stick were moved into and out of a pond at a steady rate, the entire surface of the water would be covered with waves radiating from the stick. If the number of vibrations made in each second were counted, the frequency of vibration could be determined. In ultrasound, **frequency** describes the number of oscillations per second performed by the particles of the medium in which the wave is propagating:

1 oscillation/sec = 1 cycle/sec = 1 Hz
1000 oscillations/sec = 1 kilocycle/sec = 1 kHz
1,000,000 oscillations/sec = 1 megacycle/sec = 1 MHz

The sonographer should be familiar with the units of measurement commonly used in ultrasound (Table 1-3).

Propagation of Sound through Tissue. Once sound pulses are transmitted into a body, they can be reflected, scattered, refracted, or absorbed. **Reflection** occurs whenever the pulse encounters an **interface** between tissues with different acoustic impedances (Figure 1-4). **Acoustic impedance** is the measure of a material's **resistance** to the propagation of sound. The strength of the reflection depends on the

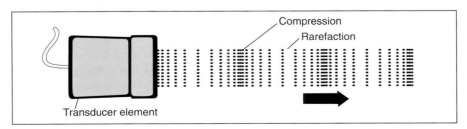

FIGURE 1-2 As the transducer element vibrates, waves undergo compression and expansion, or rarefaction, by which the molecules are pulled apart.

TABLE 1-1	Applications of Sound Frequency Ranges	
Frequency Range	**Manner of Production**	**Application**
Infrasound		
0–25 Hz	Electromagnetic vibrators	Vibration analysis of structures
Audible		
20 Hz–20 kHz	Electromagnetic vibrators, musical instruments	Communications, signaling
Ultrasound		
20–100 kHz	Air whistles, electric devices	Biology, sonar
100 kHz–1 MHz	Electric devices	Flaw detection, biology
1–20 MHz	Electric devices	Diagnostic ultrasound

Hz, Hertz; *kHz,* kilohertz; *MHz,* megahertz.

TABLE 1-3	Units Commonly Used in Ultrasound	
Quantity	**Unit**	**Abbreviation**
Amplifier gain	Decibels	dB
Area	Meters squared	m^2
Attenuation	Decibels	dB
Attenuation coefficient	Decibels per centimeter	dB/cm
Frequency	Hertz (cycles per second)	Hz
Intensity	Watts per square meter	W/m^2
Length	Meter	m
Period	Microseconds	μsec
Power	Watts	W
Pressure amplitude	Pascals	Pa
Relative power	Decibels	dB
Speed	Meters per second	m/sec
Time	Seconds	sec
Volume	Meters cubed	m^3

TABLE 1-2	Characteristic Acoustic Impedance and Velocity of Ultrasound	
Material	**Acoustic Impedance (g/cm/sec × 10)**	**Velocity (m/sec)**
Air	0.0001	331
Fat	1.38	1450
Water	1.50	1430
Blood	1.61	1570
Kidney	1.62	1560
Liver	1.65	1550
Muscle	1.70	1580
Skull	7.80	4080

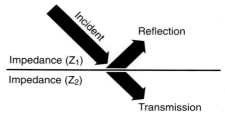

FIGURE 1-4 Reflection occurs when a sound wave strikes an interface between two objects with different acoustic impedances, causing some of the energy to be transmitted across the interface and some of it to be reflected.

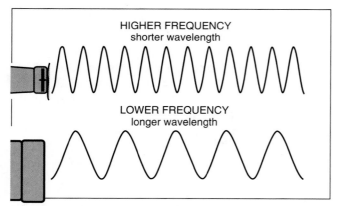

FIGURE 1-3 Wavelength is inversely related to frequency. The higher the frequency, the shorter is the wavelength and the less is the depth of penetration. The longer wavelength has a lower frequency and a greater depth of penetration.

difference in acoustic impedance between the tissues, as well as the size of the interface, its surface characteristics, and its orientation with respect to the transmitted sound pulse. The greater the acoustic mismatch, the greater is the backscatter or reflection (Figure 1-5). Large, smooth interfaces are called

specular reflectors. If specular reflectors are aligned perpendicular to the direction of the transmitted pulse, they reflect sound directly back to the active crystal elements in the transducer and produce a strong signal. Specular reflectors that are not oriented perpendicular to the sound produce a weaker signal. **Scattering** refers to the redirection of sound in multiple directions. This produces a weak signal and occurs when the pulse encounters a small acoustic interface or a large interface that is rough (Figure 1-6). **Refraction** is a change in the direction of sound that occurs when sound encounters an interface between two tissues that transmit sound at different speeds. Because the sound frequency remains constant, the **wavelength** changes to accommodate differences in the speed of sound in the two tissues. The result of this change in wavelength is a redirection of the sound pulse as it passes through the interface. **Absorption** describes the loss of sound energy secondary to its conversion to thermal energy. This is greater in soft tissues than in fluid and greater in bone than in soft tissues. Absorption is a major cause of acoustic shadowing.

Piezoelectric Crystals. When a ceramic **crystal** is electronically stimulated, it deforms and vibrates to produce the sound pulses used in diagnostic sonography (Figure 1-7).

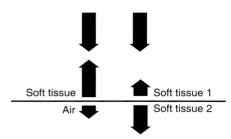

FIGURE 1-5 Acoustic impedance. If the difference between two materials is small, most of the energy in a sound wave will be transmitted across an interface between them, and the reflected echo will be weak. If the difference is large, little energy will be transmitted; most will be reflected.

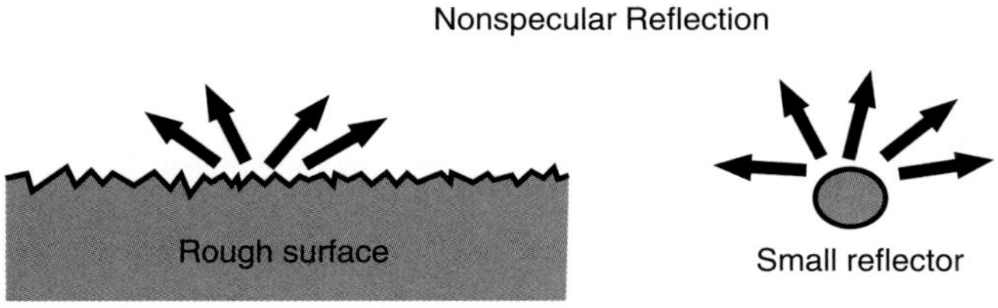

Nonspecular Reflection

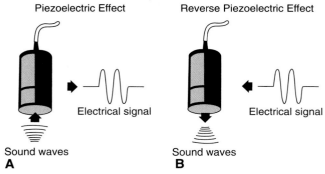

FIGURE 1-6 Scattering. Nonspecular reflectors reflect, or scatter, the sound wave in many directions.

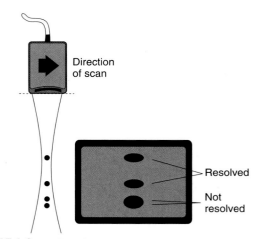

FIGURE 1-7 Piezoelectric effect. A, In certain crystals, when a sound wave is applied perpendicular to its surface, an electric charge is created. **B,** If the element is exposed to an electric shock, it will begin to vibrate and transmit a sound wave.

Pulse duration is the time that a piezoelectric element vibrates after electrical stimulation. Each pulse consists of a band of frequencies referred to as *bandwidth*. The center frequency produced by a transducer is the resonant frequency of the crystal element and depends on the thickness of the crystal. The echoes that return to the transducer distort the crystal elements and generate an electric pulse that is processed into an image. The higher-amplitude echoes produce a greater crystal deformation and generate a larger electronic voltage, which is displayed as a brighter pixel. These 2D images are known as *B-mode*, or brightness mode, images.

Image Resolution. Resolution is the ability of an imaging process to distinguish adjacent structures in an object and is an important measure of image quality. The resolution of the

ultrasound image is determined by the size and configuration of the transmitted sound pulse. Resolution is always considered in three dimensions: axial, lateral, and azimuthal. **Axial resolution** (Figure 1-8) refers to the ability to resolve objects within the imaging plane that are located at different depths along the direction of the sound pulse. This depends on the direction of the sound pulse, which, in turn, depends on the wavelength. Because wavelength is inversely proportional to frequency, the higher-frequency probes produce shorter pulses and better axial resolution, but with less penetration. These probes are best for superficial structures such as thyroid, breast, and scrotum. **Lateral resolution** (Figure 1-9) refers to the ability to resolve objects within the imaging plane that are located side by side at the same depth from the transducer. Lateral resolution can be varied by adjusting the **focal zone** of the transducer, which is the point at which the beam is the narrowest. **Azimuthal** (elevation) **resolution**

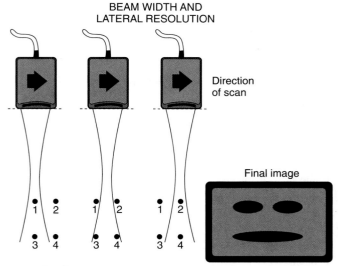

FIGURE 1-8 Axial resolution. Axial resolution refers to the minimum distance between two structures positioned along the axis of the beam where both structures can be visualized as separate objects.

BEAM WIDTH AND
LATERAL RESOLUTION

FIGURE 1-9 Lateral resolution. Lateral resolution is determined by beam width. If two reflectors are closer together than the diameter or width of the transducer, they will not be resolved.

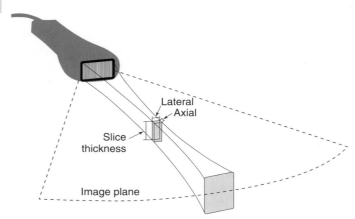

FIGURE 1-10 **Azimuthal resolution.** Slice thickness refers to the thickness of the section in the patient that contributes to the echo signals on any one image.

refers to the ability to resolve objects that are the same distance from the transducer but are located perpendicular to the plane of imaging. Azimuthal resolution is also related to the thickness of the tomographic slice (Figure 1-10). **Slice thickness** is usually determined by the shape of the crystal elements or the characteristics of fixed acoustic lenses.

Attenuation. **Attenuation** is the sum of acoustic energy loss resulting from absorption, scattering, and reflection. It refers to the reduction in intensity and amplitude of a sound wave as it travels through a medium as some of the energy is absorbed, reflected, or scattered (Figure 1-11, *A*). Thus as the sound beam travels through the body, the beam becomes progressively weaker. In human soft tissue, sound is attenuated at the rate of 0.5 dB/cm per million hertz. If air or bone is coupled with soft tissue, more energy will be attenuated. Attenuation through a solid calcium interface, such as a gallstone, will produce a posterior shadow to the ultrasound beam with sharp borders on the ultrasound image (Figure 1-11, *B*).

With the exception of air-tissue and bone interfaces, the differences in acoustic impedance in biologic tissues are so slight that only a small component of the ultrasound beam is reflected at each interface. The lung and bowel have a detrimental effect on the ultrasound beam, causing poor transmission of sound. Therefore anatomy beyond these two areas cannot be imaged because of air interference. Bone conducts sound at a much faster speed (4080 m/sec) than soft tissue. Recall that the normal transmission of sound through soft tissue travels at 1540 m/sec. Much of the sound beam is absorbed or scattered as it travels through the body, undergoing progressive attenuation. The sound is reflected according to the acoustic impedance, which is related to tissue density. Most of the sound is passed into tissues deeper in the body and is reflected at other interfaces. Because acoustic impedance is the product of the velocity of sound in a medium and the density of that medium, acoustic impedance increases if the density or propagation speed increases.

Transducer Selection

A **transducer** is a device that converts energy from one form to another. Figure 1-12 illustrates the single-element

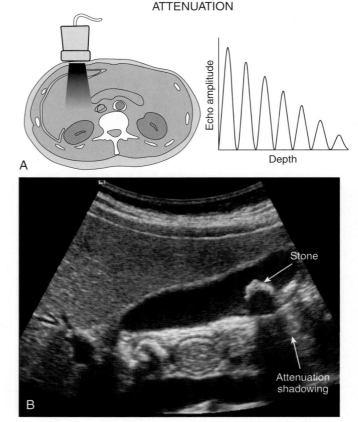

FIGURE 1-11 **Attenuation. A,** As the sound travels through the abdomen, it becomes attenuated, as some of it is reflected, scattered, and absorbed. **B,** Large gallstone causing attenuation (shadowing) beyond the calcified stone.

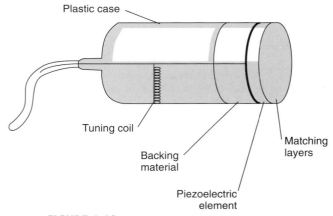

FIGURE 1-12 Single-element transducer design.

transducer design. Most of the transducers used today are not a single element, but rather a combination of elements that form an array. The transducer array scan head contains multiple small piezoelectric elements, each with its own electrical circuitry. These elements are very small in diameter, which greatly reduces beam divergence. A reduction in beam divergence leads to beam steering and focusing. The focus of the array transducers occurs on reception and on transmission (Figure 1-13). The focusing is done dynamically during

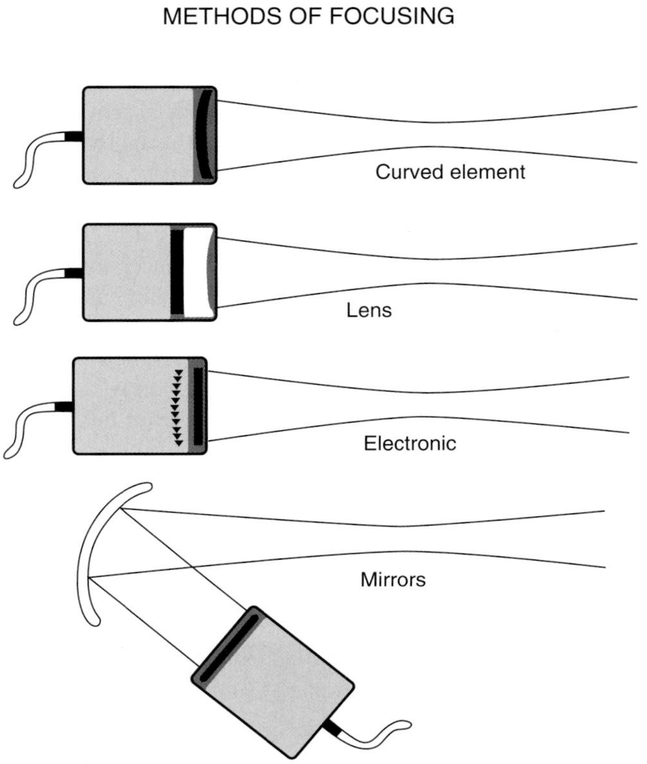

METHODS OF FOCUSING

Curved element

Lens

Electronic

Mirrors

FIGURE 1-13 Focusing effectively narrows the ultrasound beam. Multiple methods may be used to achieve this effect.

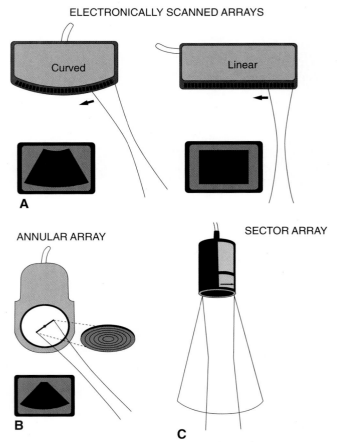

ELECTRONICALLY SCANNED ARRAYS

Curved

Linear

A

ANNULAR ARRAY

SECTOR ARRAY

B

C

FIGURE 1-14 Comparison of transducer models. **A,** Electronically scanned arrays may be curved or linear. **B,** Annular array has a larger diameter with multiple rings of focus. **C,** Sector array with multiple small elements within the transducer face.

reception. Shortly after pulse transmission, the received focus is set close to the transducer. As time elapses and the echoes from the distant targets return, the focal distance is gradually lengthened. Some instruments have multiple transmit focal zones to allow better control of the resolution of the beam at certain depths of field in the image.

The type of transducer selected for a particular examination (Figure 1-14) depends on several factors: the type of examination, the size of the patient, and the amount of fatty or muscular tissue present. High-frequency linear array probes are generally used for smaller structures (carotid artery, thyroid, scrotum, or breast). The abdomen is usually scanned with a multifocused curved array and/or a sector array; the frequency will depend on the size of the patient. Most abdominal probes are multifrequency (broadband) probes, allowing the sonographer to select the low frequency for technically difficult patients. An echocardiographic examination is performed with a multifocused broadband phased-sector array transducer to allow the smaller probe to scan in between the ribs. The transesophageal studies are obtained with the specialized smaller transesophageal probe, which is inserted into the patient's esophagus to image detailed anatomy of the cardiac structures. Obstetric and gynecologic scans are usually performed with a multifocused linear or curved array transducer. The transvaginal probe is used to scan intercavity areas in the female pelvis.

Multielement Transducer. These transducers contain groups of small crystal elements arranged in a sequential fashion.

The transmitted sound pulses are created by the summation of multiple pulses from many different elements. The timing and sequence of activation are altered to steer the transmitted pulses in different directions while focusing at multiple levels.

Sector Phased-Array Transducer. With this transducer, every element in the array participates in the formation of each transmitted pulse. The sound beams are steered at varying angles from one side of the transducer to the other to produce a sector format. The transducer is smaller and is better able to scan in between ribs (especially useful in echocardiography). The transducer permits a large, deep field of view. The limitations of this transducer are a reduced near field focus and a small superficial field of view (Figure 1-15).

Linear-Array Transducer. The linear-array transducer activates a limited group of adjacent elements to generate each pulse. The pulses travel in the same direction (parallel) and are oriented perpendicular to the transducer surface, resulting in a rectangular image. The pulses may also be steered to produce a trapezoidal image (Figure 1-16). This transducer provides high resolution in the near field. The transducer is quite large and cumbersome for accessing all areas and is used more often in obstetric ultrasound.

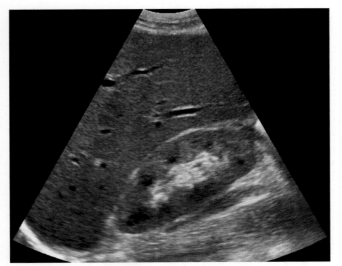

FIGURE 1-15 Small sector array has small footprint to get in between ribs, but visualization of the near field is limited.

Curved-Array Transducer. The curved-array transducer uses the linear-array transducer with the surface of the transducer reformed into a curved convex shape to produce a moderately sized sector-shaped image with a convex apex. This allows for a wider far field of view, with slightly reduced resolution. This type of probe can be formatted into many different applications with varying frequencies for use in the abdomen and in obstetric ultrasound (see Figure 1-16).

Intraluminal Transducer. These transducers are very small and can be placed into different body lumens that are close to the organ of interest. Much higher frequencies are used with high resolution. Elimination of the body adipose tissue greatly enhances image quality. The drawback of a high-frequency transducer is a limited depth of field. These transducers have been labeled as transvaginal and endorectal when used to image the female organs and rectum, respectively (Figure 1-17, *A*). Cardiologists have used the transesophageal probe to produce exquisite views of the cardiac valvular apparatus (Figure 1-17, *B*). Interventional physicians

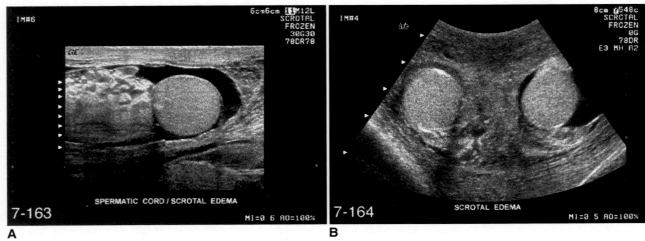

FIGURE 1-16 Comparison of linear array **(A)** versus curved array **(B)** images of the scrotal sac. The linear array produces a "rectangular" image display, whereas the curved array shows a wide "pie" curve display.

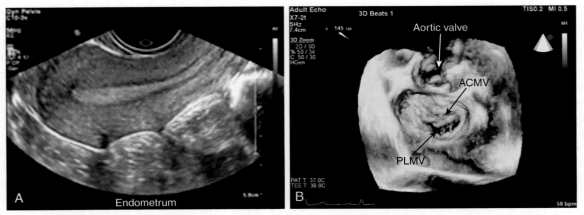

FIGURE 1-17 **A,** Endovaginal probe may provide 90- to 120-degree sector field of view of the normal uterus with the endometrial stripe. **B,** Transesophageal 3D image of the mitral valve apparatus from the "surgeon's view," looking from the head down. *ALMV,* Anterior leaflet mitral valve; *PLMV,* posterior leaflet mitral valve.

have used the tiny intraarterial probes that fit onto the end of a catheter in order to see intracoronary and intravascular detail.

Pulse-Echo Display Modes

A-Mode (Amplitude Modulation). A-mode, or amplitude modulation, produces a one-dimensional image that displays the amplitude strength of the returning echo signals along the vertical axis and the time (distance) along the horizontal axis. The amplitude display represents the time or distance it takes the beam to strike an interface and return the signal to the transducer. The greater the reflection at the interface, the taller the amplitude spike will appear (Figure 1-18).

B-Mode (Brightness Modulation). The B-mode, or brightness modulation, method displays the intensity (amplitude) of an echo by varying the brightness of a dot to correspond to echo strength. **Gray scale** is an imaging technique that assigns to each level of amplitude a particular shade of gray to visualize the different echo amplitudes. The B-mode is the basis for all real-time imaging in ultrasound (Figure 1-19). In B-mode imaging, the ultrasound beam is sent in various directions into the region of interest to be scanned. Each beam interrogates the reflectors along a different line. The echo data picked up along the beam line are displayed in a B-mode format. The B-mode display "tracks" the ultrasound beam line as it scans the region, "sketching out the 2D image" of the body. As many as 200 beam lines may be used to construct each image.

M-Mode (Motion Mode). The M-mode, or motion mode, displays time along the horizontal axis and depth along the vertical axis to depict movement, especially in cardiac structures (Figure 1-20). M-mode is used to record a graphic representation of wall motion, cardiac valvular motion, posterior cardiac wall motion, or fetal heart rhythm.

Real-time. **Real-time** imaging provides a dynamic presentation of multiple image frames per second over selected

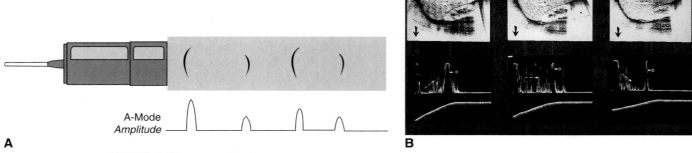

FIGURE 1-18 A, Amplitude is shown along the vertical axis, and time is shown along the horizontal axis. **B,** Earlier instrumentation used the A-mode display to help determine proper settings for the 2D image. The bottom images show the A-mode and time gain compensation scale below.

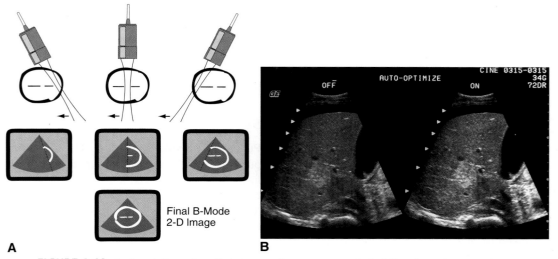

FIGURE 1-19 A, Acquisition of multiple image planes over a period of time is made to produce a B-mode image. **B,** B-mode image of the liver with a hemangioma in the center of the right lobe. The auto-optimize control is used in the right-hand display to show improved focus.

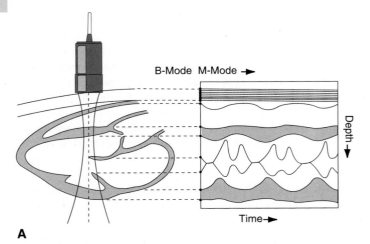

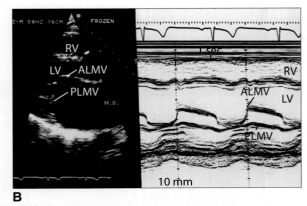

FIGURE 1-20 A, M-mode imaging. From the B-mode image, one line of site may be selected to record a motion image of a moving structure over time and distance. **B,** The M-mode is recorded through the stenotic mitral valve to show decreased opening and closing of the valve leaflet over time. On the M-mode, the vertical scale represents depth, and the space between the markers represents time. The distance between these two markers is 1 second. *ALMV,* Anterior leaflet mitral valve; *LV,* left ventricle; *PLMV,* posterior leaflet mitral valve; *RV,* right ventricle.

areas of the body. The **frame rate** is dependent on the frequency and depth of the transducer and depth selection. Typical frame rates are 30 frames per second or less. The principal barrier to higher scanning speeds is the speed of sound in tissue, dictating the time required to acquire echo data for each beam line. All of ultrasound imaging now is acquired with real-time acquisition. These images may be stored in a "cine" loop or single frame image. The **temporal resolution** refers to the ability of the system to accurately depict motion.

Harmonic Imaging

Sound waves contain many component frequencies. Harmonics are those components whose frequencies are integral multiples of the lowest frequency (the "fundamental" or "first harmonic"). Harmonic imaging involves transmitting at frequency f and receiving at frequency $2f$, the second harmonic. Because of the finite bandwidth constraints of transducers,

the transducer insonates at half of its nominal frequency (e.g., 3 MHz for a 6 MHz transducer) in harmonic mode and then receives at its nominal frequency (6 MHz in this example). The harmonic beams generated during pulse propagation are narrower and have lower side-lobe artifacts than the fundamental beam. The strength of the harmonics generated depends on the amplitude of the incoming beam. Therefore the image-degrading portions of the fundamental beam (i.e., scattered echoes, reverberations, and slice-thickness side lobes) are much weaker than the on-axis portions of the beam and generate weaker harmonics.

Harmonic formation increases with depth, with few harmonics being generated within the near field of the body wall. Therefore filtering out the fundamental frequency and creating an image from the echoes of the second harmonic should result in an image that is relatively free of the noise formed during the passage of sound through the distorting layers of the body wall.

Three-Dimensional and Four-Dimensional Ultrasound

Conventional ultrasound offers a 2D visualization of anatomic structures with the flexibility of visualizing images from different orientations or "windows" in real-time. The sonographer acquires these 2D images in at least two different scanning planes and then forms a 3D image in his or her head. Technical developments in technology now allow ultrasound images to be acquired on their *x*, *y*, and *z* axes, manually realigned, and then reconstructed into a 3D "en face" format. This technique has been useful in reconstructing the fetal face, ankle, and extremities in the second- and third-trimester fetus (Figure 1-21, *A*). The use of 3D reconstruction in echocardiography has provided improved information to the clinician and surgeon in diagnosing valvular heart problems and in accurate intracardiac device placement (Figure 1-21, *B*).

Three-dimensional ultrasound (3DU) has continued to develop, with improvements in resolution and accuracy. Data for the 3DU are acquired as a stack of parallel cross-sectional images with the use of a conventional ultrasound system or as a volume with the use of an electronic array probe. These images can be reconstructed in a variety of formats to produce the desired image. Four-dimensional ultrasound is the real-time motion of the 3DU image.

System Controls for Image Optimization

Pulse-Echo Instrumentation. The critical component of the pulse-echo instrument is the B-mode (2D) imager. The beam former includes the electronic transmitter and the receiver. The transmitter supplies electrical signals to the transducer for producing the sound beam. The transducer may be connected to the transmitter and receiver through a beam-former system. Echoes picked up by the transducer are applied to the receiver. At this point, the echoes are amplified and processed into a suitable format for display. An image memory (scan converter) retains data for viewing or storage on digital media (Figure 1-22).

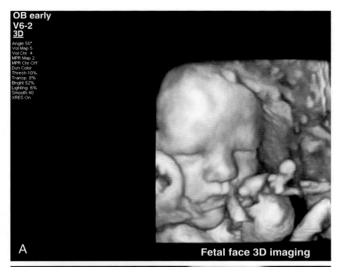

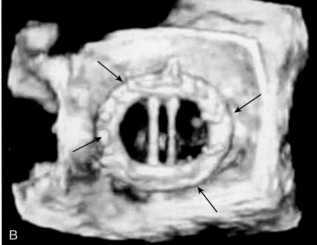

FIGURE 1-21 **A,** Three-dimensional reconstruction of the fetal face. **B,** 3D reconstruction of a mechanical mitral valve (arrows) from the surgeon's view.

reflection and less distortion of the crystal than a similar interface in the near tissues. To compensate for this attenuation of sound in the deeper tissues, the sound is "electronically amplified" after the sound returns to the transducer. The receiver **gain** allows the sonographer to amplify or boost the echo signals. It may be compared with the volume control on a radio—as one increases the volume, the sound becomes louder. The acoustic exposure to the patient is not changed when the receiver gain is increased. If the gain is set too high, artifactual low-level "echo noise" will be displayed throughout the image. Fluid or normal vascular structures should be anechoic (without echoes); if the gain is set too high, low-level artifactual echoes will be noted in these structures.

Recall the discussion of how the signal is absorbed, reflected, and attenuated as the beam traverses the body. The depth of the interface is determined by the amount of time it takes for the transmitted sound pulse to return to the transducer. The **time gain compensation (TGC)** control, sometimes referred to as *depth gain compensation (DGC),* allows the sonographer to manually amplify the receiver gain gradually at specific depths (Figure 1-23). Thus the echoes well seen in the near field may be reduced in amplitude, whereas the echoes in the far field may be amplified or increased with changing the TGC controls. The TGC control will be continually adjusted during the sonographic examination to highlight or display various signals within the body. In the abdomen, the liver is a great organ to set the TGC controls as the organ should be homogeneous from the near field (close to the transducer) to the far field (furthest from the transducer).

Focal Zone. The focal zone control allows the transducer to focus the transmitted sound at different depths (Figure 1-24). It is usually indicated on the side of the image as single or multiple arrowheads and may be adjusted in depth to focus on specific areas of interest. As multilevel focusing is used, a decrease in the frame rate will occur.

Field of View. This control allows the sonographer to adjust the depth and width of the image. The larger or deeper field of view will directly cause the frame rate to decrease. Depth is displayed as centimeters on the side of the image. Width adjusts the horizontal axis of the image and may be used to reduce side-lobe artifacts.

Reject. The reject control eliminates both electronic noise and low-level echoes from the display. This control is important to understand as the sonographer attempts to "clean up" the image artifacts, because one must be careful

Power Output. The power output determines the strength of the pulse that is transmitted into the body. The returning echoes are stronger when the transmitted pulse is stronger, and thus the image is "brighter." The power output is displayed as a decibel (dB) or as a percent of maximum.

Gain. Once the sound wave strikes the body, sound attenuation occurs with each layer the beam transverses, causing an interface in the deep tissues to produce a weaker

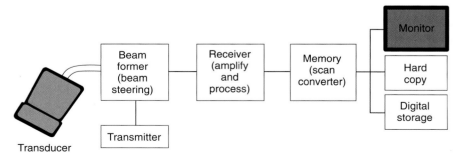

FIGURE 1-22 Components of an ultrasound system.

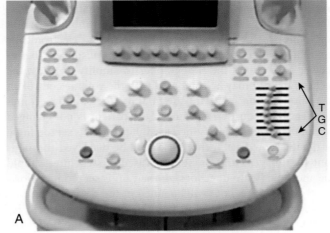

TIME GAIN COMPENSATION (TGC)

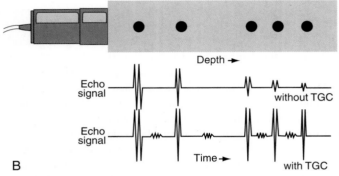

FIGURE 1-23 A, Ultrasound control panel that shows the time gain compensation (TGC) controls along the right side of the panel. **B,** The TGC allows the sonographer to amplify the receiver gain gradually at specific depths to adjust for attenuation.

not to eliminate important low-level information that may be significant in the clinical diagnosis.

Dynamic Range. The **dynamic range** of a device is the range of input signal levels that produce noticeable changes in the output of the device. The dynamic range capabilities vary among different ultrasound machines. The sonographer usually notes the low dynamic range as one of high contrast (echocardiography and peripheral vascular), whereas the high dynamic range shows more shades of gray and lower contrast (abdominal and obstetric).

Doppler Ultrasound

Two basic modes of transducer operation are used in medical diagnostic applications: continuous wave and pulsed wave. Whereas real-time 2D instrumentation uses only the pulse-echo amplitude of the returning echo to generate gray-scale information, Doppler instrumentation uses both continuous and pulse-wave operations.

Doppler Effect. The Doppler effect is the apparent change in frequency of sound or light waves emitted by a source as it moves away from or toward an observer (Figure 1-25). Sound that reflects off a moving object undergoes a change

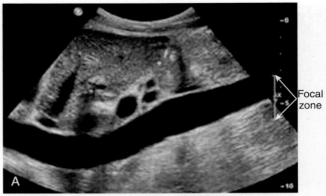

FOCAL ZONE CHARACTERISTICS

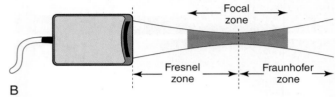

FIGURE 1-24 A, The focal zone (arrows) should be placed at the area of interest, which in this case is the inferior vena cava. **B,** The **near field (Fresnel zone)** is the area closest to the transducer. The **far field (Fraunhofer zone)** is farthest from the transducer.

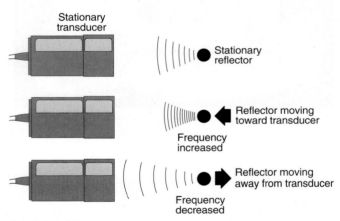

FIGURE 1-25 The Doppler effect refers to a change in frequency of a sound wave when the source or the listener is moving relative to the other.

in frequency. Objects moving toward the transducer reflect sound at a higher frequency than that of the incident pulse, and objects moving away reflect sound at a lower frequency. The difference between the transmitted and the received frequency is called the Doppler *frequency shift*. This Doppler effect is applied when the motion of laminar or turbulent flow is detected within a vascular structure. When the source moves toward the listener, the perceived frequency is higher than the emitted frequency, thus creating a higher-pitched sound. If the sound moves away from the listener, the perceived frequency is lower than the transmitted frequency, and the sound will have a lower pitch.

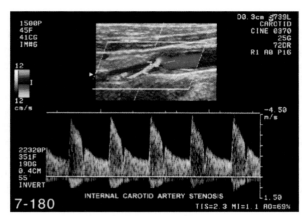

FIGURE 1-26 Color Doppler with spectral wave shows stenosis of the internal carotid artery and increased velocity through the area of stenosis.

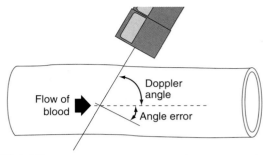

FIGURE 1-27 The closer the Doppler angle is to zero, the more accurate is the flow velocity. Thus the more parallel the transducer is to flow, the more accurate is the velocity.

In the medical application of the Doppler principle, the frequency of the reflected sound wave is the same as the frequency transmitted only if the reflector is stationary. If the red blood cell (RBC) moves along the line of the ultrasound beam (parallel to flow), the Doppler shift is directly proportional to the velocity of the RBC. If the RBC moves away from the transducer in the plane of the beam, the fall in frequency is directly proportional to the velocity and direction of RBC movement (Figure 1-26). The frequency of the echo will be higher than the transmitted frequency if the reflector is moving toward the transducer, and lower if the reflector is moving away.

Doppler Shift. The difference between the receiving echo frequency and the frequency of the transmitted beam is called the **Doppler shift.** This change in the frequency of a reflected wave is caused by relative motion between the reflector and the transducer's beam. Generally the Doppler shift is only a small fraction of the transmitted ultrasound frequency.

The Doppler shift frequency is proportional to the velocity of the moving reflector or blood cell. The frequency at which a transducer transmits ultrasound influences the frequency of the Doppler shift. The higher the original, or transmitted, frequency, the greater is the shift in frequency for a given reflector velocity. The returning frequency increases if the RBC is moving toward the transducer and decreases if the blood cell is moving away from the transducer. The Doppler effect produces a shift that is the reflected frequency minus the transmitted frequency. When interrogating the same blood vessel with transducers of different frequencies, the higher-frequency transducer will generate a larger Doppler shift frequency.

The angle that the reflector path makes with the ultrasound beam is called the **Doppler angle.** As the Doppler angle increases from 0 to 90 degrees, the detected Doppler frequency shift decreases. At 90 degrees, the Doppler shift is zero, regardless of flow velocity. The frequency of the Doppler shift is proportional to the cosine of the Doppler angle. The beam should be parallel to flow to obtain the maximum velocity. *The closer the Doppler angle is to zero, the more accurate*

is the flow velocity (Figure 1-27). If the angle of the beam to the reflector exceeds 60 degrees, velocities will no longer be accurate.

Spectral Analysis. Blood flow through a vessel may be laminar or turbulent (Figure 1-28). **Laminar** flow is the normal pattern of vessel flow, which occurs at different velocities, as flow in the center of the vessel is faster than it is at the edges. When the range of velocities increases significantly, the flow pattern becomes turbulent. The audio of the Doppler signal enables the sonographer to distinguish laminar flow from turbulent flow patterns. The process of **spectral analysis** allows the instrumentation to break down the complex multifrequency Doppler signal into individual frequency components.

The spectral display shows the distribution of Doppler frequencies versus time (Figure 1-29). This is displayed as velocity on the vertical axis and time on the horizontal axis. Flow toward the transducer is displayed above the baseline, and flow away from the transducer is displayed below the baseline.

When the area of the vessel that is examined contains RBCs moving at similar velocities, they will be represented on the spectral display by a narrow band. This area under the band is called the "window." As flow becomes more turbulent or disturbed, the velocity increases, producing **spectral broadening** on the display. A very stenotic (high-flow

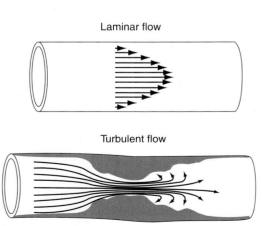

FIGURE 1-28 Laminar flow is smooth and has uniform velocity, whereas turbulent flow has multiple flow velocity characteristics.

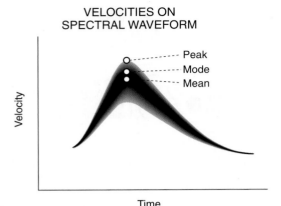

VELOCITIES ON
SPECTRAL WAVEFORM

FIGURE 1-29 The spectral display shows the distribution of Doppler frequencies versus time.

velocity) lesion would cause the window to become completely filled in.

Continuous Wave Doppler. **Continuous wave (CW) Doppler** uses two piezoelectric elements: one for sending and one for receiving. The sound is transmitted continuously rather than in short pulses. Continuous wave is used to record the higher velocity flow patterns, usually above 2 m/sec, and is especially useful in cardiology (Figure 1-30). Unlike pulsed wave Doppler, CW Doppler cannot pinpoint exactly where along the beam axis flow is occurring, as it samples all of the flow along its path. In the example of a five-chamber view of the heart, a sample volume placed in the left ventricular outflow tract will sample all the flow along that "line" to include the flows in the outflow tract and in the ascending aorta.

Pulsed Wave Doppler. **Pulsed wave (PW) Doppler** is used for lower velocity flow and has one crystal that pulses to transmit the signal while also listening or receiving the returning signal. The PW Doppler uses brief bursts of sound like those used in echo imaging. These bursts are usually of a longer duration and produce well-defined frequencies. The sonographer may set the **gate,** or Doppler window, to a specific area of interest in the vascular structure so interrogated. This means that a specific area of interest may be examined at the point the gate or sample volume is placed. For example, in a longitudinal view of the abdominal aorta, the sample volume may be placed directly in the middle of the aortic flow, and recordings only from that particular area "within the gate or window" will be measured (Figure 1-31).

With pulsed Doppler, for accurate detection of Doppler frequencies to occur, the Doppler signal must be sampled at least twice for each cycle in the wave. This phenomenon is known as the **Nyquist limit.** When the Nyquist limit is exceeded, an artifact called *aliasing* occurs. **Aliasing** presents on the spectral display as an apparent reversal of flow direction and a "wrapping around" of the Doppler spectral waveform. The highest velocity, therefore, may not be accurately demonstrated when aliasing occurs; this usually happens when the flows are greater than 2 m/sec. One can avoid aliasing by changing the Doppler signal from pulsed wave to continuous wave to record the higher velocities accurately.

Color Flow Doppler. **Color flow Doppler** is sensitive to Doppler signals throughout an adjustable portion of the area of interest. A real-time image is displayed with both gray scale and color flow in the vascular structures. Color flow Doppler is able to analyze the phase information, frequency, and amplitude of returning echoes.

Velocities are quantified by allocating a pixel to flow toward the transducer and flow away from the transducer. Each velocity frequency change is allocated a color. Color maps may be adjusted to obtain different color assignments for the velocity levels; signals from moving red blood cells are assigned a color (red or blue) based on the direction of

FIGURE 1-30 The CW sample volume (SV) is placed in the left ventricular outflow tract (see dotted line through the color jet). The high-velocity flow of aortic insufficiency above the baseline is recorded with a continuous wave (CW) transducer. The normal aortic flow pattern is noted below the baseline.

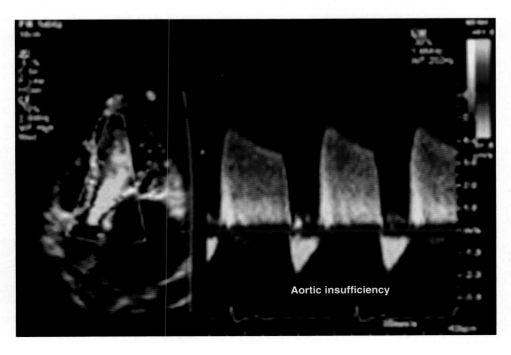

Aortic insufficiency

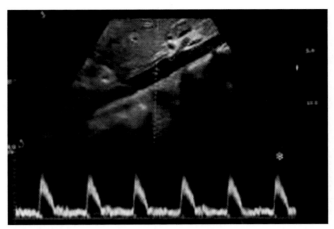

FIGURE 1-31 The pulsed wave transducer is useful for flow velocities less than 2 m/sec as seen in this abdominal aorta. The sample volume is place in the midpoint of the aorta.

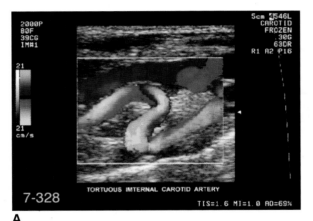

A

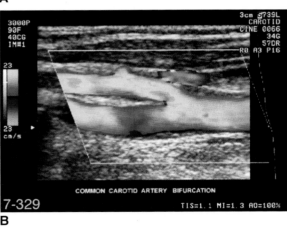

B

FIGURE 1-32 Color Doppler has been helpful to outline the direction and velocity of flow. The color box **(A)** shows which color assignment has been made for the image. The color toward the transducer is blue. **B,** This image shows that the color bar has assigned red to flow toward the transducer.

the phase shift (i.e., the direction of blood flow toward or away from the transducer) (Figure 1-32). Flow velocity is indicated by color brightness: The higher the velocity, the brighter is the color. Aliasing also occurs in color flow imaging when Doppler frequencies exceed the Nyquist limit,

just as in spectral Doppler. This appears as a wrap-around of the displayed color. The velocity scale (pulse repetition frequency, discussed later in this chapter) may be adjusted to avoid aliasing. Color arising from sources other than moving blood is referred to as flash artifact or ghosting.

Power Doppler. Power Doppler estimates the power or strength of the Doppler signal rather than the mean frequency shift. Although the Doppler detection sequence used in power Doppler is the same as that used in frequency-based color Doppler, once the Doppler shift has been detected, the frequency components are ignored in lieu of the total energy of the Doppler signal. The color and hue relate to the moving blood volume rather than to the direction or the velocity of flow (Figure 1-33).

This principle provides power Doppler several advantages over color Doppler imaging. In power Doppler, low-level noise is assigned as a homogeneous color background, even when the gain is increased. With color Doppler, the higher gains produce noise in the signal that obscures the image. The Doppler angle is not affected in power Doppler; with color Doppler the angle is critical in determining the exact flow velocity. The downside of power Doppler is that it provides no information

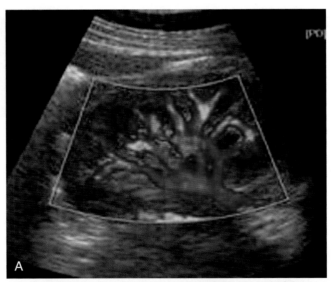

A

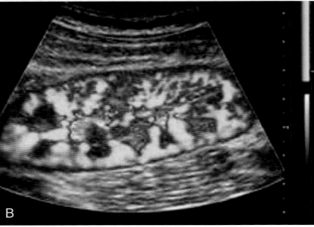

B

FIGURE 1-33 Power Doppler of the kidney: **(A)** transverse and **(B)** longitudinal.

PULSING CHARACTERISTICS

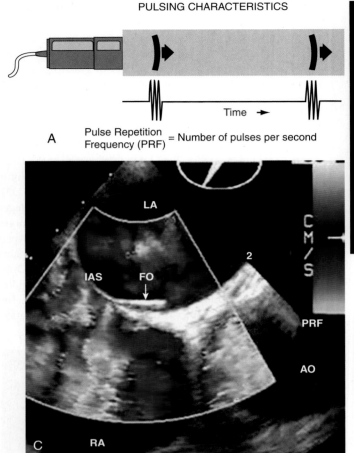

A   Pulse Repetition Frequency (PRF) = Number of pulses per second

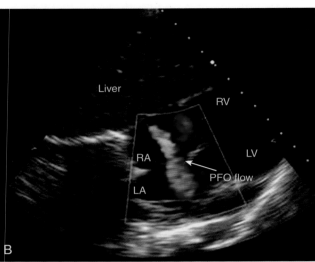

FIGURE 1-34 A, The pulse repetition frequency (PRF) may be adjusted in Doppler applications to record the lower or higher velocity signals. **B,** Power Doppler shows a communication across the patent foramen ovalae (FO), but does not provide the direction of flow. **C,** As the PRF is reduced from the 60s to the 30s, the low-flow PFO may be seen to cross from the left atrium (LA) into the right atrium (RA). *Ao,* Aorta; *IAS,* interatrial septum.

about the direction or velocity of blood flow, and it is susceptible to flash artifact (zones of intense color that result from motion of soft tissues and motion of the transducer).

Doppler Optimization

Transducer Frequency. The Doppler frequency shift is proportional to the transmitted frequency. Therefore higher-frequency probes also result in stronger reflections from RBCs. Remember that the higher-frequency probes are not sensitive to deeper structures; therefore multiple probes may be necessary, depending on the type of ultrasound examination.

Gain. Doppler gain is the receiver end amplification of the Doppler signal. This can be applied to either the waveform itself or to the color Doppler image. The Doppler gain is usually increased to the maximum limit where "noise" scatter is seen in the background. The gain is then slowly decreased until that noise disappears. The Doppler gain is independent of the gray-scale gain.

Scale. Scale allows the sonographer to expand or reduce the range of depth of the returning signal.

Baseline. The baseline may be moved up or down to image the maximal velocity of the returning signal.

Power. Power refers to the strength of the transmitted ultrasound pulse. The stronger pulse will produce stronger reflections that are more easily detected. Power will affect both gray-scale and Doppler images. Increasing the power may be helpful in the deeper structures, but increasing power increases patient exposure and may cause increased artifacts.

For these reasons, power controls generally are not modified as frequently by the sonographer as the other controls.

Pulse Repetition Frequency. The **pulse repetition frequency (PRF)** refers to the number of sound pulses transmitted per second. A high PRF results in a high Doppler scale (to record higher velocities, e.g., aortic stenosis), whereas a lower PRF results in a lower Doppler scale (to record lower velocities, e.g., venous return or low-flow states). The PRF is adjusted for the higher flows to eliminate aliasing (Figure 1-34).

Wall Filter. The wall filter allows the sonographer to eliminate artifactual or unwanted signals arising from pulsating vessel walls or moving soft tissues. This filter allows frequency shifts above a certain level to be displayed while lower-frequency shifts are not displayed.

 Key Pearls

- Ultrasound refers to instrumentation; sonography refers to the imaging technique; echocardiography refers to cardiac imaging.
- A sonographer is a member of the allied heath professions who has received specialized education in diagnostic medical sonography and has successfully completed the national boards given by the American Registry of Diagnostic Medical Sonography.

- A sonologist is a physician who has received specialized training in ultrasound and has successfully completed the national boards granted by their respective specialty.
- Diagnostic ultrasound is portable, is economical, and does not use radiation.
- Diagnostic ultrasound uses short sound pulses at frequencies of 1 to 20 million cycles/sec that are transmitted into the body to examine soft tissue anatomic structures.
- Velocity of propagation is constant for a given tissue and not affected by the frequency or wavelength of the pulse.
- Sound waves travel slowly through gas, at intermediate speed through liquids, and quickly through solids.
- The decibel unit is used to measure the intensity, amplitude, and power of an ultrasound wave.
- Power is measured in watts or milliwatts.
- Frequency describes the number of oscillations per second performed by the particles of the medium in which the wave is propagating.
- Once sound pulses are transmitted into a body, they can be reflected, scattered, refracted, or absorbed.
- Acoustic impedance is the measure of a material's resistance to the propagation of sound.
- Resolution is the ability of an imaging process to distinguish adjacent structures in an object and is an important measure of image quality (axial, lateral, and azimuthal resolution).
- Attenuation is the sum of acoustic energy loss resulting from absorption, scattering, and reflection.
- Transducers are selected for a particular examination (multielement, phased array, sector array, linear array, curved array, intraluminal).
- Pulsed echo display modes include A-mode, M-mode, B-mode, real-time mode, harmonic mode, and three- and four-dimensional modes.
- System controls for image optimization include power output, gain, TGC, focal zone, field of view, reject, and dynamic range.
- The Doppler effect is the apparent change in frequency of sound or light waves emitted by a source as it moves away from or toward an observer.
- The difference between the receiving echo frequency and the frequency of the transmitted beam is called the Doppler shift.
- Doppler may be measured using either continuous wave or pulsed wave analysis.
- Color Doppler is able to analyze the phase information, frequency, and amplitude of returning echoes.
- Power Doppler estimates the power or strength of the Doppler signal rather than the mean frequency shift.
- Doppler optimization is controlled by transducer frequency, gain, scale, baseline, power, PRF, and wall filter.

BIBLIOGRAPHY

American College of Radiology: ACR practice guideline for performing and interpreting diagnostic ultrasound examinations. Revised 2006. Available at www.acr.org.

Baker DW, Watkins D: A phase coherent pulse Doppler system for cardio-vascular measurement. In *Proceedings of the 20th Annual Conference of Engineering Medicine Biologists* 27:2, 1967.

Bom N, Lance CT, Honkoop J, Hugenholtz PG: Ultrasonic viewer for cross-sectional analyses of moving cardiac structures, *BioMed Eng* 6:500, 1971.

Campbell S: An improved method of fetal cephalometry by ultrasound, *Br J Obstet Gynaecol* 75:568-576, 1968.

Campbell S, Wilkin D: Ultrasonic measurement of the fetal abdomen circumference in the estimation of fetal weight, *Br J Obstet Gynaecol* 82:687-689, 1975.

Craig M: *Essentials of sonography and patient care*, ed 2, Philadelphia, 2006, Saunders.

Curie JP: Développement par pression de l'électricite polaire dans les cristaux hémièdres à faces inclinées, *CR Acad Sci* (Paris) 91:294, 1880.

Curry R, Tempkin B, editors: *Sonography: introduction to normal structure and function*, ed 2, Philadelphia, 2004, Saunders.

Donald I: Clinical applications of ultrasonic techniques in obstetrical and gynaecological diagnosis, *Br J Obstet Gynaecol* 69:1036, 1962.

Dussik KT: On the possibility of using ultrasound waves as a diagnostic aid, *Neurol Psychiat* 174:153-168, 1942.

Edler I, Hertz CH: The use of ultrasonic reflectoscope for the continuous recording of the movements of heart walls, *K Fysiogr Sallsk Lund Forh* 24:40, 1954.

Firestone FA: The supersonic reflectoscope, an instrument of inspecting the interior of solid parts by means of sound waves, *J Acoust Soc Am* 17:287-299, 1945.

Griffith JM, Herny WL: A sector scanner for real-time two-dimensional echocardiography, *Circulation* 49:1147, 1974.

Holmes JH, Howry DH, Posakony GJ, Cushman CR: The ultrasonic visualization of soft tissue structures in the human body, *Trans Am Clin Climatol Assoc* 66:208-223, 1954.

Howry DH: Development of an ultrasonic diagnostic instrument, *Am J Phys Med* 37:234, 1958.

Kossoff G, Carpenter D, Robinson D, Garrett WJ: A new multi-transducer water coupling echoscope. In *Proceedings of the 2nd European Congress on Ultrasonics in Medicine*, May 12-16, 1975, Munich, Germany.

Kossoff G, Garrett WJ, Radovanovich G: *Gray scale echography in obstetrics and gynecology*, Sydney, Australia, 1973, Commonwealth Acoustic Laboratories. Report No. 59.

Langévin MP: Les ondes ultrasonores, *Rev Gen Elect* 23:626, 1928.

Ludwig GD, Bolt RH, Hueter TF, Ballantine HT: Factors influencing the use of ultrasound as a diagnostic aid, *Trans Am Neurol Assoc* 51:225-228, 1950.

Middleton WD, Kurtz AB, Hertzberg BS: *Ultrasound: the requisites*, ed 2, St Louis, 2004, Mosby.

Miner NS: Basic principles. In Sanders RC, editor: *Clinical sonography*, Boston, 2001, Little, Brown.

Nelson TR, Downey DD, Pretorius DH, et al: *Three-dimensional ultrasound*, Philadelphia, 1999, Lippincott Williams & Wilkins.

Omoto R, Namekawa K, Kasai C: A prototype device incorporating a new technology for visualizing intracardiac flow, *Jpn Circ J* 47:191, 1983.

Reid JM, Spencer MP: Ultrasonic Doppler technique for imaging blood vessels, *Science* 176:1235-1236, 1972.

Robinette WB: Ultrasound contrast agents: an overview, *J Diagn Med Sonogr* 13:29S, 1997.

Taylor KJW, Carpenter DA, Hill CR, McCready VR: Gray scale ultrasound imaging: the anatomy and pathology of the liver, *Radiology* 119:415-423, 1976.

von Ramm OT, Thurstone FL: Cardiac imaging using a phased array system (I. System design), *Circulation* 53:258-262, 1976.

Wild JJ, French LA, Neal D: Detection of cerebral tumours by ultrasonic pulses, *Cancer* 4:705, 1950.

Woo JSK: A short history of the development of ultrasound in obstetrics and gynecology. Available at www.ob-ultrasound.net/history.html.

Zagzebski J, Parks J: Ultrasound physics and instrumentation, advanced ultrasound seminars, 1997. Private printing from private course.

CHAPTER
2

Essentials of Patient Care for the Sonographer

Marveen Craig

OBJECTIVES

On completion of this chapter, you should be able to:
- Define patient-focused care
- Discuss the basic patient care techniques covered in this chapter
- Describe patient transfer techniques
- Discuss infection control and isolation techniques
- Demonstrate the ability to respond to common medical emergencies
- Describe how to assist patients with special needs
- Define patient rights and HIPAA

OUTLINE

A Sonographer's Obligations
  Patient-Focused Care
Basic Patient Care
  Vital Signs
Patients on Strict Bed Rest
  Bedpans and Urinals
  Emesis Basins
Patients with Tubes and Tubing
  Intravenous Therapy
  Nasogastric Suction Tubes
  Catheters
  Oxygen Therapy
  Wounds, Drains, and Dressings
  Ostomies
Patient Transfer Techniques
  Body Mechanics

Moving Patients Up in Bed
Assisting Patients to and from the Scanning Table
Wheelchair Transfers
Stretcher Transfers
Infection Control
  Standard Precautions
  Additional Precautions
  Nosocomial Infections
Isolation Techniques
Emergency Medical Situations
  Choking
  Cardiopulmonary Resuscitation
  Basic Cardiac Life Support
Professional Attitudes
  Reestablishing Patient-Focused Care

Assisting Patients with Special Needs
  Crying Patients
  Pediatric Patients
  Adolescent Patients
  Elderly Patients
  Culturally Diverse Patients
Evaluating Patient Reactions to Illness
  Terminal Patients
Patient Rights
  Patients' Bill of Rights
  Health Insurance Portability and Accountability Act (HIPAA)

KEY TERMS

Apnea
Arrhythmia
Body mechanics
Bradycardia
Cyanosis
Dyspnea
Heimlich maneuver
Hypertension

Hypotension
Intravenous (IV) therapy
Isolated systolic hypertension
Nasal cannula
Nasal catheter
Nosocomial infections
Ostomy
Oximetry

Patient-focused care (PFC)
Prehypertension
Pulse
Pulse pressure
Respiration
Standard precautions
Tachycardia
Vital signs

As a sonographer in training, the majority of your studies will focus on anatomic and clinical knowledge, as well as the technical skills necessary to produce diagnostic ultrasound images. But another important area of study includes the basic patient care you will be expected to provide in clinical practice. The goal of this chapter is to prepare you to provide that care confidently, proficiently, and safely to the patients entrusted to your care.

A SONOGRAPHER'S OBLIGATIONS

As a sonographer, you have four main obligations: to your patients; to your sonologist, department, or institution; to the profession; and to yourself. Compassion, patience, and the desire to help people are qualities that will help you meet your obligations to your patients. Meeting the obligations to your sonologist and institution requires the ability to produce high-quality diagnostic studies, to project self-confidence and maturity, and to practice good interpersonal skills. A profession in diagnostic medical sonography requires you to act professionally at all times, to pass your registry examinations, and thereafter to continue your education to keep abreast of the growth and changes in the field. To achieve all of these goals, you have an important obligation to maintain good physical and mental health by practicing proper nutrition, engaging in adequate exercise, and getting the rest and relaxation you need.

Patient-Focused Care

Florence Nightingale advocated focusing on the patient, rather than on the disease, as a way to recognize the many unique dimensions of the sick and wounded. By distinguishing patient care from medicine, Nightingale established the value of nurses and created the earliest patient advocates.

The most important facet of being a sonographer is seeing the patient as the primary focus of your efforts. Despite personal or philosophical concerns, you must be considerate of the patient's age, cultural traditions, personal values, and lifestyle. Good patient care goes beyond procedural skills. It includes communicating with patients and allowing them to express their individual problems, fears, and frustrations. It also requires you to cooperate with other departments and facilities and health care professionals in order to deliver the best and most complete patient care through a team effort.

Patient-focused care (PFC) represents a national movement to recapture the respect and goodwill of the American public. It is the beginning of a larger objective to ensure that every patient receives the best possible medical care. The patient-focused approach encourages sonographers to relate to patients as people with needs, who are to be respected and cared for in a mature and dignified manner.

BASIC PATIENT CARE

Vital Signs

Vital signs are the observable and measurable signs of life and include the following: pulse, respiratory rate, body temperature, and blood pressure. Vital signs are monitored as indicators of how a patient's body is functioning and to establish a baseline for further study. Changes in age and medical condition can alter the normal vital sign ranges. Box 2-1 provides a concise, age-related reference for normal vital signs. It is essential to take careful and accurate measurements of each of the vital signs, as well as to include observations about the patient's skin color and any comments patients make about how they feel or how they react while in your care.

Sonographers are not routinely required to assess vital signs unless performing specific ultrasound studies (e.g., cardiovascular, obstetric) or in an emergency situation. When they do, the focus is on pulse, respiration, and blood pressure.

BOX 2-1 | Normal Vital Signs

Adult
Oral temperature: 96.8° F–99.5° F
Normal pulse: 60–100 bpm
Normal respirations: 12–20 breaths/min
Normal blood pressure range: 100–139 mm Hg diastolic;
    60–89 mm Hg systolic

Adolescent
Oral temperature: 97.5° F–98.6° F
Pulse: 55–90 bpm
Respirations: 12–20 breaths/min
Blood pressure: 121/70 mm Hg

School-Age Child
Oral temperature: 97.5° F–98.6° F
Pulse: 60–100 bpm
Respirations: 16–20 breaths/min
Blood pressure: 107/64 mm Hg

Preschool Child
Axillary temperature: 97.5° F–98.6° F
Pulse: 70–110 bpm
Respirations: 16–22 breaths/min
Blood pressure: 95/57 mm Hg

Toddler
Axillary temperature: 97.5° F–98.6° F
Pulse: 80–120 bpm
Respirations: 20–30 breaths/min
Blood pressure: 92/55 mm Hg

One-Year-Old
Axillary temperature: 97.0° F–99.0° F
Pulse: 90–130 bpm
Respirations: 20–40 breaths/min
Blood pressure: 90/56 mm Hg

Newborn
Axillary temperature: 97.7° F–99.5° F
Pulse: 120–160 bpm
Respirations: 30–60 breaths/min
Blood pressure: 73/55 mm Hg systolic

Data from *Mosby's expert physical exam handbook: rapid inpatient and outpatient assessments*, ed 3, St. Louis, 2009, Mosby; and Silvestri LA: *Saunders comprehensive review for the NCLEX-RN examination*, ed 4, Philadelphia, 2008, Saunders.
bpm, Beats per minute.

Practicing how to perform vital sign measurements on yourself or others will help you sharpen your skills before the need arises.

Pulse. When the heart actively pumps, blood is forced into large and small arteries during contractions of the left ventricle. The amount of force created when blood hits the arterial walls produces an advancing pressure wave that causes the arterial walls to expand. This expansion produces the feeling of a pulse that can be felt in the abdomen, wrists, neck, inside of the elbow, ankles, feet, scalp, behind the knee, and near the groin (peripheral pulses). The places where the pulse is measured are named after the artery that is palpated in that area. Any artery that passes over bone can be used to find the pulse, but the arteries that are most commonly used for recording the pulse are the radial and carotid arteries.

The **pulse** offers an easy and effective way to measure heart rate and is recorded as beats per minute (bpm). The beat of the pulse should be evaluated for rate, rhythm, and regularity, as well as for strength and tension (Table 2-1). Normal adult pulse rates should be between 60 and 100 bpm

TABLE 2-1	Pulse Patterns	
Pulse Type	**Rhythm: Rate**	**Factors Involved**
Normal adult female	Steady: 60–100 bpm	
Normal adult male	Steady: 55–95 bpm	
Arrhythmia	Irregular: uneven intervals between beats	Hypoxia Low potassium Occasional premature beats are normal
Tachycardia	Rapid: >100 bpm	Activity or exercise Acute pain Alcohol Anemia Anxiety Asthma medications Atropine Decongestants Extreme heat Fever Heart disease Hyperthyroidism Stimulants (e.g., caffeine, amphetamines, diet pills, cigarettes) Stress
Bradycardia	Steady: <60 bpm	Antiarrhythmics Beta-blockers Digitalis Heart disease Hypothyroidism Well-conditioned athletes

Data from Mosby's *PDQ for LPN*, ed 2, St. Louis, 2008, Mosby; and Pagana KD, Pagana TJ: *Mosby's manual of diagnostic and laboratory tests*, ed 3, St. Louis, 2006, Mosby.
bpm, Beats per minute.

and should have a regular rhythm (see Box 2-1). However, there are some normal variations. For example, rates in children, women, and the elderly are slightly higher than they are for adult males, whereas rates in athletes in good condition are slightly lower.

An increased pulse volume sounds full and bounding, whereas a decreased volume sounds weak and thready. Any irregular heartbeat is termed an **arrhythmia** or *dysrhythmia*. The following conditions may cause arrhythmias:

- Strenuous exercise
- Strong emotions
- Fever
- Pain
- Coronary artery disease
- Electrolyte imbalances in the blood (such as sodium or potassium)
- Changes in heart muscle
- Injury from a heart attack
- Healing process after heart surgery

Among the most common arrhythmias are tachycardia and bradycardia (see Table 2-1). **Tachycardia** is defined as a heart rate of more than 100 bpm. This finding may only be temporary, caused by exertion or nervousness, or it may be secondary to cardiac disease.

A heart rate of fewer than 60 bpm is **bradycardia** and may arise from disease in the heart's electrical conduction system. Examples include sinus node dysfunction and heart block. However, it is important to remember that irregular heart rhythms can also occur in "healthy" hearts as a normal physical response. In normal adults, the strength of the pulse should be full and strong, a factor that is influenced by arterial wall elasticity, blood volume, and the mechanical actions of the heart. If no abnormalities are detected, the pulse should be counted for 30 seconds and multiplied by 2. If irregularities are noted, the pulse should be counted for a full minute.

When taking a pulse, first explain the procedure to the patient and then have the patient bend his elbow with his arm at his side, palm side down. The radial artery can be located by placing the index, middle, and ring fingers on the anterior surface of the thumb side of the patient's hand (Figure 2-1). Gentle pressure should be applied to avoid obstructing blood flow. Never use your thumb to take the patient's pulse, as the strong pulse within your own thumb may be confused with that of the patient's. Using your finger, gently feel for the radial artery on the inner side of the wrist. When found, record the pulse rate and anything you notice about the pulse, such as its being weak, strong, or missing beats. If an irregularity is detected, determine whether it occurs in a pattern or is random.

If the radial pulse is difficult to count, try the carotid artery. To find the carotid artery, place your fingers just below the angle of the patient's mandible (Figure 2-2).

Pulse Oximetry. **Oximetry** is a convenient, noninvasive method of monitoring blood oxygen levels. For a variety of reasons, this information is useful to determine whether the heart, lungs, and blood are working synchronously to deliver oxygen to various parts of the body. A low blood oxygen reading can be a sign of an illness or injury.

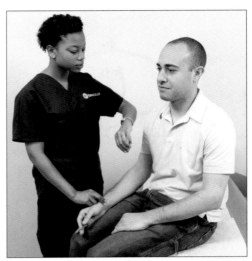

FIGURE 2-1 Taking a radial pulse. Never use the thumb to feel the patient's pulse.

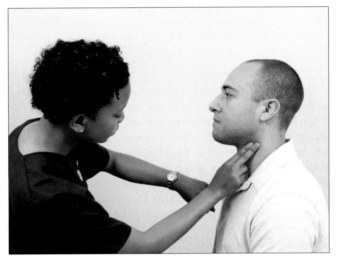

FIGURE 2-2 To locate the carotid pulse point, place your fingers just below the angle of the mandible.

The test is performed by using an oximeter, a specially designed photoelectric device that measures the difference between levels of the red pigment hemoglobin, which carries oxygen in the blood. The most commonly used oximeters are called *pulse oximeters* because they respond only to pulsations such as those of the pulsating capillaries in the area to be tested (Figure 2-3). One end of the device is attached like a clothespin to the end of the patient's index finger or earlobe. The index finger is usually selected, but a smaller finger may be used if the index finger is too large to accommodate the clip. The other end of the oximeter is attached to a monitor so that the patient's oxygenation level can be seen at all times. The patient's hand should be positioned at heart level to eliminate venous pulsations and to promote accurate readings.

The amount of oxygen in the blood is given as a percentage. A normal reading for a person breathing room air is in the high 90s. A reading of 90% or less will trigger visual and audible alarms, requiring immediate action.

Pulse oximetry cannot offer a profile of blood gas analysis nor can it act as a substitute for taking a blood sample and examining its content. The oximeter acts purely as an indicator that something somewhere is interfering with the oxygenation of blood levels and that further investigation is required. The test may not be accurate in certain conditions such as when a patient has very low blood pressure or very poor heart function, or with conditions that can change blood color (e.g., exposure to carbon monoxide). A variety of factors may cause readings to be lower than expected:

- The patient's wearing of nail polish
- Improper positioning of the probe
- Excessive movement by the patient
- Hypothermia or cold injury to the extremities
- Anemia
- Chronic obstructive pulmonary disease (COPD)
- Carbon monoxide poisoning
- Shock associated with blood loss or poor perfusion

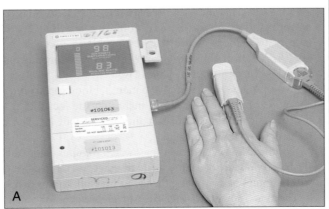

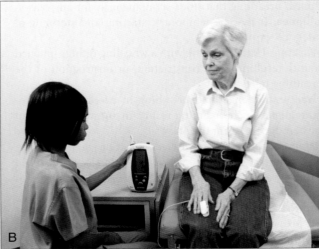

FIGURE 2-3 Pulse oximeters are used to detect problems with blood oxygen levels before clinical signs appear. **A,** Portable pulse oximeter with digit probe. **B,** The pulse oximeter sensor is attached to the patient's finger to measure the oxygen saturation levels in the blood.

| BOX 2-2 | Evaluating Patient Respiration |

Rate. The number of respirations per minute.
Rhythm. The regular rate of breathing and a symmetric movement of the chest.
Depth. The amount of air taken in with each respiration (e.g., normal, shallow, deep).
Character. The quality of respiration (quiet, labored, wheezing, coughing).

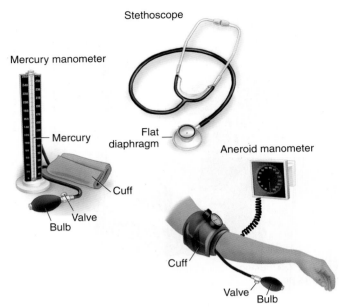

FIGURE 2-4 Instruments for measuring blood pressure. Mercury and aneroid types of manometers and accessories (stethoscope and cuff).

Respiration. **Respiration,** or breathing, is the process of inhaling and exhaling air. Its primary function is to obtain oxygen for use by the body's cells and to eliminate the cells' production of carbon dioxide.

Normal breathing is quiet, is effortless, and has a regular rhythm. In an adult at rest, respiration occurs at a rate of 12 to 20 breaths per minute. However, the normal rates change depending on age and condition (see Table 2-1). Measuring respiration for less than a full minute may lead to inaccuracies.

When assessing a patient's respiratory rate, the rhythm, depth, and character of the respiration also should be noted (Box 2-2). Any injuries to the lungs, chest muscles, or diaphragm will affect breathing. Note whether the patient needs to sit up or stand up to breathe easily as opposed to lying down. Any difficulty in breathing (**dyspnea**) or changes in the patient's color (pallor or **cyanosis**) should be noted.

To count respirations, note the number of inhalations per minute. Counting respirations is often done while continuing to hold the patient's wrist—after the pulse has been counted—to prevent patients from being aware that you are monitoring their breathing. Aware patients sometimes force a change in their respirations.

In addition to counting the respiratory rate, it is important to note whether the patient has any difficulty in breathing. Breathing problems can take many forms, including the following:

- *Dyspnea.* A shortness of breath or the feeling of not getting enough air, which may leave a person gasping.
- *Apnea.* Breathing that stops spontaneously for any reason is **apnea.** It may be temporary, starting and stopping at intervals, or prolonged.
- *Wheezing.* Hard breathing with a whistling or high-pitched sound, resulting from constriction, or obstruction of the breathing tubes.
- *Hyperventilation.* Rapid breathing in excess of body requirements. Such breathing results in an excessive loss of carbon dioxide from the body.
- *Respiratory arrest.* A life-threatening stoppage of breathing that requires emergency medical assistance. It is caused either by an excessive loss of oxygen or by an increase of excessive carbon dioxide in the blood.

Blood Pressure. One of the most important vital signs is blood pressure. Blood pressure is the pressure exerted by circulating blood against the walls of the blood vessels. As the blood travels away from the heart, the pressure of the circulating blood *decreases,* spreading through arteries and capillaries, and back toward the heart through the veins.

Unless qualified, the term *blood pressure* generally refers to the brachial arterial pressure in the major blood vessel of the upper arm. The manual measurement of blood pressure is usually performed with a sphygmomanometer, blood pressure cuff, and stethoscope. The blood pressure cuff consists of an air pump, a pressure gauge, and a rubber cuff (Figure 2-4). The instrument measures the blood pressure in units called millimeters of mercury (mm Hg). Electronic blood pressure monitors may also be used to measure heart rate or pulse.

Two numbers, systolic and diastolic, are recorded when measuring blood pressure. The higher number is the *systolic* pressure, which occurs when the ventricles contract to pump blood to the body. The lower number is the *diastolic* pressure, which occurs near the end of the cardiac cycle when the ventricles are filling with blood. Both numbers are important and are written as a fraction: the top number is the systolic number and the bottom number is the diastolic number. Both the systolic and diastolic pressures are recorded as mm Hg, representing how high the mercury column is raised by the pressure of the blood. A normal, resting blood pressure in an adult is 115 mm Hg systolic and 75 mm Hg diastolic, and it would be written as 115/75 mm Hg.

When manually taking a patient's blood pressure, you should explain the procedure, including the fact that it will take several minutes and that the patient will feel the cuff tighten and then deflate.

For the most accurate readings, wait 5 minutes before taking the blood pressure of a patient who is quiet and relaxed. Wait 15 to 30 minutes before taking the blood pressure of a patient who has been actively exercising. The proper protocol for obtaining a blood pressure includes the following steps (Figure 2-5):

- If the patient is sitting, be sure she has both feet on the floor.

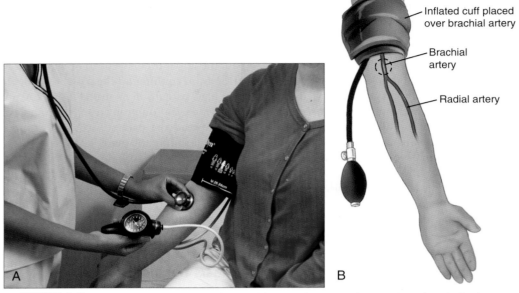

FIGURE 2-5 A, The blood pressure cuff should be snugly wrapped approximately 1 inch above the bend of the arm. **B,** The stethoscope should be placed over the brachial artery at the bend of the arm.

- The brachial artery in the upper arm is the usual site for manually taking a blood pressure. Move any clothing out of the way to be able to put the blood pressure cuff on properly.
- Place the cuff above the elbow, making sure it is about an inch above the elbow.
- You should be able to put only one finger under a cuff that is tightened correctly.
- Position the patient's arm, placing it on a table, a desk, or the bedside.
- Choose a stethoscope with a flat-style diaphragm for taking blood pressures. Place the stethoscope earpieces into your ears; then feel for the brachial artery pulsation (usually found at the crease of the elbow) and place the diaphragm there.
- Squeezing the balloon, rapidly inflate the cuff to about 200 mm Hg, or until no sound is heard. If you inflate too slowly, you will get a false reading.
- Loosen the valve slowly (no faster than 5 mm Hg/sec) to let some air out and listen for the first heartbeat. Check the position of the pointer of the dial. This first sound is the systolic reading.
- Continue deflating the cuff slowly. Check the position of the pointer for the diastolic number. The last audible sound is the diastolic reading.
- Release the cuff and record both readings as a fraction (e.g., 110/70).

The sound produced by a normal heart is heard as a *lub-dub*. Every time you hear this sound, it means the heart is contracting once. When you hear the *lub* sound, the atrioventricular valves are closing. The *dub* sound represents the pulmonic and aortic valves.

Always use a blood pressure cuff that is correctly sized for the patient. Cuffs that are too small may yield readings 10 to 50 mm Hg too high, falsely indicating hypertension.

On occasion, blood pressure may be measured in the main artery of the ankle. The ratio of the blood pressure measured at the ankle—to the brachial blood pressure—gives the ankle brachial pressure index (ABPI).

Hypertension. High blood pressure, or **hypertension,** directly increases the risk of coronary heart disease and stroke. When blood pressure is high, the arteries may have increased resistance against the flow of blood, causing the heart to pump harder.

According to the National Institutes of Health (NIH), high blood pressure for adults is defined as 140 mm Hg or greater systolic pressure and 90 mm Hg or greater diastolic pressure. In 2003 the NIH guidelines for hypertension were updated and a new blood pressure category, **prehypertension,** was added. The blood pressure readings associated with prehypertension are 120 mm Hg to 139 mm Hg systolic pressure and 80 mm Hg to 89 mm Hg diastolic pressure.

These numbers should be used only as guides, because a single elevated blood pressure measurement is not necessarily an indication of a problem. Multiple blood pressure measurements over several days or weeks are necessary before the diagnosis of hypertension is made and treatment initiated.

Isolated Systolic Hypertension. Isolated systolic hypertension exists when the systolic pressure is above 140 mm Hg, with a diastolic pressure that is still below 90 mm Hg. This condition primarily affects older people. It is characterized by an increased pulse pressure. **Pulse pressure** is the difference between the systolic and diastolic blood pressures.

When the systolic pulse pressure measurement is elevated—without an elevation of the diastolic pressure—there is an increase in the pulse pressure. Hardening of the arteries contributes to the pulse pressures associated with isolated systolic high blood pressure.

Previously thought to be harmless, a high pulse pressure is now considered a precursor of health problems and potential end-organ damage. Patients with this type of hypertension have a 2 to 4 times greater risk for enlarged heart, heart attack, and stroke. At the opposite end of the spectrum is **hypotension,** or abnormally low blood pressure. Pressure that falls too far below 90/60 mm Hg normal blood pressure is considered hypotension.

Blood pressure readings can be affected by a variety of factors, including cardiovascular disorders, neurologic conditions, kidney and urologic disorders, obesity, and some medications.

PATIENTS ON STRICT BED REST

Occasionally, patients on bed rest are brought to the ultrasound laboratory for diagnostic testing. For these patients, a full bladder can be very uncomfortable, making it difficult to remain still during scanning. Unless a full urinary bladder is needed for the study, always ask patients if they need to void before starting any lengthy procedures and be prepared with the proper equipment (a urinal, bedpan, or wheelchair, and bathroom facilities).

Bedpans and Urinals

There are two types of bedpans. Fracture pans have a flat lip in the front that makes them easy to slide under a patient who has problems lifting the pelvis for bedpan placement. The regular bedpan is somewhat larger and deeper, with a rounded lip designed to support the buttocks (Figure 2-6). Single-use disposable containers (including bedpans and urinals) are now available in many short-stay hospital departments. There are special disposal containers for these bedpans and urinals that accept both the container and contents to minimize handling.

Assisting with Patient Elimination. When assisting with patient elimination, assemble the supplies you will need, don protective gloves, and follow the procedure as outlined in Box 2-3. Be sure the patient is adequately covered for privacy. When helping female patients with a bedpan, the upper torso needs to be slightly elevated to prevent urine from running up the patient's back. You may need to help male patients use a urinal if they are unable to do so by themselves. Put on protective gloves and explain the procedure. Spread the patient's legs, lifting the sheet with one hand and sliding the penis into the urinal with the other. It may be necessary to hold the urinal in position until the patient is finished. Always check the chart before emptying bedpans or urinals to see if there is an order for a specimen collection or if urinary intake and output need to be measured. The nursing staff should indicate this and provide the correct container.

Emesis Basins

Vomiting often accompanies illness or injury. Emesis basins are kidney-shaped containers that are used to collect the vomit (emesis). (Emesis basins are also sometimes used to collect the runoff from medical procedures involving the application of liquid to the body.) If a patient is nauseated, place an emesis basin below his chin and against his neck to collect any vomit. After the patient finishes vomiting, offer him a glass of water to rinse his mouth and a tissue to dry his face.

It is important to observe the emesis with respect to its color and odor and for the presence of undigested food. Emesis that is dark brown or reddish brown may be evidence of undigested blood and should be reported. Do not dispose of the emesis until you have been cleared to do so. Check the chart for any orders to collect the emesis for laboratory study. If the order exists, place the emesis in the proper specimen container and see that it is delivered to the laboratory. Once the emesis has been removed, the basin, which may be made of stainless steel or plastic, should be cleansed or properly discarded, if disposable.

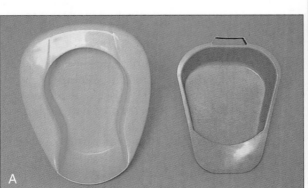
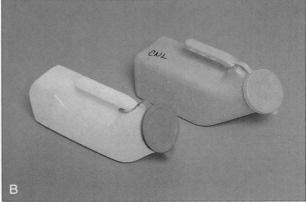

FIGURE 2-6 A, Regular bedpan *(left)* and fracture bedpan *(right).* **B,** Types of male urinals.

BOX 2-3	Assisting Patients with the Bedpan or Urinal

- Assemble the equipment: bedpan with cover; toilet tissue, disposable moist towelettes, and a sheet.
- Wash your hands, and then don disposable gloves.
- Explain the procedure and the purpose.
- Ask the patient to bend the knees and raise the hips.
- Assist the patient by lifting with one hand under the small of the back while you slide the bedpan under the patient's buttocks with your other hand.
- Ask the patient to call when finished. Elevate the side rails of the bed or stretcher, leaving the toilet tissue within reach.
- Provide the patient with privacy.
- When the patient is finished, provide a moist towelette for the patient's hands.
- Ask the patient to raise his or her hips, and then remove the bedpan.
- Cover the bedpan and place it aside until the patient is settled and secure.
- If blood is present in *either stool or urine*, record your observation.
- Dispose of the contents in the toilet (or specimen container if necessary). Remove and dispose of your gloves and repeat hand washing.

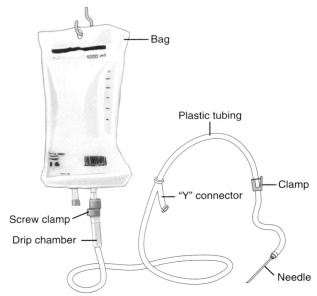

FIGURE 2-7 IV equipment. Plastic tubing leads from a solution-filled bag at one end and connects to a needle at the other end. Clamping the tubing controls the rate of flow.

PATIENTS WITH TUBES AND TUBING

The most common types of tubing that sonographers encounter when working with hospital patients are the following:
- Intravenous (IV) infusion tubing
- Nasogastric suction tubing
- Urinary catheters
- Nasal catheters/cannulae used for oxygen administration

Sonographers are generally not responsible for starting any of the procedures that use such equipment, but they are required to know how to handle and care for patients who have such tubes in place.

Intravenous Therapy

The practice of giving liquid substances directly into a vein is called **intravenous (IV) therapy.** The IV route is the fastest way to deliver fluids and medications. IV therapy is often used to correct dehydration or electrolyte imbalances or to deliver medications or blood transfusions. Fluids can be administered intermittently or continuously, with the continuous method called an *IV drip.*

Figure 2-7 shows the chief components of a standard IV infusion set: a prefilled, sterile plastic bag of fluids. There is an attached drip chamber that makes it easy to see the rate of flow and allows the fluid to flow one drop at a time. A long sterile tube with a clamp leads from the drip chamber to the insertion site of the IV. The clamp regulates or stops the flow. The IV "line" is attached to a short catheter that is inserted

into a peripheral vein. For adult patients, arm and hand veins are commonly used; for infants, the scalp veins are sometimes used.

Patients who are receiving IV fluids may come to the ultrasound department with either a standard IV set or possibly an electronic flow regulator in place. Once the patient is transferred to the scanning table, it is important to check the height of the IV fluid container. It should always be 18 to 20 cm above the level of the patient's vein. An IV container placed too high may cause too rapid a flow rate and fluid may infiltrate into the surrounding tissues. Conversely, if the container is placed too low, blood may flow back into the catheter or tubing and may clot, causing the fluid to stop flowing.

If the needle is accidentally dislodged, the IV fluid may enter the surrounding tissue rather than the vein. The patient may complain of discomfort, and you may observe swelling (edema) of the tissues around the injection site. Clamp off the flow and notify the nursing staff for instructions and to determine whether you should continue the study.

Medication pumps (electronic flow regulators) are often used for patient-controlled pain medications, parenteral nutrition, and the continuous administration of medicine (Figure 2-8). These regulators will emit a warning sound when the solution supply is low, when flow is interrupted, or when the battery power of the pump is too weak. If an alarm sounds while you are scanning, avoid the temptation to work rapidly to complete the study and have the patient returned to ward. If this situation arises, call the nursing service immediately for instructions.

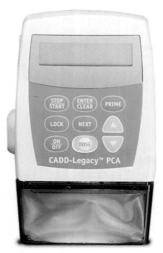

FIGURE 2-8 Patient-controlled analgesia pump. *(Courtesy Smiths Medical, ASD, Inc.)*

Nasogastric Suction Tubes

A nasogastric suction tube (NG tube) is a flexible tube made of rubber or plastic (Figure 2-9). An NG tube is passed through the nose and down through the nasopharynx and esophagus into the stomach to (1) remove the contents of the stomach, including air; (2) decompress the stomach; and (3) remove small solid objects or fluid, such as poison, from the stomach. NG tubes can also be used to instill medications and put substances such as nutrients directly into the stomach when a patient cannot take food or drink by mouth.

If used for drainage, the NG tube is usually attached to a collector bag placed below the level of the patient's stomach, thus using gravity to empty the stomach contents. If used for continuous drainage, the drainage bag is placed below the

level of the patient's stomach and suction drainage is employed. When patients connected to mechanical suction machines come to the ultrasound department, there are rules for working with them:

- Never pull on the tube when moving the patient.
- Check for leaks in both the NG tube and suction equipment. If found, report them immediately.
- Never raise or open the drainage bottle.
- Never disconnect the tubing.
- If the amount of material being suctioned rapidly increases, report it immediately.
- If the patient begins to gag or vomit while the tube is in place, report it immediately.

Catheters

Urinary catheters are used for removing fluids from the body. They are thin, sterile tubes that are inserted into the bladder as a way to manage urinary incontinence or urinary retention, to collect sterile fluid for laboratory diagnosis, and to fill the bladder before imaging studies (Figure 2-10, *A*).

Catheters come in a large variety of sizes, types, and materials (latex, silicone, and Teflon). The most commonly used catheter is the Foley catheter, a flexible latex tube that has openings in the tip and below the opening; the tubing inflates on demand like a small balloon. Once placed properly, the balloon is inflated with sterile water to effectively occlude the cervix of the bladder where the urethra begins and to prevent the catheter from sliding out of the bladder. Urine flows through the openings in the catheter tubing and into the tubing itself, instead of through the urethra and out of the urinary meatus. The urine drains into a collecting bag (Figure 2-10, *B*).

When catheterized patients are transferred from wheelchairs or stretchers to the scanning table, the collecting bag

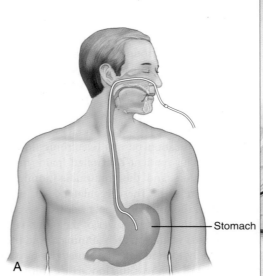

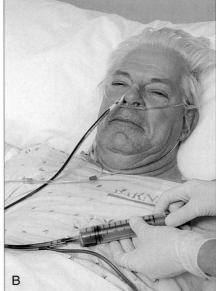

FIGURE 2-9 A, A nasogastric (NG) tube is inserted through one nostril and down through the esophagus until it reaches the stomach. **B,** A syringe can be used to suction the stomach contents.

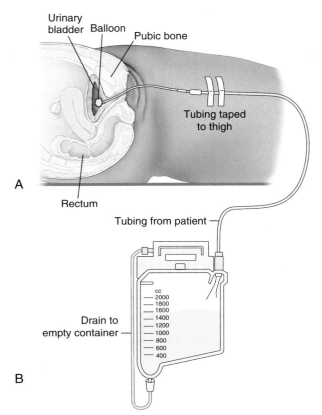

FIGURE 2-10 Catheterization equipment. **A,** A plastic/rubber urinary catheter is inserted through the urethra and into the bladder. **B,** Urine drains into a container.

must be held below the level of the patient's bladder. This will prevent urine in the tube or bag from being siphoned back into the bladder, which would cause patient discomfort and give bacteria potential access to the bladder. Because it can be left in the bladder for a period of time, the Foley catheter is also called an indwelling catheter. A sterile urinary catheterization kit needs to be provided if the patient must be catheterized while in the ultrasound department. A doctor or medical assistant is normally called to insert the Foley catheter.

Oxygen Therapy

Oxygen therapy is an essential treatment for many conditions. Its primary purpose is to decrease the work of breathing for patients experiencing respiratory difficulties. Oxygen should be treated as a drug whose dosage or concentration is ordered by a physician. There are important safety issues involving the use of oxygen. Although oxygen itself cannot burn, it will ignite and burn if it comes in contact with any combustible substance (even a spark). When large concentrations of oxygen are present, ignition could cause an explosion.

A variety of oxygen systems exist to provide either high-flow or low-flow oxygen delivery. The type of system selected depends on the concentration of oxygen needed and the age and the activity level of the patient. Oxygen systems consist of three main parts: (1) a container, (2) a breathing device (mask or cannula), and (3) a connecting tube.

Oxygen tanks have different parts:
- A pressure gauge to show how much oxygen is left in the tank
- A flowmeter to control the rate of oxygen coming out of the tank
- A humidifier bottle, where water is mixed with the oxygen and the oxygen is warmed before delivery to prevent the membranes of the patient's nose, mouth, and throat from becoming too dry

Portable oxygen systems deliver compressed oxygen in either large tanks on a cart or in smaller cylinders that can be rolled on a small cart. The large tanks are used for patients who require high flow rates of oxygen over extended periods. The smaller cylinders are used during patient transportation or for short duration needs. Ambulatory patients who require continuous oxygen generally use an over-the-shoulder strap or a rolling stand to hold the cylinder.

For scanning laboratories equipped with in-room piping, both oxygen and suction are usually provided through wall outlets. Figure 2-11 illustrates the appearance of an oxygen flowmeter. The dial on the side is used to adjust the flow rate, which is indicated by the level of the small ball shown near the center of the gauge.

Whether patients come to the ultrasound department with a tank or a cylinder, or will be using in-wall systems, there are special safety precautions to follow:
- Do not transport any oxygen tank unless it is secured to a tank/cylinder cart.
- Secure the tank in an upright position and away from any heat source because of the risks of combustion. This includes electrical equipment, such as heating pads and radios.

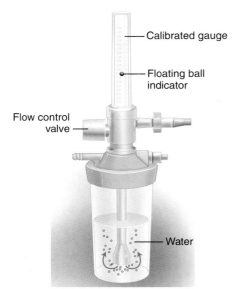

FIGURE 2-11 Schematic drawing of a typical wall-mounted oxygen flowmeter. Water levels must be kept high enough to bubble as oxygen flows through the flowmeter.

- No one should smoke where oxygen is being used.
- Any combustible material, such as alcohol, perfumes, and propane, must be kept away from oxygen tanks.
- Do not place a cylinder beside a patient when transporting the patient by stretcher.

Nasal Cannulae and Nasal Catheters. Delivery of oxygen to the patient requires tubing connected to the oxygen source on one end and attached at the other end to a patient's mask, **nasal cannula,** or a tent. Nasal cannulae are usually used to deliver low-to-medium concentrations of oxygen in situations when precise accuracy is not required. The patient-end of the nasal cannula is placed into each of the patient's nostrils and held in place by an elastic band around the patient's head (Figure 2-12, *A*).

A **nasal catheter** (oropharyngeal catheter) is a piece of tubing that is longer than a cannula. It is inserted through the nostril and into the back of the patient's mouth. This method provides more effective oxygen delivery and is used when the patient must have additional oxygen at all times. The nasal catheter is fastened to the patient's forehead or cheek by a piece of adhesive tape to hold it steady, and it must be long enough with enough slack to allow the patient to move around comfortably.

Oxygen Masks. There are a variety of oxygen masks for delivering oxygen to patients with specific needs. The simple mask is used to provide short-term therapy; it delivers both oxygen and humidity. This type of oxygen mask is typically made of transparent material that conforms to the patient's face. It is held in place by an elastic strap that is fitted over nose, mouth, and chin (Figure 2-12, *B*). The reservoir mask is a low-flow device identified by the presence of a bag, which must remain constantly inflated by one-third. There are several types: partial rebreather and non-rebreather masks. The partial rebreather mask delivers oxygen concentrations of 40% to 60%. Openings in the mask allow the patient to inhale room air if the oxygen source fails. The non-rebreather mask delivers the highest possible oxygen concentrations (60% to 90%) because the patient only breathes air from the bag. It is effective for short-term therapy (Figure 2-12, *C*).

Both masks cover the nose and mouth of the patient and are attached with an elastic band around the patient's head. These masks have an attached reservoir bag that is inflated approximately two-thirds full of oxygen before placing it on the patient. Sonographers should especially note the level of inflation on the non-rebreather mask, because if the bag completely deflates, the patient no longer has a source of air to breathe.

The Venturi mask is a high-flow mask designed to administer precisely controlled low oxygen concentrations, but with variable airflow to produce a constant oxygen concentration regardless of breathing rate. This is accomplished by a Venturi device and is identified by the presence of a hard plastic adapter with large "windows" on either side.

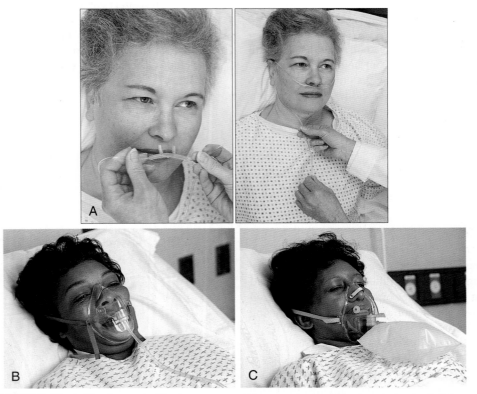

FIGURE 2-12 A, Nasal cannula. The two prongs of the cannula should be inserted a short distance into the patient's nostrils. An elastic headband behind the ears is used to keep the cannula in place. **B,** A simple oxygen face mask should cover the nose and mouth of the patient. **C,** Reservoir, or partial rebreathing, mask. This low-flow device is equipped with an inflatable bag.

The following precautions should be observed whenever working with patients receiving oxygen therapy:

- Observe all fire regulations in effect at your institution.
- Check the flowmeter to be sure oxygen is being delivered to the patient. The water level in the humidifying chamber should be high enough so that it bubbles as the oxygen goes through it.
- Be sure the tubing connected to the oxygen source is taped to the patient to help keep it from accidentally being pulled when moving the patient.
- Make sure the patient is not lying on the tubing or that it is not kinked, which can slow or stop the oxygen flow.
- In most hospitals, inhalation therapy or respiratory therapy departments are responsible for the patient's treatment. They should be called to make any needed adjustments after checking with the patient's physician or nurse.

Wounds, Drains, and Dressings

Some postsurgical patients sent for abdominal ultrasound studies may have wound drains in place. A wound drain is created by inserting a wick inside of the wound to provide drainage. It is important not to pull or dislodge the drain whenever positioning, scanning, or transferring the patient. For wounds that are actively draining, a gauze pad can be taped over the area until the scan is completed.

If the wound is situated within the scanning field, sterile technique is required to scan over the open wound. After gloving, apply sterile gel to the wound area and cover it with thin plastic film. Next, more sterile gel should be applied over the film to create an airless contact between the transducer and the wound area.

Some wounds may be covered by a dressing to protect them from injury or infection. If it becomes necessary to remove the dressing to gain scanning access, you should always check with the nursing staff before removing or replacing any dressings. It is important to determine whether wound precautions are in place, because if they are, the nursing staff is responsible for changing any dressings. If the dressings are considered nonsterile, the procedure for changing dressings is as follows:

- Wash hands and don gloves.
- Use sterile scanning gel to prevent wound infection.
- Remove the old dressing carefully to avoid dislodging any scabs or causing any pain.
- Remove the soiled dressing and dispose of it properly.
- Apply a clean dressing, using paper tape if possible.
- Report the presence of bleeding, drainage or foul odor.
- Report any patient complaints such as pain, itching, or burning.

Ostomies

Ostomies are sometimes created for patients with certain health conditions or diseases. Patients with colostomies or ileostomies have undergone surgical resection of the colon in which the distal end of the remaining functioning bowel

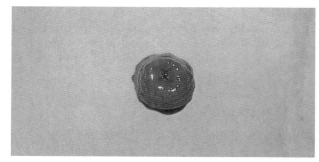

FIGURE 2-13 Typical colostomy stoma.

terminates in an artificial opening in the abdominal wall called a *stoma*. A stoma appears as a small hole surrounded by a ring of mucosal tissue (Figure 2-13). This opening may be temporary or permanent, depending on the patient's condition.

Ostomy patients must wear an external bag or pouch to collect liquefied fecal matter. The disposable ostomy bags are attached to the skin with a double-faced adhesive substance that seals the bag to the skin. The bags are equipped with a clamp or other closure device to keep the bag closed and secure between emptyings. Ostomy bags require frequent changing because of the constant flow of fecal material.

Another product designed for the ostomy patient's use is a stoma cap or cover to be placed on the stoma when the stoma is not actively draining. The cover or cap is attached to the skin in the same fashion as the ostomy bag. If your department schedules ostomy patients, keeping a small supply of the following items on hand is encouraged:

- New bags
- Plastic bags for disposal
- Closure clamps
- Water or bag-cleaning solution
- Washcloths and towels
- Toilet or bedpan
- Gloves
- Facial tissues
- Paper tape

Changing an ostomy bag requires clean rather than sterile technique. After gloving, remove and discard the old bag. Gently wipe the stoma and the peristomal skin with a facial tissue. Carefully wash and dry the peristomal skin, then apply a closure clamp if necessary. If desired, apply paper tape in a picture-frame fashion to the edges of the bag for additional security. The patient should be encouraged to stay quietly in position for about 5 minutes to improve adherence of the bag. Record the date and time of bag removal and replacement and the character of the drainage (color, amount, type, and consistency).

PATIENT TRANSFER TECHNIQUES

Patient safety is a prime component of patient care. Equally important is sonographer safety. Some of the most common injuries among members of the health care team are severe musculoskeletal strains. Sonographers can avoid many injuries with conscious use of body mechanics in their everyday activities, work activities, and especially when performing patient transfers. By protecting themselves from injury, they are also protecting their patients.

Body Mechanics

The term **body mechanics** refers to using the correct muscles to complete a task safely, efficiently, and without undue strain on any joints or muscles.

The basic principles of body mechanics require the following:

- Maintaining a stable center of gravity by keeping your center of gravity low, keeping your back straight, and bending at the hips and knees.
- Maintaining a strong base of support by keeping your feet apart, placing one foot slightly ahead of the other with toes pointed in the direction of activity, and then flexing your knees to absorb jolts and turning with your feet, instead of your hips.
- Maintaining a center of gravity by keeping your back straight and keeping any objects that are being lifted close to your body.
- Maintaining proper body alignment through good posture: Tuck in your buttocks, pull your abdomen in and up, keep your back flat, your head up, and your chin in as you keep your weight forward and supported on the outside of your feet (Figure 2-14).

Sonographers benefit greatly from using correct body mechanics when lifting and reaching. Their first consideration should be whether the object or patient is too heavy to lift alone. The potential for injury to themselves and their patients can be avoided by enlisting the help of another person.

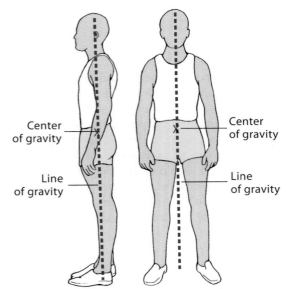

FIGURE 2-14 Correct body alignment when standing. Before lifting, feet should be placed shoulder width apart, with weight evenly distributed to provide a strong support base.

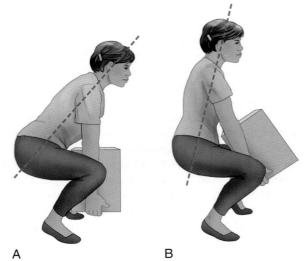

FIGURE 2-15 Proper body mechanics for lifting. **A,** Keep the back straight. When lifting, use the large muscles of the thigh instead of the smaller muscles of the back. **B,** Before the lift, tighten abdominal and pelvic muscles, tuck buttocks in, and keep head and chest up.

Lifting should be done using the strong leg muscles—not the back—and lifting straight upward in one smooth motion (Figure 2-15). When reaching, it is important to stand directly in front of the object or patient and to avoid any twisting or stretching motions. One of the most common causes of muscle strains or tears, as well as skeletal injuries, is stooping by bending at the waist.

The techniques of body mechanics are important if you will be walking patients or lifting or moving them via wheelchair or stretcher. In many hospitals, using wheeled transport is a strict policy when moving patients from one place to another. It is a safety precaution based on the possibility that ambulatory patients could become weak or faint while traveling from their room to the ultrasound department. For patients who can sit and stand comfortably, a wheelchair may be sufficient for transfer, but patients who cannot stand or walk alone should only be transferred by stretcher.

Active toddlers and infants are usually transported in their crib. The high sides provide better safety than side rails on a stretcher. An added advantage is that if the child must be unattended for any period of time, he or she will be safe. On rare occasions, patients whose condition makes it painful or difficult to move may come to the ultrasound department in a bed.

When preparing to transfer patients, always check with the nursing station to obtain the patient's chart and ask if there are any special instructions before or during transfer. The transfer equipment should be checked for safety and function. Sonographers assigned to transfer patients also are responsible for checking safety straps, buckles, brakes, and side rails (if a stretcher is used). If any extra equipment must accompany a patient (IV stands, urine bags, etc.), check with the nursing station before disconnecting any equipment or moving the patient. Once the patient is cleared for transfer, identify yourself to the patient and explain the reason for the transfer. Then ask the patient's name and check her identification (ID) bracelet to verify her identity.

Moving Patients up in Bed

First assess the patient's size and condition. If the patient is alert and cooperative and you are confident that you do not need help, follow these steps:

- Explain to the patient that on the count of 3, you are going to shift him up in bed.
- Lower the side rails to the level of the patient's shoulders.
- Move close to the side of the bed, keeping your back straight, knees bent, and one foot forward to provide a base of support.
- Ask the patient to bend his knees with his feet placed firmly on the bed.
- Place your hand and arms under the patient's hips while keeping your back straight, knees bent, and feet apart.
- Count to 3 and pull the patient up to the head of the bed, while he pulls with his arms and pushes with his feet.

If the patient is very large or unable to assist you, it will be easier to slide the patient up in bed by using a draw sheet and the help of another person (Figure 2-16):

- Ask the patient to bend her knees, then slide a draw sheet under her hips and buttocks.
- Put the head of the bed down.
- Grasp the draw sheet, pointing one of your feet in the direction in which you are moving toward the patient.
- Lean in the direction of the move, using your legs and body weight.
- On the count of 3, both of you slide the draw sheet toward the head of the bed.
- Reposition the patient comfortably and raise bedside rails if the patient is to remain in bed.

Assisting Patients to and from the Scanning Table

- When dealing with an ambulatory patient, if necessary, simply provide the patient with a gown and a private area in which to change.
- While the patient is changing, place a step stool near the middle of the scanning table and arrange the pillows, linens, and any supplies you will be using.
- When the patient is ready, escort him to the table and help him up and into the proper position for scanning.
- Once the examination is completed, help the patient down from the table and back to the changing area (Figure 2-17).

Wheelchair Transfers

It is always important to have everything ready for patient transfers before you begin. If you are moving the patient from the bed to a wheelchair, you may require the patient's help, so clear communication is essential. If patients are unable to help, you will need two people to make the transfer.

When working alone, first position and lock the wheelchair close to the bed and facing the foot of the bed. Then remove the armrest nearest the bed and swing away both leg rests (Figure 2-18):

- Adjust the bed to its lowest position to make it easy for the patient to step down to the floor.
- Sit the patient up by putting one arm under the patient's neck, with your hand supporting her shoulder blade, and putting the other hand under the patient's knees.
- Swing the patient's legs over the edge of the bed, helping her to sit up.

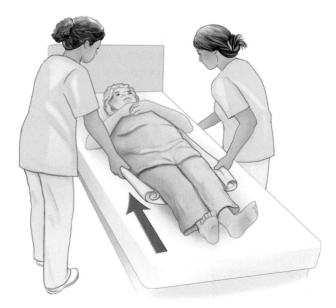

FIGURE 2-16 Using a lifting/turning sheet to move helpless patients. It is advisable to slide or pull rather than to lift. With the help of a colleague, this technique affords the safest way to move patients who are heavy or unable to help themselves.

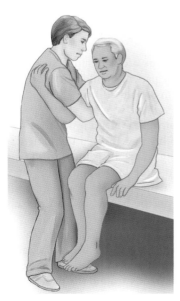

FIGURE 2-17 Assisting patients to and from a bed or scanning table. The sonographer should provide support under the arms of the patient and rotate or shift his or her weight as the person is brought closer to the sonographer.

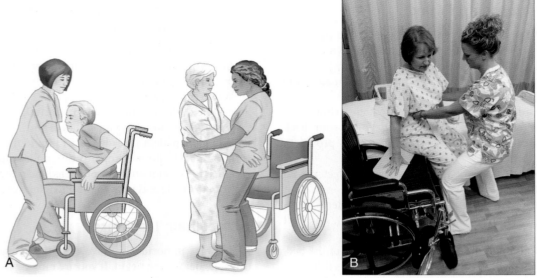

FIGURE 2-18 A, When moving patients to and from a wheelchair, bend at the knees and hips when lowering or raising the patient. Keep your shoulders level with the patient's shoulders and enlist the patient's help, if possible, by having the patient support his or her own weight when rising from or sitting down into the wheelchair. **B,** A friction-reducing device may be used to transfer a patient from the bed to the wheelchair.

- Place your arms around the torso of the patient for support. Put one arm of the patient over your shoulder or on your hip, while her other arm is extended with her hand flat on the bed to help support the position.
- Ask the patient to scoot to the edge of the bed until her feet are on the floor.
- Widen the distance of your feet with your right foot forward and left foot back, to easily shift your weight as you lift the patient.
- Put your arms around the patient's chest and clasp your hands behind her back. If available, you may also use a transfer belt around the patient's waist to provide a firmer handhold.
- While your arms are still supporting the patient's torso, one arm of the patient should still be on your shoulder and her other arm should still be extended, palm flat on the bed.
- Position your right foot alongside the patient's left foot to provide stability and to keep the patient's foot and knee from buckling when she is lifted to a standing position.
- Slightly bend your knees and lean your body forward. Instruct the patient to get ready to push the arm that is extended on the bed as you lift her up to a standing position.
- Count to 3, as you assist the patient to a standing position while she is pushing off the bed at the same time.
- Have the patient pivot toward the chair as you continue clasping your hands around the patient.
- Stand in front of the patient, keeping your knees bent and your feet about 12 inches apart.
- Make sure the backs of the patient's legs are against the chair seat. A helper can stabilize the wheelchair or the

patient from behind. Always be sure the wheelchair is locked.
- As the patient bends toward you, bend your knees and lower the patient down and toward the back of the wheelchair.

Stretcher Transfers

Patient safety is the primary concern when moving patients from a bed to a stretcher. Remember not to lift at the expense of your own back. If you move the patient's legs first, you can decrease the stress on your back. If at all possible, enlist the aid of a second person to help in making the move.

- Put the head of the bed down and adjust the bed height.
- Put a plastic slide board (or plastic trash bag) between the sheet and the draw sheet, beneath one edge of the patient's torso.
- Move the patient's legs closer to the edge of the bed.
- Instruct the patient to cross his arms across his chest, and then explain the move to the patient.
- For a two-person transfer, grasp the draw sheet on both sides of the bed (Figure 2-19).
- Adjust the bed slightly higher than the stretcher and then position the stretcher, locking it in place.
- Move the patient's legs onto the stretcher and have the helper kneel on the bed while holding onto the draw sheet.
- On the count of 3, grasp the draw sheet and slide the patient onto the stretcher.
- Raise the stretcher side rails, and unlock the brakes.
- See that the patient is comfortable and modestly covered.

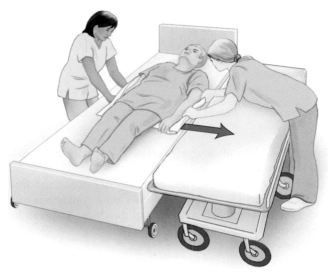

FIGURE 2-19 Transferring patients from bed to stretcher. Use of a "pulling sheet" is recommended whenever transferring patients who cannot help themselves.

INFECTION CONTROL

In the early 1800s, people believed that fresh air and sunlight were all that was needed to kill germs, and those working in the medical profession were not much more enlightened. Physicians spent little time washing their hands; a patient's skin was seldom cleansed before surgery; instruments were simply rinsed off between operations; and sponges were routinely reused. That all changed when Joseph Lister decided to spray carbolic acid on wounds, dressings, and surgical instruments. This one simple act significantly reduced postsurgical deaths. Not until the early 1900s would nurses began using gloves—not to protect the patients but to protect their hands against the harsh chemicals used during surgery. It would take many years for the medical profession to realize that wearing gloves also protects patients and to begin routinely using them as barriers to infection.

Standard Precautions

In the 1980s, the outbreak of human immunodeficiency virus/acquired immunodeficiency syndrome (HIV/AIDS) triggered the development of *universal precautions* to fight the ravaging disease. It would be another decade before the Centers for Disease Control and Prevention (CDC) would establish *standard precautions* and *additional precautions* to expand the universal precautions' guidelines by including additional body fluids and sites to the earlier protocols. These precautions apply to *all* patients regardless of their diagnoses and even if they appear asymptomatic.

It is extremely important to observe standard precautions when performing ultrasound studies on outpatients as well as inpatients.

Standard precautions are the basic infection-control guidelines used to reduce the risks of infection spread through the following three transmission modes: airborne infection, droplet infection, and contact infection.

BOX 2-4 | Infectious Materials

- Blood
- Semen
- Vaginal secretions
- Cerebrospinal fluid
- Synovial fluid
- Pleural fluid
- Pericardial fluid
- Amniotic fluid
- Saliva in dental procedures
- Any body fluid visibly contaminated with blood
- Mixtures of fluids where you cannot differentiate among body fluids
- Unfixed human tissue or organs (other than intact skin)
- Certain cell tissue or organ cultures and mediums

The most important weapon against the spread of infection is proper hand washing, followed by the use of barriers (gloves, gowns, and masks) and the proper handling and disposal of infectious waste materials. You should wash your hands whenever you come in contact with the following substances:

- Blood.
- All body fluids: secretions, excretions, and contaminated items—even if blood is not visible. The only body fluid exception is perspiration.
- Broken skin.
- Mucous membranes (inside the mouth, nose, and eyelids).
- Dried blood or dried bloody fluids.

Box 2-4 lists infectious materials you should be aware of. Included in the standard precautions are the following important protocols.

Hand Washing

- Wash your hands after touching blood, body fluids, or contaminated items—*whether or not gloves are worn.*
- Wash your hands after removing gloves, between patient contacts, and whenever indicated, to avoid transfer of microorganisms to other patients or the environment.
- It may be necessary to wash hands between tasks and procedures on the same patient, to prevent cross-contamination of different body sites.
- Use plain soap for routine hand washing and an antimicrobial agent or waterless agent for specific situations (e.g., to control outbreaks or for hyperendemic infections).

Gloves

- Wear clean, nonsterile gloves when touching blood, body fluids, secretions, excretions, and contaminated items.
- Put on clean gloves just before touching mucous membranes and nonintact skin.
- Change gloves between tasks and procedures on the same patient after contacting material that may contain a high concentration of microorganisms.
- Remove gloves promptly after use, before touching noncontaminated items and surfaces, and before going to another patient.
- Wash hands immediately to avoid transfer of microorganisms to other patients or environments.

Masks, Eye Protection, and Face Shields

- Wear a mask, eye protection, and face shields whenever performing procedures likely to generate splashes or sprays of blood, body fluids, secretions, and excretions.

Gown

- Wear a clean, nonsterile gown to protect skin and clothing from blood and body fluids during procedures or patient care activities likely to generate splashes or sprays of blood, body fluids, secretions, and excretions.
- Remove dirty gowns and gloves as soon as possible, and then wash your hands to avoid transfer of microorganisms to other patients or environments.

Patient-Care Equipment

- Handle used patient-care equipment that is soiled with blood, body fluids, secretions, and excretions in a way that prevents skin and mucous membrane exposure, contamination of clothing, and transfer of microorganisms to other patients and environments.
- If disposable items are used, they must be disposed of properly and never used again. Ensure that reusable equipment is not used for another patient unless it has been properly cleaned and reprocessed.
- Thoroughly clean the transducer after every patient with the Steri-septic cleaner.

Linens

- Handle, transport, and process used linen soiled with blood, body fluids, secretions and excretions in a way that prevents skin and mucous membrane exposures and contamination of clothing and that avoids transfer of microorganisms to other patients and environments.
- A patient's used linens should not be shaken, but rolled up and placed into a laundry hamper or bag for cleaning. Always hold the used linens away from your clothes.

Environmental Control

- Keep the work environment as clean as possible, especially after any spills.
- Be sure your institution has adequate procedures for routine care, cleaning, and disinfection of environmental surfaces, beds, or side rails.
- Equipment (blood pressure cuffs, basins, bedpans, or wheelchairs) should be cleansed according to your institution's policies.

For your own safety, change your uniform or laboratory coat daily, and bathe or shower daily, paying special attention to hair and body areas not covered by clothing. By keeping your hair covered or pinned, you will reduce the chance of it coming in contact with the blood or body fluids of patients. This is especially true with longer hair that can brush against open wounds, if not properly secured. Wash your hair daily to remove germs and debris. It is important to know what your facility's infection procedures are (Box 2-5).

Additional Precautions

Recognizing that some patients require more than basic methods of infection control, the CDC developed extra guidelines known as *additional precautions*. These are

---

BOX 2-5	What Are Your Facility's Infection Procedures?

- To whom should you report?
- Who determines the source of exposure?
- How do *you* get care?
- Who performs follow-up?

---

divided into disease categories related to specific transmission patterns:

1. *Airborne transmission.* Germs capable of floating airborne for long periods of time are often very contagious and can travel long distances. Some of the diseases spread by airborne transmission include the following:
   - Tuberculosis
   - Measles
   - Chickenpox
   - Shingles

   If you are immune to diseases such as measles or chickenpox, you can work with infected patients without concern for becoming infected with the disease. However, you must still follow all infection control precautions ordered for that patient.

2. *Droplet transmission.* Germs that are too heavy to remain airborne can drop quickly. Diseases spread via droplet transmission include the following:
   - Mumps
   - Measles (rubella)
   - Whooping cough (pertussis)
   - Pneumonia
   - Meningitis (specific forms)
   - Strep throat

   Because droplets are too heavy to float, they usually do not travel more than 3 feet. They are most commonly spread by coughing, sneezing, and talking. Patients on droplet precautions may be placed in private rooms and wear surgical masks if they are around uninfected people for short time periods. You should wear a surgical mask when working within 3 feet of these patients.

3. *Contact transmission.* Germs spread directly or indirectly by touching the germ include the following diseases:
   - Methicillin-resistant *Staphylococcus aureus* (MRSA)
   - *Escherichia coli*
   - Wound infections
   - Flu
   - Impetigo
   - Pinkeye
   - Scabies
   - Hepatitis A

   One of the most serious of these diseases is the MRSA infection. MRSA is a form of staph bacteria that live on the skin and nasal passages of a third of the world's population. These bacteria are resistant to certain broad-spectrum antibiotics. MRSA infections can be divided into two categories: (1) community-acquired infections and (2) hospital-acquired infections. The primary differences between them are that community-acquired forms typically produce skin infections, whereas the hospital-acquired forms can develop into more serious lung and bloodstream infections. MRSA is primarily spread on the hands of health care workers and infected persons. Draining wounds and infected discharge are other methods of transmission.

It is not possible to eliminate MRSA in health care settings, because new patients, visitors, and employees will reintroduce the infection. The best defense against MRSA in hospital settings is hand washing and the proper use of barrier devices. Proper maintenance of restrooms, soap and towel dispensers, and proper room cleansing also are essential to preventing the spread of infection.

Risk factors for MRSA are greatest among health care workers and patients in hospital and assisted living settings. MRSA skin infections may resemble boils or spider bites with a painful, red, and swollen ring of skin surrounding the bite. Pus drainage may occur. If MRSA spreads to other body areas (e.g., lungs or into the bloodstream), more serious symptoms may develop, such as fatigue, fever, chills, and shortness of breath.

Whereas mild infections are often treated with oral antibiotics, more serious infections, which travel in the bloodstream, frequently require intravenous antibiotic therapy (e.g., Vancomycin, Septra, or Bactrim).

As mentioned, there are two forms of infection contact: direct contact, which refers to touching the skin of an infected person, and indirect contact, which refers to touching an object that has been touched by an infected person. Examples of contact transmission include the following:

- Changing the clothes/gown of a patient infected with staph germs without wearing gloves
- Failing to change gloves between patients

Patients on contact precautions may be isolated from other patients. When caring for such patients, you may need to do the following:

- Glove before entering the patient's room.
- Change gloves during patient contact, especially after touching highly contaminated items.
- Remove gloves before leaving the patient's room and wash your hands immediately.
- Gown while in contact with the patient and remove the gown right before leaving the patient area.
- Discard disposable items and disinfect equipment used on patients with a contact infection.

Biohazardous waste—refuse that has been contaminated with germs, such as discarded dressings, used needles, contents of bedpans or urinals, and so on—should be bagged and labeled. In some cases, items may need to be double bagged. Used sharps must always be placed in puncture-proof containers.

4. *Blood-borne transmission.* Blood-borne diseases are those spread when the blood of an infected person comes in contact with the blood of another person. HIV/AIDS and hepatitis are two of the most common diseases spread by blood-borne transmission.

Nosocomial Infections

Hospital-acquired infections are known as **nosocomial infections.** Contracted as a result of medical treatment, they usually manifest within the first 48 hours of treatment. The most common of these are urinary tract infections, pneumonia, and surgical incision site infections. The patients at most risk are those whose general health is compromised: intensive care unit and neonatal intensive care unit patients and immunocompromised patients who are already fighting or at risk for infection. Transmission of nosocomial infections occurs through the following means:

- *Direct contact.* Person to person.
- *Indirect contact.* Touching an infected surface or a surface treated with improperly sterilized equipment.
- *Droplet infection.* Via sneezing and coughing.
- *Airborne transmission.* Via sneezing and coughing.
- Common vehicle transmission. Resulting from food, water, or medical devices.
- *Vector transmission.* As a result of contact or bites from an insect or animal.

The symptoms of nosocomial infection should be suspected when patients develop fever and other symptoms not associated with their primary complaint. Prevention of nosocomial infections relies on following stringent quality infection control procedures.

Preventive Measures. Do not underestimate the importance of personal protective equipment (PPE). Many health care workers who become ill are unsure of the proper order in which PPE should be donned and removed. The CDC recommends the following:

- Put on PPE before contact and generally before entering the patient's room.
- Once PPE is on, use it carefully to avoid contamination.
- Keep your hands away from your face.
- Work from clean to dirty areas.
- Limit the surfaces you touch.
- Change the PPE when torn or heavily contaminated.

Basic PPE Protocols. The proper way to don a gown is to select the appropriate size and type. With the opening at the back, secure the gown at the neck and waist. If the gown is too small to provide full coverage, wear two—the first with the opening in the front and the second placed over it with the opening in the back.

To don a mask, place it over the nose, mouth, and chin. Fit the flexible nose pieces over the bridge of your nose, and then secure it on the head with ties or elastic.

Gloves should be the last of the PPE to be applied. Extend your hands into the gloves and stretch the gloves to cover the wrist of an isolation gown. Tuck the cuffs of the gown securely in place under each glove. Adjust the gloves for comfort and dexterity (Figure 2-20).

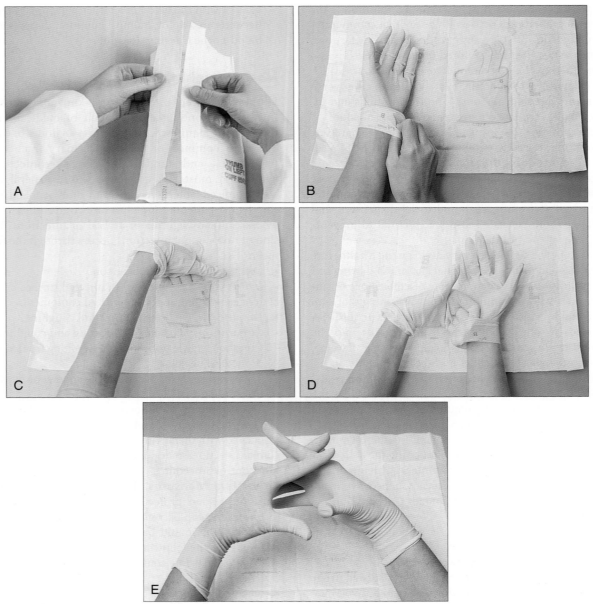

FIGURE 2-20 Open gloving. The sonographer should perform hand hygiene. Choosing the correct size glove is important. **A,** Remove outer glove package and lay it on a clean, flat surface just above waist level. Open package, keeping gloves on wrapper's inside surface. **B,** Glove the dominant hand first. With thumb and first two fingers of nondominant hand, grasp edge of cuff of glove for dominant hand. Touch only the glove's inside surface. Carefully pull the glove over the dominant hand, leaving cuff and being sure cuff does not roll up wrist. **C,** With gloved dominant hand, slip fingers underneath second glove's cuff. **D,** Carefully pull second glove over nondominant hand. Do not allow fingers and thumb of gloved dominant hand to touch any part of exposed nondominant hand. Keep thumb of dominant hand abducted back. **E,** After second glove is on, interlock hand. The cuffs usually fall down after application.

Once the patient care tasks are completed, carefully remove the PPE and discard it properly. Immediately wash your hands. While removing gloves, gowns, or masks, the goal is to avoid contaminating yourself or the environment. The outside front of gloves and masks are considered contaminated, regardless of their appearance. The outside front and sleeves of a gown are considered contaminated. Where to remove PPE depends on the type of equipment and the patient category of isolation. If only gloves are worn, they may be discarded in the patient's room. When a gown and full PPE are used, they should be discarded at the door of the patient's room or in an anteroom and in a designated container.

To remove a gown, unfasten the ties and peel the gown away from your neck and shoulders. Turn the outside toward the inside, then fold or roll the gown into a bundle and discard it in a designated receptacle. To remove a mask, *do not touch the front of it.* First, untie the bottom, then the top ties. Lift the mask away from your face and discard in a designated receptacle. To remove gloves, grasp the outer edge near the wrist. Peel the glove away from the hand, turning the glove inside out. Hold it in the opposite glove, then slide an ungloved finger under the wrist of the remaining glove and peel it off from the inside, creating a "bag" for both used gloves. Discard properly and again perform hand washing after using and discarding the PPE.

Preparing a Sterile Field. Medical aseptic technique is designed to rid an area or object of pathogenic microorganisms. Aseptic technique is commonly used in procedures that involve puncturing the skin or when placing objects into normally sterile body cavities. These are the recommended principles to follow:

- All materials in a sterile field *must be sterile* and *all objects added* to a sterile field *must also be sterile.* When placing hands into a sterile field, they must be covered with sterile gloves.
- Any sterile field that has been compromised by punctures, tears, or moisture is considered contaminated.

- Once a sterile package is opened, a 1-inch border around the edge is considered unsterile.
- If there are any questions or doubts about an object's sterility, the object should be considered unsterile.
- Movement around or in the sterile field must not compromise or contaminate the sterile field. Never reach across a sterile field and never turn your back on a sterile field. Bring all tables used in the procedure up to waist level to avoid bending over the field.
- Most procedures today use disposable equipment wrapped in paper or plastic.
- Always read the directions on the package in advance of the actual procedure.

Nondisposable equipment from central supply is usually double-wrapped in cloth and sealed with tape stating the expiration dates or with an indicator tape of a predetermined color, confirming sterilization. All such packs are wrapped in a standardized fashion and should be opened as outlined here (Figure 2-21):

- Place the pack on a clean surface within reach of the physician.
- Just before the procedure begins, break the seal and open the pack.

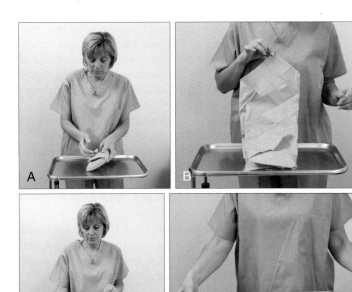

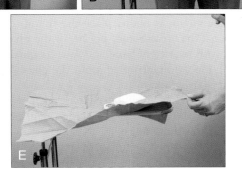

FIGURE 2-21 Preparing a sterile field. **A, B,** Open the first corner away from yourself. **C,** Open one side by grasping a corner tip. **D,** Open the second side in the same manner. **E,** Pull the remaining corner toward yourself. If there is an inner wrap, it should be opened in the same manner.

- Unfold the first corner *away* from you; then unfold the two sides.
- Pull the front fold down toward you and drop it without touching the inner surface. If there is an inner wrap, open it in the same manner.
- A sterile field has now been established. Any nondisposable items (wrapped separately) may now be added to the sterile field.
- Stand back from the table and grasp the object through the wrapping, using one hand. With the other hand, unseal the wrappings, allowing them to fall down over your wrist.
- Hold the edges of the wrapper with your free hand and drop the object onto the sterile field without dropping the wrapper.
- Add any disposable items (sponges, gloves, etc.). These will be supplied in "peel down" paper wraps. Separate the paper layers of the wraps. Invert the package and let the object fall onto the sterile field.
- If a liquid medium is to be added, read the label carefully and position the liquid toward your hand.
- Open the spout and squirt a few drops into a wastebasket or sink to wash the container lip.
- Pour the required amount into the sterile receptacle on the tray.
- Items in the sterile field may be manipulated with sterile forceps. Replace the forceps with the tips in the sterile field and the handles protruding toward you, to use again.
- If the procedure is delayed, do not open the pack. If it has already been opened, cover it at once with a sterile drape or discard it.

After the procedure is completed, don gloves and thoroughly clean all reusable items before returning the pack to central supply. Discard disposable items, placing needles in Sharps containers and the remainder in a biohazard bag.

ISOLATION TECHNIQUES

Before the development of universal precautions, the diagnosis or even the suspicion of communicable disease resulted in patient isolation. Formerly, hospital isolation procedures were adopted that were either disease specific or category specific, which included seven different types of isolation. With the advent of standard precautions and additional precautions, the following isolation techniques evolved:

1. *Blood-borne isolation techniques.* In addition to standard precautions, patients who contaminate the environment or cannot be expected to assist in maintaining appropriate hygiene or environmental control should be placed in a private room.
2. *Airborne precautions.* When working with patients known to have or suspected of having serious illnesses that are transmitted by droplet nuclei, you should always wear respiratory protection, especially when entering the room of a patient suspected of having tuberculosis.

EMERGENCY MEDICAL SITUATIONS

Each year thousands of emergency medical situations end in death because the victim did not receive immediate and proper first aid. This section focuses on the two medical emergencies that sonographers are most likely to encounter during their work with patients. In addition, being proficient in performing emergency measures can make a critical difference in the lives of your family and all other people with whom you interact outside of your daily work activities.

Choking

Choking typically results from a blockage of the upper airway by food or other objects, preventing normal breathing. In some cases, victims can dislodge the object by coughing; however, if this is not possible, choking becomes a medical emergency requiring fast, appropriate action. When someone with a completely blocked airway begins to choke, no oxygen can enter the lungs. Brain cells, which are extremely sensitive to oxygen deprivation, will begin to die within 4 to 6 minutes. If first aid is not initiated quickly, brain death can occur in as little as 10 minutes.

The universal sign of choking is that of clutching the throat while having difficulty breathing. At times, the victim's attempts to inhale may produce a high-pitched sound. The symptoms can rapidly progress to cyanosis and loss of consciousness. Even partial air exchange (involving a partial obstruction) should be treated as a complete airway obstruction.

To assist a choking victim, you must be ready to perform the **Heimlich maneuver.** This emergency treatment involves the application of sudden, upward pressure on the upper abdomen (abdominal thrusts) to create an artificial "cough" and force foreign objects from the windpipe. There are separate techniques for adults and children over 1 year of age and for babies under the age of 1.

The Heimlich maneuver (abdominal thrusts) for adults and children over age 1: If the victim can breathe, speak, and cough, *do not interfere.* If the victim cannot breathe, cough, or speak, begin the Heimlich maneuver (Figure 2-22):
- Stand behind the victim.
- Make a fist and place it below the rib cage and above the navel of the victim.
- Grasp your fist with your other hand.
- Give 6 to 10 quick, sharp thrusts backward and upward.
- If the victim is obese, place the thumb of your left fist against the breastbone—not below the rib cage. Grasp the fist with your right hand and squeeze quickly, four times.
- Continue, uninterrupted, until the object is dislodged or help arrives.
- When the object is dislodged, seek medical help at once.

To clear the airway of a choking infant under the age of 1 year, follow these steps:
- *Do not proceed* if the infant is coughing forcefully or has a strong cry, as this can dislodge the object on its own.

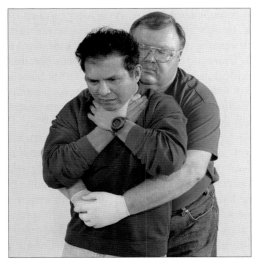

FIGURE 2-22 The Heimlich maneuver (abdominal thrusts) may be applied to choking patients either in the standing or in the supine position. The victim here is giving the universal sign of choking, with the hands crossed over the throat.

- *Do not grasp or pull the object out* if the choking infant is conscious.
- *Do not perform these steps* if the child has stopped breathing for other reasons such as asthma, allergic reaction, or a blow to the head.
- Assume a seated position and lay the infant face down along your forearm, which is resting on your thigh (Figure 2-23, *A*).
- Hold the child's head lower than its body.
- Thump the infant gently but firmly five times on the middle of the back between the shoulder blades, using the heel of your hand. The combination of gravity and back blows should release the blocking object.
- If the objection does not dislodge by itself, turn the infant face up on your forearm with its head lower than its body (Figure 2-23, *B*).
- Using two fingers placed in the center of the breastbone between the nipples, give five quick chest compressions.
- Continue five back blows and five chest thrusts until the object is dislodged.
- If breathing does not resume or the child loses consciousness, call for emergency medical help.
- If the object is dislodged, seek medical help to prevent complications that can arise from the choking or from the first aid provided.

If the victim is unconscious and breathing, follow these steps:
- Place the child down on its back.
- Place the heel of one hand (fingers pointing in the direction of the child's head) against the middle of the child's abdomen, just above the navel and well below the sternum.
- Place the other hand on top of the first hand. Using both hands, administer five thrusts, pressing inward and upward. Each thrust should be a separate and distinct effort to dislodge the object.

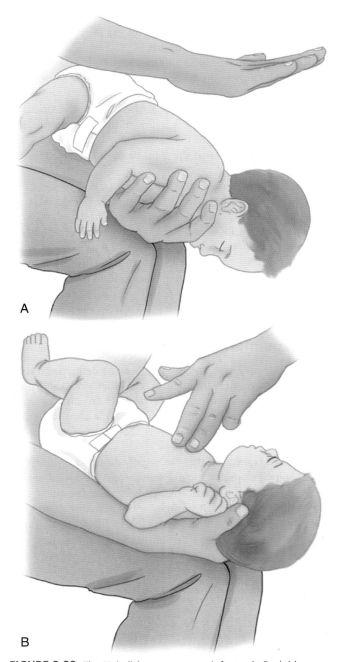

FIGURE 2-23 The Heimlich maneuver on infants. **A,** Back blows are administered between the shoulder blades to an infant supported on the arm and thigh. **B,** Chest thrusts are administered in the same position as for cardiac compressions, using two or three fingers.

- Maintain your heel hand contact with the abdomen between thrusts.
- If the object is visible, perform a finger sweep by grasping the child's tongue and jaw, lifting upward to pull the tongue away from the back of the child's throat and the lodged object.
- Using the index finger of your other hand, slide the finger inside the baby's cheek and use a sweeping, hooking action across the interior of the mouth, to the other cheek.

- If the object is within reach, you can dislodge it, grasp it, and remove it. *Do not force the object deeper,* which can happen easily in young children.

To clear the airway of an unconscious person:

- Lower the person on his or her back, onto the floor.
- Clear the airway.
- If there is a visible blockage at the back of the throat or high in the throat, reach a finger into the mouth and sweep out the cause of the blockage.
- Be careful not to push the food or object deeper into the airway.
- Begin cardiopulmonary resuscitation (CPR) as described next, if the object remains lodged and the person does not respond after you take these measures. The chest compressions used in CPR may dislodge the object, so remember to recheck the mouth periodically.

Only perform finger sweeps on unconscious victims, as the action could cause a conscious person to gag or vomit. If the victim is obese or in advanced pregnancy, performing a chest thrust would be safer.

Cardiopulmonary Resuscitation

Cardiopulmonary resuscitation (CPR) can be defined as a combination of emergency life-saving techniques aimed at restarting lung and heart function in patients in cardiac arrest (breathing and heartbeat have stopped). CPR is most successful when an irregular heartbeat is the cause of the cardiac arrest.

The heart is a muscle that can rapidly deteriorate when oxygenated blood stops flowing to the brain and other vital organs. The goal of CPR is to maintain circulation and breathing until emergency help arrives. It is important to note that if done improperly, CPR can result in serious injury. Therefore it should not be performed unless a person has stopped breathing and does not demonstrate signs of circulation (normal breathing, coughing, or movement in response to rescue breathing).

CPR measures include chest compressions to pump blood out of the heart and into the body and rescue breathing. Time is the critical factor when initiating CPR, because death can occur within 8 to 10 minutes. Approximately 95% of sudden cardiac arrest victims will die without treatment, but given CPR assistance, the survival rate triples.

For 50 years, CPR consisted of the combination of artificial blood circulation with chest compressions and lung ventilation. However, in March 2010 the American Heart Association and the European Resuscitation Council reversed their previous positions and endorsed the effectiveness of chest compressions alone—without artificial respiration—for adult victims who collapse suddenly in cardiac arrest.

Providing basic life support requires an orderly progression of activities. The American Heart Association coined the phrase *Think ABC: Airway, Breathing, and Circulation* as an easily remembered reminder of that progression.

Persons untrained in CPR should provide hands-only, uninterrupted chest compressions (two per second) until trained professionals arrive. They should not attempt rescue breathing. For the person with training come the options to alternate between 30 chest compressions and two rescue breaths or to perform only chest compressions.

The first step in administering CPR is to evaluate the situation and check the patient for consciousness by tapping or gently shaking the victim's shoulder and loudly asking, "Are you OK?" *Do not shake victims* if there is a possibility of a neck or spinal injury. If there is no response and you are alone, call out for help. If other people are present, send them for help.

Adult CPR

- Roll the victim onto his back and pull him slowly toward you.
- Open his airway by putting the palm of your hand on his forehead and gently tilting his head back (Figure 2-24, *A*).

FIGURE 2-24 Methods of artificial ventilation. **A,** Backward head-tilt position. **B,** Mouth-to-mouth resuscitation technique.

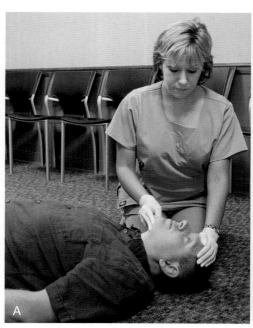
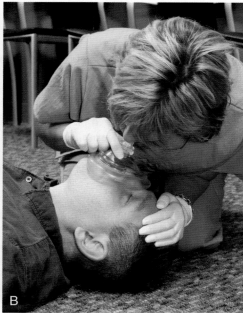
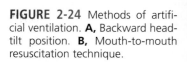

- With your other hand, gently lift his chin.
- Check for normal breathing by looking, listening, and feeling, for no more than 10 seconds. Gasping is not normal breathing.
- Initiate chest compressions by locating the sternal notch. Place the heel of your other hand on the notch, next to your fingers.
- Remove your hand from the notch and put it on top of the other hand, keeping your fingers off the chest.
- Position your shoulders over your hands and compress the breastbone 2 inches. Push hard and push fast.
- Perform two compressions per second.
- Do four cycles of compressions and breaths, rechecking the pulse after 1 minute.
- If no pulse is found, continue CPR until help arrives.
- If the victim has not responded after five cycles (about 2 minutes) and an automatic external defibrillator (AED) is available, apply it and follow the prompts.
- Alternate one shock and resume CPR starting with chest compressions for 2 minutes before administering a second shock.

Child CPR. For children ages 1 through 8, the CPR procedure is essentially the same as that for an adult. The only differences are these:

- If you are alone, perform five cycles of compressions and breaths for about 2 minutes before calling for help or using an AED.
- Use only one hand to perform chest compressions.
- Breathe more gently.
- If there is no response after 2 minutes (five cycles) and an AED is available, use pediatric pads and follow the prompts. If no pediatric pads are available, use the adult pads.
- Continue until the child moves or help arrives.

Infant CPR. Infant cardiac arrests occur primarily from lack of oxygen such as might result from drowning or choking. Perform first aid for choking if you know the infant has an airway obstruction. Perform CPR if you do not know why the infant is not breathing:

- Assess the situation by stroking the baby and watching for a response such as movement. *Do not shake the child.*
- If there is no response and you are the only rescuer, do CPR for 2 minutes before calling for help.
- If other persons are available, have one of them call for help immediately while you attend to the infant.
- Place the baby on its back on a firm flat surface such as a table, the floor, or the ground.
- Open the airway by gently tipping the head back and lift the chin with your other hand.
- Check for breathing for no more than 10 seconds, by putting your ear near the infant's mouth. Look for chest motion, listen for breath sounds, and feel for breath on your cheek and ear.
- If the chest still does not rise, check the infant's mouth to make sure no foreign material is inside. If you see such an object, sweep it out with your finger. If the airway appears blocked, perform the same first aid indicated for a choking infant.
- Begin chest compressions to restore circulation.

Barrier Devices. As a result of the risk of exposure to infectious diseases, many CPR practitioners prefer to use barrier devices when providing artificial respiration. The barrier device is of no help to the victim; it is solely used to protect the practitioner. Such devices are designed to restrict the airflow in one direction and prevent direct contact between the mouths of the victim and the rescuer. There are two commonly used CPR barrier devices. One consists of a single sheet of thin plastic; the other is a larger pear-shaped plastic apparatus that will form a seal around the mouth (Figure 2-24, *B*).

After opening an airway and checking for any obstructions, the CPR barrier device should be positioned over the victim's mouth. Two quick rescue breaths are then directed into the CPR barrier. The device is removed, and a cycle of chest compressions should be performed. After approximately 30 chest compressions, the barrier device should be replaced and two more rescue breaths given. The cycle is repeated as outlined previously. As soon as the victim shows signs of recovery such as a cough or a gasp, the CPR barrier must be removed to give the victim adequate space to breathe. In some instances, vomiting will occur. Time should never be wasted trying to locate a barrier device because it will delay the onset of CPR. The lack of a barrier device should not prevent you from performing CPR in an emergency situation, as the threat of infectious diseases is relatively small.

Basic Cardiac Life Support

Automatic External Defibrillators. An *automatic external defibrillator (AED)* is a portable device used to diagnose cardiac rhythms and to detect the absence of them (Figure 2-25). In the latter case, it is used to administer an electrical shock to reestablish a normal cardiac rhythm. AEDs are very effective, even when used by individuals with only a limited amount of training, and many public places (schools, malls, gyms, airports, sports venues, and large office buildings) are beginning to have them available. The devices use audio and visual prompts to guide users through the process. Built-in computers assess the patient's heart rhythm, judge whether defibrillation is necessary, and administer the shock.

Before using an AED unit, check for signs of life. Never use an AED on a person who is breathing and has a pulse. If the victim's chest is not rising and there is no pulse, send someone for help and to bring back an AED unit, if one is available. Before using an AED unit, make sure the surroundings are safe. Tell people to step back, and then follow the prompts given by the AED machine:

- Place one pad on the upper right side of the victim's chest and one on the lower left.
- The AED unit will diagnose the heart rhythm and indicate if a shock is needed.
- Only apply shock if there is no pulse and the unit instructs you to do so.
- Continue CPR until another shock command is issued.
- If only one shock was needed, simply follow the unit's commands until help arrives.

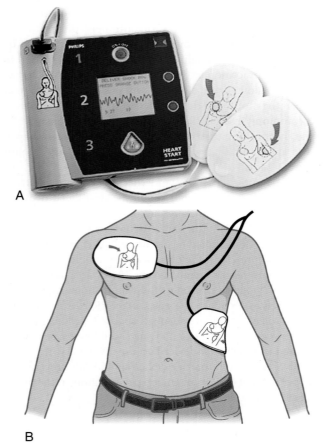

A

B

FIGURE 2-25 **A,** Automated external defibrillator (AED). **B,** Connect the adhesive pads to the AED cables, and then apply the pads to the patient's chest at the upper-right sternal border and the lower-left ribs over the cardiac apex.

PROFESSIONAL ATTITUDES

Professionalism is composed of attitudes and behaviors. Often we behave in a manner to achieve optimal outcomes in our professional tasks and interactions. Whether it is attitudes or behaviors, how we interact with patients will have a significant effect on their reactions to us and their willingness to work together to improve their medical conditions.

The first step in caring for our patients is in how we communicate with them. Accurate communications is essential not only for the immediate situation but also for ongoing patient care. The way to establish rapport with our patients is by showing respect and by listening and responding to them, as well as by giving instructions. Nonverbal communication is a process of communicating by sending and receiving wordless messages through body language, gesture, facial expression, eye contact, physical proximity, and touching. Patients will not entirely trust information given them when the body language and the verbal language of the speaker are not harmonious. The following suggestions are helpful in making sure that your patients fully understand you:

- Make eye contact with the patients to demonstrate that they have your full attention and to see that they are listening to you attentively.
- Sit rather than stand. Looking down on patients when communicating with them is intimidating. Sitting also will make the conversation seem less rushed and more respectful.
- Maintain a relaxed posture when speaking to patients. Do not cross your arms over your chest, as that gesture indicates negativity.
- Use a calm, steady voice whenever communicating sensitive or important information. Patients will be more receptive to a lower, softer voice than a shrill one.
- Do not speak rapidly or use medical jargon because it will overwhelm your patients.
- Ask comprehensive questions that require a mixture of responses from the patient rather than just a yes or a no.
- If you explain a diagnosis or give instructions, be sure to ask if the patient understands. Many patients will say yes, but after additional conversation, you should be able to determine whether they *really* do understand.

Reestablishing Patient-Focused Care

A patient is someone in need. Patients come to us because they have health problems, and our job is to assist them. The move toward patient-focused care comes at a time when it is important to stem the tide against the long trend of turning health care into a business by treating patients as *clients* or *users* and by focusing primarily on *cost-cutting* and *maximizing productivity*. The term *patient* should be defended. It implies suffering over time. Patients should be treated with dignity and as individuals, and they should be empowered to make choices about their own care. This can only be done if they are not hurried along, if they are provided information in a form they can understand, and if their views are listened to. It is hoped that among all health professionals, the return to this kind of focus will rekindle the long-admired traits of caring, compassion, and respect and encourage a sharing of skills to enhance the patient's existence.

ASSISTING PATIENTS WITH SPECIAL NEEDS

Although much of your studies focus on the art and science of producing valuable diagnostic studies, another important dimension to being a sonographer is that of assessing not only your patients' illnesses or diseases but also any special needs that they may have. This section provides suggestions on how to deal with many types of patients, including the elderly, those with sensory challenges, and culturally diverse patients whose religious and ethnic backgrounds may run counter to our own.

Crying Patients

People respond to news in many different ways. Part of your job is to comfort patients. You may not have to *do* anything if your patient is crying. Sometimes, the best thing is just being with them, sending the message that at times it is alright to cry. Sharing a burden with someone else can make bad news tolerable. If you acknowledge the situation in a calm manner, you communicate to the patient that you are concerned about him or her and that although there may be nothing you can do to fix the situation, you would like to offer what help you can. If you do not know what to do, ask. Ask the patient what would be most helpful at that moment. You may have a great opportunity to heal, even if you cannot cure.

Pediatric Patients

Small children may have difficulty expressing themselves when in unfamiliar surroundings. Usually, however, they respond to a smile and a firm and gentle touch. The following tips may make it easier for you to effectively work with the pediatric patient:

- Ask the child's name and use that familiar name throughout the examination.
- Allow the child to take a favorite toy into the ultrasound laboratory to promote a sense of security.
- Reassure a small child by talking to him in a cheerful voice, even though he may not understand all that you say.
- Remain calm, cheerful, and unhurried to give the child the opportunity to respond to the strange surroundings and frightening machines in a medical setting.

Children over the age of 4 or 5 respond differently because they are able to share information and may be able to cooperate more fully. Practice the following suggestions when dealing with this age-group:

- Children fear the loss of control. By giving them simple options such as getting onto the scanning table by themselves, or with your help, their feeling of control may be restored.
- Never tell a child, "This won't hurt very much." The only word the child will hear is *hurt.*
- Always explain what you are going to do and why you need to do it, in words that the child can understand.

- If the child asks questions, answer them simply. Do not force information on children, as it only makes them apprehensive.
- Keep directions simple and honest and assure the child that you will work as fast as you can.
- When dealing with a disruptive child or one who refuses to follow directions, set limits such as "You must lie still" or "You may not get down."

If you have been patient, and reasonable attempts are not working, ask for help. If hospital policies permit, immobilize the child gently but firmly, and complete the examination as quickly as possible.

Adolescent Patients

Working with adolescent patients can be challenging and will require creativity, flexibility, and openness. Young adolescents often try to act like adults, while hiding the fact that they are confused or frightened. In this age-group, modesty and privacy are very important. You can earn the adolescent patient's trust by adopting a friendly and nonjudgmental approach and being sensitive to their concerns about privacy and confidentiality.

Elderly Patients

Patients should be treated according to their clinical needs rather than their age. However, we must also acknowledge that aging does have adverse effects on the systems of the body (Box 2-6) and allowances must be made for those who may have multiple health issues, as well as patterns of disease and responses to treatment that differ from those of younger patients. Patients over age 85 represent the fastest growing segment of our population and are most vulnerable to adverse outcomes. It is important that you become competent and comfortable in dealing with an older patient, especially the

---

BOX 2-6	The Effects of Aging on the Body

Sensory
The development of nearsightedness and cataracts increases sensitivity to light, glare, and the risk of falling.

Cardiovascular
As systolic blood pressure rises, elderly patients are at increased risk of stroke, if untreated. As their cardiovascular reserves decline, they become more likely candidates for congestive heart failure or orthostatic hypotension.

Pulmonary
Older patients with pulmonary disease, rather than aging changes alone, will experience atrophy of the respiratory muscles and a decline in the elasticity of their lungs.

Genitourinary
Reduced bladder capacity and residual urine increase the incidences of nocturia and functional incontinence in the elderly patient.

Gastrointestinal
Loss of teeth can lead to poor nutrition or malnutrition. Declining liver function increases the chance of drug toxicity with respect to drugs

metabolized by the liver. Peristalsis declines and, with it, diet and fluid intake suffer.

Musculoskeletal
Muscle mass declines 30% with age, thereby decreasing muscle strength, bulk, and endurance. Bone density declines in both men and women may yield fractures. Degeneration of joints produces pain and increased falls.

Neurologic
Neurologic decline is more profound after age 75 and may manifest as slowed reaction times, accidents, and falls, as well as a decline in the responsiveness of the autonomic nervous system.

Immune System
The skin's ability to serve as a protective barrier begins to decline. Cellular immune responses decline, increasing the risk of infection. Cough reflexes decline, increasing the risk of pneumonia and influenza and prolonged recovery times.

Homeostatic Responses
Postural hypotension predisposes to falls. Thirst mechanisms decline, producing dehydration.

frail elder with an unstable disability for whom even the smallest event may affect the ability to function on a daily basis.

Some elderly patients may be incontinent, immobile, unstable, confused, and even display dementia as a result of their diseases. Box 2-7 lists strategies for dealing with some of the more common physical limitations of older patients. Be aware that older patients often experience a rapid onset of illness coupled with an increase in complications and delayed recovery because they lack physiologic reserves. Diseases of the elderly tend to be chronic and progressive, evolving over a long period of time. Minor insults can produce major problems, and the more coexisting health issues an elderly patient has and the more medications he or she must take lead to higher risks and more rapid deterioration.

Culturally Diverse Patients

Culture has a profound effect on our attitudes and the way in which we communicate and perceive others. There are more than 100 ethnic groups and more than 500 American Indian groups in the United States, making it one of the most culturally diverse countries in the world. Studies have shown that patients from other cultures feel alienated by the language and communication barriers of the dominant culture and by their strong allegiance to family and folk medicine. Any alienation they feel in their daily life is carried over into their perceptions and experiences with the health care system. Box 2-8 outlines some cultural differences you may encounter in a clinical setting.

Culturally appropriate care is that which respects individuality, creates mutual understanding, caters to spiritual needs,

---

| BOX 2-7 | **Strategies for Dealing with Physical Limitations of the Elderly Patient** |

Vision and Hearing Problems
Provide good lighting. Ask patients if they wear corrective lenses or hearing aids.

Slowed Physical Pace
Aging produces a tendency to proceed at one's own pace. Most elderly patients respond poorly to a feeling of being pushed or hurried.

Mental Confusion
Older patients may not understand why they find themselves in unfamiliar surroundings. Medication, illness, senility, or injury may be the reason for mental confusion. However, Alzheimer's disease or organic brain syndrome may also play a role. Treating elderly patients calmly, patiently, and with respect will help them maintain their sense of identity and increases their desire to be cooperative.

Patients who appear confused respond best to familiar situations. Use the patient's full name and ask questions about his or her past (e.g., where the patient was born, etc.). Such questions give patients a sense of comfort because their distant memories may be much clearer than their short-term memory.

| BOX 2-8 | **Cultural and Language Differences among Multicultural Patients** |

Gestures
- Gestures commonly used in the United States may have different meanings or be offensive to patients of different cultures. For example, using a finger or hand to indicate *come here* is a gesture used in some cultures to summon dogs. Pointing with one finger may also be considered rude. In Asian cultures, the entire hand is used to point to something.

Touch
- In American culture, patting a child's head is considered friendly or affectionate. However, many Asians consider touching someone's head inappropriate, as the head is believed to be a sacred part of the body.
- Physical contact while speaking may lead to discomfort because touching may be viewed as too intimate. Do not put your arm around the patient's shoulder or touch the person's face or hold his or her hand. Shaking hands on meeting is acceptable, but only momentarily.
- In the Middle East, the left hand is reserved for bodily hygiene and should not be used to touch another part or to transfer objects.
- In Muslim cultures, touch between individuals of the opposite gender is generally considered inappropriate.

Eye Contact
- Americans interpret eye contact as attentiveness and honesty. In many cultures (Hispanic, Asian, Middle Eastern, and Native American), however, eye contact is considered disrespectful or rude, especially from children. Lack of eye contact does not mean that a person is not paying attention.

- Women, in particular, may avoid eye contact with men because it can be seen as a sign of sexual interest.

Babies
- Admiring babies and young children and commenting on how cute they are is avoided in Hmong and Vietnamese cultures for fear that these comments will be overheard by a spirit who will try to steal the baby or otherwise cause it some harm.

Personal Space
- The average acceptable personal distance varies from culture to culture. Americans tend to require more personal space than people in other cultures and will back away if they feel that their personal space has been invaded.
- In many Hispanic cultures, personal and physical spaces are not emphasized and an individual may stand less than a foot away from another when conversing. In these cultures, it is considered rude to step back.

Time
- Many Hispanic cultures have a relaxed attitude toward time. Tardiness or last-minute changes are perfectly acceptable, as things will get done "in good time."

Speaking
- Americans value courtesy when engaging in discussions. They will wait until there is an opportune time to state their views or ask questions.
- Taking turns when speaking is not always the rule in many foreign cultures. People will interrupt conversations, and often many people will speak simultaneously.

and maintains dignity. One universal principle germane to this topic is that health professionals may have to challenge their own assumptions and develop an understanding of the many cultures and subcultures with which they may deal on a daily basis. The starting point for improving any service is to understand the expectations of its users and to manage areas of conflict between personal and institutional values and individual patients' cultural requirements. The following suggestions are intended to help both you and your culturally diverse patients:

- Document any request to be treated by only male or female staff.
- Thoroughly explain the procedure that you need to conduct, including which body parts you will need to touch and the reason for examining them.
- Understand that there may be a cultural reluctance to discuss certain topics, particularly if you, or an interpreter, are not of the same gender as the patient.
- Use words—not gestures—to convey your meaning (see Box 2-8). Gestures acceptable in one culture may be offensive in others.
- Be aware of the personal wishes of patients regarding their condition. In some cultures, medical decisions are only made by the family.
- Respect the patient's privacy at all times. Some patients may prefer to converse or pray in private with family members while in your department.
- Respect the patient's dietary requirements, and be aware that some patients may be fasting for religious reasons at certain times.
- Respect the patient's dress requirements as decreed by the individual's faith.

Asking a patient's views about his or her illness or condition can be culturally and clinically valuable as it may reveal health beliefs and the names of diseases with which you are unfamiliar. The following list of questions may be useful when working with multicultural patients:

- What do you call your problem? Does it have a special name?
- What caused your problem?
- Why do you think it started when it did?
- How does your sickness affect you? How severe is it?
- What problems has your sickness caused you?
- What have you done to treat your sickness?
- What results do you hope to achieve?

As we interact with others of different cultures, there is no good substitute for receptiveness to interpersonal feedback, good observation skills, effective questions, and plain common sense.

EVALUATING PATIENT REACTIONS TO ILLNESS

When patients are ill, they are under stress and many emotional pressures. Fear of pain, prolonged illness, or death and feeling a loss of control are just a few. Being able to recognize the signs and symptoms of stress and identify how the patient is coping is essential to providing effective care. Some patient fears are so great that they will avoid seeking professional help.

Beside concerns about their bodies, patients have worries that their illness may separate them from their loved ones, create financial problems, and isolate them from other people. The latter fear is particularly reinforced by not having questions answered by medical staff and being subjected to staff that talk too fast or fail to explain the reasons for tests or treatments.

Patients go through many emotional and psychological changes with regard to personal illness:

- *Denial or disbelief.* Patients may avoid, refuse, or *forget* needed care or appointments.
- *Acceptance.* During the acceptance phase, some patients may become dependent on the health care team as they focus attention on their symptoms and illness.
- *Recovery.* Depending on how much a patient's lifestyle must change as a result of the illness, the patient will eventually begin to recover, rehabilitate, or convalesce.

The patient will go through a process of resolving perceived loss or impairment of normal function.

Fear is one of the greatest emotional responses to illness and may actually produce symptoms such as tachycardia, dry mouth, constipation/diarrhea, hypertension, increased perspiration, and a flight-or-flight reaction. Anxiety is another major reaction and can lead to fatigue, insomnia, urinary urgency, diarrhea or constipation, nausea, anorexia, and excessive perspiration. Ultimately, patients experience stress or tension. When the body is stressed by physical, psychological, or physiologic changes, it attempts to rid itself of the cause of the stress and the patient may develop ulcers, hair loss, or insomnia. Increasing feelings of helplessness may lead some patients to become overly dependent while searching for help and understanding. The overly dependent patient may also become fearful or angry.

Though as a sonographer you may not often be involved in the long-term care of your patients, you must understand that there are as many reactions to illness as there are patients. You also must learn that kindness, courtesy, and understanding will help your patients go through the illness with a minimum of stress and anxiety.

Terminal Patients

Despite the fact that we all realize our mortality, there is no easy way to discuss death. To strong and healthy patients, death is a frightening thought and many consciously put that reality out of mind. Terminally ill patients have many of the same basic needs as those of other patients: spiritual, psychological, cultural, economic, and physical. What makes these patients different is a sense of urgency to resolve the majority of their needs within a limited amount of time.

Accepting mortality and mourning loss are complicated processes. Not every patient will experience, in order, the oft-quoted five stages of dying—denial, anger, bargaining, depression, and acceptance—that were first introduced in Elisabeth Kübler-Ross's book *On Death and Dying* (1969). And for some, the stage of acceptance may never be reached. Patients traditionally view death from the perspective of their own cultural heritage, and many seek comfort and support in religious faith. Patients who do learn to accept their imminent deaths often feel the need to get their affairs in order as part of their preparation for dying, and they may want to use you as a sounding board for their plans. On the other hand, it is sometimes the case that the patient's family needs more emotional support than the patient does.

Caucasian Anglo-European culture expects a dying patient to show peaceful acceptance of his or her prognosis, and the bereaved are expected to show grief. Patients who belong to other ethnic groups may demonstrate a very different response, crying loudly and inflicting pain on themselves. Death affects not only the individual patient but also family, friends, staff, and even other patients. For this reason, it is essential that all members of the health care team understand the process of dying and its possible effects on those left behind. Your partnership with your patients and their families will provide a unique insight into their values, spirituality, and relationship dynamics that will be especially helpful at the end of life.

PATIENT RIGHTS

Patients' Bill of Rights

When patients seek health care, they expect that they have certain rights, including the rights to open and honest communication, respect for their person and their values, and sensitivity to any differences that may affect their care. In 2004 the American Hospital Association replaced an earlier Patients' Bill of Rights with a plain-language brochure called *The Patient Care Partnership: Understanding Expectations, Rights and Responsibilities*. This document is available in eight different languages (English, Arabic, Simplified Chinese, Traditional Chinese, Russian, Spanish, Tagalog, and Vietnamese).

The brochure outlines how patients have a right to do the following:

- Be treated with respect
- Make a treatment choice
- Refuse treatment
- Obtain their medical records
- Protect privacy of their medical records
- Have informed consent
- Make decisions about end-of-life care

Patients also must understand that that they have a responsibility to do the following:

- Maintain healthy habits
- Be respectful to providers
- Be honest with providers
- Comply with treatment plans

- Prepare for emergencies
- Read behind the headlines
- Make decisions responsibly

Unlike our nation's Bill of Rights, few of the patients' rights are clearly spelled out, except those relating to privacy and access to medical records. Compounding the problem, there are a number of rights that patients believe they have, but which are, in fact, not rights, such as access to health care and the right to *total* privacy of medical records. Patients also must understand the rights they do *not* have, so it will be easier for them to get the care and outcomes that they seek.

Health Insurance Portability and Accountability Act (HIPAA)

The Health Insurance Portability and Accountability Act of 1996 (HIPAA) established new standards for the uses of health care information. HIPAA created three types of standards: privacy, security, and administrative simplification (e.g., transaction standards). Together, these regulations affect the day-to-day functioning of the nation's hospitals, medical providers, and medical community. They affect virtually every department of every entity that provides or pays for health care.

HIPAA has created national standards to protect individuals' medical records and other personal health information. It does the following:

- Gives patients more control over their health information
- Sets boundaries on the use and release of health records
- Establishes appropriate safeguards that health care providers and others must achieve to protect the privacy of health information
- Holds violators accountable with civil and criminal penalties that can be imposed if they violate patients' privacy rights
- Strikes a balance when public responsibility supports disclosure of some forms of data (i.e., in the case of protecting public health)

For patients, the HIPAA act means the following:

- Being able to make informed choices when seeking care and reimbursement for care, based on how personal health information may be used
- Being able to find out how their information may be used and about certain disclosures of their information that have been made
- Generally, obtaining the right to examine and obtain a copy of their own health records and request corrections
- Empowering individuals to control certain uses and disclosures of their health information

For sonographers, the HIPAA act means the following:

- Putting patient information away after hours
- Taking files out of sight of any lingering staff and custodians
- Setting screensavers on computers for the shortest time possible

- Taking care that other patients do not overhear any conversations (including phone conversations)
- Removing patient identification from any scans that will be used for publication or presentation
- Keeping any patient charts filed with the names facing the wall to ensure that passersby or visitors to the ultrasound area cannot see the names or any information on the charts
- Honoring patient requests that students, other observers, medical personnel, and families leave the room during their sonography examination
- Explaining to patients the hospital or department policies regarding the rights of friends and family to view their ultrasound procedure
- Meeting the patient's expectation of a pleasant physical and emotional environment where comfort, safety, and respect as an individual are ensured

The following links to the Patients' Bill of Rights and HIPAA should be reviewed for any updates:

- www.cc.nih.gov/participate/patientinfo/legal/bill_of_rights.shtml
- www.hhs.gov/ocr/privacy/hipaa/understanding/consumers/index.html

Providing competent and excellent patient care in today's health care environment is challenging, both because today's patients are often better informed and more demanding and because many are newcomers to the United States who bring with them different cultural and religious views on how they should be treated. Patients expect reliable care, prompt responses to their requests, and assurances that they will be safe under a sonographer's care. They expect not only proficiency, but empathy.

The modern sonographer must meet a growing list of needs while competently and efficiently carrying out his or her sonographic duties. Most diagnostic medical sonography programs do a good job of educating and training students in the scientific and technical aspects of sonography. However, they must also focus equal attention on helping sonography students to develop a humanistic approach when dealing with their patients. They must also stress the critical importance of continuing education after graduation, to stay current with the rapid and exciting developments that are a hallmark of diagnostic medical sonography.

 Key Pearls

- The patient is the primary focus of the sonographer.
- Vital signs are the observable and measureable signs of life and include the following: pulse, respiratory rate, body temperature, and blood pressure.
- The sonographer should be aware of how to meet the patient's needs: bedpans and urinals, emesis basins, tubes and tubing management, and oxygen.
- Body mechanics is essential to performing the daily routine in a health care environment.
- Infection control is a standard precaution to preventing the spread of disease.
- The sonographer should have a working knowledge of basic life support and be able to react to any emergent situation.
- Empathy, understanding, and compassion are essential to care for the variety of patients.
- The sonographer must be compliant with the Patient's Bill of Rights and HIPAA requirements.

BIBLIOGRAPHY

Craig M: *Essentials of sonography and patient care*, ed 3, St. Louis, 2010, Elsevier.

Ehrlich RA: *Patient care in radiography*, ed 7, St. Louis, 2008, Mosby.

Mosby's expert 10-minute physical examinations, St. Louis, 1997, Mosby.

Pellico LH: *Handbook of clinical skills*, Springhouse, PA, 1997, Springhouse.

Silvestri LA: *Saunders comprehensive review for the NCLEX-RN examination*, ed 3, Philadelphia, 2005, W.B. Saunders.

Ergonomics and Musculoskeletal Issues in Sonography

Carolyn Coffin, Joan P. Baker

OBJECTIVES

On completion of this chapter, you should be able to:
- Discuss the history of work-related musculoskeletal disorders in sonography
- Define OSHA and discuss its role in sonography
- Define common types of work-related injury for sonographers and know what causes them
- Describe and apply "best practices" in sonography
- Outline the costs of occupational injury to yourself and your employer

OUTLINE

History of Ergonomics
    History of Work-Related Musculoskeletal Disorders in Sonography
    History of the Occupational Safety and Health Administration's Involvement in Sonography
Injury Data in Sonography
    Definitions
    Surveys

    Risk Factors
    Mechanisms of Injury
    Types of Injury
Industry Awareness and Changes
    Ergonomically Designed Ultrasound Systems
    Administrative Controls
    Personal Protective Equipment/ Professional Controls

Work Practice Changes
    Gripping the Transducer
    Wrist Flexion and Extension
    Twisting Your Neck
    Abduction of Your Scanning Arm
    Transducer Cable Management
    Trunk Twisting
    Reaching
    Exercise
Economics of Ergonomics

KEY TERMS

Bursitis
Carpal tunnel
Cubital tunnel
de Quervain's disease
Epicondylitis (lateral and medial)
Ergonomics

Occupational Safety and Health (OSH) Act
Rotator cuff injury
Spinal degeneration
Tendonitis
Tenosynovitis

Thoracic outlet syndrome
Trigger finger
Work-related musculoskeletal disorder (WRMSD)

HISTORY OF ERGONOMICS

Broadly defined, **ergonomics** is the science of designing a job to fit the individual worker. One of its primary goals is increasing productivity and decreasing injury by modifying products, tasks, and environments to better fit people.

The term *ergonomics* comes from the Greek words *ergon*, meaning *work*, and *nomos*, meaning *study of* or *natural laws*. The word first entered the modern lexicon when Wojciech Jastrzebowski used it in his 1857 philosophical tract titled *The Science of Work, Based on the Truths Taken from the Natural Science*. The association between work activities and musculoskeletal injuries has been documented for centuries. Bernardino Ramazinni (1633–1714) was the first physician to write about work-related injuries and illnesses in his 1700 publication *De Morbis Artificum (Diseases of Workers),* which he researched by visiting the workplaces of his patients.[1]

In the early 1900s, industry production was still largely dependent on human power and motion, rather than on machines, and ergonomic concepts were developing to improve worker productivity. Frederick Winslow Taylor pioneered the "scientific management" method, which sought to improve worker efficiency by discovering the optimum way to do any given task. Frank and Lillian Gilbreth expanded upon Taylor's methods in the early 1900s with their time and motion studies aimed at improving efficiency by eliminating unnecessary steps and motion.

The assembly line developed by Ford Motor Company between 1908 and 1915 was heavily influenced by the emerging field of ergonomics. In assembly line manufacturing, parts are added to a product in a sequential, well-planned manner to create a finished product much faster than with handcrafting-type methods. Although assembly line production improved productivity in the Ford Motor Company, it also reduced the need for workers to move throughout their workday and thus resulted in static work postures.

World War II brought about a greater interest in human-machine interaction, a natural result of the development of new and complex machines and weaponry. It was not only observed that the success of the machine depended on its operator but also that the design of the machine influenced how successful its operator was. It was important that equipment fit the size of the soldier and that controls were logical and easy to understand. After World War II, the equipment design focus expanded to include worker safety as well as productivity.

In the decades since the war, the field of ergonomics has continued to flourish and diversify with the advent of the Space Age and the Computer Age.

History of Work-Related Musculoskeletal Disorders in Sonography

Awareness of pain and discomfort associated with the occupation of sonography surfaced around 1980 just before the widespread use of real-time scanners. The most common complaint was shoulder pain in the sonographer's scanning arm. The increasing number of complaints reached the attention of Marveen Craig, a well-known sonographer, educator, and author. Craig published an article in 1985 summarizing the results of a survey done of 100 sonographers who had between 5 and 20 years of scanning experience.[2] The survey respondents complained of stress and burnout, vision problems that improved when images switched from black on white to white on black, infections, and allergies. Electric shock was not uncommon, especially when doing bedside studies and when removing transducers from the articulated arm of static scanners. Muscle strain involving the wrist, base of the thumb, and shoulder was also reported. Sonographers complained of heavy transducers and cables, and carpal tunnel syndrome claimed its first victim. The term *sonographer's shoulder* came into use.

In the early 1980s, ultrasound systems underwent a complete redesign to real-time two-dimensional scanners, and although articulated arm scanners were used for many more years, real-time scanners were slowly introduced to most faculties.

As more real-time systems came into use, sonographer's shoulder appeared to diminish. However, this decline lasted only 10 years, and by 1995 the Society of Diagnostic Medical Sonography (SDMS) started receiving increasingly more and varied complaints. In 1997 an extensive 125-question survey was developed by the Health Care Benefit Trust of Vancouver Canada (HBT), in collaboration with the SDMS, the Canadian Society of Diagnostic Medical Sonography (CSDMS), and the British Columbia Ultrasound Society (BCUS). Through this survey, the incidence of work-related musculoskeletal disorder (WRMSD) was found to be 81% in the United States and 87% in Canada, for a combined average incidence in North America of 84%.[3,4]

In 2008 a follow-up survey was conducted, and the incidence increased from 81% to 90% in the United States. Several variables may account for this increase: aging workforce, increased awareness of WRMSD among sonographers, and increased willingness by sonographers to report injury.

History of the Occupational Safety and Health Administration's Involvement in Sonography

In 1970 Congress passed the federal **Occupational Safety and Health (OSH) Act**. The purpose of the OSH Act is to ensure, as far as possible, that every working man and woman in the nation has safe and healthful working conditions. Employers may be subjected to civil and sometimes criminal penalties if they violate this act.[5]

The OSH Act is administered by the Occupational Safety and Health Administration (OSHA) of the U.S. Department of Labor, although individual states had the option to create their own agency to enforce the act. Approximately 50% of the states opted to be regulated by the federal OSHA. The other states created their own agencies, which operate under a "state plan." For example, California has a state plan and created its own agency, Cal/OSHA, to enforce safety regulations within that state.[5]

Where industry-specific guidelines do not exist within the OSH Act, the general duty clause can be used. Lawyers representing injured sonographers seeking legal recourse refer to this clause. The criteria for applying the general duty clause are as follows:

- No acceptable standard for an industry
- Exposure to hazard that causes serious physical harm
- Hazard is recognized by the industry
- Feasible abatement method exists to correct the hazard

Section 5B of the general duty clause states that each employee shall comply with occupational safety and health standards and all rules, regulations, and orders issued pursuant to this act that are applicable to his or her own actions and conduct.[6]

It is under the provisions of paragraph 5A(1) that the OSH Act addresses ergonomic disorders. The language in paragraph 5B gives the impression that the employee holds significant responsibility for complying with health and safety standards; however, the employer bears most of the responsibility for compliance in the eyes of OSHA.[6]

Over the years, OSHA has used many different labels for occupational injury:

- Cumulative trauma disorder (CTD)
- Repetitive motion injury (RMI)
- Overuse syndrome
- Repetitive strain injury (RSI)
- Musculoskeletal strain injury (MSI)

The term **work-related musculoskeletal disorder (WRMSD)** is currently in use. WRMSD incidents are defined as injuries that result in (1) restricted work, (2) days away from work, (3) symptoms of musculoskeletal disorder (MSD) that remain for 7 or more days, and (4) MSD requiring medical treatment beyond first aid.

According to Liberty Mutual, which collects data on WRMSD and the associated costs, repetitive motion injuries cost U.S. industries $2.3 billion per year. Ultrasound examination specialties such as echocardiography, high-risk obstetrics, and to a lesser extent vascular sonography involve repetitive motion.

Liberty Mutual also reports that 95% of chief executive officers support workplace safety. Benefits include improved employee health. Indirect costs such as morale, productivity, and hiring of replacement staff are significantly reduced, whereas direct costs such as wage replacement and medical expenses are avoided.[7]

Over the years, the Department of Labor received numerous requests from workers' unions to create a way for employees to deal with their WRMSDs. This resulted in the development of an Alliance Program, which enables organizations to work with OSHA to prevent workplace injuries by educating and leading employers and their employees in advancing workplace safety and health.

In May 2003 an International Ultrasound Industry Consensus Conference was hosted by the SDMS to develop injury risk–reducing standards to address the problem of WRMSDs in sonography. Twenty-six organizations represented by 32 participants attended the conference with the goal of discussing how they might design new platforms and procedures that incorporate better ergonomics. The industry standards address the role of employees and employers, educators, medical facilities, and equipment manufacturers in reducing the impact of these injuries on the workforce and are intended to assist all stakeholders in making informed decisions.

Separately, but at the same time, administrators addressed the issues of workload, scheduling, and room size, while sonographers discussed best practices, education, and training. The need for accredited programs to include curriculum related to ergonomics and injury prevention, as well as certifying bodies testing knowledge of risk factors, was covered.

INJURY DATA IN SONOGRAPHY

Definitions

WRMSDs are injuries of muscles, tendons, and joints that are caused by or aggravated by workplace activities. These injuries are the main reason for long-term absence among health care workers,[8] accounting for up to 60% of all workplace illnesses. Survey data have shown that more than 80% of sonographers have some form of MSD that can be attributed to their work activities.

Surveys

Table 3-1 outlines the numerous surveys that have been conducted on the incidence of this injury in sonography. These surveys have produced other data relevant to the study of occupational injury in ultrasound, and their results support the presence of risk factors in the sonography profession. A number of other factors contribute to reported injury rates, including worker awareness; unwillingness to work in pain; busier patient schedules; job dissatisfaction; an aging workforce; and computerization of the workplace.

A positive relationship has been demonstrated between the severity of WRMSDs and the performance of repetitive work tasks or tasks that require forceful movements, with or without repetitive motion.[9] Increased use of technology has resulted in workers' being able to accomplish the same work tasks with fewer movements. Thus the relationship between

TABLE 3-1	Surveys of Work-Related Musculoskeletal Disorders				
Author	**Year**	**Number Surveyed**	**Number Responded**	**Incidence**	**Scope**
Vanderpool	1993	225	101	86%	Random ARDMS
BCUS	1994	232	211	91%	BC Canada
SDMS	1995	3000	983	81%	Random ARDMS
CSDMS	1995	Unknown	427	87%	Canada
Smith	1997	220	113	80%	National cardiac
Wihlidal	1997	156	96	89%	Alberta Canada
Gregory	1998	Unknown	197	77.8%	Australia
Magnavita	1999	2670	2041	74%	Italy MDs
McCullough	2002	Unknown	295	82%	United States
Ransom	2002	Unknown	300	89%	United Kingdom
Sound Ergonomics	2008	5800	3,244	90%	United States

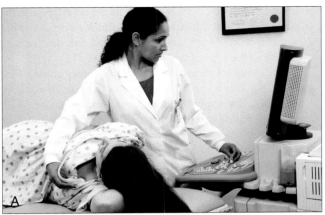 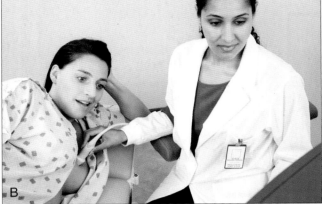

FIGURE 3-1 A, Bad ergonomics. Right-handed cardiac scanning is likely to cause injury to the sonographer because of the abduction of the arm over the patient's back, the hyperflexion of the right wrist, and the need to lean to the right and twist the neck to view the monitor. Moreover, it is the obese patient population that requires this type of test, making the level stretching and twisting even worse. **B,** Good ergonomics. It is difficult to reduce these risk factors, but one way is to turn the patient around to perform the study. *(Courtesy Siemens Healthcare, Ultrasound USA Division.)*

the user and the workstation equipment has become "frozen," and the worker is often forced into a static posture. This combination of repetitive motions and prolonged static postures results in musculoskeletal discomfort and eventually injury.

Risk Factors

Risk factors include forceful exertions, awkward postures and prolonged static postures, repetitive motions, "pinch" grip, and exposure to environmental factors such as extreme heat, cold, humidity, or vibrations (Figure 3-1). The accumulated exposure to one or more of these risk factors over time leads to injury, because repeated exposure interferes with the ability of the body to recover. WRMSDs cause pain, inflammation, swelling, deterioration of tendons and ligaments, and spinal degeneration. Muscles and joints are further stressed once their support structures are weakened.

Mechanisms of Injury

Sustained awkward postures can cause imbalances between the muscles that move and the muscles that stabilize. Repeatedly rotating the head, neck, and trunk causes one set of muscles to become stronger and shorter and the opposing muscles to become weaker and elongated. Asymmetric forces are exerted on the spine causing misalignment (Figure 3-2). Nerve entrapment syndromes can result from increased muscle and tendon pressure on major nerves that run behind tightened muscles. Tasks that require the worker to continually lean forward or to bend the head down or laterally are examples of these types of postures. Prolonged static postures, whether sitting or standing, increase the load on soft tissues and the compressive forces on the spine. Additionally, the contraction of more than 50% of the body's muscles is required to maintain static postures.[10] Human physiology depends on movement, which promotes normal muscle

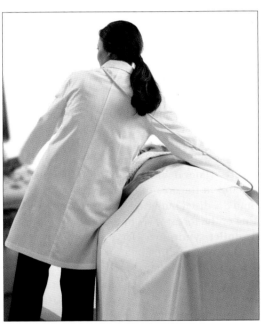

FIGURE 3-2 Asymmetric forces are exerted on the spine when more weight is put on one side of body. This means that the head must be turned farther to view the monitor, resulting in a twisted neck. *(Courtesy Philips Healthcare, Ultrasound, North America.)*

contraction and relaxation. Muscle activity circulates blood to carry nutrients to and remove toxins from muscles. Awkward and static postures cause muscles to continuously be contracted; therefore they cannot receive oxygen or get rid of toxins.[11]

Types of Injury

Tendonitis and tenosynovitis. Inflammation of the tendon and the sheath around the tendon. These often occur together.

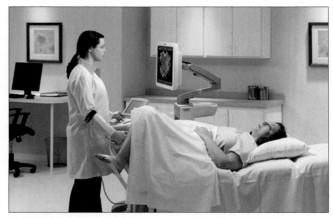

FIGURE 3-3 Epicondylitis can result from repeated twisting of the forearm, a motion performed when scanning transvaginally from the patient's side. Twisting of the forearm can be reduced or avoided by scanning from the foot of the table with the patient in leg supports (stirrups). *(Courtesy Sound Ergonomics, LLC, Kenmore, Washington.)*

de Quervain's disease. Specific type of tendonitis involving the thumb that can result from gripping the transducer.

Carpal tunnel. Entrapment of the median nerve as it runs through the carpal bones of the wrist. This results from repeated flexion and extension of the wrist and also from mechanical pressure against the wrist.

Cubital tunnel. Entrapment of the ulnar nerve as it runs through the elbow. This can result from repeated twisting of the forearm and mechanical pressure against the elbow when you rest it on the examination table while scanning.

Epicondylitis (lateral and medial). Inflammation of the periosteum in the area of the insertion of the biceps tendon into the distal humerus. This can result from repeated twisting of the forearm (Figure 3-3).

Thoracic outlet syndrome. Nerve entrapment can occur at different levels, resulting in a variety of symptoms.

Trigger finger. Inflammation and swelling of the tendon sheath in a finger entraps the tendon and restricts motion of the finger.

Bursitis (shoulder). Inflammation of the shoulder bursa from repeated motion.

Rotator cuff injury. Repeated motion results in fraying of the rotator cuff muscle tendons. This injury increases with age and is even more prevalent when work-related stresses are added. Repeated arm abduction contributes to this injury by restricting blood flow to the soft tissues of the shoulder.

Spinal degeneration. Intervertebral disc degeneration results from bending and twisting and improper seating.

INDUSTRY AWARENESS AND CHANGES

The increase in MSDs in industry led to research into the causes and to legislation in the United States regulating the design of office furniture and duration of video terminal work. Appropriate ergonomic adaptations have been found to effectively reduce the risk of MSD symptoms. Adapting a

workstation to each person and his or her work requirements ensures that it functions as intended. Productivity is increased if an employee's work area is arranged for the individual worker and the type of work being done.

Developing solutions to occupational injury among sonographers requires a combined effort on the part of equipment companies, employers, and sonographers. Because MSD is caused by multiple factors, injury prevention requires solutions from many sources as well. By taking a multidisciplinary approach, significant improvements can be made in the risk for work-related injury in the sonography profession.

Mitigating risk for injury involves a strategy for control. The first solutions to consider are engineering solutions, which involve a change in the physical features of a workplace. This is the preferred method for control because it can effectively eliminate the workplace hazard. However, these solutions also tend to be the most expensive initially.[7]

When engineering controls are not feasible or cost prohibitive, administrative controls can be implemented. These solutions are not as effective as engineering controls and include changes in workplace policies, changes in patient scheduling and sonographer rotations, and the implementation of rest breaks. Administrative controls lessen the duration and frequency of exposure to an injury risk.[7]

The least effective control is the use of personal protective equipment (PPE) or professional practices. This method addresses best practices and the use of arm support devices. The sonographer is still exposed to the risk factor, but the exposure is somewhat reduced.[7]

Over the years, the major ultrasound equipment manufacturers addressed the issue of occupational injury by redesigning the platform of their systems. This involved changing the aspects of the system's control panel, monitors, and transducers. As a result, many features of today's ultrasound systems are designed with ergonomics in mind.

Ergonomically Designed Ultrasound Systems

The well-designed ultrasound system should be easily mobile and have brakes. The control panel should be height adjustable and should swivel. The monitor should also be height adjustable, independent of the control panel, and should turn and tilt. Controls should be easy to access without overreaching. Transducers should not be too wide, which causes stretching of the fingers, or too narrow, which causes a "pinch grip." Transducer cables should be thin, flexible, and lightweight, and the transducer cable should be supported during an examination. In addition, transducers should be easy to activate with readily accessible connecting ports and storage.

Other engineering controls involve the workstation, which includes the examination table and the chair and accessories (Figure 3-4). An electronically height adjustable examination table is an important component of an ergonomically designed workstation. It should be specialty specific by providing options that adapt it for use in certain procedures. Examples would be a drop section for apical cardiac views or

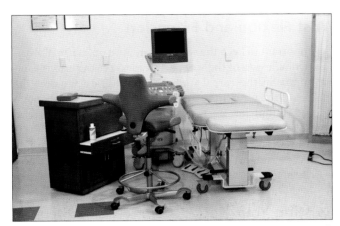

FIGURE 3-4 An ultrasound workstation with an ergonomically designed table and chair. *(Courtesy Oakworks Medical, Inc., New Freedom, Pennsylvania.)*

stirrups for obstetric/gynecologic examinations. If the sonographer sits to scan, a height-adjustable chair with an appropriate height range is equally as important as the examination table. The sonographer also should be able to support his or her arms while scanning and have an examination room that is large enough to allow for a flexible setup. The room must have appropriate lighting to avoid glare on the monitor and reduce eyestrain.

Administrative Controls

Patient examinations should be carefully scheduled to prevent repetition of the same type of examination back to back. It is important to perform a variety of examinations, allowing different muscles to fire. The schedule should allow enough time between examinations for muscle recovery. Examination gloves should have textured fingers to prevent the need to grip the transducer too tightly. Take short "mini" breaks during examinations to relax muscles, especially in the

shoulder and neck. If it is necessary to perform bedside examinations, make sure that the ultrasound system can be moved easily and has a small footprint. Try to share bedside examinations with other staff, and do these examinations only when absolutely necessary, not because it is just more convenient. Bedside examinations should be reserved for those patients whose condition prohibits transporting them.

Provide separate monitors so that the patient and the sonographer do not have to share the monitor mounted on the system. Provide ergonomically designed scanning rooms to reduce the risk of injury to the sonographer, including appropriately adjustable ancillary equipment.

Personal Protective Equipment/Professional Controls. You are the only person who can control your work postures and behaviors, some of which may be injury producing (Figure 3-5). You must take responsibility for your postural alignment and take the time to arrange the examination room equipment to suit you and the study you are performing. Best practices address how to prevent or reduce your exposure to known risk factors. Be aware of what causes pain and make changes in technique and postures immediately:

- Minimize sustained bending, twisting, reaching, lifting, and transducer pressure.
- Avoid awkward postures.
- Alternate sitting and standing throughout examinations.
- Vary scanning techniques and transducer grips.
- Adjust all equipment to suit each user's size.
- Have accessories on hand before beginning the examination.
- Use appropriate measures to reduce arm abduction.
- Avoid forward and backward reach.
- Instruct the patient to move as close to you as possible.
- Adjust the height of the table and chair.
- Use support for your arms.
- Relax your muscles periodically throughout the day.
- Stretch your hand, wrist, shoulder muscles, and spine.
- Take mini breaks during the procedure.
- Take meal breaks separate from work-related tasks.

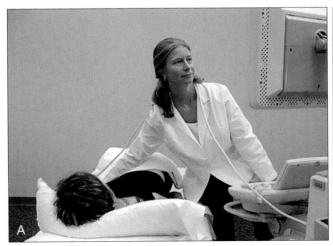
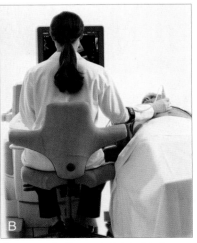

FIGURE 3-5 A, You must take responsibility for your postural alignment. **B,** Sit up straight with the top of the monitor level with your eyes and arm's length away. Support your feet on the ring of the chair, and support your forearm on a cushion. *(A, Courtesy Susan Rantz Stephenson. B, Courtesy Philips Healthcare, Ultrasound, North America.)*

- Using the 20-20-20 rule, refocus your eyes every 20 minutes on an object about 20 feet from you for 20 seconds.
- Vary procedures, tasks, and skills as much as reasonably possible.
- Use correct body mechanics when moving patients, wheelchairs, beds, stretchers, and ultrasound systems.
- Report and document any persistent pain to your employer, and seek competent medical advice.
- Maintain a good level of physical fitness in order to perform the demanding work tasks required.
- Collaborate with employers on staffing solutions that allow sufficient time away from work.

WORK PRACTICE CHANGES

Gripping the Transducer

Use mild transducer pressure. Avoid the temptation to be "image driven"—sacrificing your body for a "pretty picture" that does not affect the diagnosis. It is unnecessary to grip the transducer tightly. This might be no more than a bad habit and you may be unaware that you are doing it. This is also a difficult habit to break, as it is as natural as holding a pen.

Manufacturer improvements, such the lightweight flexible cables, can reduce the weight and torque that the transducer produces on the scanning hand. If they are available in your department, use lightweight transducers. Keeping the transducer handle free of excess gel will also reduce the amount of force needed to grip the transducer. It is also important to use gloves that fit properly. Gloves that are too large require more muscle force to grip than gloves that fit. Additionally, it takes 40% more effort to hold a transducer in a pinch grip versus a power grip. Therefore it is important to learn different ways to hold the transducer that allow you to use more of your hand rather than your fingers.

Wrist Flexion and Extension

It is important to keep the wrist in a neutral or "normal" position. Dorsiflexion of the wrist can lead to pressure and resultant injury in the carpal tunnel. This position requires the muscles of the forearm to fire continuously. When transporting the equipment, push from the legs, not the arms and wrists, keeping your wrists in a neutral position. Avoid resting your wrist on the keyboard while scanning or typing. Be sure to support your forearm while scanning to reduce muscle fatigue of the forearm, neck, and shoulder.

Twisting Your Neck

This position produces increased pressure on the intervertebral discs and should be minimized as much as possible. Position the ultrasound system so that it is as close to the examination table as possible with the monitor facing you to reduce neck twisting. Do not share the monitor with the patient. An external monitor for patient viewing is strongly recommended. Also remember to keep your shoulders relaxed as much as possible, rolling them periodically during the scan to release your neck muscles.

Abduction of Your Scanning Arm

The main reason for shoulder pain associated with right-handed scanning is due to the abduction of the shoulder. Shoulder abduction must be reduced to 30 degrees or less (Figure 3-6). Lower the examination table or elevate the chair to achieve the correct posture. The sonographer must also position the patient by having him or her move to the edge of the examination table so that the patient's side is touching the sonographer's right hip to further reduce abduction and reach. One study showed that decreasing the angle of abduction from 75 degrees to 30 degrees and supporting the forearm on

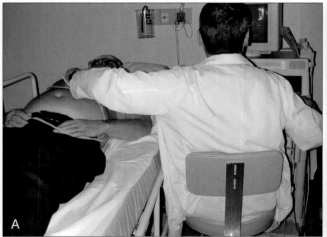
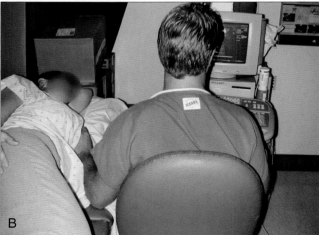

FIGURE 3-6 **A,** Bad ergonomic practice in left-handed cardiac scanning. **B,** Good ergonomics. In left-handed cardiac scanning, it is easy to adjust the height of the chair up and the table down to reduce the angle of abduction to 30 degrees or less. This often requires that you bring the patient to the edge of the table. *(Courtesy Sound Ergonomics, LLC, Kenmore, Washington.)*

support cushions could achieve a reduction of up to 88% in muscle activity of the shoulder. Sonographers who are short in stature may have to stand to scan. It may also be helpful to sit for part of the scan and stand for other parts, as long as the equipment is readjusted to suit the two different positions. Support your scanning arm by placing support cushions or a rolled-up towel under your elbow.

Transducer Cable Management

Current transducers inherently create torque on the wrist forcing the muscles of the hand and forearm to fire constantly to counteract the drag. Cable braces can be used to hold and support the cable of ultrasound transducers. This takes the strain off the operator's hand and forearm created by the imbalance of the transducer and cable, significantly reducing torque on the wrist. Additionally, cable braces can alleviate the need to grip as tightly or the need to put the cable around your neck or between your hip and the table. This latter position creates issues of spinal alignment and weight imbalance.

Trunk Twisting

Trunk twisting is often necessary in small rooms where equipment cannot be optimally positioned to reduce twisting. Sonographers with poor scanning technique also exhibit this posture (Figure 3-7). If you stand to scan, have your weight evenly distributed over both feet so that your spine remains straight. If you are uncertain as to whether you have the habit of leaning on one leg, ask a colleague to watch you scan and observe your spine position. When seated, use your abdominal muscles to support your trunk, and sit upright with good postural alignment. This often takes some practice but can be more readily achieved by using a specially designed chair that puts you into a more natural position. These chairs have a saddle-type seat and are ideal for maintaining the natural lordosis of the spine. Another option is an air-filled cushion, which forces you to maintain a stable, more neutral, position by engaging your abdominal muscles to help you balance on the cushion.

Reaching

This occurs when you reach for the controls while scanning with the opposite hand. To reduce reach, the ultrasound system must be brought as close as possible to you. Frequently used controls should be in the middle of the control panel, so that regardless of the hand used to manipulate them, they can be adjusted without causing strain. If you sit to scan, you must be able to fit your legs under the control panel in order to position the system close enough. Be sure your feet are fully supported when sitting, either on the system, the floor, the chair, or a footstool. If this is not possible, it may be better to stand while scanning. Do not get into the habit of leaving your nonscanning arm in an extended position over the control panel, especially over the freeze frame control.

All these work practices also apply to your computer workstation and the Picture Archiving and Communication

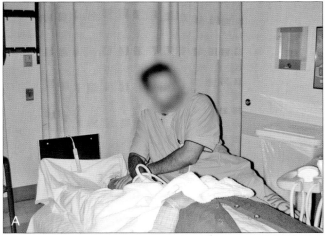

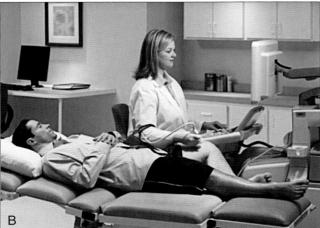

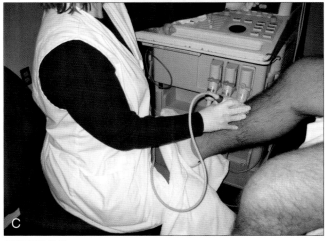

FIGURE 3-7 A, Ultrasound performed for evaluation of deep vein thrombosis (DVT) can be very injury producing if not performed correctly. **B,** When scanning the patient's left leg, turn the patient so that the left leg is closest to you. **C,** This is the most ergonomic way to perform a scan for the evaluation of DVT if you have a mobile patient. (A, C, *Courtesy Sound Ergonomics, LLC, Kenmore, Washington.* B, *Courtesy Siemens Healthcare Ultrasound, USA Division.*)

Systems (PACs) station. These environments are part of your workday and can be another source for injury. The heights of the computer monitor, work desk, and chair should all be adjustable. The keyboard should be positioned to minimize reach and maximize a neutral wrist posture.

Exercise

Sonographers should also learn and perform a regular maintenance exercise program designed to strengthen and stretch the shoulders, arms, hands, and trunk (Figure 3-8).

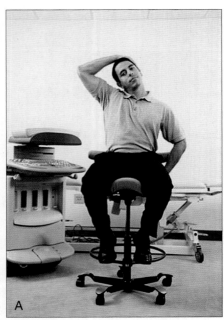

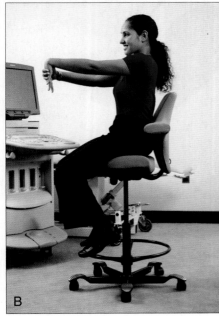

FIGURE 3-8 Simple stretches and exercises such as these done throughout the day for a few minutes can make a significant difference to your health and well-being. *(Courtesy Siemens Healthcare Ultrasound, USA Division.)*

ECONOMICS OF ERGONOMICS

The cost of occupational injury to both the employer and the employee is phenomenal. The losses to the employer encompass not only the medical costs of an injury, but also the cost of replacement staff, workers' compensation, and loss of revenue. The loss of experienced professionals and a skilled, stable workforce also affects productivity. The cost to the worker includes not only monetary hardship, but also the possibility of permanent injury, chronic pain, and loss of profession.

Acute and chronic MSDs are the most prevalent workplace injury in all industries. The Bureau of Labor Statistics states that more than 300,000 MSDs are reported annually. They account for 56% of the work-related illnesses reported to OSHA and are responsible for 640,000 lost workdays. MSDs are also the most costly of all occupational problems, accounting for the majority of workers' compensation costs. The costs related to occupational musculoskeletal disorders are both direct and indirect. MSDs cost $60 billion overall per year and to businesses, $5 billion to $20 billion per year in direct costs. These costs include workers' compensation and medical expenses, the latter of which are increasing 2.5 times faster than any other benefit cost:

- Approximately $1 of every $3 of workers' compensation costs are spent on occupational MSDs.
- Employers pay $15 billion to $20 billion per year in workers' compensation costs for lost workdays.
- The mean cost per cause of upper extremity WRMSD is $8070 versus a mean cost of $4075 per case for all types of work-related injury. With regard to incurred claim costs (which include indemnity and medical payments), the average for all claims is $10,105, but for carpal tunnel syndrome, it is $13,263.
- Indirect costs are 3 to 5 times higher, reaching approximately $150 billion per year. These include absenteeism, staff replacement and retraining, and loss of productivity or quality.
- The cost of hiring temporary replacement staff is between $130,000 and $166,000 per year. The estimated average cost to find and hire a new sonographer is $10,000.
- If an ultrasound examination room is down because of the loss of worker time, the loss of chargeable income is equal to $4500 per day, $22,500 per week, or $1,170,000 per year in lost revenue.

The cost of equipping a sonography examination room is minimal compared with addressing a workers' compensation injury. The quality of the patient's examination may also suffer if the sonographer is in pain while performing the examination. Quality diagnostic images take time to produce, and sonographers should not feel rushed to produce images because of scheduling conflicts or pain.

Accessory equipment that can mitigate injury risk includes the following:

- *A height-adjustable stool.* Cost: $750 reimbursement on two to three patient studies.

- *A set of support cushions.* Cost: $250 reimbursement on one patient study.
- *An ergonomic examination table.* Cost: $7400 reimbursement from 2 days' work.

It is very important that work-related injuries be reported immediately to occupational health or risk management departments. These injuries should be recorded on OSHA logs. Failure to do this may result in denial of claims.

Key Pearls

- The term **work-related musculoskeletal disorder (WRMSD)** incidents are defined as injuries that result in (1) restricted work, (2) days away from work, (3) symptoms of musculoskeletal disorder (MSD) that remain for 7 or more days, and (4) MSD requiring medical treatment beyond first aid.
- WRMSDs are injuries of muscles, tendons, and joints that are caused by or aggravated by workplace activities.
- Risk factors include forceful exertions, awkward postures and prolonged static postures, repetitive motions, "pinch" grip, and exposure to environmental factors such as extreme heat, cold, humidity, or vibrations.
- Sustained awkward postures can cause imbalances between the muscles that move and the muscles that stabilize.
- Adapting a workstation to each person and his or her work requirements ensures that it functions as intended. Productivity is increased if an employee's work area is arranged for the individual worker and the type of work being done.
- You are the only person who can control your work postures and behaviors, some of which may be injury producing.
- Best practices address how to prevent or reduce your exposure to known risk factors.

- Be aware of what causes pain and make changes in technique and postures immediately.
- The cost of occupational injury to both the employer and the employee is phenomenal. The losses to the employer encompass not only the medical costs of an injury, but also the cost of replacement staff, workers' compensation, and loss of revenue.

REFERENCES

1. Ergoweb Inc.: History. Available at www.ergoweb.com/resources/reference/history.cfm.
2. Craig M: Sonography: an occupational health hazard? *J Diagnostic Medical Sonographers* 1(3):121-126, 1985.
3. Pike I, Russo A, Berkowitz J, et al: The prevalence of musculoskeletal disorders among diagnostic medical sonographers, *J Diagnostic Medical Sonographers*, 13(5):219-227, 1997.
4. Murphy C, Russo, A: *An update on ergonomic issues in sonography (Canada) healthcare benefit trust*, British Columbia, 2000, Employee Health and Safety Services Steering Committee.
5. U.S. Department of Labor: The Occupational Safety and Health Administration: a history of its first thirteen years, 1971-1984. Available at www.dol.gov/oasam/programs/history/mono-osha13introtoc.htm.
6. U.S. Department of Labor, Occupational Safety and Health Administration: OSH Act of 1970. Sec. 5. Duties. Available at www.osha.gov/pls/oshaweb/owadisp.show_document?p_id=3359&p_table=OSHACT.
7. Society of Diagnostic Medical Sonography: *Industry standards for the prevention of work-related musculoskeletal disorders in sonography*, May 2003. Available at www.sdms.org/pdf/wrmsd2003.pdf.
8. Bongers PM, deWinter CR, Kompier MAJ, Hildebrandt VH: Psychosocial factors at work and musculoskeletal disease, *Scand J Work Environ Health* 19(5):297-312, 1993.
9. Barr AE, Safadi FF, Gorzelany I, et al: Repetitive, negligible force reaching in rates induces pathological overloading of upper extremity bones, *J Bone Miner Res* 18(11):2023-2032, 2003.
10. Valachi B, Valachi K: Mechanisms leading to musculoskeletal disorders in dentistry, *J Am Dent Assoc*, (134):1344-1350, October 2003.
11. Kroemer K, Grandjean E: *Fitting the task to the human*, ed 5, Philadelphia, 2000, Taylor & Francis.

Anatomic and Physiologic Relationships within the Abdominopelvic Cavity

Sandra L. Hagen-Ansert

OBJECTIVES

On completion of this chapter, you should be able to:
- Define and use terms for anatomic directions
- Discuss the body systems and their functions
- Know the terms for the body planes
- Describe and locate the abdominal quadrants and regions
- List the organs located in each major body cavity
- Identify and locate the abdominal viscera and other abdominal structures and spaces

OUTLINE

From Atom to Organism
Metabolism
Homeostasis
Vital Signs
Body Systems
The Circulatory System: Blood Composition and Function

The Gastrointestinal System
The Genitourinary System
Anatomic Relationships within the Abdominopelvic Cavities
The Abdominal Cavity
The Retroperitoneal Cavity
The Pelvic Cavity

Abdominopelvic Membranes and Ligaments
Potential Spaces in the Body

KEY TERMS

Acidic
Alkaline
Anemia
Anterior pararenal space
Ascites
Bile
Diaphragm
Dysuria
Erythrocytes
Hematochezia
Hematocrit
Homeostasis
Hypertension
Hypotension
Inguinal ligament

Intertubercular plane
Lateral arcuate ligament
Left crus of the diaphragm
Lesser sac
Leukocytes
Linea semilunaris
Medial arcuate ligament
Metabolism
Morison's pouch
Parietal peritoneum
Pelvic cavity
Perirenal space
Peritoneal cavity
Peritoneal recesses
Plasma

Polycythemia
Posterior pararenal space
Rectouterine pouch
Rectus abdominis muscle
Right crus of the diaphragm
Scrotal cavity
Subcostal plane
Superficial inguinal ring
Tachycardia
Thrombocytes
Transpyloric plane
Urinary incontinence
Vesicouterine pouch
Viscera
Visceral peritoneum

To understand the complexity of the human body and how the parts work together to function as a whole truly is to gain an appreciation of anatomy and physiology. The science of body structure (anatomy) and the study of body function (physiology) are intricately related, for each structure of the human body system carries out a specific function. Anatomy and physiology can take many forms: Gross anatomy studies the body by dissection of tissues; histology studies parts of body tissues under the microscope; embryology studies development before birth; and pathology is the study of disease processes.

FROM ATOM TO ORGANISM

A review of the composition of the human body begins with an understanding that all materials consist of chemicals. The basic units of all matter are tiny invisible particles called *atoms.* An atom is the smallest component of a chemical element that retains the characteristic properties of that element. Atoms can combine chemically to form larger particles called *molecules.* For example, two atoms of hydrogen combine with one atom of oxygen to produce a molecule of water.

The next level of complexity in the human body is a microscopic unit called a *cell.* Although they share common traits, cells can vary in size, shape, and specialized function. In the human body, atoms and molecules associate in specific ways to form cells, and trillions of different types of cells are found within the body. All cells have specialized tiny parts called *organelles,* which carry on specific activities. These organelles consist of aggregates of large molecules, including those of such substances as proteins, carbohydrates, lipids, and nucleic acids. One organelle, the *nucleus,* serves as the information and control center of the cell.

Cells that are organized into layers or masses that have common functions are known as *tissue.* The four primary types of tissue in the body are muscle, nervous, connective, and epithelial tissues. Groups of different tissues combine to form *organs*—complex structures with specialized functions, such as the liver, pancreas, or kidneys. One organ may have more than one type of tissue (e.g., the heart mainly consists of muscle tissue, but it is also covered by epithelial tissue and contains connective and nervous tissue).

A coordinated group of organs are arranged into organ or *body systems.* For example, the digestive system consists of the mouth, esophagus, stomach, intestines, liver, gallbladder, and pancreas. Body systems make up the total part or *organism* that is the human body.

Metabolism

All physical and chemical changes that occur within the body are referred to as **metabolism.** The metabolic process is essential to digestion, growth and repair of the body, and conversion of food energy into forms useful to the body. Other metabolic processes maintain the routine operations of the nerves, muscles, and other body parts.

Homeostasis

The anatomic structures and functions of all body parts are directed toward maintaining the life of the organism. To sustain life, an organism must have the proper quantity and quality of water, food, oxygen, heat, and pressure. Maintenance of life depends on the stability of these factors. **Homeostasis** is the ability to maintain a steady and stable internal environment. Stressful stimuli, or *stressors,* disrupt homeostasis.

Vital Signs

Vital signs are medical measurements used to ascertain how the body is functioning. These measurements include body temperature and blood pressure and rates and types of pulse and breathing movements. A close relationship has been noted between these signs and the homeostasis of the body, as vital signs are the result of metabolic activities.

BODY SYSTEMS

A body system consists of a group of tissues and organs that work together to perform specific functions. Each system contributes to the dynamic, organized, and carefully balanced state of the body. The sonographer should be familiar with at least the integumentary, lymphatic, skeletal, endocrine, muscular, respiratory, and nervous systems of the body. The remaining systems—circulatory, digestive, urinary, and reproductive—should be thoroughly understood by the sonographer. Table 4-1 lists the components and functions of human body systems.

The Circulatory System: Blood Composition and Function

Knowledge of the circulatory system is fundamental to understanding human physiology. The circulation of blood throughout the body serves as a vital connection to the cells, tissues, and organs to maintain a relatively constant environment for cell activity. Blood is composed of **plasma** and "formed elements." The *plasma* is broken down into 7% proteins (albumins, globulins, and fibrinogen), 91% water, and 2% other solutes (ions, nutrients, waste products, gases, regulatory substances) (Figure 4-1). The "formed elements" are comprised of platelets, leukocytes (neutrophils, lymphocytes, monocytes, eosinophils, and basophils), and erythrocytes.

Blood Composition. Plasma makes up 55% of the total blood volume and consists of about 92% water. The remaining 8% comprises numerous substances suspended or dissolved in this water. Hemoglobin of the red cells accounts for two thirds of the blood proteins, with the remaining consisting of plasma proteins. These include serum albumin, globulin, fibrinogen, and prothrombin.

Serum album constitutes 53% of the total plasma proteins. It is produced in the liver and serves to regulate blood volume. Globulin can be separated into alpha, beta, and gamma globulin. The latter is involved in immune reactions in the body's defense against infection. Fibrinogen is concerned with coagulation of blood. Prothrombin is produced in the liver and participates in blood coagulation. Vitamin K is essential for prothrombin production.

Functions of the Blood. The blood is responsible for a variety of functions, including transportation of oxygen and nutrients, defense against infection, and maintenance of pH. The red blood cells, white blood cells, and platelets are continually being destroyed so the body must make new ones to replace the destroyed cells every second. Two kinds of connective tissue make blood cells for the body: myeloid

TABLE 4-1	Systems in the Human Body	
System	**Components**	**Functions**
Integumentary	Skin, hair, nails, sweat glands	Covers and protects tissues, regulates body temperature, supports sensory receptors
Skeletal	Bones, cartilage, joints, ligaments	Supports the body, provides framework, protects soft tissues, provides attachments for muscles, produces blood cells, stores inorganic salts, provides calcium storage
Muscular	Skeletal, cardiac, smooth muscle	Moves parts of skeleton, provides locomotion, pumps blood, aids movement of internal materials, produces body heat
Nervous	Nerves and sense organs, brain, and spinal cord	Receives stimuli from external and internal environment, conducts impulses, integrates activities of other systems
Endocrine	Pituitary, adrenal, thyroid, pancreas, parathyroid, ovaries, testes, pineal, and thymus gland	Regulates body chemistry and many body functions
Lymphatic	Lymph nodes	Returns tissue fluid to the blood, carries specific absorbed food molecules, defends the body against infection
Circulatory	Heart, blood vessels, blood, lymph and lymph structures	Moves the blood through the vessels and transports substances throughout the body
Respiratory	Lungs, bronchi, and air passageways	Exchanges gases between blood and external environment
Digestive	Mouth, tongue, teeth, salivary glands, pharynx, esophagus, stomach, liver, gallbladder, pancreas, small and large intestines	Receives, breaks down, and absorbs food and eliminates unabsorbed material from the body
Urinary	Kidney, bladder, ureters	Excretes waste from the blood, maintains water and electrolyte balance, and stores and transports urine
Reproductive	Testes, scrotum, spermatic cord, vas deferens, ejaculatory duct, penis, epididymis, prostate, uterus, ovaries, fallopian tubes, vagina, breast	Reproduction; provides for continuation of the species

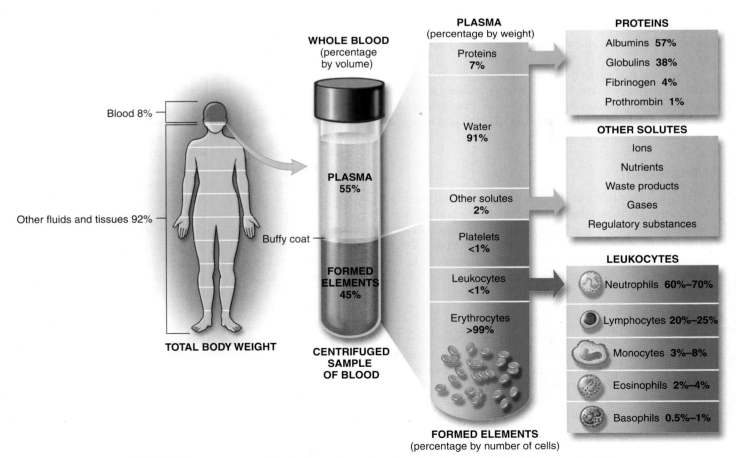

FIGURE 4-1   Components of blood. Approximate values for the components of blood in a normal adult.

tissue (red bone marrow) and lymphatic tissue (lymph nodes, thymus, spleen). The formation of new blood cells is called *hemopoiesis*. As the blood cells mature, they move into the circulatory vessels.

Acidic versus Alkaline. Blood is thicker than water and therefore flows more slowly than water. The specific gravity of blood may be calculated by comparing the weight of blood versus water; with water being 1.00, blood is in the range of 1.045 to 1.065. The hydrogen ion and the hydroxyl ion are found within water. When a solution contains more hydrogen than hydroxyl ions, it is called an **acidic** solution. Likewise, when it contains more hydroxyl ions than hydrogen ions, it is referred to as an **alkaline** solution. This concentration of hydrogen ions in a solution is called the pH, with the scale ranging up to 14.0.

In water, an equal concentration of both ions exists; water is thus a neutral solution, or 7.0 on the pH scale. Human blood has a pH of 7.34 to 7.44, being slightly alkaline. A blood pH below 6.8 is a condition called *acidosis;* blood pH above 7.8 is known as *alkalosis*. Both conditions can lead to serious illness and eventual death unless proper balance is restored. To help in this process, blood plasma is supplied with chemical compounds called *buffers*. These buffers can act as weak acids or bases to combine with excess hydrogen or hydroxyl ions to neutralize the pH. Plasma is the basic supporting fluid and transporting vehicle of the blood. It constitutes 55% of the total blood volume.

The volume of blood in the body depends on the body surface area; however, the total volume may be estimated as approximately 9% of total body weight. Therefore blood volume is approximately 5 quarts in a normal-sized man.

The red blood cells (**erythrocytes**), white blood cells (**leukocytes**), and platelets (**thrombocytes**) make up the remainder of the blood. The percent of the total blood volume containing these three elements is called the **hematocrit**. Normally, the hematocrit is 45% of the total blood volume with plasma accounting for the remaining 55%.

Complete Blood Count. The differential complete blood count (CBC) is a laboratory blood test that evaluates and states specific values for all these subgroups of white blood cells.

Red Blood Cells. Red blood cells (RBCs) are disc-shaped, biconcave cells without a nucleus. They are formed in the bone marrow and are the most prevalent of the formed elements in the blood. Their primary role is to carry oxygen to the cells and tissues of the body. Oxygen is picked up by a protein in the red cell called *hemoglobin*. Hemoglobin releases oxygen in the capillaries of the tissues. The function of *erythrocyte* is to provide oxygen and carbon dioxide transport.

The production of RBCs is called *erythropoiesis*. Their life span is approximately 120 days. Vitamin B_{12} is necessary for complete maturity of the RBCs. The inner mucosal lining of the stomach secretes a substance called the *intrinsic factor,* which promotes absorption of vitamin B_{12} from ingested food. **Anemia** is an abnormal condition where the blood lacks either a normal number of red blood cells or normal concentration of hemoglobin. If too many RBCs are produced, **polycythemia** results.

As old RBCs are destroyed in the liver, part of the hemoglobin is converted to bilirubin, which is excreted by the liver in the form of **bile.** When excessive amounts of hemoglobin are broken down, or when biliary excretion is decreased by liver disease or biliary obstruction, the plasma bilirubin level rises. This rise in plasma bilirubin results in a yellow-skin condition termed *jaundice.*

White Blood Cells. White blood cells (WBCs) are the body's primary defense against infection. WBCs lack hemoglobin, are colorless, contain a nucleus, and are larger than RBCs. White cells are extremely active and move with an ameboid motion, often against the flow of blood. They can pass from the bloodstream into intracellular spaces to phagocytize foreign matter found between the cells. A condition called *leukopoiesis* is WBC formation stimulated by the presence of bacteria.

Leukocytes. Neutrophils, lymphocytes, monocytes, eosinophils, and basophils are in the group of leukocytes. Their function is to ingest and destroy bacteria with the formation of pus. The functions of the leukocytes are as follows:

- Neutrophil and monocyte: immune defense—phagocytosis
- Lymphocyte: antibody production and cellular immune response
- Eosinophil: defense against irritants that cause allergies; phagocytosis
- Basophil: inflammatory response; contain heparin and control clotting

Lymphocytes and Monocytes. The lymphocytes are WBCs formed in lymphatic tissue. They enter the blood by way of the lymphatic system and contain antibodies responsible for delayed hypersensitivity reactions. Monocytes are large white cells capable of phagocytosis and are quite mobile. Their numbers are few, and they are produced in the bone marrow.

White Blood Cells. White cells have two main sources: (1) red bone marrow (granulocytes) and (2) lymphatic tissue (lymphocytes). When an increase in the white cells arises from a tumor of the bone marrow, it is called *myelogenous leukemia* and is noted as an increase in granulocytes. On the other hand, an increase in WBCs caused by overactive lymphoid tissue is called *lymphatic leukemia,* with an increase in lymphocytes. In bacterial infections, the white cells increase in number (leukocytosis), with most of the increase noted in the neutrophils. A decrease in the total white cell count (leukopenia) is a result of a viral infection.

Thrombocytes. Thrombocytes, or blood platelets, are formed from giant cells in the bone marrow. They initiate a chain of events involved in blood clotting together with a plasma protein called *fibrinogen*. Thrombocytes are destroyed by the liver and have a life span of 8 days.

The Gastrointestinal System

The gastrointestinal (GI) system consists of two major divisions: the GI tract and the accessory organs. The GI tract is a hollow tube that begins at the mouth and ends at the anus. About 25 feet long, the GI tract includes the pharynx, esophagus, stomach, small intestine, and large intestine (Figure 4-2). Accessory GI organs include the liver, pancreas, gallbladder,

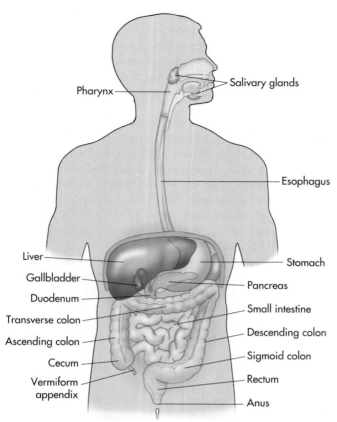

Pharynx

Salivary glands

Esophagus

Liver

Gallbladder

Duodenum

Transverse colon

Ascending colon

Cecum

Vermiform appendix

Stomach

Pancreas

Small intestine

Descending colon

Sigmoid colon

Rectum

Anus

FIGURE 4-2 The digestive system includes the mouth, pharynx, esophagus, stomach, small intestine, large intestine, rectum, and anus.

and bile ducts and will be discussed in detail in their respective chapters. The abdominal aorta and the gastric and splenic veins also aid the GI system.

Major functions of the GI system include ingestion and digestion of food and elimination of waste products. GI complaints can be especially difficult to assess and evaluate because the abdomen has so many organs and structures that may influence pain and tenderness.

Normal Findings for the GI System
Visual Inspection
- Skin is free from vascular lesions, jaundice, surgical scars, and rashes.
- Faint venous patterns (except in thin patients) are apparent.
- Abdomen is symmetric, with a flat, round, or scaphoid contour.
- Umbilicus is positioned midway between the xiphoid process and the symphysis pubis, with a flat or concave hemisphere.
- No variations in the color of the patient's skin are detectable.
- No bulges are apparent.
- The abdomen moves with respiration.

Guidelines for GI Assessment
Temperature. Fever may be a sign of infection or inflammation.

Pulse. **Tachycardia** may occur with shock, pain, fever, sepsis, fluid overload, or anxiety. A weak, rapid, and irregular pulse may point to hemodynamic instability, such as that caused by excessive blood loss. Diminished or absent distal pulses may signal vessel occlusion from embolization associated with prolonged bleeding.

Respirations. Altered respiratory rate and depth can result from hypoxia, pain, electrolyte imbalance, or anxiety. Respiratory rate also increases with shock. Increased respiratory rate with shallow respirations may signal fever and sepsis. Absent or shallow abdominal movement on respiration may point to peritoneal irritation.

Blood Pressure. Decreased blood pressure may signal compromised hemodynamic status, perhaps from shock caused by GI bleed. Sustained severe **hypotension** results in diminished renal blood flow, which may lead to acute renal failure. Moderately increased systolic or diastolic pressure may occur with anxiety or abdominal pain. **Hypertension** can result from vascular damage caused by renal disease or renal artery stenosis. A blood pressure drop of greater than 30 mm Hg when the patient sits up may indicate fluid volume depletion.

Common Signs and Symptoms of GI Diseases and Disorders. The most significant signs and symptoms related to gastrointestinal diseases and disorders are abdominal pain, diarrhea, bloody stools, nausea, and vomiting (Table 4-2).

Abdominal Pain. Abdominal pain usually results from a GI disorder, but it can be caused by a reproductive, genitourinary, musculoskeletal, or vascular disorder; use of certain drugs; or exposure to toxins.
- Constant, steady abdominal pain suggests organ perforation, ischemia, inflammation, or blood in the peritoneal cavity.
- Intermittent and cramping abdominal pain suggests the patient may have an obstruction.
- Ask if the pain radiates to other areas or if eating relieves the pain.
- Abdominal pain may arise from the abdominopelvic viscera, the parietal peritoneum, or the capsule of the liver, kidney, or spleen, and may be acute or chronic, diffuse or localized.
- Visceral pain develops slowly into a deep, dull, aching pain that is poorly localized in the epigastric, periumbilical, or hypogastric region.
- Mechanisms that produce abdominal pain, including stretching or tension of the gut wall, traction on the peritoneum or mesentery, vigorous intestinal contraction, inflammation, or ischemia, may cause sensory nerve irritation.

Diarrhea. Diarrhea is usually a primary sign of intestinal disorder. Diarrhea is an increase in the volume, frequency, and liquidity of stools compared with the patient's normal bowel habits. It varies in severity and may be acute or chronic.
- Acute diarrhea may result from acute infection, stress, fecal impaction, or use of certain drugs.

TABLE 4-2	Signs and Probable Indications of Gastrointestinal Diseases and Disorders
Signs or Symptoms	**Probable Indication**
Abdominal Pain	
Localized abdominal pain, described as steady, gnawing, burning, aching, or hunger-like, high in the midepigastrium slightly off center, usually on the right	Duodenal ulcer
Pain begins 2–4 hours after a meal	
Ingestion of food or antacids brings relief	
Changes in bowel habits	
Heartburn or retrosternal burning	
Pain and tenderness in the right or left lower quadrant, may be sharp and severe on standing or stooping	Ovarian cyst
Abdominal distention	
Mild nausea and vomiting	
Occasional menstrual irregularities	
Slight fever	
Referred, severe upper abdominal pain, tenderness, and rigidity that diminish with inspiration	Pneumonia
Fever, shaking, chills, aches, and pains	
Blood-tinged or rusty sputum	
Dry, hacking cough	
Dyspnea	
Diarrhea	
Diarrhea occurs within several hours of ingesting milk or milk products	Lactose intolerance
Abdominal pain, cramping, and bloating	
Flatus	
Recurrent bloody diarrhea with pus or mucus	Ulcerative colitis
Hyperactive bowel sounds	
Cramping lower abdominal pain	
Occasional nausea and vomiting	
Hematochezia	
Moderate to severe rectal bleeding	Coagulation disorders
Epistaxis (nosebleed)	
Purpura (skin rash resulting from bleeding into the skin from small blood vessels)	
Bright-red rectal bleeding with or without pain	Colon cancer
Diarrhea or ribbon-shaped stools	
Stools may be grossly bloody	
Weakness and fatigue	
Abdominal aching and dull cramps	
Chronic bleeding with defecation	Hemorrhoids
Painful defecation	
Nausea and Vomiting	
May follow or accompany abdominal pain	Appendicitis
Pain progresses rapidly to severe, stabbing pain in the right lower quadrant (McBurney sign)	
Abdominal rigidity and tenderness	
Constipation or diarrhea	
Tachycardia	
Nausea and vomiting of undigested food	Gastroenteritis
Diarrhea	
Abdominal cramping	
Hyperactive bowel sounds	
Fever	
Headache with severe, constant, throbbing pain	Migraine headache
Fatigue	
Photophobia	
Light flashes	
Increased noise sensitivity	

- Chronic diarrhea may result from chronic infection, obstructive and inflammatory bowel disease, malabsorption syndrome, an endocrine disorder, or GI surgery.
- The fluid and electrolyte imbalance may precipitate life-threatening arrhythmias or hypovolemic shock.

Hematochezia. **Hematochezia** is the passage of bloody stools and may be a sign of GI bleeding below the ligament of Treitz. It may also result from a coagulation disorder, exposure to toxins, or a diagnostic test. It may lead to hypovolemia.

Nausea and Vomiting. Nausea is a sensation of profound revulsion to food or of impending vomiting. Vomiting is the forceful expulsion of gastric contents through the mouth that is often preceded by nausea.

- Nausea and vomiting may occur with fluid and electrolyte imbalance; infection; metabolic, endocrine, labyrinthine, and cardiac disorders; use of certain drugs; surgery; and radiation.
- Nausea and vomiting may also arise from severe pain, anxiety, alcohol intoxication, overeating, or ingestion of distasteful food or liquids.

The Genitourinary System

It is important to recognize that a disorder of the genitourinary system can affect other body systems. For example, ovarian dysfunction can alter endocrine balance, or kidney dysfunction can affect the production of certain hormones that regulate RBC production.

The urinary system consists of the kidneys, ureters, bladder, and urethra (Figure 4-3). The primary functions of the urinary system are the formation of urine and the maintenance of homeostasis. These functions are performed by the kidneys. Kidney dysfunction can cause trouble with concentration, memory loss, or disorientation. Progressive chronic kidney failure can also cause lethargy, confusion, disorientation, stupor, convulsions, and coma. Observation of the patient's vital signs may give indication of hypertension, which may be related to renal dysfunction if the hypertension is uncontrolled.

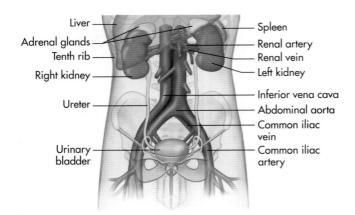

FIGURE 4-3 The urinary system includes the kidneys, ureters, bladder, and urethra.

Anatomy of the Genitourinary System

Kidneys. The kidneys are highly vascular organs that function to produce urine and maintain homeostasis in the body. The two bean-shaped organs of the kidneys are located in the retroperitoneal cavity along either side of the vertebral column. The peritoneal fat layer protects the kidneys. The right kidney lies slightly lower than the left because it is displaced by the liver. Each kidney contains about 1 million nephrons. Urine gathers in the collecting tubules and ducts and eventually drains into the ureters, then the bladder, and through the urethra (via urination).

Ureters. The ureters are 25 to 30 cm long. The narrowest part of the ureter is at the ureteropelvic junction. The other two constricted areas occur as the ureter leaves the renal pelvis and at the point it enters into the bladder wall. The ureters carry urine from the kidneys to the bladder by peristaltic contractions that occur 1 to 5 times per minute.

Bladder. The bladder is the vessel where urine collects. Bladder capacity ranges from 500 to 1000 ml in healthy adults. Children and older adults have less bladder capacity. When the bladder is empty, it lies behind the symphysis pubis; when it is full, it becomes displaced under the peritoneal cavity and serves as an excellent "window" for the sonographer to view the pelvic structures.

Urethra. The urethra is a small duct that carries urine from the bladder to the outside of the body. It is only 2.5 to 5 cm long and opens anterior to the vaginal opening. In the male, the urethra measures about 15 cm as it travels through the penis.

Common Signs and Symptoms Related to Urinary Dysfunction. The most common symptom of urinary dysfunction for both women and men is urinary incontinence. For women, a common symptom is dysuria, which often means a urinary tract infection. For men, common signs of urinary dysfunction include urethral discharge and urinary hesitancy. Tables 4-3 and 4-4 summarize the most common symptoms and probable causes of urinary dysfunction for women and men, respectively.

Dysuria. **Dysuria** is painful or difficult urination and is commonly accompanied by urinary frequency, urgency, or hesitancy. This symptom usually reflects a common female disorder of a lower urinary tract infection (UTI).

Pertinent questions for the patient would include how long the patient has noticed the symptoms, whether anything precipitates them, if anything aggravates or alleviates them, and where exactly the discomfort is felt. You might also ask if the patient has undergone a recent invasive procedure such as a cystoscopy or urethral dilation.

Urinary Incontinence. **Urinary incontinence** is the uncontrollable passage of urine. Incontinence results from a bladder abnormality or a neurologic disorder. A common urologic sign may involve large volumes of urine or dribbling. This condition would be important for the sonographer if a full bladder were required. It may be difficult for the patient to hold large enough volumes of fluid to fill the bladder for proper visualization.

TABLE 4-3	Signs and Probable Indications of Urinary Dysfunction in Women	
Signs or Symptoms		**Probable Indication**
Dysuria		
Urinary frequency		Cystitis
Nocturia		
Straining to void		
Hematuria		
Perineal or low-back pain		
Fatigue		
Low-grade fever		
Dysuria throughout voiding		Urinary system obstruction
Bladder distention		
Diminished urinary stream		
Urinary frequency and urgency		
Sensation of bloating or fullness in the lower abdomen or groin		
Urinary urgency		Urinary tract infection
Hematuria		
Cloudy urine		
Bladder spasms		
Feeling of warmth or burning during urination		
Urinary Incontinence		
Urge or overflow incontinence		Bladder cancer
Hematuria		
Dysuria		
Nocturia		
Urinary frequency		
Suprapubic pain from bladder spasms		
Palpable mass on bimanual examination		
Overflow incontinence		Diabetic neuropathy
Painless bladder distention		
Episodic diarrhea or constipation		
Orthostatic hypotension		
Syncope		
Dysphagia		
Urinary urgency and frequency		Multiple sclerosis
Visual problems		
Sensory impairment		
Constipation		
Muscle weakness		

TABLE 4-4	Signs and Probable Indications of Urinary Dysfunction in Men	
Signs or Symptoms		**Probable Indication**
Scrotal Swelling		
Swollen scrotum that is soft or unusually firm		Hernia
Bowel sounds may be heard in the scrotum		
Gradual scrotal swelling		Hydrocele
Scrotum may be soft and cystic or firm and tense		
Painless		
Round, nontender scrotal mass on palpation		
Glowing when transilluminated		
Scrotal swelling with sudden and severe pain		Testicular torsion
Unilateral elevation of the affected testicle		
Nausea and vomiting		
Urethral Discharge		
Purulent or milky urethral discharge		Prostatitis
Sudden fever and chills		
Lower back pain		
Myalgia (muscle pain)		
Perineal fullness		
Arthralgia		
Urinary frequency and urgency		
Cloudy urine		
Dysuria		
Tense, boggy, very tender, and warm prostate palpated on digital rectal examination		
Opaque, gray, yellowish, or blood-tinged discharge that is painless		Urethral neoplasm
Dysuria		
Eventual anuria		
Scant or profuse urethral discharge that is thin and clear, mucoid, or thick and purulent		Urethritis
Urinary hesitancy, frequency, and urgency		
Dysuria		
Itching and burning around the meatus		
Urinary Hesitancy		
Reduced caliber and force of urinary stream		Benign prostatic hyperplasia
Perineal pain		
Feeling of incomplete voiding		
Inability to stop the urine stream		
Urinary frequency		
Urinary incontinence		
Bladder distention		
Urinary frequency and dribbling		Prostate cancer
Nocturia		
Dysuria		
Bladder distention		
Perineal pain		
Constipation		
Hard, nodular prostate palpated on digital rectal examination		
Dysuria		Urinary tract infection
Urinary frequency and urgency		
Hematuria		
Cloudy urine		
Bladder spasms		
Costovertebral angle tenderness		
Suprapubic, low back, pelvic, or flank pain		
Urethral discharge		

Male Urethral Discharge. Male urethral discharge is discharge from the urinary meatus that may be purulent, mucoid, or thin; sanguineous or clear. It usually develops suddenly. The patient may have other signs of fever, chills, or perineal fullness. Previous history of prostate problems, sexually transmitted disease, or UTIs may be associated with this condition.

Male Urinary Hesitancy. Male urinary hesitancy is a condition that usually arises gradually with a decrease in urinary stream. When the bladder becomes distended, the discomfort increases. Often prostate problems, previous UTI or obstruction, or neuromuscular disorders are associated with this condition.

ANATOMIC RELATIONSHIPS WITHIN THE ABDOMINOPELVIC CAVITIES

The human body includes many cavities. These body cavities contain the internal organs, or **viscera.** The two principal body cavities are the dorsal cavity and the ventral cavity (Figure 4-4). The bony dorsal cavity may be subdivided into the *cranial cavity,* which holds the brain, and the *vertebral* or *spinal canal,* which contains the spinal cord. The ventral cavity is located near the anterior body surface and is subdivided into the *thoracic cavity* and the *abdominopelvic cavity.*

The thoracic and abdominopelvic cavities are separated by a broad muscle called the **diaphragm.** The diaphragm forms the floor of the thoracic cavity. Divisions of the thoracic cavity are the pleural sacs, each containing a lung, with the mediastinum between them. Within the mediastinum lie the heart, the thymus gland, and part of the esophagus and trachea. The heart is surrounded by another cavity called the *pericardial sac.*

The *retroperitoneal space* lies on the posterior abdominal wall behind the parietal peritoneum. It extends from the twelfth thoracic vertebra and the twelfth rib to the sacrum and the iliac crests.

The Abdominal Cavity

The abdominal cavity is a cavity within the abdomen that is lined with serous membrane, the peritoneum. It is bounded superiorly by the diaphragm; anteriorly by the abdominal wall muscles; posteriorly by the vertebral column, ribs, and iliac fossa; and inferiorly by the pelvis. It is continuous with the pelvic cavity to form the abdominopelvic cavity.

To identify specific abdominal structures or to refer to an area of pain, the abdominopelvic cavity may be divided into four quadrants and nine abdominal regions. The quadrant is determined by a midsagittal plane and a transverse plane that passes through the umbilicus. The four quadrants are the right upper quadrant (RUQ), left upper quadrant (LUQ), right lower quadrant (RLQ), and left lower quadrant (LLQ).

The abdominopelvic cavity is commonly divided into nine regions by two vertical and two horizontal lines. The surface landmarks of the anterior abdominal wall help to define the specific abdominal regions (Figure 4-5, *A*). Each vertical line passes through the mid-inguinal point (i.e., the point that lies on the inguinal ligament halfway between the pubic symphysis and the anterior superior iliac spine). The upper horizontal line, referred to as the **subcostal plane,** joins the lowest point of the costal margin on each side of the body. The lowest horizontal line, the **intertubercular plane,** joins the tubercles on the iliac crests. The **transpyloric plane** is a horizontal plane that passes through the pylorus, the duodenal junction, the neck of the pancreas, and the hilum of the kidneys. The nine abdominal regions (Figure 4-5, *B*) are as follows: (1) upper abdomen/right hypochondrium, (2) epigastrium, (3) left hypochondrium, (4) middle abdomen/right lumbar, (5) umbilical, (6) left lumbar, (7) lower abdomen/right iliac fossa, (8) hypogastrium, and (9) left iliac fossa. See Chapter 5, Box 5-1, for a list of additional

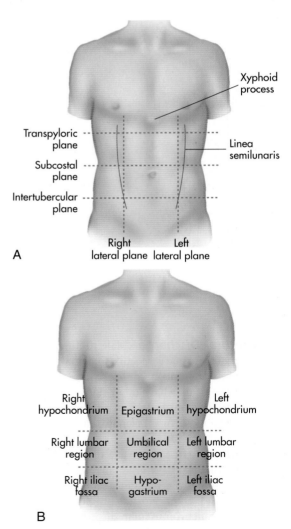

A, Surface landmarks of the anterior abdominal wall.

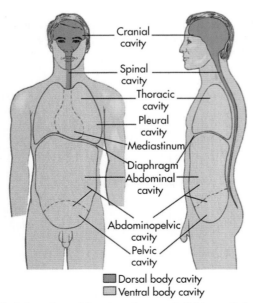

FIGURE 4-4 Body cavities. Locations and divisions of the dorsal and ventral body cavities as viewed from anterior and lateral.

FIGURE 4-5 A, Surface landmarks of the anterior abdominal wall. **B,** Nine regions of the abdominal wall.

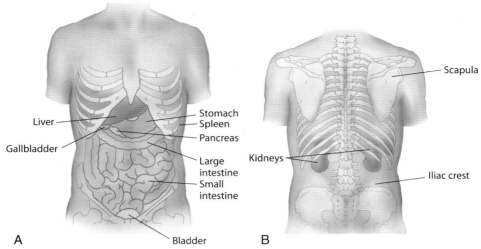

FIGURE 4-6 A, Basic abdominal landmarks and viscera viewed from anterior. **B,** Landmarks of the posterior torso.

terms that the sonographer is likely to encounter when identifying specific body regions or structures.

Visceral Organs of the Abdominal Cavity. The visceral organs within the abdominal cavity include the liver, gallbladder, spleen, pancreas, adrenal glands, kidneys and ureters, stomach, small and large intestines (except sigmoid colon and rectum), bladder and uterus, and prostate gland (Figure 4-6). Throughout the ultrasound examination, the sonographer will observe respiratory and positional variations in the abdominal viscera as they occur from patient to patient.

Liver. The liver lies posterior to the lower ribs, with most of the right lobe in the right hypochondrium and epigastrium; the left lobe lies in the epigastrium/left hypochondrium.

Gallbladder. The fundus of the gallbladder usually lies opposite the tip of the right ninth costal cartilage.

Spleen. The spleen lies in the left hypochondrium under cover of the ninth, tenth, and eleventh ribs. Its long axis corresponds to the tenth rib, and in adults it usually does not project forward of the midaxillary line.

Pancreas. The pancreas lies in the epigastrium. The head usually lies inferior and to the right (in the lap of the duodenum), the neck lies on the transpyloric plane, and the body and tail lie superior and to the left (hilum of the spleen).

Adrenal Glands. The adrenal glands lie along the superior medial border of the kidneys.

Kidneys and Ureters. The right kidney lies slightly lower than the left. Each kidney moves about 2 cm in a vertical direction during full respiratory movement of the diaphragm. The hilus of the kidney lies on the transpyloric plane, about three finger-widths from the midline.

Stomach. The stomach usually lies in the LUQ transpyloric plane between the esophagus and the small intestine.

Small Intestine. This tubular organ extends from the pyloric sphincter to the beginning of the large intestine.

Large Intestine. The large intestine extends from the small intestine to the anal canal.

Bladder and Uterus. The bladder and uterus lie in the lower pelvis in the hypogastric plane.

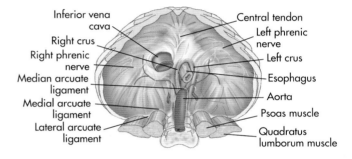

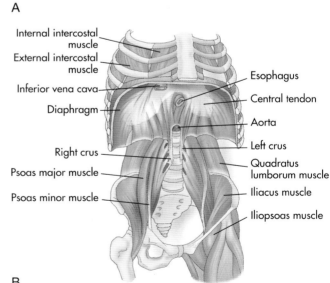

FIGURE 4-7 A, Inferior view of the diaphragm. **B,** Anterior view of the diaphragm. Note the posterolateral extension of the diaphragm along the rib cage.

Prostate Gland. The prostate gland lies in the lower pelvic in the hypogastric plane between the neck of the bladder above and the urogenital diaphragm below.

Other Abdominal Structures

Diaphragm. The diaphragm is a dome-shaped muscle that separates the thorax from the abdominal cavity (Figure 4-7). Its muscular component arises from the margins of the thoracic outlet. The **right crus of the diaphragm** arises from the sides of the bodies of the first three lumbar vertebrae; the **left crus of the diaphragm** arises from the sides of the bodies of the first two lumbar vertebrae.

Lateral to the crura, the diaphragm arises from the medial and lateral arcuate ligaments. The **medial arcuate ligament** is the thickened upper margin of the fascia covering the anterior surface of the psoas muscle. It extends from the side of the body of the second lumbar vertebra to the tip of the transverse process of the first lumbar vertebra. The medial arcuate ligament connects the medial borders of the two crura as they cross anterior to the aorta.

The **lateral arcuate ligament** is the thickened upper margin of the fascia covering the anterior surface of the quadratus lumborum muscle. It extends from the tip of the transverse process of the first lumbar vertebra to the lower border of the twelfth rib.

The diaphragm inserts into a central tendon. The superior surface of the tendon is partially fused with the inferior surface of the fibrous pericardium. Fibers of the right crus surround the esophagus to act as a sphincter to prevent regurgitation of gastric contents into the thoracic part of the esophagus.

Abdominal Wall. Superiorly, the abdominal wall is formed by the diaphragm. Inferiorly, it is continuous with the pelvic cavity through the pelvic inlet. Anteriorly, the wall is formed above by the lower part of the thoracic cage and below by several layers of muscles: rectus abdominis, external oblique, internal oblique, and transversus abdominis (Figure 4-8). The **linea alba** is a fibrous band that stretches from the xiphoid to the symphysis pubis. It is wider at its superior end and forms a central anterior attachment for the muscle layers of the abdomen. It is formed by the interlacing of fibers of the aponeuroses of the right and left oblique and transversus abdominis muscles.

Posteriorly, the abdominal wall is formed at the midline by five lumbar vertebrae and their discs (Figure 4-9). Posterolaterally, it is formed by the twelfth ribs, upper part of the bony pelvis, psoas muscles, quadratus lumborum muscles, and aponeuroses of the origin of the transversus abdominis muscles.

Laterally, the wall is formed above by the lower part of the thoracic wall, including the lungs and pleura, and below by

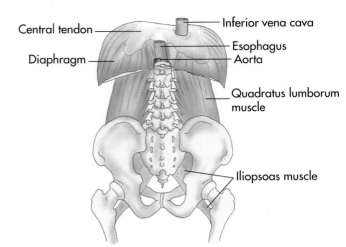

FIGURE 4-9 Posterior view of the diaphragm and abdominal muscles.

the external and internal oblique muscles and the transversus abdominis muscles.

Abdominal Muscles

External Oblique Muscle. The external oblique muscle arises from the lower eight ribs and fans out to be inserted into the xiphoid process, the linea alba, the pubic crest, the pubic tubercle, and the anterior half of the iliac crest (Figure 4-10, *A*).

The **superficial inguinal ring** is a triangular opening in the external oblique aponeurosis and lies superior and medial to the pubic tubercle. The spermatic cord or the round ligament of the uterus passes through this opening.

The **inguinal ligament** is formed between the anterior superior iliac spine and the pubic tubercle, where the lower border of the aponeurosis is folded backward on itself. The lateral part of the posterior edge of the inguinal ligament gives origin to part of the internal oblique and transverse abdominal muscles.

Internal Oblique Muscle. The internal oblique muscle lies very deep to the external oblique muscle (Figure 4-10, *B*). Most of its fibers are aligned at right angles to the external oblique muscle. It arises from the lumbar fascia, the anterior two thirds of the iliac crest, and the lateral two thirds of the inguinal ligament. The muscle inserts into the lower borders of the ribs and their costal cartilages, the xiphoid process, the linea alba, and the pubic symphysis. The internal oblique has a lower free border that arches over the spermatic cord or the round ligament of the uterus and then descends behind it to be attached to the pubic crest and the pectineal line. The lowest tendinous fibers are joined by similar fibers from the transversus abdominis to form the conjoint tendon.

Transversus Muscle. The transversus muscle lies deep to the internal oblique muscle, and its fibers run horizontally forward (Figure 4-10, *C*). The muscle arises from the deep surface of the lower six costal cartilages (interlacing with the diaphragm), the lumbar fascia, the anterior two thirds of the iliac crest, and the lateral third of the inguinal ligament. It

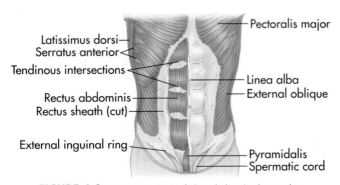

FIGURE 4-8 Anterior view of the abdominal muscles.

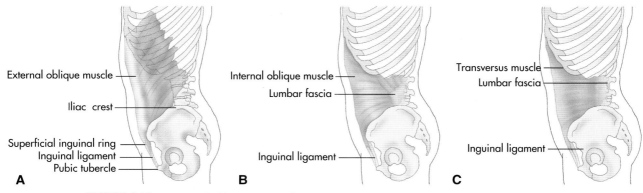

FIGURE 4-10 **A,** External oblique muscle of the anterior and lateral abdominal wall. **B,** Internal oblique muscle of the anterior and lateral abdominal wall. **C,** Transversus muscle of the anterior and lateral abdominal wall.

inserts into the xiphoid process, the linea alba, and the pubic symphysis.

Rectus Sheath. The **rectus abdominis muscle** is a sheath formed by the aponeuroses of the muscles of the lateral group (Figure 4-11). The rectus muscle arises from the front of the symphysis pubis and from the pubic crest. It inserts into the fifth, sixth, and seventh costal cartilages and the xiphoid process. On contraction, the lateral margin forms a palpable curved surface, termed the **linea semilunaris,** which extends from the ninth costal cartilage to the pubic tubercle. The anterior surface of the rectus muscle is crossed by three tendinous intersections and is firmly attached to the anterior wall of the rectus sheath.

Linea Alba. The linea alba is a fibrous band stretching from the xiphoid to the symphysis pubis (see Figure 4-8). It is wider above than below and forms a central anterior attachment for the muscle layers of the abdomen. It is formed by the interlacing of the aponeuroses of the right and left oblique muscles and transversus abdominis muscles.

Back Muscles. The deep muscles of the back help to stabilize the vertebral column. They also influence the posture and curvature of the spine. These muscles have the ability to extend, flex laterally, and rotate all or part of the vertebral column.

The Retroperitoneal Cavity

The retroperitoneal cavity contains the pancreas, kidneys, ureters, adrenal glands, aorta, inferior vena cava, bladder, uterus, and prostate gland. The ascending and descending colon and most of the duodenum are also located in the retroperitoneum.

Aorta. The aorta lies anterior to the spine, slightly to the left of the midline in the abdomen. The distal abdominal aorta bifurcates into the right and left common iliac arteries opposite the fourth lumbar vertebra on the intercristal plane.

Inferior Vena Cava. The inferior vena cava is formed by the confluence of the right and left common iliac veins. The inferior vena cava lies to the right of the spine to empty blood from the abdominopelvic cavity and lower extremities into the right atrium.

Retroperitoneal Spaces. The **anterior pararenal space** (Figure 4-12) is located between the anterior surface of the renal fascia (Gerota's fascia) and the posterior area of the peritoneum. Within this area are the ascending and descending colon, the pancreas, and the duodenum. The **posterior pararenal space** is found between the posterior renal fascia and the muscles of the posterior abdominal wall. Only fat and vessels are found within this space. The **perirenal space** is located directly around the kidney and is completely enclosed by renal fascia. Within this space lie the kidneys, adrenal glands, lymph nodes, blood vessels, and perirenal fat.

The Pelvic Cavity

The lower portion of the abdominopelvic cavity below the pelvic brim is the **pelvic cavity** (see Figure 4-4). The pelvis is

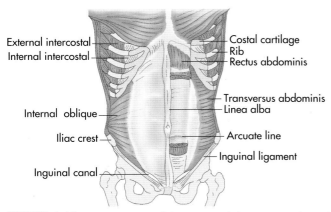

FIGURE 4-11 Anterior view of the rectus abdominis muscle and rectus sheath.

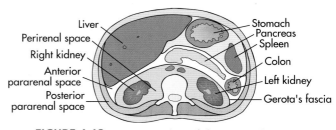

FIGURE 4-12 Transverse view of the retroperitoneum.

divided into a pelvis major (false pelvis) and a pelvis minor (true pelvis). The pelvis major is part of the abdominal cavity proper and lies between the iliac fossae, superior to the pelvic brim. The pelvis minor (which actually contains the pelvic cavity) is found inferior to the brim of the pelvis. The cavity of the pelvis minor is continuous at the pelvic brim with the cavity of the pelvis major.

The pelvic cavity contains several pelvic organs: part of the large intestine, the rectum, the urinary bladder, and the reproductive organs. In the female, the peritoneum descends from the anterior abdominal wall to the level of the pubic bone onto the superior surface of the bladder. The peritoneum covers the fundus and body of the uterus and extends over the posterior fornix and the wall of the vagina.

In the male, the peritoneum is reflected onto the upper part of the posterior surface of the bladder and the seminal vesicles, forming the rectovesical pouch. Also in the male, the pelvic cavity has a small outpocket called the **scrotal cavity,** which contains the testes.

False Pelvis. The false pelvis is bound posteriorly by the lumbar vertebrae, laterally by the iliac fossae and iliacus muscles, and anteriorly by the lower anterior abdominal wall. The sacral promontory and the iliopectineal line form the boundary between the false pelvis and the true pelvis to delineate the boundary of the abdominal and pelvic cavities.

The uterus lies anterior to the rectum and posterior to the bladder and divides the pelvic peritoneal space into anterior and posterior pouches. The anterior pouch is termed the **vesicouterine pouch,** and the posterior pouch is called the **rectouterine pouch,** or the pouch of Douglas (Figure 4-13). The rectouterine pouch is a common location for accumulation of fluids, such as pus or blood.

The fallopian tubes extend laterally from the fundus of the uterus and are enveloped by a fold of peritoneum known as the broad ligament. This ligament arises from the floor of the pelvis and contributes to the division of the peritoneal space into anterior and posterior pouches.

True Pelvis. The true pelvis protects and contains the lower parts of the intestinal and urinary tracts and the reproductive organs. The true pelvis has an inlet, an outlet, and a cavity and is bounded posteriorly by the sacrum and coccyx (Figure 4-14). The anterior and lateral margins are formed by the pubis, the ischium, and a small portion of the ilium. A muscular "sling" consisting of the coccygeus and levator ani muscles forms the inferior boundary of the true pelvis and separates it from the perineum.

The true pelvis is divided into anterior and posterior compartments. The anterior compartment contains the bladder and reproductive organs. The posterior compartment contains the posterior cul-de-sac, rectosigmoid muscle, perirectal fat, and presacral space.

The walls of the pelvis are formed by bones and ligaments, which are partially lined by muscles covered with fascia and parietal peritoneum. The pelvis has anterior, posterior, and lateral walls and an inferior floor. The obturator internus muscle lines the lateral pelvic wall. These muscles are symmetrically aligned along the lateral border of the pelvis with a concave medial border (see Figure 4-14).

The psoas and iliopsoas muscles lie along the posterior and lateral margins of the pelvis major (Figure 4-15). The fan-shaped iliacus muscles line the iliac fossae in the false pelvis. The psoas and iliacus muscles merge at their inferior portions

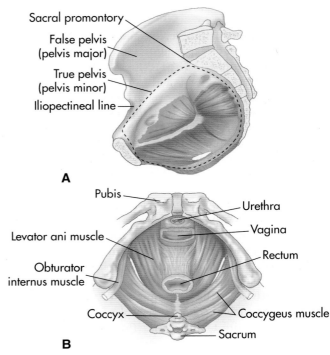

A

B

FIGURE 4-14 A, Lateral view of the pelvis, demonstrating the true pelvis and the false pelvis. **B,** Inferior view of the pelvic diaphragm muscles.

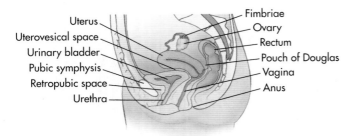

FIGURE 4-13 Midsagittal view of the female pelvis.

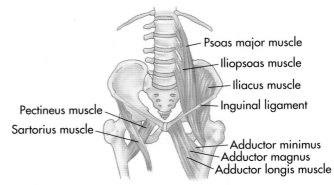

FIGURE 4-15 Anterior view of the psoas and iliopsoas muscles.

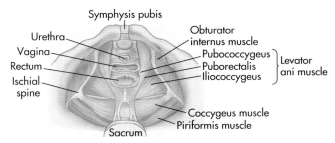

FIGURE 4-16 View of the female pelvic floor shows the levator ani, coccygeus, and piriformis muscles.

to form the iliopsoas complex. The posterior border of the iliopsoas lies along the iliopectineal line and may be used as a separation landmark of the true pelvis from the false pelvis.

The piriformis muscles form the posterior pelvic wall (Figure 4-16). The pelvic floor stretches across the pelvis and divides it into the main pelvic cavity, which contains the pelvic viscera, and the perineum below. The levator ani muscles and pubococcygeus muscles form the pelvic diaphragm. The coccygeus muscles are rounded, concave muscles that lie more posterior than the obturator internus muscles.

Perineum. The pelvic diaphragm is formed by the levatores ani and coccygeus muscles. The perineum has the following surface relationships: The pubic symphysis is anterior; posterior is the tip of the coccyx; and lateral are the ischial tuberosities. The region is divided into two triangles formed by joining the ischial tuberosities with an imaginary line. The posterior triangle is the anal triangle, and the anterior triangle is the urogenital triangle.

Abdominopelvic Membranes and Ligaments

The major membranes and ligaments within the abdominopelvic cavity include the peritoneum, the mesentery, omentum, greater and lesser sacs, epiploic foramen, and peritoneal ligaments.

Peritoneum. The peritoneum is a serous membrane lining the walls of the abdominal cavity and clothing the abdominal viscera (Figure 4-17). The peritoneum is formed by a single layer of cells called the *mesothelium*, which rests on a thin layer of connective tissue. If the mesothelium is damaged or removed in any area (such as in surgery), the danger is that two layers of peritoneum may adhere to each other and form an adhesion. This adhesion may interfere with the normal movements of the abdominal viscera.

The peritoneum is divided into two layers. The **parietal peritoneum** is the portion that lines the abdominal wall but does not cover a viscus; the **visceral peritoneum** is the portion that covers an organ (Figure 4-18). The **peritoneal cavity** is the potential space between the parietal and visceral peritonea. This cavity contains a small amount of lubricating serous fluid to help the abdominal organs move on one another without friction. With certain pathologies, the potential space of the peritoneal cavity may be distended into an actual space containing several liters of fluid. This accumulation of fluid is known as **ascites.** Other fluid substances, such as blood from a ruptured

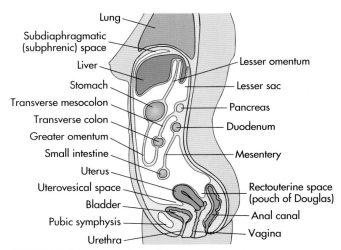

FIGURE 4-17 Lateral view of the peritoneum (*white area,* peritoneal cavity).

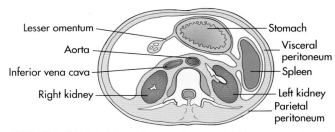

FIGURE 4-18 Axial view of the peritoneum (*white area,* peritoneal cavity).

organ, bile from a ruptured duct, or fecal matter from a ruptured intestine, also may accumulate in this cavity.

The peritoneal cavity forms a completely closed sac in the male; in the female, communication with the exterior occurs through the fallopian tubes, uterus, and vagina. Retroperitoneal organs and vascular structures remain posterior to the cavity and are covered anteriorly with peritoneum. These include the urinary system, aorta, inferior vena cava, colon, pancreas, uterus, and bladder. The other abdominal organs are located within the peritoneal cavity.

Mesentery. A mesentery is a two-layered fold of peritoneum that attaches part of the intestines to the posterior abdominal wall and includes the mesentery of the small intestine, the transverse mesocolon, and the sigmoid mesocolon.

Omentum. The omentum is a two-layered fold of peritoneum that attaches the stomach to another viscous organ. The greater omentum is attached to the greater curvature of the stomach and hangs down like an apron in the space between the small intestine and the anterior abdominal wall (Figure 4-19). The greater omentum is folded back on itself and is attached to the inferior border of the transverse colon. The lesser omentum slings the lesser curvature of the stomach to the undersurface of the liver (Figure 4-20). The gastrosplenic omentum ligament connects the stomach to the spleen.

Greater and Lesser Sacs. The peritoneal cavity may be divided into two parts known as the greater and lesser sacs.

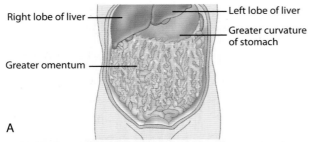

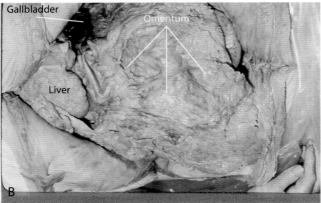

FIGURE 4-19 **A,** Anterior view of the greater omentum. **B,** Gross anatomy with the anterior abdominal flap open to demonstrate the extent of the omentum.

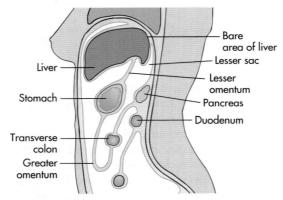

FIGURE 4-20 Sagittal view of the lesser omentum.

FIGURE 4-21 Upper abdominal dissection, with part of the left lobe of the liver and the lesser omentum removed to show the area of the epiploic foramen. Posterior to the foramen lie the celiac trunk, portal vein, bile duct, and related structures; this is one of the most important regions in the abdomen.

The greater sac is the primary compartment of the peritoneal cavity and extends across the anterior abdomen and from the diaphragm to the pelvis.

The **lesser sac** is an extensive peritoneal pouch located behind the lesser omentum and stomach (Figure 4-21). It extends upward to the diaphragm and inferior between the layers of the greater omentum. The left margin is formed by the spleen and the gastrosplenic and lienorenal ligaments. The right margin of the lesser sac opens into the greater sac through the epiploic foramen.

Epiploic Foramen. The epiploic foramen, the opening to the lesser sac in the abdomen, includes the following boundaries: anteriorly, the free border of the lesser omentum containing the common bile duct, hepatic artery, and portal vein; posteriorly, the inferior vena cava; superiorly, the caudate process of the caudate lobe of the liver; and inferiorly, the first part of the duodenum (see Figure 4-21).

Ligament. The peritoneal ligaments are two-layered folds of peritoneum that attach the lesser mobile solid viscera to the abdominal walls. For example, the liver is attached by the falciform ligament to the anterior abdominal wall and to the undersurface of the diaphragm (Figure 4-22). The ligamentum teres lies in the free borders of this ligament. The peritoneum leaves the kidney and passes to the hilus of the spleen as the posterior layer of the lienorenal ligament. The visceral peritoneum covers the spleen and is reflected onto the greater curvature of the stomach as the anterior layer of the gastrosplenic ligament.

Potential Spaces in the Body

Subphrenic Spaces. The subphrenic spaces are the result of the complicated arrangement of the peritoneum in the region of the liver (Figure 4-23). The right and left anterior subphrenic spaces lie between the diaphragm and the liver, one on each side of the falciform ligament. The sonographer should become very familiar with the right posterior subphrenic space that lies between the right lobe of the liver, the right kidney, and the right colic flexure. This is also called **Morison's pouch**. It is a frequent location

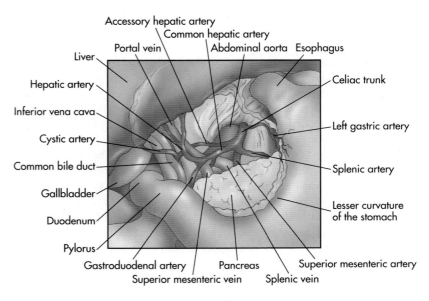

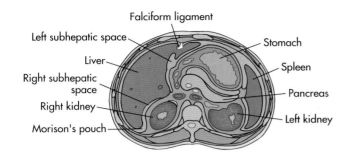

A

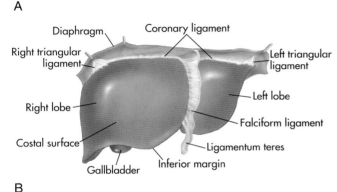

B

FIGURE 4-22 A, Transverse view of the falciform ligament. **B,** Anterior view of the falciform ligament.

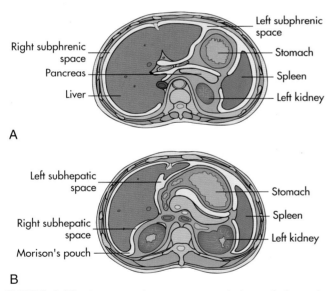

A

B

FIGURE 4-23 The supracolic compartment is located above the transverse colon and contains the right and left subphrenic spaces and the right and left subhepatic spaces. **A,** Transverse view of the subphrenic spaces. **B,** Transverse view of the subhepatic spaces.

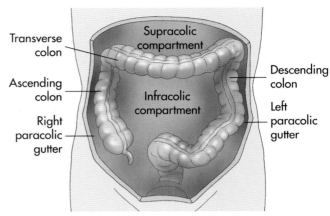

FIGURE 4-24 The infracolic compartment is found below the transverse colon. The right and left paracolic gutters are troughlike spaces located lateral to the ascending and descending colon.

for fluid collections, such as ascites, blood, and infection, to accumulate.

Peritoneal Recesses. The omental bursa normally has some empty places. Parts of the peritoneal cavity near the liver are so slitlike that they are also isolated. These areas, known as **peritoneal recesses,** are clinically important because infection may collect in them. Two common sites are where the duodenum becomes the jejunum and where the ileum joins the cecum.

Paracolic Gutters. The arrangement of the ascending and descending colon, the attachments of the transverse mesocolon, and the mesentery of the small intestine to the posterior abdominal wall result in the formation of four paracolic gutters (Figure 4-24). The clinical significance of these gutters is their ability to conduct fluid materials from one part of the body to another. Materials such as abscess, ascites, blood, pus, bile, or metastases may be spread through this network.

The gutters are on the lateral and medial sides of the ascending and descending colon. The right medial paracolic gutter is closed off from the pelvic cavity inferiorly by the mesentery of the small intestine. The other gutters are in free communication with the pelvic cavity. The right lateral paracolic gutter communicates with the right posterior subphrenic space. The left lateral gutter is separated from the area around the spleen by the phrenicocolic ligament.

Inguinal Canal. The inguinal canal is an oblique passage through the lower part of the anterior abdominal wall. In the male, it allows structures to pass to and from the testes to the abdomen (Figure 4-25). In the female, it permits passage of the round ligament of the uterus from the uterus to the labium majus.

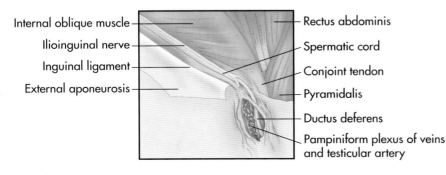

FIGURE 4-25 Right inguinal canal, spermatic cord, ductus deferens, and pampiniform plexus.

Key Pearls

- Understand the complexity of the body—atom, molecules, cells, organs, body systems, to organism.
- All physical and chemical changes that occur within the body are referred to as *metabolism.*
- *Homeostasis* is the ability to maintain a steady and stable internal environment.
- Vital signs are medical measurements used to ascertain how the body is functioning.
- The circulation of blood throughout the body serves as a vital connection to the cells, tissues, and organs to maintain a relatively constant environment for cell activity.
- Understand the composition of blood (plasma, hemoglobin).
- The blood is responsible for a variety of functions, including transportation of oxygen and nutrients, defense against infection, and maintenance of pH.
- Define the function of the red and white blood cells.
- The GI system consists of two major divisions: the GI tract (pharynx, esophagus, stomach, small intestine, and large intestine) and the accessory organs.
- Major functions of the GI system include ingestion and digestion of food and elimination of waste products.
- The most significant signs and symptoms related to GI diseases and disorders are abdominal pain, diarrhea, bloody stools, nausea, and vomiting.
- The urinary system consists of the kidneys, ureters, bladder, and urethra.
- The primary functions of the urinary system are the formation of urine and the maintenance of homeostasis.
- The two principal body cavities are the dorsal cavity and the ventral cavity.
- The ventral cavity is located near the anterior body surface and is subdivided into the *thoracic cavity* and the *abdominopelvic cavity.*
- The *retroperitoneal space* lies on the posterior abdominal wall behind the parietal peritoneum.
- The abdominal cavity is a cavity within the abdomen that is lined with serous membrane, the peritoneum.

- The visceral organs within the abdominal cavity include the liver, gallbladder, spleen, pancreas, adrenal glands, kidneys and ureters, stomach, small and large intestines (except sigmoid colon and rectum), bladder and uterus, and prostate gland.
- The retroperitoneal cavity contains the pancreas, kidneys, ureters, adrenal glands, aorta, inferior vena cava, bladder, uterus, and prostate gland. The ascending and descending colon and most of the duodenum are also located in the retroperitoneum.
- The pelvis is divided into a pelvis major (false pelvis) and a pelvis minor (true pelvis).
- The major membranes and ligaments within the abdominopelvic cavity include the peritoneum, the mesentery, omentum, greater and lesser sacs, epiploic foramen, and peritoneal ligaments.
- The subphrenic spaces are the result of the complicated arrangement of the peritoneum in the region of the liver.
- The sonographer should become very familiar with the right posterior subphrenic space that lies between the right lobe of the liver, the right kidney, and the right colic flexure. This is also called *Morison's pouch.*
- The omental bursa normally has some empty places, known as *peritoneal recesses,* and are clinically important because infection may collect in them.
- The arrangement of the ascending and descending colon, the attachments of the transverse mesocolon, and the mesentery of the small intestine to the posterior abdominal wall result in the formation of four paracolic gutters.

BIBLIOGRAPHY

McMinn RMH, Gaddum-Rosse P, Hutchings RT, Logan BM: *McMinn's functional and clinical anatomy*, St. Louis, 1995, Mosby.

Netter F: *The CIBA collection: digestive system*, vol 3, West Caldwell, NJ, 1989, CIBA.

Snell RS: *Clinical anatomy*, ed 7, Baltimore, 2004, Lippincott Williams & Wilkins.

Swobodnik W, Herrmann M, Altwein J: *Atlas of ultrasound anatomy: normal anatomy as the basis of sonographic diagnosis*, New York, 1991, Thieme Medical Publishers.

Comparative Sectional Anatomy of the Abdominopelvic Cavity

Sandra Hagen-Ansert

OBJECTIVES

On completion of this chapter, you should be able to:
- List the body planes in the abdomen
- Define the abdominal structures in the transverse and sagittal planes
- Know the abdominal quadrants and regions of the body

- Discuss the difference between a coronal image and a sagittal image
- Compare and contrast computed tomography and ultrasound

OUTLINE

Planes or Body Planes
Abdominal Quadrants and Regions

Sectional Anatomy
  Transverse Plane

Longitudinal Plane

KEY TERMS

Aorta
Caudate lobe
Celiac axis
Common femoral arteries
Confluence of the splenic and portal veins
Coronal
Crus of the diaphragm
Falciform ligament
Femoral veins
Gastroduodenal artery
Hepatic artery
Hepatic vein

Iliac arteries
Iliac veins
Inferior mesenteric artery
Inferior vena cava
Intertubercular plane
Left gastric artery
Left portal vein
Left renal artery
Ligamentum venosum
Longitudinal
Morison's pouch
Portal confluence
Psoas major muscles

Right and left renal veins
Right renal artery
Sagittal
Splenic artery
Splenic hilum
Splenic vein
Subcostal plane
Superior mesenteric artery
Superior mesenteric vein
Transpyloric plane
Transverse

It is important that sonographers understand other imaging modalities, especially computed tomography (CT) and magnetic resonance imaging (MRI), which most frequently complement sonography. No longer does each of the various imaging modalities operate within a "silo," independent of each other. Instead, many diagnostic algorithms require two or more imaging modalities to be employed, and diagnosis requires that specific comparisons be made between them. In this way, ultrasound now interacts extensively with CT and other imaging methods to optimize the workup of a patient. Many patients referred to ultrasound for evaluation of a potential abnormality have already been imaged by another modality, which has detected an abnormality but was unable to characterize it or vice versa. Understanding what each modality has to offer is of prime importance in crafting the multimodality imaging workup for any particular problem.

It is also becoming more common for physicians to follow up an abnormality—even one that has been previously characterized—by using another imaging method such as ultrasound. Ultrasound is often preferred over CT, which involves ionizing radiation, or MRI, which is both time consuming and costly. To effectively meet the patient's needs, the sonographer must be able to tailor his or her examination appropriately so as to exploit the unique strengths of ultrasound and to minimize its limitations. The sonographer must also understand how the ultrasound examination in each setting may be influenced or guided by findings from previous CT or other studies.

The various imaging modalities ultimately depict and evaluate the same abnormalities, and they are generally equivalent in identifying the physical size and shape of pathologic lesions. However, each modality approaches the problem from a different standpoint, using differing physical properties of the normal tissue and pathologic lesions to derive image contrast and resolve important details. Ultrasound and MRI both have a safety advantage in that they do not use ionizing radiation. CT scanning and general diagnostic (x-ray) imaging, on the other hand, both image the body by use of ionizing radiation, often in significant doses. The radiation for both CT and x-ray is produced by an external source and tends to produce sharp images with high anatomic detail.

The purpose of this chapter is to introduce the sonographer to sectional anatomy compared with CT images and ultrasound images.

PLANES OR BODY SECTIONS

The ability of the sonographer to understand anatomy as it relates to cross-sectional, coronal, oblique, and sagittal projections is critical to performing a quality sonographic examination. Normal anatomy has many variations in size and position, and the sonographer must be able to demonstrate these findings on the sonogram. A thorough understanding of anatomy as it relates to anteroposterior relationships and variations in sectional anatomy is required and is essential in three-dimensional analysis and reconstruction. The sonographer images the body in multiple planes, which include, but are not limited to, the following: transverse, sagittal, longitudinal, and coronal (Figure 5-1).

- **Transverse.** The transverse plane is horizontal to the body. This plane divides the body or any of its parts into upper and lower portions.

- **Sagittal.** The sagittal plane is a lengthwise plane running from front to back. It divides the body or any of its parts into right and left sides, or two equal halves; this is known as the midsagittal plane.
- **Longitudinal.** The longitudinal plane is parallel to the long axis of the body or part.
- **Coronal.** The coronal plane is a lengthwise plane running from side to side, dividing the body into anterior and posterior portions.

ABDOMINAL QUADRANTS AND REGIONS

To identify specific abdominal structures or to refer to an area of pain, the abdominopelvic cavity may be divided into four quadrants and nine abdominal regions. The quadrant is determined by a midsagittal plane and a transverse plane that pass through the umbilicus. The four quadrants include the right upper quadrant (RUQ), left upper quadrant (LUQ), right lower quadrant (RLQ), and left lower quadrant (LLQ).

The abdominopelvic cavity is commonly divided into nine regions by two vertical and two horizontal lines. The surface landmarks of the anterior abdominal wall help to define the specific abdominal regions (Figure 5-2). Each vertical line passes through the mid-inguinal point (i.e., the point that lies on the inguinal ligament halfway between the pubic symphysis and the anterior superior iliac spine). The upper horizontal line, referred to as the **subcostal plane,** joins the lowest point of the costal margin on each side of the body. The lowest horizontal line, the **intertubercular plane,** joins the tubercles on the iliac crests. The **transpyloric plane** is a horizontal plane that passes through the pylorus, the duodenal junction, the neck of the pancreas, and the hilum of the kidneys. The nine abdominal regions (Figure 5-3) are as follows: (1) upper abdomen/right hypochondrium, (2) epigastrium,

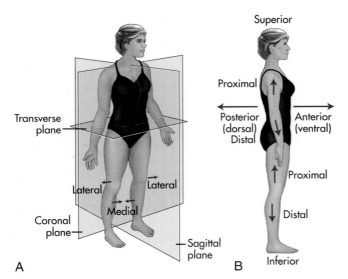

FIGURE 5-1 A, Anterior view of the body in the anatomic position. Note the directions and body planes. **B,** Lateral view of the body.

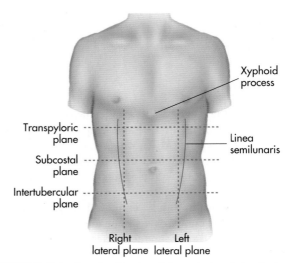

FIGURE 5-2 Surface landmarks of the anterior abdominal wall.

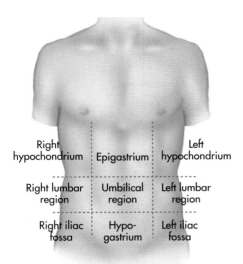

FIGURE 5-3 Regions of the abdominal wall.

BOX 5-1	Terms for Common Body Regions and Structures

Abdominal: Portion of trunk below the diaphragm
Axillary: Area of armpit
Brachial: Arm
Celiac: Abdomen
Cervical: Neck region
Costal: Ribs
Femoral: Thigh; the part of the lower extremity between the hip and the knee
Groin/inguinal: Depressed region between the abdomen and the thigh
Leg: Lower extremity, especially from the knee to the foot
Lumbar: Loin; the region of the lower back and side, between the lowest rib and the pelvis
Mammary: Breasts
Pelvic: Pelvis; the bony ring that girdles the lower portion of the trunk
Perineal: Region between the anus and the pubic arch; includes the region of the external reproductive structures
Popliteal: Area behind the knee
Thoracic: Chest; the part of the trunk below the neck and above the diaphragm

(3) left hypochondrium, (4) middle abdomen/right lumbar, (5) umbilical, (6) left lumbar, (7) lower abdomen/right iliac fossa, (8) hypogastrium, and (9) left iliac fossa. Box 5-1 provides a list of additional terms that the sonographer is likely to encounter when identifying specific body regions or structures.

SECTIONAL ANATOMY

The sonographer must have a solid knowledge of gross and sectional anatomy and of the many anatomic variations that may occur in the body. The sonographer should carefully evaluate organ and vascular relationships to neighboring structures, rather than memorize where in the abdomen a particular structure "should" be: It is better to recall the location of the gallbladder as anterior to the right kidney and medial to the liver than to remember than it is found 6 cm above the umbilicus.

The sonographer should also reflect on the anatomic variations that are present in each individual. Keep in mind that the descriptors given here may vary somewhat from the examples shown for CT and ultrasound. Images were selected to highlight the anatomy described; CT is a composite image of the transverse plane, whereas most ultrasound images focus on a particular organ.

Transverse Plane

The transverse sectional illustrations (see Figures 5-4 through 5-18) are presented in descending order from the dome of the diaphragm to the symphysis pubis. The sonographer should review the relationship of each organ to its neighboring structures, while proceeding in a caudal direction. Specific detail is listed below each illustration, and a thumbnail sketch of expected anatomy is outlined here:

Dome of the liver (Figure 5-4): The **splenic artery (SA)** enters as the **splenic vein (SV)** leaves the splenic hilum. The abdominal portion of the esophagus lies to the left of the midline and opens into the stomach through the cardiac orifice. The liver extends to the left mammillary line. The **falciform ligament (FL)** extends into the diaphragm.

Level of the caudate lobe (Figure 5-5): The right **hepatic vein** enters the lateral margin of the **inferior vena cava (IVC)**. The fundus of the stomach is shown with the hepatogastric and gastrocolic ligaments. The lesser omental cavity is posterior to the stomach. The upper border of the splenic flexure of the colon is seen. The **caudate lobe** of the liver is anterior to the IVC and is demarcated by the **ligamentum venosum (LV)**. The body and tail of the pancreas are seen near the splenic hilum. The adrenal glands are lateral to the **crus of the diaphragm.**

Level of the caudate lobe and celiac axis (Figure 5-6): The **celiac axis (CA)** (branches into **left gastric artery [LGA]**, splenic artery, and **hepatic artery**) should be found near this section as it arises from the anterior wall of the **aorta.** The transverse and descending colons are shown inferior to the splenic flexure. The caudate lobe of the liver is shown. The body of the pancreas is anterior to the splenic vein. Both kidneys and the adrenal glands are shown lateral to the spine and crus of the diaphragm. The IVC is shown anterior to the crus, and the aorta is posterior to the crus of the diaphragm.

Level of the superior mesenteric artery and pancreas (Figure 5-7): The **psoas major muscles** are lateral to the spine. The **right renal artery** is shown posterior to the IVC. The **left renal artery** would arise from the posterolateral

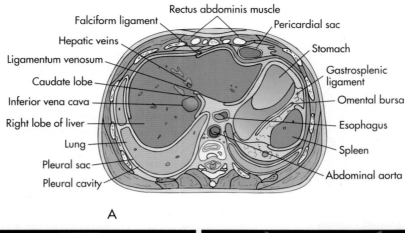

A

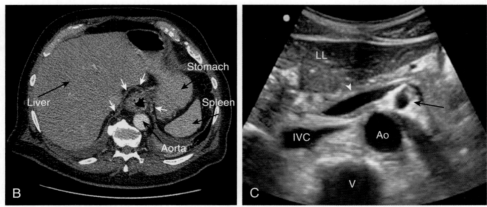

FIGURE 5-4 **A,** Cross section of the abdomen at the level of the tenth intervertebral disk. The lower portion of the pericardial sac is seen. The splenic artery enters the spleen, and the splenic vein emerges from the splenic hilum. The abdominal portion of the esophagus lies to the left of the midline and opens into the stomach through the cardiac orifice. The liver extends to the left mammillary line. The falciform ligament extends into the section above this. The spleen is shown to lie alongside the ninth rib. **B,** CT transverse section through the liver, stomach, spleen, and aorta. **C,** Focused ultrasound image showing the splenic vein *(small arrow),* superior mesenteric artery *(large arrow),* aorta *(Ao),* inferior vena cava *(IVC),* all anterior to the vertebral column *(V).*

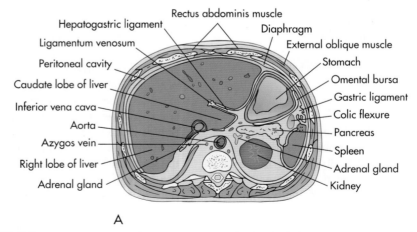

A

FIGURE 5-5 **A,** Cross section of the abdomen at the level of the eleventh thoracic disk. The hepatic vein is shown to enter the inferior vena cava. The renal artery and the vein of the left kidney are shown. The left branch of the portal vein is seen to arch upward to enter the left lobe of the liver. The upper part of the stomach is shown with the hepatogastric and gastrocolic ligaments. The lesser omental cavity is posterior to the stomach. The upper border of the splenic flexure of the colon is seen. The caudate lobe of the liver is in this section. The tail and body of the pancreas are shown anterior to the left kidney. The spleen is shown to lie along the left lateral border. The adrenal glands are lateral to the crus of the diaphragm.

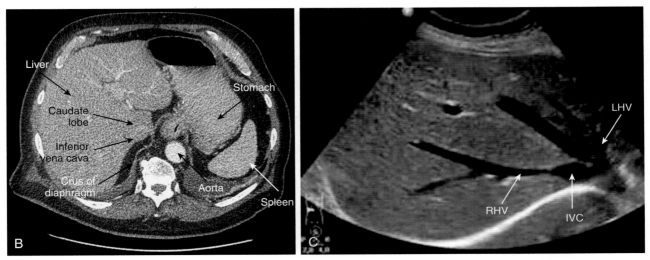

FIGURE 5-5, cont'd   B, CT transverse section through the liver, caudate lobe, stomach, spleen, aorta, inferior vena cava, and crus of the diaphragm. **C,** Focused transverse ultrasound image near the dome of the liver demonstrating the three hepatic veins as they empty into the IVC. Left hepatic vein *(LHV),* right hepatic vein *(RHV),* inferior vena cava *(IVC).*

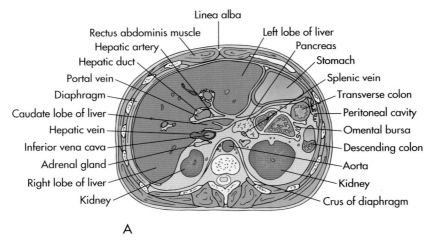

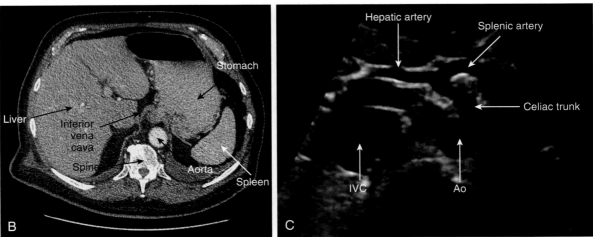

FIGURE 5-6   A, Cross section of the abdomen at the level of the twelfth thoracic vertebra. The celiac axis arises in the middle of this section from the anterior abdominal aorta. The right renal artery originates at this level. The hepatic vein is shown to enter the inferior vena cava. The greater curvature of the stomach and the pylorus are shown. The transverse and descending colon are shown inferior to the splenic flexure. The caudate lobe of the liver is well seen. The body of the pancreas, both kidneys, and the lower portions of the adrenal glands are shown. **B,** CT transverse image showing the liver, stomach, spleen, aorta, inferior vena cava, and spine. **C,** Focused ultrasound image demonstrating the celiac trunk and its branches as it arises from the anterior aortic wall. The IVC is shown to the right of the aorta.

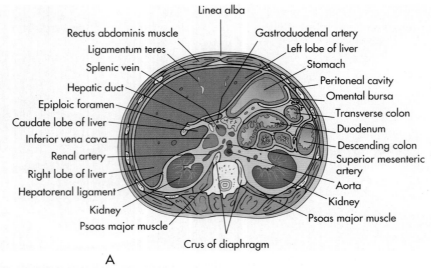

A

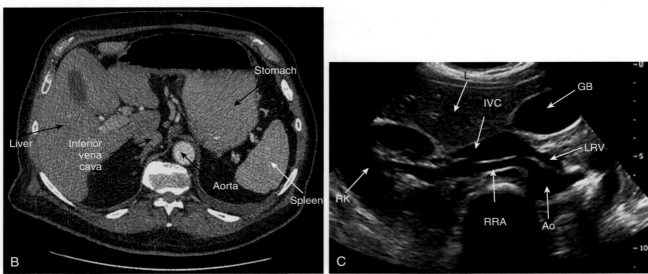

B   C

FIGURE 5-7 A, Cross section of the abdomen at the first lumbar vertebra. The psoas major muscle is seen. The crura of the diaphragm are shown on either side of the spine. The right renal artery is seen. The left renal artery arises from the lateral wall of the aorta. Both renal veins enter the inferior vena cava. The portal vein is seen to be formed by the union of the splenic vein and the superior mesenteric vein. The lower portions of the stomach and the pyloric orifice are seen, as is the superior portion of the duodenum. The duodenojejunal flexure and the descending and transverse colon are shown. The greater omentum is very prominent. The small, nonperitoneal area of the liver is shown anterior to the right kidney. The round ligament of the liver and the umbilical fissure, which separates the right and left lobes of the liver, are seen. The neck of the gallbladder (not shown) is found just inferior to this section, between the quadrate and caudate lobes of the liver. The cystic duct is cut in two places. The hepatic duct lies just anterior to the cystic duct. The cystic and hepatic ducts unite in the lower part of the section to form the common bile duct. The pancreatic duct is found within the pancreas at this level. Both kidneys are seen just lateral to the psoas muscles. **B,** CT transverse section through the right lobe of the liver, stomach, spleen, aorta, and inferior vena cava. **C,** Focused ultrasound image demonstrating the gallbladder *(Gb),* liver *(L),* right kidney *(RK),* right renal artery *(RRA)* arising from the aorta to the kidney, and left renal vein *(LRV)* as it leaves the hilus of the kidney to cross anterior to the aorta and empty into the IVC.

wall of the aorta; the **right and left renal veins** are inferior to the renal arteries. The **portal confluence** (also called the **confluence of the splenic and portal veins**) is formed by the splenic vein and the **superior mesenteric vein.** The superior portion of the duodenum is shown posterior to the stomach. Part of the transverse colon is shown. The hepatic duct is anterior to the portal vein.

Level of the gallbladder and right kidney (Figure 5-8): The kidneys are lateral to the psoas muscles. The **gastroduodenal artery (GDA)** lies along the anterolateral border of the head of the pancreas, and the duodenum surrounds the lateral border. The stomach and transverse colon fill the left upper quadrant, and the liver fills the right upper quadrant.

The gallbladder is medial to the liver. The common bile duct is seen along the posterior lateral border of the pancreatic head.

Level of the liver, gallbladder, and right kidney (Figure 5-9): The **inferior mesenteric artery** originates from the abdominal aorta at this level. The greater omentum is shown on the left side of the abdomen. The descending and ascending portions of the duodenum lie between the aorta and the superior mesenteric artery and vein. The gallbladder is seen along the medial border of the right lobe of the liver. Both lower poles of the kidneys are seen lateral to the psoas muscles.

Level of the right lobe of the liver (Figure 5-10): The lower portion of the right lobe of the liver and the duodenum are shown.

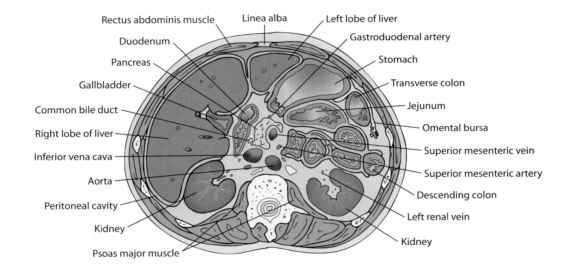

A

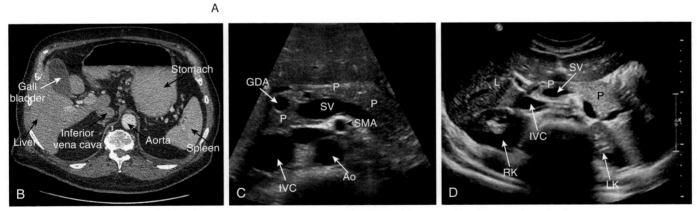

FIGURE 5-8 A, Cross section of the abdomen at the level of the second lumbar vertebra. The lower portion of the stomach is found in this section, and the hepatic flexure of the colon is seen. The lobes of the liver are separated by the round ligament. The left lobe of the liver ends at this level. The head and neck of the pancreas drape around the superior mesenteric vein. Both kidneys and the psoas muscles are shown. **B,** CT transverse section at the level of the liver, gallbladder, stomach, spleen, aorta, and inferior vena cava. **C,** Focused ultrasound image of the aorta *(Ao),* inferior vena cava *(IVC),* superior mesenteric artery *(arrow),* splenic vein *(SV),* pancreas *(P),* and gastroduodenal artery *(GDA).* **D,** Ultrasound transverse image at the same level showing right and left kidney, liver, IVC, pancreas.

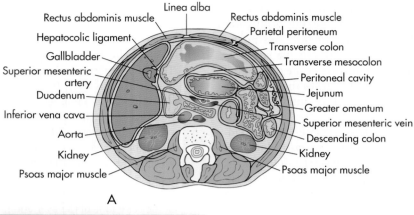

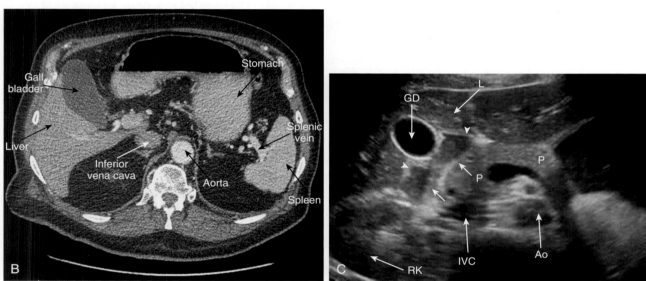

FIGURE 5-9 **A,** Cross section of the abdomen at the level of the third lumbar vertebra. The inferior mesenteric artery originates from the abdominal aorta at this level. The greater omentum is shown mostly on the left side of the abdomen. The descending and ascending portions of the duodenum lie between the aorta and the superior mesenteric artery and vein. The fundus of the gallbladder lies in the lower portion of this section. The lower poles of both kidneys lie lateral to the psoas muscles. **B,** CT transverse section at the level of the gallbladder, liver, stomach, splenic vein, spleen, aorta, and inferior vena cava. **C,** Focused ultrasound imaged at the lower right lobe of the liver (L), gallbladder (Gb), duodenum (arrows), right kidney (RK), pancreas (P), aorta (Ao), and inferior vena cava (IVC).

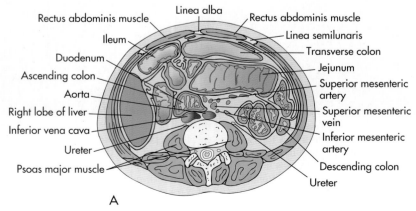

FIGURE 5-10 **A,** Cross section of the abdomen at the level of the third lumbar disk. The lower portion of the duodenum is shown. The lower margin of the right lobe of the liver is seen along the right lateral border.

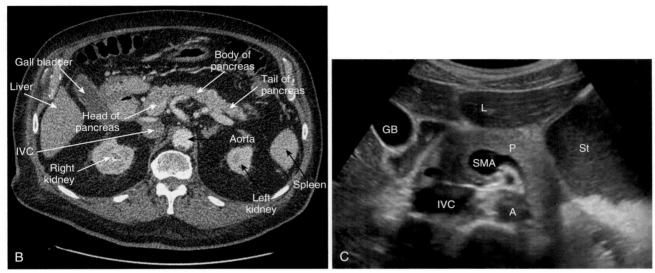

FIGURE 5-10, cont'd B, CT transverse section at the lower right lobe of the liver, gallbladder, pancreas, spleen, aorta, kidneys, and IVC. **C,** Focused ultrasound of the midabdomen that shows the left lobe of the liver *(L)*, gallbladder *(Gb)*, pancreas *(P)*, stomach *(St)*, superior mesenteric vein *(SMV)*, aorta *(Ao)*, and inferior vena cava *(IVC)*.

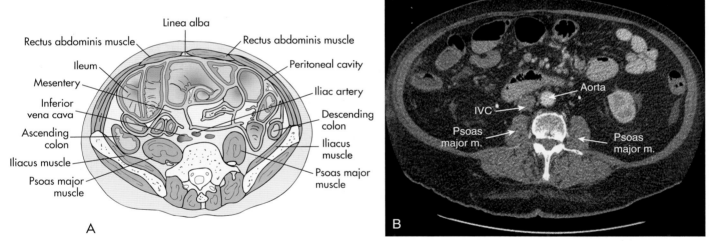

FIGURE 5-11 A, Cross section of the abdomen at the level of the fifth lumbar vertebra. It cuts the ileum through the upper part of the iliac fossa and passes just above the wings of the sacrum. The gluteus medius and iliacus muscles are shown. The right common iliac artery bifurcates into the external and internal iliac arteries. The common iliac veins are shown to unite to form the inferior vena cava. The lower part of the greater omentum is shown in this section. **B,** CT transverse section of the bowel, aorta, IVC, and psoas muscles.

Level of the bifurcation of the aorta (Figure 5-11): The psoas major muscles are lateral to the spine. The **iliac arteries** are anterior to the spine. The common **iliac veins** unite to form the inferior vena cava.

Level of the external iliac arteries (Figure 5-12): The external iliac arteries are well seen. The ileum is seen throughout this level, and the mesentery terminates at this level.

Level of the external iliac veins (Figure 5-13): The internal and external iliac veins have united to form the common iliac vein.

Level of the male pelvis (Figure 5-14): The external iliac arteries become the **common femoral arteries** in this section. The **femoral veins** become the external iliac veins. The cecum and rectum are seen.

Level of the male pelvis (Figure 5-15): The pelvic muscles are shown; the rectum is seen in the midline. The trigone of

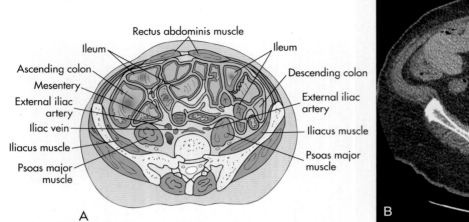

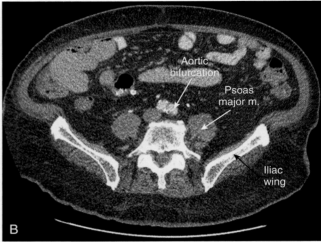

FIGURE 5-12 A, Cross section of the pelvis taken at the lower margin of the fifth lumbar vertebra and disk. The gluteus minimus muscle is shown on this section, as are the right external and internal iliac arteries. The left common iliac artery branches into the external and internal arteries. The ileum is seen throughout this level, and the mesentery terminates at this level. **B,** CT transverse section that shows the aortic bifurcation, psoas muscles, and iliac wing.

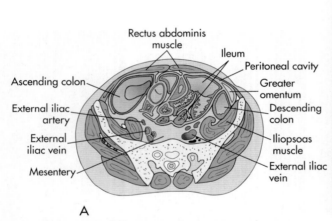

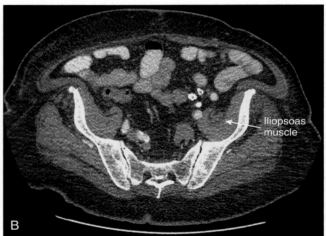

FIGURE 5-13 A, Cross section of the pelvis taken at the level of the sacrum and the anterior superior spine of the ilium. The gluteus maximus muscle appears on both sides. The internal and external iliac veins have united to form the common iliac vein. The ileum is seen throughout this section. **B,** CT transverse section through the lower abdomen and iliopsoas muscle.

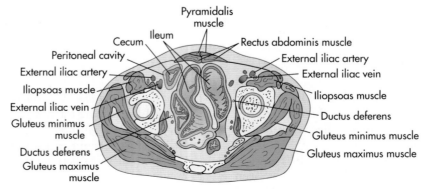

FIGURE 5-14 Cross section of the pelvis taken above the margins of the fifth anterior pair of sacral foramina and head of the femur. The external iliac arteries become the femoral arteries in this section. The femoral veins become the external iliac veins.

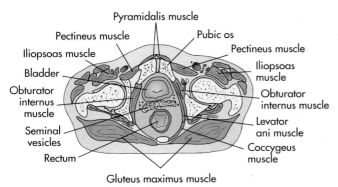

FIGURE 5-15 Cross section of the pelvis at the level of the coccyx, the spine of the ischium, the femur, and the greater trochanter. This cross section passes through the coccyx, spine of the ischium, acetabulum, head of the femur, greater trochanter, pubic symphysis, and upper margins of the obturator foramen. The gemellus inferior and superior, coccygeus, and levator ani muscles are shown. The rectum is seen in the midline. The trigone of the bladder and the urethral orifice are well shown, and the seminal vesicles and the ampulla of the vasa deferentia can be identified. The ejaculatory ducts enter the urethra in the lower portion of this section.

the bladder and urethral orifice are shown, and the seminal vesicles and the ampulla of the vasa deferentia can be identified. The ejaculatory ducts enter the urethra in the lower portion of this section.

Level of the male pelvis (Figure 5-16): The rectum, prostate gland, penis, and corpus cavernosum are seen.

Level of the female pelvis (Figure 5-17): The bladder is anterior to the uterus. The pouch of Douglas is posterior to the uterus, anterior to the rectum. The ovaries are seen along the fundal border of the uterus.

Level of the female pelvis (Figure 5-18): The pelvic diaphragm muscles are shown.

Longitudinal Plane

The longitudinal sectional illustrations (see Figures 5-19 through 5-29) are presented from the right abdominal border, proceeding across the abdominal wall to the left border.

Level of the right lobe of the liver (Figure 5-19): The right lobe of the liver, diaphragm, omentum, and muscles are shown.

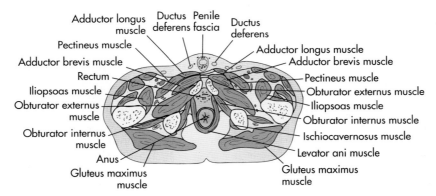

FIGURE 5-16 Cross section of the pelvis at the tip of the coccyx, inferior ramus of the pubis, and neck of the femur. This cross section passes below the tip of the coccyx, upper portion of the tuberosity of the ischium and inferior ramus of the pubis, neck of the femur, and lower portion of the greater trochanter. The rectum, penis, and corpus cavernosum are seen.

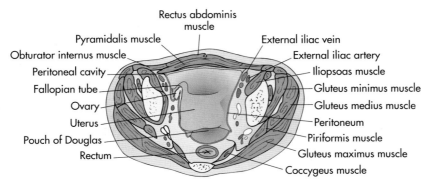

FIGURE 5-17 This cross section is a section through the female pelvis just below the junction of the sacrum and coccyx, through the anterior inferior spine of the ilium and the greater sciatic notch. The uterine artery and vein and the ureter are shown dissected beyond the uterine wall. The bladder is anterior to the uterus. The ovaries are cut through their midsections on this level.

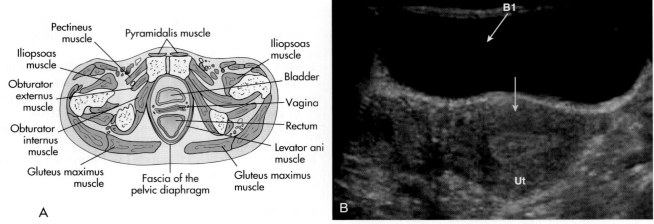

FIGURE 5-18 A, Cross section of the female pelvis taken through the lower part of the coccyx and the spine of the ischium. The superior gemellus muscles and the pectineus muscle appear in this section, and the coccygeus muscle terminates here. The gluteus maximus, gluteus minimus, and gluteus medius muscles all begin their insertions in the lower part of this section. The external os of the cervix is shown. The ureters empty into the bladder at the base. **B,** Ultrasound of the pelvis shows the distended urinary bladder *(Bl),* uterus *(ut),* and endometrium *(arrow).*

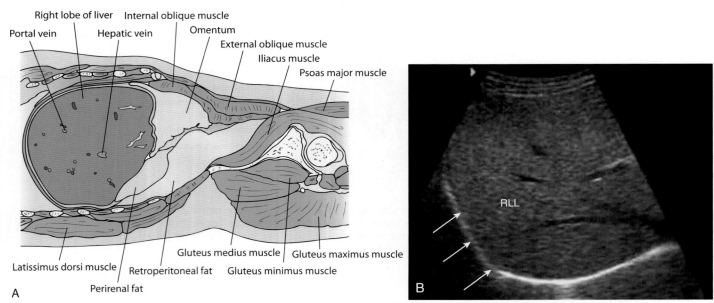

FIGURE 5-19 A, Sagittal section of the abdomen taken along the right lateral abdominal border. **B,** Longitudinal ultrasound, right lobe liver *(RLL),* diaphragm *(arrows).*

Level of the liver and gallbladder (Figure 5-20): The diaphragm, right lobe of the liver, gallbladder, and perirenal fat area are shown. The costodiaphragmatic recess is seen superior to the diaphragm.

Level of the liver, gallbladder, and right kidney (Figure 5-21): The diaphragm, right lobe of the liver, gallbladder, and right kidney are seen. The perirenal fat and fascia are shown surrounding the kidney. **Morison's pouch** is found anterior to the kidney and posterior to the inferior right lobe of the liver. The caudate lobe of the liver is beginning to show.

Level of the liver, caudate lobe, and psoas muscle (Figure 5-22): The diaphragm, right lobe of the liver, caudate lobe, and neck of the gallbladder are seen.

Level of the liver, duodenum, and pancreas (Figure 5-23): The portal vein and cystic duct are shown. The duodenum wraps around the head of the pancreas.

Level of the liver, inferior vena cava, pancreas, and gastroduodenal artery (Figure 5-24): The gastroduodenal artery is the anterior border of the head of the pancreas. The **left portal vein** is shown to enter the left lobe of the liver.

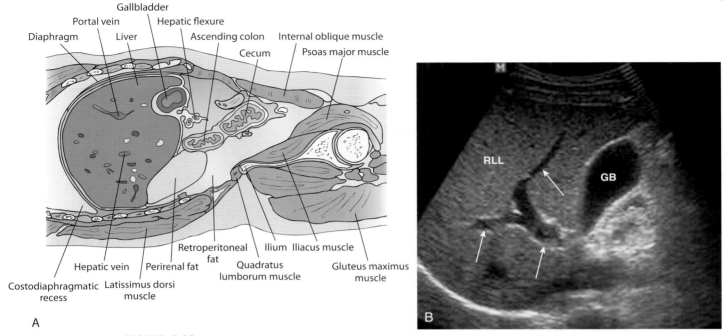

FIGURE 5-20 **A,** Sagittal section of the abdomen 8 cm from the midline. **B,** Longitudinal ultrasound of the right lobe liver *(RLL),* portal vein *(arrows),* and gallbladder *(Gb).*

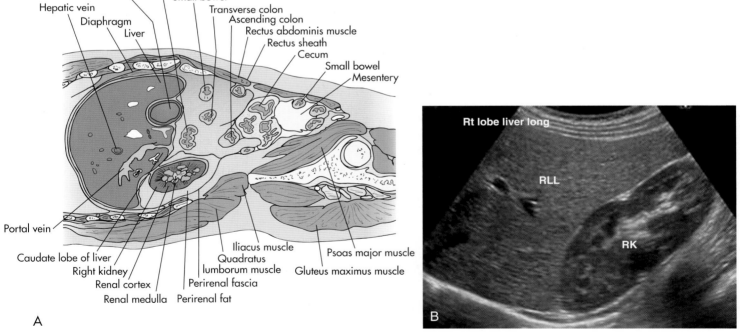

FIGURE 5-21 **A,** Sagittal section of the abdomen 7 cm from the midline. **B,** Longitudinal ultrasound of right lobe liver *(RLL),* right kidney *(RK).*

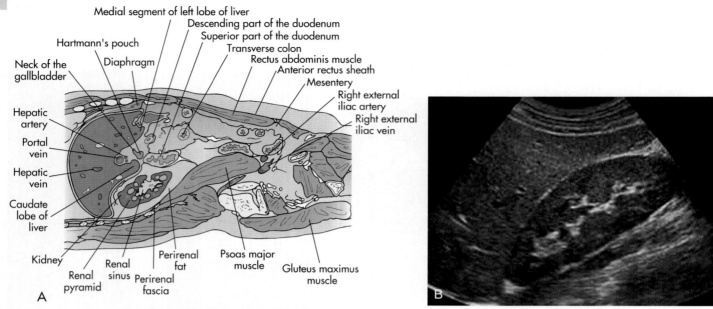

FIGURE 5-22 **A,** Sagittal section of the abdomen 6 cm from the midline. **B,** Longitudinal ultrasound of right lobe liver *(RLL)* with patient in full inspiration to image entire right kidney *(RK).*

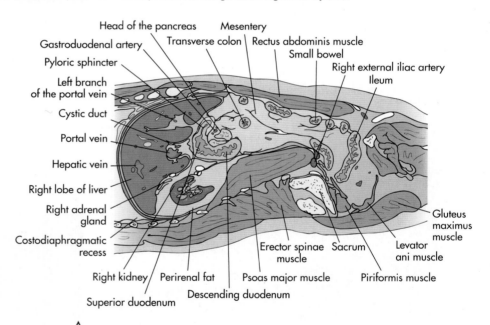

FIGURE 5-23 **A,** Sagittal section of the abdomen 5 cm from the midline. **B,** Longitudinal ultrasound of the left lobe liver *(LLL).*

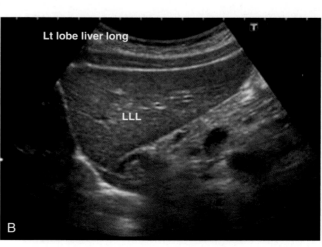

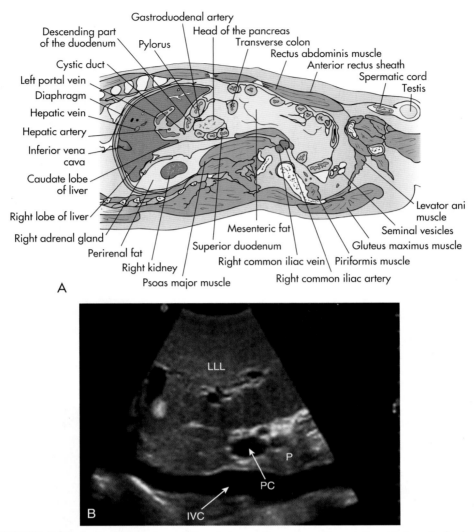

FIGURE 5-24 A, Sagittal section of the abdomen 3 cm from the midline. **B,** Longitudinal ultrasound of the left lobe liver *(LLL)*, portal confluence *(Pc)*, pancreas *(P)*, and inferior vena cava *(IVC)*.

Level of the inferior vena cava, left lobe of the liver, and pancreas (Figure 5-25): The inferior vena cava is shown along the posterior border of the liver. The pancreas lies anterior to the inferior vena cava and inferior to the portal vein.

Level of the hepatic vein and inferior vena cava, pancreas, and superior mesenteric vein (Figure 5-26): The superior mesenteric vein flows anterior to the uncinate portion of the pancreas and posterior to the body. The middle hepatic vein empties into the inferior vena cava. The falciform ligament is seen along the anterior border of the abdomen.

Level of the crus of the diaphragm and caudate lobe (Figure 5-27): The caudate lobe is seen posterior to the ligamentum venosum. The aorta is starting to come into view.

Level of the aorta and superior mesenteric artery (Figure 5-28): The **superior mesenteric artery (SMA)** arises from the anterior border of the aorta. The pancreas is seen anterior to the SMA; the splenic artery and vein form the posterior border. The left renal vein is posterior to the SMA and anterior to the aorta. The area of the lesser sac is shown.

Level of the spleen and left kidney (Figure 5-29): The spleen is shown just below the diaphragm in the left upper quadrant. The left kidney is inferior to the spleen. The tail of the pancreas lies anterior to the kidney and inferior to the **splenic hilum.**

CT coronal image of the abdomen shows the liver, right kidney, spleen, and left kidney. Note the perinephric fat pad surrounding the kidneys (Figure 5-30).

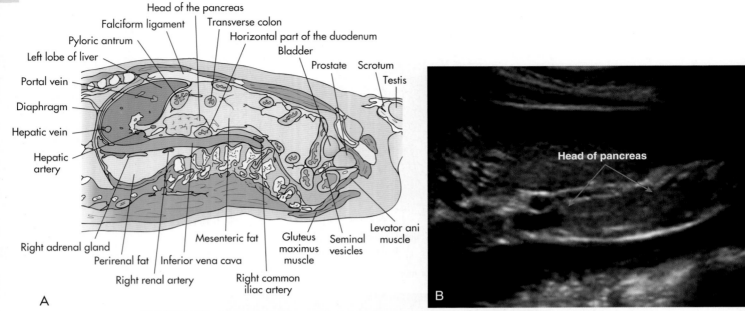

FIGURE 5-25 A, Sagittal section of the abdomen 2 cm from the midline. **B,** Longitudinal ultrasound of the left lobe liver *(LLL),* head of pancreas *(arrows),* and inferior vena cava *(IVC).*

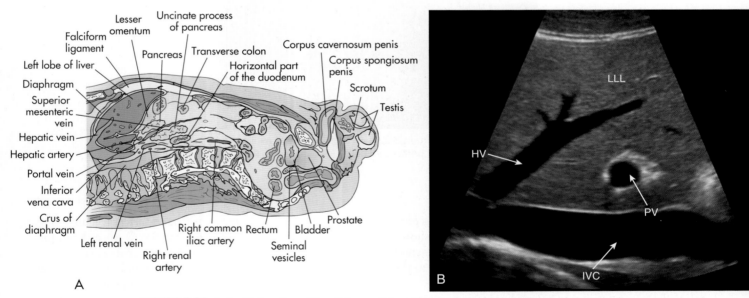

FIGURE 5-26 A, Sagittal section of the abdomen 0.5 cm from the midline. **B,** Longitudinal ultrasound of the patient in full inspiration shows the left lobe liver *(LLL),* inferior vena cava *(IVC),* portal vein *(PV),* and hepatic vein *(HV).*

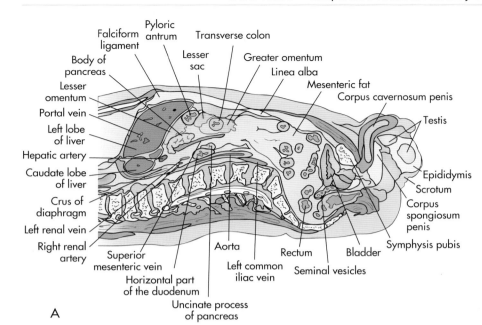

Pyloric
antrum
Falciform
ligament
Body of
pancreas
Lesser
sac
Lesser
omentum
Transverse colon
Portal vein
Greater omentum
Left lobe
of liver
Linea alba
Hepatic artery
Mesenteric fat
Caudate lobe
of liver
Corpus cavernosum penis
Crus of
diaphragm
Testis
Left renal vein
Epididymis
Right renal
artery
Scrotum
Superior
mesenteric vein
Corpus
spongiosum
penis
Horizontal part
of the duodenum
Aorta
Symphysis pubis
Uncinate process
of pancreas
Left common
iliac vein
Rectum
Seminal vesicles
Bladder

A

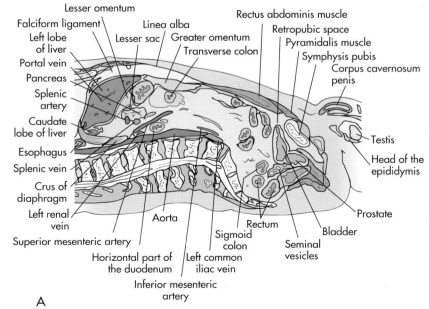

B

FIGURE 5-27 **A,** Sagittal section of the abdomen 0.2 cm from the midline. **B,** Longitudinal ultrasound of the left lobe liver *(LLL)*, caudate lobe *(arrows)*, portal confluence *(Pc)*, and inferior vena cava *(IVC)*.

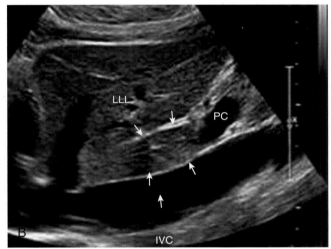

Lesser omentum
Falciform ligament
Linea alba
Rectus abdominis muscle
Left lobe
of liver
Lesser sac
Retropubic space
Portal vein
Greater omentum
Pyramidalis muscle
Pancreas
Transverse colon
Symphysis pubis
Splenic
artery
Corpus cavernosum
penis
Caudate
lobe of liver
Esophagus
Testis
Splenic vein
Head of the
epididymis
Crus of
diaphragm
Left renal
vein
Prostate
Aorta
Superior mesenteric artery
Rectum
Bladder
Horizontal part of
the duodenum
Sigmoid
colon
Left common
iliac vein
Seminal
vesicles
Inferior mesenteric
artery

A

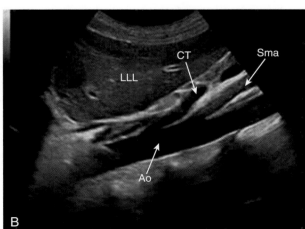

B

FIGURE 5-28 **A,** Midline sagittal section of the abdomen. **B,** Longitudinal ultrasound of the left lobe liver *(LLL)*, aorta *(Ao)*, celiac trunk *(ct)*, and superior mesenteric artery *(sma)*.

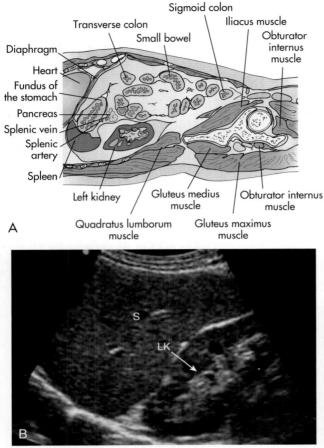

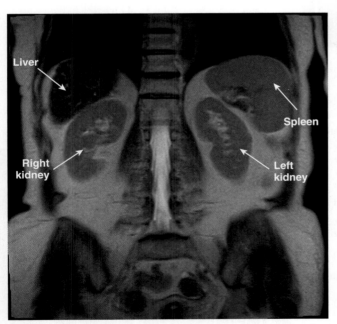

FIGURE 5-29 A, Sagittal section of the abdomen along the left abdominal border. **B,** Longitudinal ultrasound of the prominent spleen *(S)* and left kidney *(LK).*

 Key Pearls

- Ultrasound is often preferred over CT, which involves ionizing radiation, or MRI, which is both time consuming and costly.
- Each modality (ultrasound, CT, MRI) approaches the problem from a different standpoint, using differing physical properties of the normal tissue and pathologic lesions to derive image contrast and resolve important details.
- Ultrasound and MRI both have a safety advantage in that they do not use ionizing radiation.
- CT scanning and general diagnostic (x-ray) imaging, on the other hand, both image the body by use of ionizing radiation, often in significant doses.
- The transverse plane is horizontal to the body. This plane divides the body or any of its parts into upper and lower portions.
- The sagittal plane is a lengthwise plane running from front to back. It divides the body or any of its parts into right and left sides, or two equal halves; this is known as the midsagittal plane.
- The longitudinal plane is parallel to the long axis of the body or part.
- The coronal plane is a lengthwise plane running from side to side, dividing the body into anterior and posterior portions.
- To identify specific abdominal structures or to refer to an area of pain, the abdominopelvic cavity may be divided into four quadrants and nine abdominal regions.
- The four quadrants are the right upper quadrant (RUQ), left upper quadrant (LUQ), right lower quadrant (RLQ), and left lower quadrant (LLQ).
- The nine abdominal regions are as follows: (1) upper abdomen/right hypochondrium, (2) epigastrium, (3) left hypochondrium, (4) middle abdomen/right lumbar, (5) umbilical, (6) left lumbar, (7) lower abdomen/right iliac fossa, (8) hypogastrium, and (9) left iliac fossa.

BIBLIOGRAPHY

Moses KP, Banks JC, Nava PB, Petersen D: *Atlas of clinical gross anatomy,* St. Louis, 2005, Elsevier Mosby.

Swobodnik W, Herrmann M, Altwein J: *Atlas of ultrasound anatomy: normal anatomy as the basis of sonographic diagnosis,* New York, 1991, Thieme Medical Publishers.

FIGURE 5-30 CT coronal view of the midabdominal cavity demonstrated the liver, spleen, kidneys, and pararenal fat.

Basic Ultrasound Imaging: Techniques, Terminology, and Tips

Sandra L. Hagen-Ansert

The production of a high-quality sonographic image is an "art" that demands many talents of the sonographer: a high degree of manual dexterity and hand-eye coordination; the ability to conceptualize two-dimensional (2D) information into a three-dimensional (3D) format; and a thorough understanding of anatomy, physiology, pathology, instrumentation, artifact recognition, and transducer characteristics. The sophistication of ultrasound systems requires a greater understanding of the physical principles of ultrasound and computers than ever before. Moreover, sonographers should be able to incorporate

Doppler techniques, color flow mapping, tissue harmonics, strain analysis, and 3D imaging to provide an enhanced understanding of anatomy and physiology as it relates to hemodynamic blood flow and reconstruction.

Although one-on-one, hands-on training in a clinical setting is an essential part of the sonographer's experience of producing high-quality scans, this chapter will take you on a journey toward mastering the foundations of abdominal scanning. Correlation of ultrasound images with sectional anatomy is critical for producing consistent, quality images.

The approach to general abdominal ultrasound will be presented in this chapter. Specific organ protocols will be presented in their respective chapters. You may find the protocol for an abdominal scan to differ slightly between ultrasound departments; the key is to develop a protocol that is within the national practice guidelines, such as American Institute of Ultrasound in Medicine (AIUM) or American College of Radiology (ACR) and to consistently maintain such protocol for all patients. The protocol presented here is generic and may be adapted to the particular laboratory situation. Also included in this chapter are special scanning techniques and specific applications of abdominal scanning.

BEFORE YOU BEGIN TO SCAN PATIENTS

Remember that your ultimate goal as a sonographer is to produce diagnostic images that can be interpreted by the physician to answer a clinical question. To create images that are diagnostically useful, you must be familiar with ultrasound instrumentation and the clinical considerations of the patient examination. Clinical considerations include knowing which patient position should be used for specific examinations, transducer selection and scanning techniques, patient breathing techniques, and how to perform a sonographic survey of the abdomen.

Be sure you are very familiar with various types of ultrasound equipment. Know where the operator's manual is and how to find what you need in the manual. (Every manufacturer places the power supply in a different position, so make sure you know how to turn the machine on and off.) Become familiar with the transducers available for each machine, how to activate the transducers, and how to change transducers; some of the plug-in formats take some practice to master. Know where the critical knobs are that operate the ultrasound instrumentation (e.g., time gain compensation [TGC], power, gain, depth, angle, focus, Doppler, color flow). Know where the annotate text keys are for labeling the image. If the ultrasound equipment is new to you, it may be a good idea for one sonographer to work the controls while the other images the patient until you become comfortable with the equipment.

It is highly recommended that the student sonographer practice in a supervised laboratory setting (away from patients) or with one of the anatomic mannequin/ultrasound models before beginning to work with patients. This way, the student sonographer can become familiar with the ultrasound equipment by scanning phantoms or even "building" his or her own phantoms to be scanned.

The next step should be for one student to scan the other students in the sonography laboratory. This allows the actual experience of feeling how "cold that gel really is" when applied to the abdomen and knowing what the probe feels like with different individual scan techniques. (Most laboratories are equipped with gel warmers to avoid that patient discomfort.) The student can see firsthand how a *light* touch does not make as pretty an image as a moderate touch with the transducer adjacent to the skin and may experience the agony of the heavy hand as it scrapes across the rib cage. The student will also learn how much scanning gel is the right amount: If it drips down your wrist and onto your clothes, it is too much gel.

Controlled supervised scanning should also emphasize how important it is for the patient to take in a breath or suspend breathing so the highest quality images are obtained. A recommended patient breathing technique tip is to have the patient inhale through the nose to reduce the amount of air going into the stomach. *Breathing is probably the weakest learning link for the student.* Careful control of respiration is critical for making a beautiful scan versus an image that is not easy to interpret.

The student sonographer should also begin to learn the specific protocols required for each examination. Nationally recognized protocols for all areas of ultrasound have been developed by the American College of Radiology (www.acr.org) and the American Institute of Ultrasound in Medicine (www.aium.org) for ultrasound examinations. Likewise, the American Congress of Obstetricians and Gynecologists (www.acog.org) has developed ultrasound protocols for the female patient. The American Society of Echocardiography (www.asecho.org) has developed extensive guidelines for all areas in echocardiography. The Society for Vascular Ultrasound (www.svt.org) has established protocols and guidelines for specific vascular examinations. Each of these protocols can be found on the websites of the respective organizations.

Students may be overwhelmed at first with the detail these protocols require and may not completely remember all the steps in the protocols when they first begin their clinical scanning experience. Some equipment manufacturers have built a "Smart Examination Protocol" into the equipment; once activated, the system will direct the sonographer to the next required view. Suggested steps to help the student master the protocols are included in the workbook that accompanies this textbook.

Orientation to the Clinical Laboratory

A new student in the clinical ultrasound laboratory may be overwhelmed at first with the control panel on the ultrasound system, the hand-eye coordination required to produce an image, and the protocol required for the particular examination. The following suggestions may make your entrance into the clinical world a little smoother:

- Know all of the ultrasound equipment in your laboratory. This means that every free minute should be spent with the equipment, finding the correct knobs necessary to perform the examination. Know where the depth, gain, 2D, color, M-mode, harmonics, and TGC controls are located.
- Know where the operator's manuals are for each piece of equipment so you may have a reference for troubleshooting.
- Find out what protocols are used for each examination. Most departments have a "Standard Manual of Protocols" for all their examinations.

- Understand how to read the patient order, find out what question the ordering physician needs to have answered, and know which items in the patient records are relevant for patient identification.
- When you call for patients, be sure to check their ID with at least two identifiers (i.e., name and birth date, doctor who ordered the examination, type of examination ordered).
- Introduce yourself and explain briefly the procedure you are going to do. Also explain the procedure the department will follow to notify the patient's physician of the results of the examination.
- Always keep your conversation professional. Remember that you need to focus on the examination.
- Discuss the case only with your mentor or with the physician responsible for interpreting the study.

Written Order for the Examination

An electronic or written order by the health care provider will indicate the reason for the ultrasound examination. This order should contain the appropriate clinical information relevant to the patient in order to provide the necessary information from the ultrasound procedure to the clinician.

Documentation for the Ultrasound Examination

Accurate documentation must be made for the ultrasound procedure. There should be a permanent record of the examination and its interpretation available on the electronic medical record or written format. The images obtained from the examination should be recorded in a retrievable format (i.e., PACS system or disc). Communication of the results must be maintained between the providing physician and the ordering physician.

Scanning Techniques

Ultrasound can distinguish multiple interfaces between soft tissue structures of different acoustic densities. The strength of the echoes reflected depends on the acoustic interface and the angle at which the sound beam strikes the interface. The sonographer must determine which patient "window" is best to record optimal ultrasound images, and which transducer size best fits into that window. The curved array transducer provides a large field of view, but in some patients this transducer may be too large to fit in between the ribs to provide adequate contact for accurate reflection of the sound wave. The smaller footprint transducer allows the sonographer to scan between intercostal spaces with the patient in a supine, coronal, decubitus, or upright position, but limits the near field of view. It is not unusual to use multiple transducers on one patient to complete the examination, as transducers are available in multiple sizes and frequencies.

Patient Preparation

It is recommended that the patient fast for 8 hours before the ultrasound examination of the abdomen. Fasting helps to reduce the interference that may be caused from gas overlying the midline abdominal structures. It will also ensure that the gallbladder will be fully distended. If the patient has eaten, it is still possible to perform the general ultrasound examination; however, visualization of all structures may not be as clear.

Patient Positions

The general abdominal examination is performed initially with the patient in the supine position. Additional views may require the oblique, lateral decubitus, prone, and occasionally upright positions for examination of specific areas of interest (Figure 6-1). For example, the gallbladder may be examined with the patient in the supine, oblique, or lateral decubitus positions. These positions will be discussed in more detail in the specific chapters.

Transducer Selection

Know the various transducers available for each ultrasound system, and know which transducers are used for specific examinations (Figure 6-2). The curved array transducer provides a large pie sector and is used for the survey of the abdomen. The linear array transducer provides a rectangular image of the structure, such as the abdominal aorta or inferior vena cava. The sector array provides a small pie sector of the area. The sector array is useful to find a "window" in

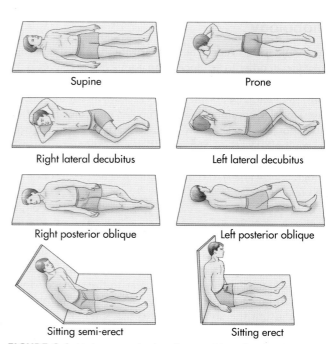

FIGURE 6-1 Various standard patient positions for the ultrasound examination.

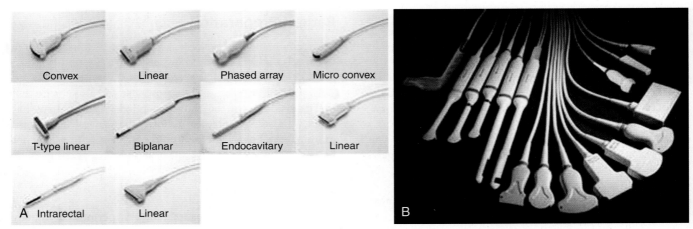

FIGURE 6-2 Transducer designs in multiple shapes and sizes are used for specific ultrasound examinations. **A,** Transducer design ranges from very small to the larger curved array probes. **B,** An array of transducer sizes and frequencies may be used in a general ultrasound department.

between the intercostal spaces to image the liver and biliary system. It is also used extensively to image the cardiac structures. The endocavity or endovaginal transducer is a high-frequency crystal mounted on a longer handle. The transducer is used in female pelvic and male pelvic examinations. If the endocavity transducer is used, the sonographer needs to be familiar with the decontamination process for the transducer. This process is discussed further in Chapter 42.

The size of the patient will influence which megahertz transducer will be used. Generally speaking, the lower-frequency transducer has better penetration and is used for the adult abdomen, whereas the high-frequency probe has higher resolution with improved axial resolution and is used for more superficial structures such as the thyroid or breast.

Knobology

The sonographer needs to be familiar with the ultrasound control panel in order to produce an anatomic image (Figure 6-3). The primary controls include the depth, gain (TGC, lateral gain), frequency, focal zone, modes (2D, M-mode, 3D, pulsed wave Doppler, continuous wave Doppler, and color Doppler), annotation, and calculation package. Each of these controls has multiple layers of software (tissue harmonics, dynamic compression range, frame rate, scale, baseline, etc.) that the sonographer will learn to manipulate in order to produce the high-quality image.

Transducer Positions

The sonographer will use multiple wrist actions throughout the study. Remember that the beam is ideally reflected when the transducer is perpendicular to the surface. However, the body has many angles, curves, and rib interferences, causing the sonographer to use intercostal spaces, subcostal windows, multiple degrees of angulation, and many rotations of the transducer to obtain anatomic images (Figure 6-4).

There are multiple scanning motions that the sonographer needs to master throughout the examination: *sweep, slide, rock, fan,* and *rotate.* These movements may be large (macro) or small (micro). The **macro movement** of the probe is used with the sweep and slide motion in which the probe is moved greater than 1 cm. Macro movement also occurs if the fan or rock motion changes the angle of insonation by more than 15 degrees in either direction. The **micro movement** of the probe is used with the sweep and slide motion in which the probe is moved less than 1 cm. Micro movement likewise occurs if the fan or rock motion changes the angle of insonation by less than 15 degrees in either direction. It is important to perform only one motion at a time. The movement should be similar every time you have the same scanning window to consistently produce an image.

In a survey of the abdomen, the sonographer will initially use the **sweep** motion. This requires the transducer to remain in one area while using a large wrist motion with the probe perpendicular to the skin surface to sweep through the abdomen. It is used to locate and interrogate an area of interest or to evaluate the scan windows of abdominal structures before the scan protocol is begun.

The **slide** motion is used when the transducer is physically moved along the abdomen, such as a longitudinal movement to follow the course of the abdominal aorta into the bifurcation of the iliac arteries.

Once an area of interest is located, the sonographer may pause over the structure and slowly **rock** or pivot the transducer back and forth or up and down to image the area completely or to follow the anatomic structure. This is when the "cine" frame capture is useful to record the motion. This may be used in demonstrating the junction of the common bile duct and cystic duct or in tracking the communication of the hepatic artery as it arises from the celiac trunk.

A smaller version of the sweep motion is the **fan** motion, which is used when the transducer is minutely swept, pivoting on a point of interest. This may be useful in the superficial

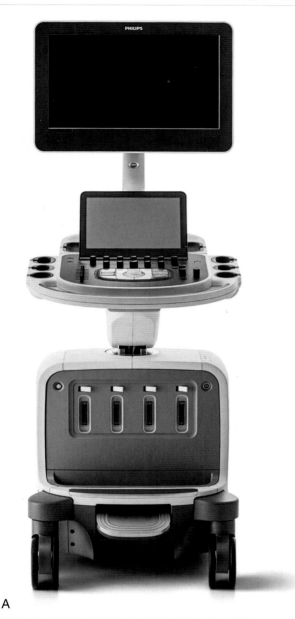

A

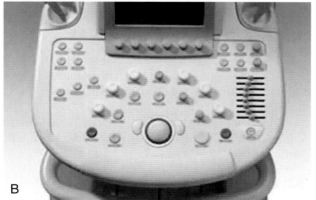

B

FIGURE 6-3 A, Ultrasound system demonstrates portability and ergonomic features for the sonographer. (Philips EPIQ 7 ultrasound system. Used with permission from Philips.) **B,** Example of the control panel of an ultrasound system. The pods on the right-hand side control the TGC. Other central controls include gain, depth, filter, scale, mode selection, zoom, calipers, and gray-scale maps.

Perpendicular
The transducer is straight up and down.

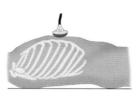

Subcostal
The transducer is angled superiorly just beneath the inferior costal margin.

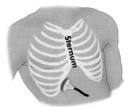

Intercostal
The transducer is between the ribs. It can be perpendicular, subcostal, or angled.

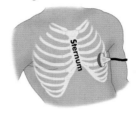

Angled
The transducer is angled superiorly, inferiorly, or right and left laterally at varying degrees.

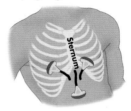

Rotated
The transducer is rotated varying degrees to oblique the scanning plane.

FIGURE 6-4 The sonographer must use a number of different transducer positions and angulations to complete the ultrasound examination.

structures such as the breast when differentiation is needed between the duct and the invasive lesion within the duct.

The **rotate** motion is useful to navigate between the ribs or to change from transverse to longitudinal planes, where the transducer is held in one area and rotated 90 degrees to the opposite plane. Rotate is also used in smaller increments as the transducer is slowly turned around the area of interest.

Annotation

Ultrasound images are labeled as *transverse* or *longitudinal* for a specific organ, such as the liver, gallbladder, pancreas, spleen, or uterus. The smaller organs that can be imaged on a single plane, such as the kidney, are labeled as *long-midline, -lateral,* or *-medial,* whereas the transverse scans are labeled as *transverse-low, -middle,* or *-high.*

All transverse supine scans are oriented with the liver on the left of the monitor; this means that the sonographer will be viewing the body from the feet up to the head ("optimistic view") (Figure 6-5). Longitudinal scans display the patient's head to the left and feet to the right of the screen and use the xiphoid, umbilicus, or symphysis to denote the midline of the scan plane (Figure 6-6).

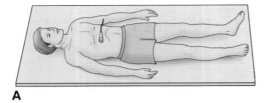

A

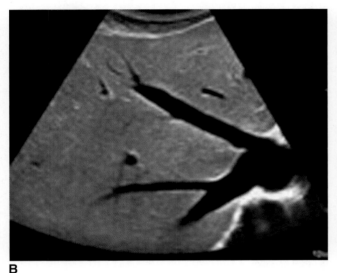

B

FIGURE 6-5 **A,** The curved array probe is held in a transverse position just under the costal margin with a steep angulation to be perpendicular to the dome of the liver. Patient is supine. **B,** All transverse supine scans are oriented as looking up from the feet, with the liver on the left side of the screen (right side of the patient is on the left of the screen).

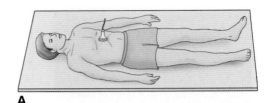

A

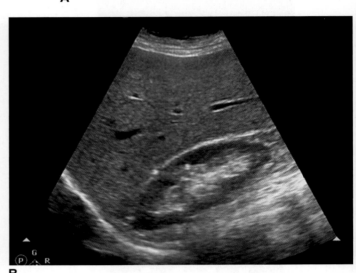

B

FIGURE 6-6 **A,** The curved array probe has been rotated 180 degrees to perform a sagittal scan of the abdomen. **B,** The longitudinal scans for the abdomen and pelvis are oriented with the patient's head toward the left of the screen and feet toward the right.

All scans should be appropriately labeled for future reference, including the patient's name, date, and anatomic position. Body position markers are available on many ultrasound machines and may be used in place of written labels.

The position of the patient should be described in relation to the scanning table (e.g., a right decubitus would mean the right side down; a left decubitus would indicate the left side down). If the scanning plane is oblique, the sonographer should merely state that it is an oblique view without specifying the exact degree of obliquity.

Artifacts

Sonographers need to learn about ultrasound artifacts early in their learning curve. There are a few primary artifacts that sonographers should recognize as they begin their scanning experience: reverberation, mirror, side lobe, and shadowing (Figure 6-7). *Reverberation* artifacts occur between the transducer and a strong reflector such as the rib causing multiple linear lines equidistant apart. A *mirror* artifact is a form of reverberation that shows structures that exist on one side of a strong reflector as being present on the other side as well; for example, the liver/diaphragm interface may show "liver" tissue in the pleural space. *Side lobe* artifacts are beams that propagate from a single

transducer element in directions different from the primary beam, such as those produced by bone or gas. *Shadowing* is the reduction in echo amplitude from reflectors that lie behind a strongly reflecting or attenuating structure; for example, calcified gallstone will cause a "shadow" posterior to the stone. Artifacts found in ultrasound images are discussed in more detail in Chapter 7.

INDICATIONS FOR ABDOMINAL SONOGRAPHY

The AIUM has listed multiple indications for an abdominal sonogram that include, but are not limited to, the following:
- Signs or symptoms that may be referred from the abdominal and/or retroperitoneal region such as jaundice or hematuria
- Generalized abdominal, flank, or back pain
- Palpable mass or organomegaly
- Abnormal laboratory values or abnormal findings on other imaging modalities
- Follow-up of known or suspected abnormalities in the abdomen or retroperitoneum
- Search for metastatic disease or occult primary neoplasm
- Evaluation of suspected congenital abnormalities

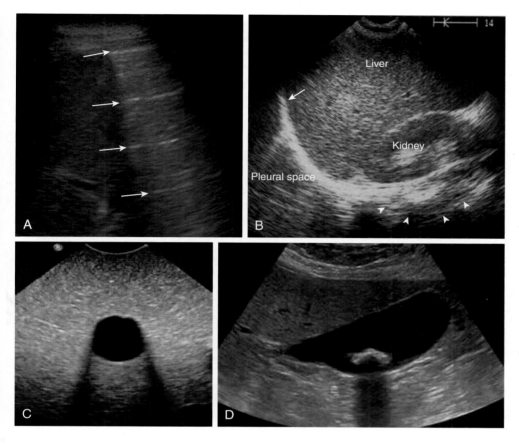

FIGURE 6-7 Artifacts. **A,** *Reverberation* artifacts occur between the transducer and a strong reflector such as the rib causing multiple linear lines equidistant apart. **B,** A *mirror* artifact is a form of reverberation that shows structures that exist on one side of a strong reflector as being present on the other side as well; for example, the liver/diaphragm interface may show "liver" tissue in the pleural space. **C,** *Side lobe* artifacts are beams that propagate from a single transducer element in directions different from the primary beam, such as those produced by bone or gas. **D,** *Shadowing* is the reduction in echo amplitude from reflectors that lie behind a strongly reflecting or attenuating structure; for example, calcified gallstone will cause a "shadow" posterior to the stone.

- Trauma to the abdomen or retroperitoneum
- Pretransplant and posttransplant evaluation
- Invasive procedure localization
- Localization for free or loculated peritoneal, pleural, or retroperitoneal fluid
- Suspicion of hypertrophic pyloric stenosis or intussusception
- Evaluation of a urinary tract infection

The request for an abdominal or retroperitoneal sonographic examination needs to provide sufficient information to demonstrate the medical necessity of the examination with allowance for proper performance and interpretation.

The documentation that must be met for medical necessity includes the following items: (1) patient signs and symptoms and (2) previous history pertinent to the examination requested. Additional information such as the specific reason for the examination or a provisional diagnosis would be helpful and may aid in the proper performance and interpretation of the examination. This will allow the sonographer to tailor the examination to answer the question from the ordering physician.

ULTRASOUND TERMINOLOGY

The sonographer is responsible for reviewing the patient's request for the ultrasound examination and for discussing any specific requests with the referring physician. Therefore a familiarity with basic medical terminology and abbreviations is necessary. Common medical and ultrasound abbreviations are listed on the inside covers of this book for quick reference.

One of the sonographer's primary responsibilities is the identification and description of normal and abnormal anatomy. The following list of terms is universally accepted and will help the sonographer describe the results obtained from various ultrasound examinations:

Anechoic or sonolucent: opposite of echogenic; without internal echoes; the structure is fluid filled and transmits sound easily (Figure 6-8, *A*). Examples: vascular structures, distended urinary bladder, gallbladder, and amniotic cavity.

Echogenic or hyperechoic: opposite of anechoic; echo-producing structure; reflects sound with a brighter intensity (Figure 6-8, *B*). Examples: gallstone, renal calyx, bone, fat, fissures, and ligaments.

Enhancement, increased through-transmission: sound that travels through an anechoic (fluid-filled) substance and is not attenuated; brightness is increased directly beyond the posterior border of the anechoic structure compared with the surrounding area—this is "enhancement" (see Figure 6-8, *A*).

Fluid-fluid level: interface between two fluids with different acoustic characteristics; this level will change with patient position. Example: dermoid tumor with fluid level.

Heterogeneous: not uniform in texture or composition (Figure 6-8, *C*). Example: Many tumors have characteristics of both decreased and increased echogenicity.

Homogeneous: opposite of heterogeneous; completely uniform in texture or composition (Figure 6-8, *D*). Example: The textures of the liver, thyroid, testes, and myometrium are generally considered homogeneous.

Hypoechoic: low-level echoes within a structure (Figure 6-8, *E*). Examples: lymph nodes and fibroma.

Infiltrating: usually refers to a diffuse disease process or metastatic disease (Figure 6-8, *F*). Examples: carcinoid or sarcoid infiltration.

Irregular borders: Borders are not well defined, are ill defined, or are not present (Figure 6-8, *G*). Examples: abscess, thrombus, and metastases.

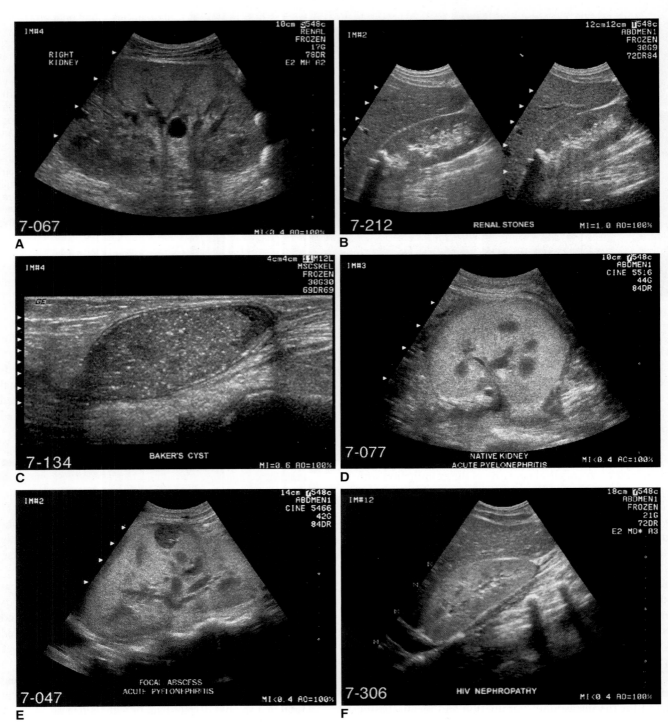

FIGURE 6-8 A, Anechoic (simple cyst). **B,** Echogenic (stone with shadowing). **C,** Heterogeneous (Baker cyst with mixture of fluid, debris, and bright echo reflectors). **D,** Homogeneous (renal parenchyma). **E,** Hypoechoic (hemorrhagic cyst). **F,** Infiltrating (HIV systemic disease process involving the kidney).

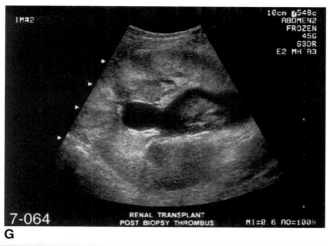

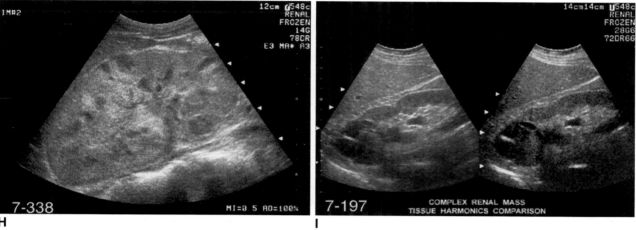

FIGURE 6-8, cont'd **G,** Irregular borders (thrombus within the renal pelvis). **H,** Isoechoic (one half of renal parenchyma has lower level echoes). **I,** Loculated (complex renal mass with septations).

Isoechoic: very close to the normal parenchyma echogenicity pattern (Figure 6-8, *H*). Example: metastatic disease.

Loculated mass: well-defined borders with internal echoes; the septa may be thin (likely benign) or thick (likely malignant) (Figure 6-8, *I*).

Shadowing: The sound beam is attenuated by a solid or calcified object. This reflection or absorption may be partial or complete; air bubbles in the duodenum may cause a "dirty shadow" to occur secondary to reflection; a stone would cause a sharp shadow posterior to its border (see Figure 6-8, *B*).

IDENTIFYING ABNORMALITIES

Careful evaluation for the presence of pathology is incorporated into the general abdominal protocol. The sonographer needs to be able to demonstrate the normal anatomic structures, as well as the pathology that may invade or surround such structures. The abnormality is identified and evaluated according to a number of criteria, including the border definition, internal texture, tissue characteristics,

---

BOX 6-1	Ultrasound Criteria for Identifying Abnormal Structures

Border. Border of the structure may be smooth and well defined, or irregular.

Texture. Texture (parenchyma) of the structure may be homogeneous or heterogeneous.

Characteristic. Characteristic of an organ or of a mass is said to be anechoic, hypoechoic, isoechoic, hyperechoic, or echogenic to the rest of the parenchyma.

Transmission. Transmission of sound may be increased, decreased, or unchanged. An anechoic mass (fluid-filled cyst) will show increased transmission of sound, whereas a dermoid tumor (composed of muscle, teeth, and bone) will show decreased transmission.

---

and transmission of sound, which are listed in Box 6-1 and illustrated in Figure 6-9.

Pathology may be further identified by the internal composition as cystic, complex, or solid (Box 6-2). A cystic mass has a well-defined, smooth border; internally the lesion is anechoic with increased through sound transmission beyond

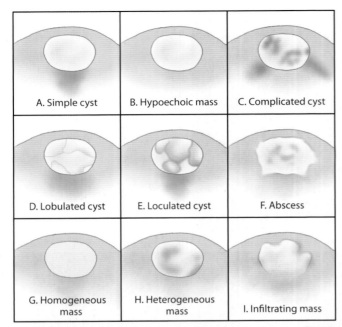

FIGURE 6-9 Ultrasound criteria for describing a mass. **A,** Simple cyst: smooth borders, anechoic, increased transmission. **B,** Hypoechoic mass: few to low-level internal echoes, smooth border, no increased transmission. **C,** Complicated cyst: mixed pattern of cystic and solid, fluid, debris, and blood; transmission may or may not increase. **D,** Lobulated cyst: well defined with thin septa, increased transmission. **E,** Loculated cyst: well defined with thick septa. **F,** Abscess: may have irregular borders, debris within, transmission may or may not be increased. **G,** Homogeneous mass: uniform texture within. **H,** Heterogeneous mass: nonuniform texture within. **I,** Infiltrating mass: distorted architecture, irregular borders, decreased transmission.

BOX 6-2	**Abnormal Structures That Affect Transmission**

Cyst. Has smooth, well-defined borders, anechoic, increased through-transmission (see Figure 6-10).
Complex. Has characteristics of both a cyst and a solid structure (see Figure 6-11).
Solid. Irregular borders, internal echoes, decreased through-transmission (see Figure 6-11).

its posterior border (Figure 6-10). A solid mass has irregular borders, internal echoes (echogenic), and decreased through-transmission (Figure 6-11). A complex mass has characteristics of both a cyst and a solid lesion. Transmission characteristics are determined by how easily the sound is able to transmit through the mass. Transmission is altered depending on what the mass is composed of pathologically. Throughout the chapters of this text, gross pathologic specimens will be included to provide the sonographer with a better understanding of these principles.

ANATOMIC DIRECTIONS

The anatomic position assumes that the body is standing erect, the eyes are looking forward, and the arms are at the sides with

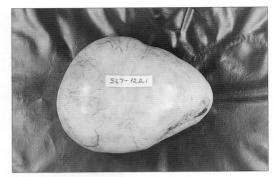

FIGURE 6-10 Gross pathology of a simple ovarian cyst showing well-defined smooth borders; straw-colored fluid was found inside the mass.

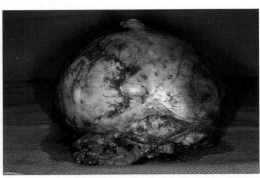

FIGURE 6-11 Gross pathology of a solid ovarian mass with irregular borders; the mass was filled with complex tissue.

the palms and toes directed forward. Refer to Figure 5-1 for the five anatomic directions of the body discussed here.

1. **Superior/inferior.** The top of the head is the most superior point of the body. The inferior point of the body is the bottom of the feet. All anatomic structures are designated relative to these two terms. The liver is considered to be superior to the bladder because the liver is closer to the head. The gallbladder is inferior to the diaphragm because it is closer to the feet. Other terms that are interchanged with *superior* are *cephalic* and *cranial* (toward the head). *Caudal* (toward the tail) is sometimes used instead of *inferior.*

2. **Anterior/posterior.** The front (belly) surface of the body is anterior, or *ventral.* The back surface of the body is posterior, or *dorsal.* This concept is very important to sonographers and to their understanding of sectional anatomy. If the patient is lying supine (face up), the aorta is anterior to the vertebral column. The right kidney is posterior to the head of the pancreas.

3. **Medial/lateral.** The body axis is an imaginary line from the center of the top of the head to the groin. *Medial* is described as the superior-inferior body axis as it goes right through the midline of the body. Structures are said to be medial if they are closer to the midline of the body than to another structure (e.g., the hepatic artery is medial to the common duct). The structure is *lateral* if it is toward the side of the body (e.g., the adnexae are lateral to the uterus).

4. **Proximal/distal.** When a structure is closer to the body midline or point of attachment to the trunk, it is described

as *proximal* (e.g., the hepatic duct is proximal to the common bile duct). *Distal* means farther from the midline or point of attachment to the trunk (e.g., the sphincter of Oddi is distal to the common bile duct).

5. **Superficial/deep.** Additionally, structures may be identified as being superficial or deep. Structures located close to the surface of the body are *superficial*. The rectus abdominis muscles are superficial to the transverse abdominis muscles. Structures located farther inward (away from the body surface) are *deep*.

CRITERIA FOR AN ADEQUATE SCAN

With the use of real-time ultrasound, it is sometimes difficult to become oriented to all of the anatomic structures on a frozen image; it is therefore critical to obtain as many landmarks of the anatomy as possible in a single image. Make every effort to avoid rib interference to eliminate artifactual ring-down, attenuation, or reverberation noise that may distort anatomic information. Most abdominal surveys are performed with the curved array multihertz transducer. The small-footprint sector transducer allows the sonographer to scan in between the ribs, but limits near-field visualization. Variations in the patient's respirations may also help eliminate rib interference and improve image quality. The sonographer can easily see in real-time how much interference is caused by patient breathing and can ask the patient to take in a breath and hold it, or to stop breathing at critical points to capture particular parts of the anatomy. Observing the image form in real-time allows the sonographer see what effect respiration will have on the image. If the left upper quadrant is not adequately imaged, the patient may be given water in an effort to fill the stomach. As the patient is rolled into a right decubitus position, the fluid flows from the body of the stomach to fill the antrum and duodenum, allowing the tail of the pancreas and great vessels to be imaged.

GENERAL ABDOMINAL ULTRASOUND PROTOCOLS

It is the responsibility of the sonographer to ensure that patients are afforded the highest-quality care possible during their sonographic examination. This entails identifying the patient properly, ensuring confidentiality of information and patient privacy, providing proper nursing care, and maintaining clean and sanitary equipment and examination rooms.

Initial Survey of the Abdomen

The upper abdomen is imaged with high-resolution real-time ultrasound equipment. As discussed previously, the transducer may be a sector or curved linear array or, in many cases, a combination of the two. The frequency of the transducer used depends on the size, muscle, and fat composition of the patient. Generally, a broad-bandwidth transducer is used, with variations of 2.25 to 7.5 MHz, depending on the size of the patient and the depth of field. All organs are routinely imaged in at least two planes: transverse and longitudinal.

The baseline abdominal ultrasound examination may include the complete abdomen and/or retroperitoneal space, a signal organ, or several organs. A combination of structures may be imaged because of their location or function. For example, the upper abdominal scan includes a survey of the liver and porta hepatis, vascular structures, biliary system, pancreas, kidneys, spleen, and para-aortic area. A functional focused scan may include the liver, gallbladder, and bile ducts. A follow-up or focused examination is generally performed once a complete baseline scan has been made. An established protocol (such as established by the AIUM) should be used. The baseline upper abdominal ultrasound examination includes a survey of the liver and porta hepatis, vascular structures, biliary system, pancreas, kidneys, spleen, and para-aortic area. If variations in anatomy or pathology are seen, multiple views are obtained over the area of interest.

Before you begin the protocol for the specific examination, take a minute to survey the abdomen by using the sweep motion. It is useful to ask the patient to take in a deep breath for this survey. This will give you an opportunity to see how the patient images appear with "routine" instrument settings, to observe where the organs are in relationship to the patient's respiration pattern, and to see if the patient has a good "scanning window" in the supine position, or if the patient position needs to be moved into a decubitus or upright position.

In a general abdominal survey, ask the patient to take in a deep breath; begin at the level of the xiphoid in the midline with the transducer angled steeply toward the patient's head (cephalic), so as to be perpendicular to the diaphragm (Figure 6-12). With the transducer fixed at the xyphoid, slowly angle the transducer inferiorly to "sweep" through the liver, gallbladder, head of the pancreas, and right kidney. The transducer may then be redirected in the same manner, only angled toward the left shoulder with a gradual angulation made inferiorly, to see the stomach, spleen, pancreas, and left kidney. Likewise, a quick survey of the abdomen may be done with the transducer in the midline sagittal position (Figure 6-13). Remember to ask the patient to take in a

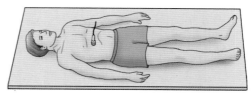

FIGURE 6-12 Most abdominal ultrasound examinations are performed initially in the supine position. The curved array probe is shown in the transverse position.

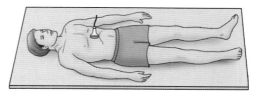

FIGURE 6-13 Longitudinal scan. The probe has now been rotated to the midline sagittal position.

breath and hold it. Image the aorta first with the vertebral column posterior to the aorta. Then slowly angle the transducer to the right to image the dilated inferior vena cava (suspended respiration allows the inferior vena cava to fill with blood returning to the heart) and liver. Continue to angle toward the right to image the right lobe of the liver, gallbladder, and right kidney. If adequate penetration is seen with balanced TGC and overall gain adjustments, you can proceed with the routine protocol for the abdominal study.

Transverse Scans

In the transverse plane, the sonographer should adjust the depth of the field of view with the depth knob on the ultrasound system control panel. The gain should be adjusted so the homogeneous liver parenchyma is uniform in texture. The homogeneous echogenicity of the liver parenchyma should be compared with the right kidney. The echogenic "horseshoe-shaped" contour of the vertebral column should be well delineated to ensure adequate sound penetration is present through the abdominal structures without obstruction from bowel gas interference.

With the patient in deep inspiration, the posterior border of the liver should be imaged as the transducer is angled in a cephalic direction and slowly swept from the diaphragm/dome of the liver to its inferior edge (Figure 6-14). This will ensure that the TGC is correctly adjusted with a gradual increase with depth of tissue to the posterior border

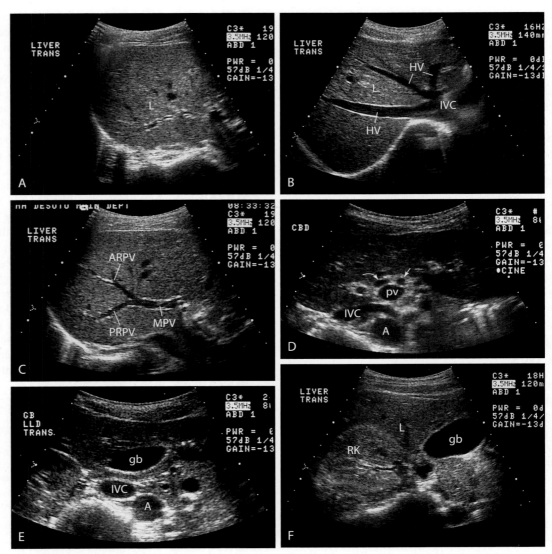

FIGURE 6-14 A, Transverse image of the right lobe of the liver *(L)* at the liver/lung interface. **B,** Transverse image at the dome of the liver *(L)* in full inspiration to demonstrate the hepatic veins *(HV)* flowing into the inferior vena cava *(IVC)*. **C,** Transverse image of the liver, main portal vein *(MPV)*, and right portal vein with bifurcation of anterior *(ARPV)* and posterior *(PRPV)* branches. **D,** Transverse image of portal tried in the center of the image: portal vein *(pv)* with common bile duct *(curved arrow)* anterior and lateral; hepatic artery *(arrow)* anterior and medial; inferior vena cava *(IVC)*; and aorta *(A)*. **E,** Transverse decubitus image of liver, gallbladder *(gb)*, inferior vena cava *(IVC)*, and aorta *(A)*. **F,** Transverse image of liver *(L)*, gallbladder *(gb)*, and right kidney *(RK)*.

of the liver. The overall gain should be adjusted to provide a uniform homogeneous liver parenchyma throughout. If too many echoes are seen "outside the liver," the overall gain should be decreased. If the near gain or TGC is set too low, the anterior surface of the liver will not be delineated. The liver should be evaluated for focal and/or diffuse abnormalities. The vascular structures within the liver should be well demonstrated to include the hepatic veins, main portal vein with right and left branches, and inferior vena cava. The right, left, and caudate hepatic lobes should be demonstrated. The right hemidiaphragm and pleural space may be seen posterior to the right lobe of the liver with steep cephalic angulation of the transducer.

In addition to the supine views, the gallbladder and biliary system will require additional oblique, decubitus, and upright views to demonstrate the anatomy (Figure 6-15). It is critical that the patient be on nothing-by-mouth status for at least 8 hours before the examination to permit adequate distention

of the normally functioning gallbladder. Intrahepatic ducts may be evaluated by obtaining images of the liver and portal veins. The intrahepatic ducts may be evaluated by obtaining views of the liver demonstrating the right and left branches of the portal vein; these ducts are not well seen until they are dilated.

All areas of the pancreas should be evaluated (head, body, tail). The distal common bile duct in the pancreatic head should also be evaluated—this is best seen on the transverse view (Figure 6-16). If the pancreas is not clearly seen, oral contrast agents or water may be administered to provide better visualization.

The aorta, inferior vena cava, and other vascular structures should be well seen anterior to the vertebral column as echo-free, or anechoic, structures (Figure 6-17). The aorta is usually found as the pulsatile vessel slightly to the left of midline. The inferior vena cava is found slightly to the right of midline and varies with inspiration and expiration.

The spleen and flow velocities in the splenic vein and artery should be assessed with the patient in a steep decubitus position. The parenchyma of the spleen may be compared with the echogenicity of the left kidney (Figure 6-18). With deep inspiration, the sonographer should be able to see the movement of the diaphragm and the left pleural space.

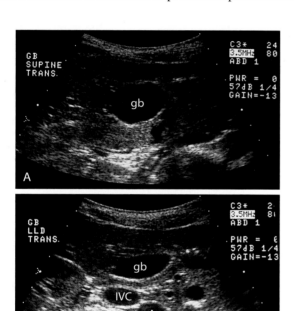
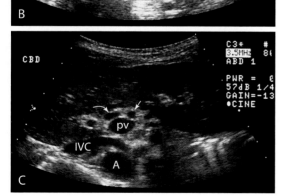

FIGURE 6-15 A, Transverse image of gallbladder (gb). **B,** Transverse decubitus image of gallbladder (gb), inferior vena cava (IVC), and aorta (A). **C,** Transverse image of portal triad in the center of the image; portal vein (pv) with common bile duct (curved arrow) anterior and lateral; hepatic artery (arrow) anterior and medial, inferior vena cava (IVC), and aorta (A).

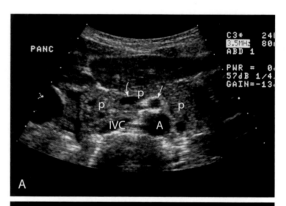
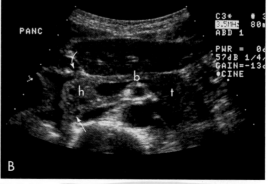

FIGURE 6-16 A, Transverse image of pancreas (p) as it lies anterior to superior mesenteric artery (arrow) and vein (curved arrow). The aorta (A) and inferior vena cava (IVC) are anterior to the horseshoe shape of the spine. **B,** Transverse image of head (h), body (b), and tail (t) of the pancreas. The gastroduodenal artery (curved arrow) is the anterolateral border of the head; the common bile duct (arrow) is the posterolateral border of the head.

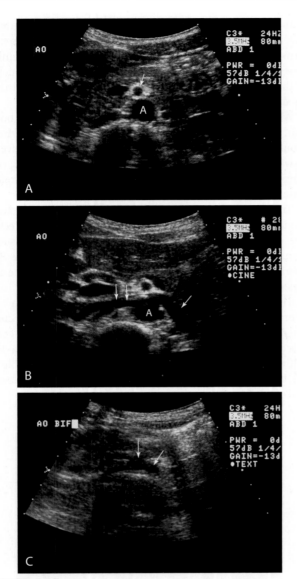

FIGURE 6-17 A, Transverse image of the high abdominal aorta *(A)* at the level of the superior mesenteric artery *(arrow).* **B,** Transverse image of the midabdominal aorta *(A)* at the level of the renal vessels (left renal artery—*one arrow;* right renal artery—*two arrows).* **C,** Transverse image of the distal aorta at the bifurcation *(arrows).*

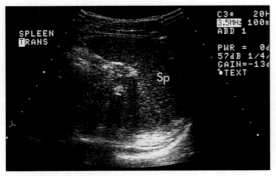

FIGURE 6-18 Transverse image of spleen *(Sp).*

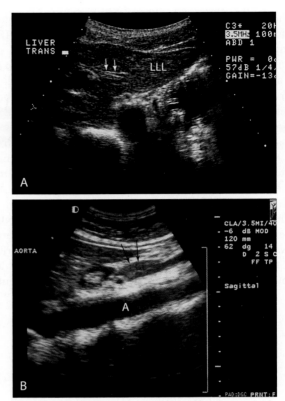

FIGURE 6-19 A, Transverse image of the left lobe of liver *(LLL)* and left portal vein *(arrows).* The air-filled stomach *(St)* is seen posterior and lateral to the left lobe of the liver. **B,** Longitudinal image of the body of the pancreas *(arrows)* anterior to the aorta *(A).* The bull's-eye target represents the antrum of the stomach, superior to the pancreas and anterior to the aorta *(curved arrow).*

The sonographer should be aware of the fluid-filled stomach, antrum of the stomach, and duodenum in the left upper quadrant (Figure 6-19). Bowel structures may be evaluated for wall thickening, dilation, hypertrophy, or other pathology. Normal bowel should compress with gentle pressure. The sonographer may note peristalsis within the bowel.

The kidneys, adrenals, and urinary bladder are well imaged with ultrasound. The renal cortex and renal pelvis should be assessed, and the renal length recorded. Doppler velocities of the renal vascular structures may be assessed to identify stenosis or thrombosis (Figure 6-20). The patient may be rolled into a decubitus or prone position to better image the kidneys.

Longitudinal Scans

All of the anatomic structures (liver and vascular structures, gallbladder, pancreas, kidneys, aorta, inferior vena cava, spleen, and gastrointestinal organs) visualized in the transverse views should also be demonstrated in the longitudinal plane. To obtain the longitudinal plane, the transducer should be rotated 90 degrees.

The diaphragm should be well defined as a linear bright line superior to the dome of the liver (Figure 6-21). The liver parenchyma should be homogeneous and uniform throughout, except for the anechoic portal and hepatic veins. The liver should

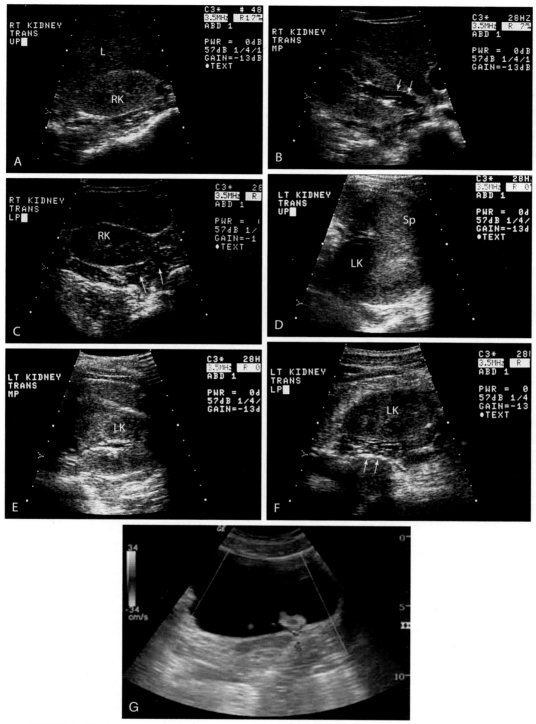

FIGURE 6-20 A, Transverse image of upper pole of right kidney *(RK);* liver *(L).* **B,** Transverse image of middle of right kidney with the renal vein *(arrows).* **C,** Transverse image of lower pole of right kidney *(RK).* The psoas muscle is medial to the kidney *(arrows).* **D,** Transverse image of upper pole of left kidney *(LK)* and spleen *(Sp).* **E,** Transverse image of middle of left kidney *(LK).* **F,** Transverse image of lower pole of left kidney *(LK)* and psoas muscle *(arrows).* **G,** Transverse image of full urinary bladder with color flow of ureteral jets.

be imaged from the midline to the far right lateral border. The curved array transducer will display the greatest area of the liver. To image the liver completely, the probe should be placed in the midline below the xyphoid process and slowly angled toward the right lobe of the liver as the patient takes in a deep breath (Figure 6-22). If the gain is adjusted to maximum without adequate uniform penetration, a lower frequency setting may be selected to provide increased sensitivity. The larger vascular structures (aorta and inferior vena cava) should be well outlined as hollow tubular structures with the patient in deep inspiration.

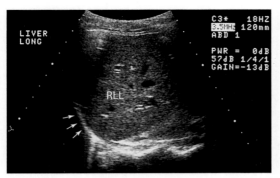

FIGURE 6-21 Longitudinal image of lateral segment of the right lobe of liver *(RLL)* and vascular structures; diaphragm *(arrows)*.

The abdominal aorta and inferior vena cava may be demonstrated in their long axis with the probe in the midline of the abdomen. A slight angulation to the patient's left will demonstrate the pulsatile abdominal aorta, with the anterior branches of the celiac artery and superior mesenteric artery (Figure 6-23). With the patient in deep inspiration, the transducer should be angled slightly to the patient's right of the midline to demonstrate the inferior vena cava as it drains the lower abdomen to empty into the right atrium of the heart (Figure 6-24).

The gallbladder and common bile duct may be seen in the right upper quadrant of the abdomen with the patient in deep inspiration (Figure 6-25). The portal vein serves as a useful posterior landmark to locate the common bile duct.

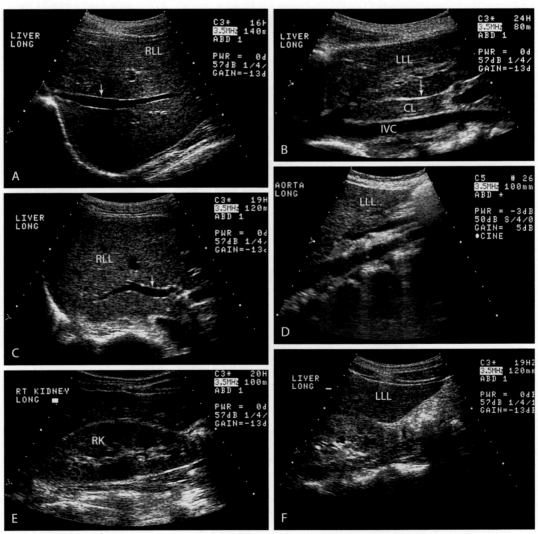

FIGURE 6-22 A, Longitudinal image of right lobe of liver *(RLL)* and right hepatic vein *(arrow)*. This long-axis view is used to measure the long axis of the liver from the diaphragm to the tip. **B,** Longitudinal image of left lobe of liver *(LLL)*, caudate lobe *(CL)*, ligamentum venosum *(arrow)*, and inferior vena cava *(IVC)*. **C,** Longitudinal oblique image of right lobe of liver *(RLL)* and right portal vein *(arrow)*. **D,** Longitudinal image of tip of left lobe of liver *(LLL)*. **E,** Longitudinal image of right kidney *(RK)*. **F,** Longitudinal image of left lobe of liver *(LLL)*.

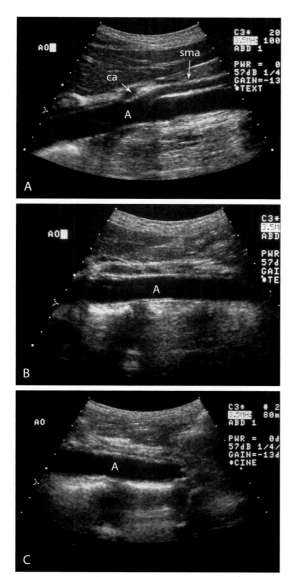

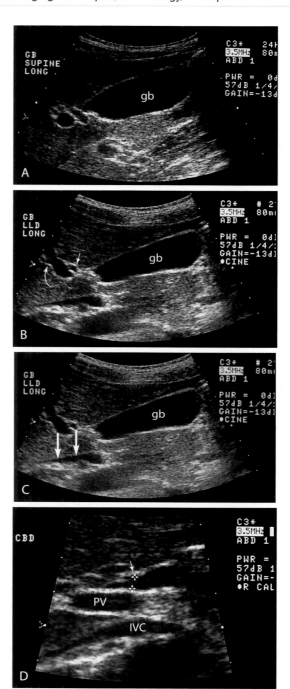

FIGURE 6-23 A, Longitudinal image of the aorta *(A)* with celiac axis *(ca)* and superior mesenteric artery *(sma)*. **B,** Longitudinal image of the proximal aorta *(A)* anterior to the spine. **C,** Longitudinal image of the distal aorta *(A)*.

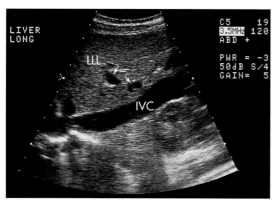

FIGURE 6-24 Longitudinal image of left lobe of liver *(LLL),* portal vein *(arrows),* and inferior vena cava *(IVC).*

FIGURE 6-25 A, Longitudinal image of gallbladder *(gb),* including neck. **B,** Longitudinal image of gallbladder *(gb),* main lobar fissure *(arrow),* and portal vein *(curved arrow).* **C,** Longitudinal image of the pancreas (posterior to the gallbladder) with the common bile duct *(arrows)* beginning to move posterior to join the pancreatic duct. **D,** Longitudinal image of common bile duct *(arrow)* anterior to portal vein *(PV)* that lies anterior to the inferior vena cava *(IVC).*

The right and left kidneys are demonstrated anterior to the psoas muscle along the flanks of the midabdomen with the patient in deep inspiration (Figure 6-26). The entire organ should be demonstrated on the sonogram. The homogeneous spleen is anatomically found lateral to the upper pole of the left kidney. Occasionally this structure may be seen with the

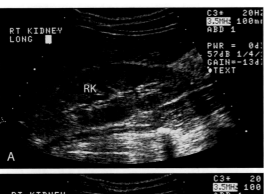

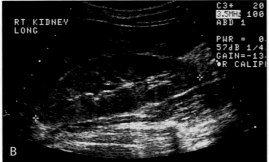

FIGURE 6-26 A, Longitudinal image of right kidney *(RK)*. **B,** Longitudinal image of left kidney *(LK)* with measurement of long axis.

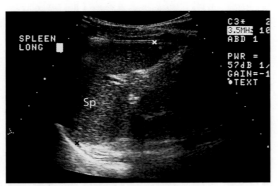

FIGURE 6-27 Longitudinal image of spleen *(Sp)*. The long axis is measured from the crossbars.

patient in a supine position; however, the best image is with the patient in a steep lateral position on an echo bed with a drop-down door so the sonographer may image the spleen from the inferior border of the spleen to the upper border/diaphragm interface (Figure 6-27).

ABDOMINAL DOPPLER

Doppler ultrasound has been used for many decades to evaluate cardiovascular flow patterns. As in other areas of ultrasound, many improvements have been made to the technology, such as the development of pulsed wave Doppler, spectral analysis of the returning waveform, power Doppler, and color flow mapping. These advances in Doppler instrumentation, combined with high-resolution imaging of the vessels, have led to "duplex scanning equipment," which combines these modalities into a single probe.

Doppler is used to ascertain the presence or absence of flow. It can be used to differentiate vessels from nonvascular structures with confusingly similar images (e.g., common duct from hepatic artery, arterial aneurysm from a cyst). The determination and direction of flow may also be of diagnostic value. Once the presence and direction of flow have been determined, spectral analysis of the flow gives further information on flow velocity and turbulence. Increased velocity and post-stenotic turbulence may be seen in vascular stenosis. In postoperative patients, increased turbulence alone may be present at the site of a graft anastomosis with the native vessel. Evaluation of the shape of the waveform, with comparison of the systolic and diastolic components, may yield information on increased vascular impedance, as is seen in renal transplant rejection. Doppler may also be useful in determining whether a mass is vascular or avascular.

Doppler Scanning Techniques

Normal routine longitudinal, transverse, coronal, and oblique scans of vascular structures are used to produce adequate images. Doppler techniques supplement the routine examination by permitting blood flow within those vessels to be detected and characterized. Flow toward the transducer is positive, or above baseline, whereas flow away from the transducer is negative, or below baseline (Figure 6-28). Arterial flow pulsates with the cardiac cycle and shows its maximal peak during the systolic part of the cycle. Venous flow shows no pulsatility and has lower flow velocity than arterial structures. A phasic pattern may be seen in the hepatic veins (near the heart) that is associated with overload of the right ventricle.

As seen in echocardiography, many abdominal vessels have characteristic waveforms. If the sample volume can be directed parallel to the flow, quantification of peak gradients can be estimated. However, given the tortuous course of most abdominal vascular structures, this can be very difficult in the abdomen.

Pulsed wave (PW) Doppler is the most common instrumentation used to evaluate the lower-velocity abdominal flow patterns. PW Doppler allows placement of the small sample volume within the vascular structure of interest by means of a trackball movement. If the velocities are lower than 3 m/sec and the probe is parallel to the vascular flow profile, accurate hemodynamic information may be obtained.

Aorta

- Doppler flow in the pulsatile aorta demonstrates arterial signals in the patent lumen. If the vessel were occluded, no arterial signals would be recorded (Figure 6-29).
- Aortic dissection and pseudoaneurysms: Flow, often with two distinct patterns, can be seen in the true and false lumens by Doppler ultrasound. The development of a pseudoaneurysm as a complication of an aortic graft procedure may be difficult to determine if pulsations are present or transmitted through the aortic wall. Doppler ultrasound may be useful to detect flow within the pseudoaneurysm.

Inferior Vena Cava and Hepatic Vein

- Decreased velocity: The Doppler waveform recorded in the inferior vena cava and hepatic veins shows a lower flow than is found in arterial structures. The flow is increased in the presence of thrombus formation (Figure 6-30).

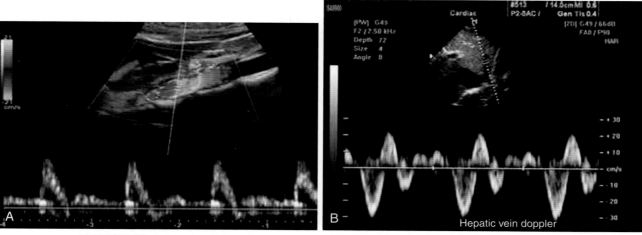

FIGURE 6-28 **A,** Doppler tracing of the abdominal aorta demonstrates a high systolic peak with a relatively low diastolic component on the spectral tracing. **B,** Pulsed wave (PW) Doppler tracing of the middle hepatic vein shows a continuous undulating low-flow profile representing blood flow from the hepatic vein into the inferior vena cava.

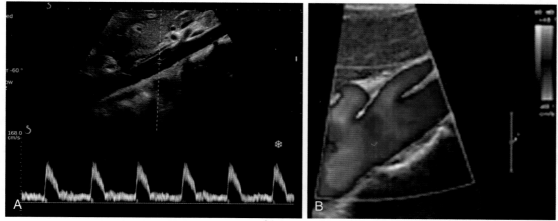

FIGURE 6-29 **A,** The sample volume is placed in the midabdominal aorta to record the Doppler velocity profile. The flow is positive, above the baseline. There is a high systolic component and a small diastolic component. **B,** Color Doppler of the abdominal aorta, celiac trunk, and superior mesenteric artery.

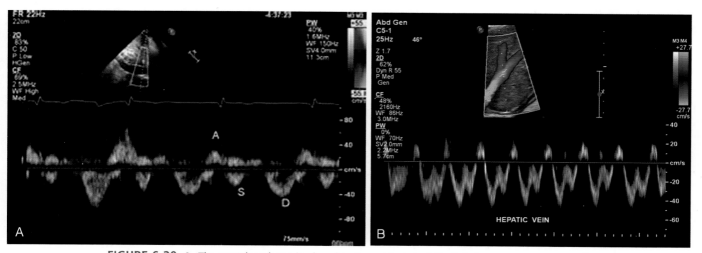

FIGURE 6-30 **A,** The sample volume is placed in the midpoint of the inferior vena cava to record a small atrial reversal (A), a systolic component (S), and a diastolic component (D). **B,** A similar flow pattern is noted in the hepatic veins.

Portal Venous System

- Doppler flow patterns can be used to diagnose varices or collaterals in the **portal venous system** (Figure 6-31).
- Doppler flow patterns can be used to evaluate changes in flow patterns that occur in the course of portal hypertension.
- As liver function improves, normal hepatopetal flow is restored.
- If pressures worsen, shunting away from the liver may be increased.
- If a shunt is present in the porta hepatis, Doppler may be useful to determine the patency of the shunt.

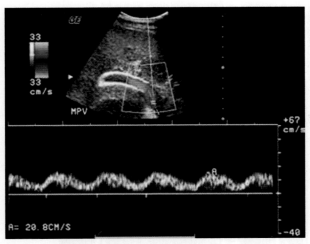

FIGURE 6-31 The sample volume is placed in the portal vein. Venous flow shows no pulsatility and has lower flow velocity than arterial structures.

 Key Pearls

- Know all of the ultrasound equipment in your laboratory and understand the knobology.
- Know where the operator's manuals are for each piece of equipment so you may have a reference for troubleshooting.
- Know the protocols for each examination.
- Understand how to read the patient order, find out what question the ordering physician needs to have answered, and know which items in the patient records are relevant for patient identification.
- Know the difference between curved array and sector array probes.
- Understand the transducer movements and how they may affect the image.
- Know the indications for abdominal sonography.
- Identify the ultrasound terminology and anatomic directions.
- Explain how to perform an initial survey of the abdomen.
- Identify the general protocol for an abdominal sonographic examination.
- Understand basic Doppler concepts, hemodynamics, and flow patterns within the abdominal vascular structures.

BIBLIOGRAPHY

American Institute of Ultrasound in Medicine: AIUM practice guideline for documentation of an ultrasound examination, *J Ultrasound Med* 33:2219-2224, 2014.

American Institute of Ultrasound in Medicine: Ultrasound examination of the abdomen and/or retroperitoneum, 2012. Available at www.aium.org.

Block B: *Color atlas of ultrasound anatomy*, New York, 2004, Thieme.

Curry R, Tempkin B: *Sonography: introduction to normal structure and function*, ed 3, St. Louis, 2010, Mosby.

Kremkau F: *Diagnostic ultrasound: principles and instruments*, ed 8, Philadelphia, 2011, Saunders.

Imaging and Doppler Artifacts*

Frederick W. Kremkau

OBJECTIVES

On completion of this chapter, you should be able to:
- List ways in which sonographic gray-scale images can present anatomic structures incorrectly
- List ways in which spectral and color Doppler displays can present motion and flow information incorrectly
- Describe how specific artifacts can be recognized
- Explain how artifacts can be handled to avoid the pitfalls and misdiagnoses that they can cause

OUTLINE

KEY TERMS

Aliasing
Comet tail
Enhancement
Grating lobes
Mirror-image artifact
Noise

Nyquist limit
Range ambiguity
Refraction
Resonance
Reverberation
Ring-down artifact

Section-thickness artifacts
Shadowing
Speckle
Speed error

In sonographic imaging, an artifact is the appearance of anything that does not properly present the structures or motion imaged. An artifact is caused by some problematic aspect of the imaging technique. Some artifacts are helpful. They should be used to advantage in the diagnostic imaging process. Others hinder proper interpretation and diagnosis. These artifacts must be avoided or handled properly when encountered.

Artifacts in sonography occur as apparent structures that are one or more of the following:
- Not real
- Missing

- Misplaced
- Of improper brightness, shape, or size

Some artifacts are produced by improper equipment operation or settings (e.g., incorrect gain and compensation settings). Others are inherent in the sonographic and Doppler methods and can occur even with proper equipment and technique.

PROPAGATION

The assumptions in the design of sonographic instruments are that sound travels in straight lines, that echoes originate from objects located on the beam axis, that the amplitudes of returning echoes are related directly to the echogenicity of the objects that produced them, and that the distance to echogenic objects is proportional to the round-trip travel

---

*This chapter is adapted from Forsberg F, Kremkau FW: Artifacts. Chapter 6 in Kremkau FW: *Sonography: principles and instruments*, ed 9, Philadelphia, 2016, WB Saunders.

time (13 μsec/cm of depth). If any of these assumptions is violated, an artifact occurs.

Section-Thickness Artifacts

Axial and lateral (detail) resolutions are artifactual because a failure to resolve means a loss of detail, and two adjacent structures may be visualized as one. These artifacts occur because the ultrasound pulse has finite length and width in the scan plane. Increasing frequency improves both resolutions, whereas focusing improves lateral (Figure 7-1, *A*). The beam width perpendicular to the scan plane (the third dimension in Figure 7-1, *B*) results in **section-thickness artifacts,** for example, the appearance of false debris in what should be echo-free areas (Figure 7-1, *C* and *D*). These artifacts occur because the interrogating beam has finite thickness as it scans through the patient. Echoes are received that originate not only from the center of the beam but also from off-center. These echoes are all collapsed into a thin (zero-thickness) two-dimensional image that is composed of echoes that have come from a not-so-thin tissue volume scanned by the beam. Section-thickness artifact is also called slice-thickness or partial-volume artifact.

Speckle

Apparent image resolution can be deceiving. The detailed echo pattern often is not related directly to the scattering properties of tissue (called *tissue texture*) but rather is the result of the interference effects of the scattered sound from the distribution of scatterers in the tissue. There are many scatterers in the ultrasound pulse at any instant as it travels through tissue. Their echoes can combine constructively or destructively. The result varies as the beam is scanned through the tissue, producing the pattern of bright and dark spots. This phenomenon is called acoustic **speckle** (Figure 7-2).

Reverberation

Multiple reflection, or **reverberation,** can occur between the transducer and a strong reflector (Figure 7-3). The multiple echoes may be sufficiently strong to be detected by the instrument and to cause confusion on the display (additional echoes that do not represent additional structures). The process by which they are produced is shown in Figure 7-3, *B*. This results in the display of additional reflectors that are not real (Figure 7-4). The multiple reflections are placed beneath the real reflector at separation intervals equal to the separation between the transducer and the real reflector. Each subsequent reflection is weaker than prior ones, but this diminution is counteracted at least partially by the attenuation compensation (time gain compensation [TGC]) function. Reverberations can also originate between two anatomic reflecting surfaces. When closely spaced, they appear in a form called *comet tail* (Figure 7-5, *A-I*).

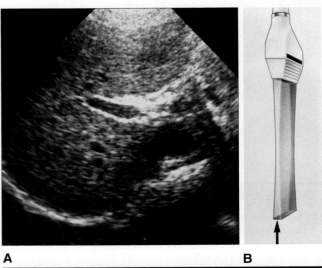

A   B

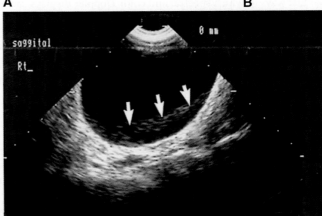

C

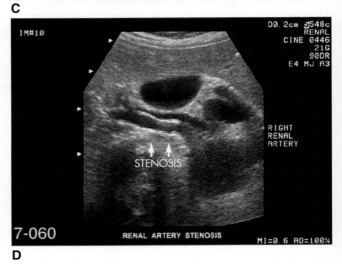

D

FIGURE 7-1 A, Without focusing, there is lateral smearing in this abdominal image. **B,** The scan "plane" through the tissue is really a three-dimensional volume. Two dimensions (axial and lateral) are in the scan plane, but there is a third dimension (called section thickness or slice thickness). The third dimension *(arrow)* is collapsed to zero thickness when the image is displayed in two-dimensional format. **C,** An ovarian cyst that should be echo-free has an echogenic region *(arrows)*. These off-axis echoes are a result of scan-plane section thickness. **D,** Section-thickness artifact appears as low-level echoes within hypoechoic structures.

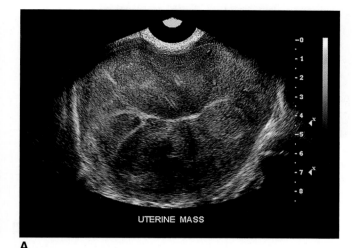

UTERINE MASS

A

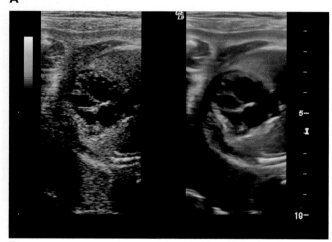

B

FIGURE 7-2 A, The typically grainy appearance of this ultrasound image is not primarily the result of detail resolution limitations but rather of speckle. Speckle is the interference pattern resulting from constructive and destructive interference of echoes returning simultaneously from many scatterers within the propagating ultrasound pulse at any instant. **B,** Approaches to speckle reduction (right image compared with the left) are implemented in modern instruments.

Comet tail, a particular form of reverberation, is a series of closely spaced, discrete echoes. Figure 7-6 shows an artifact that appears similar but is fundamentally different. Discrete echoes cannot be identified here because continuous emission of sound from the origin appears to be occurring. This continuous effect, termed **ring-down artifact,** is caused by a resonance phenomenon associated with the presence of a collection of gas bubbles. **Resonance** is the condition in which a driven mechanical vibration is of a frequency similar to a natural vibration frequency of the structure. The bubbles are stimulated into vibration by the incident ultrasound pulse. They then pulsate (expand and contract) for several cycles, acting as a source of ultrasound, producing a continuous stream of ultrasound that

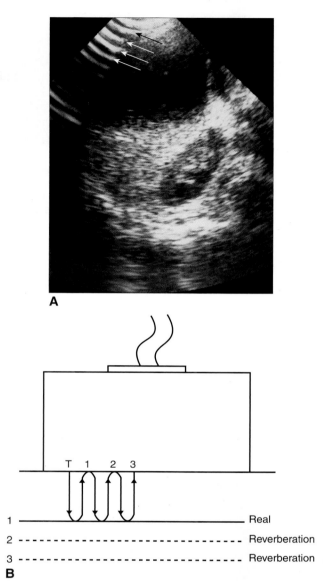

A

B

FIGURE 7-3 A, Reverberation artifact appearing as multiple presentations of a rib *(arrows).* **B,** The behavior in **A** is explained as follows: A pulse (T) is transmitted from the transducer. A strong echo is generated at the rib and is received *(1)* at the transducer, allowing correct imaging of the object. However, the echo is reflected partially at the transducer so that a second echo *(2)* is received, as well as a third (3) and possibly more. Because these echoes arrive later, they appear deeper on the display, where there are no reflectors. The lateral displacement of the reverberating sound path is for figure clarity. In fact, the sound travels down and back the same path repeatedly.

progresses distal to the bubble collection as the echo stream returns.

Mirror-Image Artifact

The **mirror-image artifact,** also a form of reverberation, shows structures that exist on one side of a strong reflector as being present on the other side as well. Figure 7-7 explains how this happens and shows examples. Mirror-image artifacts are

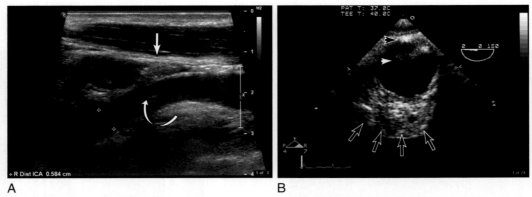

FIGURE 7-4 A, Reverberation *(curved arrow)* appearing in the carotid artery. This is a second echo from the proximal echogenic layer *(straight arrow).* **B,** Transesophageal scan of ascending a orta shows reverberation *(white arrowhead)* as the second echo from the proximal margin *(black arrowhead).* Enhancement *(arrows)* is also evident.

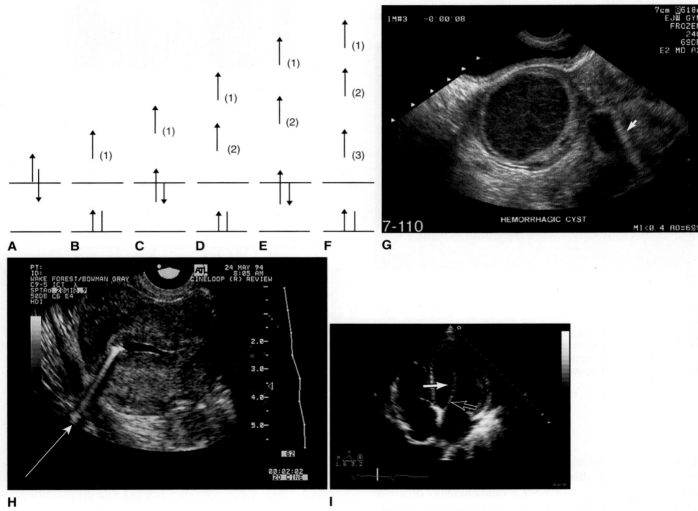

FIGURE 7-5 Generation of comet-tail artifact (closely spaced reverberations). Action progresses in time from left to right. **A,** An ultrasound pulse encounters the first reflector and is reflected partially and is transmitted partially. **B,** Reflection and transmission at the first reflector are complete. Reflection at the second reflector is occurring. **C,** Reflection at the second reflector is complete. Partial transmission and partial reflection are again occurring at the first reflector as the second echo passes through. **D,** The echoes from the first *(1)* and second *(2)* reflectors are traveling toward the transducer. A second reflection (repeat of **B**) is occurring at the second reflector. **E,** Partial transmission and reflection are again occurring at the first reflector. **F,** Three echoes are now returning—the echo from the first reflector *(1),* the echo from the second reflector *(2),* and the echo from the third reflector *(3)*—that originated from the back side of the first reflector **(C)** and reflected again from the second reflector **(D).** A fourth echo is being generated at the second reflector **(F). G,** Comet tail appears as a strong acoustic interface *(arrow)* from gas-filled bowel. **H,** Comet tail *(arrow)* from bubbles in an intrauterine saline injection. **I,** Apical four-chamber view of comet tail artifact *(top left arrow)* in the left ventricle. Artifact is connected to the anterior mitral leaflet *(lower right arrow).*

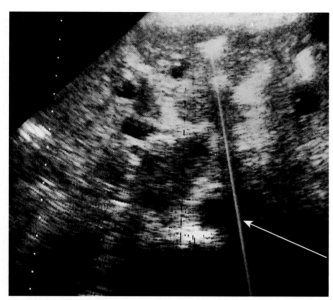

FIGURE 7-6   Ring-down artifact *(arrow)* from air in the bile duct.

common around the diaphragm and pleura because of the total reflection from air-filled lung. They occasionally occur in other locations (Figure 7-7, *C*). Sometimes the mirrored structure is not in the unmirrored scan plane.

Refraction

Refraction of light enables lenses to focus and distorts the presentation of objects, as shown in Figure 7-8. Refraction can cause a reflector to be positioned improperly (laterally) on a sonographic display (Figure 7-9). This is likely to occur, for example, when the transducer is placed on the abdominal midline (Figure 7-10), producing doubling of single objects. Beneath are the rectus abdominis muscles, which are surrounded by fat. These tissues present refracting boundaries because of their different propagation speeds.

Grating Lobes

Side lobes are beams that propagate from a single transducer element in directions different from the primary beam. **Grating lobes** are additional beams emitted from an array transducer that are stronger than the side lobes of individual elements (Figure 7-11). Side and grating lobes are weaker than the primary beam and normally do not produce echoes that are imaged, particularly if they fall on a normally echogenic region of the scan. However, if grating lobes encounter a strong reflector (e.g., bone or gas), their echoes may well be imaged, particularly if they fall within an anechoic region. If so, they appear in incorrect locations (Figure 7-12).

Speed Error

Propagation **speed error** occurs when the assumed value for propagation speed (1.54 mm/μsec, leading to the

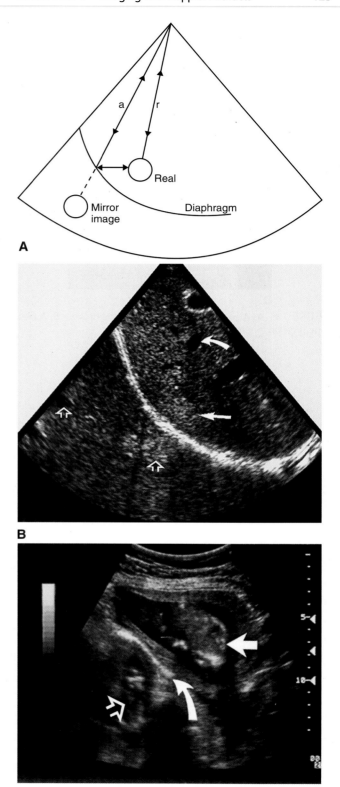

FIGURE 7-7   **A,** When pulses encounter a real hepatic structure directly (scan line *r*), the structure is imaged correctly. If the pulse first reflects off the diaphragm (scan line *a*) and the echo returns along the same path, the structure is displayed on the other side of the diaphragm. **B,** A hemangioma *(straight arrow)* and vessel *(curved arrow)* with their mirror images *(open arrows)*. **C,** A fetus *(straight arrow)* also appears as a mirror image *(open arrow)*. The mirror *(curved arrow)* is probably echogenic muscle.

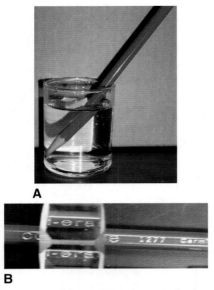

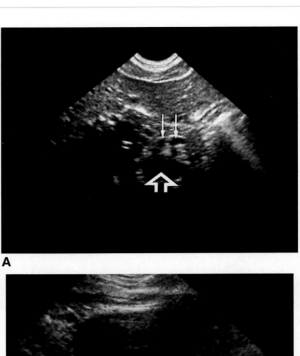

A

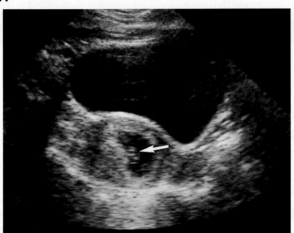

B

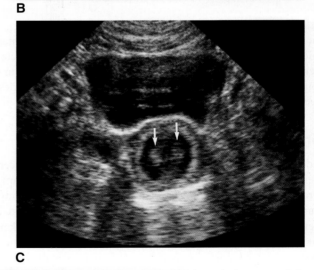

C

FIGURE 7-8 **A,** A pencil in water appears to be broken. **B,** A pencil beneath a prism appears to be split into two.

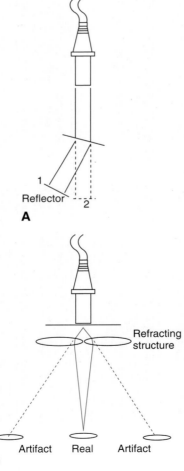

FIGURE 7-9 Refraction **(A)** results in improper positioning of a reflector on the display. The system places the reflector at position 2 (because that is the direction from which the echo was received) when in fact the reflector is actually at position 1. **B,** One real structure is imaged as two artifactual objects because of the refracting structure close to the transducer. If unrefracted pulses can propagate to the real structure, a triple presentation (one correct, two artifactual) will result.

FIGURE 7-10 **A,** Refraction (probably through the rectus abdominis muscle) has widened the aorta *(open arrow)* and produced a double image of the celiac trunk *(arrows).* Refraction may cause a single gestation **(B)** to appear as a double gestation **(C).**

13 μsec/cm round-trip travel-time rule) is incorrect. If the propagation speed that exists over a path traveled is greater than 1.54 mm/μsec, the calculated distance to the reflector is too small, and the display will place the reflector too close to the transducer (Figure 7-13). This occurs because

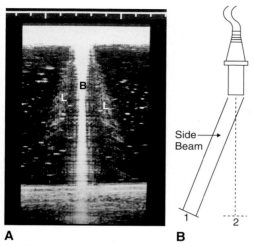

A   **B**

FIGURE 7-11 A, The primary beam *(B)* and grating lobes *(L)* from a linear array transducer. **B,** A side lobe or grating lobe can produce and receive a reflection from a "side view."

the increased speed causes the echoes to arrive sooner. If the actual speed is less than 1.54 mm/µsec, the reflector will be displayed too far from the transducer (Figure 7-14) because the echoes arrive later. Refraction and propagation speed error also can cause a structure to be displayed with incorrect shape.

Range Ambiguity

In sonographic imaging, it is assumed that for each pulse all echoes are received before the next pulse is emitted. If this were not the case, error could result (Figures 7-15 and 7-16). The maximum depth imaged correctly by an instrument is determined by its pulse repetition frequency (PRF). To avoid **range ambiguity,** PRF automatically is reduced in deeper imaging situations. This also causes a reduction in frame rate. Sometimes two artifacts combine to present even more challenging cases. An example involving range ambiguity is shown in Figure 7-17.

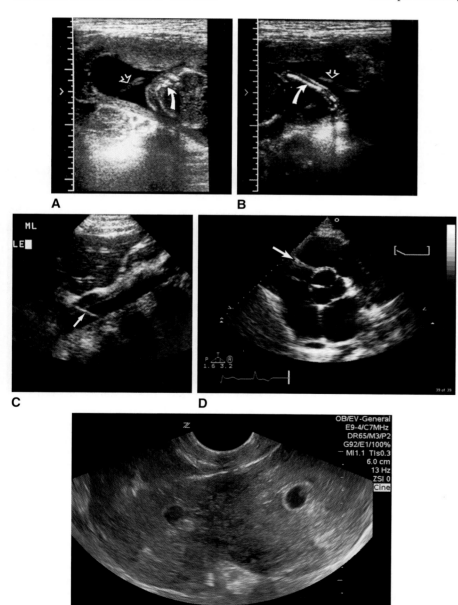

FIGURE 7-12 Grating lobes in obstetric scans can produce the appearance of amniotic sheets or bands. **A, B,** Grating lobe duplication *(open arrows)* of fetal bones *(curved arrows)* resembles amniotic bands or sheets. **C,** Artifactual grating lobe echoes *(arrow)* cross the aorta. **D,** Grating lobe *(arrow)* in the cardiac right ventricle. **E,** At first glance, this seems to be a mirror-image artifact, similar to what is seen in abdominal imaging (Figure 6-7). However, it is not for two reasons: (1) There is no apparent echogenic mirror. (2) The repeat on the left side is not horizontally reversed as would be the case with mirroring. Rather, it is a less echogenic repeat of what is on the right. Therefore this is grating-lobe duplication. Such duplications appear laterally and with less brightness than the correct presentation. (Part E courtesy David Bahner, MD, RDMS, Ohio State University, College of Medicine.)

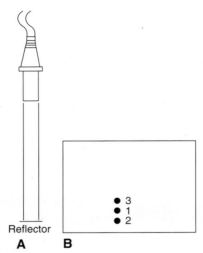

FIGURE 7-13 The propagation speed over the traveled path **(A)** determines the reflector position on the display **(B)**. The reflector is actually in position *1*. If the actual propagation speed is less than that assumed, the reflector will appear in position *2*. If the actual speed is more than that assumed, the reflector will appear in position *3*.

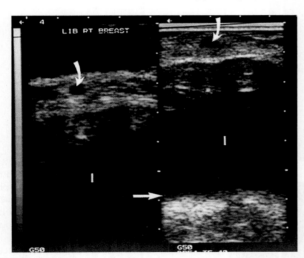

FIGURE 7-14 The low propagation speed in a silicone breast implant *(I)* causes the chest wall *(straight arrow)* to appear deeper than it should. Note that a cyst *(curved arrows)* is shown more clearly on the left image than on the right because a gel standoff pad has been placed between the transducer and the breast, moving the beam focus closer to the cyst.

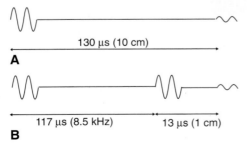

FIGURE 7-15 A, An echo (from a 10-cm depth) arrives 130 μsec after pulse emission. **B,** If the pulse repetition period were 117 μsec (corresponding to a pulse repetition frequency of 8.5 kHz), the echo in **A** would arrive 13 μsec after the next pulse was emitted. The instrument would place this echo at a 1-cm depth rather than the correct value. This range location error is known as the range-ambiguity artifact.

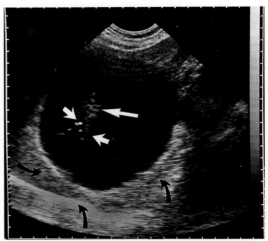

FIGURE 7-16 A large renal cyst (diameter about 10 cm) has artifactual range-ambiguity echoes within it *(white arrows)*. They are generated from structure(s) below the display. These deep echoes arrive after the next pulse is emitted. Because the time from the emission of the last pulse to echo arrival is short, the echoes are placed closer to the transducer than they should be. Echoes arrive from much deeper (later) than usual in this case because the sound passes through the long, low-attenuation paths in the cyst. These echoes may have come from bone or far body wall. Low attenuation in the cyst is indicated by the strong echoes (enhancement) below it *(curved black arrows)*.

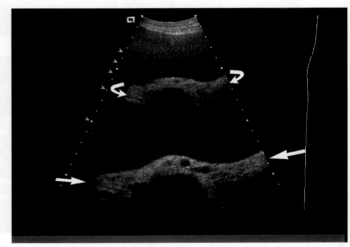

FIGURE 7-17 A large pelvic cyst produces a large echo-free region in this scan. A structure is located at a depth of about 13 cm *(straight arrows)*. Located in the anechoic region at a depth of about 6 cm is a structure *(curved arrows)* shaped like that at 13 cm. How could this artifact appear closer than the actual structure, implying that these echoes arrived earlier than those from the correct location? It turns out that the artifact is actually a combination of two phenomena: reverberation and range ambiguity. The artifact seen is a reverberation from the deep structure and the transducer. But a reverberation should appear at twice the depth of the actual structure—that is, at about 26 cm. However, the arrival of the reverberation echoes occurs about 78 μsec after the next pulse is emitted so that they are placed at a 6-cm depth. Single artifacts are difficult enough. Fortunately, combinations like this occur infrequently.

ATTENUATION

Another assumption in anatomic imaging is that the brightness (gray level) of the displayed echo is a proportional representation of the echogenicity of the object producing the echo. If this assumption is violated, echo strengths are presented improperly on the display. This artifact occurs primarily in two forms, shadowing and enhancement.

Shadowing

Shadowing is the reduction in echo amplitude from reflectors that lie behind a strongly reflecting or attenuating structure. A strongly attenuating or reflecting structure weakens the sound distal to it, causing echoes from the distal region to be weak and thus to appear darker, like a shadow. Of course, the returning echoes also must pass through the attenuating structure, adding to the shadowing effect. Examples of shadowing structures include calcified plaque, bone, and stone (Figure 7-18). Shadowing also can occur beyond the edges of objects that are not necessarily strong attenuators (Figure 7-19). In this case, the cause may be the defocusing action of a refracting curved surface. Alternatively, it may be attributable to destructive interference caused by portions of an ultrasound pulse passing through tissues with different propagation speeds and subsequently getting out of phase. In either case, the intensity of the beam decreases beyond the edge of the structure, causing echoes to be weakened.

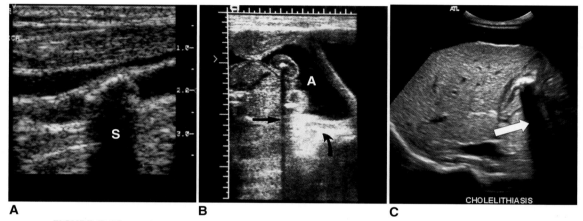

FIGURE 7-18 A, Shadowing from a high-attenuation calcified plaque in the common carotid artery. **B,** Shadowing *(straight arrow)* from a fetal limb bone and enhancement *(curved arrow)* caused by the low attenuation of amniotic fluid through which the ultrasound travels. **C,** Shadowing *(arrow)* from gallstones.

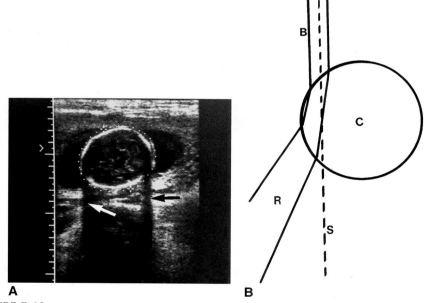

FIGURE 7-19 A, Edge shadows *(arrows)* from a fetal skull. **B,** As a sound beam *(B)* enters a circular region *(C)* of higher propagation speed, it is refracted, and refraction occurs again as it leaves. This causes spreading of the beam with decreased intensity. The echoes from region R are presented deep to the circular region in the neighborhood of the dashed line. Because of beam spreading, these echoes are weak and thus cast a shadow *(S)*.

Continued

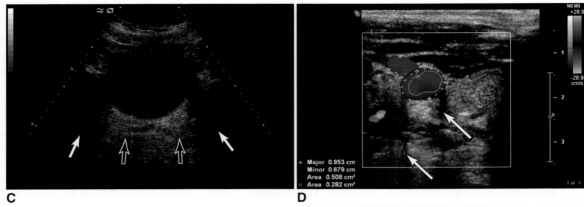

C **D**

FIGURE 7-19, cont'd C, Enhancement *(black arrows)* and edge shadows *(white arrows)* from pediatric bladder. **D,** Transverse carotid scan showing edge shadows *(arrows).*

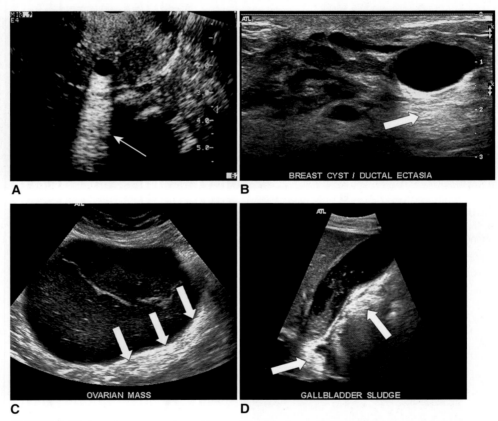

A **B**

BREAST CYST / DUCTAL ECTASIA

OVARIAN MASS

GALLBLADDER SLUDGE

C **D**

FIGURE 7-20 A, Enhancement *(arrow)* beyond a cervical cyst. **B** to **D,** Examples of enhancement *(arrows).*

Enhancement

Enhancement is the strengthening of echoes from reflectors that lie behind a weakly attenuating structure (Figure 7-20; also see Figures 7-16 and 7-18, *B*). Shadowing and enhancement result in reflectors being placed on the image with amplitudes that are too low and too high, respectively. Brightening of echoes also can be caused by the increased intensity in the focal region of a beam because the beam is narrow there. This is called *focal enhancement* or *focal banding* (Figure 7-21, *A*). Banding can also be caused by incorrect gain and TGC settings (Figure 7-21, *B*). Shadowing and enhancement are

often useful for determining the nature of masses and structures. Shadowing is reduced with spatial compounding because several approaches to each anatomic site are used, allowing the beam to "get under" the attenuating structure. This is useful with shadowing because it can uncover structures (especially pathologic ones) that were not imaged because they were located in the shadow.

Noise

Noise, generated internally or from external influences, also can produce artifacts (Figure 7-22).

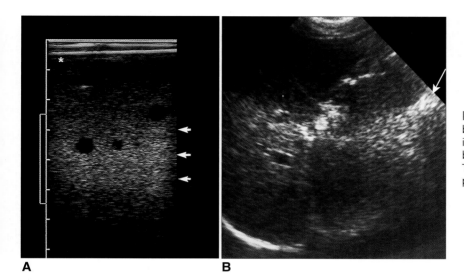

FIGURE 7-21 A, Focal banding *(arrows)* is the brightening of echoes around the focus, where intensity is increased by the narrowing of the beam. **B,** Banding *(arrow)* caused by incorrect TGC settings. The midfield gain is too high compared with near- and far-field gain.

Aliasing

Aliasing is the most common artifact encountered in Doppler ultrasound. The word *alias* comes from Middle English *elles,* Latin *alius,* and Greek *allos,* which mean *other* or *otherwise.* Contemporary meanings for the word include (as an adverb) *otherwise called* or *otherwise known as* and (as a noun) *an assumed or additional name.* Aliasing in its technical use indicates improper representation of information that has been sampled insufficiently. An optical form of temporal aliasing occurs in motion pictures when wagon wheels appear to rotate at various speeds and in reverse direction. Similar behavior is observed when a fan is lighted with a strobe light. Depending on the flashing rate of the strobe light, the fan may appear stationary or rotating clockwise or counterclockwise at various speeds.

Nyquist Limit

Pulsed wave Doppler instruments are sampling instruments. Each emitted pulse yields a sample of the desired Doppler shift. The upper limit to Doppler shift that can be detected properly by pulsed instruments is called the **Nyquist limit.** If the Doppler-shift frequency exceeds one half the PRF (which, for Doppler functions, is normally in the 5 to 30 kHz range), temporal aliasing occurs. Improper Doppler shift information (improper direction and improper value) results. Higher PRFs (Table 7-1) permit higher Doppler shifts to be detected but also increase the chance of the range-ambiguity artifact occurring. Continuous wave Doppler instruments do not experience aliasing, but neither do they provide depth localization. Figure 7-23 illustrates aliasing in the popliteal artery and in the heart of a normal subject. This figure also illustrates how aliasing can be corrected, reduced, or eliminated (Box 7-1) by increasing PRF, increasing Doppler angle (which decreases the Doppler shift for a given flow), or by *baseline shift.* The latter is an electronic cut-and-paste technique that moves the misplaced aliasing peaks over to their proper location. The technique is successful as long as there are no legitimate Doppler shifts in the region of the aliasing. If there are legitimate Doppler shifts, they will be moved over to an inappropriate location along with the aliasing

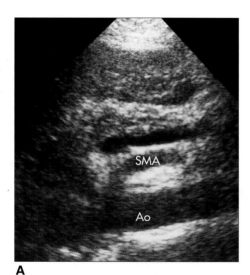

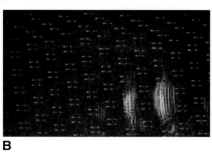

FIGURE 7-22 A, Noise is seen with "fill-in" of anechoic vascular structures. *Ao,* Aorta; *SMA,* superior mesenteric artery. **B,** Interference (repeating white specks) from nearby electronic equipment.

SPECTRAL DOPPLER

Several artifacts are encountered in Doppler ultrasound, yielding incorrect presentations of Doppler flow information, either in spectral or in color Doppler form. The most common of these is aliasing. Others include spectrum mirror image and those that also occur in anatomic imaging.

TABLE 7-1	Aliasing and Range-Ambiguity Artifact Values	
Pulse Repetition Frequency (kHz)	Doppler Shift Above Which Aliasing Occurs (kHz)	Range Beyond Which Ambiguity Occurs (cm)
5.0	2.5	15
7.5	3.7	10
10.0	5.0	7
12.5	6.2	6
15.0	7.5	5
17.5	8.7	4
20.0	10.0	3
25.0	12.5	3
30.0	15.0	2

In Figure 7-23, *A,* the vertical axis is calibrated in Doppler-shift frequency units so that we can see that aliasing occurs at Doppler shifts greater than 1.75 kHz. The aliased peaks add another 1.25 kHz of Doppler shift, so the correct peak systolic shift is 3 kHz. With the higher PRF in Figure 7-23, *C,* this result is confirmed. Thus at the lower PRF, the peak shift can be determined and baseline shifting is not necessary (but *is* convenient). However, if the peaks were buried in other portions of the Doppler signal (as in Figure 7-23, *H*), baseline shifting would not help, but a higher PRF (most convenient method), a larger Doppler angle, or a lower operating frequency would. Aliasing occurs with the pulsed system because it is a sampling system; that is, a pulsed system acquires samples of the desired Doppler shift frequency from which it must be synthesized. If samples are taken often enough, the correct result is achieved. Figure 7-24 shows temporal sampling of a signal. Sufficient sampling yields the correct result. Insufficient sampling yields an incorrect result.

peaks. (This would happen if the baseline were shifted farther down in Figure 7-23, *E.*) Baseline shifting is not helpful if the desired information (e.g., peak systolic Doppler shift) is buried in another portion of the spectral display, as in Figure 7-23, *H.* Other approaches to eliminating aliasing include changing to a lower-frequency Doppler transducer (Figure 7-23, *F* and *G*) or switching to continuous wave operation (Figure 7-23, *H* and *I*). The common and convenient solutions to aliasing are first shifting the baseline and then increasing PRF if necessary in extreme cases.

The Nyquist limit, or Nyquist frequency, describes the minimum number of samples required to avoid aliasing. At least two samples per cycle of the desired Doppler shift must be obtained for the image to be presented correctly. For a complicated signal, such as a Doppler signal containing many frequencies, the sampling rate must be such that at least two samples occur for each cycle of the highest frequency present. To restate this rule, if the highest Doppler-shift frequency

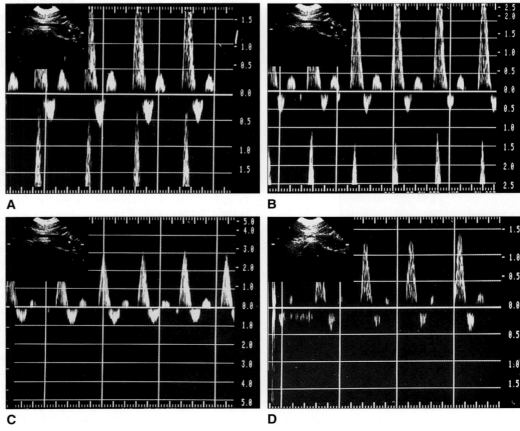

FIGURE 7-23 A, Aliasing in the popliteal artery. **B,** Pulse repetition frequency (PRF) is increased. **C,** The PRF is increased further. **D,** Doppler angle is increased with original PRF.

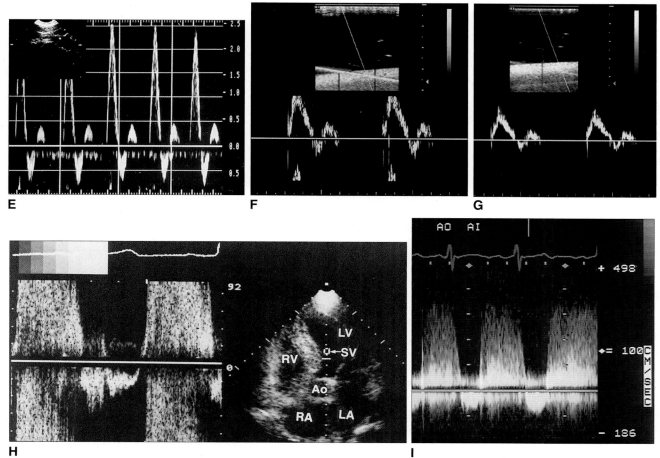

FIGURE 7-23, cont'd E, Baseline is shifted down with original PRF. **F,** Aliasing is occurring with an operating frequency of 6 MHz. **G,** When operating frequency is reduced to 4 MHz, the Doppler shifts are reduced to less than the Nyquist limit, thereby eliminating the aliasing seen in **F. H,** The sample volume *(SV)* is placed in the left-ventricular outflow tract. There is aortic insufficiency that causes the Doppler shifts to exceed the Nyquist limit producing aliasing. *Ao,* aorta; *LA,* left atrium, *LV,* left ventricle; *RA,* right atrium; *RV,* right ventricle. **I,** Using continuous wave *(CW)* ultrasound eliminates the aliasing because there is no sampling.

BOX 7-1	Methods of Correcting, Reducing, or Eliminating Aliasing

Shift the baseline.*
Increase the pulse repetition frequency.*
Increase the Doppler angle.
Use a lower operating frequency.
Use a continuous wave device.

*These are the most convenient and commonly used. Both are required in extreme cases.

present in a signal exceeds one half the PRF, aliasing will occur (see Figure 7-24).

Lesser-used correction methods include increasing the Doppler angle (which reduces the Doppler shift), reducing the operating frequency, and switching to continuous wave operation. Continuous wave operation, because it is not pulsed, is not a sampling mode, and is thus not subject to aliasing. However, it does not have range selectivity ability.

Range Ambiguity

In attempting to solve the aliasing problem by increasing the PRF, one can encounter the range-ambiguity problem. As described previously under the propagation group, this problem occurs when a pulse is emitted before all the echoes from the previous pulse have been received. When this happens, early echoes from the last pulse are received simultaneously with late echoes from the previous pulse. The instrument is unable to determine whether an echo is an early one (superficial) from the last pulse or a late one (deep) from the previous pulse. To solve this difficulty, the instrument simply assumes that all echoes are derived from the last pulse and that these echoes have originated from depths determined by the 13 μsec/cm rule. As long as all echoes are received before the next pulse is sent out, this is true. However, with high PRFs, this may not be the case. Doppler flow information therefore may come from locations other than the assumed one (the gate location). In effect, multiple gates or sample volumes are operating at different depths. Table 7-1 lists, for various PRFs, the ranges beyond which ambiguity occurs. Multiple sample volumes are shown on the display to indicate this condition.

FIGURE 7-24 In this spectral display, the presentation above the baseline is correct (unaliased, five samples per cycle), whereas the systolic peaks appear incorrectly below the baseline (aliased, one sample per cycle).

Mirror Image

A mirror image of a Doppler spectrum can appear on the opposite side of the baseline when, indeed, flow is unidirectional and should appear only on one side of the baseline. This is an electronic duplication of the spectral information. The duplication can occur when Doppler gain is set too high, causing overloading in the amplifier and leakage, called *crosstalk,* of the signal from the proper-direction channel into the opposite-direction channel (Figure 7-25).

Noise

Doppler spectra have a speckle quality to them that is similar to that observed in sonography. Internally generated electronic noise appears if Doppler gain is set too high (Figure 7-26, *A*).

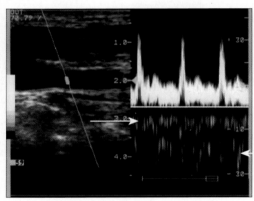

FIGURE 7-25 High gain produces a mirror image *(arrows)* of the carotid artery spectrum below the baseline.

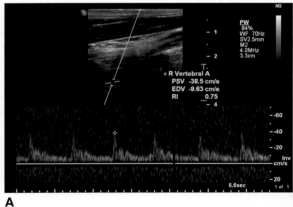

A

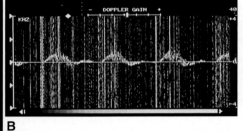

B

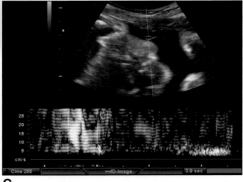

C

FIGURE 7-26 A, Doppler gain is set too high, causing noise to appear on the spectral display. **B,** Interference from nearby electrical equipment clouds the spectral display with electric noise (the vertical "snow" lines). **C,** Interference (wavy horizontal lines in the spectral display) from an external source.

Electromagnetic interference from nearby equipment can cloud the spectral display with lines or "snow" (Figure 7-26, *B* and *C*).

COLOR DOPPLER

Artifacts observed with color Doppler imaging are two-dimensional color presentations of artifacts that are seen in gray-scale sonography and Doppler spectral displays. They are incorrect presentations of two-dimensional motion information, the most common of which is aliasing. However,

others occur, including anatomic mirror image, Doppler angle effects, shadowing, and clutter.

Aliasing

Aliasing occurs when the Doppler shift exceeds the Nyquist limit (Figure 7-27). The result is incorrect flow direction on the color Doppler image (Figure 7-28). Increasing the flow speed range (which is actually an increase in PRF) can solve the problem (Figure 7-29). However, too high a range can

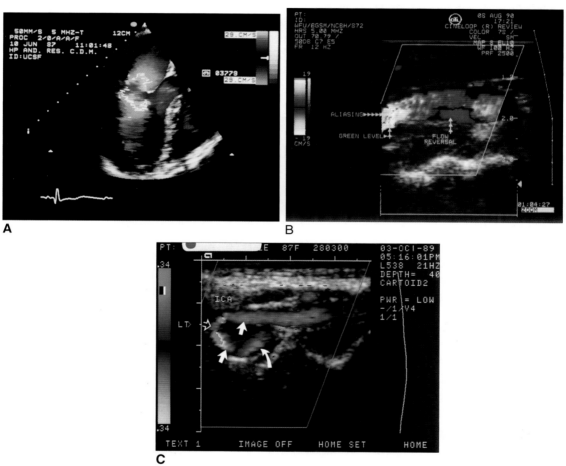

FIGURE 7-27 A, A transesophageal cardiac color Doppler image of the long axis in diastole. The blue colors in the left atrium *(upper)* and left ventricle *(lower)* represent blood traveling away from the transducer, but where the flow speeds exceed the Nyquist limit (29 cm/sec), aliasing occurs and the yellow and orange colors have replaced the blue colors. **B,** Color Doppler presentation of common carotid artery flow, including flow reversal and aliasing. The two can be distinguished because the boundary between the different directions with flow reversal passes through the baseline *(black),* whereas the aliasing boundary passes through the upper and lower extremes of the color bar *(white).* In this particular color bar assignment, the maximum positive Doppler shifts are assigned the color green, so that a thin green region shows the exact boundary where aliasing occurs. The aliasing occurs in the distal portion of the vessel because it is curving down, reducing the Doppler angle between the flow and the scan lines. **C,** In a tortuous internal carotid artery, negative Doppler shifts are indicated in the red regions *(solid straight arrows).* Two regions of positive Doppler shifts *(blue)* are seen *(open arrow* and *curved arrow).* In the latter, legitimate flow toward the transducer is indicated. In the former, the flow away from the transducer has yielded high Doppler shifts (because of a small Doppler angle; i.e., flow is approximately parallel to scan lines), which produces a color shift to the opposite side of the map because of aliasing. The boundaries from and to normal negative Doppler shifts into and out of the aliased region are bright yellow and cyan from the ends of the color bars. The transition from unaliased negative Doppler shift into unaliased positive Doppler shift (near bottom) is black, representing the baseline of the color bar. The flow direction is counterclockwise.

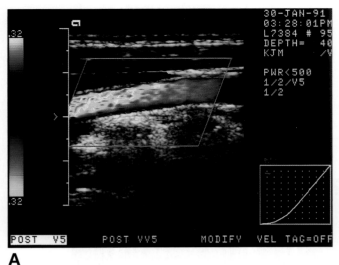

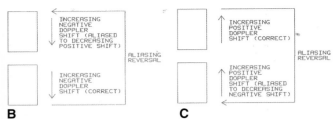

FIGURE 7-28 A, Positive *(blue)* Doppler shifts are shown in the arterial flow in this image. **B,** These are actually negative Doppler shifts that have exceeded the lower Nyquist limit (converted here to the equivalent flow speed: −0.32 m/sec) and are wrapped around to the positive portion of the color bar **(C).** Positive shifts that exceed the +0.32 m/sec limit would alias to the negative side.

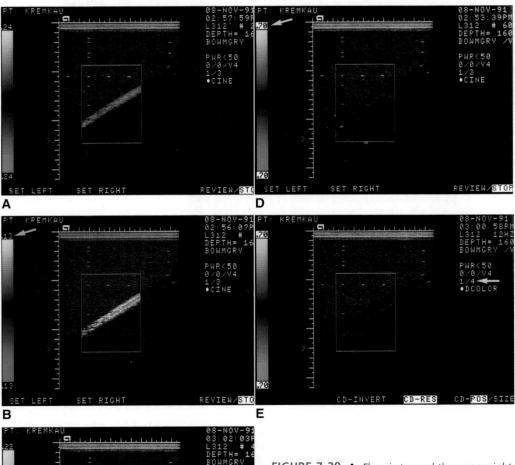

FIGURE 7-29 A, Flow is toward the upper right, producing positive Doppler shifts. **B,** The pulse repetition frequency and Nyquist limit (0.13, *arrow*) are too low, resulting in aliasing (negative Doppler shifts) at the center of the flow in the vessel. **C,** With the same pulse repetition frequency setting as in **B,** the aliasing has been corrected by shifting the baseline *(arrow)* down 10 cm/sec below the center of the color bar. **D,** The Nyquist limit setting (0.70, *arrow*) is too high, causing the detected Doppler shifts to be well down the positive scale, producing a dark red appearance. **E,** With the Nyquist limit set as in **D,** an increase in the wall filter setting *(arrow)* eliminates what little color flow information there was in **D.**

cause loss of flow information, particularly if the wall filter is set high (Figure 7-29, *D* and *E*). Baseline shifting can decrease or eliminate the effect of aliasing (Figure 7-29, *C*), as in spectral displays.

Mirror Image, Shadowing, Clutter, and Noise

In the mirror (or ghost) artifact (Figure 7-30), an image of a vessel and source of Doppler-shifted echoes can be duplicated on the opposite side of a strong reflector (e.g., pleura or diaphragm). This is a color Doppler extension of gray-scale mirror. Shadowing is the weakening or elimination of Doppler-shifted echoes beyond a shadowing object, just as occurs with non–Doppler-shifted (gray-scale) echoes (Figure 7-31). Clutter results from tissue, heart wall or valve, or vessel wall motion (Figure 7-32). Such clutter is eliminated by wall filters. Doppler angle effects include zero Doppler shift when the Doppler angle is 90 degrees, as

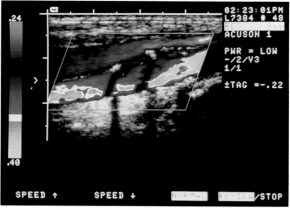

FIGURE 7-31 Shadowing from calcified plaque follows the gray-scale scan lines straight down while following the angled color scan lines parallel to the sides of the parallelogram.

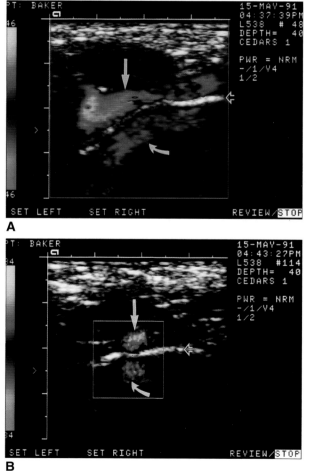

FIGURE 7-30 Color Doppler imaging of the subclavian artery *(straight arrow)* in longitudinal **(A)** and transverse **(B)** views. The pleura *(open arrow)* causes the mirror image *(curved arrow)*.

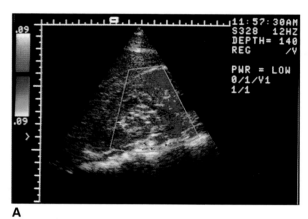

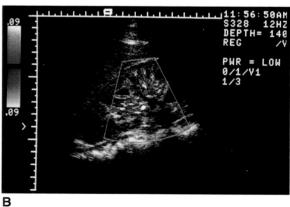

FIGURE 7-32 A, Clutter from tissue motion (caused by respiration) obscures underlying blood flow in the renal vasculature. **B,** An increased wall filter setting removes the clutter, revealing the underlying flow.

well as the change of color in a straight vessel viewed with a sector transducer. Noise in the color Doppler electronics can mimic flow, particularly in hypoechoic or anechoic regions (Figure 7-33). The "twinkling" artifact (Figure 7-34) has been observed at strongly reflecting scattering surfaces.

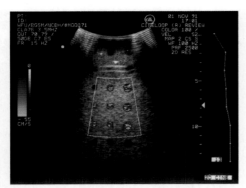

FIGURE 7-33 Color appears in echo-free (cystic) regions of a tissue-equivalent phantom. The color gain has been increased sufficiently to produce this effect. The instrument tends to write color information preferentially in areas where non–Doppler-shifted echoes are weak or absent.

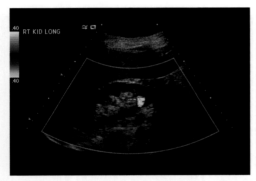

FIGURE 7-34 Twinkling artifact associated with a renal stone.

It is thought to occur with complications in the phase detection process of Doppler detection when a finite number of strong scatterers is encountered.

SUMMARY

This chapter has discussed several ultrasound imaging and flow artifacts, which are listed in Table 7-2, along with their causes. In some cases, the names of the artifacts are identical to their causes.

- Shadowing and enhancement are useful in interpretation and diagnosis.
- Other artifacts can cause confusion and error.
- Artifacts seen in two-dimensional imaging are evidenced in three-dimensional imaging also, sometimes in unusual ways.
- All of these artifacts can hinder proper interpretation and diagnosis and so must be avoided or handled properly when encountered.
- A proper understanding of artifacts and how to deal with them when they are encountered enables sonographers and sonologists to use them to advantage while avoiding the pitfalls that they can cause.

TABLE 7-2	Artifacts and Their Causes
Artifact	**Cause**
Axial resolution	Pulse length
Comet tail	Reverberation
Grating lobe	Grating lobe
Lateral resolution	Pulse width
Mirror image	Multiple reflection
Refraction	Refraction
Reverberation	Multiple reflection
Ring down	Resonance
Section thickness	Pulse width
Speckle	Interference
Speed error	Speed error
Range ambiguity	High pulse repetition frequency
Shadowing	High attenuation
Edge shadowing	Refraction or interference
Enhancement	Low attenuation
Focal enhancement	Focusing
Aliasing	Low pulse repetition frequency
Spectrum mirror	High Doppler gain

 Key Pearls

- An artifact is the appearance of anything that does not properly present the structures or motion imaged.
- An artifact is caused by some problematic aspect of the imaging technique.
- Axial and lateral (detail) resolutions are artifactual because a failure to resolve means a loss of detail, and two adjacent structures may be visualized as one.
- The beam width perpendicular to the scan plane results in section-thickness artifacts, for example, the appearance of false debris in what should be echo-free areas.
- The detailed echo pattern often is not related directly to the scattering properties of tissue (called tissue texture) but rather is the result of the interference effects of the scattered sound from the distribution of scatterers in the tissue.
- The multiple reflections are placed beneath the real reflector at separation intervals equal to the separation between the transducer and the real reflector.
- Comet tail, a particular form of reverberation, is a series of closely spaced, discrete echoes.
- Ring-down artifact is caused by a resonance phenomenon associated with the presence of a collection of gas bubbles.
- Resonance is the condition in which a driven mechanical vibration is of a frequency similar to a natural vibration frequency of the structure.
- The mirror-image artifact, also a form of reverberation, shows structures that exist on one side of a strong reflector as being present on the other side as well.
- Refraction can cause a reflector to be positioned improperly (laterally) on a sonographic display.

- Side lobes are beams that propagate from a single transducer element in directions different from the primary beam.
- Grating lobes are additional beams emitted from an array transducer that are stronger than the side lobes of individual elements.
- Propagation speed error occurs when the assumed value for propagation speed (1.54 mm/μsec, leading to the 13 μsec/cm round-trip travel-time rule) is incorrect.
- Shadowing is the reduction in echo amplitude from reflectors that lie behind a strongly reflecting or attenuating structure.
- Enhancement is the strengthening of echoes from reflectors that lie behind a weakly attenuating structure.
- Aliasing is the most common artifact encountered in Doppler ultrasound.
- The upper limit to Doppler shift that can be detected properly by pulsed instruments is called the Nyquist limit.
- The Nyquist limit, or Nyquist frequency, describes the minimum number of samples required to avoid aliasing.
- Clutter results from tissue, heart wall or valve, or vessel wall motion; such clutter is eliminated by wall filters.

BIBLIOGRAPHY

Aytac SK, Ozcan H: Effect of color Doppler system on the twinkling sign associated with urinary tract calculi, *J Clin Ultrasound* 27:433-439, 1999.

Campbell SC, Cullinan JA, Rubens DJ: Slow flow or no flow? Color and power Doppler US pitfalls in the abdomen and pelvis, *RadioGraphics* 24:497-506, 2004.

Forsberg F, Kremkau FW: *Artifacts.* Chapter 6 in Kremkau FW: Sonography: principles and instruments, ed 9, Philadelphia, 2016, WB Saunders.

Mitchell C, Pozniak M, Zagzebski J, Ledwidge M: Twinkling artifact related to intravesicular suture, *J Ultrasound Med* 22:1409-1411, 2003.

Mitchell DG, Burns P, Needleman L: Color Doppler artifact in anechoic regions, *J Ultrasound Med* 9:255-260, 1990.

Nelson TR et al: Sources and impact of artifacts on clinical three-dimensional ultrasound imaging, *Ultrasound Obstet Gynecol* 16:374-383, 2000.

Pozniak MA, Zagzebski JA, Seanlan KA: Spectral and color Doppler artifacts, *RadioGraphics* 12:25-44, 1992.

Rahmouni A, Bargoin R, Herment A, et al: Color-Doppler twinkling artifact in hyperechoic regions, *Radiology* 199:269-271, 1996.

Sanders RC: *Atlas of ultrasonographic artifacts and variants*, ed 2, St. Louis, 1992, Mosby.

Waldroup LD, Kremkau FW: Artifacts in ultrasound imaging. In Goldberg BB, editor: *Textbook of abdominal ultrasound*, Baltimore, 1993, Williams & Wilkins.

PART II

Abdomen

Vascular System

Sandra L. Hagen-Ansert

OBJECTIVES

On completion of this chapter, you should be able to:

- Describe the anatomy of the arterial system, venous system, and portal venous system
- Understand the function of the circulatory system
- Recognize the sonographic findings and pathology found in the vascular structures
- Define the two types of aneurysm formation
- Explain the factors that may cause development of an aneurysm

- Identify the sonographic findings in aortic dissection
- Identify causes of pseudopulsatile abdominal masses
- Explain the sonographic findings and complications in portal hypertension
- Describe the Doppler flow patterns in arterial versus venous structures

OUTLINE

KEY TERMS

Abdominal aortic aneurysm
Anastomosis
Aorta
Arteries
Arteriosclerosis
Arteriovenous fistula
Atherosclerosis
Capillaries
Cavernous transformation of the portal vein
Common hepatic artery
Common iliac arteries
Cystic medial necrosis
Dissecting aneurysm
Doppler sample volume
Fusiform aneurysm
Gastroduodenal artery

Hepatic veins
Hepatofugal
Hepatopetal
Inferior mesenteric artery
Inferior mesenteric vein
Inferior vena cava
Left gastric artery
Left hepatic artery
Left renal artery
Left renal vein
Marfan syndrome
Nonresistive
Portal vein
Portal venous hypertension
Pseudoaneurysm
Renal vein thrombosis
Resistive

Resistive index
Right gastric artery
Right hepatic artery
Right renal artery
Right renal vein
Saccular aneurysm
Spectral broadening
Splenic artery
Splenic vein
Superior mesenteric artery
Superior mesenteric vein
Tunica adventitia
Tunica intima
Tunica media
Vasa vasorum
Veins

Knowledge of the vascular structures within the abdomen, retroperitoneum, and pelvis is extremely useful to the sonographer as landmarks for the identification of specific organ structures. To understand the origin and anatomic variations of the major arterial and venous structures, the sonographer must be able to identify the anatomy correctly on the sonographic image.

FUNCTION OF THE CIRCULATORY SYSTEM

The function of the circulatory system, along with the heart and lymphatics, is to transport gases, nutrient materials, and other essential substances to the tissues, and subsequently to transport waste products from the cells to appropriate sites for excretion.

Blood is carried away from the heart by the arteries and is returned from the tissues to the heart by the veins. Arteries divide into progressively smaller branches, the smallest of which are the arterioles. These lead into the capillaries, which are minute vessels that branch and form a network where the exchange of materials between blood and tissue fluid takes place. After the blood passes through the capillaries, it is collected in the small veins, or venules. These small vessels unite to form larger vessels that eventually return the blood to the heart for recirculation.

A typical artery in cross section consists of the following three layers (Figure 8-1):

- **Tunica intima** (inner layer), which itself consists of the following three layers: a layer of endothelial cells lining the arterial passage (lumen), a layer of delicate connective tissue, and an elastic layer made up of a network of elastic fibers.
- **Tunica media** (middle layer), which consists of elastin, smooth muscle fibers, and collagenous tissue. The media provides the strength of the aorta. Unfortunately, elastin is produced only minimally in the body. Therefore with increasing age, the elastin production is lost.
- **Tunica adventitia** (external layer), which consists of loose connective tissue with bundles of smooth muscle fibers and elastic tissue, and carries nerves and the vaso vasorum. The **vasa vasorum** comprises the tiny arteries and veins that supply the walls of blood vessels.

Specific differences exist between the arteries and the veins. The **arteries** are hollow elastic tubes that carry blood away from the heart. They are enclosed within a sheath that includes a vein and a nerve. The smaller arteries contain less elastic tissue and more smooth muscles than the larger arteries. The elasticity of the larger arteries is important in maintaining a steady blood flow. The abdominal aorta will not change in diameter with changes in respiration; however, pulsation of blood flow that corresponds to the cardiac cycle will be noted.

The **veins** are hollow collapsible tubes with diminished tunica media that carry blood toward the heart. The veins appear collapsed because they have little elastic tissue or muscle within their walls. Veins have a larger total diameter

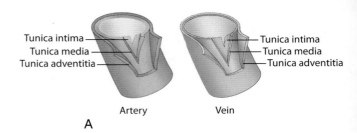

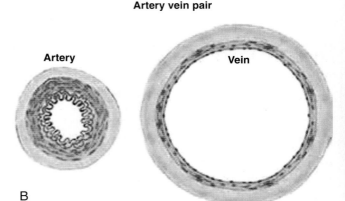

FIGURE 8-1 A, Cross section of an artery and vein showing the distinctions among the three layers of each vessel: tunica intima (inner layer), tunica media (middle layer), and tunica adventitia (external layer). **B,** Comparison between the artery and vein. Note the thin middle and inner layers of the vein compared with the artery.

than arteries, and they move blood more slowly. The veins contain special valves that prevent backflow and permit blood to flow in only one direction—toward the heart. Numerous valves are found within the extremities, especially the lower extremities, because flow must work against gravity. Venous return is also aided by muscle contraction, overflow from capillary beds, gravity, and suction from negative thoracic pressure. The sonographer may note that the inferior vena cava should dilate slightly with suspended respiration.

The **capillaries** are microscopic vessels just wide enough to let one red blood cell squeeze through. These tiny vessels connect the arterial and venous systems. Their walls have only one layer. The cells and tissues of the body receive their nutrients from fluids passing through the capillary walls; at the same time, waste products from the cells pass into the capillaries. Arteries do not always end in capillary beds; some end in anastomoses, which are end-to-end grafts between different vessels that equalize pressure over vessel length and provide alternative flow channels.

AORTA

The **aorta** is the largest principal artery of the body. It may be divided into the following five sections: (1) root of the aorta, (2) ascending aorta and arch, (3) descending aorta, (4) abdominal aorta and abdominal aortic branches, and (5) bifurcation of the aorta into iliac arteries (Figure 8-2).

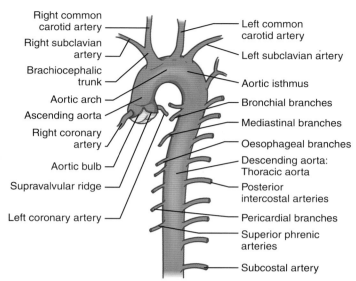

Right common carotid artery
Right subclavian artery
Brachiocephalic trunk
Aortic arch
Ascending aorta
Right coronary artery
Aortic bulb
Supravalvular ridge
Left coronary artery

Left common carotid artery
Left subclavian artery
Aortic isthmus
Bronchial branches
Mediastinal branches
Oesophageal branches
Descending aorta: Thoracic aorta
Posterior intercostal arteries
Pericardial branches
Superior phrenic arteries
Subcostal artery

FIGURE 8-2 The aorta is divided into five sections: the aortic root, the ascending aorta, the aortic arch (brachiocephalic artery, common carotid artery, and subclavian artery), the thoracic (descending) artery, and the abdominal aorta, with the bifurcation.

Root of the Aorta

The systemic circulation leaves the left ventricle of the heart by way of the aorta. The root of the aorta arises from the left ventricular outflow tract in the heart. The aortic root has three semilunar cusps that prevent blood from flowing back into the left ventricle. These cusps open with ventricular systole to allow blood to be ejected into the ascending aorta; the cusps are closed during ventricular diastole. The coronary arteries arise superiorly from the right and left coronary cusps to form the right and left coronary arteries, respectively. These coronary arteries further bifurcate to supply the vasculature of the cardiac structures. After the aorta arises from the left ventricle, it ascends posterior to the main pulmonary artery to form the ascending aorta.

Ascending Aorta

The ascending aorta arises a short distance from the ventricle and arches superiorly to form the aortic arch at the level of the sternoclavicular junction. Three arterial branches arise from the superior border of the aortic arch to supply the head, neck, and upper extremities: the brachiocephalic, left common carotid, and left subclavian arteries.

Descending Aorta

From the aortic arch, the aorta descends posteriorly along the back wall of the heart through the thoracic cavity, where it pierces the diaphragm to become the abdominal aorta. The descending (thoracic) aorta enters the abdomen through the aortic opening of the diaphragm anterior to the twelfth thoracic vertebra in the retroperitoneal space.

Abdominal Aorta

The abdominal aorta is the largest artery in the body that supplies blood to all visceral organs and to the legs. The aorta continues to flow in the retroperitoneal cavity anterior and slightly left of the vertebral column. The aorta lies posterior to the left lobe of the liver, the body of the pancreas, the gastroesophageal junction, the pylorus of the stomach, and the splenic vein (Figure 8-3). The diaphragmatic crura surrounds the proximal abdominal aorta as this vessel projects through the diaphragm into the abdominal cavity (Figure 8-4). Many branches arise from the abdominal aorta: the celiac axis, superior mesenteric, inferior mesenteric, renal, suprarenal, and gonadal arteries (Figure 8-5). At the level of the fourth lumbar vertebra (near the umbilicus), the aorta bifurcates into the right and left common iliac arteries. The aorta has four branches that supply other visceral organs and the mesentery: the celiac trunk, the superior and inferior mesenteric arteries, and the renal arteries.

The normal diameter of the abdominal aorta is evaluated at the region of the supraceliac and infrarenal locations. The diameter in men is slightly greater than in women. The proximal abdominal aorta tapers in size secondary to the three large branches (celiac, superior mesenteric, and renal arteries). In the supraceliac area, the aorta measures 2.5 to 2.7 cm in men and 2.1 to 2.3 cm in women. In the infrarenal area, the aorta measures 2.0 to 2.4 cm in men and 1.7 to 2.2 cm in women. There is gradual tapering to 1.1 to 1.5 cm in men and 1.1 to 1.3 cm in women at the bifurcation into the iliac arteries (Table 8-1). The size of the aorta will vary slightly according to body mass index; the larger the body size, the greater is the measurement of the aorta. It is also important to note that the aorta does change in size as one grows older; therefore an aorta in a younger adult measuring 1.8 cm may increase to 2.2 cm by the time the adult reaches 60 years of age.

Aorta and Iliac Artery Protocol

The aorta is examined primarily to determine the presence of aneurysmal dilation.
1. Patient preparation: nothing by mouth for at least 6 hours.
2. Transducer selection: 2.5 to 4 mHz curvilinear.
3. Patient position: supine or slightly decubitus.
4. Images and observations should include the following:
   - The aorta should be imaged in the longitudinal plane from the diaphragm to below the bifurcation at the iliac junction (Figure 8-6, *A–D*).
   - Transverse scans should be made at the level of the diaphragm, superior to the renal arteries, inferior to the renal arteries, and at the bifurcation. Scans of the iliac arteries should be made (Figure 8-6, *E–G*).
   - Lymphadenopathy should also be evaluated because the lymph nodes lie anterior to the vessels.
   - The inferior vena cava is best imaged on a longitudinal plane through the right lobe of the liver with the patient in full inspiration (Figure 8-7).
   - An alternative imaging plane is the slight decubitus view. The patient rolls onto his or her left side; the

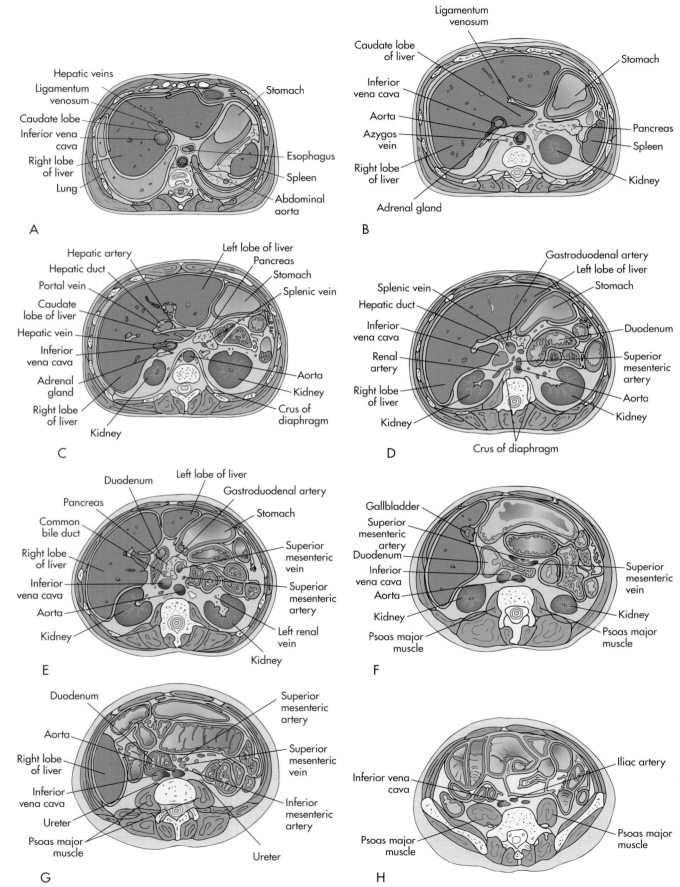

FIGURE 8-3 Multiple transverse sections through the abdominal cavity from the dome of the liver to the bifurcation of the aorta into the iliac arteries.

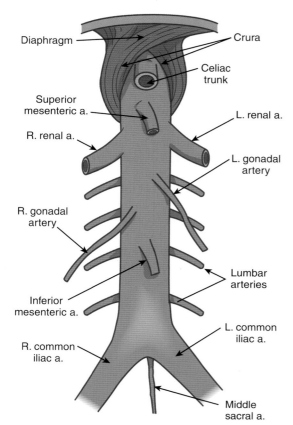

FIGURE 8-4 The abdominal aorta with multiple arterial branches. The diaphragmatic crura surrounds the proximal abdominal aorta as this vessel projects through the diaphragm into the abdominal cavity.

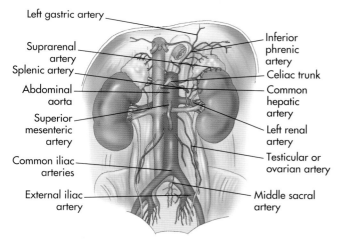

FIGURE 8-5 The abdominal arterial vascular system and its tributaries is shown in relation to the inferior vena cava.

transducer is longitudinal and is sharply angled from the right lobe of the liver to the left iliac wing. This allows the sonographer to image the inferior vena cava "anterior" to the aorta (Figure 8-8). This view usually allows the sonographer to perform a shallow sweep to follow the entrance and exit of the renal veins and arteries into the great vessels and provides an excellent

TABLE 8-1	Size of Abdominal Aorta and Iliac Branches	
	Men	**Women**
	Diameter	*Diameter*
Aorta supraceliac	2.5–2.7 cm	2.1–2.3 cm
Aorta infrarenal	2.0–2.4 cm	1.7–2.2 cm
Common iliac artery	1.1–1.5 cm	1.0–1.3 cm
Common femoral artery	0.9–1.2 cm	0.8–1.0 cm

window to perform color flow or Doppler interrogation of the renal vessels (Figure 8-9).

- Outer to outer measurements should be taken of the aorta in the longitudinal and transverse planes (Figure 8-10).

Protocol to Evaluate an Abdominal Aortic Aneurysm. An *aortic aneurysm* is defined as that with a vessel diameter greater than 3 cm or noted focal dilation of the vessel (Figure 8-11, *A* and *B*). An *iliac aneurysm* is defined as a vessel with a diameter greater than 2 cm. Aneurysms larger than 5 cm and those with documented rapid rates of expansion have an increased risk of catastrophic rupture. *The physician must be made aware of these patients before they leave the department.* If an abnormal bulging of the abdominal aorta (aneurysm) is present, the sonographer should note the following additional views:

- The aneurysm should be followed to measure the length of the dilation and to note the position of the renal arteries in relation to the aneurysm.
- The aneurysm should be measured in both transverse (depth and width) and longitudinal planes (Figure 8-11, *C* and *D*).
- Clot or thrombus formation should be carefully assessed.
- Longitudinal scans of each iliac vessel from the bifurcation to the most distal segment should be taken.
- Transverse scans of the iliacs below the bifurcation should be taken.

SONOGRAPHIC EVALUATION OF THE ABDOMINAL AORTA

In most patients, the abdominal aorta is usually one of the easiest abdominal structures to image with ultrasound because of the marked change in acoustic impedance between its elastic walls and blood-filled lumen. Sonography provides the diagnostic information needed to create an image of the entire abdominal aorta, to assess its diameter, and to visualize the presence of thrombus, calcification, or dissection within the walls.

Multiple acoustic windows may be utilized to image the aorta. The traditional view is performed with the patient in the supine position. Gas-filled loops of bowel may prevent adequate visualization of the aorta, but this can sometimes be overcome by applying gentle pressure with the transducer or by changing the angle of the transducer to move the gas out of the way. An alternative imaging plane is made when the patient is rolled into a right lateral decubitus position and scanned along the left lateral flank with the transducer directed slightly toward the spine. (Recall that the aorta will be seen directly anterior to the spine.) Other visualization problems encountered in the abdominal aortic ultrasound may occur with increased amounts of mesenteric fat in obese patients. Patients should wait to be imaged at least 24 hours after a barium study or an endoscopic evaluation, as barium or air may still be a residual impairment to adequate visualization.

Longitudinal Plane. To begin the sonographic evaluation of the abdominal aorta, the patient is usually imaged first in the longitudinal plane. The aorta is imaged as a long pulsatile tubular structure that lies just anterior and to the left of the spine (Figure 8-12). The landmarks of the left lobe of the liver and the gastroesophageal junction may be seen anterior to the aorta. Longitudinal images should include the proximal, mid, and distal aorta to the bifurcation. The image acquisition should be made with the transducer perpendicular to the abdomen, beginning at the midline with a slight angulation of the transducer to the left of the spine, from the xiphoid to well below the level of bifurcation. In the normal individual, the luminal dimension of the aorta gradually tapers as it proceeds distally in the abdomen.

A low to medium gain should be used to demonstrate the walls of the aorta without "noisy" artifactual internal echoes. These weak echoes may result from increased gain, reverberation from the anterior abdominal wall fascia or musculature, or poor lateral resolution. These factors result in echoes being recorded at the same level as those from soft tissue that surround the vessel lumen, particularly if the vessels are smaller in diameter than the transducer. Try to use different techniques of breath holding to eliminate these *artifactual* echoes. Sometimes, increased gentle pressure or change in angulation of the transducer may help displace bowel gas or may compress fatty tissue so that the transducer will be closer to the abdominal aorta. If the abdomen is very concave, the patient may be instructed to extend his or her abdomen ("push the abdomen muscle out") so as to provide a better scanning plane. Color Doppler is useful to fully demonstrate the patent lumen of the aorta, from the diaphragm (celiac axis) to the bifurcation of the aorta into the iliac arteries (see Figure 8-9).

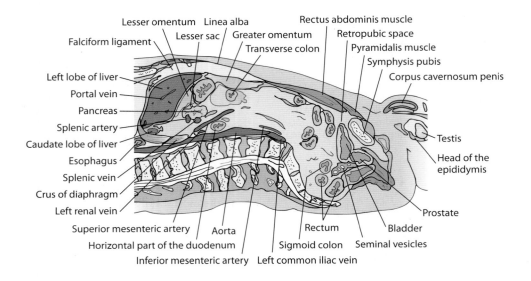

A

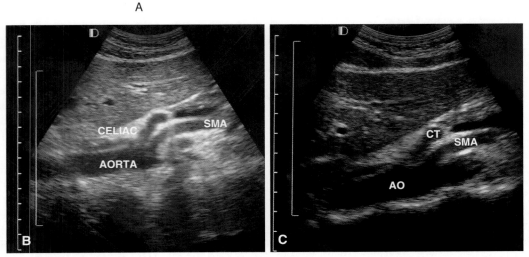

FIGURE 8-6 A, Midline sagittal section of the abdomen. The aorta is seen anterior to the vertebral column. Normal aorta protocol. **B** through **D,** Longitudinal images.

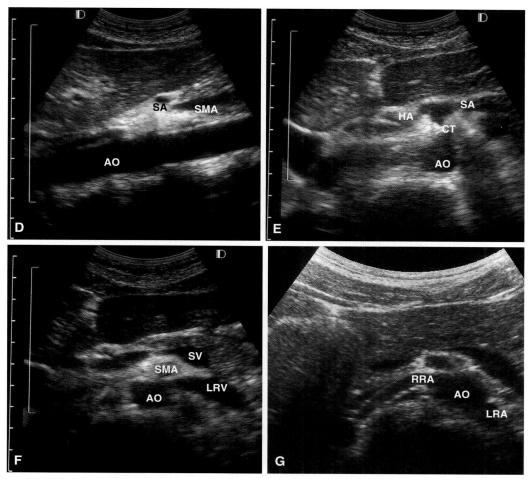

FIGURE 8-6, cont'd E through **G,** Transverse images at level of celiac trunk *(CT). AO,* Aorta; *HA,* hepatic artery; *LRA,* left renal artery; *LRV,* left renal vein; *RRA,* right renal artery; *SA,* splenic artery; *SMA,* superior mesenteric artery; *SV,* splenic vein.

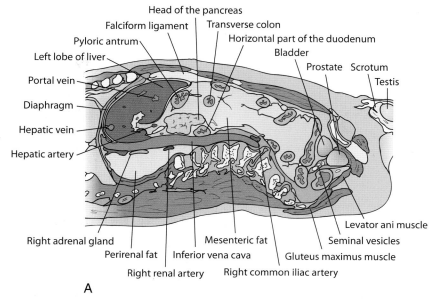

FIGURE 8-7 A, Sagittal section of the abdomen to the right of midline showing the inferior vena cava.   *Continued*

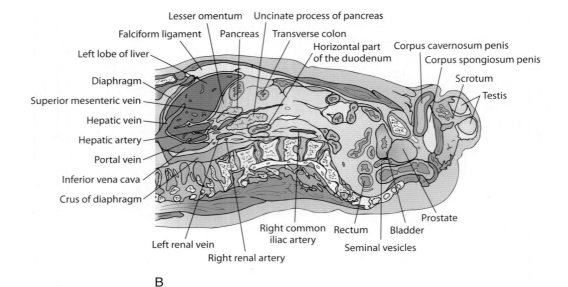

Lesser omentum   Uncinate process of pancreas
Falciform ligament   Pancreas   Transverse colon
Left lobe of liver   Horizontal part   Corpus cavernosum penis
    of the duodenum   Corpus spongiosum penis
Diaphragm   Scrotum
Superior mesenteric vein   Testis
Hepatic vein
Hepatic artery
Portal vein
Inferior vena cava
Crus of diaphragm   Prostate
    Right common   Rectum   Bladder
Left renal vein   iliac artery   Seminal vesicles
    Right renal artery

B

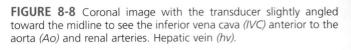

FIGURE 8-7, cont'd B, Note the drainage of the hepatic vein into the inferior vena cava at the level of the diaphragm. C, Longitudinal image of the hepatic vein (hv) and inferior vena cava (IVC). Liver (L), Portal vein (PV).

FIGURE 8-8 Coronal image with the transducer slightly angled toward the midline to see the inferior vena cava (IVC) anterior to the aorta (Ao) and renal arteries. Hepatic vein (hv).

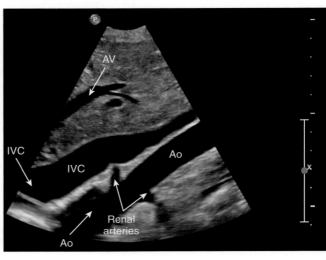

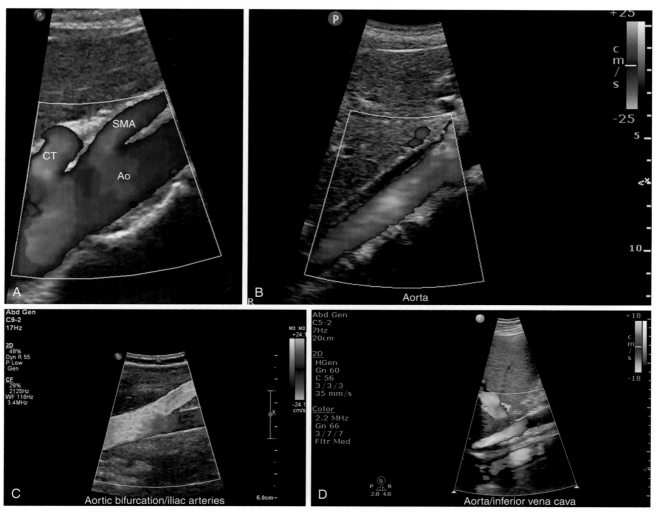

FIGURE 8-9 A, Color Doppler longitudinal image of the abdominal aorta with the celiac trunk *(ct)* and superior mesenteric artery *(sma)* arising from the anterior border. **B,** Color Doppler of the normal aorta should demonstrate a smooth, laminar flow pattern. **C,** Color Doppler of the bifurcation of the aorta into the iliac arteries. **D,** Coronal oblique view of the inferior vena cava (blue) anterior to the aorta (red).

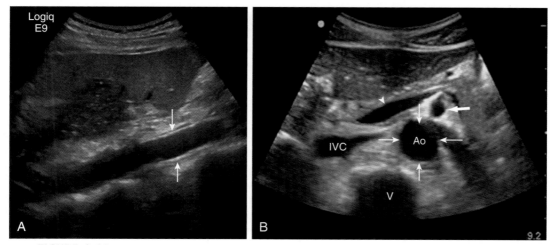

FIGURE 8-10 Outer to outer measurements should be taken of the aorta in the longitudinal **(A)** and transverse **(B)** planes. Aorta *(Ao)*, inferior vena cava *(IVC)*, splenic vein *(short arrow)*, superior mesenteric artery *(long arrow)*.

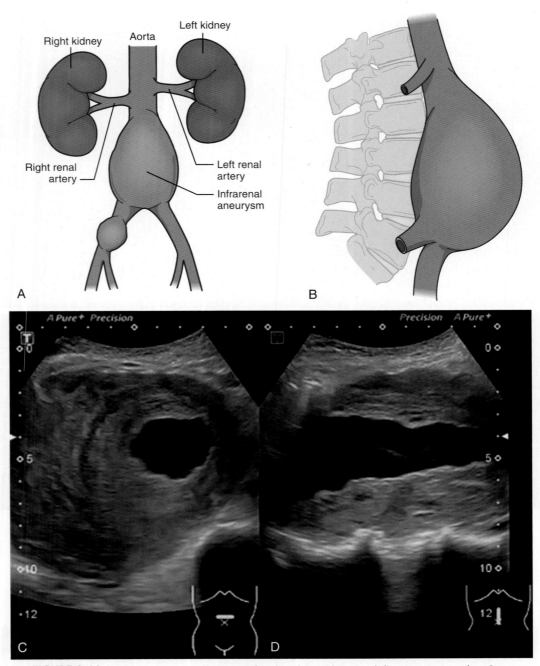

FIGURE 8-11 **A, B,** An *aortic aneurysm* is defined as that with a vessel diameter greater than 3 cm or noted focal dilation of the vessel. **C,** Transverse, and **D,** longitudinal sonographic images of the aortic aneurysm with circumferential thrombus.

Transverse Plane. In the transverse plane, the aorta is imaged as a circular structure anterior to the spine and slightly to the left of the midline (Figure 8-13). In some cases, the transverse diameter of the aorta (anterior-posterior and width) differs from that found in longitudinal measurements; thus it is important to identify and measure the vessel in two dimensions. Multiple scans should be made from the xiphoid to the bifurcation to record the dimensions of the aorta at the diaphragm, just above the renal vessels, just inferior to the renal vessels, and at the level of the bifurcation.

If the patient has a very tortuous aorta, scans may be difficult to obtain in a single longitudinal plane. During scanning in the longitudinal plane, the upper portion of the abdominal aorta may be well visualized, but the lower portion may be out of the plane of view. In this case the sonographer should obtain a complete scan of the upper segment and then should concentrate fully on the lower segment. In some patients, the aorta may stretch from the far right of the abdomen to the far left. Transverse images of the aorta may be helpful to map the course of the vessel.

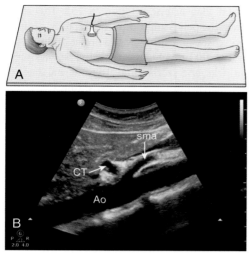

FIGURE 8-12 **A,** Longitudinal scan; the probe has been rotated from the transverse plane to the longitudinal plane. **B,** Longitudinal view of the abdominal aorta *(Ao)* with the celiac trunk *(ct)* and superior mesenteric artery *(sma)* arising from the anterior wall.

Measurement of the Aorta.

The aorta follows the anterior course of the vertebral column, and it is important that the transducer also follow a perpendicular path along the entire curvature of the spine. The anterior and posterior walls of the aorta should be easily seen as two thin pulsatile parallel lines. This facilitates measuring the anteroposterior diameter of the aorta, which in most institutions is done from the leading outer edge of the anterior wall to the leading inner edge of the posterior wall. Measurements are made at the proximal, mid, and distal aorta in the transverse and longitudinal

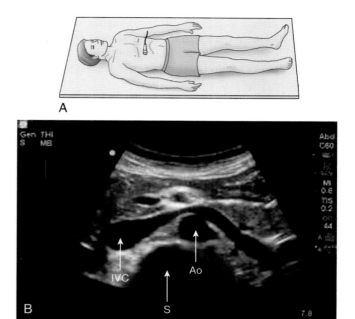

FIGURE 8-13 **A,** Transverse plane. **B,** Transverse sonographic image of the aorta *(Ao)* anterior to the spine *(S),* and to the left of the inferior vena cava *(IVC).*

plane. These measurements are made with the reduced gain setting from outer edge to outer edge at the greatest diameter.

The sonographer should be careful to identify the posterior edge of the aorta as separate from the spine when performing the measurements. Calcification of the aorta or ossification of the spine may require careful analysis to make this measurement accurate (Figure 8-14).

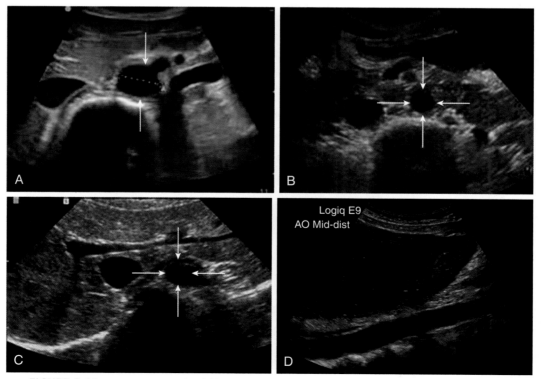

FIGURE 8-14 Measurements should be made at the **(A)** proximal abdominal aorta, **(B)** mid aorta, **(C)** distal aorta, and **(D)** longitudinal aorta.

If an aneurysm is present, the sonographer should measure and document the maximal size and location of the aneurysm. It is important to note the relationship of the dilated aortic segment in relation to the renal arteries and to note the extension into the iliac vessels.

Common Iliac Arteries

The **common iliac arteries** arise at the bifurcation of the abdominal aorta at the fourth lumbar vertebra (near the superior sacrum). These vessels further divide into the internal and external iliac arteries (Figure 8-15). The internal iliac artery enters the pelvis anterior to the sacroiliac joint, at which point it is crossed anteriorly by the ureter. It divides into anterior and posterior branches to supply the pelvic viscera, peritoneum, buttocks, and sacral canal. The external iliac artery runs along the medial border of the psoas muscle, following the pelvic brim. The inferior epigastric and deep circumflex iliac branches branch off before they pass under the inguinal ligament to become the femoral artery. The portion of the femoral artery posterior to the knee is the popliteal artery. This artery further divides into the anterior and posterior tibial arteries.

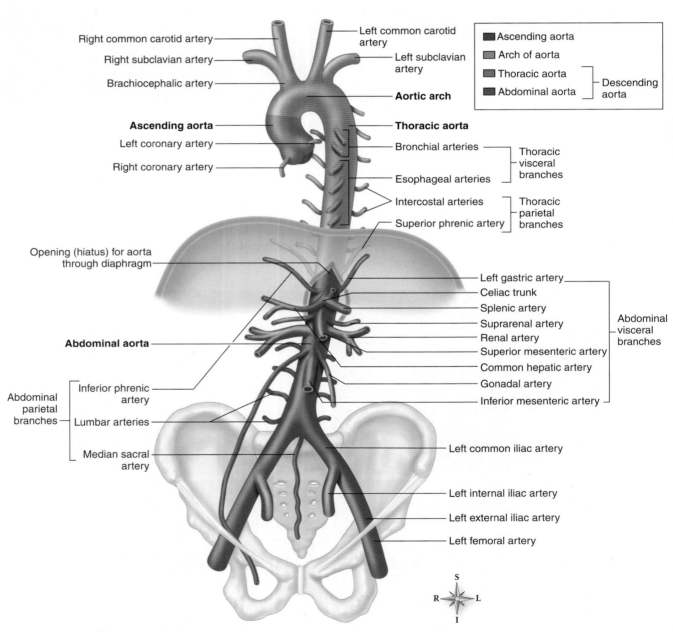

FIGURE 8-15 The common iliac arteries arise at the bifurcation of the abdominal aorta at the fourth lumbar vertebra (near the superior sacrum). These vessels further divide into the internal and external iliac arteries.

SONOGRAPHIC EVALUATION

To better visualize the iliac arteries at the aortic bifurcation, use a slight lateral decubitus position. The patient should be rotated 5 to 10 degrees from the true lateral position. The patient should be examined in deep inspiration, which projects the liver and diaphragm into the abdominal cavity and provides an acoustic window in which to image the vascular structures. Slight medial to lateral angulation of the transducer may be necessary to image the bifurcation in the longitudinal plane. With the patient rolled into this oblique plane, the inferior vena cava may be visualized anterior to the aorta (Figure 8-16, *A* and *B*). The iliac arteries should measure less than 1.2 cm in transverse anteroposterior diameter. It is common for the iliac arteries to be dilated if an aortic aneurysm is present, as most aneurysms develop inferior to the renal vessels near the bifurcation of the aorta. If the iliac artery measures greater than 3 cm, it may be considered for surgical repair.

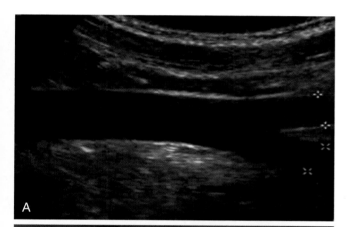

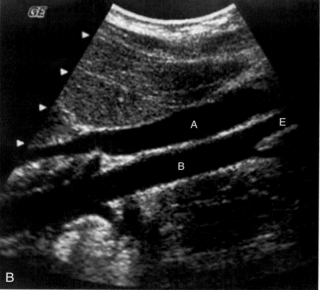

FIGURE 8-16 A, Slight oblique view of the abdominal aorta and bifurcation into the iliac arteries. **B,** Coronal view of the inferior vena cava *(A)*, aorta *(B)*, right renal artery *(C)*, left renal artery *(D)*, and iliac arteries *(E)*.

Abdominal Aortic Branches

The small phrenic arteries arise from the lateral walls of the aorta to supply the undersurface of the diaphragm. Surgical intervention or trauma to the phrenic artery may cause limited movement of the diaphragm. The celiac trunk is the first anterior branch of the aorta, arising 1 to 2 cm inferior to the diaphragm. The median arcuate ligament surrounds the aorta and has been known to compress the celiac trunk. The short celiac trunk gives rise to three smaller vessels: the splenic, common hepatic, and left gastric arteries (see Figure 8-4). The superior mesenteric artery is the second anterior branch, arising approximately 2 cm from the celiac trunk. The right renal artery and the left renal artery are lateral branches that arise just inferior to the superior mesenteric artery. The small inferior mesenteric artery arises anteriorly near the bifurcation. The distribution of these branch arteries is to the visceral organs and the mesentery.

Anterior Branches of the Abdominal Aorta

Celiac Trunk. The celiac trunk originates within the first 2 cm from the diaphragm (Figure 8-17). It is surrounded by the liver, spleen, inferior vena cava, and pancreas. After arising from the anterior wall, it immediately branches into the following three vessels: common hepatic, left gastric, and splenic arteries.

Common Hepatic Artery. The **common hepatic artery** arises from the celiac trunk and courses to the right of the abdomen at almost a 90-degree angle (see Figure 8-17). At this point, it branches into the proper hepatic artery and the gastroduodenal artery. The gastroduodenal artery courses along the upper border of the head of the pancreas, behind the posterior layer of the peritoneal bursa, to the upper margin of the superior part of the duodenum, which forms the lower boundary of the epiploic foramen (Figure 8-18). The duodenum and parts of the stomach are supplied by the **gastroduodenal artery** and the **right gastric artery.** Along with the hepatic duct and the portal vein, the common hepatic artery then ascends into the liver (through the porta hepatis), which it divides into two branches: the right and left hepatic arteries.

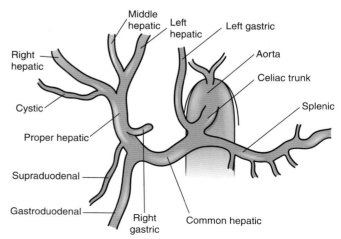

FIGURE 8-17 The celiac trunk originates within the first 2 cm from the diaphragm.

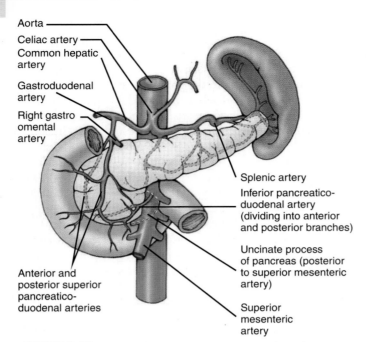

Aorta
Celiac artery
Common hepatic artery
Gastroduodenal artery
Right gastro omental artery
Anterior and posterior superior pancreatico-duodenal arteries
Splenic artery
Inferior pancreatico-duodenal artery (dividing into anterior and posterior branches)
Uncinate process of pancreas (posterior to superior mesenteric artery)
Superior mesenteric artery

FIGURE 8-18 The gastroduodenal artery courses along the upper border of the head of the pancreas, behind the posterior layer of the peritoneal bursa, to the upper margin of the superior part of the duodenum, which forms the lower boundary of the epiploic foramen.

Left and Right Hepatic Arteries. The **left hepatic artery** is a small branch supplying the caudate and left lobes of the liver. The **right hepatic artery** supplies the gallbladder via the cystic artery and the liver (see Figure 8-17).

Left Gastric Artery. The **left gastric artery** is a small branch of the celiac trunk, passing anterior, cephalic, and left to reach the esophagus and then descending along the lesser curvature of the stomach (see Figure 8-17). It supplies the lower third of the esophagus and the upper right of the stomach.

Splenic Artery. The **splenic artery** is the largest of the three branches of the celiac trunk (see Figure 8-18). From its origin, the artery takes a somewhat tortuous course horizontally to the left as it forms the superior border of the pancreas.

At a variable distance from the spleen, it divides into two branches. One of these branches, the left gastroepiploic artery, runs caudally into the greater omentum toward the right gastroepiploic artery. The other courses in a cephalic direction and divides into the short gastric artery, which supplies the fundus of the stomach, and into a number of splenic branches, which supply the spleen.

Several smaller arterial branches originate at the splenic artery as it courses through the upper border of the pancreas: the dorsal pancreatic, great pancreatic, and caudal pancreatic arteries. The dorsal or superior pancreatic artery originates from the beginning of the splenic artery or from the hepatic artery, celiac trunk, or aorta. It runs behind and within the substance of the pancreas, dividing into right and left branches. The left branch is the transverse pancreatic artery. The right branch constitutes an anastomotic vessel to the anterior pancreatic arch and also a branch to the uncinate process.

The great pancreatic artery originates from the splenic artery farther to the left and passes downward, dividing into branches that anastomose with the transverse or inferior pancreatic artery. The caudal pancreatic artery supplies the tail of the pancreas and divides into branches that anastomose with terminal branches of the transverse pancreatic artery. The transverse pancreatic artery courses behind the body and tail of the pancreas close to the lower pancreatic border. It may originate from or communicate with the superior mesenteric artery.

The distribution of the celiac trunk vessels is to the liver, spleen, stomach, pancreas, and duodenum.

SONOGRAPHIC EVALUATION

The celiac trunk may be visualized sonographically on transverse or longitudinal images (Figure 8-19). It is usually seen as a small vascular structure, arising anteriorly from the abdominal aorta just below the diaphragm. Because it is only 1 to 2 cm long, it is sometimes difficult to record unless the area near the midline of the aorta is carefully examined. Sometimes the celiac trunk can be seen to extend in a

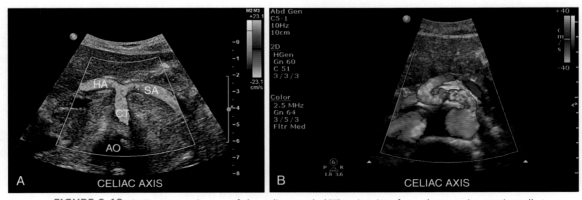

FIGURE 8-19   A, Transverse image of the celiac trunk *(CT)* as it arises from the anterior aortic wall *(AO)* and branches into splenic *(SA)* and hepatic arteries *(HA)*. **B,** Color Doppler transverse image of the aorta (red) shown to the left of the inferior vena cava (blue) and celiac trunk arising from the anterior border.

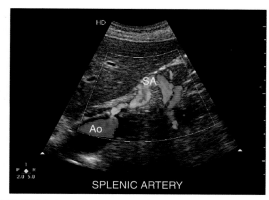

FIGURE 8-20 Transverse image of the splenic artery *(SA)* shown posterior to the left lobe of the liver and the tail of the pancreas. *Ao,* Aorta.

cephalic rather than a caudal presentation. The superior mesenteric artery is just inferior to the origin of the celiac trunk. The superior mesenteric artery may be used as a landmark in locating the celiac trunk. Transversely, one can differentiate the celiac trunk as the "wings of a seagull," arising with its short trunk before dividing into the "wings" of the hepatic and splenic arteries.

The splenic artery may be seen to flow directly from the celiac trunk toward the spleen (Figure 8-20). Because it is so tortuous, it may be difficult to follow on the transverse scan. Generally, small pieces of the splenic artery are visible as the artery weaves in and out of the left upper quadrant.

The common hepatic artery can be seen to branch anterior and to the right of the celiac trunk, where it then divides into the right and left hepatic arteries in the liver (Figure 8-21). The sonographer should be aware of the many variations in the hepatic artery branches as seen in Figure 8-22.

The left gastric artery has a very small diameter and often is difficult to visualize with ultrasound. It becomes difficult to separate from the splenic artery unless distinct structures are seen in the area of the celiac trunk branching to the left of the abdominal aorta.

Superior Mesenteric Artery. The **superior mesenteric artery** (SMA) arises from the anterior abdominal aortic wall approximately 1 cm inferior to the celiac trunk. Occasionally, the SMA may have a common origin with the celiac trunk. The SMA runs posterior to the neck of the pancreas and anterior to the uncinate process, which is anterior to the third part of the duodenum; it then branches into the mesentery and colon. The right hepatic artery is sometimes seen to arise from the superior mesenteric artery.

The SMA has the following five main branches (Figure 8-23): inferior pancreatic artery, duodenal artery, colic artery, ileocolic artery, and intestinal artery. These branch arteries supply the small bowel; each consists of 10 to 16 branches arising from the left side of the superior mesenteric trunk. They extend into the mesentery, where adjacent arteries unite with them to form loops or arcades. Their distribution is to the proximal half

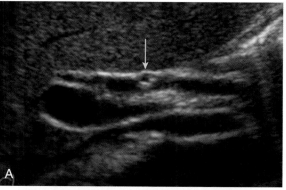

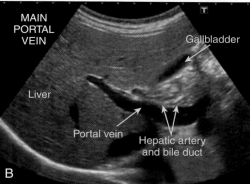

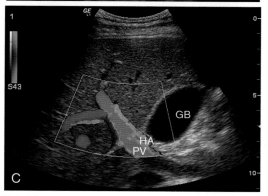

FIGURE 8-21 **A,** The common hepatic artery *(arrow)* can be seen to branch anterior and to the right of the celiac trunk, where it then divides into the right and left hepatic arteries in the liver. **B,** Transverse image of the hepatic artery and bile duct. **C,** Oblique transverse view of the portal triad: the portal vein *(PV)* is posterior, and the hepatic artery *(HA)* anterior and medial.

of the colon (cecum, ascending, and transverse) and the small intestine.

SONOGRAPHIC EVALUATION

The SMA is well seen on both transverse and longitudinal scans (Figure 8-24). As it arises from the anterior aortic wall, the SMA usually follows a parallel course along the abdominal aorta or branches off the anterior wall of the aorta at a slight angle and then follows a parallel course. Transversely, the artery can be seen as a separate small, circular structure anterior to the abdominal aorta and posterior to the pancreas. Characteristically, it is surrounded by highly reflective echoes from the retroperitoneal fascia.

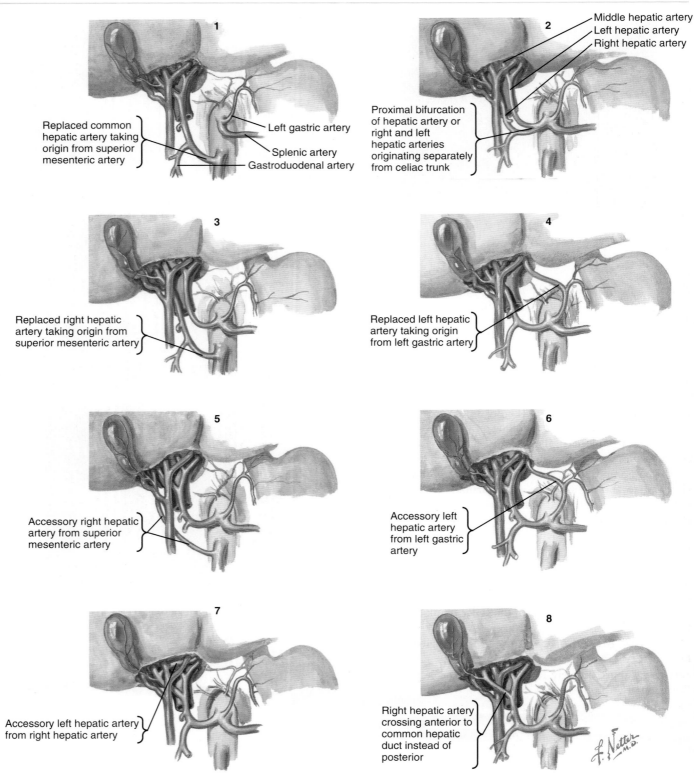

FIGURE 8-22 Illustration of the many variations in the hepatic artery branches. *(Copyright 2017 Elsevier Inc. All rights reserved. www.netterimages.com).*

Adenopathy should be considered if the angle of the superior mesenteric to the aorta is severe (greater than 15 degrees) (Figure 8-25).

Inferior Mesenteric Artery. The **inferior mesenteric artery** arises from the anterior abdominal aorta approximately at the level of the third or fourth lumbar vertebra (Figure 8-26). It proceeds to the left to distribute arterial blood to the descending colon, sigmoid colon, and rectum. It has the following three main branches: left colic, sigmoid, and superior rectal arteries. The distribution is to the left transverse colon, descending colon, sigmoid colon, and rectum.

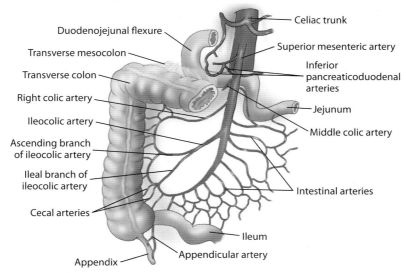

FIGURE 8-23 The superior mesenteric artery arises anteriorly from the abdominal aorta approximately 1 cm below the celiac trunk. It supplies the proximal half of the colon and small intestine.

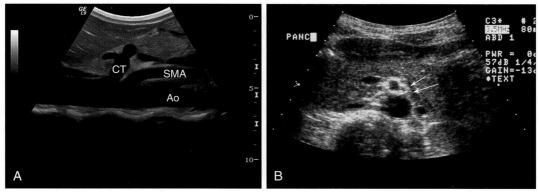

FIGURE 8-24 Superior mesenteric artery. **A,** Longitudinal image of the abdominal aorta *(Ao),* celiac trunk *(CT),* and superior mesenteric artery *(SMA)* arising from the anterior wall of the aorta. **B,** Transverse image of the superior mesenteric artery anterior to the aorta and posterior to the splenic vein *(arrows).*

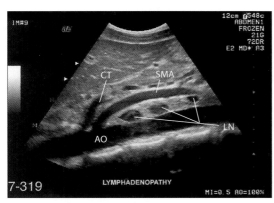

FIGURE 8-25 If the superior mesenteric artery arises at an angle steeper than 15 degrees from the aorta, lymphadenopathy should be considered, as is shown in this image with three well-defined nodes anterior to the aorta *(AO). CT,* celiac trunk; *LN,* enlarged lymph nodes; *SMA,* superior mesenteric artery.

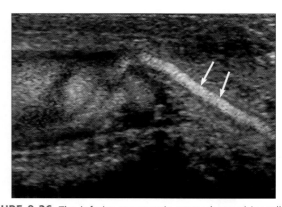

FIGURE 8-26 The inferior mesenteric artery *(arrows)* is well outlined with B-color. (B-color is the manufacturer-specific name for the ability to detect flow velocity by assigning gray-scale interpolation to flow velocity.)

SONOGRAPHIC EVALUATION

The inferior mesenteric artery is more difficult to visualize using ultrasound; when it is seen, it is generally on a longitudinal scan. It is a small tubular structure inferior to the superior mesenteric artery, which originates from the anterior wall of the aorta. On transverse scans, it is difficult to separate from small loops of bowel within the abdomen.

Splanchnic Aneurysms. The splanchnic aneurysms may be atherosclerotic, posttraumatic, mycotic, congenital, or inflammatory (Figure 8-27). A small percentage of patients with chronic pancreatitis may develop these aneurysms, which may occur in the SMA, hepatic and splenic arteries, gastroduodenal arteries, or inferior mesenteric artery. They may have mural thrombus that is well demonstrated with color Doppler.

Lateral Branches of the Abdominal Aorta

Phrenic Arteries. The phrenic arteries are paired small vessels that arise from the lateral wall of the aorta to supply the undersurface of the diaphragm.

Renal Arteries The renal arteries arise from the lateral aspect of the aorta at the level of and anterior to the first lumbar vertebra just inferior to the superior mesenteric artery (Figure 8-28). Both vessels divide into the anterior and inferior suprarenal arteries. Duplication of the renal arteries is not uncommon.

Right Renal Artery. The **right renal artery** is a longer vessel than the left; it courses from the aorta posterior to the inferior vena cava and anterior to the vertebral column in a posterior and slightly caudal direction to enter the hilus of the right kidney. The renal artery passes posterior to the renal vein before entering the renal hilus.

Left Renal Artery. The **left renal artery** courses from the aorta directly into the hilus of the left kidney.

Sonographic Findings. Both renal arteries are best seen on transverse sonograms (Figure 8-29). The right renal artery passes posterior to the inferior vena cava and anterior to the vertebral column in a posterior and slightly caudal direction. Occasionally, on longitudinal scans, a segment of the right renal artery is seen as a circular structure posterior to the inferior vena cava (Figures 8-30 and 8-31). The left renal artery takes a direct course from the aorta, anterior to the psoas muscle, to enter the renal sinus.

The coronal oblique scan of the aorta and inferior vena cava is excellent for demonstrating the origin of the renal arteries and veins (see Figure 8-30). The patient is rolled into a steep decubitus position. The transducer is directed longitudinally with its axis across the inferior vena cava and aorta in efforts to see the origin of the renal vessels. The patient should be in full inspiration to dilate the venous structures for better visualization.

Gonadal Artery. The gonadal artery arises inferior to the renal arteries and courses along the psoas muscle to the respective gonadal area (see Figure 8-11A).

Dorsal Aortic Branches

Lumbar Artery. Four lumbar arteries are usually present on each side of the aorta (see Figure 8-11A). The vessels travel lateral and posterior to supply muscle, skin, bone, and spinal cord. The midsacral artery supplies the sacrum and rectum.

Pathology of the Aorta

The sonographer may be asked to evaluate the abdominal aorta for several clinical reasons: pulsatile abdominal mass, abdominal pain radiating to the back, an abdominal bruit, or hemodynamic compromise in the lower legs. The arterial system may be affected by atheroma, aneurysm, connective tissue disorder, rupture, thrombosis, or infection.

The sonographer has several objectives to meet when performing a complete evaluation of the abdominal aorta. Recall the discussion that the entire aorta should be imaged in at least two planes (transverse and longitudinal) with appropriate measurements of the aortic diameter in the proximal, mid, and distal segments. The real advantage for the sonographer is the ability to "follow" the vessel with the transducer. If the vessel is tortuous, the transducer should be rotated or angled slightly to follow the course of the

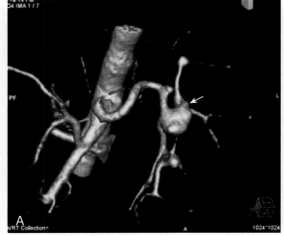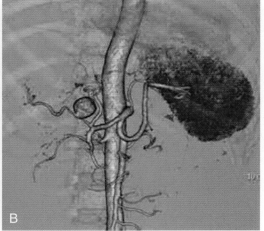

FIGURE 8-27 A, The splanchnic aneurysms may be atherosclerotic, posttraumatic, mycotic, congenital, or inflammatory. **B,** Small aneurysm of the hepatic artery.

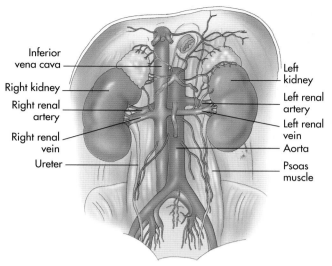

FIGURE 8-28 The kidneys and their vascular relationships.

artery. The size of the aorta increases up to 25% in the seventh and eighth decades.

It is important to distinguish between aortic ectasia and an aneurysm of the aorta. Ectasia implies the diffuse dilation of a vessel, whereas an abdominal aortic aneurysm is a region of focal enlargement (Figure 8-32). Ectasia occurs when the aorta increases both in transverse diameter and in vertical length, which causes the distal aorta to "kink," usually anterior and to the left. The aorta may be "folded," or tortuous, in its course, providing a challenge to the sonographer to follow the vessel in its entirety.

Arteriosclerosis versus Atherosclerosis. **Arteriosclerosis** occurs when the arterial vascular system becomes thick and stiff, which can lead to restriction of blood flow to the organs and tissues in the body. Normal healthy arteries are flexible and elastic. With the development of arteriosclerosis, the walls in the arteries can harden and stiffen, resulting in higher blood pressure. **Atherosclerosis** is a specific form of arteriosclerosis.

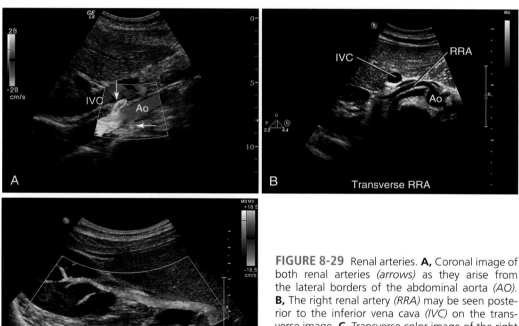

FIGURE 8-29 Renal arteries. **A,** Coronal image of both renal arteries *(arrows)* as they arise from the lateral borders of the abdominal aorta *(AO)*. **B,** The right renal artery *(RRA)* may be seen posterior to the inferior vena cava *(IVC)* on the transverse image. **C,** Transverse color image of the right renal artery.

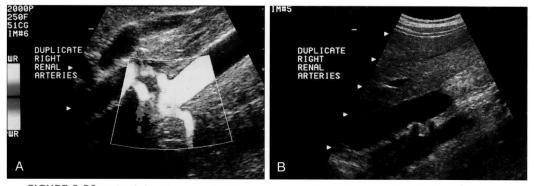

FIGURE 8-30 Color **(A)** and gray-scale **(B)** images of a patient with a duplicated right renal artery. The images are made in the right coronal oblique view.

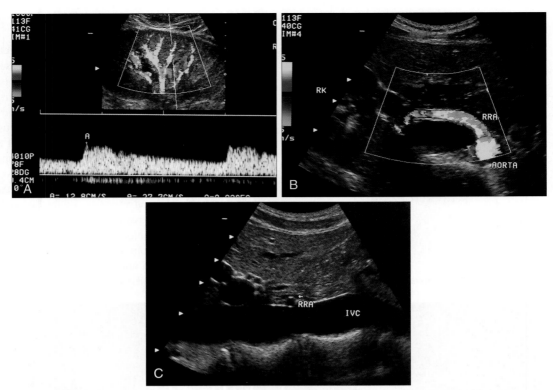

FIGURE 8-31 A–C, Variations in renal arteries. This patient has a right renal artery *(RRA)* that lies anterior (instead of posterior) to the inferior vena cava *(IVC)*. Normal spectral flow is shown in the renal parenchyma.

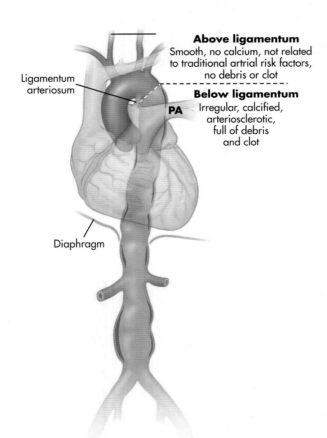

FIGURE 8-32 Ectasia (shown) implies the diffuse dilation of a vessel, whereas an abdominal aortic aneurysm is a region of focal enlargement.

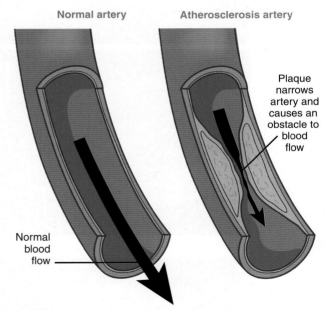

FIGURE 8-33 Arteriosclerosis occurs when the arterial vascular system becomes thick and stiff, which can lead to restriction of blood flow to the organs and tissues in the body. Atherosclerosis is a specific form of arteriosclerosis.

These terms are often used interchangeably. The buildup of fats, cholesterol, and other substances within the arterial wall (known as *plaque*) can restrict blood flow (Figure 8-33). These plaques may burst and trigger a blood clot or thrombus to form in the artery. The disease usually affects the ascending and descending aorta, but can be found in any of the arterial vessels in the body. Atherosclerosis is preventable and treatable with medication and lifestyle changes. The disease process develops gradually so patients do not have early warning symptoms until the plaque ruptures or obstructs the blood flow.

Symptoms of moderate to severe atherosclerosis depend on which arteries are affected:

- Heart—chest pain or pressure (angina)
- Brain—sudden numbness or weakness in arms or legs, difficulty speaking or slurred speech, or drooping muscles in the face
- Arms and legs—leg pain when walking or exercising (intermittent claudication)
- Kidneys—high blood pressure or kidney failure

Atherosclerosis is a slow, progressive disease. The damage builds over the years and is caused by a number of factors, which may include elevated blood pressure, high cholesterol, high triglycerides, smoking, diabetes, inflammation from systemic diseases such as arthritis or lupus, or infections. Other risk factors include family history of heart disease and lack of exercise. Once the wall of the artery is damaged, the cells clump at the injury site to build up in the inner lining of the artery. These fatty deposits harden and cause narrowing of the vessel, thus preventing the organs and tissue the proper blood supply. These fatty deposits may break off and enter the bloodstream to cause a blood clot that may embolize anywhere in the body. Arteriosclerosis is most commonly associated with the development of an aneurysm.

Abdominal Aortic Aneurysm. An **abdominal aortic aneurysm** (AAA) is a localized dilation of the abdominal aorta, usually greater than 3 cm in diameter or more than 1.5 times the diameter of the proximal aorta. The force of blood pushing against the walls of an artery combined with damage or injury to the artery's walls may cause an aneurysm. The abdominal aorta is more common than the thoracic aorta for aneurysm formation (Figure 8-34). The aneurysm may develop over years without the patient complaining of symptoms. Symptoms may not occur until the pressure of the aneurysm compresses adjacent organs, causes a blockage of blood flow, or ruptures into the abdominal or thoracic cavity. The primary risk factors for a patient with an AAA are dissection and rupture of the vessel. Dissection occurs when the force of blood pumping splits the layers of the arterial wall, allowing blood to leak in between the walls. The critical condition is when the aneurysm ruptures, causing bleeding internally. Catastrophic outcome may result from an aortic dissection or rupture. Box 8-1 summarizes the features of AAAs.

Risk factors that contribute to the development of an aneurysm include tobacco use, hypertension, and other cardiovascular disease. Other risk factors include chronic obstructive pulmonary disease and positive family history for AAA. Genetic conditions linked to AAA include Marfan syndrome and Ehlers-Danlos syndrome (Box 8-2).

AAA occurs more commonly in men over age 65 in the United States compared with women. Visualization of the abdominal aorta has traditionally been an asset in diagnosing the clinical problem. Ultrasound is very capable of demonstrating abnormalities in the diameter, length, and extent of the AAA. The majority of AAAs occur below the kidneys (infrarenal) with the remainder occurring at the level of or above the kidneys (Figure 8-35). The diagnosis of an aneurysm depends on a comparison of the aortic diameter of the suspicious area versus that of the normal area of the vessel above and below that area. The sonographer should note the relationship of the aortic aneurysm to the renal arteries. Thus not only the diameter, but also the longitudinal extent of the aneurysm as it relates to the origin of the renal vessels, should be measured. Often bowel gas may impair adequate visualization of the renal arteries; therefore a more indirect method must be used to locate the origin of the superior mesenteric artery and renal arteries. The patient should be examined

---

BOX 8-1 Features of Abdominal Aortic Aneurysms

- Most are true aneurysms—involve all three layers
- Approximately 85% are infrarenal
- Measure anteroposterior diameter on longitudinal views
- Mural thrombus is common with larger aneurysm
- Atherosclerosis—tortuosity, folding
- Aortic pseudoaneurysm—trauma
- Mycotic aneurysm—infection
- Surgery may be considered when >5 cm

BOX 8-2 Factors That May Cause the Development of an Aortic Aneurysm

1. Atherosclerosis
2. Trauma to the chest
3. Congenital defects (aortic sinus, post–coarctation of the aorta, ductus diverticulum)
4. Syphilis (involving the ascending aorta and arch)
5. Mycosis (fungal dissection)
6. Cystic medial necrosis (e.g., Marfan syndrome)
7. Inflammation of media and adventitia (e.g., rheumatic fever, polychondritis, ankylosing spondylitis)
8. Increased pressure (systemic hypertension, aortic valve stenosis)
9. Abnormal volume load (severe aortic regurgitation)

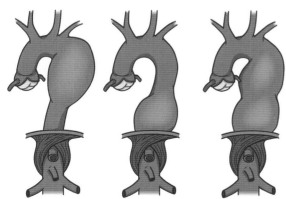

FIGURE 8-34 The abdominal aorta is more common than the thoracic aorta for aneurysm formation.

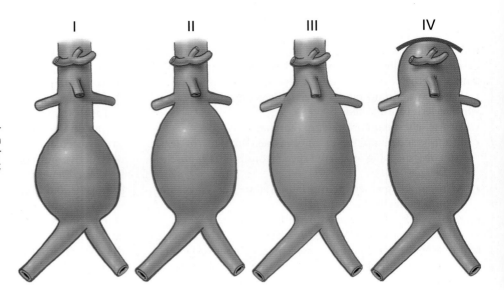

FIGURE 8-35 The majority of AAAs occur below the kidneys (infrarenal) with the remainder occurring at the level of or above the kidneys. *I,* infrarenal; *II,* juxtarenal; *III,* pararenal; *IV,* suprarenal.

from both the supine and the left flank with the patient rolled into a right lateral decubitus position. Color Doppler may be useful for producing an image of arterial flow from the lateral margins of the abdominal aorta to the kidneys.

Clinical Symptoms. Most patients with an AAA are asymptomatic. If the patient does have symptoms, they may include throbbing or deep pain in the abdomen, back, or flank area. The pain may extend into the buttocks, groin, or legs. The enlarged vessel may be found during routine physical examination or during an unrelated radiologic or surgical procedure.

Clinical symptoms of the patient with an aortic aneurysm may result from rupture or expansion of the vessel. The enlarged vessel may produce symptoms by impinging on adjacent structures, or the vessel may become occluded by direct pressure or thrombus with resulting embolism. The enlarged aneurysm may rupture into the peritoneal cavity or the retroperitoneum, causing intense back pain and a drop in hematocrit. *Grey Turner's sign* may be associated with an extensive bleed in the retroperitoneal cavity. Patients may present with satiety (becoming full easily) or nausea and vomiting. Abrupt onset of severe, constant pain in the abdomen, back, or flank that is unrelieved by positional changes is characteristic of rapid expansion or rupture of an aneurysm. Other complications may include dissection, thrombosis, distal embolism, infection, and obstruction and invasion of adjacent structures. Commonly, branch artery occlusions or stenosis may be seen in the inferior mesenteric artery or renal arteries.

The patient with an aneurysm most likely has many other medical problems as well. It is important that the clinician be able to sequentially follow the size and growth of the aneurysm noninvasively over a structured time period by sonography. Therefore it is important in these cases to measure the exact location of the aneurysm so subsequent follow-up sonographic evaluations will be accurate. The patient with an AAA measurement of less than 4 cm in diameter is generally followed every 6 months with sonography; intervention may occur once the patient becomes symptomatic. In patients with aneurysms ranging from 4 to 5 cm in diameter, surgery or endovascular aneurysm repair may be suggested if the patient is in good

health. Patients with aneurysms ranging from 5 to 6 cm may benefit from repair, especially if they have other factors for rupture (e.g., hypertension, smoking, chronic obstructive pulmonary disease). Aneurysms less than 6 cm show a very slow growth pattern (less than 0.2 to 0.5 cm/yr) and may be followed annually with sonography. Patients with aneurysms measuring 6 cm may be followed at 6-month intervals. Patients at the highest risk are those with aneurysms measuring greater than 6 to 7 cm. The risk increases with age and other medical problems (Box 8-3). There are three primary factors related to the growth rate of abdominal aneurysms: the initial size of the aortic aneurysm, the presence of cardiac disease, and the presence of beta-adrenergic blockade (blood pressure–lowering medications).

Surgical intervention may be considered if associated renal and iliac involvement is present with occlusive disease or aneurysmal development. The sonographer should measure the length of the infrarenal aortic neck, which may help determine the best surgical approach (retroperitoneal vs. transabdominal) and the location of the aortic cross clamp. Endovascular stent grafts for treatment are a less invasive approach to the repair of an aneurysm as this graft is placed through two small incisions in the abdomen.

Classification of Aneurysms. Histologically, the aneurysm may be classified as a *true aneurysm* (lined by all three layers of the aorta) or as a *false aneurysm (pseudoaneurysm)* (not lined by all three layers). A true aneurysm forms when the tensile strength of the wall decreases. A small

BOX 8-3	Size, Growth Rate, and Risk of Rupture for Abdominal Aortic Aneurysms	
Size (cm)	**Growth Rate (cm/yr)**	**Annual Rupture Risk (%)**
3.0–3.9	0.39	0
4.0–4.9	0.36	0.5–5
5.0–5.9	0.43	3–15
6.0–6.9	0.64	10–20
>7.0		20–50

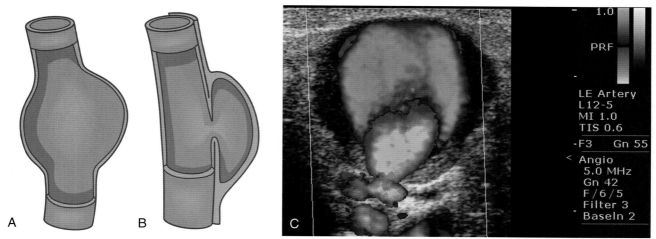

FIGURE 8-36 The aneurysm may be classified as a true aneurysm **(A)** (lined by all three layers of the aorta), or as a false aneurysm, also known as *pseudoaneurysm* **(B),** not lined by all three layers. **C,** Color Doppler of flow in a pseudoaneurysm.

percentage of true aneurysms occur secondary to underlying diseases such as Marfan syndrome, Ehlers-Danlos syndrome, and familial aortic dissection.

In the **pseudoaneurysm,** blood escapes through a hole in the intima of the vessel wall, but is contained by the deeper layers of the aorta or by adjacent tissue. In the pseudoaneurysm, the dilation is confined by two layers, only one layer, or only adjacent soft tissue. With color Doppler, blood can be seen to flow into the protuberance during systole and out during diastole (Figure 8-36). These events can occur after trauma to the vessel as a result of accident or surgery, or after an interventional cardiac catheterization or angiography procedure. Ultrasound evaluation of the pulsatile mass is conducted, with color Doppler showing communication between the artery and the vein. Compression of the mass with a linear transducer at 20-minute compression intervals may allow the lesion to close if the communication is small. Sometimes it takes several compressions (20 minutes on and 20 minutes off) to completely close the communication. Color flow allows the sonographer to see whether the communication is closed. Pseudoaneurysms that are unable to be closed with this technique may require surgical intervention, as they may become a source of emboli, the site of increased chance of infection secondary to abnormal communication of blood flow, or a cause of local pressure effects. In addition, they can rupture, which may result in exsanguination.

Descriptive Terms for an Abdominal Aortic Aneurysm.
An aneurysm may be described as fusiform or saccular (Figure 8-37). The idiopathic abdominal aneurysm is a true aneurysm that most commonly develops inferorenally (in more than 85% of patients). It usually begins below the renal arteries (inferior to the superior mesenteric artery) and extends to the bifurcation of the aorta at the iliac arteries.

The most common presentation of an atherosclerotic aneurysm is a **fusiform aneurysm** of the distal aorta at the aortic bifurcation (see Figure 8-11). The fusiform aneurysm represents a gradual transition between normal and abnormal and extends over the length of the aorta to resemble a "football-like" shape. Sonography displays atherosclerosis of the vessel

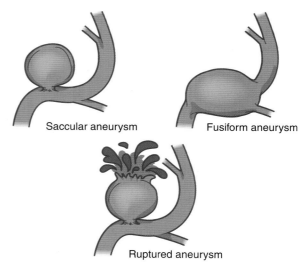

FIGURE 8-37 Illustration of the types of aneurysms: saccular, fusiform, and ruptured.

as decreased pulsations of the aortic walls, with bright echoes reflecting the degree of thickening and calcification. These aneurysms often extend into the iliac vessels in the pelvis.

A **saccular aneurysm** shows a sudden transition between normal and abnormal and is somewhat spherical and larger (5 to 10 cm) than fusiform aneurysms. This type of aneurysm is connected to the vascular lumen by a mouth that varies in size but may be as large as an aneurysm. It may be partially or completely filled with mural thrombus (see Figure 8-37). The sonographer must carefully follow the course of such an aneurysm to differentiate it from a retroperitoneal mass or lymphadenopathy. Pulsations are usually diminished secondary to clot formation.

A large aneurysm may compress its neighboring structures. Compression of the common bile duct may cause obstruction; compression of the renal artery can cause hypertension and renal ischemia. Retroperitoneal fibrosis with an aneurysm may involve the ureter, causing hydronephrosis. The left kidney is more frequently affected than the right.

The abdominal aneurysm may extend into the iliac arteries. The sonographer should examine both iliac arteries in at least two planes. At the level of the bifurcation, the iliac vessels may be seen as circular, pulsatile vessels just anterior to the spine. The oblique longitudinal scan is used to produce an image of the vessel in its entire length. Normal iliac arteries usually measure less than 1 cm in diameter.

Inflammatory Aortic Aneurysm. This type of aneurysm is a variant in which the wall of the aneurysm is thickened and surrounded by fibrosis and adhesions of a type similar to those found in retroperitoneal fibrosis. These patients present with a higher surgical risk. Clinically, they present with pain that may mimic a retroperitoneal hemorrhage. A rare condition is the development of a mycotic aneurysm secondary to infection. The most common infections result from septic emboli, streptococci, staphylococci, and *Salmonella*. The infection may produce a focal abscess that appears as a complex fluid collection with irregular borders.

Rupture of Aortic Aneurysm. The rupture of an aortic aneurysm is catastrophic, with a mortality rate of 50%. The diameter alone may not be an accurate prediction of rupture risk, as smaller aortic diameters may rupture and larger diameter aortas may remain stable. The wall stress may influence the risk of rupture (when the wall stress exceeds the wall strength). The diameter rate of change may influence the rupture risk.

The classic symptoms of a ruptured aortic aneurysm are excruciating abdominal pain, shock, and an expanding abdominal mass. Rupture of the aorta is a surgical emergency, and computed tomography (CT) is the first choice for imaging to obtain the most information in the shortest time. CT is not hampered by bowel gas and allows a rapid overview of the abdominal pelvic structures. The operative mortality rate for such ruptures is very high. The rupture may extend into the perirenal space with displacement of renal hilar vessels, effacement of the aortic border, and silhouetting of the lateral psoas border at the level of the kidney (Figure 8-38). The most common site for rupture is the lateral wall inferior to the renal vessels. Hemorrhage into the posterior pararenal space accounts for loss of visualization of the lateral psoas muscle merging inferior to the kidney and may also displace the kidney. The iliac aneurysm may rupture into the rectosigmoid colon, iliac vein, or ureter.

Sonographic Findings. Recall that the normal average measurement for a male adult abdominal aorta is usually less than 3 cm, with measurement taken perpendicular to the vessel from outer layer–to–outer layer walls. (This measurement correlates with the measurement made by the surgeon.) The sonographer should search for focal dilation of the abdominal aorta or lack of normal tapering distally. The anterior and posterior borders are often better imaged than the lateral borders. The adventitia is slightly echogenic; however, with atherosclerosis the walls may become increasingly echogenic with calcification. When an aneurysm is detected, the presence of a mural thrombus should be evaluated. A mural thrombus usually occurs along an anterior or anterolateral wall. The thrombus is often poorly attached and friable and may be a source for distal emboli. Thrombus within an aneurysm is shown ultrasonically as medium- to low-level echoes (Figure 8-39). Generally, increased sensitivity is likely to highlight the low-level echoes from the thrombus. These echoes

Abdominal Aortic Aneurysm with Fatal Rupture

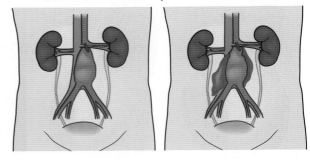

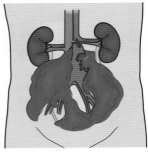

FIGURE 8-38 Illustration of the retroperitoneal collection of blood that results from an abdominal aortic rupture.

should be seen in both planes on more than one scan to be separated from low-level reverberation echoes. A chronic thrombotic clot is easier to see with sonography because of the bright calcification that appears as thick, echogenic echoes, sometimes with posterior shadowing. The amount of thrombus in a vessel has no relation to the risk of rupture.

The sonographer should note the maximum length, width, and transverse dimension of the aortic aneurysm. Documentation of the shape (fusiform or saccular) and location of the aneurysm in relation to the renal arteries is important. Extension of the aneurysm into the iliac arteries should also be noted. Measurements of length × width × height should be included in the report. A description of wall thickening, the presence of calcification, blood flow, soft plaque, or calcified plaque should also be included in the report. Careful evaluation of the presence or absence of an aortic dissection should be noted. Because the aneurysm may often affect the renal vessels, both kidneys should be analyzed. (Measure the renal size and exclude pelvocaliectasis.) If hypertrophy of one or both kidneys occurs, a full Doppler evaluation of the renal vessels should be conducted to rule out renal artery stenosis.

Aortic Dissection. A defect in the vessel intimal wall must exist along with internal weakness for a dissection to occur. Dissection of the aorta may occur secondary to **cystic medial necrosis** (weakening of the arterial wall), to hypertension, or to the inherited disease **Marfan syndrome.** Individuals with this disorder are extremely tall, lanky, and double-jointed; a progressive stretching disorder exists in all arterial vessels, especially in the aorta, causing abnormal dilation, weakened walls, and eventual dissection, rupture, or both. Color flow Doppler may be used to detect flow into the false channel.

Three classifications of aortic dissection are based on the DeBakey model (Figure 8-40). Types I and II involve the

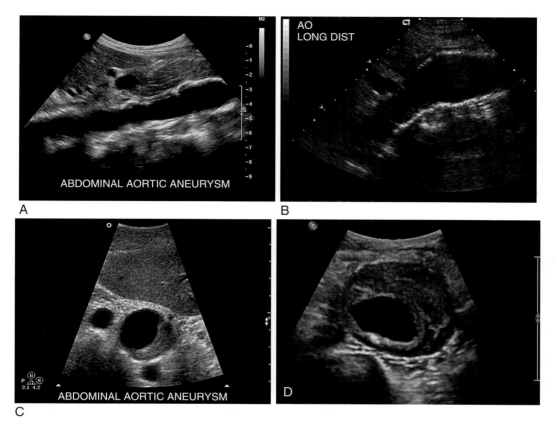

FIGURE 8-39 Abdominal aortic aneurysm. **A,** Longitudinal image of a small abdominal aortic aneurysm extending superior to the bifurcation. **B,** Sagittal image of a large abdominal aortic aneurysm; the largest diameter of the aneurysm should be measured. **C,** Multiple echoes within represent thrombus formation. **D,** Transverse image of a large AAA with thrombus along the anterolateral boarders *(arrows)*.

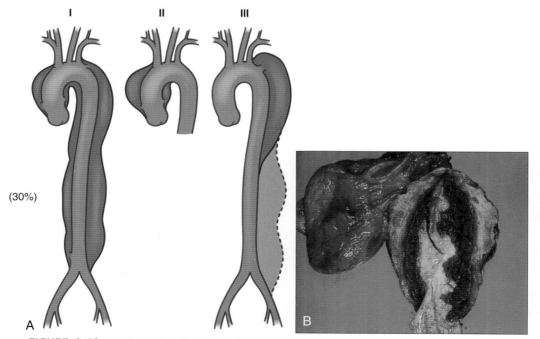

FIGURE 8-40 A, Three classifications of aortic dissection are based on the DeBakey model. Types I and II involve the ascending aorta and the aortic arch; type III involves the descending aorta at a level inferior to the left subclavian artery. **B,** Dissecting aneurysm of the thoracic aorta. The blood has filled the space formed by the separation of the intima and media of the aorta.

ascending aorta and the aortic arch; type III involves the descending aorta at a level inferior to the left subclavian artery. A high incidence of mortality is associated with type I and II dissections because of possible obstruction at the origin of the coronary arteries and possible obstruction of blood into the head and neck vessels. The lowest mortality rate is associated with the type III dissection, which begins inferior to the left subclavian artery with possible extension into the abdominal aorta.

The type I dissection begins at the root of the aorta and may extend the entire length of the arch, descending to the aorta and into the abdominal aorta. This is the most dangerous, especially if the dissection spirals around the aorta, cutting off the blood supply to the coronary, carotid, brachiocephalic, and subclavian vessels. The third type of dissection (type III) begins at the lower end of the descending aorta and extends into the abdominal aorta. This may be critical if the dissection spirals around to impede the flow of blood into the renal vessels. Less than 5% of dissections occur primarily in the abdomen.

A **dissecting aneurysm** may be detected with sonography, although CT is generally the preferred imaging choice in emergent situations. The patient may be known to have an aortic or thoracic aneurysm, and presents clinically with sudden excruciating chest pain radiating to the back that develops as the result of a dissection. These critical patients may go into shock very quickly, and CT is generally ordered to obtain the most information in the shortest amount of time. However, the patient who presents with some of these symptoms and is stable may have a slow leak aneurysm. These stable patients are appropriately imaged with sonography. The sonographer should look for a dissection "flap" or recent channel, with or without frank aneurysmal dilation. This flap is well demonstrated with M-mode as a fluttering within the lumen at different phases of the cardiac cycle. The dissection of blood occurs along the laminar planes of the aortic media with formation of a blood-filled channel within the aortic wall (Figure 8-41). Color Doppler will demonstrate flow in both channels (true and false lumens) with the flow rate differing between the channels.

When the dissection develops, hemorrhage may occur between the middle and outer thirds of the media. An intimal tear is considered if the tear is found in the ascending portion of the arch. This type of dissection extends proximally toward the heart and distally, sometimes to the iliac and femoral arteries. A small number of dissections do not have an obvious intimal tear. Extravasation may completely encircle the aorta or may extend along one segment of its circumference, or the aneurysm may rupture into any of the body cavities.

Aortic Graft. An abdominal aortic aneurysm may be surgically repaired with a flexible graft material attached to the end of the remaining aorta. The synthetic material used for a graft produces bright textured echo reflections compared with those from normal aortic walls. After surgery, the attached walls may swell at the site of attachment and form another aneurysm or pseudoaneurysm (Figure 8-42). Other complications of prosthetic grafts include hematoma, infection, and degeneration of graft material.

Newer surgical techniques now repair the aneurysm with an endovascular graft treatment. The graft may be anastomosed in an end-to-side or end-to-end manner. These grafts would be placed within the aorta, at the level of the aorta and iliac artery, or within the femoral artery (Figure 8-43). Further development in techniques has placed the grafts in the aortofemoral and juxtarenal positions. Complications of these grafts resulted in endoleak formations that were immediate, without outflow, and persistent. The type of graft used, the technique of graft insertion, and the aortic anatomic features all affected the rate of endoleaks.

The sonographer should carefully examine the upper and lower ends of the anastomoses with both real-time and color Doppler. During evaluation of the graft, the sonographer should look for stenosis at the ends of the graft, aneurysm formation, or pseudoaneurysm development. Doppler evaluation of the distal vessels should be conducted to ensure that adequate blood flow is available. Fluid collections (i.e., hematoma, lymphocele, seroma, or abscess formation) may develop at the graft site.

Iliac and Thoracic Aneurysms

Iliac Aneurysm. A very small percentage of patients (less than 5%) with an abdominal aneurysm will also have an iliac

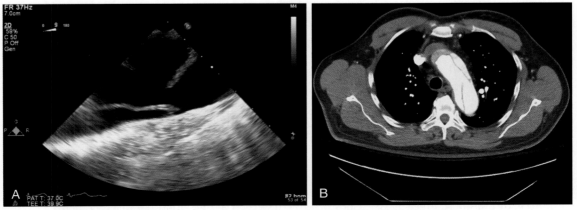

FIGURE 8-41 Aortic dissection, type I, was seen in this patient. The dissection began in the ascending aorta and extended into the aortic arch.

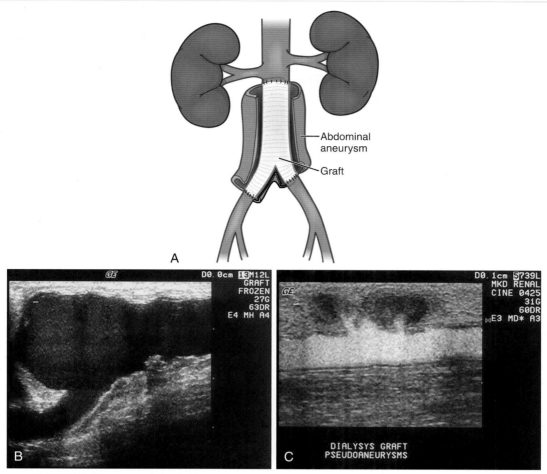

FIGURE 8-42 **A,** An abdominal aortic aneurysm may be surgically repaired with a flexible graft material attached to the end of the remaining aorta. **B** and **C,** Complications of graft repair of aneurysms may result in new aneurysm formation **(A)** or pseudoaneurysm formation **(B).**

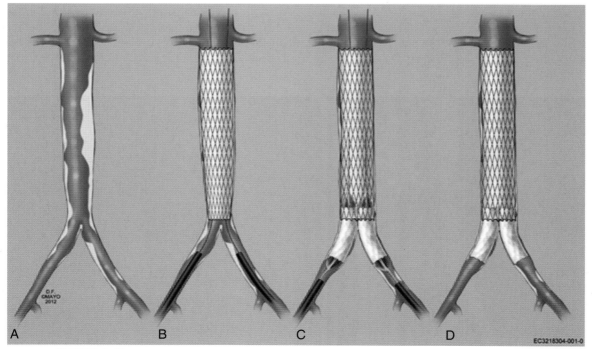

FIGURE 8-43 Illustration of the endovascular graft. The graft may be anastomosed in an end-to-side or end-to-end manner. These grafts would be placed within the aorta, at the level of the aorta and iliac artery, or within the femoral artery. *(Used with permission of Mayo Foundation for Medical Education and Research. All rights reserved.)*

aneurysm. These may occur at the bifurcation of the common iliac artery or in the external iliac just distal to the bifurcation.

Thoracic Aneurysm. If an aneurysm extends beyond the diaphragm into the thoracic aorta, it may be difficult to follow with ultrasound because of lung interference with the sound beam. Several attempts may be necessary to demonstrate this thoracic aneurysm. The transducer should be sharply angled in the longitudinal plane from the anterior abdomen at the xiphoid toward the sternal notch to allow visualization of the distal thoracic aorta. Another technique allows the sonographer to place the transducer along the left of the sternum to make a longitudinal parasternal scan over the long axis of the heart. The thoracic aorta should be seen as the pulsatile structure posterior to the cardiac structures. A third alternative is to scan posteriorly along the patient's back to the left of the spine with the patient sitting upright or prone. The transducer should be angled slightly medially and placed in a sagittal plane along the left intercostal space. This is very effective if the thoracic aorta is deviated slightly to the left of the spine. Scalloped reverberations from the ribs will be recorded, with the luminal echoes of the thoracic aorta directly posterior.

Pseudopulsatile Abdominal Masses. Masses other than an aortic aneurysm that can simulate a pulsatile abdominal mass include retroperitoneal tumor, huge fibroid uterus, or para-aortic nodes. Because the mass is adjacent to the aorta, pulsations are transmitted from the aorta to the mass. Next to an abdominal aneurysm, the most common cause for a pulsatile abdominal mass is enlarged retroperitoneal lymph nodes. This mass is usually the result of lymphoma in the middle-aged patient. On ultrasound, the nodes are homogeneous masses surrounding the aorta. The aortic wall may be poorly defined because of the close acoustic impedance of the nodes and the aorta. The sonographer should also look for splenomegaly. A retroperitoneal sarcoma may present as a pulsatile mass; it may extend into the root of the mesentery and give rise to a larger intraperitoneal component. The echodensity depends on the tissue type that predominates; fatty lesions are more echodense than fibrous or myomatous lesions.

Arteriovenous Fistula. An **arteriovenous fistula** is not a common finding with sonography. Most fistulas are acquired secondary to trauma. Some may develop as a complication of arteriosclerotic aortic aneurysms. Clinical signs that the patient may have an arteriovenous fistula include low back and abdominal pain, progressive cardiac decompensation, a pulsatile abdominal mass associated with a bruit, and massive swelling of the lower trunk and lower extremities. Clinical signs are explained on the basis of the altered hemodynamics produced by a high-velocity shunt leading to increased blood volume, venous pressure, and cardiac output with cardiac failure and cardiomegaly. If lower trunk and leg edema is present, along with a dilated inferior vena cava, an arteriovenous fistula should be suspected. If the fistula is large, the vein becomes very distended. A normal inferior vena cava measures less than 2.0 cm in its anteroposterior dimension. Right-sided heart disease or failure may also cause inferior vena cava distention.

Splanchnic Aneurysm. The splanchnic aneurysms may be atherosclerotic, posttraumatic, mycotic, congenital, or inflammatory. A small percentage of patients with chronic pancreatitis may develop these aneurysms, which may occur in the SMA, hepatic and splenic arteries, gastroduodenal arteries, or inferior mesenteric artery. They may have mural thrombus that is well demonstrated with color Doppler.

Renal Arterial Disease

Renal Artery Stenosis. Renal artery stenosis may present clinically as hypertension. The stenosis is due to atherosclerotic disease or fibromuscular hyperplasia. Color and spectral Doppler are used to investigate the renal vessels for increased velocity flow patterns representative of obstruction of flow into the kidney (Figure 8-44). Recall that the right renal artery arises from the kidney and travels posterior to the inferior vena cava to enter the medial wall of the abdominal aorta. The left renal artery has a more direct course from the kidney to the lateral wall of the aorta.

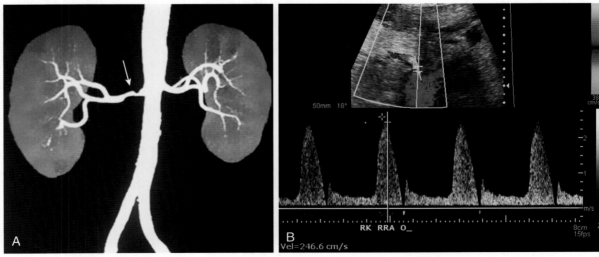

FIGURE 8-44 A, Contrast CT image depicting renal artery stenosis *(arrow).* **B,** Spectral Doppler tracing of a patient with renal artery stenosis showing high flow velocity.

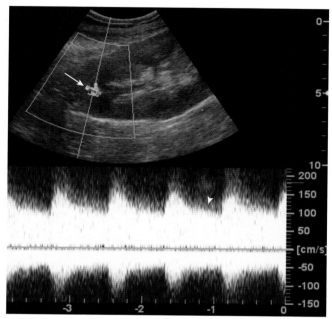

FIGURE 8-45 In the aneurysmal type of arteriovenous fistula, a vascular lesion should be suspected when the presence of a thrombus is noted in the periphery of a mass *(long arrow)* with a tubular anechoic lumen with pulsations *(short arrow).*

Thus the renal arteries may be difficult to align parallel with the Doppler beam to obtain a correct velocity measurement.

Renal Arteriovenous Fistulas. Renal arteriovenous fistulas can be congenital or acquired. Congenital arteriovenous fistulas may be of the cirsoid type or the aneurysmal type. Acquired fistulas occur secondary to trauma, surgery, or inflammation or are associated with a neoplasm, such as renal cell carcinoma.

The sonographer will find multiple anechoic tubular structures feeding the malformation with an enlarged renal artery and vein, confirming increased blood flow to the kidney (Figure 8-45). It may look like hydronephrosis or a parapelvic cyst in association with a dilated inferior vena cava. The diagnosis is made by identifying one or more channels that enter the mass, suggesting that the lesion is related to the renal vasculature. The sonographer should look for pulsations. The fistula has a characteristic sonographic appearance of a cluster of tubular anechoic structures within the kidney; it is supplied by an enlarged renal artery and is drained by a dilated renal vein. In the aneurysmal type of fistula, a vascular lesion should be suspected when the presence of a thrombus is noted in the periphery of a mass with a tubular anechoic lumen with pulsations. Occasionally, renal cell carcinoma is associated with arteriovenous shunting, resulting from invasion of larger arteries and venous structures.

INFERIOR VENA CAVA

The **inferior vena cava** (IVC) is formed by the union of the common iliac veins posterior to the right common iliac artery at the level of the fifth lumbar vertebra (Figure 8-46). The IVC ascends vertically through the retroperitoneal space on the right side of the aorta posterior to the liver,

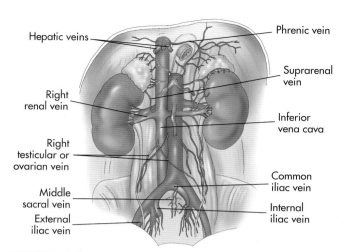

FIGURE 8-46 The inferior vena cava is formed by the union of the common iliac veins posterior to the right common iliac artery at the level of the fifth lumbar vertebra.

piercing the central tendon of the diaphragm at the level of the eighth thoracic vertebra to enter the right atrium of the heart. Its entrance into the lesser sac separates it from the portal vein (Figure 8-47). Caudal to the renal vein entrance, the IVC shows posterior "hammocking" through the bare area of the liver (Figure 8-48).

The tributaries of the IVC include the following:
- Three anterior hepatic veins
- Three lateral tributaries: the right suprarenal vein (the left suprarenal vein drains into the left renal vein), the renal veins, and the right testicular or ovarian vein

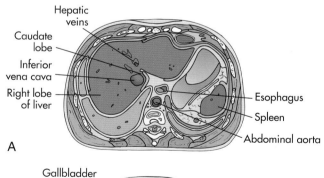

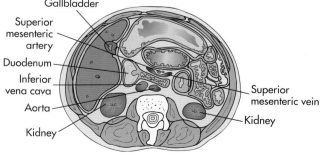

FIGURE 8-47 **A,** Cross section of the abdomen at the level of the tenth intervertebral disk. **B,** Cross section of the abdomen at the first lumbar vertebra.

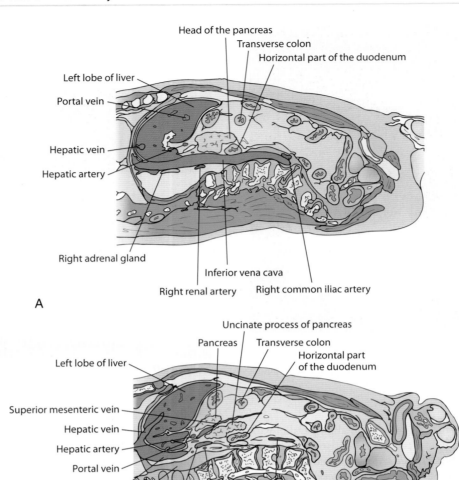

FIGURE 8-48 A, Sagittal section of the abdomen 3 cm from the midline. **B,** Sagittal section of the abdomen 2 cm from the midline.

- Five lateral abdominal wall tributaries: the inferior phrenic vein and the four lumbar veins
- Three veins of origin: the two common iliac veins and the median sacral vein

The IVC is a large, collapsible vein that returns blood from the abdomen, pelvis, and lower limbs through the system's major tributaries into the right atrium of the heart. The superior vena cava drains the head, neck, thoracic cavity, and upper extremities and is discussed in Chapter 38. The walls of the cava are much thinner than those of the aorta because the pressure of blood flow is much lower.

Sonographic Findings. The IVC serves as a landmark for many other abdominal structures and should be routinely visualized on all examinations. The intrahepatic portion of the cava is seen by using the liver as an acoustic window (Figure 8-49). Beyond the liver border, the cava may become obscured by overlying bowel gas. The complete IVC is imaged on a sagittal scan. Beginning at the midline of the abdomen, the transducer should be angled slightly to the right with a slight oblique tilt until the entire vessel is seen. The patient should be instructed to hold his or her breath; this causes the patient to perform a slight Valsalva maneuver toward the end of inspiration, which dilates the IVC. The inferior vena cava may expand to 2.5 cm in diameter with this maneuver. With expiration, venous return improves, and therefore the caval diameter decreases. Both cardiac and respiratory pulsations are transmitted in the IVC to produce a phasic pattern similar to the pattern in the peripheral veins. The diameter of the IVC will depend on the patient's age and body mass. The normal adult inferior vena cava size should measure less than 2.2 cm with greater than 50% respiratory collapse.

The pulsatile aorta is easily differentiated from the IVC as the IVC travels in a horizontal course with its proximal portion

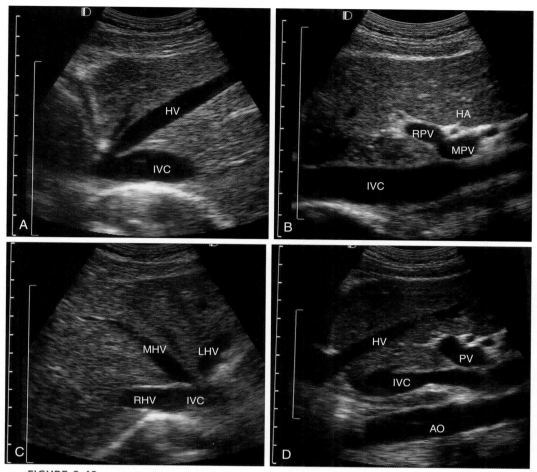

FIGURE 8-49 Normal inferior vena cava protocol. **A** and **B,** Longitudinal images. **A,** The hepatic vein *(HV)* drains into the inferior vena cava *(IVC)* at the diaphragm. **B,** The IVC is the posterior border of the portal vein. *HA,* Hepatic artery; *MPV,* main portal vein; *RPV,* right portal vein. **C,** Transverse image: The three hepatic veins are shown to drain into the IVC at the dome of the liver. *LHV,* Left hepatic vein. **D,** Oblique coronal image: The patient is rolled into a slight oblique position (right side up). The transducer is angled from the midclavicular line toward the midline of the abdomen to see the IVC "anterior" to the abdominal aorta *(AO).*

curving slightly anterior as it pierces the diaphragm to empty into the right atrial cavity (Figure 8-50). The aorta, on the other hand, follows the curvature of the spine, with its distal portion lying more posterior, before bifurcating into the iliac vessels. The lumen of the cava should be anechoic, although with slow flowing blood, the lumen becomes slightly more echogenic with *swirling* of the blood seen in real-time.

On transverse scans, the almond-shaped IVC serves as a landmark for localizing the splenic vein, which is generally found anterior and slightly medial to the cava as it crosses in a horizontal path from the spleen to form the portal vein (Figure 8-51). On longitudinal scans, the IVC serves as a landmark for the portal vein, which is located just anterior to the anterior wall of the midpoint of the inferior vena cava (Figure 8-52).

The inferior vena cava is also useful in identifying the echogenic pancreas and small common bile duct (Figure 8-53). The head of the pancreas is seen just inferior to the portal vein and anterior to the IVC as it makes a slight impression or

indentation on the anterior wall of the cava. The common duct is seen anterior to the portal vein as it dips posterior to enter the head of the pancreas.

Inferior Vena Cava Abnormalities

Congenital Abnormalities. The IVC is formed by three pairs of cardinal veins in the retroperitoneum; these veins undergo sequential development and regression. The posterior cardinal veins appear at 6 weeks and form no part of the cava, but may be part of the anomalies (Figure 8-54). The subcardinal veins appear at 7 weeks to produce the prerenal segment of the IVC. The supracardinal system at 8 weeks produces the postrenal segment of the IVC. The supracardinals form the azygos and hemiazygos system above the diaphragm. The anastomosis between the subcardinal and supracardinal systems forms the renal veins. The normal left cardinal system involutes, and the right consists of the posterior infrarenal vein, supracardinal vein, renal segment,

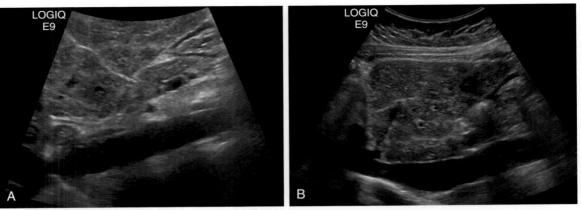

FIGURE 8-50 A, The pulsatile aorta is easily differentiated from the inferior vena cava **(B)** as the IVC travels in a horizontal course with its proximal portion curving slightly anterior as it pierces the diaphragm to empty into the right atrial cavity.

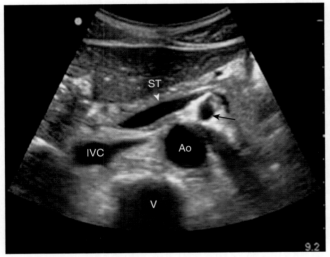

FIGURE 8-51 On transverse scans, the almond-shaped inferior vena cava serves as a landmark for localizing the splenic vein *(short arrow)*, which is generally found anterior and slightly medial to the cava as it crosses in a horizontal path from the spleen to form the portal vein. Superior mesenteric artery *(long arrow)*, aorta *(Ao)*, inferior vena cava *(IVC)*, vertebral body *(V)*.

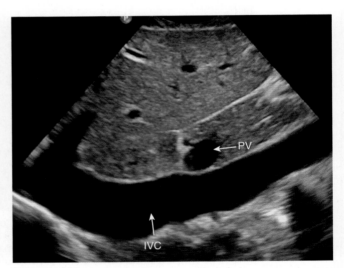

FIGURE 8-52 On longitudinal scans, the inferior vena cava serves as a landmark for the portal vein *(PV)*, which is located just anterior to the anterior wall of the midpoint of the inferior vena cava *(IVC)*.

anterior suprarenal subcardinal vein, and the confluence of hepatic veins. Abnormalities in development of the IVC include a *double inferior vena cava* and an *absent inferior vena cava* (Figure 8-55).

Double Inferior Vena Cava. Double IVC has an incidence of less than 3%. The size of the two vessels can be the same or may vary, depending on the dominant side. In the most common type, the left IVC joins the left renal vein, which crosses the midline at its normal level to join the right IVC. The left IVC does not continue above the left renal vein. Less commonly, the right IVC joins the left IVC to join the hemiazygos.

Infrahepatic Interruption of the Inferior Vena Cava. This condition results from failure of union of the hepatic veins and the right subcardinal vein, which can include azygos or, less commonly, hemiazygos continuation. The azygos veins consist of the main azygos vein, the

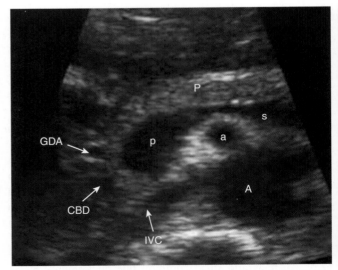

FIGURE 8-53 The inferior vena cava is also useful in identifying the echogenic pancreas and small common bile duct *(CBD)*, gastroduodenal artery *(GDA)*. Portal vein *(p)*, splenic vein *(s)*, superior mesenteric artery *(a)*, aorta *(A)*.

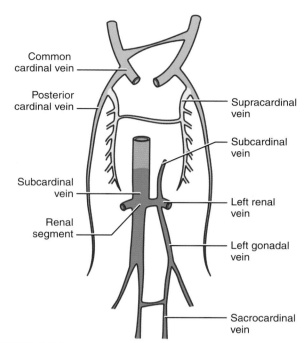

FIGURE 8-54 The inferior vena cava is formed by three pairs of cardinal veins in the retroperitoneum; these veins undergo sequential development and regression. The posterior cardinal veins appear at 6 weeks and form no part of the cava, but may be part of the anomalies.

inferior hemiazygos vein, and the superior hemiazygos vein (Figure 8-56). They drain blood from the posterior parts of the intercostal spaces, the posterior abdominal wall, the pericardium, the diaphragm, the bronchi, and the esophagus. Interruption of the IVC connection to the heart is associated with acyanotic and cyanotic congenital heart disease, abnormalities of cardiac position, and abdominal situs with asplenia and polysplenia.

■ *Sonographic Findings.* In patients with an interruption of the IVC, the azygos vein continuation is identical to or larger than the IVC, which passes along the aorta medial to the right crus of the diaphragm. The hepatic veins drain into an independent confluence that passes through the diaphragm to enter the right atrium. A membranous obstruction of the IVC may simulate infrahepatic interruption of the cava with azygos continuation. A web or membrane obstructs the IVC at the level of the diaphragm and leads to chronic congestion of the liver with centrilobular and periportal fibrosis.

The following three types of obstruction occur:
- A thin membrane at the level of the entrance to the right atrium
- An absent segment of the IVC without characteristic conical narrowing
- Complete obstruction secondary to thrombosis

Clinically, patients present in the third to fourth decade of life with portal hypertension. Ultrasound shows obstruction at the diaphragm and dilation of the azygos system. On longitudinal scans, it is very difficult to identify the presence of the IVC. The azygos system is dilated on the right side of the midline, "acting" as the IVC.

Inferior Vena Cava Dilation or Compression. In patients with right ventricular failure, the IVC does not collapse with inspiration or expiration. Dilation of the IVC may be noted in several pathologies, including right ventricular heart failure (Figure 8-57), congestive heart disease, constrictive pericarditis, tricuspid disease, and right heart obstructive tumors. Tumor or thrombus may be found in the IVC and may cause obstruction of blood returning into the right atrium. In patients with hepatomegaly, the IVC and hepatic veins are dilated; increased pressure is transmitted through the sinusoids, resulting in portal vein distention. If severe cirrhosis is present, the sinusoids may be unable to transmit pressure, and the portal veins will not distend.

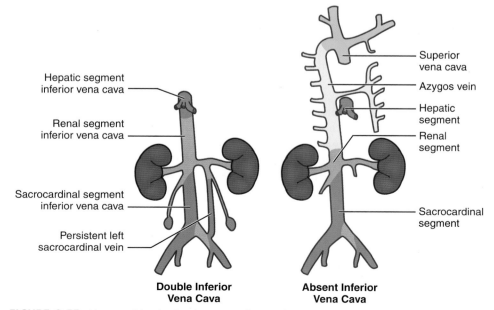

FIGURE 8-55 Abnormalities in development of the inferior vena cava include a double inferior vena cava and an absent inferior vena cava.

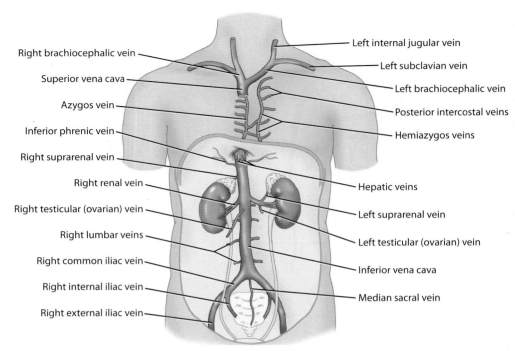

FIGURE 8-56 The azygos veins consist of the main azygos vein, the inferior hemiazygos vein, and the superior hemiazygos vein.

Right brachiocephalic vein
Superior vena cava
Azygos vein
Inferior phrenic vein
Right suprarenal vein
Right renal vein
Right testicular (ovarian) vein
Right lumbar veins
Right common iliac vein
Right internal iliac vein
Right external iliac vein

Left internal jugular vein
Left subclavian vein
Left brachiocephalic vein
Posterior intercostal veins
Hemiazygos veins
Hepatic veins
Left suprarenal vein
Left testicular (ovarian) vein
Inferior vena cava
Median sacral vein

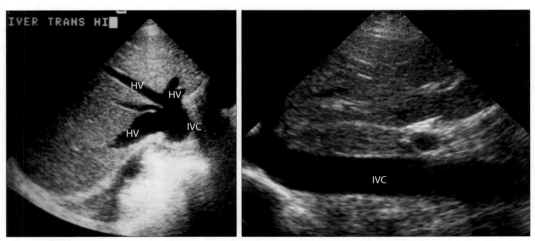

FIGURE 8-57 Transverse and sagittal scans of a patient in right ventricular heart failure show a dilated inferior vena cava *(IVC)* and hepatic veins *(HV)*.

Compression of the IVC may be seen in later stages of pregnancy as the enlarged uterus compresses the vena cava. Over time, this compression will produce edema of the ankles and feet and temporary varicose veins. Other forms of caval compression may arise from malignant retroperitoneal tumors, hepatic neoplasm, or pancreatic mass. The presence of thrombus within the vessel should be evaluated, especially in patients with a known renal tumor.

Inferior Vena Cava Tumors, Thrombus, and Filters. It is important for the sonographer to identify the entire IVC; bowel gas can make the distal cava difficult to identify.

Locations of Inferior Vena Cava

Hepatic Portion of Inferior Vena Cava. Masses posterior to the hepatic portion of the IVC are the right adrenal, neurogenic,

and hepatic. With enlargement of the liver, the cava is compressed rather than displaced. A localized liver mass would produce posterior, lateral, or medial displacement of the IVC, whereas a mass in the posterior caudate lobe and right lobe may elevate the cava.

Pancreatic Portion of the Inferior Vena Cava. The middle, or pancreatic, portion of the IVC may elevate the cava from abnormalities of the right renal artery, right kidney, lumbar spine, or lymph node masses.

Small Bowel (Lower) Segment. Lumbar spine abnormalities or lymph nodes would elevate the IVC.

Sonographic Findings. The IVC may become obstructed by tumor formation (Figure 8-58). The ultrasound appearance of the tumor is of single or multiple echogenic nodules along

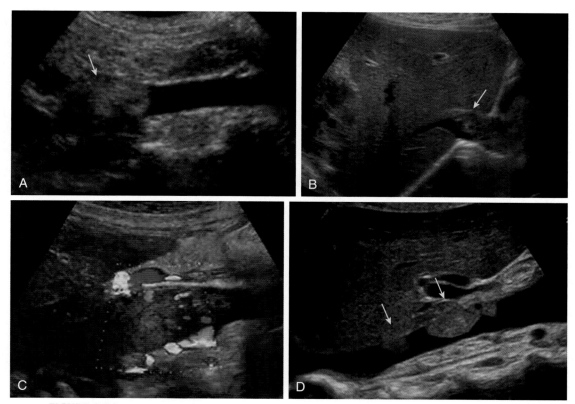

FIGURE 8-58 The inferior vena cava may become obstructed by tumor formation. **A,** Longitudinal and **B,** transverse view of the inferior vena cava filled with tumor *(arrow).* **C,** Color Doppler shows the tumor obstructing the flow of blood in the inferior vena cava. **D,** Longitudinal image of tumor formation within the inferior vena cava.

the wall. The cava may be distended and filled with a tumor. The most common tumor is renal cell carcinoma, usually from the right kidney. Wilms' tumor is also seen extending into the IVC and right atrium. Other less common tumors are retroperitoneal liposarcoma, leiomyosarcoma, pheochromocytoma, osteosarcoma, and rhabdomyosarcoma. Benign tumors, such as angiomyolipoma, can have venous involvement.

Inferior Vena Cava Thrombosis. Complete thrombosis of the IVC is life-threatening. Patients present with leg edema, low back pain, pelvic pain, gastrointestinal complaints, and renal and liver abnormalities (Figure 8-59). Thrombosis within the IVC appears as a homogeneous echo mass. Color Doppler is useful to determine whether the vessel is occluded.

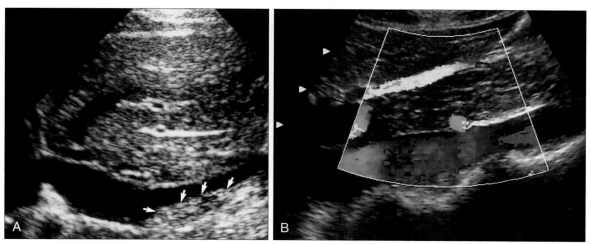

FIGURE 8-59 A, Longitudinal image of the inferior vena cava with a tumor lying along the posterior wall *(arrows).* **B,** Color flow Doppler will delineate the patency of the inferior vena cava in the event of tumor or thrombus formation.

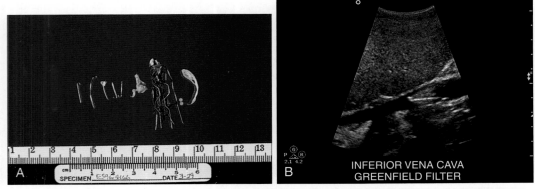

FIGURE 8-60 A, Surgical specimen of the vena cava filter. **B,** Longitudinal image of the filter in place within the inferior vena cava.

Inferior Vena Cava Filters. The most common origin of pulmonary emboli is venous thrombosis from the lower extremities. Surgical and angiographic placement of transvenous filters into the cava has been used to prevent recurrent embolization in patients who cannot tolerate anticoagulants (Figure 8-60). The preferred location of the filter is in the iliac bifurcation below the renal veins. The filter is a tubular wire mesh that is implanted into the IVC to trap small emboli that may cause problems in the heart or the lungs. After placement, some filters can migrate cranially or caudally and perforate the cava, producing a retroperitoneal bleed. Filters can also perforate the duodenum, aorta, ureter, and hepatic vein.

Lateral Tributaries to the Inferior Vena Cava

Renal Veins. Five or six branches of the renal vein unite to form the main renal vein. The right and left main renal veins arise anterior to the renal arteries at their respective sides of the IVC at the level of L2 (Figure 8-61).

Left Renal Vein. The **left renal vein** arises medially to exit from the hilus of the kidney. It flows from the left kidney posterior to the superior mesenteric artery and anterior to the aorta to enter the lateral wall of the IVC (Figure 8-62). Above the entry of the renal veins, the IVC enlarges because of the increased volume of blood returning from the kidneys. The left renal vein is larger than the right renal vein. It accepts branches from the left adrenal, left gonadal, and lumbar veins. Best images are seen on the transverse views; the left renal vein is an anechoic tubular structure that originates from the medial hilum of the left kidney, courses posterior to the SMA, and anterior to the aorta to enter the medial wall of the IVC. The left renal vein is visualized as a small circular structure coursing between the SMA and the aorta on the longitudinal image.

Right Renal Vein. The **right renal vein** is best seen on transverse images as it flows directly from the hilum of the right kidney into the posterolateral aspect of the IVC (Figure 8-63). It seldom accepts tributaries; the right adrenal and right gonadal veins enter the IVC directly.

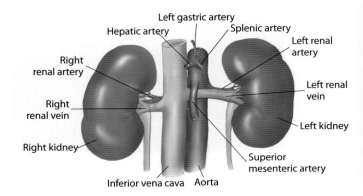

A

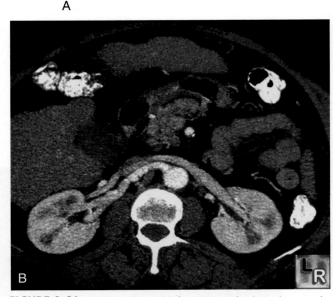

B

FIGURE 8-61 A, The right and left main renal veins arise anterior to the renal arteries at their respective sides of the inferior vena cava at the level of L2. **B,** Transverse CT of the left renal vein arising from the hilum of the kidney, crossing anterior to the aorta to enter the inferior vena cava. The right renal artery may be seen to leave the medial wall of the aorta, posterior to the left renal vein, into the right renal hilum.

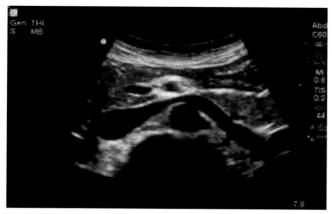

FIGURE 8-62 The left renal vein *(LRV)* is well seen as it leaves the renal hilus and flows anterior to the aorta *(A)* and posterior to the superior mesenteric artery *(SMA)* to enter the lateral wall of the inferior vena cava *(IVC)*.

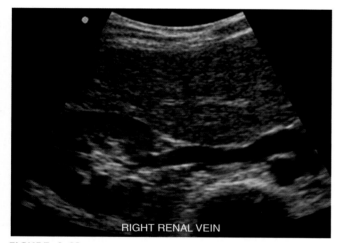

FIGURE 8-63 The right renal vein is best seen on transverse images as it flows directly from the hilum of the right kidney into the posterolateral aspect of the inferior vena cava.

Renal Vein Obstruction. Renal vein obstruction is seen in the dehydrated or septic infant. It may also be seen in adults with multiple renal abnormalities (nephrotic syndrome, shock, renal tumor, kidney transplant, or trauma). Left renal vein obstruction may result from the spread of such nonrenal

malignancies as carcinoma of the pancreas or lung, or lymphoma. A retroperitoneal tumor can occlude the left renal vein by direct extension into the vein lumen or compression of the lumen by a contiguous mass.

Clinical Signs. The patient presents with flank pain, hematuria, flank mass, and proteinuria. The condition may be associated with maternal diabetes and transient high blood pressure.

Sonographic Findings. Sonography may be used to confirm that a palpable flank mass is kidney and to exclude hydronephrosis and multicystic kidney as causes of a nonfunctioning kidney (Figure 8-64). In infants with renal vein obstruction, enlarged kidneys without cysts are seen. Medium echoes or "clumps" of echoes may be randomly scattered within the kidney, with surrounding echo-free spaces. The parenchymal anechoic areas are the result of hemorrhage and infarcts. The renal pattern progresses to atrophy over 2 months. Late findings include increased parenchymal echoes, loss of corticomedullary junction, and decreased renal size.

Renal Vein Thrombosis. Renal vein thrombosis is the formation of a clot in the vein that drains blood from the kidneys, ultimately leading to a reduction in the drainage of one or both kidneys and the possible migration of the clot to other parts of the body (Figure 8-65). Thrombosis most commonly affects newborns with blood clotting abnormalities or dehydration and adults with nephrotic syndrome.

If the following findings are present on sonography, renal vein thrombosis may be diagnosed:
1. Direct visualization of thrombi in the renal vein and IVC
2. Demonstrated renal vein dilation proximal to the point of occlusion
3. Loss of normal renal structure
4. Increased renal size (acute phase) (Figure 8-66)
5. Decreased flow or no flow shown on Doppler

Clinical Signs. The patient presents with pain, nephromegaly, hematuria, or thromboembolic phenomena elsewhere in the body. A variety of lesions may be associated with this abnormality.

Gonadal Veins. The gonadal veins (testicular and ovarian) course anterior to the external and internal iliac veins and continue cranially and retroperitoneally along the psoas muscle until their terminus. The left gonadal vein usually enters

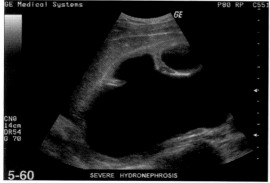

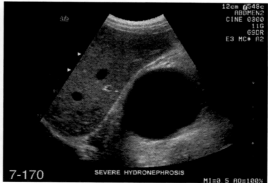

FIGURE 8-64 Hydronephrosis of the right kidney.

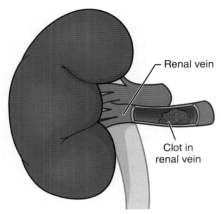

FIGURE 8-65 Renal vein thrombosis is the formation of a clot in the vein that drains blood from the kidneys, ultimately leading to a reduction in the drainage of one or both kidneys and the possible migration of the clot to other parts of the body.

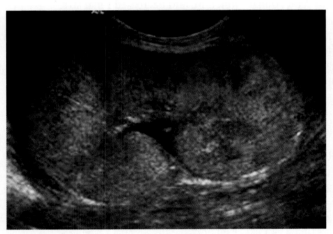

FIGURE 8-66 Renal transplant demonstrates an enlarged kidney and loss of normal renal structure secondary to renal vein thrombosis.

the left renal vein or the left adrenal vein, which empties into the IVC. The right gonadal vein enters the IVC on the anterolateral border above the entrance of the lumbar veins.

Suprarenal Veins. The right suprarenal vein arises from the suprarenal gland and usually drains directly into the IVC. The left arises from the suprarenal gland and drains into the left renal vein.

Anterior Tributaries to the Inferior Vena Cava

Hepatic Veins. The **hepatic veins** are the largest visceral tributaries of the IVC. They originate between the segments of the liver and drain posteriorly into the IVC at the level of the diaphragm (Figure 8-67). The hepatic veins return unoxygenated blood from the liver. The veins collect blood from the three minor tributaries within the liver: the right hepatic vein drains the right lobe of the liver, the middle hepatic vein drains the caudate lobe, and the left hepatic vein drains the left lobe of the liver. The

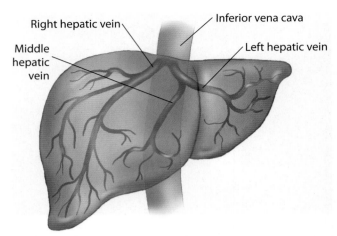

FIGURE 8-67 The hepatic veins are divided into three components: right, middle, and left. They all drain into the inferior vena cava at the level of the diaphragm.

middle and left hepatic veins may fuse before emptying into the IVC.

Sonographic Findings. The hepatic veins are best visualized on longitudinal scans of the liver as they drain into the IVC at the level of the diaphragm (Figure 8-68, *A* and *B*). Transverse scans obtained with a cephalic angle of the transducer at the level of the xiphoid often show at least two of the three veins draining into the IVC (Figure 8-68, *C* and *D*). The hepatic veins resemble the "bunny" or "reindeer" sign on the sonogram.

Distinguishing hepatic veins from other vascular structures requires recognition of their anatomic patterns. Hepatic veins drain cephalad toward the diaphragm and then dorsomedial toward the IVC. Hepatic veins increase in caliber as they approach the diaphragm. Unlike portal veins, they are not surrounded by bright acoustic reflections, although a slight amount of acoustic enhancement may be seen along their posterior border.

Hepatic veins demonstrate a triphasic and pulsatile flow pattern that reflects the transmitted cardiac pulsations (Figure 8-69). Patients with cirrhosis and portal hypertension will lose this pulsatile pattern, and patients in right-sided heart failure will show increased pulsations.

PORTAL VENOUS SYSTEM

Portal Vein

The **portal vein** is formed posterior to the pancreas by the union of the superior mesenteric vein and splenic veins at the level of L2. Its trunk is 5 to 7 cm in length (Figure 8-70, *A* and *B*). The portal vein courses posterior to the first portion of the duodenum and then between the layers of the lesser omentum to the porta hepatis, where it bifurcates into its hepatic branches. It carries blood from the intestinal tract to the liver by means of its two main branches: the right and left portal veins. It drains blood from the gastrointestinal tract; from the lower end of the esophagus to the upper end of the anal canal;

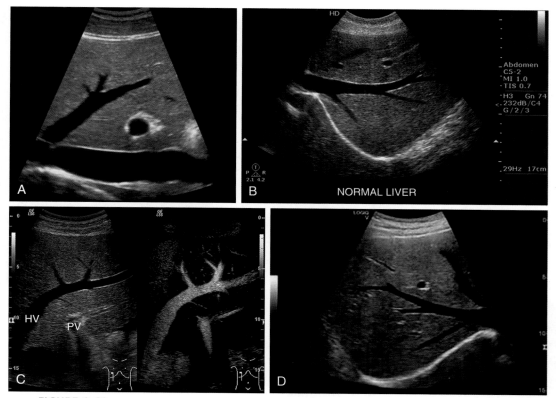

NORMAL LIVER

HV PV

FIGURE 8-68 A–C, Longitudinal image of the hepatic vein draining into the inferior vena cava at the level of the diaphragm. **D,** Transverse images of the right, middle, and left hepatic veins.

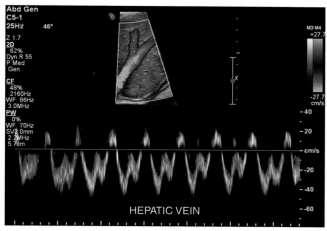

HEPATIC VEIN

FIGURE 8-69 Hepatic veins demonstrate a triphasic and pulsatile flow pattern that reflects the transmitted cardiac pulsations.

and from the pancreas, gallbladder, bile ducts, and spleen. The portal vein has an **anastomosis** with the esophageal veins, rectal venous plexus, and superficial abdominal veins. The portal venous blood traverses the liver and drains into the IVC via the hepatic veins.

The liver receives a dual blood supply from the portal vein and the hepatic artery. The portal vein supplies up to one half of the oxygen requirements of the hepatocytes because of its great flow, even though it carries incompletely oxygenated (less than 80%) venous blood from the intestines and spleen.

The portal triad contains branches of the portal vein, hepatic artery, and bile duct contained within a connective tissue sheath that gives the portal vein an echogenic wall as seen on liver sonographic images.

Sonographic Findings. The portal vein is clearly seen on both transverse and sagittal scans (Figure 8-71). On transverse scans, the main portal vein is a thin-walled circular structure, generally lateral and somewhat anterior to the IVC. It is often possible to record the splenic vein as it crosses the midline of the abdomen to join the superior mesenteric vein to form the main portal trunk. Thus a long section of the splenic vein can be visualized. Often the right or left portal vein can be seen branching from the portal trunk to enter the hilum of the liver.

Portal veins become smaller as they progress into the liver from the porta hepatis. Large radicles situated near or approaching the porta hepatis are portal veins, not hepatic veins. The portal veins are characterized by high-amplitude acoustic reflections that presumably arise from the fibrous tissues surrounding the portal triad as it courses through the liver substance.

The right and left portal veins course transversely through the liver; thus transverse scans display their longest extent (Figure 8-71, *B*). The right portal vein is most consistently demonstrated on the sonogram. Anatomically, any intraparenchymal segment of the portal venous system lying to the right of the lateral aspect of the IVC is a branch of the right portal system. The right portal vein has an anterior branch

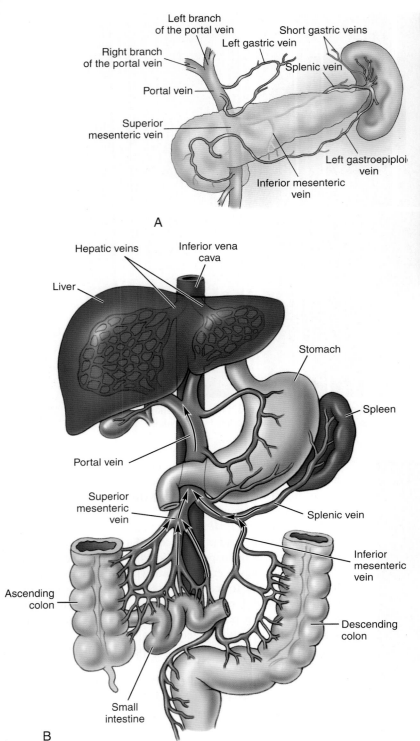

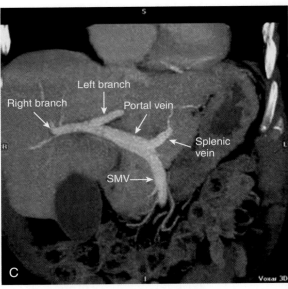

FIGURE 8-70 A, The superior and inferior mesenteric veins join the splenic vein to form the portal vein. **B,** The portal vein *(PV)* is formed posterior to the pancreas by the union of the superior mesenteric vein and splenic veins at the level of L2. **C,** CT contrast image of the portal system. Splenic vein *(SV)*, inferior mesenteric vein *(imv)*, superior mesenteric vein *(smv)*, right portal vein *(RPV)*, left portal vein *(LPV)*, right posterior segment *(RPS)*, right anterior segment *(RAS)*.

that lies centrally within the anterior segment of the right lobe and a posterior branch that lies centrally within the posterior segment of the right lobe.

The left portal vein has a narrow-caliber trunk and may be seen coursing transversely through the left hepatic lobe from a posterior to an anterior position (Figure 8-71, *C*). The main portal vein is well seen as a circular anechoic structure to the IVC. The portal radicle may have many different variations;

therefore, it is important to become familiar with their patterns to be able to distinguish them from dilated biliary radicles.

Splenic Vein

The **splenic vein** is a tributary of the portal circulation. It begins at the hilum of the spleen, where it is formed by the union of several veins. It is subsequently joined by the short

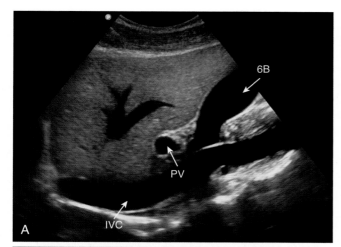

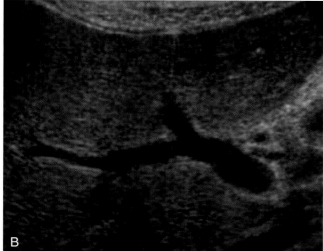

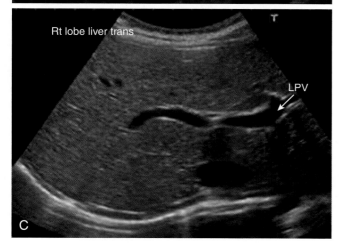

FIGURE 8-71 A, Longitudinal image of the portal vein *(PV)* anterior to the inferior vena cava *(IVC)*. Gallbladder *(Gb)*. **B,** Transverse image of the main portal vein with bifurcation into the right posterior and anterior branches. **C,** Transverse image of the left portal vein *(LPV)*.

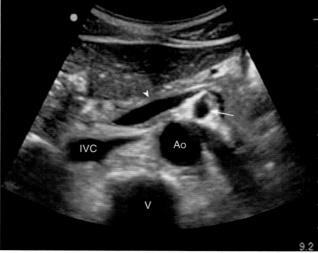

FIGURE 8-72 The splenic vein *(short arrow)* is best visualized in the transverse plane as it crosses the upper abdomen from the hilum of the spleen to join the superior mesenteric vein to form the portal vein slightly to the right of midline. Superior mesenteric artery *(long arrow)*, aorta *(Ao)*, inferior vena cava *(IVC)*.

gastric and left gastroepiploic veins (see Figure 8-70, *A*). The splenic vein runs along the posteromedial border of the pancreas. It joins the superior mesenteric vein posterior to the neck of the pancreas to form the portal vein. Additional veins from the pancreas and inferior mesenteric vein drain into the splenic vein. The splenic vein drains blood from the stomach, spleen, and pancreas.

■ ***Sonographic Findings.*** The splenic vein is best visualized in the transverse plane as it crosses the upper abdomen from the hilum of the spleen to join the superior mesenteric vein to form the portal vein slightly to the right of midline (Figure 8-72). The splenic vein crosses anteriorly to the aorta and the IVC and generally relates to the medial and posterior borders of the pancreatic body and tail. Its course is variable, so small degrees of obliquity with the transducer may be necessary to image the vein entirely. It is usually smaller than the superior mesenteric vein and the main portal vein. The larger diameter of the portal vein is the result of the influx of blood from the superior mesenteric vein. An obvious widening is demonstrated at the junction of the portal and splenic veins.

On sagittal scans, the splenic vein can be visualized posterior to the left lobe of the liver and anterior to the major vascular structures. The pancreas may be seen inferior and slightly anterior to the vein (Figure 8-73). When splenomegaly is present, it is often possible to identify the origin of the splenic vein at the splenic hilum.

Superior Mesenteric Vein

The **superior mesenteric vein** is also a tributary to the portal vein (see Figure 8-70). It begins at the ileocolic junction and runs cephalad along the posterior abdominal wall within the root of the mesentery of the small intestine to the right of the superior mesenteric artery. The superior mesenteric vein passes anterior to the third part of the duodenum and posterior to the neck of the pancreas, where it joins the splenic vein to form the main portal vein. It also receives tributaries that correspond to the branches of the superior

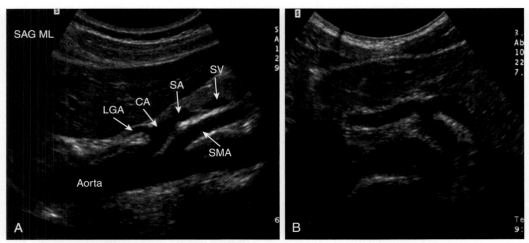

FIGURE 8-73 A, Longitudinal and **B,** transverse images of the splenic vein.

mesenteric artery, where it is joined by the inferior pancreaticoduodenal vein to the right gastroepiploic vein from the right aspect of the greater curvature of the stomach. The superior mesenteric vein drains blood from several smaller veins: the middle colic vein (transverse colon), the right colic vein (ascending colon), and the pancreatic duodenal vein.

◼ *Sonographic Findings.* The superior mesenteric vein is somewhat variable in its anatomic location. Generally, it is anterior to the IVC and to the right of the superior mesenteric artery. The superior mesenteric vein drains into the main portal vein (with the splenic vein); therefore, the sonographer should not be able to demonstrate these three structures together on a single transverse scan (Figure 8-74). The superior mesenteric vein is the posterior border of the neck of the pancreas and the anterior border of the uncinate process of the pancreatic head.

On sagittal scans, the vein is seen as a long, tubular structure anterior to the IVC. With correct oblique angulation of the transducer, the path of the superior mesenteric vein can be followed as it enters the portal system.

The following points help to distinguish the superior mesenteric artery from the vein:

- The superior mesenteric vein is of larger caliber than the artery.
- Real-time identification of the confluence of the superior mesenteric vein–portal vein or superior mesenteric artery is possible as the superior mesenteric artery originates directly from the anterior wall of the abdominal aorta.

Inferior Mesenteric Vein

The **inferior mesenteric vein** drains the left third of the colon and upper colon and ascends retroperitoneally along the left psoas muscle. It begins midway down the anal canal as the superior rectal vein (see Figure 8-70). It runs cranially in the posterior abdominal wall on the left side of the inferior mesenteric artery and duodenojejunal junction to join the splenic vein posterior to the pancreas. It receives many tributaries along its way, including the left colic vein. The inferior mesenteric vein drains several tributaries: the

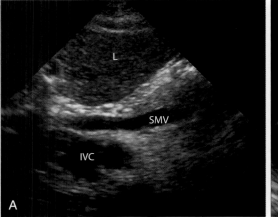 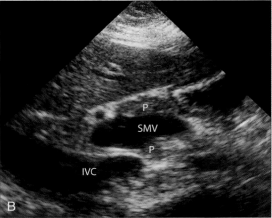

FIGURE 8-74 A and **B,** Sagittal images of the superior mesenteric vein *(SMV)* as it lies anterior to the uncinate process of the pancreas *(P)* and posterior to the body. *IVC,* inferior vena cava; *L,* liver.

left colic vein (descending colon), the sigmoid vein (sigmoid colon), and the superior rectal vein (upper rectum).

Sonographic Findings. The inferior mesenteric vein is difficult to recognize on ultrasound because of its anatomic location and small diameter. It is generally covered by the small bowel and has no major vascular structures posterior to it to aid in its recognition.

ABDOMINAL DOPPLER TECHNIQUES

Doppler ultrasound is a useful clinical tool for diagnosing many disease processes. The following paragraphs present an overview of abdominal applications that have been used with color flow detection and pulsed Doppler techniques. Doppler has helped detect the presence or absence of blood flow, the direction of blood flow, and flow disturbance patterns. It has also been used in tissue characterization and waveform analysis.

Blood Flow Analysis

Presence or Absence of Flow. Doppler ultrasound frequently is used to differentiate vessels from nonvascular structures. For example, to distinguish the common bile duct from the hepatic artery, look for absence of flow in the common duct; to distinguish the hepatic artery from the splenic artery, look for direction of flow; to differentiate an aneurysm from a pancreatic pseudocyst, look for slow flow in the aneurysm; to differentiate dilated intrahepatic bile ducts and prominent hepatic artery, again look for absence of flow in the bile duct.

Direction of Flow. In patients who develop **portal venous hypertension,** the portal blood flow becomes **hepatofugal** (away from the liver) instead of **hepatopetal** (toward the liver). This may occur secondary to portal venous shunts or varices. The sonographer detects a high-velocity flow pattern at the site of the shunt with a turbulent flow pattern on color Doppler.

Disturbance of Flow. A flow disturbance (increased velocity or obstruction of flow) may result from the formation of an atheroma, arteriovenous fistula, pseudoaneurysm, or aneurysmal dilation.

Tissue Characterization. Research is currently under way in the area of tissue characterization. Doppler is thought to be capable of characterizing tissue because of the specific perfusion patterns characteristic of some tissues or states of tissue activity. Hepatocellular carcinomas of the liver appear to have a specific pattern. Pseudoaneurysms of peripancreatic arteries have turbulent flow patterns. Pancreatic tumors may have specific flow patterns.

Doppler Waveform Analysis. The shape of the waveform provides information on the vascular impedance of the organ the vessel supplies. Spectral analysis tells the velocity and turbulence of blood flow.

Nonresistive versus Resistive Vessels. **Nonresistive** vessels have a high diastolic component and supply organs that need constant perfusion, such as the internal carotid artery, the

hepatic artery, and the renal artery. **Resistive** vessels have very little or even reversed flow in diastole and supply organs that do not need a constant blood supply, such as the external carotid and the iliac and brachial arteries.

Peak systole is compared with minimum diastole to quantify a vessel's impedance. This ratio is the **resistive index.**

Spectral display shows us the following:

$x =$ Time is depicted on the horizontal axis.
$y =$ Doppler shift frequency (velocity) is on the vertical axis (flow toward the transducer equals positive shift, or above baseline; flow away from the transducer equals negative shift, or below baseline).
$z =$ Gray scale indicates the quantity of blood flowing at a given velocity. More red blood cells produce a brighter gray-scale assignment.

Plug flow is a pattern of blood flow, typically seen in large arteries, in which most cells are moving at the same velocity across the entire diameter of the vessel. In other vessels, the different velocities are the result of friction between the cells and arterial walls. A "clear window" under systole is typical of plug flow. When plug flow is present, the volume of blood flow can be calculated.

Doppler Technique

Unlike visualization of the heart, in which high-velocity flows are present, visualization of abdominal vessels requires very sensitive Doppler instrumentation. Abdominal vessels generally have low velocity and flow. This segment provides a brief overview of Doppler techniques the beginning student should become familiar with.

Methods. Doppler is performed as part of the routine real-time examination. The patient should be fasting and should suspend respirations for the best color and pulsed **Doppler sample volume** to be obtained. The Doppler sample volume (sometimes referred to as the Doppler "gate") should be adjusted to encompass but not exceed the diameter of the vessel. If the sample volume exceeds the diameter, noise and ghost echoes may appear. This occurs because a too wide Doppler gate causes interference from surrounding vessels and structures.

The sonographer has the ability to control the velocity of the returning echoes to prevent the alias pattern by using a lower-frequency transducer or changing from pulsed wave to continuous wave. Another feature of Doppler is that the beam records only accurate velocity patterns when the beam is parallel to the flow (the angle of flow can be changed up to 60 degrees and still be accurate). The more perpendicular the beam is to the flow, the less signal is recorded; it falls to zero velocity when the beam is directly perpendicular to the flow. Thus Doppler causes the sonographer to be creative in attempting to record accurate velocity flow patterns. The patient must be rolled into various obliquities with different angulations of the transducer to be parallel to many vascular structures.

Color Doppler is a relatively new and exciting modality that makes it easier to localize and identify smaller vessels from the biliary tree, or lymphadenopathy or other pathology. Colors are arbitrarily assigned on all equipment and refer to the direction of flow. If red is assigned as a positive flow signal, all flow toward the transducer is coded in various shades of red, depending on returning velocity. If blue is assigned a negative flow signal, the flow away from the transducer is coded in various shades of blue. The sonographer may select the particular color scheme to be used; some laboratories choose to code all positive-flow patterns red and negative-flow patterns blue. Other laboratories code all arterial flows red and venous flows blue.

Doppler Flow Patterns in the Abdominal Arterial Vessels

Box 8-4 lists Doppler flow patterns in the abdominal arteries.
Aorta. The patient should be scanned in the longitudinal plane (Figure 8-75). The flow pattern of the proximal abdominal aorta above the renal arteries shows a high systolic peak and a relatively low diastolic component. Little **spectral broadening** (turbulence) is evident. A clear window under systole means that plug flow is present. The distal abdominal aorta below the renal arteries shows flow with a small reversed component present during diastole. The closer the sonographer approaches the common iliac vessels, the greater the reverse component becomes. This occurs because of the high impedance of peripheral circulation in the leg as it becomes triphasic, crossing the baseline three times.
Celiac Axis. The sonographer should scan transversely to search for the seagull sign, celiac trunk, hepatic artery, and splenic artery. If they cannot be seen, the sonographer should

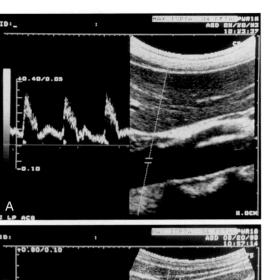

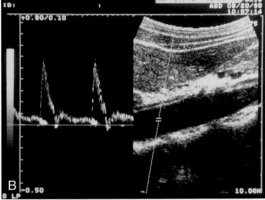

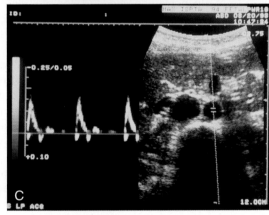

FIGURE 8-75 A, Sagittal scans of normal flow in the abdominal aorta. **B,** The flow pattern of the proximal aorta above the renal arteries shows a high systolic peak and a relatively low diastolic component. **C,** Transverse view.

scan longitudinally. Typically, spectral analysis of the celiac trunk shows systolic flow with spectral broadening (turbulence) in diastole (Figure 8-76, *A*). No change in the flow pattern is observed after meals.
Hepatic Artery. The hepatic artery is the most variable of all abdominal arteries. It has been reported that 12% of the population has a replaced hepatic artery arising from the superior mesenteric artery (Figure 8-76, *B*). Two thirds of patients have a right hepatic artery that crosses posterior to the common bile duct or right hepatic duct, whereas the left hepatic artery crosses anterior to the left hepatic duct. Flow

---

BOX 8-4	Doppler Flow Patterns in Abdominal Arteries

Aorta
- Flow varies at different levels
- Proximal aorta has high systolic/low diastolic flow
- Distal demonstrates triphasic flow

Celiac Axis
- Some spectral broadening
- Unchanged after meals

Hepatic Artery
- Spectral broadening
- Crucial in heart transplants

Splenic Artery
- Very turbulent flow pattern
- Very prone to aneurysm

Superior Mesenteric Artery
- Highly resistive in fasting patient
- Nonresistive in nonfasting patient

Renal Artery
- Nonresistive
- Spectral broadening

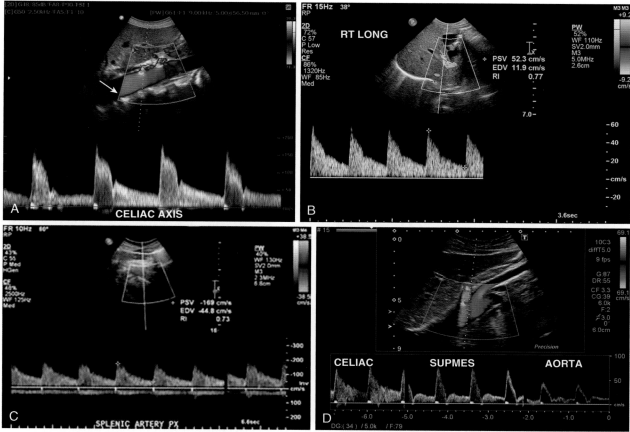

FIGURE 8-76 A, Longitudinal image of the Doppler flow obtained from the celiac axis. **B,** Flow in the hepatic artery in diastole persists because of the low vascular impedance of the liver. **C,** The splenic artery shows the greatest turbulence of all the celiac branches, probably because of its tortuosity. **D,** The superior mesenteric artery is a highly resistive vessel (with decreased diastolic flow) in the fasting state, with little or no flow in diastole.

in diastole persists because of the low vascular impedance of the liver. Similar waveforms are seen in the main hepatic and intrahepatic arteries. Typically, more spectral broadening occurs during systole and diastole.

Splenic Artery. The splenic artery shows the greatest turbulence of all the celiac branches, probably because of its tortuosity (Figure 8-76, *C*). Aneurysms of the celiac branches have been described most commonly in the splenic branch. Patients with chronic pancreatitis are particularly prone to these. The sonographer should always apply Doppler to pancreatic pseudocysts; their appearance is very similar to that of vascular aneurysms.

Superior Mesenteric Artery. Typically, the SMA is a highly resistive vessel (with decreased diastolic flow) in the fasting state, with little or no flow in diastole (see Figure 8-76, *D*). However, after a meal, the pattern of the SMA changes to a low-resistive waveform demonstrating enhanced diastolic flow. Doppler analysis of the SMA has the potential to diagnose mesenteric arterial occlusion and abdominal angina.

Renal Artery. The main renal artery has a low-impedance (nonresistive) pattern with significant diastolic flow—usually

30% to 50% of peak systole (Figure 8-77). Continuous diastolic flow provides continuous perfusion of the kidneys. Spectral broadening occurs in systole and diastole. Segmental, interlobar, and arcuate arteries demonstrate a pattern similar to that of the main renal artery. However, the flow is progressively dampened in the periphery and shows reduced velocity patterns. It may be very hard to demonstrate renal artery stenosis in a native kidney because of the difficulty involved in seeing the vessel at its origin and in its entirety (Figure 8-78). Renal artery occlusion can be declared only when the artery is unquestionably imaged. The sonographer should be careful because with complete obstruction of the native artery as collateral arterial pathways may be mistaken for a patent renal artery. At least 30% of the population has multiple renal arteries, which makes it more difficult to rule out obstruction.

Doppler Flow Patterns in the Abdominal Venous Vessels

Box 8-5 lists Doppler flow patterns in the abdominal veins.

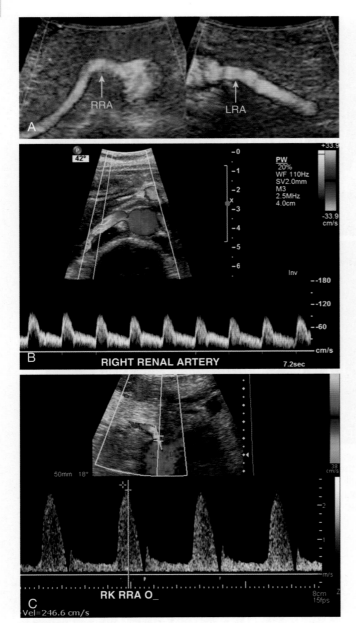

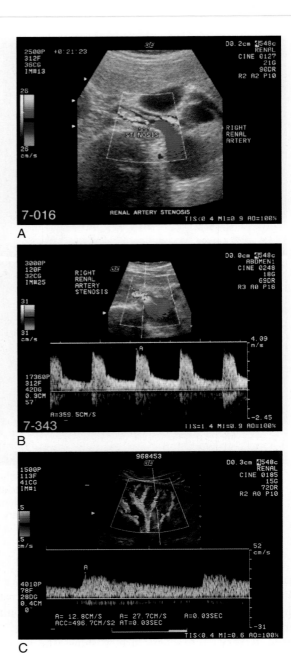

FIGURE 8-77 A, Power Doppler flow in the renal arteries. **B,** Normal right renal artery flow velocity. **C,** High-velocity flow profile in a patient with renal artery stenosis.

FIGURE 8-78 A, High-velocity jet shown in the right renal artery. **B,** Spectral waveform shows increased velocity of more than 4 m/sec, representing renal artery stenosis. **C,** With color Doppler, flow analysis may be made out to the peripheral renal arteries.

Renal Vein. The renal vein shows a variable flow pattern similar to that found in the IVC (Figures 8-79 and 8-80). The sonographer should closely evaluate the renal veins in any patient with a suspected tumor or renal obstructive lesion as this tumor may invade outside the renal capsule into the venous pathway. In the patient with a renal transplant, the sonographer should always search for a patent renal vein postoperatively. Complications of occlusion of the renal vein may cause a blockage in the vascular pathway; the kidney then reacts as though it is in rejection (i.e., laboratory values are abnormal for urea, nitrogen, creatinine, and protein).

Inferior Vena Cava and Hepatic Veins. The IVC and hepatic veins present a complex waveform, which flows

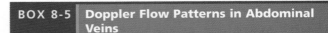

BOX 8-5	**Doppler Flow Patterns in Abdominal Veins**

Renal Vein
- Variable flow much like the inferior vena cava
- Evaluate with transplants

Inferior Vena Cava and Hepatic Veins
- Vary with respiration
- Flow above and below the baseline, reflux from right atrium

Portal Vein
- Hepatopetal flow
- Continuous flow pattern; varies slightly with respirations

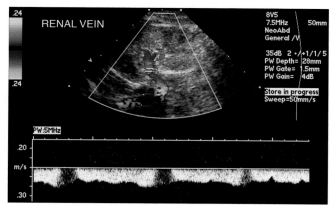

FIGURE 8-79 Normal flow velocity of the renal vein.

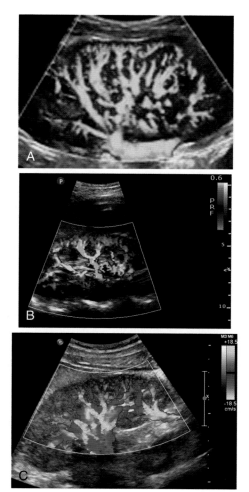

FIGURE 8-80 A, Power Doppler of the normal flow in a renal transplant kidney. B, Color power angiogram of renal flow. C, Color Doppler of an accessory renal artery.

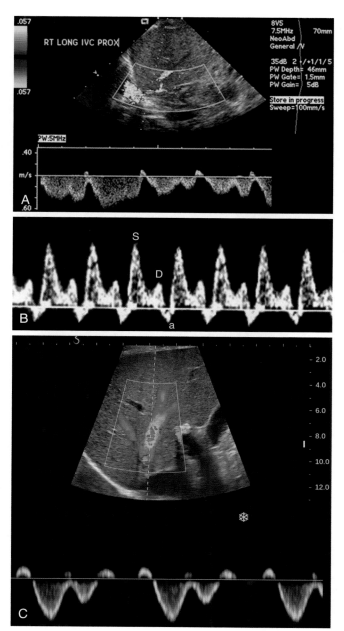

FIGURE 8-81 A, The inferior vena cava and hepatic veins present a complex waveform, which flows above and below the baseline, reflecting reflux of blood from the right atrium during systole and variations with the respiratory cycle. B, Hepatic vein flow is triphasic, with systolic (S), diastolic (D), and atrial (a) components. C, Color Doppler of normal hepatic vein flow.

above and below the baseline, reflecting reflux of blood from the right atrium during systole and variations with the respiratory cycle (Figure 8-81). The sonographer should always look at the cava and renal veins for tumor invasion when a renal cell carcinoma is observed.

Portal Vein. In the normal superior mesenteric vein and splenic vein, flow is hepatopetal (toward the liver) (Figures 8-82 and 8-83). The portal vein shows a relatively continuous flow at low velocities, which may vary slightly with respirations. Portal vein thrombosis can be easily diagnosed with sonography. A direct sign is visualization of a thrombus. Indirect signs include the loss of normal portal venous landmarks, dilation of the superior mesenteric vein and splenic vein, and venous collaterals in the porta hepatis (**cavernous transformation of the portal vein**).

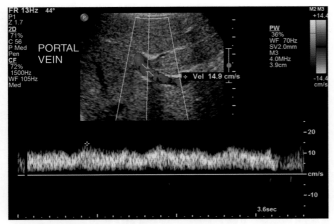

FIGURE 8-82 Portal vein flow is monophasic and hepatopetal.

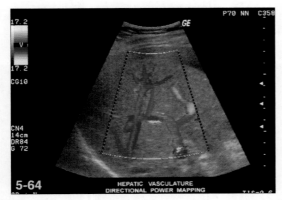

FIGURE 8-83 Color Doppler of the portal flow within the liver.

Pulsed Doppler adds to these findings; lack of Doppler signals from the lumen indicates absence of blood flow. In cirrhotic patients, thrombosis is often suspected when ascites suddenly worsens. Consequently, in these patients, special attention must be paid to the portal vein to identify a thrombus. It is often difficult to visualize the portal vein in such patients.

 Key Pearls

- The function of the circulatory system, along with the heart and lymphatics, is to transport gases, nutrient materials, and other essential substances to the tissues, and subsequently to transport waste products from the cells to appropriate sites for excretion.
- Blood is carried away from the heart by the arteries and is returned from the tissues to the heart by the veins.
- Veins have a diminished tunica media compared with the arteries.
- The aorta may be divided into the following five sections: (1) root of the aorta, (2) ascending aorta and arch, (3) descending aorta, (4) abdominal aorta and abdominal aortic branches, and (5) bifurcation of the aorta into iliac arteries.

- The diaphragmatic crura surrounds the proximal abdominal aorta as this vessel projects through the diaphragm into the abdominal cavity.
- The normal diameter of the abdominal aorta is evaluated at the region of the supraceliac and infrarenal locations.
- Measurements are made at the proximal, mid, and distal aorta in the transverse and longitudinal plane.
- The common iliac arteries arise at the bifurcation of the abdominal aorta at the fourth lumbar vertebra (near the superior sacrum). These vessels further divide into the internal and external iliac arteries.
- The short celiac trunk gives rise to three smaller vessels: the splenic, common hepatic, and left gastric arteries.
- The right renal artery and the left renal artery are lateral branches that arise just inferior to the superior mesenteric artery.
- The common hepatic artery branches into the proper hepatic artery and the gastroduodenal artery.
- The left hepatic artery is a small branch supplying the caudate and left lobes of the liver. The right hepatic artery supplies the gallbladder via the cystic artery and the liver.
- Several smaller arterial branches originate at the splenic artery as it courses through the upper border of the pancreas: the dorsal pancreatic, great pancreatic, and caudal pancreatic arteries.
- The superior mesenteric artery arises from the anterior abdominal aortic wall approximately 1 cm inferior to the celiac trunk.
- The right renal artery is a longer vessel than the left; it courses from the aorta posterior to the inferior vena cava and anterior to the vertebral column in a posterior and slightly caudal direction to enter the hilus of the right kidney.
- The left renal artery courses from the aorta directly into the hilus of the left kidney.
- Ectasia implies the diffuse dilation of a vessel, whereas an abdominal aortic aneurysm is a region of focal enlargement.
- Arteriosclerosis occurs when the arterial vascular system becomes thick and stiff, which can lead to restriction of blood flow to the organs and tissues in the body.
- An *aortic aneurysm* is defined as that with a vessel diameter greater than 3 cm or noted focal dilation of the vessel.
- The primary risk factors for a patient with an AAA are dissection and rupture of the vessel.
- Grey Turner's sign may be associated with an extensive bleed in the retroperitoneal cavity.
- An aneurysm may be classified as a true aneurysm (lined by all three layers of the aorta) or as a false aneurysm (pseudoaneurysm) (not lined by all three layers).
- The fusiform aneurysm represents a gradual transition between normal and abnormal and extends over the length of the aorta to resemble a "football-like" shape.
- A saccular aneurysm shows a sudden transition between normal and abnormal and is somewhat spherical and larger (5 to 10 cm) than fusiform aneurysms.

- Three classifications of aortic dissection are based on the DeBakey model. Types I and II involve the ascending aorta and the aortic arch; type III involves the descending aorta at a level inferior to the left subclavian artery.
- An abdominal aortic aneurysm may be surgically repaired with a flexible graft material attached to the end of the remaining aorta.
- Masses other than an aortic aneurysm that can simulate a pulsatile abdominal mass include retroperitoneal tumor, huge fibroid uterus, or para-aortic nodes.
- The inferior vena cava is formed by the union of the common iliac veins posterior to the right common iliac artery at the level of the fifth lumbar vertebra.
- In patients with right ventricular failure, the inferior vena cava does not collapse with inspiration or expiration.
- Masses posterior to the hepatic portion of the inferior vena cava are the right adrenal, neurogenic, and hepatic.
- The middle, or pancreatic, portion of the inferior vena cava may elevate the cava from abnormalities of the right renal artery, right kidney, lumbar spine, or lymph node masses.
- The right and left main renal veins arise anterior to the renal arteries at their respective sides of the inferior vena cava at the level of L2.
- Renal vein thrombosis is the formation of a clot in the vein that drains blood from the kidneys, ultimately leading to a reduction in the drainage of one or both kidneys and the possible migration of the clot to other parts of the body.
- The hepatic veins are the largest visceral tributaries of the inferior vena cava. They originate between the segments of the liver and drain posteriorly into the inferior vena cava at the level of the diaphragm.
- The right hepatic vein drains the right lobe of the liver, the middle hepatic vein drains the caudate lobe, and the left hepatic vein drains the left lobe.
- The portal vein is formed posterior to the pancreas by the union of the superior mesenteric vein and splenic veins at the level of L2.
- The portal vein has an anastomosis with the esophageal veins, rectal venous plexus, and superficial abdominal veins.
- The liver receives a dual blood supply from the portal vein and the hepatic artery.
- The portal triad contains branches of the portal vein, hepatic artery, and bile duct contained within a connective tissue sheath that gives the portal vein an echogenic wall as seen on liver sonographic images.
- Portal veins become smaller as they progress into the liver from the porta hepatis.
- The right and left portal veins course transversely through the liver; thus transverse scans display their longest extent.
- The splenic vein is a tributary of the portal circulation. It begins at the hilum of the spleen, where it is formed by the union of several veins.
- The superior mesenteric vein is also a tributary to the portal vein.
- Doppler ultrasound frequently is used to differentiate vessels from nonvascular structures.
- In patients who develop portal venous hypertension, the portal blood flow becomes hepatofugal (away from the liver) instead of hepatopetal (toward the liver).
- A flow disturbance (increased velocity or obstruction of flow) may result from the formation of an atheroma, arteriovenous fistula, pseudoaneurysm, or aneurysmal dilation.
- Spectral analysis tells the velocity and turbulence of blood flow.
- Nonresistive vessels have a high diastolic component and supply organs that need constant perfusion, such as the internal carotid artery, the hepatic artery, and the renal artery.
- Resistive vessels have very little or even reversed flow in diastole and supply organs that do not need a constant blood supply, such as the external carotid and the iliac and brachial arteries.
- The flow pattern of the proximal abdominal aorta above the renal arteries shows a high systolic peak and a relatively low diastolic component.
- Two thirds of patients have a right hepatic artery that crosses posterior to the common bile duct or right hepatic duct, whereas the left hepatic artery crosses anterior to the left hepatic duct.
- The splenic artery shows the greatest turbulence of all the celiac branches, probably because of its tortuosity.
- Typically, the superior mesenteric artery is a highly resistive vessel (with decreased diastolic flow) in the fasting state, with little or no flow in diastole.
- The main renal artery has a low impedance (nonresistive) pattern with significant diastolic flow—usually 30% to 50% of peak systole.
- The inferior vena cava and hepatic veins present a complex waveform, which flows above and below the baseline, reflecting reflux of blood from the right atrium during systole and variations with the respiratory cycle.
- The renal vein shows a variable flow pattern similar to that found in the inferior vena cava.
- In the normal superior mesenteric vein and splenic vein, flow is hepatopetal (toward the liver).
- The portal vein shows a relatively continuous flow at low velocities, which may vary slightly with respirations.

CHAPTER 9

Liver

Sandra L. Hagen-Ansert

OBJECTIVES

On completion of this chapter, you should be able to:
- Describe normal anatomy of the liver, including vascular supply and relational landmarks
- List the functions of the liver
- Describe the liver function tests and their relevance to hepatic disease
- Discuss the sonographic evaluation of the liver in the sagittal, transverse, and decubitus planes
- List the clinical signs, sonographic features, and differentials for the pathology discussed in this chapter

OUTLINE

Anatomy of the Liver
    Normal Anatomy
    Lobes of the Liver
    Vascular Supply
Physiology and Laboratory Data of the Hepatobiliary System
    Hepatic Physiology
    Hepatic versus Obstructive Disease
    Hepatic Metabolic Functions
    Hepatic Detoxification Functions

Bile
Liver Function Tests
Sonographic Evaluation of the Liver
    Liver and Porta Hepatis
        Protocol
    Normal Sonographic Anatomy and Texture
    Sagittal Plane
    Transverse Plane
    Lateral Decubitus Plane

Pathology of the Liver
    Developmental Anomalies
    Diffuse Disease
    Hepatic Vascular Flow Abnormalities
    Diffuse Abnormalities of the Liver Parenchyma
    Focal Hepatic Disease
    Infectious Disease of the Liver
    Hepatic Tumors

KEY TERMS

Alanine aminotransferase (ALT)
Alkaline phosphatase
Aspartase aminotransferase (AST)
Bare area
Bilirubin
Blood urea nitrogen (BUN)
Bull's-eye (target) lesions
Caudate lobe
Collateral circulation
Diffuse hepatocellular disease
Epigastrium
Extrahepatic
Falciform ligament

Hepatocellular disease
Hepatocyte
Hepatofugal
Hepatopetal
Hyperglycemia
Hypoglycemia
Intrahepatic
Left hypochondrium
Left lobe of the liver
Left portal vein
Ligamentum teres
Ligamentum venosum
Liver function tests

Main lobar fissure
Main portal vein
Metastatic disease
Neoplasm
Obstructive disease
Pyogenic abscess
Right hypochondrium
Right lobe of the liver
Right portal vein
Transjugular intrahepatic portosystemic shunt (TIPS)

The liver is the largest organ in the abdominal cavity, measuring approximately 21 to 22.5 cm in its greatest transverse diameter, 13 to 17.5 cm in its greatest vertical height, and 10 to 12.5 cm in its anteroposterior depth, weighing approximately 1200 to 1600 g in the adult. The size and texture of the liver parenchyma make it very accessible to sonographic evaluation. The parenchyma of the normal liver is used to evaluate other organs and glands in the body—that is, the kidneys are equally echogenic or less echogenic than the liver, the spleen has about the same to slightly more echogenicity than the liver, and the pancreas is as echogenic as or slightly more echogenic than the liver. The size and shape of the liver determine the quality of the sonographic examination performed. For example, the prominent left lobe of the liver facilitates visualization of the pancreas, which is situated just inferior to the border of the left lobe, whereas if the right lobe extends just below the costal margin, it may facilitate visualization of the gallbladder and right kidney.

ANATOMY OF THE LIVER

Normal Anatomy

The liver occupies almost all of the **right hypochondrium,** the greater part of the **epigastrium,** and the **left hypochondrium** as far as the mammillary line. The contour and shape of the liver vary according to the patient's habitus and lie. Its shape is also influenced by the lateral segment of the left lobe and the length of the right lobe of the liver. The liver lies inferior to the diaphragm. The ribs cover the greater part of the right lobe (usually a small part of the right lobe is in contact with the abdominal wall). In the epigastric region, the liver extends several centimeters below the xiphoid process. Most of the left lobe is covered by the rib cage (Figure 9-1).

The fundus of the stomach lies posterior and lateral to the left lobe of the liver and may frequently be seen on transverse sonograms. The remainder of the stomach lies inferior to the liver and is best visualized on sagittal sonograms. The duodenum lies adjacent to the right lobe and medial segment of the left lobe of the liver. The body of the pancreas is usually seen just inferior to the left lobe of the liver. The posterior border of the liver contacts the right kidney, inferior vena cava, and aorta. The diaphragm covers the superior border of the liver (Figure 9-2, A).

The liver is suspended from the diaphragm and anterior abdominal wall by the falciform ligament and from the diaphragm by the reflections of the peritoneum.

Most of the liver is covered by peritoneum, but a large area rests directly on the diaphragm; this is called the **bare area** (Figure 9-2, B). The subphrenic space between the liver (or spleen) and the diaphragm is a common site for abscess formation. The right posterior subphrenic space lies between the right lobe of the liver, the right kidney, and the right colic flexure (Figure 9-2, C). The lesser sac is an enclosed portion of the peritoneal space posterior to the liver and stomach. This sac communicates with the rest of the peritoneal space at a point near the head of the pancreas. It also may be a site for abscess formation. The right subhepatic space is located inferior to the right lobe of the liver and includes Morison's pouch, which lies between the posterior aspect of the right lobe and the upper pole of the right kidney.

The posterior borders of the liver are in contact with the inferior vena cava, the gallbladder and cystic duct, the portal vein confluence, the hepatic artery, the right kidney, and the colon (Figure 9-2, D).

Projections of the liver may be altered by some disease states. Tumor infiltration, cirrhosis, or a subphrenic abscess often causes inferior displacement, whereas ascites, excessive dilation of the colon, or abdominal tumors can elevate the liver. Retroperitoneal tumors may move the liver slightly anterior.

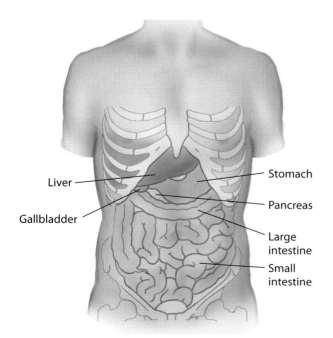

FIGURE 9-1 Anteroposterior view of the abdomen shows the right lobe of the liver covered by the ribs. The left lobe of the liver lies in the midline just posterior to the tip of the sternum. The stomach lies posterior and lateral to the left lobe of the liver.

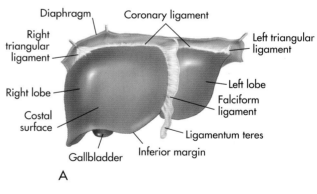

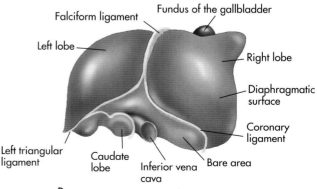

FIGURE 9-2 **A,** Anterior view of the liver. The right lobe is the largest of the four lobes of the liver. **B,** Superior view of the liver. The left lobe of the liver lies in the epigastric and left hypochondriac regions. *Continued*

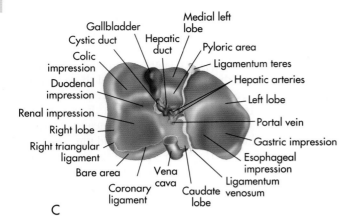

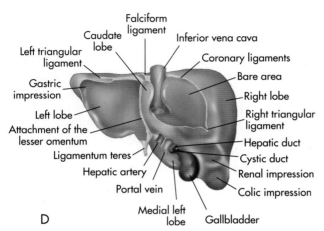

FIGURE 9-2, cont'd **C,** Inferior view of the visceral surface of the liver. **D,** Posterior view of the diaphragmatic surface of the liver. The caudate lobe is located on the posterosuperior surface of the right lobe, opposite the tenth and eleventh thoracic vertebrae. The medial segment is also called the quadrate lobe.

Lobes of the Liver

The liver has been divided into four anatomic lobes: the left, right, quadrate, and caudate, with the falciform ligament separating the left from the right lobe. However, functional divisions have more value from a surgical perspective. The functional division between the left and right lobes is based upon the vasculature, not the falciform ligament. The vascular supply and drainage divide the liver into regions that can be resected independently. The middle hepatic vein and the ascending section of the left portal vein divide the liver, functionally into a left lobe and a right lobe. This dividing line tends to be near the left edge of the inferior vena cava and the gallbladder fossa. The quadrate lobe is functionally part of the medial segment of the left lobe, which lies between the middle hepatic vein and the left hepatic vein. Using these functional divisions, the falciform ligament now belongs to the left lobe. It runs along the medial left lobe close to the border with the lateral left lobe. The following descriptions consider the anatomic/morphologic lobes of the liver. The sonographer not only should know these anatomic lobes, but also understand the locations in the liver based on functional divisions, which is explained in the Couinaud hepatic segment section.

Right Lobe. The right hypochrondrium contains the **right lobe of the liver,** which is six times larger than the left lobe. Anatomically, the right lobe appears to be separated from the left lobe by the falciform ligament on its *anterior* surface and main lobar fissure. However, functionally the middle hepatic vein runs vertically between the left medial segment and right anterior segment. Its *inferior* and *posterior* surfaces are marked by three fossae: the porta hepatis, the gallbladder fossa, and the inferior vena cava fossa. The right lobe contains an anterior and posterior segment; the right hepatic vein runs horizontally between the right anterior and posterior segments. A congenital variant, Riedel's lobe, can sometimes be seen as an anterior projection of the liver and may extend to the iliac crest.

Left Lobe. The **left lobe of the liver** lies in the epigastric and left hypochondriac regions (see Figure 9-2, *B*). The left intersegmental fissure divides the left lobe into medial and lateral segments; the left hepatic vein runs horizontally between the medial and lateral segments. Its upper surface is convex and molded onto the diaphragm (see Figure 9-2, *C* and *D*). The left lobe is bound posterior by the porta hepatis, medially by the fossa for the gallbladder, and laterally by the fossa for the umbilical vein. The size of the left lobe of the liver varies considerably; a more prominent left lobe will allow the sonographer to image the pancreas and vascular structures anterior to the spine. There are two fissures in the left lobe: the fissure for the ligamentum teres and the ligamentum venosum.

Caudate Lobe. The **caudate lobe** is a small lobe situated on the posterior surface of the left lobe, with the inferior vena cava as its posterior border and the fissure for the ligamentum venosum its anterior border (see Figure 9-2, *D*). The hepatic boundary of the superior recess of the lesser sac is formed by the left margin of the caudate lobe. A small papillary process that extends obliquely and laterally from the caudate lobe is called the *caudate process.* This small projection courses between the portal vein and inferior vena cava toward the right lobe of the liver. This process may appear separate from the caudate lobe and thus be mistaken for a mass such as pancreatic tumor or enlarged lymph node.

Vascular Anatomy and Intersegmental Segments. Understanding the vascular relationships within the hepatic segments is crucial for the surgical approach. It is important to note the hepatic veins' course between the lobes and interlobar/intersegmental segments. The hepatic veins may be visualized with the patient in full inspiration in a transverse image of the liver with a cephalic angulation of the probe. The *right hepatic vein* courses within the *right intersegmental fissure* to divide the right lobe into anterior and posterior segments. The *middle hepatic vein* courses within the main lobar fissure to separate the anterior segment of the right lobe from the medial segment of the left lobe. The *left intersegmental fissure* separates the medial segment of the left lobe from the lateral segment. This fissure is further divided into *cranial, middle,* and *caudal* sections. The *left hepatic vein* forms the boundary of the cranial third, the ascending branch of the left portal vein represents the middle third, and the fissure for the ligamentum teres forms the most caudal division of the left lobe. The major branches of the *portal veins* run centrally within the segments (intrasegmental) with the exception of the ascending portion of the left portal vein, which runs in the left intersegmental fissure.

Couinaud's System of Hepatic Nomenclature. Although the liver has been divided into four anatomic lobes with the falciform ligament "separating the left from the right lobe," Couinaud's system of hepatic nomenclature (Box 9-1) provides the functional division between the right and left lobes based on the vasculature, not the falciform ligament, for hepatic surgical resections. The vascular supply and drainage divide the liver into regions that can be resected independently. The middle hepatic vein and the ascending section of the left portal vein divide the liver, functionally, into a left lobe and a right lobe (Figure 9-3). This dividing line tends to be near the left edge of the inferior vena cava and the gallbladder fossa. The quadrate lobe is functionally part of the medial segment of the left lobe which lies between the middle hepatic vein and the left hepatic vein. Using these functional divisions, the falciform ligament now belongs to the left lobe, which runs along the medial left lobe, close to the border with the lateral left lobe.

By using the Couinaud system, the sonographer should be able to precisely isolate the location of a lesion for the surgical team. The description of the liver segments is based on the portal and hepatic venous segments, with each segment having its own blood supply, lymphatics, and biliary drainage. Each of the eight segments has a central branch or branches of the portal vein that is bounded by a hepatic vein. The right, middle, and left hepatic veins divide the liver longitudinally into four

sections. Each of these sections is further divided transversely by an invisible plane through the right and left portal veins.

The Couinaud system divides the left lateral, right anterior, and right posterior segments into superior and inferior subsegments and maintains the caudate lobe and the medial left segment as single segments.

This is how the eight segments are divided and numbered (a separate portal venous branch supplies each of these subsegments):

  I. Caudate lobe may receive branches of both the right and left portal veins and may have one or more hepatic veins draining into the inferior vena cava
 II. Left lateral superior
III. Left lateral inferior
 IV. Left medial superior (a) and inferior (b)
  V. Right anterior inferior
 VI. Right posterior inferior
VII. Right posterior superior
VIII. Right anterior superior

Ligaments and Fissures. There are several important ligaments and fissures to remember in the liver: Glisson's capsule, main lobar fissure, falciform ligament, ligamentum teres (round ligament), and ligamentum venosum. These ligaments and fissures appear echogenic or hyperechoic because of the presence of collagen and fat within and around the structures.

The liver is covered by a thin connective tissue layer called *Glisson's capsule.* This capsule completely surrounds the liver and is thickest around the inferior vena cava and portal hepatis. The *hepatoduodenal ligament* contains the main portal vein, the proper hepatic artery, and the common duct. The **main lobar fissure** is the boundary between the right and left lobes of the liver. On the longitudinal scan, it may be seen as a hyperechoic line extending from the portal vein to the neck of the gallbladder (Figure 9-4, *A*). The sonographer uses this ligament to find the gallbladder on the longitudinal scan, especially when it is packed with stones and not well imaged. The **falciform ligament** extends from the umbilicus to the diaphragm in a parasagittal plane and contains the ligamentum

---

BOX 9-1 | Hepatic Segmental Anatomy

Segment I: Caudate lobe
Segments II and III: Left superior and inferior lateral segments
Segments IVa and IVb: Medial segments of the left lobe
Segments V and VI: Caudal to the transverse plane
Segments VII and VIII: Cephalad to the transverse plane

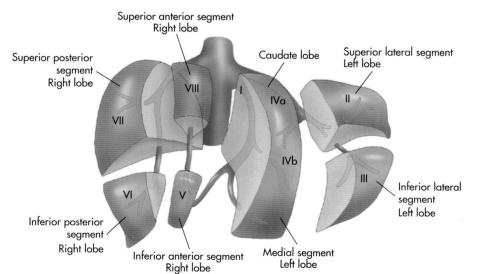

FIGURE 9-3 Couinaud's hepatic segments divide the liver into eight segments. The three hepatic veins are the longitudinal boundaries. The transverse plane is defined by the right and left portal pedicles. The caudate lobe (segment I) is situated posteriorly. Segment I includes the caudate lobe. Segments II and III include the left superior and inferior lateral segments. Segments IVa and IVb include the medial segment of the left lobe. Segments V and VI are caudal to the transverse plane. Segments VII and VIII are cephalad to the transverse plane.

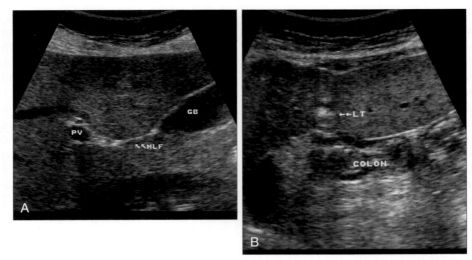

FIGURE 9-4 A, Main lobar fissure *(MLF)* extends between the long axis neck of the gallbladder *(GB)* and the main portal vein *(PV)* on the longitudinal image. **B,** Falciform ligament extends from the umbilicus to the diaphragm in a longitudinal plane.

teres. In the anteroposterior axis, the falciform ligament extends from the right rectus muscle to the bare area of the liver, where its echogenic reflections separate to contribute to the hepatic coronary ligament and attach to the undersurface of the diaphragm. The **ligamentum teres** appears as a bright echogenic focus on the sonogram and is seen as the rounded termination of the falciform ligament (Figure 9-4, *B*). The fissure for the **ligamentum venosum** separates the left lobe from the caudate lobe (Figure 9-5). On ultrasound, it may be seen just inferior to the dome of the liver as a linear horizontal line just anterior to the caudate lobe and inferior vena cava. The caudate lobe, ligamentum venosum, portal vein, and left lobe

of the liver may be seen on the longitudinal plane over the area of the inferior vena cava.

Vascular Supply

The liver receives blood supply from the portal veins and hepatic artery. The portal vein conveys about 70% to 80% of the blood to the liver, and the remaining 20% to 30% is oxygenated blood conveyed to the liver via the hepatic artery. The right lobe of the liver receives blood primarily from the intestine, whereas the left lobe and caudate lobes receive blood from the stomach and the spleen.

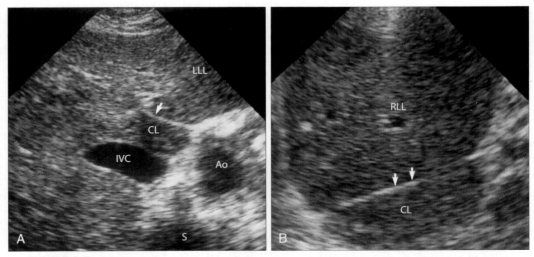

FIGURE 9-5 Ligamentum venosum. A, Transverse image high in the liver shows the spine *(S),* aorta *(AO),* and inferior vena cava *(IVC).* The caudate lobe *(CL)* is anterior to the inferior vena cava *(IVC)* and is separated from the left lobe of the liver *(LLL)* by the ligamentum venosum *(arrow).* **B,** Longitudinal oblique image through the right lobe of the liver *(RLL)* shows the ligamentum venosum *(arrows)* and caudate lobe *(CL).*

The venous blood supply from the greater part of the gastrointestinal tract and its accessory organs drains into the liver through the portal venous system. The proximal tributaries drain directly into the portal vein, but the veins forming the distal tributaries correspond to the branches of the celiac artery and superior and inferior mesenteric arteries.

Hepatic Portal Vein. The portal vein drains blood from the gastrointestinal tract from the lower third of the esophagus to midway down the anal canal; it also drains blood from the spleen, pancreas, and gallbladder. The portal vein enters the liver and breaks up into sinusoids, from which blood passes into the hepatic veins that empty into the inferior vena cava. The portal venous system is a reliable indicator of various ultrasonic tomographic planes throughout the liver (Figure 9-6).

The portal triad consists of the portal vein, hepatic artery, and bile duct. The portal vein is contained within a connective tissue sheath that provides an echogenic structure on the sonographic image to distinguish it from the hepatic vein.

Main Portal Vein. The **main portal vein** approaches the porta hepatis in a rightward, cephalic, and slightly posterior direction within the hepatoduodenal ligament. It comes in contact with the anterior surface of the inferior vena cava near the porta hepatis and serves to locate the liver hilum (Figure 9-7). It then divides into two branches: the right and left portal veins.

Right Portal Vein. The **right portal vein** is the larger of the two branches and requires a more posterior and more caudal transducer approach. It usually is possible to identify the anterior and posterior divisions of the right portal vein on sonography (Figure 9-8). The right portal vein has an anterior

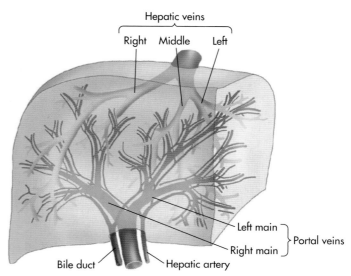

FIGURE 9-6 **Vascular system of the liver.** The liver receives blood supply from the portal veins and hepatic artery. The venous blood supply from the greater part of the gastrointestinal tract and its accessory organs drains into the liver through the portal venous system. The portal triad consists of the portal vein, hepatic artery, and bile duct. There are essentially three major components of the hepatic veins: right, middle, and left, which drain into the inferior vena cava.

branch that lies centrally within the anterior segment of the right lobe and a posterior branch that lies within the posterior segment of the right lobe.

Left Portal Vein. The **left portal vein** lies more anterior and cranial than the right portal vein. The main portal vein is seen to elongate at the origin of the left portal vein (Figure 9-9). The vessel lies within a canal containing large amounts of

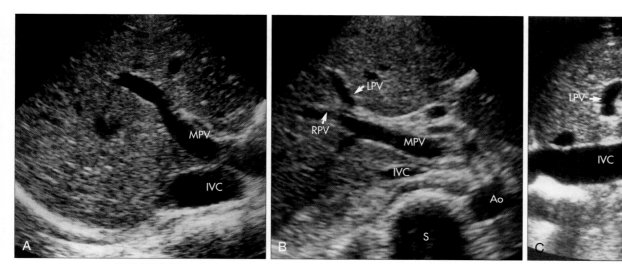

FIGURE 9-7 **Main portal vein. A,** Transverse image of the main portal vein *(MPV)* as it enters the liver. *IVC,* Inferior vena cava. **B,** Transverse image of the main portal vein *(MPV)* as it bifurcates into right *(RPV)* and left *(LPV)* branches. *AO,* Aorta; *IVC,* inferior vena cava; *S,* spine. **C,** Longitudinal image just to the right of midline shows the inferior vena cava *(IVC),* main portal vein *(MPV),* and left portal vein *(LPV).*

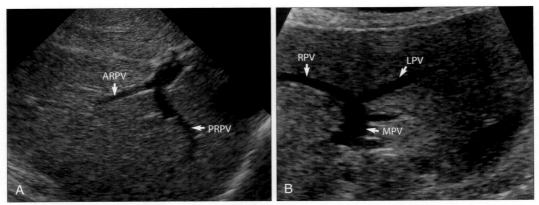

FIGURE 9-8 **Right portal vein. A,** Transverse image of the right portal vein as it bifurcates into the anterior *(ARPV)* and posterior *(PRPV)* branches. **B,** Transverse image of the main portal vein *(MPV)* as it bifurcates into right *(RPV)* and left *(LPV)* branches.

connective tissue, which results in the visualization of an echo-genic linear band coursing through the central portion of the lateral segment of the left lobe. The left portal vein courses anterior to the caudate lobe initially and then travels anteriorly in the left intersegmental fissure to divide the medial and lateral segments of the left lobe.

Hepatic Arteries. The hepatic artery arises from the celiac trunk to supply the liver. The right and left branches of the hepatic artery accompany the portal veins (Figure 9-10).

Hepatic Veins. The blood is perfused within the liver parenchyma through the hepatic sinusoids before it enters the terminal hepatic venules, which unite to form the larger hepatic veins. There are essentially three major components of the hepatic veins: right, middle, and left, which drain into the inferior vena cava (Figure 9-11; also see Figure 9-6). The *right hepatic vein* is the largest, courses in the right intersegmental fissure, and enters the right lateral aspect of the inferior vena cava. The right hepatic vein separates the anterior and posterior lobes of the right lobe. Often it is possible to identify a long horizontal branch of the right hepatic vein coursing between the anterior and posterior divisions of the right portal vein.

The *middle hepatic vein* courses in the main lobar fissure and enters the anterior or right anterior surface of the inferior vena cava. The middle hepatic vein commonly forms a common trunk with the left hepatic vein.

The *left hepatic vein,* which is the smallest, enters the left anterior surface of the inferior vena cava. The left hepatic vein forms the most cephalad boundary between the medial and lateral segments of the left lobe.

Distinguishing Characteristics of Portal and Hepatic Veins. The best way to distinguish the hepatic from the portal vessels is to trace their points of entry to the liver. The hepatic vessels flow into the inferior vena cava, whereas the splenic vein and superior mesenteric vein join to form the portal venous system. A continuous sector scanning sweep allows the sonographer to make this assessment within a few seconds. Hepatic veins course between the hepatic lobes and segments (Figure 9-12, *A*). The portal veins are larger at their origin as they emanate from the porta hepatis. Portal veins have more echogenic borders than the hepatic veins because they have a thicker collagenous sheath (Figure 9-12, *B*).

Intrahepatic Vessels and Ducts. The portal veins carry blood to the liver, whereas the hepatic veins drain the

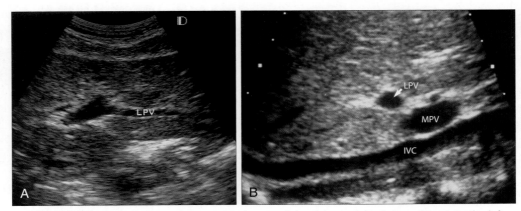

FIGURE 9-9 **Left portal vein. A,** Transverse image of the right portal vein branching into the left portal vein *(LPV)* as it flows into the left lobe of the liver. **B,** Longitudinal image just to the right of midline shows the inferior vena cava *(IVC)*, the main portal vein *(MPV)*, and the left portal vein *(LPV)*.

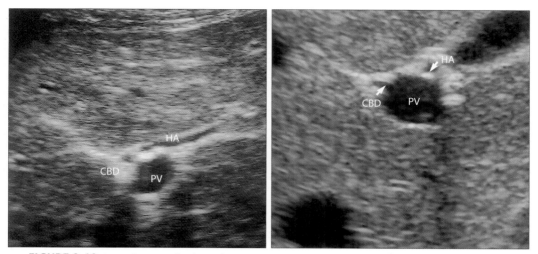

FIGURE 9-10 Hepatic artery *(HA)* may be seen anterior and medial to the portal vein on an oblique transverse image; this is known as the *portal triad. Arrow,* Hepatic artery; *CBD,* common bile duct; *PV,* portal vein.

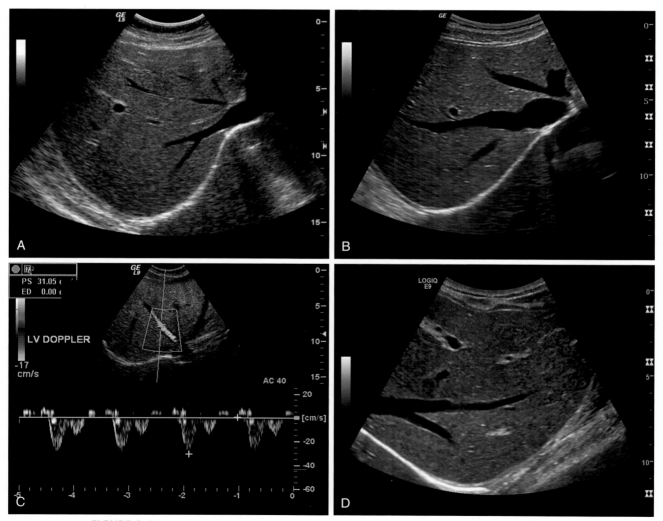

FIGURE 9-11 Hepatic veins. A and **B,** Transverse images at the dome of the liver show the hepatic veins as they empty into the inferior vena cava *(IVC).* **C,** Transverse Doppler evaluation of the middle hepatic vein as it empties into the inferior vena cava. **D,** Longitudinal image of the hepatic veins draining into the inferior vena cava.

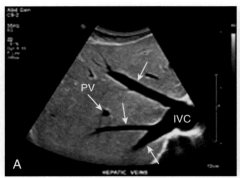
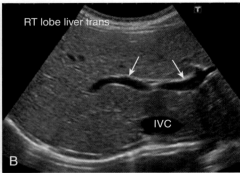

FIGURE 9-12 Portal versus hepatic veins. A, The hepatic veins *(arrows)* are larger as they drain into the inferior vena cava *(IVC)* before entering the right atrium. **B,** The portal veins *(pv)* have more echogenic borders than the hepatic veins. *IVC,* Inferior vena cava.

blood from the liver into the inferior vena cava. The hepatic arteries carry oxygenated blood from the aorta to the liver. The bile ducts transport bile, manufactured in the liver, to the duodenum.

PHYSIOLOGY AND LABORATORY DATA OF THE HEPATOBILIARY SYSTEM

The liver, bile ducts, and gallbladder constitute the hepatobiliary system, which performs metabolic and excretory functions essential to physical well-being. Although sonography is an important clinical tool for detecting anatomic changes associated with hepatobiliary disease, accurate sonographic evaluation can be accomplished only when other diagnostic information (e.g., signs, symptoms, and laboratory results) is considered in conjunction with the sonographic findings. The task of correlating these clinical and ultrasound data falls primarily to the sonologist. However, the sonographer must also understand the entire clinical picture to be able to plan and properly perform the ultrasound examination. It is necessary, therefore, that the sonographer be aware of the normal and abnormal physiology of the hepatobiliary system. This section is intended as a primer of hepatobiliary physiology, with particular attention to physiologic alterations that commonly occur in hepatobiliary disease.

Hepatic Physiology

The liver has many functions, including metabolism, digestion, storage, and detoxification (Box 9-2). The liver is a major center of metabolism, which may be defined as the physical and chemical process whereby foodstuffs are synthesized into complex elements, complex substances are transformed into simple ones, and energy is made available for use by the organism. Through the process of digestion, the liver expels these waste products from the body via its excretory product, bile, which also plays an important role in fat absorption. **Bilirubin** is a pigment released when the red blood cells are broken down. The liver is a storage site for several compounds used in a variety of physiologic activities throughout the body. In hepatobiliary disease, each of these functions may be altered, leading to abnormal physical, laboratory, and sonographic findings. Finally, the liver is also a center for

BOX 9-2	Primary Functions of the Liver

Metabolism
- *Carbohydrate.* The liver converts glucose to glycogen and stores it; when glucose is needed, it breaks down the glycogen and releases glucose into the blood.
- *Protein.* The liver performs many important functions in metabolism of proteins, fats, and carbohydrates. It manufactures many of the plasma proteins found in the blood. The liver converts excess amino acids to fatty acids and urea. It also removes nutrients from the blood and phagocytizes bacteria and worn-out red blood cells.

Digestion
The liver secretes bile, which is important in the digestion of fats. Bilirubin, a pigment released when red blood cells are broken down, is excreted in the bile.

Storage
The liver stores iron and certain vitamins.

Detoxification
The liver detoxifies many drugs and poisons that enter the body.

detoxification of the waste products of metabolism accumulated from other sources in the body and foreign chemicals (usually drugs) that enter the body.

Hepatic versus Obstructive Disease

Diseases affecting the liver may be classified as *hepatocellular,* when the liver cells or hepatocytes are the immediate problem, or *obstructive,* when bile excretion is blocked. Viral hepatitis is an example of hepatocellular liver disease: The virus attacks liver cells and damages or destroys them, resulting in an alteration of liver function. In obstructive disorders, the flow of bile from the liver is blocked at some point, and the liver malfunctions as a secondary result of the blockage.

The differentiation between **hepatocellular disease** and **obstructive disease** is of considerable importance clinically. Hepatocellular diseases are treated medically with supportive measures and drugs; obstructive disorders are usually treated surgically. In some cases the distinction between hepatocellular and obstructive disease can be made through clinical laboratory tests, but often the laboratory findings are equivocal. Sonography has been of great benefit because it allows the physician to accurately separate hepatocellular and obstructive causes of liver disease.

Hepatic Metabolic Functions

Raw materials in the form of carbohydrates (sugars), fats, and amino acids (basic components of proteins) are absorbed from the intestine and transported to the liver via the circulatory system. In the liver, these substances are converted chemically to other compounds or are processed for storage or energy production. The following sections are brief discussions of the liver's metabolic functions and of how liver disease can disturb these functions.

Carbohydrates. Sugars may be absorbed from the blood in several forms, but only glucose can be used by cells throughout the body as a source of energy. The liver functions as a major site for conversion of dietary sugars into glucose, which is released into the bloodstream for general use. The body requires only a certain amount of glucose at any one time. Excess sugar is converted by the liver to glycogen (a starch), which may be stored in the liver cells or transported in the blood to distant storage sites. When dietary sugar is unavailable, the liver converts glycogen released from storage into glucose; it can also manufacture glucose directly from other compounds, including proteins or fats, when other sources of glucose have been depleted. Thus the liver helps to maintain a steady state of glucose in the bloodstream.

In severe liver disease, unless glucose is administered intravenously, the body may become glucose deficient (**hypoglycemia**), with profound effects on the function of the brain and other organs. Uncontrolled increases in blood glucose (**hyperglycemia**) may occur in severe liver disease if a large dose of glucose is administered, because the liver fails to convert the excess glucose to glycogen.

Fats. The liver is also a principal site for metabolism of fats, which are absorbed from the intestine in the form of monoglycerides and diglycerides. Dietary fats are converted in the hepatocytes to lipoproteins, in which form fats are transported throughout the body to sites where they are stored or used by other organs. Conversely, stored fats may be transported to the liver and converted into energy, yielding glucose or other substances, such as cholesterol.

In severe liver disease, abnormally low blood levels of cholesterol may be noted because the liver is the principal site for cholesterol synthesis. Furthermore, failure of hepatic conversion of fat to glucose in liver disease may contribute to hypoglycemia. A striking histologic manifestation of many forms of hepatocellular disease is the so-called *fatty liver*. On gross pathologic examination, the fatty liver has a yellow color and feels greasy to the touch; on microscopic study, globules of fat (primarily triglycerides) crowd the hepatocytes. The cause of fat accumulation in the liver cells is poorly understood, but it is believed to result from failure of the

hepatocytes to manufacture special proteins, called *lipoproteins,* that coat small quantities of fat, making the fat soluble in plasma and allowing for its release into the bloodstream. Fatty liver is a nonspecific finding that may be seen in a variety of conditions including viral hepatitis, alcoholic liver disease, obesity, diabetes, pregnancy, and exposure to toxic chemicals.

Proteins. The liver produces a variety of proteins, either indirectly from amino acids absorbed from the gut or directly from raw materials stored within the body. Albumin, in particular, is produced in great quantities. In the bloodstream, it functions as a transport medium for some kinds of molecules. Because it is nonionic, it also functions to draw water into the vascular system from tissue spaces; therefore it helps to maintain oncotic pressure within the vascular system. When the liver is chronically diseased, clinical laboratory results may reveal a significant lowering of the serum albumin, a condition called *hypoalbuminemia.* The accompanying loss of osmotic pressure in the vascular system allows fluid to migrate into the interstitial space, resulting in edema (swelling) in dependent areas, such as the lower extremities. In patients with severe liver disease, especially advanced cirrhosis, ascites also develops. Hypoalbuminemia may account in part for the ascites, but the development of ascites is principally caused by portal hypertension.

In addition to being the primary source of albumin synthesis, the liver is the principal source of proteins necessary for blood coagulation, including fibrinogen (factor I), prothrombin (factor II), and factors V, VII, IX, and X. In liver disease, decreased production of these proteins may lead to inadequate blood coagulation and uncontrollable hemorrhage. Commonly such hemorrhages occur into the bowel after rupture of a dilated vein or development of an ulcer. These hemorrhages are often the immediate or contributing cause of death. Deficiencies of clotting factors II, VII, IX, and X also may result from failure of intestinal absorption of vitamin K, which is a precursor (raw material) required for synthesis of these factors. Vitamin K is a fat-soluble vitamin (as are vitamins D, A, and E) and is absorbed only from the intestine in solution with fat.

Fat absorption is severely limited in cases of bile duct obstruction because of the absence of bile salts (discussed later), which severely reduces the absorption of fat-soluble vitamins. Ultimately the deficiency of vitamin K lowers the amount of the previously mentioned factors and coagulation is retarded. Deficiency of prothrombin and other vitamin K–dependent factors can be corrected in cases of obstruction through parenteral administration of vitamin K.

In hepatocellular disease, administration of vitamin K may improve the coagulopathy but frequently does not restore normal clotting function because the primary problem is hepatocyte dysfunction.

Clotting deficiencies related to liver disease may be detected with several laboratory tests. Of particular interest are the prothrombin time (pro time) and partial thromboplastin time (PTT) tests. The results of these tests are presented as percentages of the time required for certain coagulation steps to occur in the patient's blood compared with normal blood. Longer periods (lower percentages) indicate greater degrees of abnormality in each of these tests.

Hepatic Enzymes. Enzymes are protein catalysts used throughout the body in all metabolic processes. Because the liver is a major center of metabolism, large quantities of enzymes are present in hepatocytes, and these enzymes leak into the bloodstream when the liver cells are damaged or destroyed by disease. The presence of increased quantities of enzymes in the blood is a sensitive indicator of a hepatocellular disorder.

In hepatobiliary disease the enzymes **aspartate aminotransferase (AST), alanine aminotransferase (ALT),** and **alkaline phosphatase** are of particular interest. Serum levels of all three of these enzymes are increased in both hepatocellular disease and biliary obstruction, but the patterns of elevation may help differentiate hepatocellular from obstructive causes (Table 9-1). In biliary obstruction, elevation of AST and ALT is usually mild (serum levels typically do not exceed 300 units). However, in severe hepatocellular destruction, such as acute viral or toxic hepatitis, a striking elevation of AST and ALT may be seen (levels frequently exceed 1000 units).

Marked elevation of alkaline phosphatase, on the other hand, is typically associated with biliary obstruction or the presence of mass lesions in the liver (e.g., metastatic disease or abscesses). Low levels of alkaline phosphatase are unusual in obstruction, and high levels (greater than 15 Bodansky units) are uncommon in hepatocellular disorders. Alkaline phosphatase is such a sensitive indicator of obstruction that it may become elevated before the serum bilirubin in cases of acute obstruction. Hence, a disproportional increase of alkaline phosphatase relative to bilirubin always suggests obstruction. Elevation of serum alkaline phosphatase may be the only abnormal laboratory finding in metastatic disease.

Whereas the pattern of enzyme abnormality may strongly suggest hepatocellular disease or obstruction in some cases, it may not allow this distinction to be made in others because obstruction may be superimposed on preexisting hepatocellular disease or unrelieved obstruction may cause hepatocellular damage. Confusion in interpretation of serum enzyme abnormalities may also occur when AST, ALT, or alkaline phosphatase is released from diseased tissues other than the liver. For example, AST and ALT are increased with damage to heart and skeletal muscle, and alkaline phosphatase is elevated in bone disease and in normal pregnancies. ALT is somewhat more specific for liver disease than AST; therefore elevation of ALT above AST suggests a hepatic cause.

Hepatic Detoxification Functions

The liver is a major location for detoxification of waste products of energy production and other metabolic activities occurring throughout the body. It is also the principal site of breakdown of foreign chemicals, such as drugs. Although these functions fall under the general definition of metabolism and could therefore be grouped in the preceding section, it is useful for instructional purposes to think of these functions as separate categories of hepatic activity.

Ammonium, a toxic product of nitrogen metabolism, is converted to nontoxic urea in the liver, which is practically the only site where this conversion occurs. Urea is subsequently eliminated from the body by the kidneys. The level of urea in the blood is measured as the **blood urea nitrogen (BUN),** and in severe liver disease (acute or chronic) the BUN may be abnormally low because of falloff of urea production. The exhaled breath of patients with severe liver disease may have a fruity or pungent odor (known as *fetor hepaticus*) because of ammonium (NH_4) accumulation. More important, the concentration of NH_4 in the blood may rise to toxic levels and cause brain dysfunction (including confusion, coordination disturbances, tremor, and coma).

Gastrointestinal hemorrhage frequently leads to the accumulation of toxic levels of NH_4 in the blood. Blood lost into the intestine is broken down by bacteria into nitrogen-containing substances, which are absorbed into the bloodstream. The failing liver may therefore be presented with a large amount of NH_4 that it cannot detoxify; coma may result and is frequently a precursor to death if the patient does not succumb to the direct effects of blood loss. Thus failure of ammonium detoxification is a serious consequence of liver failure.

Bilirubin Detoxification. Bilirubin, the breakdown product of hemoglobin, is also an important substance detoxified in the liver. Along with detoxification, the liver also excretes bilirubin into the gut via the biliary tree. Red blood cells survive an average of 120 days in the circulatory system; they are then trapped and broken down by reticuloendothelial cells, primarily within the spleen. Hemoglobin released from the red cells is converted to bilirubin within the reticuloendothelial system and is then released into the bloodstream. The bilirubin molecules become attached to albumin in the blood and are transported to the

TABLE 9-1	Comparison of Laboratory Abnormalities in Hepatocellular Disease and Biliary Obstruction				
Condition	**Bilirubin**	**Serum Albumin**	**AST**	**ALT**	**Alkaline Phosphatase**
Hepatocellular disease	Minimal to severe increase	Decreased	Moderate to severe increase	Moderate to severe increase	Minimal to moderate increase
Obstruction	Severe increase	Normal	Mild increase	Mild increase	Severe increase

ALT, Alanine aminotransferase; *AST,* aspartate aminotransferase.

liver, where the following metabolic steps take place in the hepatocytes:

1. *Uptake.* The bilirubin is separated from albumin, probably at the cell membrane, and is taken within the hepatocytes.
2. *Conjugation.* The bilirubin molecule is combined with two glucuronide molecules, forming bilirubin diglucuronide.
3. *Excretion.* The bilirubin molecule is actively transported across the cell membrane into the bile canaliculi, which are the microscopic "headwaters" of the biliary system. Bilirubin released from the hepatocytes passes through the bile ducts with other components of bile and is delivered to the bowel, where most bilirubin diglucuronide is excreted into the feces. (A small portion is broken down into urobilinogen by intestinal bacteria, absorbed into the portal system, and reexcreted by the liver.)

Measurement of the concentration of bilirubin in the blood is a standard laboratory test for hepatocellular disease. The following two fractions of bilirubin are measured: the direct-acting fraction, which reacts chemically in an aqueous medium and consists of conjugated bilirubin, and the indirect-acting fraction, which consists of unconjugated bilirubin released from the reticuloendothelial system. Indirect bilirubin reacts only in a nonaqueous (alcohol) medium. The total bilirubin is the sum of the direct-acting and the indirect-acting fractions and normally does not exceed 1 mg/100 ml of serum. In hematologic diseases associated with abrupt breakdown of large numbers of red blood cells (hemolytic anemias, transfusion reactions), the liver may receive more bilirubin from the reticuloendothelial system than it can detoxify. The level of indirect, or unconjugated, bilirubin therefore is elevated.

In biliary obstruction, the hepatocytes pick up bilirubin and conjugate it with glucuronide molecules but cannot dispose of it. The conjugated form is then regurgitated into the bloodstream, with resultant elevation of the direct-acting bilirubin fraction. The indirect-acting bilirubin may also rise slightly in biliary obstruction, but the direct bilirubin predominates.

The direct, or conjugated, form also predominates in hepatocellular disease. Excretion of bilirubin is the step most readily affected when the hepatocytes are damaged; therefore the diseased hepatocytes continue to take in and conjugate bilirubin but are unable to excrete it. As in biliary obstruction, the accumulated conjugated bilirubin is regurgitated into the blood.

The direct and indirect patterns may be summarized as in Table 9-2.

Elevation of serum bilirubin results in jaundice, which is a yellow coloration of the skin, sclerae, and body secretions. Jaundice is a nonspecific finding seen in massive blood breakdown, hepatocellular disease, or biliary obstruction. Chemical separation of bilirubin into direct and indirect fractions helps to specify a hepatocellular or hematologic cause for jaundice. Furthermore, if jaundice results from liver disease, the level of bilirubin may help to separate hepatocellular disease from obstruction because it is uncommon for the total bilirubin to rise above 35 mg/100 ml of serum with obstruction.

Hormone and Drug Detoxification. The liver breaks down several hormones that otherwise would accumulate in the body. For example, failure to metabolize estrogen in men with chronic hepatocellular disease, such as cirrhosis, causes gynecomastia (breast enlargement), testicular atrophy, and changes in body-hair patterns. Reduced detoxification of the hormone glucagon, which is an insulin antagonist, occurs in liver disease and may contribute to the fluctuations in blood sugar levels seen in severe hepatic disorders. The liver is also the primary location for breakdown of medications and other foreign chemicals administered orally or parenterally. It is of particular concern that doses of medications be reduced to compensate for the loss of this function in patients with severe liver disease; otherwise, accumulation of drugs may lead to overdosage.

Bile

Bile is the excretory product of the liver. It is formed continuously by the hepatocytes, collects in the bile canaliculi adjacent to these cells, and is transported to the gut via the bile ducts (Figure 9-13). The principal components of bile are water, bile

TABLE 9-2	Direct and Indirect Patterns of Bilirubin	
Condition	**Direct Bilirubin Predominates**	**Indirect Bilirubin Predominates**
Hemolysis		X
Hepatocellular disease	X	
Biliary obstruction	X	

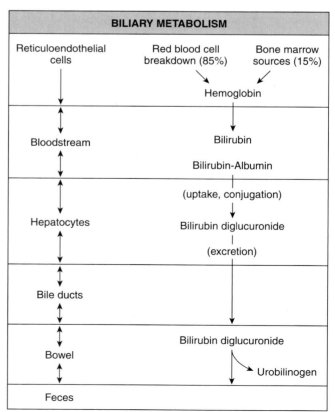

FIGURE 9-13 Biliary metabolism.

salts, and bile pigments (primarily bilirubin diglucuronide). Other components include cholesterol, lecithin, and protein. The primary functions of bile are the emulsification of intestinal fat and the removal of waste products excreted by the liver.

Fats are absorbed into the portal blood and intestinal lymphatics in the form of monoglycerides and triglycerides by the action of the intestinal mucosa, but efficient absorption occurs only when the fat molecules are suspended in solution through the emulsifying action of bile salts. As emulsifiers, bile salts act like nonionic detergents to suspend fats in solution within the watery medium of the intestinal contents. Both hepatocellular disease and biliary obstruction affect the amount of bile salts available for fat absorption, but obstruction generally has the more profound effect. Absence of bile salts may lead to steatorrhea (fatty stools), but a more important effect is failure of absorption of the fat-soluble vitamins (D, A, K, and E). As previously noted, vitamin K is an essential precursor for hepatic production of several clotting factors; the absence of this vitamin leads to bleeding tendencies in patients with hepatobiliary disease.

Bile Pigments. Bile pigments are the principal cause of ultrasonic scattering in echogenic bile, although cholesterol crystals may also contribute to this finding. The presence of echogenic bile indicates stasis, but this stasis is not always pathologic and may simply result from prolonged fasting.

Liver Function Tests

Liver function tests are a group of laboratory tests established to analyze how the liver is performing under normal and diseased conditions. In patients with known liver disease, a number of laboratory tests are used to help in the diagnosis, including the following:

- Aspartate aminotransferase (AST)
- Alanine aminotransferase (ALT)
- Lactic acid dehydrogenase (LDH)
- Alkaline phosphatase (alk phos)
- Bilirubin (indirect, direct, and total)
- Prothrombin time
- Albumin and globulins

Aspartate Aminotransferase. Aspartate aminotransferase (AST) is an enzyme present in tissues that have a high rate of metabolic activity, one of which is the liver. As a result of death or injury to the producing cells, the enzyme is released into the bloodstream in abnormally high levels. Any disease that injures the cells causes an elevation in AST levels. This enzyme is also produced in other high-metabolic tissues, so an elevation does not always mean liver disease is present. Significant elevations are characteristic of acute hepatitis and cirrhosis. The level is also elevated in patients with hepatic necrosis, acute hepatitis, and infectious mononucleosis.

Alanine Aminotransferase. Alanine aminotransferase (ALT) is more specific than AST for evaluating liver function. This enzyme is slightly elevated in acute cirrhosis, hepatic metastasis, and pancreatitis. There is a mild to moderate increase in obstructive jaundice. Hepatocellular disease and infectious or toxic hepatitis produce moderate to highly increased levels. In alcoholic hepatitis, AST is higher.

Lactic Acid Dehydrogenase. Lactic acid dehydrogenase is found in the tissues of several systems, including the kidneys, heart, skeletal muscle, brain, liver, and lungs. Cellular injury and death cause this enzyme to increase. This test is moderately increased in infectious mononucleosis and mildly elevated in hepatitis, cirrhosis, and obstructive jaundice. Its primary use is in detection of myocardial or pulmonary infarction.

Alkaline Phosphatase. Alkaline phosphatase is produced by the liver, bone, intestines, and placenta. It may be a good indicator of intrahepatic or extrahepatic obstruction, hepatic carcinoma, abscess, or cirrhosis. In hepatitis and cirrhosis the enzyme is moderately elevated.

Bilirubin. Bilirubin is a product of the breakdown of hemoglobin in tired red blood cells. The liver converts these byproducts into bile pigments, which, along with other factors, are secreted as bile by the liver cells into the bile ducts. The following are three ways this cycle can be disturbed:

- An excessive amount of red blood cell destruction
- Malfunction of liver cells
- Blockage of ducts leading from cells

These disturbances cause a rise in serum bilirubin, which leaks into the tissues and thus gives the skin a jaundiced, or yellow, coloration.

Indirect bilirubin is unconjugated bilirubin. Elevation of this test result is seen with increased red blood cell destruction (anemias, trauma from a hematoma, or hemorrhagic pulmonary infarct).

Direct bilirubin is conjugated bilirubin. This product circulates in the blood and is excreted into the bile after it reaches the liver and is conjugated with glucuronide. Elevation of direct bilirubin is usually related to obstructive jaundice (from stones or neoplasm).

Specific liver diseases may cause an elevation of both direct and indirect bilirubin levels, but the increase in the direct level is more marked. These diseases are hepatic metastasis, hepatitis, lymphoma, cholestasis secondary to drugs, and cirrhosis.

Prothrombin Time. Prothrombin is a liver enzyme that is part of the blood clotting mechanism. The production of prothrombin depends on adequate intake and use of vitamin K. The prothrombin time is increased in the presence of liver disease with cellular damage. Cirrhosis and metastatic disease are examples of disorders that cause prolonged prothrombin time.

Albumin and Globulins. Assessment of depressed synthesis of proteins, especially serum albumin and the plasma coagulation factors, is a sensitive test for metabolic derangement of the liver. In patients with hepatocellular damage, a low serum albumin suggests decreased protein synthesis. A prolonged prothrombin time indicates a poor prognosis. Chronic liver diseases commonly show an elevation of gamma globulins.

SONOGRAPHIC EVALUATION OF THE LIVER

Evaluation of the hepatic structures is one of the most important procedures in sonography for many reasons. The normal homogeneous parenchyma of the liver allows imaging of the neighboring anatomic structures in the upper abdomen.

Echo amplitude, attenuation, transmission, and parenchymal textures may be sonographically assessed with proper evaluation of the hepatic structures. The patient should be instructed to fast for at least 6 to 8 hours in an effort to eliminate bowel gas and ensure distention of the gallbladder. The liver is examined with the patient in a supine or right anterior oblique position, usually with deep inspiration to allow the liver to move inferior to the rib cage. The liver is then examined in a transverse, coronal, subcostal oblique, and sagittal view to completely survey the organ. The left lobe of the liver is imaged from the subxyphoid window with the transducer angled slightly cephalic. The right lobe of the liver may be imaged from both a subcostal and intercostal approach. The intercostal space is generally most effective with the patient supine with normal respiration to avoid interference from the right lung base. The patient may be instructed to place his or her arm above the head, which helps to open the intercostal spaces and allow better probe connection to image the hepatic parenchyma. Rib shadowing may also be minimized by using a smaller transducer face, or scanning obliquely in a plane parallel to the long axis of the intercostal spaces. If adequate windows are not available through the subxyphoid or intercostal window, the subcostal approach may be used. This approach required the patient to be rolled slightly into a left lateral decubitus or left posterior oblique position to allow the liver to shift medial and inferior, thus providing a better window for visualization. Keep in mind that the transducer should be angled in a superior enough position to fully image the dome of the liver and the diaphragm.

Within the homogeneous liver parenchyma lie the thin-walled hepatic veins, the brightly reflective portal veins, the hepatic arteries, and the hepatic duct (Figure 9-14). Color flow Doppler imaging is useful in determining the direction of flow of the portal and hepatic veins in relation to the Doppler probe. The portal flow is shown to be **hepatopetal** (toward the liver), whereas the hepatic venous flow is **hepatofugal** (away from the liver). The portal vein serves as the landmark to locate the smaller hepatic duct and artery. Near the porta hepatis, the hepatic duct can be seen along the anterior lateral border of the portal vein, whereas the hepatic artery can be seen along the anterior medial border (Figure 9-15). With color Doppler, the hepatic artery would show flow toward the liver, whereas the ductal system would show no flow.

The system gain should be adjusted to adequately penetrate the entire right lobe of the liver as a smooth, homogeneous echo-texture pattern (Figure 9-16, *A* and *B*). Adequate sensitivity (gain) must be adjusted to image the normal smooth liver parenchyma. If too much gain is used, the electronic "noise" or "snow" is produced that appears as low-level echoes in the background of the image (e.g., outside the liver

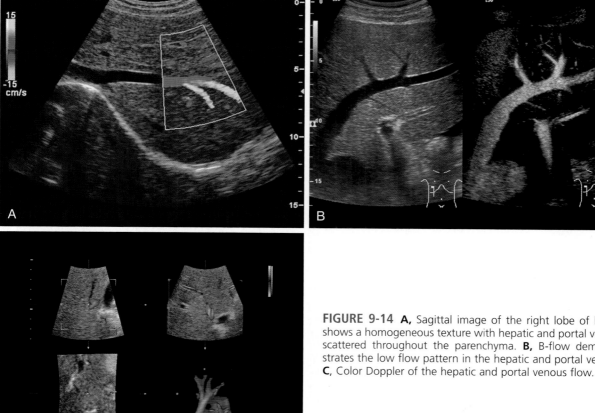

FIGURE 9-14 A, Sagittal image of the right lobe of liver shows a homogeneous texture with hepatic and portal veins scattered throughout the parenchyma. **B,** B-flow demonstrates the low flow pattern in the hepatic and portal veins. **C,** Color Doppler of the hepatic and portal venous flow.

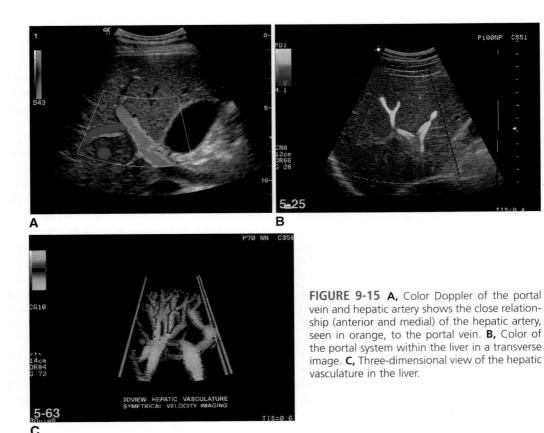

FIGURE 9-15 **A,** Color Doppler of the portal vein and hepatic artery shows the close relationship (anterior and medial) of the hepatic artery, seen in orange, to the portal vein. **B,** Color of the portal system within the liver in a transverse image. **C,** Three-dimensional view of the hepatic vasculature in the liver.

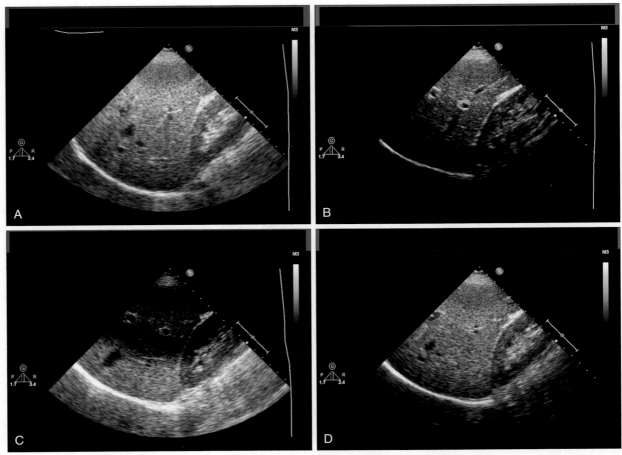

FIGURE 9-16 **A,** Longitudinal image of the liver shows equal distribution of echoes from anterior to posterior, which means the gain and time gain compensation settings are correct. **B,** Incorrect gain settings show the lack of echoes in the distal (posterior) lobe of the liver. **C,** Incorrect near-field gain settings eliminate texture information in more than half of the liver. **D,** Depth of field set correctly at 15 cm with a balanced time gain compensation (TGC) to balance the near and far fields.

parenchyma, above the diaphragm, or within the vascular structures). The ultrasound manufacturers have made it possible to preselect various preprocessing and postprocessing controls to allow the sonographer to emphasize or highlight various aspects of the liver parenchyma. This setting is automatically visible on the monitor once the equipment is turned on or the "reset" button is depressed.

The time gain compensation (TGC) should be adjusted to balance the far-gain and the near-gain echo signals. The easiest way to do this is to hold the transducer over a deep segment of the right lobe of the liver. The far TGC pods should gradually be increased with a smooth motion of the index finger until the posterior aspect of the liver is clearly visible. The near-field TGC pods should be adjusted (usually decreased) to distinguish the anterior wall and muscles, the anterior hepatic capsule, and the near field of the hepatic parenchyma.

The depth should be adjusted so the posterior right lobe is positioned at the lower border of the screen (Figure 9-16, C and D). The electronic focus on the equipment is positioned near the posterior border of the liver, or the multiple focus points may be positioned equidistant throughout the liver to

further enhance the hepatic parenchyma. The multifocal technique causes the frame rate to decrease and thus causes a "slower sweep" of the real-time image (Figure 9-17). If the patient cannot take a deep breath, the sonographer may choose not to use the multiple-frequency focus with decreased frame rate. In most patients who can suspend their respiration for a variable amount of time, this multifocal technique works well because the liver is a nondynamic organ and does not need a high frame rate to obtain a quality image.

The appropriate transducer depends on the patient's body habitus and the clinical request for the ultrasound examination. The transducer frequency depends on the body habitus and size. The average adult abdomen usually requires at least a broadband 2.5- to 5-MHz frequency, whereas the more obese adult may require a lower frequency transducer. Slender adults and young children may require a higher frequency; the neonate may need an even higher-frequency, 7.5- to 12-MHz transducer.

Generally, a wider "pie" sector or curved linear array transducer is the most appropriate to optimally image the near field of the abdomen (Figure 9-18). This transducer is especially useful in detecting liver abscesses or metastases. To

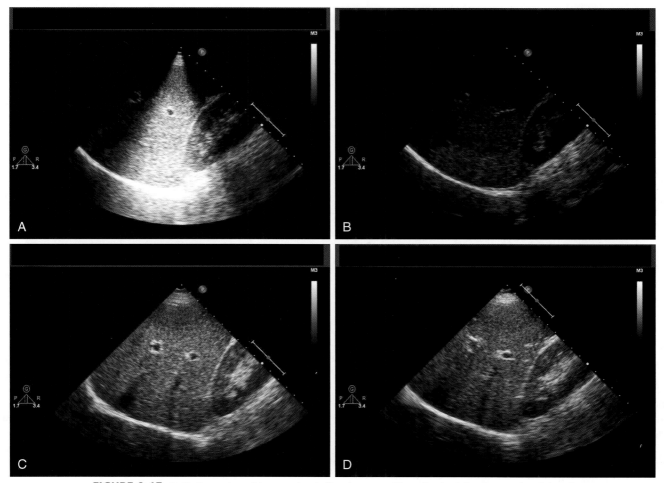

FIGURE 9-17 A–C, Examples of incorrect gain/focal zone settings (look at the line to the right of the image). The focal zone should be set to encompass the total area of interest or to "clean up" the far-field echoes to increase sharpness. **D,** Shadowing from the portal veins or variations in breathing may cause image distortion.

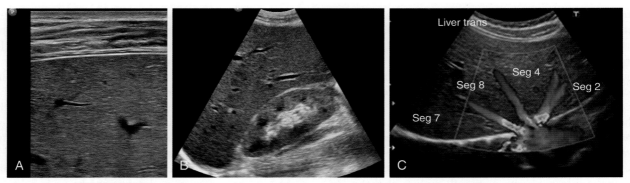

FIGURE 9-18 A, Linear array with excellent visualization of the near field of the liver, **B,** Small sector probe limits the near field of view, and **C,** Curved array versus sector changes the near field of focus and the focal zone in the far field.

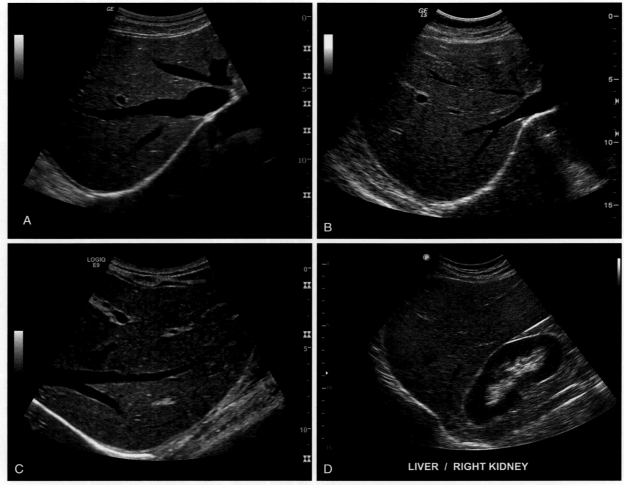

FIGURE 9-19 Transverse (**A** and **B**) and longitudinal (**C** and **D**) images should show adequate gain, time gain compensation, depth, and landmarks within the liver (ligaments, vascular structures, and spine).

image the far field better, a sector or curved array transducer with a longer focal zone is used. Often the transducers are interchanged throughout the examination to obtain the ideal image pattern.

Adequate scanning technique demands that each patient be examined with the following assessment criteria (Figure 9-19):

1. The size of the liver in the longitudinal plane approximately 15 cm

2. Parenchyma—homogeneous
3. The liver texture is greater than the right kidney, less than the pancreas and spleen
4. The presence of hepatic vascular structures, ligaments, and fissures
5. Surface—smooth

The basic instrumentation should be adjusted in the following parameters:

1. Time gain compensation

2. Overall gain
3. Transducer frequency and type
4. Depth and focus

Liver and Porta Hepatis Protocol

The liver is examined as part of a comprehensive sonographic evaluation of the abdomen. Abnormalities that can be evaluated include cirrhosis, fatty infiltration, hepatomegaly, portal hypertension, primary and metastatic tumors, abscess formation, and trauma. Color and pulsed wave (PW) Doppler are used to assess the hepatic vascular system. (Table 9-3)

1. Patient preparation: nothing by mouth (NPO) for at least 6 to 8 hours.
2. Transducer selection: 2.5 to 4 MHz curvilinear/sector, or 3 to 5 MHz curvilinear.
3. Patient position: supine and decubitus as necessary.
4. Images and observations should include the following:
   - Compare echogenicity of the liver parenchyma to the renal parenchyma.
   - Hepatic veins, portal veins, and inferior vena cava.
   - Ligamentum teres should be identified in the left lobe of the liver.
   - The dome of the right lobe of the liver should be surveyed with the patient in deep inspiration.
   - The right hemidiaphragm and right pleural gutter.
   - The main lobar fissure, as it projects from the right portal vein to the neck of the gallbladder.
   - Liver size in a parasagittal scan demonstrating the diaphragm and tip of the right lobe of the liver should be measured.
   - The size of any demonstrated masses should be imaged in two planes.

The presence of ascites (including the four quadrants of the abdomen) should be evaluated and recorded.

Doppler of the vascular structures in the liver if pathology is present:
- Assessment of the patency and direction of flow of the main, right, and left portal veins.
- Assessment of the patency of the right, middle, and left hepatic veins.

- Assessment of the patency of the umbilical vein (recanalized umbilical vein) or other collateral vessels.
- Assessment of the patency of surgically or angiographically placed shunts.
- Performance of pulsed Doppler analysis of the hepatic artery with resistance measurements.

Normal Sonographic Anatomy and Texture

The upper border of the liver is usually found at the fifth intercostal space at the midclavicular line. The lower border of the liver may extend to slightly below the costal margin. The length of the liver may be assessed in the midclavicular line, usually measuring approximately 15.5 cm. On occasion, a normal tongue-like variant, Reidel's lobe, may be seen as an extension of the right lobe. The normal texture of the liver is homogeneous with fine, low-level echoes. Compared with the renal cortex of the kidneys, the liver texture is minimally hyperechoic to isoechoic. Compared with the texture of the spleen, the liver is hypoechoic.

Sagittal Plane

The sagittal plane offers an excellent window to visualize the hepatic structures (Figure 9-20). With the patient in full inspiration, the transducer may be swept from the base of the costal margin (with slight to medium pressure) in a cephalic direction to record the liver parenchyma from the anterior abdominal wall to the diaphragm.

Scan I. With the transducer perpendicular to the abdominal wall, the initial scan should be made slightly to the left of the midline to record the left lobe of the liver and the abdominal aorta. The left hepatic and portal veins may be seen as small circular structures in this view (Figure 9-21, A).

Scan II. With the probe still perpendicular, as the sonographer scans slightly to the right of midline, a larger segment of the left lobe and the inferior vena cava may be seen posteriorly. In this view, it is useful to record the inferior vena cava as it is dilated near the end of inspiration. The left or middle hepatic vein may be imaged as it drains into the inferior vena cava near the level of the diaphragm. The area of the porta hepatis is shown anterior to the inferior vena cava as the superior mesenteric vein and splenic vein converge to form the main portal vein. The common bile duct may be seen just anterior to the main portal vein. The head of the pancreas may be seen just inferior to the liver and main portal vein, and anterior to the inferior vena cava (Figure 9-21, B).

Scan III. The next image should be made slightly lateral to this sagittal plane to record part of the right portal vein and right lobe of the liver. The caudate lobe is often seen in this view (Figure 9-21, C).

Scans IV, V, and VI. The next five scans should be made with the sweep movement of the probe (from the abdominal wall to the diaphragm) in small increments through the right lobe of the liver (Figure 9-21, D–H). The last scan is usually made to assess the right kidney and lateral segment of the right lobe of the liver. The liver texture is compared

Organ	Scan Plane	Anatomy
Liver	Trv Rt lobe/(dome) hepatic veins	Rt lobe/lung Lt lobe/lt portal vein Lt lobe/caudate lobe Rt lobe/portal veins (main, rt) Rt lobe/gallbladder/kidney
	Long	Lt lobe/aorta Lt lobe/caudate lobe/IVC Rt lobe/dome (diaphragm) Rt lobe/lung Rt lobe/portal vein Rt lobe/kidney (measure rt lobe)

TABLE 9-3 Abdominal Ultrasound Protocol: Liver

IVC, inferior vena cava; *Long*, longitudinal; *Lt*, Left; *Rt*, right; *Trv*, transverse.

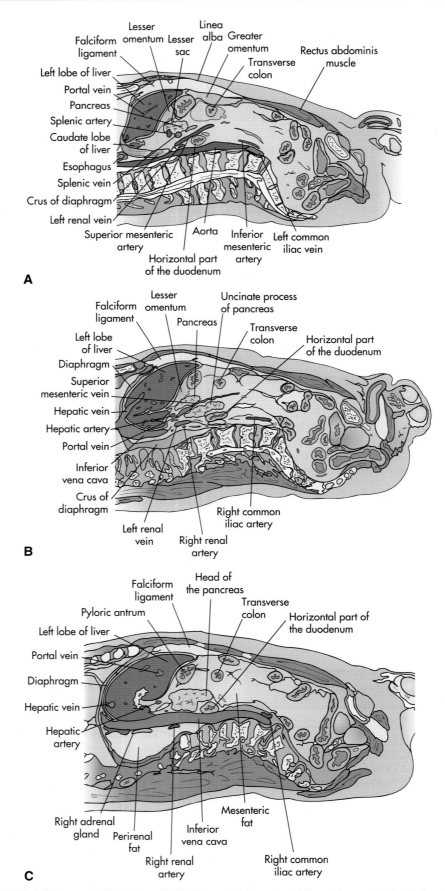

FIGURE 9-20 Longitudinal plane. A, Midline sagittal section of the abdomen. **B,** Sagittal section of the abdomen. **C,** Sagittal section of the abdomen 3 cm from the midline.

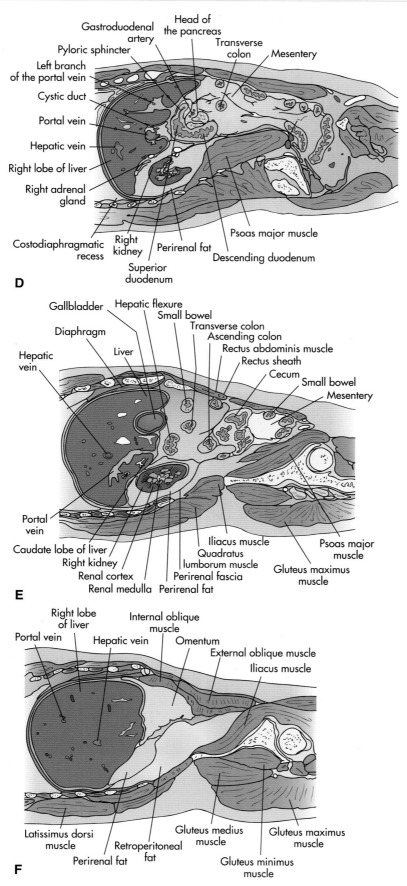

FIGURE 9-20, cont'd D, Sagittal section of the abdomen 5 cm from the midline. **E,** Sagittal section of the abdomen 7 cm from the midline. **F,** Sagittal section of the abdomen taken along the right abdominal border.

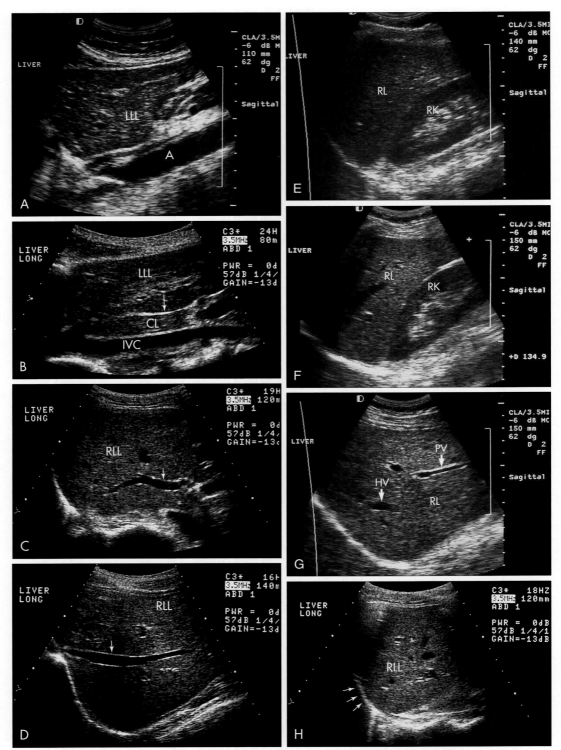

FIGURE 9-21 Longitudinal images. A, *Midline,* left lobe liver, aorta. **B,** *Midline (right)* left lobe liver, inferior vena cava, portal vein, caudate lobe. **C,** *Midline with right lateral angle:* right lobe liver, right kidney. **D,** *Midline with right lateral angle:* right lobe liver, hepatic vein *(arrow).* **E,** *Midsubcostal with right lateral angle:* right lobe liver, hepatic vein, right kidney. **F,** *Midsubcostal with right lateral angle:* right lobe liver, hepatic vein, right kidney. **G,** *Midsubcostal sweep to identify hepatic and portal veins.* **H,** Longitudinal image of the lateral segment of the right lobe liver *(RLL),* diaphragm *(arrows).*

with the renal parenchyma. The normal liver parenchyma should have a softer, more homogeneous texture than the dense medulla and hypoechoic renal cortex. Liver size may be measured with the probe in the midclavicular line extending from the inferior tip of the liver to the dome/diaphragm interface. Generally this measurement is less than 15 cm, with 15 to 20 cm representing the upper limits of normal. Hepatomegaly is present when the liver measurement exceeds 20 cm.

Transverse Plane

Multiple transverse scans are made across the upper abdomen to record specific areas of the liver (Figure 9-22). The transducer

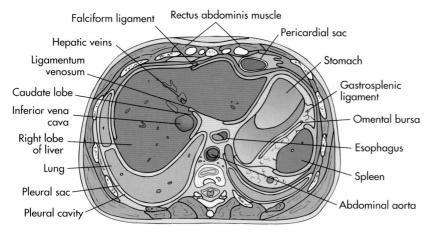

A

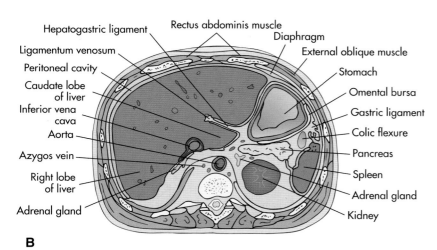

B

FIGURE 9-22 **Transverse plane. A,** Cross section of the abdomen at the level of the tenth intervertebral disk. **B,** Cross section of the abdomen at the level of the eleventh thoracic disk. **C,** Cross section of the abdomen at the level of the 12th thoracic vertebra.

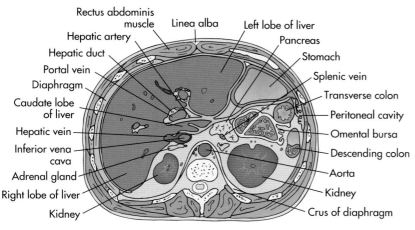

C

Continued

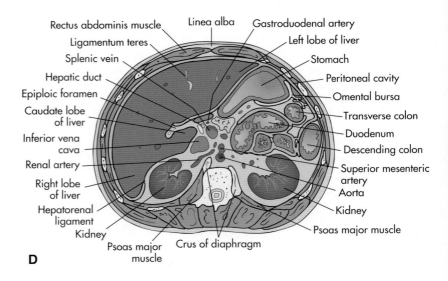

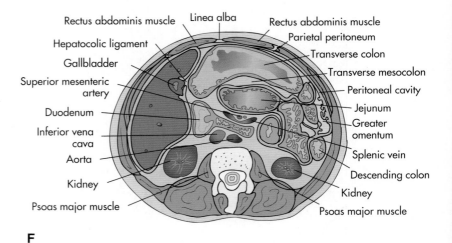

FIGURE 9-22, cont'd D, Cross section of the abdomen at the first lumbar vertebra. **E,** Cross section of the abdomen at the level of the second lumbar vertebra. **F,** Cross section of the abdomen at the level of the third lumbar vertebra.

should be angled in a steep cephalic direction to be as parallel to the diaphragm as possible. The patient should be in full inspiration to obtain adequate detail of the liver parenchyma, vascular architecture, and ductal structures.

Scan I. The initial transverse image is made with the transducer inferior to the costal margin at a steep angle perpendicular to the diaphragm (Figure 9-23, *A*). The patient should be in deep inspiration to adequately record the dome of the liver, the inferior vena cava, and three hepatic veins as they drain into the cava. This pattern has sometimes been referred to as the "reindeer sign" or "Playboy bunny" sign.

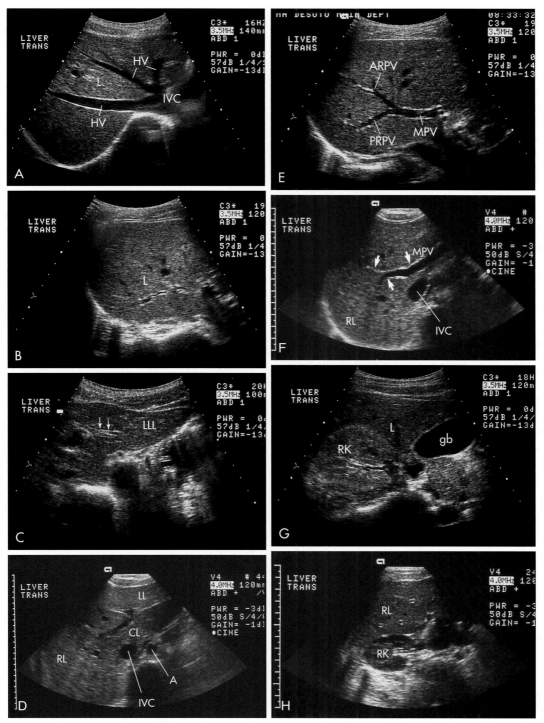

FIGURE 9-23 Transverse images. A, *Subcostal with cephalic angle:* right lobe liver *(RL),* hepatic veins *(arrows),* inferior vena cava *(IVC).* **B,** *Subcostal with steeper cephalic angle:* left lobe liver, left portal vein *(arrow),* ligamentum venosum *(arrows),* caudate lobe *(CL).* **C,** *Slow caudal inferior sweep from dome:* caudate lobe *(CL),* left lobe *(LL),* right lobe *(RL)* of liver, left and right portal veins, IVC, and aorta *(Ao).* **D,** *Slow caudal inferior sweep from dome:* right lobe liver *(RL),* main portal vein *(MPV),* right portal vein with branches *(RPV),* and IVC. **E,** *Deep inspiration, subcostal over* right lobe liver *(RL).* **F,** *Deep inspiration, subcostal over* right lobe liver *(RL)* and right kidney *(RK).* **G,** Slight caudal sweep through right lobe liver to area of gallbladder (gb) and right kidney (RK). **H,** Slight caudal sweep through right lobe liver right kidney (RK).

Scan II. The probe should be steeply angled toward the diaphragm to image the dome of the liver (Figure 9-23, *B*).

Scan III. The transducer is then directed slightly inferior to the point described in scan I to record the left portal vein as it flows into the left lobe of the liver (Figure 9-23, *C*).

Scan III. The porta hepatis is seen as a tubular structure within the central area of the liver. The bifurcation of the portal vein into the left or right portal vein can be identified. The caudate lobe is shown anterior to the inferior vena cava (Figure 9-23, *D*).

Scan IV. The next two images should show the right portal vein as it divides into the anterior and posterior segments of the right lobe of the liver. The gallbladder may be seen in this scan as an anechoic structure medial to the right lobe and anterior to the right kidney (Figure 9-23, *E* and *F*).

Scans V and VI. These two scans are made through the lower segment of the right lobe of the liver. The right kidney is the posterior border (Figure 9-23, *G*). Usually intrahepatic vascular structures are not clearly identified in these views (Figure 9-23, *F*).

Lateral Decubitus Plane

Left Posterior Oblique/Right Anterior Oblique. The left posterior/right anterior oblique image requires that the patient roll slightly to the left. A 45-degree sponge or pillow may be placed under the right hip to support the patient. This view allows better visualization of the lower right lobe of the liver, usually displacing the duodenum and transverse colon to the midline of the abdomen, out of the field of view. Transverse, oblique, or longitudinal scans may be made in this position.

Left Lateral Decubitus. If the previously described scans do not allow adequate visualization of the liver and vascular structures, the lateral decubitus position may be used. If the body habitus allows the transducer to image between the intercostal spaces, additional views may be obtained of the dome of the liver and medial segment of the left lobe of the liver.

PATHOLOGY OF THE LIVER

Evaluation of the liver parenchyma includes the assessment of its size, configuration, homogeneity, and contour. Liver volume can be determined from serial scans in an effort to detect subtle increases in size or hepatomegaly. The development and clinical utility of three-dimensional ultrasound in determining organ volumes is currently under clinical investigation at many academic institutions.

As in other organ systems, the hepatic parenchymal pattern changes with disease processes. Hepatocellular disease affects the hepatocytes and interferes with liver function enzymes. Cirrhosis, ascites, or fatty liver patterns may be detected with the ultrasound examination. In an effort to provide a differential diagnosis for the clinician, intrahepatic, extrahepatic, subhepatic, and subdiaphragmatic masses may be outlined and their internal composition recognized as specific echo patterns.

Subsequent sections discuss the pathology of liver disease in the following categories: developmental anomalies, diffuse disease, functional disease, infectious disease, benign disease, malignant disease, and vascular problems.

Developmental Anomalies

Agenesis. Agenesis of the liver is incompatible with life. There have been reported cases of agenesis of the right, left, or caudate lobes. When this occurs, hypertrophy of the other lobes develops.

Anomalies of Position. The liver may be found in other locations in two conditions: situs inversus, in which the organs are reversed, with the liver on the left and spleen on the right; or in a congenital diaphragmatic hernia or omphalocele, where varying amounts of liver tissue may herniate into the thorax or outside the abdominal cavity.

Accessory Fissures. True accessory fissures are uncommon and caused by infolding of peritoneum. The inferior accessory hepatic fissure is a true accessory fissure that stretches inferiorly from the right portal vein to the inferior surface of the right lobe of the liver.

Vascular Anomalies. The hepatic artery may have many variations as it arises from the celiac axis. At least 45% of patients may have the following variations: (1) replaced left hepatic artery originating from the left gastric artery, (2) replaced right hepatic artery originating from the superior mesenteric artery, and (3) replaced common hepatic artery originating from the superior mesenteric artery.

Variations in the portal venous anatomy are uncommon but include atresias, strictures, and obstructing valves. On the other hand, variations in the branching of the hepatic veins are common, with the most common being when the accessory vein drains the superoanterior segment of the right lobe. It may empty into the middle hepatic vein or join the right hepatic vein.

Diffuse Disease

Diffuse hepatocellular disease affects the hepatocytes and interferes with liver function. The **hepatocyte** is a parenchymal liver cell that performs all the functions ascribed to the liver. This abnormality is measured through the series of liver function tests. The hepatic enzyme levels are elevated with cell necrosis. With cholestasis (i.e., interruption in the flow of bile through any part of the biliary system, from the liver to the duodenum), the alkaline phosphatase and direct bilirubin levels increase. Likewise, when there are defects in protein synthesis, there may be elevated serum bilirubin levels and decreased serum albumin and clotting factor levels.

There are many subcategories of diffuse parenchymal disease, including fatty infiltration, acute and chronic hepatitis, early alcoholic liver disease, and acute and chronic cirrhosis. See Table 9-4 for clinical findings, sonographic findings, and differential considerations for diffuse hepatic disease.

Fatty Infiltration Fatty infiltration of the liver is an acquired, reversible disorder of metabolism, resulting in an

TABLE 9-4	Liver Findings: Diffuse Disease	
Clinical Findings	**Sonographic Findings**	**Differential Considerations**
Fatty Infiltration		
Normal to ↑ hepatic enzymes ↑ Alk phos ↑ Direct bilirubin	↑ Echogenicity ↑ Attenuation Impaired visualization of borders of portal/hepatic structures (secondary to increased attenuation) Hepatomegaly May be patchy, inhomogeneous Focal sparing	Hepatitis Cirrhosis Metastases
Acute Hepatitis		
↑ AST, ALT ↑ Bilirubin Leukopenia	Nonspecific and variable Normal to slightly ↑ Echogenicity ↑ Brightness of portal vein borders Hepatosplenomegaly ↑ Thickness of gallbladder wall	Fatty liver
Chronic Hepatitis		
↑ AST, ALT ↑ Bilirubin Leukopenia	Coarse hepatic parenchyma ↑ Echogenicity ↓ Visualization brightness of portal triad Fibrosis may produce soft shadowing	Cirrhosis Fatty liver
Cirrhosis		
↑ Alk phos ↑ Direct bilirubin ↑ AST, ALT Leukopenia	Coarse liver parenchyma with nodularity ↑ Echogenicity ↑ Attenuation ↓ Vascular markings with acute cirrhosis Hepatosplenomegaly with ascites Shrunken liver with chronic cirrhosis (also ↑ nodularity) Regeneration of hepatic nodules Portal hypertension	Fatty liver Hepatitis
Glycogen Storage Disease		
Disturbance of acid-base balance	Hepatomegaly ↑ Echogenicity ↑ Attenuation von Gierke's adenoma (round, homogeneous)	Focal nodular hyperplasia Fatty liver
Hemochromatosis		
↑ Iron levels in blood	↑ Echogenicity throughout liver	Cirrhosis

Alk phos, Alkaline phosphatase; *ALT,* alanine aminotransferase; *AST,* aspartate aminotransferase.

intracellular accumulation of triglycerides within hepatocytes. Fatty infiltration implies increased lipid accumulation in the hepatocytes and results from major injury to the liver or a systemic disorder leading to impaired or excessive metabolism of fat. Fatty infiltration is a benign process and may be reversible with correction of the process, although it has been shown that fatty infiltration of the liver is the precursor for significant chronic disease in a percentage of patients. The patient is usually asymptomatic, although some patients may present with jaundice, nausea and vomiting, and abdominal tenderness or pain. Common causes of fatty liver include obesity, alcohol abuse, cholesterol-lowering medications, diabetes, and certain chemotherapy agents. Box 9-3 lists the common findings of fatty liver.

BOX 9-3	Causes of Fatty Liver

Obesity
Excessive alcohol intake (alcohol stimulates lipolysis)
Poorly controlled hyperlipidemia
Diabetes mellitus
Excess corticosteroids
Pregnancy
Total parenteral hyperalimentation (nutrition)
Severe hepatitis
Glycogen storage disease
Cystic fibrosis
Pharmaceutical
Chronic illness

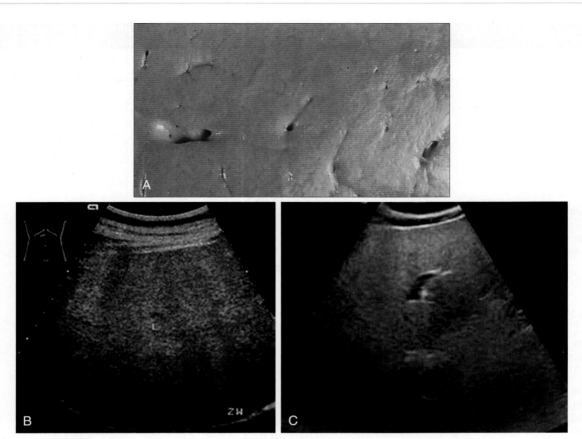

FIGURE 9-24 A, Gross appearance of the fatty liver. **B,** Fatty infiltration of the liver appears in a variety of patterns that depend on the amount and distribution of fat in the liver parenchyma. **C,** The portal vein structures may be difficult to visualize because of the increased attenuation, which in turn causes a decrease in penetration of the sound beam.

◢ *Sonographic Findings.* Fatty infiltration of the liver appears in a variety of patterns that depend on the amount and distribution of fat in the liver parenchyma (Figure 9-24). Fatty infiltration most commonly appears in a diffuse distribution and results in uniform increased echogenicity of the liver. Thus comparison of the liver parenchyma to the kidney is very useful in determining if fatty infiltration is present. The pancreas may also be used to judge the fatty infiltration pattern as its parenchyma is more echogenic that the liver. If the liver appears more "hyperechoic" than the pancreas, fatty infiltration should be considered. Localized enlargement of the lobe affected by fatty infiltration is evident. The portal vein structures may be difficult to visualize because of the increased attenuation of the ultrasound beam. The increased attenuation also causes a decrease in penetration of the sound beam, which may be a clue for the sonographer to think of fatty liver disease. The liver is so dense that "typical" gain settings do not allow penetration to the posterior border of the liver. It thus becomes more difficult to see the outline of the portal vein and hepatic vein borders. Authors have stated that this increase in echo texture may result from increased collagen content of the liver or increase in lipid accumulation. The following three grades of liver texture have been defined in sonography for classification of fatty infiltration:

- *Mild.* The mild form will present with minimal diffuse increase in hepatic echogenicity with normal visualization

of the diaphragm and intrahepatic vascular borders (Figure 9-25, *A*).
- *Moderate.* Moderate fatty infiltration shows increased echogenicity with slightly impaired visualization of the diaphragm and intrahepatic vascular borders (Figure 9-25, *B*).
- *Severe.* The severe form presents with a marked increase in echogenicity of the liver parenchyma, decreased penetration of the posterior segment of the right lobe of the liver, and decreased to poor visualization of the diaphragm and hepatic vessels (Figure 9-25, *C*).

Focal Fatty Infiltration and Focal Fatty Sparing. Fatty infiltration is not always uniform throughout the liver parenchyma; in fact, regions of increased echogenicity are present within a normal liver parenchyma. It is not uncommon to see patchy distribution of hypoechoic masses (fat) within a dense, fatty infiltrated liver parenchyma, especially in the right lobe of the liver. It is important to note that the fat does not displace normal intrahepatic vascular architecture. The margins of the fatty tissue may appear nodular, round, or interdigitated with the normal hepatic tissue. Fatty infiltration has the ability to resolve rapidly.

The other characteristic of fatty infiltration is focal sparing. This condition should be suspected in patients who have "masslike" hypoechoic areas in typical locations in a liver that is otherwise increased in echogenicity. The most

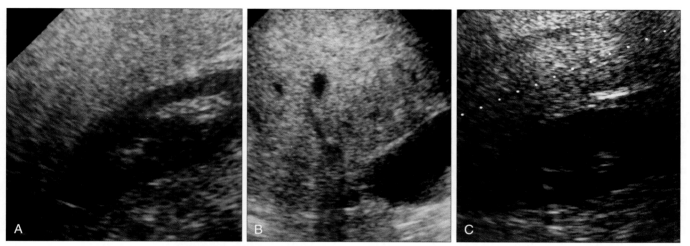

FIGURE 9-25 **Fatty infiltration. A,** Grade I. **B,** Grade II. **C,** Grade III.

common areas are anterior to the gallbladder or the portal vein and the periportal region of the medial segment of the left lobe of the liver (Figure 9-26). Focal subcapsular fat may be found in diabetic patients receiving insulin in peritoneal dialysate.

Viral Hepatitis. Hepatitis is considered to result from infection by a group of viruses that specifically target the hepatocytes. Hepatitis is the general name for inflammatory and infectious disease of the liver, of which there are many causes. The disease may result from a local infection (viral hepatitis), from an infection elsewhere in the body (e.g., infectious mononucleosis or amebiasis), or from chemical or drug toxicity. Mild inflammation impairs hepatocyte function, whereas more severe inflammation and necrosis may lead to obstruction of blood and bile flow in the liver and impaired liver cell function.

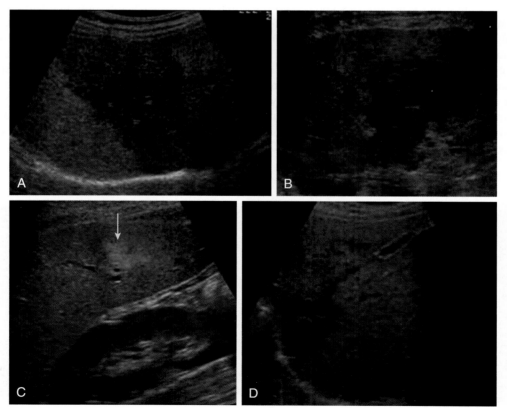

FIGURE 9-26 **Focal sparing secondary to fatty infiltration.** This condition should be suspected in patients who have masslike hypoechoic areas in typical locations in a liver that is otherwise increased in echogenicity.

Patients with hepatitis may initially present with flulike and gastrointestinal symptoms, including loss of appetite, nausea, vomiting, and fatigue. Viral hepatitis may be fatal with secondary acute hepatic necrosis or chronic hepatitis, which may lead to portal hypertension, cirrhosis, and hepatocellular carcinoma (HCC).

There are many distinct hepatitis viruses that have been identified that are beyond the scope of this chapter. The more common hepatitis A, B, and C will be discussed. Hepatitis A is found worldwide and is spread primarily by fecal contamination, because the virus lives in the alimentary tract. In developing countries, the disease is endemic and the infection occurs very early in life. Hepatitis A is an acute infection that leads to either complete recovery or death from acute liver failure. Hepatitis B is caused by the type B virus, which exists in the bloodstream and can be spread by transfusions of infected blood or plasma or through the use of contaminated needles. Hepatitis B is of the greatest risk to health care workers because of the nature of transmission. This virus is also found in body fluids, such as saliva and semen, and may be spread by sexual contact. Hepatitis C virus (HCV) is diagnosed by the presence in blood of the antibody to HCV (anti-HCV).

Acute Hepatitis. In acute hepatitis, without complications, the clinical recovery usually occurs within 4 months. Complications of hepatitis involving damage to the liver may range from mild disease to massive necrosis and liver failure. The pathologic changes seen include the following: (1) liver cell injury, swelling of the hepatocytes, and hepatocyte degeneration, which may lead to cell necrosis; (2) reticuloendothelial and lymphocytic response with Kupffer cells enlarging; and (3) regeneration.

Sonographic Findings. The liver texture may appear normal or the sonographer may note that the portal vein borders are more echogenic than usual (known as the "starry sky" sign), the liver parenchyma is slightly more echogenic than normal, and attenuation may be present (Figure 9-27). Hepatosplenomegaly is present, and the gallbladder wall is markedly thickened with contraction of the gallbladder lumen.

Chronic Hepatitis. Chronic hepatitis exists when there is clinical or biochemical evidence of hepatic inflammation that extends beyond 6 months. Causes include viral, metabolic, autoimmune, or drug induced. In chronic active hepatitis, there are more extensive changes than in chronic persistent hepatitis, with inflammation extending across the limiting plate, spreading out in a perilobular fashion, and causing piecemeal necrosis, which is frequently accompanied by fibrosis. Patients may present with nausea, anorexia, weight loss, tremors, jaundice, dark urine, fatigue, and varicosities. Chronic persistent hepatitis is a benign, self-limiting process. Chronic active hepatitis usually progresses to cirrhosis and liver failure.

Sonographic Findings. On ultrasound examination the liver parenchyma is coarse with decreased brightness of the portal triads, but the degree of attenuation is not as great as is seen in fatty infiltration (Figure 9-28). The liver does not increase in size with chronic hepatitis. Fibrosis may be evident, which may produce "soft shadowing" posteriorly.

Cirrhosis. Cirrhosis is a chronic degenerative disease of the liver in which the hepatic lobes are covered with fibrous tissue, the parenchyma degenerates, and the lobules are infiltrated with fat. The essential feature is simultaneous parenchymal necrosis, regeneration, and diffuse fibrosis resulting in disorganization of lobular architecture (Figure 9-29). Cirrhosis may be classified as micronodular (nodules 0.1 to 1 cm in diameter) or macronodular (nodules up to 5 cm in diameter). The process of cirrhosis is chronic and progressive, with liver cell failure and portal hypertension as the end stage. Micronodular cirrhosis is most commonly the result of chronic alcohol abuse, whereas macronodular cirrhosis is caused by chronic viral hepatitis or other infection. Other causes of cirrhosis include biliary cirrhosis, Wilson's disease, primary sclerosing cholangitis, and hemochromatosis.

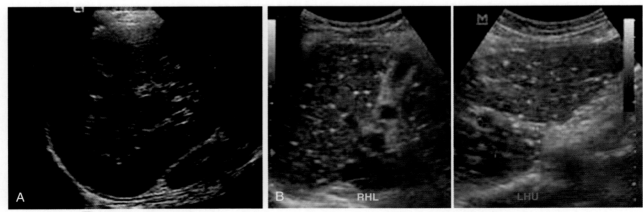

FIGURE 9-27 Hepatitis. The liver texture may appear normal or the portal vein borders are more echogenic than usual (known as the "starry sky" sign), the liver parenchyma is slightly more echogenic than normal, and attenuation may be present.

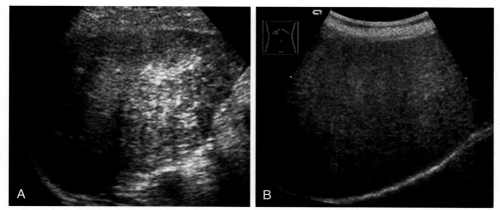

FIGURE 9-28 Chronic hepatitis. The liver parenchyma is coarse with decreased brightness of the portal triads; however, the degree of attenuation is not as great as is seen in fatty infiltration.

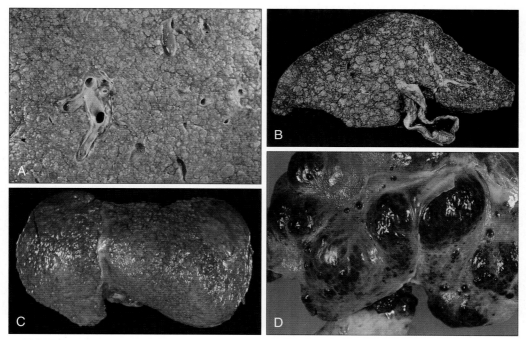

FIGURE 9-29 A, Gross pathology of alcoholic cirrhosis with high degree of fat content. **B,** Biliary cirrhosis (liver is nodular). **C,** Micronodular cirrhosis (nodules are small with uniform size). **D,** Macronodular cirrhosis.

Patients with acute cirrhosis may seem asymptomatic or may have symptoms that include nausea, flatulence, ascites, light-colored stools, weakness, abdominal pain, varicosities, and spider angiomas. The classic clinical presentation of a patient with cirrhosis is hepatomegaly, jaundice, and ascites. Chronic cirrhosis patient symptoms include nausea, anorexia, weight loss, jaundice, dark urine, fatigue, or varicosities. Chronic cirrhosis may progress to liver failure and portal hypertension.

Sonographic Findings. The sonographic diagnosis of cirrhosis may be challenging. In the early stage of cirrhosis, hepatomegaly is the first sonographic finding. As the cirrhosis becomes more severe, the liver volume decreases in the right lobe, with enlargement of the left and caudate lobes. The

evaluation of the ratio of the caudate lobe width to the right lobe width (C/RL) has been used as an indicator of cirrhosis. A C/RL value of 0.65 is considered indicative of cirrhosis. (This measurement is useful if abnormal, but not as sensitive when it is normal.)

Specific findings may include increased echogenicity and coarsening of the hepatic parenchyma secondary to fibrosis and surface nodularity (Figure 9-30). This evaluation is subjective and depends on appropriate gain settings (both time gain compensation and overall gain). Increased attenuation may be present, with decreased vascular markings. The amount of fatty infiltration will certainly influence the amount of echogenicity and attenuation. Hepatosplenomegaly may be present with ascites surrounding the liver. In

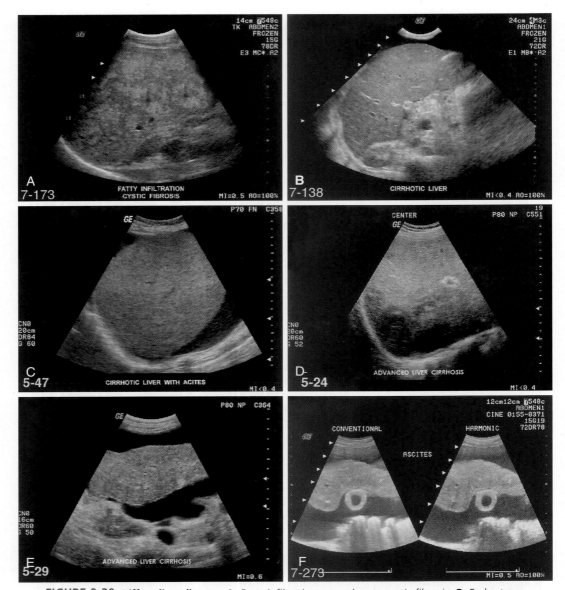

FIGURE 9-30 **Diffuse liver disease. A,** Fatty infiltration secondary to cystic fibrosis. **B,** Early stages of cirrhosis: hepatomegaly, decreased vasculature. **C,** Cirrhotic liver with ascites. **D,** Advanced cirrhosis with attenuation. **E,** Late-stage cirrhosis with shrunken liver, ascites. **F,** Late-stage cirrhosis with thick gallbladder wall, ascites, shrunken liver.

addition, there may be atrophy of the right and left medial lobes of the liver.

Chronic cirrhosis may show surface nodularity of the liver edge, especially well demonstrated if ascites is present. The use of a higher frequency, linear array transducer may allow the sonographer to demonstrate the surface of the liver. The hepatic fissures may be accentuated. The isoechoic regenerating nodules may be seen throughout the liver parenchyma. Portal hypertension may be present with or without abnormal Doppler flow patterns. Patients who have cirrhosis have an increased incidence of hepatoma tumors within the liver parenchyma.

Regenerating nodules represent regenerating hepatocytes surrounded by a fibrosis septa. They are "isoechoic" to the

liver parenchyma and thus may be indistinguishable from normal liver texture. Dysplastic nodules or adenomatous hyperplastic nodules are larger than the regenerating nodules and are considered premalignant. These nodules contain well-differentiated hepatocytes, portal venous blood supply, and atypical or frankly malignant cells. Color Doppler is used to image the portal venous blood supply.

Doppler Characteristics of Cirrhosis. Doppler evaluation of the hepatic veins is useful to detect the presence of altered flow dynamics. The hepatic vein velocity waveform reflects the hemodynamics of the right atrium. This is a triphasic pattern with two large antegrade diastolic and systolic waves and a small retrograde wave that corresponds to the atrial kick (from the heart) (Figure 9-31). Recall that the

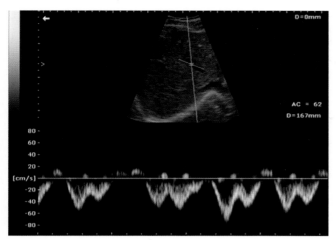

FIGURE 9-31 The hepatic vein velocity waveform reflects the hemodynamics of the right atrium as a triphasic pattern with two large antegrade diastolic and systolic waves and a small retrograde wave that corresponds to the atrial kick (from the heart).

thin walls of the hepatic veins easily receive the transfer of flow via the collaterals from the portal veins in a normal liver. In patients with compensated cirrhosis (no portal hypertension), the Doppler waveform is abnormal. Two patterns have been found in these patients with fatty infiltration of their liver: decreased amplitude of phasic oscillations with loss of reversed flow and a flattened waveform. As the cirrhosis advances, the hepatic veins develop luminal narrowing with increased velocities and turbulence of the flow patterns.

The hepatic artery waveform also shows altered flow dynamics in cirrhosis and chronic liver disease. The resistive index is blunted after a meal in patients with liver disease (Figure 9-32).

Glycogen Storage Disease. Glycogen storage disease is an inherited disease characterized by the abnormal storage and accumulation of glycogen in the tissues, especially the liver and kidneys. There are six categories of glycogen storage disease, which are divided on the basis of clinical symptoms and specific enzymatic defects. The most common is type I, or von Gierke's disease. This is a form of glycogen storage disease in which abnormally large amounts of glycogen are deposited in the liver and kidneys.

Sonographic Findings. On sonography, patients with glycogen storage disease present with hepatomegaly, increased echogenicity, and slightly increased attenuation (similar to diffuse fatty infiltration). The disease is associated with hepatic adenomas, focal nodular hyperplasia, and hepatomegaly. The adenoma presents as a well-demarcated, round, homogeneous, echogenic tumors (Figure 9-33). If the tumor is large, it may be slightly inhomogeneous.

Hemochromatosis. Hemochromatosis is a rare disease of iron metabolism characterized by excess iron deposits throughout the body. This disorder may lead to cirrhosis and portal hypertension.

Sonographic Findings. Ultrasound does not show specific findings other than hepatomegaly and cirrhotic changes. Some increased echogenicity may be seen uniformly throughout the hepatic parenchyma (Figure 9-34).

Hepatic Vascular Flow Abnormalities

Portal Hypertension. Portal hypertension is caused by increased resistance to venous flow through the liver. It is associated with cirrhosis, hepatic vein thrombosis, portal vein thrombosis, and thrombosis of the inferior vena cava. Ultrasound findings include dilation of the portal, splenic, and mesenteric veins; reversal of portal venous blood flow; and the development of collateral vessels (e.g., patent umbilical vein, gastric varices, splenorenal shunting).

The sonographic protocol for portal hypertension includes the following:
- Perform the routine abdominal imaging protocol.
- Assess for the presence of ascites.
- Obtain diameter measurements of the splenic and main portal veins on inspiration and expiration.
- Assess for the presence of collateral blood vessels (splenic hilum, porta hepatis, umbilical vein).

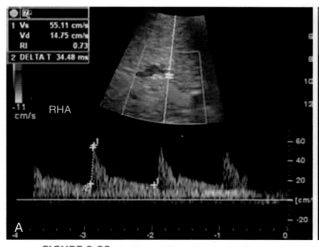
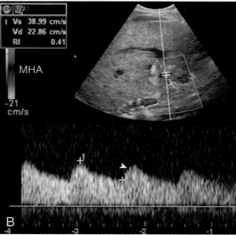

FIGURE 9-32 A, Normal hepatic arterial flow velocity. **B,** High-velocity hepatic arterial flow pattern.

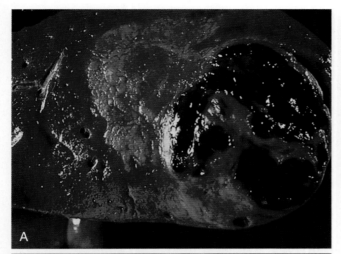

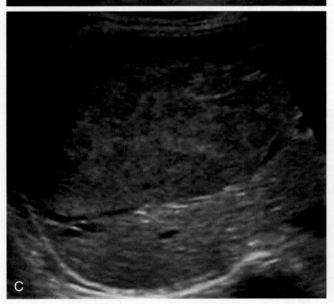

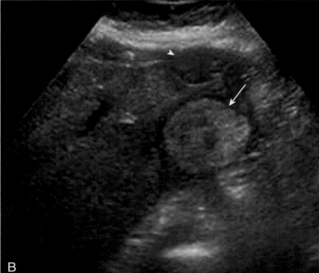

FIGURE 9-33 A, Gross pathology of hepatic adenoma with hemorrhage. **B,** The small adenoma presents as a well-demarcated, round, homogeneous, echogenic tumor. **C,** With increasing size, the adenoma may become inhomogeneous.

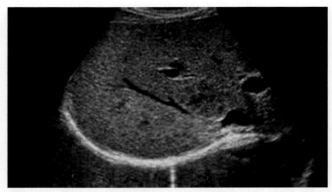

FIGURE 9-34 Hemochromatosis. Hepatomegaly with slightly increased echogenicity throughout the liver parenchyma.

- Determine the flow direction of the portal veins (main, left, and right portal veins) and splenic and superior mesenteric veins.
- Assess for the presence of splenorenal shunting.
- Assess for patency of the umbilical vein.
- Determine the patency and direction of flow in the inferior vena cava and hepatic veins.
- Assess and document the patency of surgically placed shunts.

Portal Venous Hypertension. Portal hypertension is defined as an increase in portal venous pressure or hepatic venous gradient. It exists when the portal venous pressure is above 10 mm Hg or the hepatic venous gradient is more than 5 mm Hg. Portal hypertension may be further defined by the following:

- A wedged hepatic vein pressure or direct portal vein pressure of more than 5 mm Hg greater than the inferior vena cava pressure
- Splenic vein pressure of greater than 15 mm Hg
- Portal vein pressure of greater than 30 cm H_2O

Portal hypertension is divided into presinusoidal and intrahepatic groups, depending on whether the hepatic vein wedged pressure is normal (presinusoidal) or elevated (intrahepatic). The development of increased pressure in the portal-splenic venous system is the cause of extrahepatic portal hypertension. Acute or chronic hepatocellular disease can block the flow of blood throughout the liver, causing it to back up into the hepatic portal circulation. This causes the blood pressure in the hepatic circulation to increase, thus the development of portal hypertension. In an effort to relieve the pressure, collateral veins are formed that connect to the systemic veins. These are known as varicose veins and occur most frequently in the area of the esophagus, stomach, and rectum. Rupture of these veins can cause massive bleeding that may result in death.

Intrahepatic portal hypertension is the result of diseases that affect the portal zones of the liver like primary biliary cirrhosis, schistosomiasis, congenital hepatic fibrosis, or toxic drugs. Cirrhosis is the most common cause of intrahepatic portal hypertension. Diffuse metastatic liver disease may also produce portal hypertension, as the normal architecture of the liver is replaced by the distorted vascular channels that provide increased resistance to portal venous blood flow and obstruction to hepatic venous outflow. Other causes include thrombotic diseases of the inferior vena cava and hepatic veins; constrictive pericarditis or other right-sided heart failure over time will cause centrilobular fibrosis, hepatic regeneration, and cirrhosis, all leading to subsequent portal hypertension.

Portal hypertension may also develop when hepatopetal flow (toward the liver) is impeded by thrombus or tumor invasion. The blood becomes obstructed as it passes through the liver to the hepatic veins and is diverted to collateral pathways in the upper abdomen. Box 9-4 lists the indications for portal hypertension.

Portal hypertension may develop along two pathways. One entails increased resistance to flow, and the other entails increased portal blood flow. The most common mechanism for increased resistance to flow occurs in patients with cirrhosis (Figures 9-35 and 9-36). The disease process of cirrhosis produces areas of micronodular and macronodular regeneration, atrophy, and fatty infiltration, which make it difficult for the blood to perfuse. This condition may be found in patients with liver disease or diseases of the cardiovascular system. Patients with increased portal blood flow may have an arteriovenous fistula or splenomegaly secondary to a hematologic disorder.

Collateral circulation develops when the normal venous channels become obstructed. This diverted blood flow causes embryologic channels to reopen; blood flows hepatofugally (away from the liver) and is diverted into collateral vessels. The

collateral channels may be into the gastric veins (coronary veins), esophageal veins, recanalized umbilical vein, or splenorenal, gastrorenal, retroperitoneal, hemorrhoidal, or intestinal veins (Figure 9-37). The most common collateral pathways are through the coronary and esophageal veins, as occurs in 80% to 90% of patients with portal hypertension. Varices, tortuous dilations of veins, may develop because of increased pressure in the portal vein, usually secondary to cirrhosis. Bleeding from the varices occurs with increased pressure.

The most definitive way to diagnose portal hypertension is with arteriography. Sonography may be very useful in these patients to define the presence of ascites, hepatosplenomegaly, and collateral circulation; the cause of jaundice; and the patency of hepatic vascular channels. See Table 9-5 for clinical findings, sonographic findings, and differential considerations for portal venous hypertension.

Patient Preparation and Positioning. A history should be obtained from the patient to focus on the risk factors, signs, and symptoms of hepatocellular disease. Any previous medical history relating to hepatocellular disease should be noted. Likewise, any recent surgical intervention or shunt placement within the portal venous system should be documented in the patient history worksheet. The patient is placed initially in the supine position; the patient may also be rolled into a slight left lateral decubitus position to obtain a better intercostal window. The images and Doppler evaluation may be obtained in the longitudinal, coronal, oblique, or transverse plane. Breath holding is very important in obtaining good Doppler color and spectral waveforms. Initially the sonographer should image the patient in shallow respiration to set up his or her controls and depth. Then instruct the patient to stop breathing or take in a deep breath and hold it while the Doppler images are recorded. The image may be visualized on the monitor, allowing you to see which technique works best to obtain the clearest images. It is helpful to remember that a portal vein diameter greater than 13 mm has been associated with portal hypertension. As portosystemic shunts develop, the diameter of the portal vein decreases. Secondary signs of splenomegaly, alterations in liver size, ascites, and portosystemic venous collaterals should be evaluated (Box 9-5).

BOX 9-4	Indications for Portal Hypertension

- Suspected portal hypertension secondary to liver disease
- Portal vein compression or thrombosis
- Acute onset of hepatic vein occlusion (Budd-Chiari syndrome), constrictive pericarditis, or congestive heart failure with tricuspid regurgitation
- Congenital, traumatic, or neoplastic arterioportal fistula

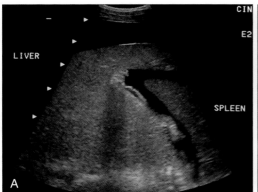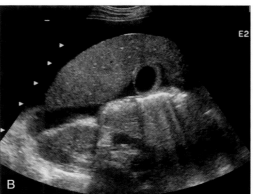

FIGURE 9-35 Portal hypertension. A, Transverse image of hepatosplenomegaly in a patient with advanced cirrhosis, decreased vasculature, and ascites. **B,** Transverse image of the thickened gallbladder wall, accentuated by the ascitic fluid.

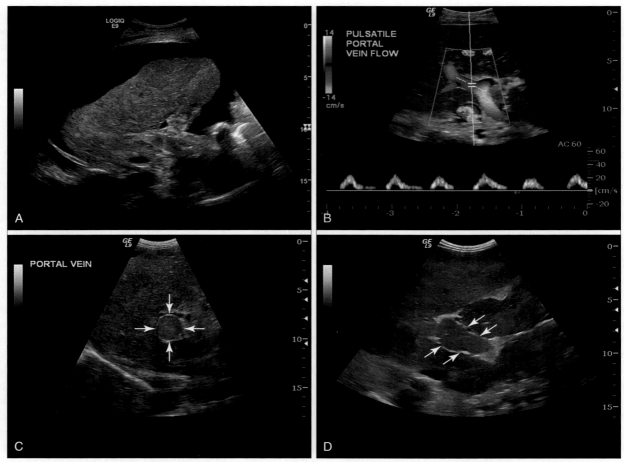

FIGURE 9-36 Portal hypertension. A, Hepatomegaly with massive ascites. The portal vein is filled with thrombus. **B,** The sonographer should search for hepatofugal flow in the portal vein. Note the nodular border of the liver. **C,** The portal vein is dilated and completely filled with thrombus *(arrows)*. **D,** Thrombosis of the main portal vein *(arrows)* with reduced flow.

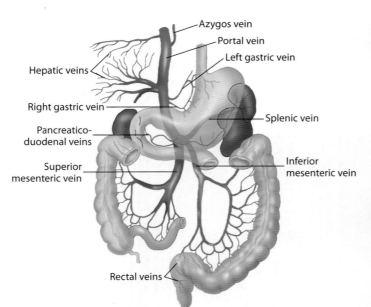

FIGURE 9-37 Collateral circulation of the extrahepatic portal circulation. The collateral channels may be into the gastric veins (coronary veins), esophageal veins, recanalized umbilical vein, or splenorenal, gastrorenal, retroperitoneal, hemorrhoidal, or intestinal veins.

TABLE 9-5	Liver Findings: Portal Venous Hypertension	
Clinical Findings	**Sonographic Findings**	**Differential Considerations**
↑ Liver enzymes	Collateral circulation/	Occlusion of vessels
Gastrointestinal	reversal of flow	
bleeding	Ascites	
Jaundice	Hepatosplenomegaly	
Hematemesis		

BOX 9-5	Major Sites of Portosystemic Venous Collaterals

- Gastroesophageal junction located between the coronary and short gastric veins and the systemic esophageal veins (may lead to fatal hemorrhage)
- Paraumbilical vein runs in the falciform ligament and connects the left portal vein to the systemic epigastric veins near the umbilicus
- Splenorenal and gastrorenal veins
- Intestinal veins
- Hemorrhoidal veins

The sonographer should keep in mind these important technical points in evaluating the patient for portal hypertension:

- The examination is performed with both imaging and Doppler evaluation of the portal system, the hepatic veins, and the hepatic arteries.
- Remember, the transducer must be *parallel* to the vessel; the Doppler angle should be less than 60 degrees to obtain the maximum peak systolic velocity.
- The evaluation of the portal venous system, hepatic veins, and hepatic artery is performed during the Doppler imaging examination.
- A Doppler examination should also evaluate flow in the extra–hepatic-portal venous system and the inferior vena cava, as well as the size of the common bile duct, liver, kidneys, and spleen.
- The pelvic cavity, flanks, and lower quadrants should be evaluated for the presence of free fluid.

Doppler Technique. Box 9-6 summarizes Doppler technique for abdominal examinations.

Color Doppler Evaluation of Collateral Circulation. Under normal circumstances, the portal venous blood traverses the liver and drains into the inferior vena cava of the

---

BOX 9-6   Doppler Technique

- The pulse repetition frequency (PRF) allows one to record lower velocities as the PRF is lowered; as the PRF is increased, the lower velocities are filtered out to record only the higher-velocity signal.
- The PRF may be changed with the scale control on the Doppler panel (look at the color bar on the left side of the monitor; the PRF will change as the "scale" on the Doppler control is changed).
- The PRF increases as imaging depth increases and decreases as depth decreases. Flow within the normal hepatic venous system is low; therefore a lower PRF is necessary to record the flow pattern. As the flow increases beyond 40 cm/sec, the PRF should be increased to prevent aliasing. (Aliasing may also be reduced by scanning at a lower frequency.)
- The Doppler sample volume should be smaller than the diameter of the lumen. If you have difficulty finding the vessel, increase the width of the sample volume to locate the flow, and then reduce the volume width to clear up the spectral waveform.
- The Doppler angle correction should be less than 60 degrees to display the peak spectral velocity.
- Wall filters help to eliminate "noise" or low-level Doppler shifts seen within the vessel.
- Pulsed wave Doppler provides quantitative information from a selected location.
- Color Doppler velocity is dependent on the direction of flow, velocity, and angle to flow. A positive Doppler shift is toward the transducer; negative shift shows flow away from the transducer. The laminar flow is distinguished from turbulent flow by varying the shades of color on the color map.
- Doppler measurements: peak systolic velocity (calculated highest velocity in cm/sec); resistive index (RI): subtract the end diastolic velocity from the peak systolic velocity and divide by the peak systolic velocity. Normal or low resistive RI measures less than 0.7.

---

systemic venous circulation by way of the hepatic veins. This is the direct route. However, other smaller communications exist between the portal and systemic systems, and they become important when the direct route becomes blocked. The sonographer should be aware of these communications that include the lower third of the esophagus; the esophageal branches of the left gastric vein (portal tributary) anastomose with the esophageal veins draining the middle third of the esophagus into the azygos veins (systemic tributary). The paraumbilical veins connect the left branch of the portal vein with the superficial veins of the anterior abdominal wall (systemic tributaries). The paraumbilical veins travel in the falciform ligament and accompany the ligamentum teres. The veins of the ascending colon, descending colon, duodenum, pancreas, and liver (portal tributary) anastomose with the renal, lumbar, and phrenic veins (systemic tributaries).

The dilated venous structures near the superior mesenteric-splenic vein confluence, the main portal vein, and the gastric veins should be evaluated (Figure 9-38). As the sonographer scans in the longitudinal plane, medial to the superior mesenteric and splenic vein confluence, the right and left gastric veins may be seen as collateral circulation. If the gastric veins are serving as collateral circulation, their diameter should be enlarged to 4 to 5 mm. Remember, the Doppler signals should be obtained from the imaging plane that allows the beam to be as parallel to the vessel as possible.

The umbilical vein may become recanalized secondary to portal hypertension. This vessel is best seen on the longitudinal plane near the midline, as a tubular structure coursing posterior to the medial surface of the left lobe of the liver (Figure 9-39). On transverse scans, a bull's-eye is seen within the ligamentum teres as the enlarged umbilical vein. Color Doppler helps the sonographer identify this vascular structure. Table 9-6 summarizes hepatic vasculature technique.

The collateral esophageal vessels are best seen in the midline transverse plane as the transducer is angled in a cephalic direction through the left lobe of the liver. The dilated gastrorenal, splenorenal, and short gastric veins are appreciated in the transverse and longitudinal planes near the splenic hilum.

As discussed earlier, the normal portal venous blood flows toward the liver, with the main portal vein flowing in a hepatopetal direction into the liver. Color Doppler will show this flow as a red or positive color pattern. The portal branches coursing posteriorly, or away from the transducer, will appear as blue, or negative, flow. Thus the right portal vein will appear blue and the left portal vein will appear red. The normal portal vein waveform is monophasic with low velocity (15 to 18 cm/sec) and varies with the patient's respiration and cardiac pulsation. The flow should be smooth and laminar. The normal diameter of the portal vein is 1.0 to 1.2 cm. With the development of portal hypertension, the flow in the portal vein loses its undulatory pattern and becomes monophasic. With severe portal hypertension, the flow becomes biphasic and finally hepatofugal (away from the liver). At this point intrahepatic arterial-portal venous shunting may also be seen.

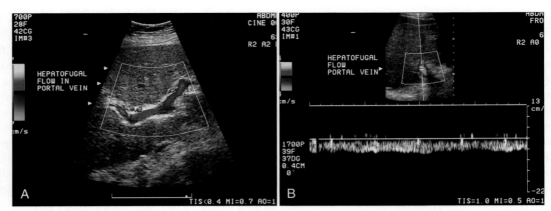

FIGURE 9-38 A, Flow reversal is shown in the main portal vein. **B,** Spectral Doppler shows flow below the baseline in the main portal vein.

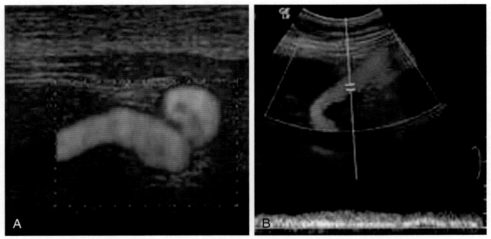

FIGURE 9-39 Color flow Doppler of the recanalized umbilical vein.

The superior mesenteric vein and splenic vein are more influenced by respiration and patient position; thus, if they appear larger, it may not be as a result of portal hypertension. Flow reversal is seen both with spectral waveform patterns below the baseline in the main portal vein and with reversed color direction. Obstruction of the portal venous system is recognized by turbulence within the vessel. Table 9-7 summarizes observations important in abdominal Doppler examinations.

Doppler Interrogation. The hepatic vessels should be imaged at four anatomic locations:
1. Midline, beneath the xiphoid for the left hepatic vein, left hepatic artery, and left portal vein
2. Midclavicular and intercostals at the porta hepatis for the main hepatic artery and main portal vein
3. Lateral and intercostals at the right lobe for the right hepatic artery and right portal vein
4. Subcostal and midclavicular for the right hepatic vein and middle hepatic vein

Portal Hypertension Secondary to Portal Vein Thrombosis. The invasion of the portal system with tumor or thrombosis may cause portal hypertension if the vessel is

significantly occluded preventing blood flow into the liver. The clinical symptoms are very different from those of intrahepatic disease; ascites is the primary complaint. The patient does not have jaundice or a tender enlarged liver. Splenomegaly and bleeding varices may be present. Portal vein thrombosis may develop secondary to trauma, sepsis, cirrhosis, or hepatocellular carcinoma (Figure 9-40). The definitive diagnosis is made with a liver biopsy and positive findings of portal hypertension.

Sonographic Findings. Portal vein thrombosis shows absence of portal flow with echogenic thrombus within the lumen of the vein, the development of portal vein collaterals, expansion of the caliber of the vein, and cavernous transformation of the vessels. The cavernous transformation of the portal vein appears as a wormlike structure in the area of the porta hepatis that completely fills with color representing the periportal collateral circulation. Acute thrombus may appear anechoic and thus be missed by the sonographer if Doppler interrogation is not performed. Malignant thrombosis of the portal vein is closely associated with hepatocellular carcinoma and is often expansive.

TABLE 9-6	**Hepatic Vasculature Technique**	
Vessel	**Image Plane**	**Technique**
Left hepatic vein (LHV)	Transverse/longitudinal	Locate the left lobe of the liver. Identify the IVC and angle steeply toward the diaphragm. The LHV and MHV should be seen as they drain into the IVC.
Left portal vein (LPV) Left hepatic artery (LHA)	Transverse, coronal, intercostal, decubitus Transverse	Locate horizontal segment of LPV, adjust transducer to obtain steepest angle for Doppler (parallel to the vessel), and zoom in on the LPV. Usually found posterior to horizontal segment of LPV. After interrogating the LPV, look for LHA with color Doppler (expand color box to cover the LPV and adjacent liver tissue). Place PW cursor/sample volume in area of LHA (suspend respiration); watch for "flashing" of signal as it comes in and out of view with respiration. Look for LHA on deep inspiration. If you cannot get the signal in the periphery of the liver, move to another location closer to the main portal vein.
Common hepatic artery (HA)	Longitudinal—porta hepatis	Use same technique as described for LHA. Transplant recipient patients: usually only able to Doppler HA at the porta hepatis. Include extrahepatic and intrahepatic segments of HA. Difficult to image site of anastomosis.
Main portal vein (MPV) Inferior vena cava (IVC)	Longitudinal—porta hepatic Longitudinal, coronal—slightly to right of midline; suspend breath; angle transducer in cephalad to caudal sweep to record flow	If shunt is present, anastomosis site is easier to identify (more prone to thrombosis); be sure to investigate the MPV proximal, within, and distal to anastomosis. May be difficult to obtain good angle because of horizontal location on transverse plane. If shunt is present, evaluate site of anastomosis carefully (proximal, within, and distal). Look carefully for presence of internal echoes that represent thrombosis. If you suspect thrombus is present, and the Doppler signal is very "choppy" with high velocity and little phasicity, the likelihood of thrombus is good. Be sure to follow the IVC all the way into the right atrium of the heart.
Splenic vein (SV) Right hepatic artery (RHA)	Transverse Transverse, anterior to right posterior portal branch	Examine SV from the splenic hilum to the portal-splenic confluence. Use same techniques as mentioned to Doppler the RPV and RHA. If you are unable to locate the RHA in the periphery of the liver, move closer to the trunk of the adjacent PV. If you cannot find the RHA at the right posterior portal branch, try looking for it at the level of the right anterior PV branch.
Right portal vein (RPV)	Anterior, intercostal approach; one rib space away from window for porta hepatis	To locate the right posterior branch of RPV, begin with the MPV at the porta hepatis. Follow the MPV into the liver until you see the RPV. The posterior branch extends posteriorly into the right lobe. It is easier to obtain a good Doppler angle if you use a more anterior intercostal approach.
Right hepatic vein (RHV)	Transverse, subcostal	Place the probe just below the level of the xiphoid with a steep angulation toward the diaphragm. Locate the IVC; the RHV will be seen in the right lobe of the liver in a horizontal plane as it empties into the IVC.
Middle hepatic vein (MHV)	Transverse, subcostal	Place the probe just below the level of the xiphoid with a steep angulation toward the diaphragm. Locate the IVC; the MHV will be seen in a vertical plane as it separates the right lobe from the left lobe of the liver as it empties into the IVC.

Portal Vein Hypertension and Portacaval Shunts. If portal hypertension becomes extensive, the portal system can be decompressed by shunting blood to the systemic venous system. Portacaval shunts for the treatment of portal hypertension may involve the anastomosis of the portal vein, because it lies within the lesser omentum, to the anterior wall of the inferior vena cava behind the entrance into the lesser sac. The splenic vein may be anastomosed to the left renal vein after removing the spleen. Basically, the three types of shunts are portacaval, mesocaval, and splenorenal. It is the responsibility of the sonographer to know specifically which type of shunt the patient has in place to image the flow patterns correctly.

The *portacaval shunt* attaches the main portal vein at the superior mesenteric vein–splenic vein confluence to the anterior aspect of the inferior vena cava. The *mesocaval shunt* attaches the middistal superior mesenteric vein to the inferior vena cava (Figure 9-41). This shunt may be difficult to image if overlying bowel gas is present. The *splenorenal shunt* attaches the splenic vein to the left renal vein. The shunt and connecting

TABLE 9-7	Doppler Observations
Hepatic Artery	
Left hepatic artery (LHA)	Low-resistance waveform; forward flow in diastolic above baseline.
Right hepatic artery (RHA)	Vessel is tortuous; flow may appear to move toward and away from the transducer.
Common hepatic artery (CHA)	Systolic window with narrow bandwidth with parabolic flow profile.
	Spectral fill-in of systolic window because of small vessel diameter.
	High-resistance waveforms may indicate veno-occlusive disease.
Portal Venous System	
Left portal vein (LPV)	Continuous, low-velocity phasic signal (phasic means that the velocity increases and decreases with respiration, giving the signal a smooth wavelike appearance).
Right portal vein (RPV)	Normal flow is termed *hepatopetal* (toward the liver).
Main portal vein (MPV)	Reversed flow is *hepatofugal* (away from the liver).
	Portal venous thrombosis or postoperative anastomosis from a liver transplant can cause an abnormal portal vein signal. This results from decreased vessel lumen size, which reduces the pressure and consequently increases the velocity of flow through the narrowed region, giving a "choppy" appearance as a result of increased velocities.
	Note: The hepatic artery and portal vein flow should be in the same direction, because the hepatic artery runs parallel with the portal vein.
Hepatic Venous System	
Left hepatic vein (LHV)	Multiphasic pulsatile flow pattern secondary to proximity of the right atrium with flow above and below the baseline caused by close proximity to the right atrium, which results in hemodynamic changes.
Right hepatic vein (RHV)	Right-sided heart failure may cause the hepatic veins to become pulsatile and dilated.
Middle hepatic vein (MHV)	Increased intrahepatic pressure or venous obstruction demonstrates a more continuous or monophasic signal.
Inferior Vena Cava	
	Continuous waveform with respiratory variations; becomes more pulsatile as it empties into the right atrium.
	Best imaged with a slight cranial-caudal sweep in the longitudinal plane with the patient in deep inspiration.
	Anastomosis from surgical transplantation may alter the normal flow into the inferior vena cava.
	Thrombosis can cause the inferior vena cava waveform to appear monophasic with high velocities ("choppy" appearance). Examine for thrombus in the renal veins as well.
	If a surgical shunt is present, be sure to check the patient's history to find out if the specific type of shunt (portal/cava or mesenteric/cava) is in place.

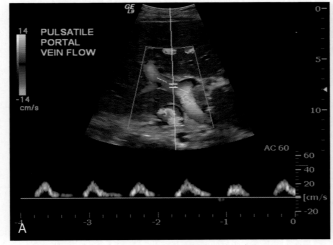 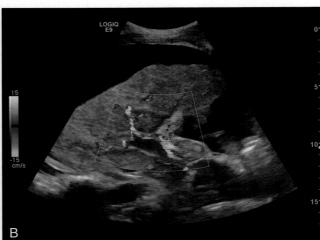

FIGURE 9-40 A, Normal portal vein flow. **B,** Portal vein thrombosis.

vessel should be documented with pulsed wave Doppler and color Doppler to determine flow patterns and patency.

Intrahepatic shunts are created percutaneously with the use of metallic expandable stents, which can be seen on ultrasound. This type of shunt is the **transjugular intrahepatic portosystemic shunt (TIPS)** (Figure 9-42). The TIPS is evaluated for patency using the liver as an acoustic window to image the flow velocity pattern within the shunt. Baseline studies are performed with color and spectral Doppler, so variations in flow patterns may be monitored before clinical symptoms are apparent. Stenosis may occur at the hepatic vein level or within the shunt.

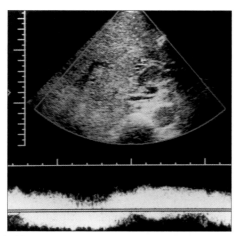

FIGURE 9-41 **Mesocaval shunt.** The mesocaval shunt attaches the middistal superior mesenteric vein to the inferior vena cava. This patient had thrombus at the distal end with to-and-fro flow reversal.

Budd-Chiari Syndrome. Budd-Chiari syndrome is an uncommon, often dramatic illness caused by thrombosis of the hepatic veins or inferior vena cava. It was first described by George Budd in 1846 and by Hans Chiari in 1899. The patient with Budd-Chiari syndrome has a poor prognosis and is characterized by abdominal pain, massive ascites, and hepatomegaly.

This condition may present acutely or as a chronic illness lasting from a few weeks to several years. Extensive hepatic vein occlusion is usually fatal within weeks or months of the onset of symptoms.

Budd-Chiari syndrome may be classified as primary or secondary on the basis of its pathophysiology. The primary type is caused by congenital obstruction of the hepatic veins or inferior vena cava by membranous webs across the upper vena cava at or just above the entrance of the left and middle hepatic veins. This lesion has been found to be most common in Asia.

The secondary type results from thrombosis in the hepatic veins or inferior vena cava. It often occurs in patients with predisposing conditions, such as prolonged use of oral contraceptives, pregnancy tumors (hepatocellular carcinoma, renal cell carcinoma, adrenal carcinoma, leiomyosarcoma of the inferior vena cava), infections, and in rare cases trauma. In approximately 25% to 30% of all cases, the exact cause is never determined.

Ascites is the most characteristic clinical feature of Budd-Chiari syndrome. Other symptoms are abdominal pain, hepatosplenomegaly, jaundice, vomiting, and diarrhea. Rarely, patients present with acute illness with abdominal pain, hepatomegaly, and shock. More commonly, patients have a vague illness and abdominal distress weeks or months in duration, followed by the

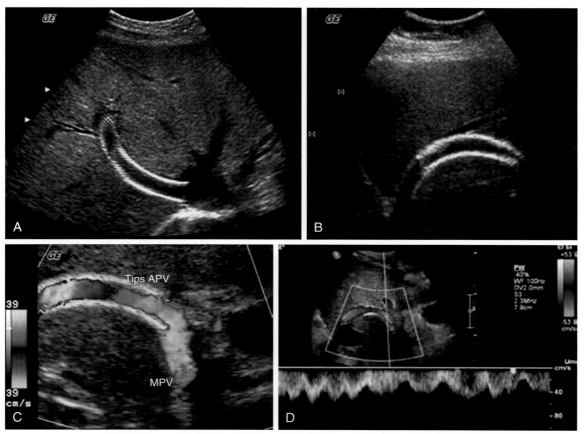

FIGURE 9-42 **Transjugular intrahepatic portosystemic shunt (TIPS).** A 50-year-old male after TIPS procedure shows patency of the stent and normal flow from the portal vein to the inferior vena cava without evidence of thrombus.

TABLE 9-8	Liver Findings: Budd-Chiari Syndrome	
Clinical Findings	Sonographic Findings	Differential Considerations
Ascites, right upper quadrant pain, hepatomegaly	↑ Caudate lobe Atrophy in right lobe of the liver	Portal hypertension

appearance of ascites and hepatomegaly. Jaundice is mild or absent. As portal hypertension increases, the spleen becomes palpable. When thrombus is found in the inferior vena cava, edema of the legs is gross and there is venous distention over the abdomen, flanks, and back. Albuminuria may be found.

Routine biochemical determinations of aminotransferases and alkaline phosphatase indicate mild or moderate impairment of hepatic function, depending on the stage of disease. See Table 9-8 for clinical findings, sonographic findings, and differential considerations for Budd-Chiari syndrome.

Sonographic Findings. Sonography is useful in imaging patients with hepatic vein thrombosis. The caudate lobe of the liver, seen in longitudinal and transverse scans, has an independent vascular supply. In Budd-Chiari syndrome the caudate lobe becomes enlarged, and there is often atrophy of the right hepatic lobe, probably as a result of sparing of caudate lobe hepatic veins when there is thrombosis of the right, middle, and left hepatic veins.

The liver appears hypoechoic in the early stages of acute thrombosis; it appears hyperechoic and inhomogeneous, with fibrosis in later stages (Figure 9-43). The middle and left hepatic veins are imaged in the transverse plane at the level of the xiphoid. The transducer is angled in a cephalad position with the patient in deep inspiration. This allows the veins to be parallel to the Doppler beam. The right hepatic vein is evaluated from a right intercostal approach. With thrombosis, the hepatic veins become enlarged. In chronic cases of Budd-Chiari syndrome, the hepatic veins are usually not visualized. Demonstration of at least one major vein may show abnormalities in the vessel suggestive of this syndrome, including stenosis, dilation, thick wall echoes, abnormal course, extrahepatic anastomoses, and thrombosis.

Doppler sonography may show altered blood-flow patterns in the hepatic veins and inferior vena cava. In normal subjects the Doppler signal in the hepatic veins is phasic in response to both the cardiac and respiratory cycles, with wide variations in flow velocity and direction. In Budd-Chiari syndrome, flow in the inferior vena cava or hepatic veins changes from phasic to absent, reversed, turbulent, or continuous. Abnormal Doppler patterns with slow, continuous flow may indicate partial obstruction. The absence of flow signals suggests subtotal or total occlusion. Turbulent flow may be observed beyond the area of stenosis. The portal venous flow pattern may also be affected with decreased velocities or reversal of flow.

Color flow Doppler is an excellent technique for evaluating the hepatic venous system. Flow direction and velocities and areas of turbulent flow can be demonstrated with color. Patency of the hepatic veins and inferior vena cava can be determined with color flow Doppler, which compares very favorably with angiography.

Diagnostic Criteria for Hepatic Vascular Imaging. See Table 9-9 for the diagnostic criteria for hepatic vascular imaging, including gray scale, Doppler, and color Doppler.

Diffuse Abnormalities of the Liver Parenchyma

Abnormalities—such as biliary obstruction, common duct stones and stricture, extrahepatic mass, and passive hepatic congestion—are discussed as each lesion is seen on the ultrasound. See Table 9-10 for clinical findings, sonographic findings, and differential considerations of diffuse abnormalities of the liver parenchyma.

Biliary Obstruction: Proximal. Biliary obstruction proximal to the cystic duct can be caused by gallstones, carcinoma of the common bile duct, or metastatic tumor invasion of the porta hepatis (Figure 9-44). Clinically the patient may be jaundiced and have pruritus (itching). Liver function tests show an elevation in the direct bilirubin and alkaline phosphatase levels.

Sonographic Findings. Sonographically, carcinoma of the common duct presents as a tubular branching with dilated intrahepatic ducts best seen in the periphery of the

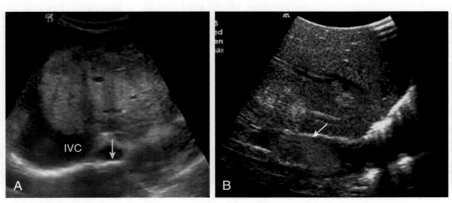

FIGURE 9-43 Budd-Chiari syndrome. Transverse image of the enlarged liver and thrombosis of the inferior vena cava *(IVC).*

TABLE 9-9 | Diagnostic Criteria for Hepatic Vascular Imaging

Interpretation	Gray Scale	Doppler	Color Doppler
Portal Veins			
Normal	No intraluminal echoes; bright, echogenic borders	Low-velocity signal with respiratory variation	Smooth fill-in of color
Thrombus	Enlarged or normal portal venous system with low-level echoes within the lumen; may appear isoechoic with the liver	Decreased low-velocity to absent Doppler waveform; look for hepatofugal flow	Decreased to absent color flow
Portal hypertension	Enlargement of the portal venous system Recanalization of the umbilical vein	Look for hepatofugal flow in portal venous system	Hepatofugal flow with good color fill of lumen
Cavernous transformation	Multiple vascular channels near the porta hepatis and/or splenic hilum Thrombosis of the extrahepatic portal vein (may be difficult to image) Look for recanalized umbilical vein	Continuous low-velocity flow	Color fills dilated collateral vessels; portal vein is difficult to fill with color
Hepatic Artery (HA)			
Normal	Follow course of portal vein to image hepatic artery anterior Enlarge image size to visualize artery Proximal HA best seen at level of celiac axis Distal HA seen in intercostal coronal view at level of MPV and CBD	Low-resistance waveform with systolic and diastolic component	Increase gain slightly to fill in vessel lumen with color
Thrombus	Increased low-level echoes within the lumen	Obstruction would cause increased velocity waveforms	Turbulence or absence of flow if complete obstruction is present
Inferior Vena Cava (IVC)			
Normal	Low-level intraluminal echoes within the lumen returning to right atrium; changes size with respiration	Continuous triphasic waveform with respiratory variations	Color fills lumen
Thrombosis	Increased echogenicity of low-level echoes filling lumen Examine renal veins for extension of thrombus	Decreased Doppler waveform secondary to degree of thrombus	Decreased color within lumen; color will outline the area of thrombus/obstruction
Right-sided heart failure	Dilation of lumen that does not change with respiration	Multiphasic, pulsatile flow	Color fills lumen of hepatic veins and inferior vena cava
Thrombosis/Budd-Chiari syndrome	Low-level echoes within the lumen of the hepatic veins; may completely restrict blood flow into the inferior vena cava Caudate lobe enlargement may be suspicious of thrombosis of hepatic veins	Decreased flow signal	Decreased color fill-in of hepatic veins; IVC may appear collapsed with decreased blood return

CBD, common bile duct; *MPV*, main portal vein

liver (Figure 9-45). It may be difficult to image a discrete mass lesion. The gallbladder is of normal size, even after a fatty meal is administered.

Biliary Obstruction: Distal. A biliary obstruction distal to the cystic duct may be caused by stones in the common duct, an extrahepatic mass in the porta hepatis, or stricture of the common duct. Clinically, common duct stones cause right upper quadrant pain, jaundice, and pruritus, as well as an increase in direct bilirubin and alkaline phosphatase.

Sonographic Findings. On ultrasound examination, the dilated intrahepatic ducts are seen in the periphery of the liver (Figure 9-46). The gallbladder size is variable, usually small. Gallstones are often present and appear as hyperechoic lesions along the posterior floor of the gallbladder, with a sharp posterior acoustic shadow. Careful evaluation of the common duct may show shadowing stones within the dilated duct.

Extrahepatic Mass. An extrahepatic mass in the area of the porta hepatis causes the same clinical signs as seen in biliary obstruction. The lesion may arise from the lymph nodes, pancreatitis, pseudocyst, or carcinoma in the head of the pancreas.

Sonographic Findings. On ultrasound examination, an irregular, ill-defined, hypoechoic, and inhomogeneous mass lesion may be seen in the area of the porta hepatis (Figure 9-47). There is intrahepatic ductal dilation, with a hydropic gallbladder.

Common Duct Stricture. Clinically the patient is jaundiced and has had a previous cholecystectomy. Laboratory values show an increase in the direct bilirubin and alkaline phosphatase levels.

Sonographic Findings. On ultrasound examination, common duct stricture presents as dilated intrahepatic ducts with absence of a mass in the porta hepatis.

TABLE 9-10	Liver Findings: Diffuse Abnormalities of the Liver Parenchyma	
Clinical Findings	**Sonographic Findings**	**Differential Considerations**
Biliary Obstruction: Proximal ↑ Direct bilirubin ↑ Alk phos	Carcinoma of common bile duct shows tubular branching with dilated intrahepatic ducts Gallbladder small to normal size; gallstones	Obstruction to distal duct Extrahepatic metastases
Biliary Obstruction: Distal ↑ Direct bilirubin ↑ Alk phos	Carcinoma of common bile duct shows tubular branching with dilated intrahepatic ducts Gallbladder small; gallstones and common duct stones	Obstruction to proximal duct Extrahepatic metastases
Extrahepatic Mass ↑ Direct bilirubin ↑ Alk phos	Irregular, ill-defined hypoechoic, heterogeneous lesion in area of porta hepatic Intrahepatic ductal dilation Hydropic gallbladder	Proximal or distal obstruction to the cystic duct Metastases
Common Duct Stricture ↑ Direct bilirubin ↑ Alk phos Previous cholecystectomy	Dilated intrahepatic ducts Absence of mass in porta hepatis	Extrahepatic mass Passive hepatic congestion
Passive Hepatic Congestion ↑ LFT	↑ IVC, HV, PV	N/A

Alk phos, Alkaline phosphatase; *HV,* hepatic vein; *IVC,* inferior vena cava; *LFT,* liver function test; *N/A,* not applicable; *PV,* portal vein.

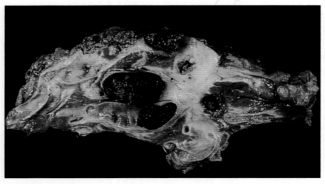

FIGURE 9-44 Gross pathology of gallstones in the hepatic duct.

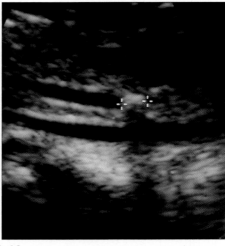

FIGURE 9-46 Obstruction distal to the cystic duct may be caused by stones in the common duct. The distal cystic duct is enlarged and obstructed by a stone at the distal end. The inferior vena cava is posterior to the duct.

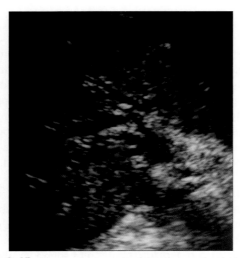

FIGURE 9-45 Obstruction proximal to the cystic duct may be secondary to pancreatic carcinoma or tumor invasion to the porta hepatis. Dilated intrahepatic ducts will result from this obstruction.

Passive Hepatic Congestion. Passive hepatic congestion develops secondary to congestive heart failure with signs of hepatomegaly. Laboratory data indicate normal to slightly elevated liver function tests.

▆ *Sonographic Findings.* On ultrasound examination, dilation of the inferior vena cava and superior mesenteric, hepatic, portal, and splenic veins is noted (Figure 9-48). The inferior vena cava normally decreases in size with expiration and increases with inspiration; however, with congestion there is little change in the size.

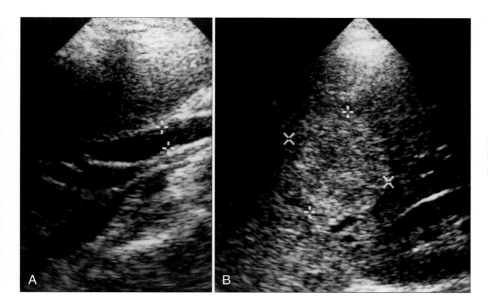

FIGURE 9-47 **A,** Sagittal scan of the dilated common duct. **B,** Sagittal scan of a mass in the porta hepatis.

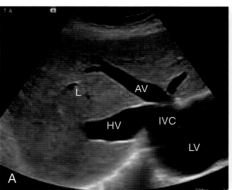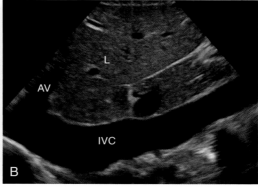

FIGURE 9-48 **A,** Transverse and **B,** longitudinal images of a patient in congestive liver failure. The inferior vena cava *(IVC)* and hepatic veins *(HV)* are dilated without respiratory collapse. Right atrium *(RA)*, liver *(L)*.

Focal Hepatic Disease

Few hepatic lesions have specific sonographic features. Therefore it is important to know the patient's clinical history and the sonographic patterns associated with various lesions. The knowledge of laboratory values in liver function tests also helps determine the hepatic lesions. The differential diagnosis for focal diseases of the liver includes cysts, abscess, hematoma, primary tumor, and metastases. See Table 9-11 for clinical findings, sonographic findings, and differential considerations for focal hepatic disease.

The sonographer should be able to differentiate whether the mass is **extrahepatic** or **intrahepatic**. Intrahepatic masses may cause the following findings on ultrasound: displacement of the hepatic vascular radicles, external bulging of the liver capsule, or a posterior shift of the inferior vena cava. An extrahepatic mass may show internal invagination or discontinuity of the liver capsule, formation of a triangular fat wedge, anteromedial shift of the inferior vena cava, or anterior displacement of the right kidney.

Cystic Lesions. *Hepatic cyst* usually refers to a solitary nonparasitic cyst of the liver. The cyst may be congenital or acquired, solitary or multiple. Patients are often asymptomatic and require no treatment. Sonographic findings of a benign cyst show the lesion to be well demarcated, thin walled, and anechoic with posterior acoustic enhancement. When the cysts become large, pain may develop as the lesion compresses the hepatic vasculature or ductal system. Fever may be present if the cyst hemorrhages and becomes infected. Once the cyst becomes infected, septations and internal echoes from the debris replace the anechoic properties. The wall may become thickened. Cystic lesions within the liver include the following: simple or congenital hepatic cysts, traumatic cysts, parasitic cysts, inflammatory cysts, polycystic disease, and pseudocysts.

Simple Hepatic Cysts. The sonographic finding of a simple hepatic cyst is usually incidental because most patients are asymptomatic. As the cyst grows, it may cause pain or a mass effect to suggest a more serious condition, such as infection, abscess, or necrotic lesion. Hepatic cysts occur more often in females than in males.

Sonographic Findings. On ultrasound examination, the cyst walls are thin, with well-defined borders, and anechoic, with distal posterior enhancement (Figure 9-49, *A*). Infrequently, cysts contain fine linear internal septa. Complications, such as hemorrhage, may occur and cause pain (Figure 9-49, *B*). Calcification may be seen within the cyst wall and may cause shadowing.

TABLE 9-11	Liver Findings: Focal Disease	
Clinical Findings	**Sonographic Findings**	**Differential Considerations**
Simple Hepatic Cysts		
N/A	Anechoic Thin walls Well-defined borders Distal posterior enhancement May have calcification	Congenital Hematoma Necrotic tumor
Polycystic Liver Disease		
Autosomal dominant 25%–50% of patients with polycystic kidney disease have hepatic cysts 60% of patients with polycystic liver disease have associated PKD	Anechoic Well-defined borders ↑ Acoustic enhancement Multiple cysts throughout liver parenchyma	Necrotic metastasis Echinococcal cyst Hematoma Abscess Hepatic cystadenocarcinoma
Pyogenic Abscess		
↑ White cell count Abnormal LFT Anemia	Variable appearance Right central lobe most common site Hypoechoic to complex to hyperechoic when fluid level present Round to oval or irregular Complex	Amebic abscess Echinococcal cyst Hepatic candidiasis
Hepatic Candidiasis		
↑ WBC Fever	Multiple small hypoechoic masses with echogenic central core "Bull's-eye" lesions "Wheel-within-wheel" pattern	Abscess Echinococcal cyst Metastases
Chronic Granulomatous Disease		
N/A	Poorly marginated Hypoechoic Posterior enhancement May have calcification/shadowing	Abscess
Amebic Abscess		
↑ Leukocytes Low fever Abdominal pain and diarrhea	Mass is variable Round or oval; lack notable borders Hypoechoic with debris	Pyogenic abscess Echinococcal cyst Hepatic candidiasis
Echinococcal Cyst		
↑ WBCs History of sheep-farming exposure	Simple to complex cysts Acoustic enhancement Oval or spherical Calcification Honeycomb appearance/"water lily" sign	Polycystic liver disease Amebic abscess Pyogenic abscess

LFT, Liver function test; *N/A*, not applicable; *PKD*, polycystic kidney disease; *WBCs*, white blood cells.

Congenital Hepatic Cysts. A solitary congenital cyst of the liver is rare and usually is an incidental lesion. This abnormality arises from developmental defects in the formation of bile ducts.

◢ ***Sonographic Findings.*** The mass is usually solitary and may vary in size from tiny to as large as 20 cm. The cyst is usually found on the anterior undersurface of the liver. It usually does not cause liver enlargement and is found in the right lobe of the liver more often than the left lobe.

Peribiliary Cysts. These tiny cysts (which range in size from 0.2 to 2.5 cm) are more commonly found in patients with severe liver disease. They are located centrally within the porta hepatis at the junction of the right and left hepatic ducts. Obstruction may occur if the cyst becomes large enough to cause biliary obstruction.

◢ ***Sonographic Findings.*** These small cysts are seen as discrete, clustered tubular-appearing cysts with thin septae that parallel the bile ducts and portal veins in the central area of the liver (Figure 9-50).

Polycystic Liver Disease. Polycystic liver disease is inherited in an autosomal dominant pattern that affects 1 in 500 individuals. At least 50% to 74% of patients with polycystic renal

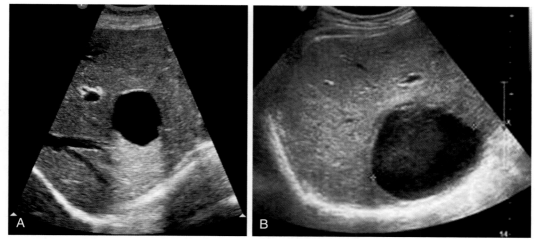

FIGURE 9-49 **A,** Solitary hepatic cyst in the left lobe of the liver shows increased through-transmission and well-defined borders. **B,** Liver cyst appears complex secondary to the hemorrhage.

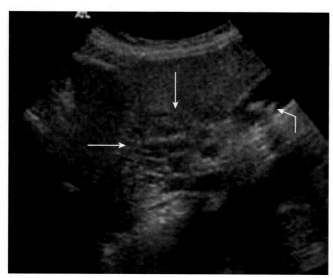

FIGURE 9-50 Peribiliary cysts are seen as discrete, clustered tubular-appearing cysts with thin septae that parallel the bile ducts and portal veins in the central area of the liver.

disease have one to several hepatic cysts. Of patients with polycystic liver disease, 60% have associated polycystic renal disease. The cysts are small, less than 2 to 3 cm, and multiple throughout the hepatic parenchyma. Cysts within the porta hepatis may enlarge and cause biliary obstruction. Histologically, they appear similar to simple hepatic cysts. It may be difficult to assess an abscess formation or neoplastic lesion in a patient with polycystic liver disease. Liver function tests are usually normal.

Sonographic Findings. On ultrasound examination, the cysts generally present as anechoic, well-defined borders with acoustic enhancement (Figure 9-51). The differential diagnosis for a cystic lesion includes the following: necrotic metastasis, echinococcal cyst, hematoma, hepatic cystadenocarcinoma, and abscess. Ultrasound may be used to direct the needle if percutaneous aspiration is necessary to obtain specific diagnostic information.

Infectious Disease of the Liver

Hepatic abscesses occur most often as complications of biliary tract disease, surgery, or trauma. The following three basic types of abscess formation occur in the liver: intrahepatic, subhepatic, and subphrenic. Clinically the patient presents with fever, elevated white cell count, and right upper quadrant pain. The search for an abscess must be made to locate solitary or multiple lesions within the liver or to search for abnormal fluid collections in Morison's pouch or in the subdiaphragmatic or subphrenic space. The following infectious processes are discussed: pyogenic abscess, hepatic candidiasis, chronic granulomatous disease, amebic abscess, and echinococcal disease.

Pyogenic Abscess. A **pyogenic abscess** is a pus-forming abscess. There are many routes for bacteria to gain access to the liver: through the biliary tree, the portal vein, or the hepatic artery; through a direct extension from a contiguous infection; or, rarely, through hepatic trauma. Sources of infection include cholangitis; portal pyemia secondary to appendicitis, diverticulitis, inflammatory disease, or colitis; direct spread from another organ; trauma with direct contamination; or infarction after embolization or from sickle cell anemia.

Clinically the patient presents with fever, pain, pleuritis, nausea, vomiting, and diarrhea. Elevated liver function tests, leukocytosis, and anemia are present. The abscess formation is multiple in 50% to 67% of patients. The most frequent organisms are *Escherichia coli* and anaerobes.

Sonographic Findings. The ultrasound appearance of a pyogenic abscess may be variable, depending on the internal consistency of the mass. The size varies from 1 cm to very large. The right central lobe of the liver is the most common site for abscess development. The abscess may be hypoechoic with round or ovoid margins and acoustic enhancement, or it may be complex, with some debris along the posterior margin and irregular walls (Figure 9-52, *A*). It may have a fluid level; if gas is present, it can be hyperechoic with dirty shadowing.

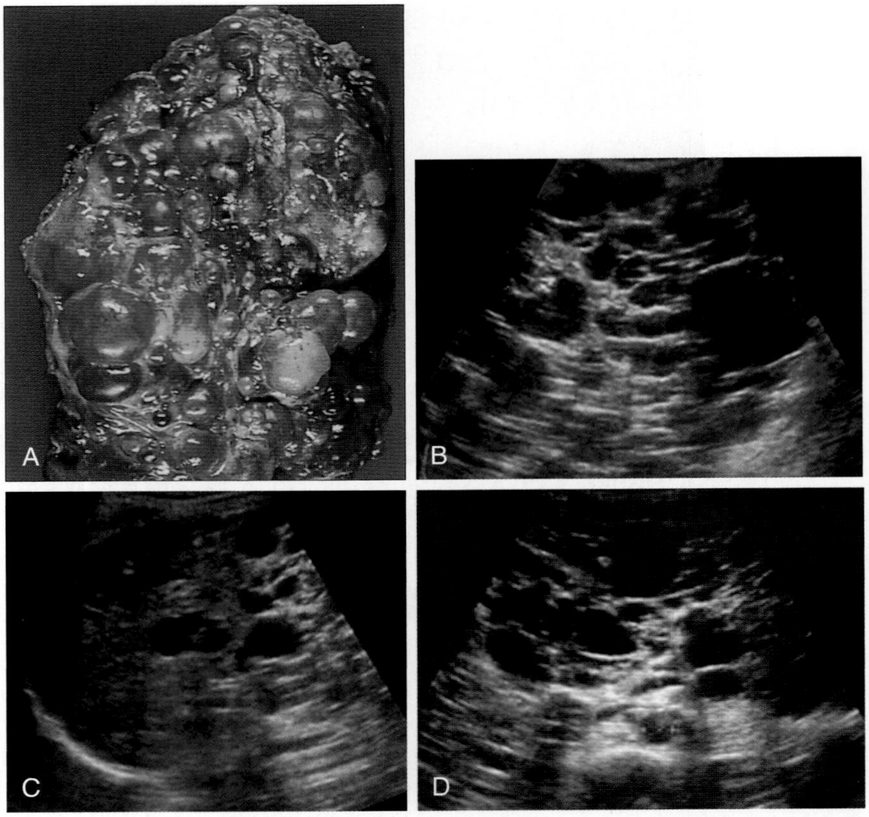

FIGURE 9-51 A, Gross pathology of polycystic liver disease. There are numerous large cysts throughout the liver parenchyma. **B–D,** Images of a liver parenchyma filled with multiple cystic lesions in patients with hepatic polycystic disease.

Hepatic Candidiasis. Hepatic candidiasis is caused by a species of *Candida*. It usually occurs in immunocompromised hosts, such as patients undergoing chemotherapy, organ transplant recipients, or individuals with human immunodeficiency virus (HIV) infection. The candidal fungus invades the bloodstream and may affect any organ, with the more perfused kidneys, brain, and heart affected the most. Clinically the patient may present with nonspecific findings, such as persistent fever in a neutropenic patient whose leukocyte count is returning to normal. Localized pain may also be present.

◗ *Sonographic Findings.* Candidiasis within the liver may present as multiple small hypoechoic masses with echogenic central cores, referred to as **bull's-eye (target) lesions** (Figure 9-52, *B*). The hyperechoic center (containing inflammatory cells) with a hypoechoic rim is present when the neutrophil counts return to normal. Other sonographic patterns have been described as "wheel-within-wheel" patterns, or multiple small hypoechoic lesions. A peripheral hypoechoic zone with an inner echogenic wheel and central hypoechoic focal necrosis may be found. The most common finding is uniformly hypoechoic. As scar formation develops, the pattern becomes echogenic. Specific diagnosis can only be made with fine-needle aspiration.

Chronic Granulomatous Disease. Chronic granulomatous disease is a genetic disorder in which phagocytes are unable to kill certain bacteria and fungi. It occurs mostly in children, with a more frequent occurrence in boys because it is a recessive trait. A pediatric patient may have recurrent respiratory infections.

◗ *Sonographic Findings.* A poorly marginated, hypoechoic mass is seen with posterior enhancement. Calcification may be present with posterior shadowing. Aspiration is necessary to specifically classify the mass as granulomatous disease.

Amebic Abscess. Amebic abscess is a collection of pus formed by disintegrated tissue in a cavity, usually in the liver, caused by the protozoan parasite *Entamoeba histolytica*. The infection is primarily a disease of the colon, but it can also spread to the liver, lungs, and brain. The parasites reach the liver parenchyma via the portal vein. Amebiasis is contracted by ingesting the cysts in contaminated water and food. The ameba usually affects the colon and cecum, and the organism remains within the gastrointestinal tract. If the organism invades the colonic mucosa, it may travel to the liver via the portal venous system. Patients may be asymptomatic or may show the gastrointestinal symptoms of abdominal pain, diarrhea, leukocytosis, and low fever.

◗ *Sonographic Findings.* The sonographic appearance of amebic abscess is variable and nonspecific. The abscess may be round or oval and lack notable defined wall echoes. The lesion is hypoechoic compared with normal liver parenchyma, with low-level echoes at higher sensitivity. There may be some internal echoes along the posterior margin secondary to debris (Figure 9-52, *C* and *D*). Distal enhancement may be seen beyond the mass lesion. Some organisms may rupture through the diaphragm into the hepatic capsule.

Echinococcal Cyst. Hepatic echinococcosis is an infectious cystic disease common in sheep-herding areas of the world, but seldom encountered within the United States. The echinococcus is a tapeworm that infects humans as the intermediate host. The worm resides in the small intestine of dogs. The ova from the adult worm are shed through canine feces into the environment,

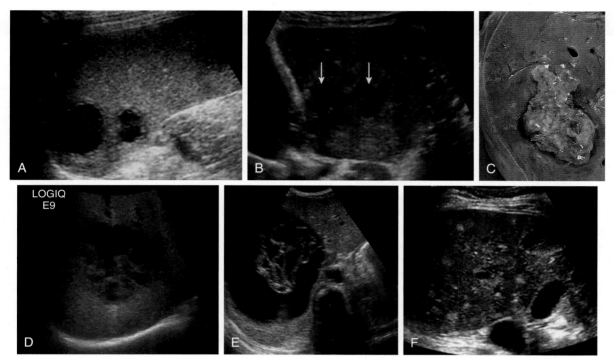

FIGURE 9-52 A and **B,** Pyogenic abscess is shown as a complex mass in the right lobe of the liver in a patient with cirrhosis, abdominal pain, and fever. The complex mass has round margins without increased through-transmission. **C,** Gross pathology of an amebic abscess. The intracavitary lesion is filled with yellow necrotic material and does not contain pus. **D,** Amebic abscess is a complex lesion, usually in the right lobe of the liver. This patient recently returned from a vacation in Mexico and presented with right upper quadrant pain and fever for 2 weeks. **E,** Echinococcal cyst. This complex mass found in the right lobe of the liver shows mixed fluid and debris components. **F,** *Pneumocystis carinii.* The sonographic pattern ranges from diffuse, tiny, nonshadowing echogenic foci to extensive replacement of the liver parenchyma by various echogenic clumps of calcification.

where the intermediate hosts ingest the eggs. After entering the proximal portion of the small intestine in humans, the larvae burrow through the mucosa, enter the portal circulation, and travel to the liver.

The echinococcal cyst has two layers: the inner layer and the outer, or inflammatory, reaction layer. The smaller, daughter cysts may develop from the inner layer. The cysts may enlarge and rupture. The cysts may also impinge on the blood vessels and lead to vascular thrombosis and infarction.

Sonographic Findings. Several patterns may occur, from a simple cyst to a complex mass with acoustic enhancement. The shape may be oval or spherical, with regularity of the walls. Calcifications may occur. Septations are frequent and include honeycomb appearance with fluid collections; "water lily" sign, which shows a detachment and collapse of the germinal layer; or "cyst within a cyst." Sometimes the liver contains multiple parent cysts in both lobes of the liver; the cyst with the thick walls occupies a different part of the liver (Figure 9-52, *E*). The tissue between the cysts indicates that each cyst is a separate parent cyst and not a daughter cyst. If a daughter cyst is found, it is specific for echinococcal disease.

Pneumocystis carinii. *Pneumocystis carinii* is the most common organism causing opportunistic infection in patients with acquired immunodeficiency syndrome (AIDS). Pneumocystis pneumonia is a common life-threatening infection in patients with HIV. *Pneumocystis carinii* affects patients undergoing

bone marrow and organ transplantation, or patients receiving chemotherapy.

Sonographic Findings. The pattern ranges from diffuse, tiny, nonshadowing echogenic foci to extensive replacement of the liver parenchyma by various echogenic clumps of calcification (Figure 9-52, *F*).

Hepatic Tumors

A **neoplasm** is any new growth of new tissue, either benign or malignant. A benign growth occurs locally but does not spread or invade surrounding structures. It may push surrounding structures aside or adhere to them. A malignant mass is uncontrolled and is prone to metastasize to nearby or distant structures via the bloodstream and lymph nodes. Thus it is important not only to recognize the tumor mass itself but also to appreciate which structures the malignancy may invade. See Table 9-12 for clinical findings, sonographic findings, and differential considerations for hepatic tumors.

Benign Hepatic Tumors

Cavernous Hemangioma. A cavernous hemangioma is the most common benign neoplasm of the liver. This spongelike tumor consisting of large, blood-filled cystic spaces is found more frequently in females. Patients are usually asymptomatic, although a small percentage may bleed, causing right upper quadrant pain. Hemangiomas enlarge

TABLE 9-12	Liver Findings: Tumors	
Clinical Findings	**Sonographic Findings**	**Differential Considerations**
Cavernous Hemangioma		
Small percentage may bleed; RUQ pain	Most are hyperechoic with enhancement	Metastasis
More frequent in women	Round or oval, well defined	Hepatoma (HCC)
	Larger masses may show necrosis, degeneration, calcification	Adenoma
		Focal nodular hyperplasia
Liver Cell Adenoma		
RUQ pain when mass bleeds	Hyperechoic with central echogenic area caused by hemorrhage	Hemangioma
		Focal nodular hyperplasia
	Solitary or multiple	Hepatoma (HCC)
	Fluid may be present	
Focal Nodular Hyperplasia		
More frequent in women younger than 40 years	Multiple, well defined with hyperechoic to isoechoic patterns	Hemangiomas
		Hepatoma (HCC)
	Frequently found in right lobe of liver	Metastases
		Adenoma
Hepatocellular Carcinoma		
70% of patients have ↑ alpha-fetoprotein level	Solitary, multiple	Hemangioma
	Infiltrative, diffuse	Metastases
Abnormalities in liver function tests, with the indications of cirrhosis	Hypoechoic, isoechoic, or hyperechoic	
	May invade hepatic veins	
	Thrombus	
Metastatic Disease		
Abnormal LFTs	Hypoechoic or echogenic mass	Abscess
Jaundice	Diffuse distortion of bull's-eye pattern	Hemangioma
Hepatomegaly	Solitary or multiple	Hepatoma (HCC)
Weight loss	Well to ill defined	Adenoma
Decreased appetite		
Lymphoma		
Abnormal LFT	Hypoechoic or diffuse patterns	Hemangioma
	Target or echogenic lesions	HCC
	Intrahepatic and lucent multiple small, discrete solid lesions without enhancement	Metastases

HCC, Hepatocellular carcinoma; *LFT,* liver function test; *RUQ,* right upper quadrant.

slowly and undergo degeneration, fibrosis, and calcification. They are found in the subcapsular hepatic parenchyma or in the posterior right lobe more than the left lobe of the liver.

Sonographic Findings. The appearance is typically a homogeneous, hyperechoic mass that is usually less than 3 cm in size with acoustic enhancement (Figure 9-53, *A* and *B*). Within the tumor are found multiple, small, blood-filled spaces separated by fibrous septations and lined with endothelial cells. The lesions are round, oval, or slightly lobulated with sharp, well-defined borders. The larger hemangiomas are more likely to appear with an atypical pattern as a result of fibrosis, thrombosis, and necrosis. Hemangiomas may become more heterogeneous as they undergo degeneration and fibrous replacement. Calcifications may occur, but are unusual. The atypical hemangioma may have a hyperechoic periphery with a hypoechoic central core producing a "reverse" target echo pattern. There is low-velocity blood flow that is too low to be detected by color Doppler. This diminished blood flow pattern may help to distinguish the hemangioma

from a malignant mass. Intravenous contrast has demonstrated peripheral puddling in the mass. Hemangiomas are generally stable over time; however, some will show regression and others may show a decrease in echogenicity. Rarely will the mass enlarge. The differential considerations for hemangioma should include metastases, hepatoma, focal fatty infiltration, and adenoma.

Focal Nodular Hyperplasia. Focal nodular hyperplasia (FNH) is the second most common benign liver mass after hemangioma. FNH is a benign tumor of the liver composed of Kupffer cells, hepatocytes, and biliary structures, but lacks the typical normal lobular hepatic features of portal triads and central veins. The mass is thought to arise from developmental hyperplastic lesions related to an area of congenital vascular formation. Hormonal influence may be present as FNH is found more commonly in women under 40 than in men. The mass is usually found as an incidental finding as the patient is asymptomatic. There is typically one well-circumscribed lesion, but there may be more than one

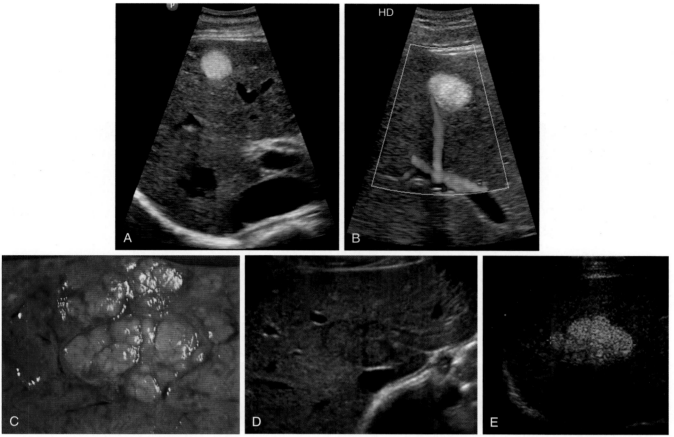

FIGURE 9-53 **A** and **B,** Cavernous hemangioma. The appearance is typically a homogeneous, hyperechoic mass that is usually less than 3 cm in size. **C,** Gross pathology of focal nodular hyperplasia with a lobular mass with a central fibrotic scar. **D,** Focal nodular hyperplasia is a subtle liver mass that may be difficult to differentiate in echogenicity from the liver parenchyma. The mass is usually isoechoic or nearly isoechoic compared with the liver parenchyma. **E,** Hepatic adenoma. This lesion is usually hyperechoic with a central hypoechoic area caused by hemorrhage.

mass; many are located along the subcapsular area of the liver, some are pedunculated, and many have a central scar from the bile ducts and prominent thick-walled arterial vessels. Bands of fibrous tissue separate the multiple nodules. The size of the mass is usually less than 5 cm in diameter. The mass may displace the normal blood vessels within the liver parenchyma.

Sonographic Findings. Focal nodular hyperplasia is a subtle liver mass that may be difficult to differentiate in echogenicity from the liver parenchyma. The mass is usually isoechoic or nearly isoechoic compared with the liver parenchyma. The sonographer may note subtle contour abnormalities and displacement of the vascular structures secondary to the mass. The central scar may be identified as a hypoechoic linear or stellate area within the center of the mass (Figure 9-53, *C* and *D*). The internal linear echoes may be seen within the lesions if multiple nodules occur together. Color Doppler may show the well-developed peripheral and central blood vessels that feed into the focal nodular hyperplasia lesion, known as the "spoke-wheel" pattern. Contrast agents may help to define the hypervascular arterial phase and the presence of stellate vessels with the tortuous feeding artery.

The differential diagnosis of FNH includes fibrolamellar carcinoma, hepatic adenoma, hepatocellular carcinoma, hemangioma, and vascular metastases.

Hepatic Adenoma. An adenoma is a rare benign tumor that consists of normal or slightly atypical hepatocytes, frequently containing areas of bile stasis and focal hemorrhage or necrosis. Tumor capsules are absent or incomplete. The lesion is found more commonly in women and has been related to oral contraceptive use. The adenoma has also been found in men taking anabolic steroids. The presence of multiple adenomas is increased in patients with type I glycogen storage disease or von Gierke's disease. Patients may present with right upper quadrant pain secondary to rupture with bleeding into the tumor. Adenomas have a low but real risk of malignant degeneration.

Sonographic Findings. The mass may have varied and nonspecific findings. The echogenicity may be hyperechoic, hypoechoic, isoechoic, or mixed. With hemorrhage, a fluid component may be seen within or around the lesion. This lesion is usually hyperechoic with a central hypoechoic area caused by hemorrhage (Figure 9-53, *E*). The lesion may be solitary and well encapsulated or multiple. If the lesion ruptures, fluid should be found in the peritoneal cavity. A hepatic adenoma may be difficult to distinguish sonographically from focal nodular hyperplasia.

Malignant Hepatic Neoplasms.   Primary malignant tumors are relatively rare in the liver. The most common tumor is hepatocellular carcinoma, sometimes referred to as hepatoma.

Tumors may also result from prolonged exposure to carcinogenic chemicals. Sonography has the advantage over other imaging modalities in defining liver texture in many different planes. This technique is especially useful in the diagnosis of malignant hepatic disease. A comparison of the different liver textures and patterns is shown in Figure 9-54.

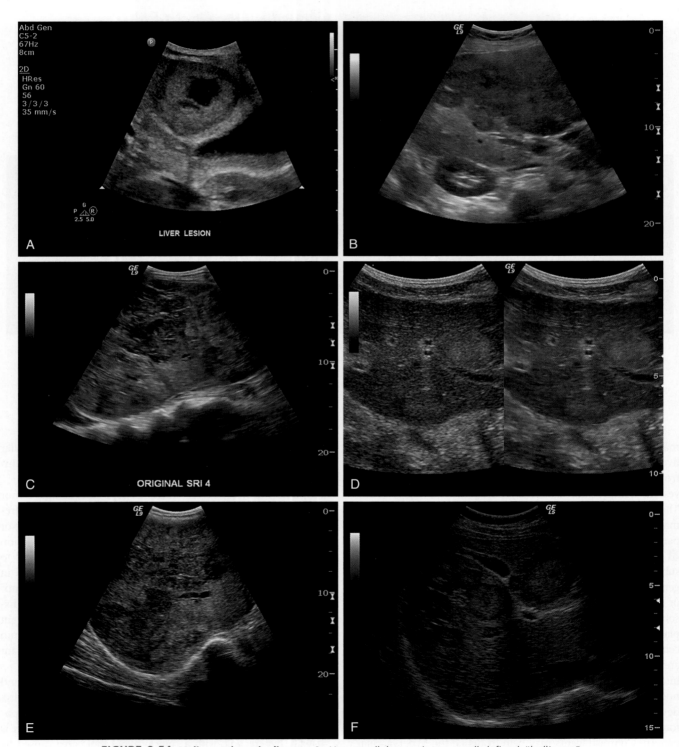

FIGURE 9-54   Malignant hepatic disease. A, Hepatocellular carcinoma: well-defined "bull's-eye" lesion. **B,** Hepatocellular carcinoma: well-defined isoechoic lesion. **C,** Necrotic hepatoma: necrotic isoechoic lesion. **D,** Advanced metastases: large isoechoic lesions. **E,** Metastases: ill-defined complex necrotic lesion. **F,** Metastases: well-defined hyperechoic lesion.

The clinical signs of liver cancer are similar to those of other hepatocellular diseases. These symptoms include nausea and vomiting, fatigue, weight loss, and hepatomegaly. Portal hypertension and splenomegaly are common.

Hepatocellular Carcinoma. As noted, hepatocellular carcinoma (HCC) is the most common primary malignant neoplasm. Although HCC can occur in patients with normal livers, it is strongly associated with chronic liver disease. The prevalence varies, depending on predisposing factors such as hepatitis B and C infection and cirrhosis. There is a high incidence of hepatocellular carcinoma in Africa, Japan, Greece, Italy, and Southeast Asia secondary to the prevalence of hepatitis and aflatoxin ingestion. In non-Asian populations, cirrhosis is the most important condition predisposing to HCC; other predisposing conditions include hemochromatosis, Wilson's disease, and type I glycogen storage disease.

The pathogenesis of hepatocellular carcinoma is related to cirrhosis (80% of patients with preexisting cirrhosis develop hepatocellular carcinoma), chronic hepatitis B virus infection, and hepatocarcinogens in foods. The tumor occurs more frequently in men. Clinically, patients with HCC usually present with a previous history of cirrhosis or hepatitis B and C, a palpable mass, hepatomegaly, appetite disorder, and fever.

The HCC may present in one of three patterns: solitary massive tumor, multiple nodules throughout the liver, or diffuse infiltrative masses in the liver. Pathologically the tumor may present as a focal lesion, an invasive lesion with necrosis and hemorrhage, or a poorly defined lesion (Figure 9-55). The carcinoma can be very invasive and has been known to invade the hepatic veins to produce Budd-Chiari syndrome. The portal venous system may also be invaded with tumor or thrombosis. Hepatocellular carcinoma has a tendency to destroy the portal venous radicle walls, with invasion into the lumen of the vessel.

Sonographic Findings. A variable sonographic appearance is noted with discrete lesions, either solitary or multiple, that are usually hypoechoic or hyperechoic. Sometimes the lesions may be isoechoic, and a thin, peripheral hypoechoic halo may surround the lesion (Figure 9-56). Another pattern presents as diffuse parenchymal involvement with inhomogeneity throughout the liver without distinct masses. Over time the mass becomes more complex and inhomogeneous with resulting fibrosis and necrosis. The last pattern is a combination of discrete and diffuse echoes. Hepatocellular carcinoma cannot be differentiated from metastases on ultrasound.

Internal echoes within the portal veins, hepatic veins, or inferior vena cava indicate tumor invasion or thrombosis within the vessel. The evaluation of the vascular structures with color Doppler helps to rule out the presence of clot or tumor invasion. Hepatic flow is abnormal if an obstruction is present. Obstruction of the portal vein may be present with thrombosis and well demonstrated with color Doppler.

Metastatic Disease. The most common form of neoplastic involvement of the liver is **metastatic disease** (Figure 9-57). The lungs and the liver are the most frequent sites of distant metastatic disease. The primary sites are the colon, breast, and lung with the majority of metastases arising from a primary colonic malignancy or a hepatoma. The incidence of hepatic metastases depends on the type of tumor and its stage at initial detection. Patients with short survival rates after initial detection of liver metastases are those with HCC and carcinoma of the pancreas, stomach, and esophagus. Patients with a more prolonged survival are those with head and neck carcinoma and carcinoma of the colon. Metastatic spread to the liver occurs as the tumor erodes the wall and travels through the lymphatic system or through the bloodstream to the portal vein or hepatic artery to the liver.

Sonographic Findings. The sonographic patterns of metastatic tumor involvement in the liver vary. It is typical to have multiple nodes throughout both lobes of the liver. The following three specific patterns have been described: (1) a well-defined hypoechoic mass, (2) a well-defined echogenic mass, and (3) diffuse distortion of the normal homogeneous parenchymal pattern without a focal mass (Figure 9-58). The hypovascular lesions produce hypoechoic patterns in the liver because of necrosis and ischemic areas from neoplastic thrombosis. Most cases of hypervascular lesions correspond to hyperechoic patterns.

The common primary masses include renal cell carcinoma, carcinoid, choriocarcinoma, transitional cell carcinoma, islet cell carcinoma, and hepatocellular carcinoma. The echogenic lesions are common with primary colonic tumors and may

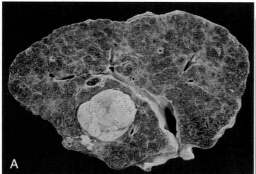
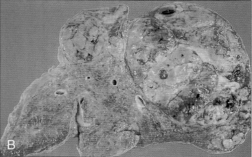

FIGURE 9-55 Gross pathology of hepatocellular carcinoma. A, The cirrhotic liver contains a solitary malignant nodule. **B,** The huge tumor is poorly demarcated from the remaining liver.

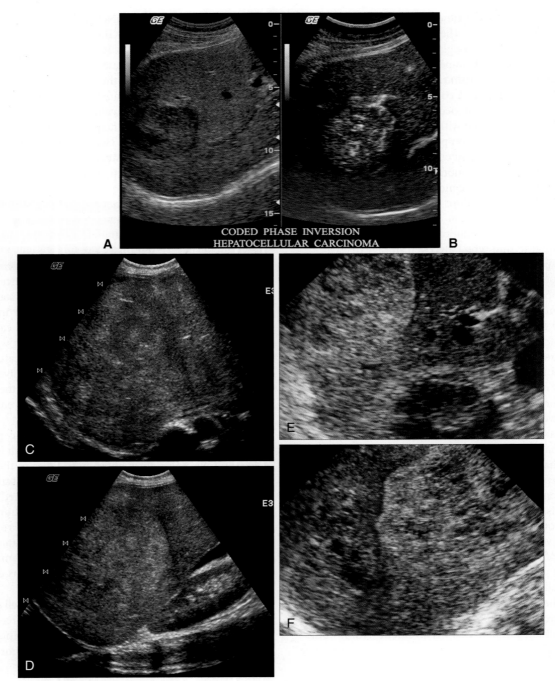

FIGURE 9-56 **A** and **B,** Hepatocellular carcinoma shows a discrete hypoechoic lesion in the right lobe of the liver. **C** and **D,** Transverse and sagittal images of the upper right quadrant show a large hepatocellular carcinoma in the right lobe of the liver. **E** and **F,** Hepatocellular carcinoma in a 58-year-old male shows hepatomegaly with diffuse abnormal lesions throughout the liver parenchyma.

present with calcification. Target types of metastases or bull's-eye patterns are the result of edema around the tumor or necrosis or hemorrhage within the tumor. Thus on sonography, the target lesion has an appearance with an echogenic or isoechoic center with a hypoechoic halo. The appearance may vary; when the halo is thin, it may represent dilated peritumoral sinusoids or compressed liver parenchyma. The proliferating tumor demonstrates a thick halo surround the

echogenic center. As the nodules increase rapidly in size and outgrow their blood supply, central necrosis and hemorrhage may result. Other conditions that may present with target lesions include HCC and lymphoma. Less common target lesions are seen in abscesses, adenomas, and FNH, and rarely hemangioma.

Hyperechoic metastases are found to occur more frequently with gastrointestinal lesions, most commonly from the colon,

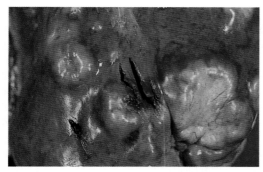

FIGURE 9-57 Metastatic carcinoma. The liver contains numerous spherical nodules, many of which show central indentation corresponding to the areas of necrosis.

and neuroendocrine tumors. Calcified metastases are most common from the colon; however, metastases from the ovary, breast, and stomach may also calcify. Cystic hepatic metastases are less frequent; these have a thick wall, thick septations, or obvious solid components.

Various combinations of these patterns can be seen simultaneously in a patient with metastatic liver disease. The first abnormality is hepatomegaly or alterations in contour, especially on the lateral segment of the left lobe. The lesions may be solitary or multiple, be variable in size and shape, and have sharp or ill-defined margins. Metastases may be extensive or localized to produce an inhomogeneous parenchymal pattern.

Ultrasound may be useful to follow patients after surgery. After a baseline hepatic ultrasound has been performed, the sonographer can assess any regression or progression of tumor and change in parenchymal pattern.

Lymphoma. Lymphomas are malignant neoplasms involving lymphocyte proliferation in the lymph nodes. The two main disorders, Hodgkin's lymphoma and non-Hodgkin's lymphoma, are differentiated by lymph node biopsy. No specific cause is known. Hepatic lymphoma usually presents in the setting of advanced disease elsewhere and is of the non-Hodgkin variety. Primary hepatic lymphoma occurs most often in the setting of an immunocompromised state such as AIDS or posttransplantation. Patients with lymphoma have hepatomegaly with a normal or diffuse alteration of parenchymal echoes. A focal hypoechoic mass is sometimes seen. The patient may present with enlarged, nontender lymph nodes, fever, fatigue, night sweats, weight loss, bone pain, or an abdominal mass. The presence of splenomegaly or retroperitoneal nodes may help confirm the diagnosis of lymphadenopathy.

Sonographic Findings. Hodgkin's lymphoma shows up as diffuse parenchymal changes in the liver. Non-Hodgkin's lymphoma may appear with target hypoechoic mass lesions. Burkitt's lymphoma lesions may appear intrahepatic and lucent. Patients with leukemia have multiple small, discrete hepatic masses that are solid with no acoustic enhancement (Figure 9-59). A bull's-eye appearance with a dense central core may be present as a result of tumor necrosis.

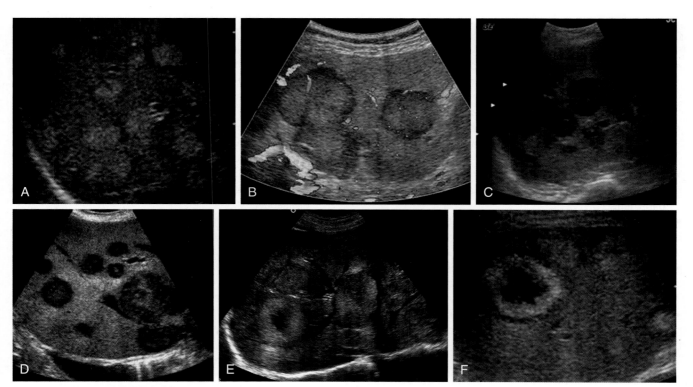

FIGURE 9-58 The sonographic patterns of metastatic tumor involvement in the liver vary. **A** and **B,** Well-defined hypoechoic mass. **C** and **D,** Well-defined echogenic mass. **E** and **F,** Diffuse distortion of the normal homogeneous parenchymal pattern without a focal mass.

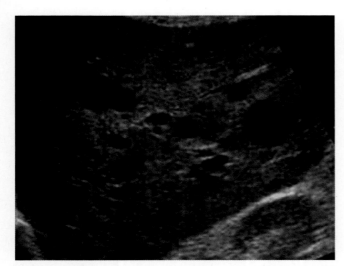

FIGURE 9-59 Lymphoma was found in this elderly male with hepatomegaly. Multiple isoechoic lesions were found throughout the liver.

In the pediatric population, the most common malignancies are neuroblastomas, Wilms' tumor, and leukemia. The neuroblastoma presents as a densely reflective echo pattern with liver involvement similar to that of a hepatoma. In patients with a Wilms' tumor, metastases generally invade the lung; however, the liver may be a secondary site. These lesions present as a densely reflective pattern with lucencies resulting from necrosis.

 Key Pearls

- The liver is the largest organ in the abdominal cavity, measuring approximately 21 to 22.5 cm in its greatest transverse diameter, 13 to 17.5 cm in its greatest vertical height, and 10 to 12.5 cm in its anteroposterior depth.
- The liver occupies almost all of the right hypochondrium, the greater part of the epigastrium, and the left hypochondrium as far as the mammillary line.
- Most of the liver is covered by peritoneum, but a large area rests directly on the diaphragm; this is called the bare area.
- The subphrenic space between the liver (or spleen) and the diaphragm is a common site for abscess formation.
- The right posterior subphrenic space lies between the right lobe of the liver, the right kidney, and the right colic flexure.
- The right subhepatic space is located inferior to the right lobe of the liver and includes Morison's pouch, which lies between the posterior aspect of the right lobe and the upper pole of the right kidney.
- Tumor infiltration, cirrhosis, or a subphrenic abscess often causes inferior displacement, whereas ascites, excessive dilation of the colon, or abdominal tumors can elevate

the liver; retroperitoneal tumors may move the liver slightly anterior.
- The liver has been divided into four anatomic lobes: the left, right, quadrate, and caudate, with the falciform ligament separating the left from the right lobe; however, functional divisions have more value from a surgical perspective (Couinaud's system of hepatic nomenclature).
- The right hypochrondrium contains the right lobe, which is six times larger than the left lobe.
- The middle hepatic vein and the ascending section of the left portal vein divide the liver functionally into a left lobe and a right lobe.
- The quadrate lobe is functionally part of the medial segment of the left lobe, which lies between the middle hepatic vein and the left hepatic vein.
- Using these functional divisions, the falciform ligament now belongs to the left lobe; it runs vertically along the medial left lobe close to the border with the lateral left lobe.
- The left intersegmental fissure divides the left lobe into medial and lateral segments; the left hepatic vein runs horizontally between the medial and lateral segments.
- There are two fissures in the left lobe: the fissure for the ligamentum teres and the ligamentum venosum.
- The caudate lobe is a small lobe situated on the posterior surface of the left lobe, with the inferior vena cava as its posterior border and the fissure for the ligamentum venosum its anterior border.
- Note the hepatic veins course between the lobes and interlobar/intersegmental segments.
- The major branches of the portal veins run centrally within the segments (intrasegmental) with the exception of the ascending portion of the left portal vein, which runs in the left intersegmental fissure.
- The Couinaud system divides the left lateral, right anterior, and right posterior segments into superior and inferior subsegments and maintains the caudate lobe and the medial left segment as single segments.
- The liver is covered by a thin connective tissue layer called Glisson's capsule.
- The main lobar fissure is seen on sonography as a hyperechoic line extending from the portal vein to the neck of the gallbladder.
- The falciform ligament extends from the umbilicus to the diaphragm in a parasagittal plane and contains the ligamentum teres.
- The fissure for the ligamentum venosum separates the left lobe from the caudate lobe.
- The portal vein conveys about 70% to 80% of the blood to the liver, and the remaining 20% to 30% is oxygenated blood conveyed to the liver via the hepatic artery.
- The venous blood supply from the greater part of the gastrointestinal tract and its accessory organs drains into the liver through the portal venous system.
- The portal triad consists of the portal vein, hepatic artery, and bile duct.

- The blood is perfused within the liver parenchyma through the hepatic sinusoids before it enters the terminal hepatic venules, which unite to form the larger hepatic veins.
- The best way to distinguish the hepatic from the portal vessels is to trace their points of entry to the liver.
- The liver has many functions, including metabolism, digestion, storage, and detoxification.
- Through the process of digestion, the liver expels these waste products from the body via its excretory product, bile, which also plays an important role in fat absorption.
- Diseases affecting the liver may be classified as *hepatocellular*, when the liver cells or hepatocytes are the immediate problem, or *obstructive*, when bile excretion is blocked.
- The liver is a major location for detoxification of waste products of energy production and other metabolic activities occurring throughout the body.
- Along with detoxification, the liver also excretes bilirubin into the gut via the biliary tree.
- Elevation of serum bilirubin results in jaundice, which is a yellow coloration of the skin, sclerae, and body secretions.
- Bile is the excretory product of the liver and is formed continuously by the hepatocytes, collects in the bile canaliculi adjacent to these cells, and is transported to the gut via the bile ducts.
- Liver function tests are a group of laboratory tests established to analyze how the liver is performing under normal and diseased conditions.
- Evaluation of the liver parenchyma includes the assessment of its size, configuration, homogeneity, and contour.
- Hepatocellular disease affects the hepatocytes and interferes with liver function enzymes.
- The hepatocyte is a parenchymal liver cell that performs all the functions ascribed to the liver.
- There are many subcategories of diffuse parenchymal disease, including fatty infiltration, acute and chronic hepatitis, early alcoholic liver disease, and acute and chronic cirrhosis.
- Fatty infiltration of the liver is an acquired, reversible disorder of metabolism, resulting in an intracellular accumulation of triglycerides within hepatocytes.
- Fatty infiltration most commonly appears in a diffuse or patchy distribution and results in uniform increased echogenicity of the liver.
- Fatty infiltration is not always uniform throughout the liver parenchyma; in fact, regions of increased echogenicity are present within a normal liver parenchyma.
- Focal sparing should be suspected in patients who have "masslike" hypoechoic areas in typical locations in a liver that is otherwise increased in echogenicity.
- Hepatitis is the general name for inflammatory and infectious disease of the liver.
- Complications of hepatitis involving damage to the liver may range from mild disease to massive necrosis and liver failure.
- On ultrasound, the patient with acute hepatitis may demonstrate a normal liver texture or the portal vein borders may be more echogenic than usual (known as the "starry sky" sign), the liver parenchyma is slightly more echogenic than normal, and attenuation may be present.
- With chronic hepatitis, the liver parenchyma is coarse with decreased brightness of the portal triads, but the degree of attenuation is not as great as is seen in fatty infiltration.
- Cirrhosis is a chronic degenerative disease of the liver in which the hepatic lobes are covered with fibrous tissue, the parenchyma degenerates, and the lobules are infiltrated with fat.
- The process of cirrhosis is chronic and progressive, with liver cell failure and portal hypertension as the end stage.
- With sonography, cirrhosis may appear as hepatomegaly, increased echogenicity, and coarsening of the hepatic parenchyma secondary to fibrosis and surface nodularity.
- Chronic cirrhosis may show surface nodularity of the liver edge, especially well demonstrated if ascites is present.
- Doppler evaluation of the hepatic veins is useful to detect the presence of altered flow dynamics.
- Glycogen storage disease is an inherited disease characterized by the abnormal storage and accumulation of glycogen in the tissues, especially the liver and kidneys.
- The most common glycogen storage disease is type I, or von Gierke's disease. On sonography, patients with glycogen storage disease present with hepatomegaly, increased echogenicity, and slightly increased attenuation.
- Hemochromatosis is a rare disease of iron metabolism characterized by excess iron deposits throughout the body. Some increased echogenicity may be seen uniformly throughout the hepatic parenchyma.
- Portal hypertension is caused by increased resistance to venous flow through the liver. It is associated with cirrhosis, hepatic vein thrombosis, portal vein thrombosis, and thrombosis of the inferior vena cava.
- Portal hypertension is divided into presinusoidal and intrahepatic groups, depending on whether the hepatic vein wedged pressure is normal (presinusoidal) or elevated (intrahepatic).
- The development of increased pressure in the portal-splenic venous system is the cause of extrahepatic portal hypertension. Acute or chronic hepatocellular disease can block the flow of blood throughout the liver, causing it to back up into the hepatic portal circulation.
- Intrahepatic portal hypertension is the result of diseases that affect the portal zones of the liver such as primary biliary cirrhosis, schistosomiasis, congenital hepatic fibrosis, or toxic drugs. Cirrhosis is the most common cause of intrahepatic portal hypertension.
- Portal hypertension may also develop when hepatopetal flow (toward the liver) is impeded by thrombus or tumor invasion.
- Collateral circulation develops when the normal venous channels become obstructed.
- If portal hypertension becomes extensive, the portal system can be decompressed by shunting blood to the systemic venous system.
- Portacaval shunts for the treatment of portal hypertension may involve the anastomosis of the portal vein, because it lies within the lesser omentum, to the anterior wall of

Continued

- the inferior vena cava behind the entrance into the lesser sac.
- The mesocaval shunt attaches the middistal superior mesenteric vein to the inferior vena cava.
- The splenorenal shunt attaches the splenic vein to the left renal vein.
- Intrahepatic shunts are created percutaneously with the use of metallic expandable stents, which can be seen on ultrasound. This type of shunt is the transjugular intrahepatic portosystemic shunt (TIPS).
- Budd-Chiari syndrome is an uncommon condition caused by thrombosis of the hepatic veins or inferior vena cava.
- Biliary obstruction proximal to the cystic duct can be caused by gallstones, carcinoma of the common bile duct, or metastatic tumor invasion of the porta hepatis.
- A biliary obstruction distal to the cystic duct may be caused by stones in the common duct, an extrahepatic mass in the porta hepatis, or stricture of the common duct.
- An extrahepatic mass in the area of the porta hepatis causes the same clinical signs as seen in biliary obstruction.
- Passive hepatic congestion develops secondary to congestive heart failure with signs of hepatomegaly and dilation of the inferior vena cava and superior mesenteric, hepatic, portal, and splenic veins.
- The differential diagnosis for focal diseases of the liver includes cysts, abscess, hematoma, primary tumor, and metastases.
- Intrahepatic masses may cause the following findings on ultrasound: displacement of the hepatic vascular radicles, external bulging of the liver capsule, or a posterior shift of the inferior vena cava.
- An extrahepatic mass may show internal invagination or discontinuity of the liver capsule, formation of a triangular fat wedge, anteromedial shift of the inferior vena cava, or anterior displacement of the right kidney.
- *Hepatic cyst* usually refers to a solitary nonparasitic cyst of the liver. The cyst may be congenital or acquired, solitary or multiple.
- Patients with polycystic liver disease may also have polycystic renal disease.
- Hepatic abscesses occur most often as complications of biliary tract disease, surgery, or trauma.
- The following three basic types of abscess formation occur in the liver: intrahepatic, subhepatic, and subphrenic.
- A pyogenic abscess is a pus-forming abscess. There are many routes for bacteria to gain access to the liver: through the biliary tree, the portal vein, or the hepatic artery; through a direct extension from a contiguous infection; or, rarely, through hepatic trauma.
- Hepatic candidiasis is caused by a species of *Candida*. It usually occurs in immunocompromised hosts, such as patients undergoing chemotherapy, organ transplant recipients, or individuals with HIV infection.
- Amebic abscess is a collection of pus formed by disintegrated tissue in a cavity, usually in the liver, caused by the protozoan parasite *Entamoeba histolytica*.

- Hepatic echinococcosis is an infectious cystic disease common in sheep herding areas of the world, but seldom encountered within the United States.
- The echinococcal cyst has two layers: the inner layer and the outer, or inflammatory, reaction layer. The smaller, daughter cysts may develop from the inner layer. The cysts may enlarge and rupture.
- A neoplasm is any new growth of new tissue, either benign or malignant.
- A benign growth occurs locally but does not spread or invade surrounding structures. It may push surrounding structures aside or adhere to them.
- A malignant mass is uncontrolled and is prone to metastasize to nearby or distant structures via the bloodstream and lymph nodes.
- Cavernous hemangioma is typically a homogeneous, hyperechoic mass that is usually less than 3 cm in size with acoustic enhancement.
- Focal nodular hyperplasia is a subtle liver mass that may be difficult to differentiate in echogenicity from the liver parenchyma (isoechoic or nearly isoechoic compared with the liver parenchyma).
- An adenoma is a rare benign tumor that consists of normal or slightly atypical hepatocytes, frequently containing areas of bile stasis and focal hemorrhage or necrosis.
- Hepatocellular carcinoma (HCC) is the most common primary malignant neoplasm.
- HCC may present in one of three patterns: solitary massive tumor, multiple nodules throughout the liver, or diffuse infiltrative masses in the liver.
- The most common form of neoplastic involvement of the liver is metastatic disease.
- The primary sites are the colon, breast, and lung with the majority of metastases arising from a primary colonic malignancy or a hepatoma.
- On sonography, the following three specific patterns are seen in metastatic disease: (1) a well-defined hypoechoic mass, (2) a well-defined echogenic mass, and (3) diffuse distortion of the normal homogeneous parenchymal pattern without a focal mass.
- Hodgkin's lymphoma shows up as diffuse parenchymal changes in the liver.
- Non-Hodgkin's lymphoma may appear with target hypoechoic mass lesions.
- Burkitt's lymphoma lesions may appear intrahepatic and lucent.
- Patients with leukemia have multiple small, discrete hepatic masses that are solid with no acoustic enhancement.

BIBLIOGRAPHY

Abdalla EK, Vauthey JN, Couinaud C: The caudate lobe of the liver: implications of embryology and anatomy for surgery, *Surg Oncol Clin North Am* 11:835-848, 2002.

Andrew A: Portal hypertension: a review, *J Diagn Med Sonography* 17:193-200, 2001.

Bernatik T, Strobel D, Hahn EG, Becker D: Detection of liver metastases: comparison of contrast-enhanced wide-beam harmonic imaging with conventional ultrasonography, *J Ultrasound Med* 20:509-515, 2001.

Bertolotto M, Catalano O: Contrast-enhanced ultrasound: past, present, and future, *Ultrasound Clin* 4:339-367, 2009.

Carr CE, Tuite CM, Soulen MC, et al: Role of ultrasound surveillance of tansjugular intrahepatic portosystemic shunts in the covered stent era, *J Vasc Interv Radiol* 17:1297-1305, 2006.

Castroagudin JF, Molina E, Abdulkader I, et al: Sonographic features of liver involvement by lymphoma, *J Ultrasound Med* 26:791-796, 2007.

Cecchetto BL, et al: Space-occupying lesions of the liver detected by ultrasonography and their relation to hepatocellular carcinoma in cirrhosis, *Liver* 12:80, 1992.

Chiou SY, Forsberg F, Fox TB, Needleman L: Comparing differential tissue harmonic imaging with tissue harmonic and fundamental gray scale imaging of the liver, *J Ultrasound Med* 26:1557-1563, 2007.

Cutcher R, Smith GS, Sen F, et al: Comparison of sonograms and liver histologic findings in patients with chronic hepatitis C virus infection, *J Ultrasound Med* 17:321-325, 1998.

Feigin RD, Glickson M, Varstending A: Familial Budd-Chiari syndrome due to membranous obstruction of the hepatic vein treated with transluminal angioplasty, *Am J Gastroenterol* 85(1):94, 1990.

Fratzer W, Fritz V, Mason RA, et al: Factors affecting liver size, *J Ultrasound Med* 22:1155-1161, 2003.

Furuse J, Matsutani S, Yoshikawa M: Diagnosis of portal vein tumor thrombus by pulsed Doppler ultrasonography, *J Clin Ultrasound* 20:439, 1992.

Gabow PA, Johnson A, Kaehny W: Risk factors for the development of hepatic cysts in autosomal dominant polycystic kidney disease, *Hepatology* 11:1033, 1990.

Gandolfi L, Leo P, Solmi L: Natural history of hepatic haemangiomas: clinical and ultrasound study, *Gut* 32:677, 1991.

Garrant P, Meire HB: Hepatic vein pulsatility assessment on spectral Doppler ultrasound, *Br J Radiol* 70:829, 1997.

Giorgio A, Francica G, de Stefano G: Sonographic recognition of intraparenchymal regenerating nodules using high frequency transducers in patients with cirrhosis, *J Ultrasound Med* 10:355, 1991.

Goyal AK, Pokharna DS, Sharma SK: Ultrasonic measurements of portal vasculature in diagnosis of portal hypertension, *J Ultrasound Med* 9:45, 1990.

Grant EG, Melany M: Doppler imaging of the liver, *J Vasc Technol* 19:277, 1995.

Hisham T, Ralls PW, Radin R, Grant E: Sonography of diffuse liver disease. *J Ultrasound Med* 21:1023-1032, 2002.

Inturri P, Rossaro L: Pathophysiology of portal hypertension, *J Vasc Technol* 19:271, 1995.

Ishak KG, Zimmerman HJ, Ray MB: Alcoholic liver disease: pathologic, pathogenetic and clinical aspects, *Alcohol Clin Exp Res* 15:45, 1991.

Kim CK, Lim JH, Lee WJ: Detection of hepatocellular carcinomas and dysplastic nodules in cirrhotic liver, *J Ultrasound Med* 20:99-124, 2001.

Kudo M, Tomita S, Minowa K: Color Doppler flow imaging of hepatic focal nodular hyperplasia, *J Ultrasound Med* 11:553, 1992.

Leung JW, Yu AS: Hepatolithiasis and biliary parasites, *Bailliere's Clin Gastroenterol* 11:681, 1997.

Li D, Hann LE: A practical approach to analyzing focal lesions in the liver, *Ultrasound Quarterly* 21:187-200, 2005.

Lin ZY, Chang W, Wang L: Doppler sonography in the differential diagnosis of hepatocellular carcinoma and other common hepatic tumors, *Br J Radiol* 65:202, 1992.

Martinoli C, Cittadini G, Conzi R: Sonographic characterization of an accessory fissure of the left hepatic lobe determined by omental infolding, *J Ultrasound Med* 11:103, 1992.

Matsui O, Kadoya M, Kameyama T: Benign and malignant nodules in cirrhotic livers: distinction based on blood supply, *Radiology* 178:493, 1991.

Middleton WD, Kurtz AB, Hertzberg BS: *Ultrasound: the requisites*, ed 2, St Louis, 2004, Mosby.

Miller WJ, Federle MP, Campbell WL: Diagnosis and staging of hepatocellular carcinoma, *Am J Roentgenol* 157:303, 1991.

Nisenbaum HL, Rowling SE: Ultrasound of focal hepatic lesions, *Semin Roentgenol* 30:324, 1995.

Numata K, Tanaka K, Kiba T: Contrast-enhanced wide-band harmonic correlation with helical computed tomographic findings, *J Diagn Med Sonography* 20:89-97, 2001.

Ong JP, Sands M, Younossi ZM: Transjugular intrahepatic portosystem shunts (TIPSS) a decade later, *J Clin Gastroenterol* 30(1):14-28, 2000.

Pompili M: Ultrasound Doppler diagnosis of Budd-Chiari syndrome, *J Clin Gastroenterol* 12:591, 1990.

Robinson KA, Middleton WD, Al-Sukaiti R, et al: Doppler sonography of portal hypertension, *Ultrasound Quarterly* 25:3-13, 2009.

Rumack CM, Wilson SB, Charboneau JW, Johnson J: *Diagnostic ultrasound*, vol 1, ed 3, St Louis, 2005, Mosby.

Sabih DE, Sabih Z, Khan A: "Congealed waterlilly" sign: a new sonographic sign of hydatid cyst, *J Clin Ultrasound* 24:297-303, 1996.

Sautereau D, Berry P, Cessot F: Hepatocellular carcinoma, *J Hepatol* 14:413, 1992.

Seeto RK, Rockey DC: Pyogenic liver abscess: changes in etiology, management, and outcome, *Medicine* 75:99, 1996.

Shapiro RS: Cryotherapy of metastatic carcinoid tumors, *Abdom Imaging* 23:314, 1998.

Shibata T: Recurrent hepatocellular carcinoma, *J Clin Ultrasound* 19:8, 1991.

Shin DS, Jeffrey RB, Desser TS: Pearls and pitfalls in hepatic ultrasonography, *Ultrasound Quarterly* 26:17-25, 2010.

Smith D: Sonographic demonstration of Couinaud's liver segments, *J Ultrasound Med* 17:375, 1998.

Snell RT: *Clinical anatomy*, ed 7, Philadelphia, 2004, Lippincott Williams & Wilkins.

Sugiura N: Portosystemic collateral shunts originating from the left portal veins in portal hypertension: demonstration by color Doppler flow imaging, *J Clin Ultrasound* 20:427, 1992.

Taylor CR, et al: Doppler ultrasound in the evaluation of cirrhotic patients, *Ultrasound Med Biol* 23:1155, 1997.

Tchelepi H, Ralls PW, Radin R, Grant E: Sonography of diffuse liver disease, *J Ultrasound Med* 21:1023-1032, 2002.

Trigaux JP: Alcoholic liver disease: value of the left-to-right portal vein ratio in its sonographic diagnosis, *Gastrointest Radiol* 16:215, 1991.

Wachsberg RH: Echogenicity of hepatic versus portal vein walls revisited with histologic correlation, *J Ultrasound Med* 16:807, 1997.

Wernecke K: The distinction between benign and malignant liver tumors on sonography: value of a hypoechoic halo, *Am J Roentgenol* 159:1005, 1992.

Wilson SR, Jang HJ, Kim TK, Burns PN: Diagnosis of focal liver masses on ultrasonography, *J Ultrasound Med* 26:775-787, 2007.

Zhou Y, Sui C, Li B, et al: Repeat hepatectomy for recurrent hepatocellular carcinoma: a local experience and a systemic review, *World J Surg Oncol* 8:55, 2010.

Gallbladder and the Biliary System

Sandra L. Hagen-Ansert

OBJECTIVES

On completion of this chapter, you should be able to:
- Describe the internal, surface, and relational anatomies of the gallbladder
- Explain the function of the gallbladder
- Differentiate the sectional anatomy of the hepatobiliary system and adjacent structures
- Describe the normal sonographic pattern of the gallbladder, cystic duct, hepatic ducts, and common bile duct
- Differentiate the sonographic appearances of the gallbladder and biliary system pathologies discussed in this chapter

OUTLINE

KEY TERMS

Adenomyomatosis
Ampulla of Vater
Bilirubin
Cholangitis
Cholecystectomy
Cholecystitis
Cholecystokinin
Choledochal cysts
Choledocholithiasis
Cholelithiasis

Cholesterolosis
Common bile duct
Common hepatic duct
Cystic duct
Gallbladder
Hartmann's pouch
Heister's valve
Hydrops
Jaundice
Junctional fold

Klatskin's tumor
Murphy's sign
Pancreatic duct
Phrygian cap
Polyps of the gallbladder
Porcelain gallbladder
Porta hepatis
Sludge
Sphincter of Oddi
Wall, echo, shadow (WES) sign

Together with the liver and pancreas, the biliary system plays a role in the digestive process. The gallbladder serves as a reservoir for bile that is drained from the hepatic ducts within the liver. Sonographic evaluation of the gallbladder and biliary system is used as a primary diagnostic tool and has proven to be effective in diagnosing various types of gallbladder disease, including the more common problems of cholelithiasis, cholecystitis, and dilation of the ductal system.

ANATOMY OF THE BILIARY SYSTEM

Normal Anatomy

The biliary apparatus consists of the right and left hepatic ducts, the common hepatic duct, the common bile duct, the pear-shaped gallbladder, and the cystic duct (Figure 10-1). The bile ducts are divided into intrahepatic and extrahepatic segments. The intrahepatic ducts run in the portal triads

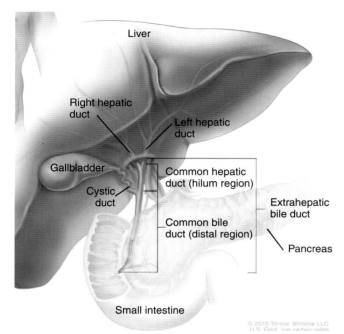

FIGURE 10-1 The biliary apparatus consists of the right and left hepatic ducts, the common hepatic duct, the common bile duct, the pear-shaped gallbladder, and the cystic duct. (© 2015 Terese Winslow LLC, U.S. Govt. has certain rights.)

along with the portal veins and hepatic arteries (Figure 10-2). The peripheral intrahepatic ducts run parallel and adjacent to the hepatic arteries and portal veins. The anterior and posterior relationship of the three structures is more variable than that of the extrahepatic ducts.

Hepatic Ducts. The extrahepatic portion of the bile ducts includes the common hepatic duct, common bile duct, and a portion of the central right and left ducts (see Figure 10-1). The right and left hepatic ducts emerge from the right lobe of the liver in the **porta hepatis** and unite to form the common

hepatic duct, which then passes caudally and medially. The hepatic duct runs parallel with the portal vein. Each duct is formed by the union of bile canaliculi from the liver lobules.

The common hepatic duct is approximately 4 mm in diameter and descends within the edge of the lesser omentum. The common hepatic duct is the segment above the cystic duct and the common bile duct is the segment below. The cystic duct may be difficult to image on sonography; therefore the sonographer may use the general term as the *proximal or distal* segments of the "common duct." The **common hepatic duct** is the bile duct system that drains the liver into the common bile duct.

Common Bile Duct. The normal **common bile duct** has a diameter of up to 6 mm. The first part of the duct lies in the right free edge of the lesser omentum (Figure 10-3). The second part of the duct is situated posterior to the first part of the duodenum. The third part lies in a groove on the posterior surface of the head of the pancreas. It ends by piercing the medial wall of the second part of the duodenum about halfway down the duodenal length. There the common bile duct is joined by the main pancreatic duct, and together they open through a small ampulla (the **ampulla of Vater**) into the duodenal wall. The end parts of both ducts (common bile duct and main **pancreatic duct**) and the ampulla are surrounded by circular muscle fibers known as the **sphincter of Oddi.**

The proximal portion of the common bile duct is lateral to the hepatic artery and anterior to the portal vein. The duct moves more posterior after it descends behind the duodenal bulb and enters the pancreas. The distal duct lies parallel to the anterior wall of the vena cava.

Within the liver parenchyma, the bile ducts follow the same course as the portal venous and hepatic arterial branches. The hepatic and bile ducts are encased in a common collagenous sheath, forming the portal triad. The hepatic artery arises from the celiac axis and travels in the depatoduodenal ligament anterior to the portal vein and medial to the common duct. On transverse views this is known as the "Mickey Mouse" sign with the portal vein as the head, the hepatic artery the left ear, and the bile duct the right ear. In most patients the right hepatic artery passes between the common duct and the portal vein; however, in a small percentage the artery passes anterior to the common duct, or there may be a variant of two hepatic arteries anterior and/or posterior to the duct. The hepatic artery can be quite tortuous, so only a small segment is usually

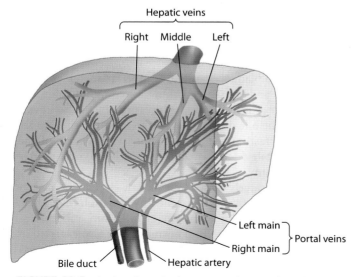

FIGURE 10-2 The intrahepatic ducts run in the portal triads along with the portal veins and hepatic arteries.

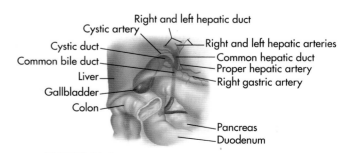

FIGURE 10-3 Relationships within the porta hepatis.

imaged. A replaced right hepatic artery that arises from the superior mesenteric artery is a normal variant that alters the anatomy of the porta hepatis. Color Doppler and tracing the vessel to its point of origin help to define the vessel.

Cystic Duct. The **cystic duct** is about 4 cm long and connects the neck of the gallbladder with the common hepatic duct to form the common bile duct. It is usually somewhat S-shaped and descends for a variable distance in the right free edge of the lesser omentum.

The Gallbladder. The **gallbladder** is a pear-shaped organ that is found on the inferior margin of the liver between the right and left lobes of the liver (Figure 10-4). Two anatomic landmarks are used to locate the gallbladder. The middle hepatic vein is in alignment with the gallbladder fossa. The interlobar fissure extends from the right portal vein to the gallbladder fossa. The gallbladder lies in the intrahepatic position, but as it migrates to the surface of the liver during embryologic development it acquires a peritoneal covering over most of its surface. The remainder of the gallbladder surface is covered with adventitial tissue that merges with the connective tissue with the liver. This potential space between the liver and the gallbladder is an area for infection or inflammation to collect. If this migration does not occur, the gallbladder remains intrahepatic or it may be enveloped in the visceral peritoneum, hanging into the lower abdomen. The gallbladder has been found to lie in various ectopic positions (suprahepatic, suprarenal, within the anterior abdominal wall, or in the falciform ligament). Failure of the gallbladder to develop is rare; this is known as *agenesis* of the gallbladder. These patients may still have the biliary ductal system, which can become inflamed or filled with stones.

The gallbladder is divided into the *fundus, body,* and *neck* (Figure 10-5). The rounded fundus usually projects below the inferior margin of the liver, where it comes into contact with the anterior abdominal wall at the level of the ninth right costal cartilage. The body generally lies in contact with the visceral surface of the liver and is directed upward, backward, and to the left. The neck becomes continuous with the cystic duct, which turns into the lesser omentum to join the right side of the common hepatic duct to form the common bile duct. The neck of the gallbladder is oriented posteromedially toward the porta hepatis. The fundus is situated lateral, caudal, and anterior to the neck.

The size and shape of the gallbladder are variable. Generally the normal gallbladder measures approximately 2.5 to 4 cm in diameter and 7 to 10 cm in length. The walls are less than 3 mm thick. Dilation of the gallbladder is known as **hydrops.**

Several anatomic variations may occur within the gallbladder to give rise to its internal echo pattern on the sonogram. The gallbladder may have a small outpouch, also known as the *infundibulum,* forming **Hartmann's pouch;** this is significant as gallstones may collect in this pouch (see Figure 10-5). Other anomalies include partial septation, complete septation (double gallbladder), and folding of the fundus (**Phrygian cap**) (Figure 10-6).

With a capacity of 50 ml, the gallbladder serves as a reservoir for bile. It also has the ability to concentrate the bile.

To aid this process, its mucous membrane contains folds that unite with each other, giving the surface a honeycomb appearance. **Heister's valve** in the neck of the gallbladder helps to prevent kinking of the duct (see Figure 10-4).

Vascular Supply

The arterial supply of the gallbladder is from the cystic artery, which is a branch of the right hepatic artery (see Figure 10-3). The cystic vein drains directly into the portal vein. Smaller arteries and veins run between the liver and the gallbladder.

PHYSIOLOGY AND LABORATORY DATA OF THE GALLBLADDER AND BILIARY SYSTEM

The primary functions of the extrahepatic biliary tract are (1) the transportation of bile from the liver to the intestine and (2) the regulation of its flow. This is an important function as the liver secretes approximately 1 to 2 liters of bile per day. When the gallbladder and bile ducts are functioning normally, they respond in a fairly uniform manner in various phases of digestion. Concentration of bile in the gallbladder occurs during a state of fasting. It is forced into the gallbladder by an increased pressure within the common bile duct, which is produced by the action of the sphincter of Oddi at the distal end of the gallbladder.

During the fasting state, very little bile flows into the duodenum. Stimulation produced by the influence of food causes the gallbladder to contract, resulting in an outpouring of bile into the duodenum. When the stomach is emptied, duodenal peristalsis diminishes, the gallbladder relaxes, the tonus of the sphincter of Oddi increases slightly, and thus very little bile passes into the duodenum. Small amounts of bile secreted by the liver are retained in the common duct and forced into the gallbladder. The contracted gallbladder appears on sonography as a thick-walled structure with a slit for the bile. It is nearly impossible to see luminal or wall abnormalities when the gallbladder is contracted.

Removal of the Gallbladder

When the gallbladder is removed, the sphincter of Oddi loses tonus, and pressure within the common bile duct drops to that of intraabdominal pressure. Bile is no longer retained in the bile ducts but is free to flow into the duodenum during fasting and digestive phases. Dilation of the extrahepatic bile ducts (usually less than 1 cm) occurs after **cholecystectomy.**

Secretion is largely caused by a bile salt–dependent mechanism, and ductal flow is controlled by secretion. Bile is the principal medium for excretion of **bilirubin** and cholesterol. The products of steroid hormones are also excreted in the bile, as are drugs and poisons (e.g., salts of heavy metals). The bile salts from the intestine stimulate the liver to make more bile. Bile salts activate intestinal and pancreatic enzymes.

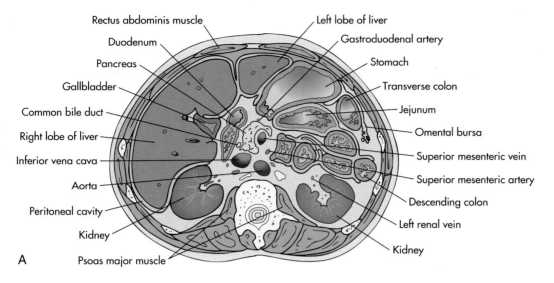

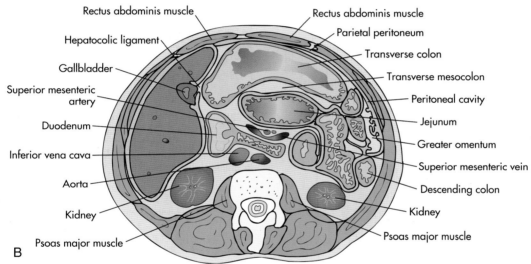

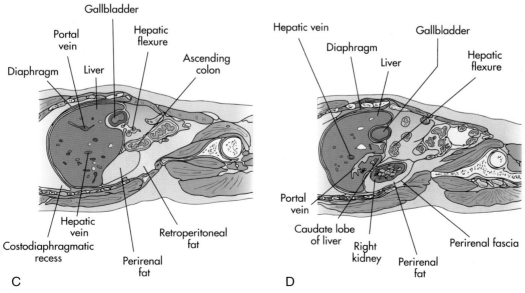

FIGURE 10-4 A and **B,** Transverse views of the right upper quadrant to include the biliary system, beginning at the level of the caudate lobe and proceeding in a caudal direction. **C** and **D,** Sagittal views of the right upper quadrant to include the biliary system beginning near the midclavicular line and moving toward the midline.

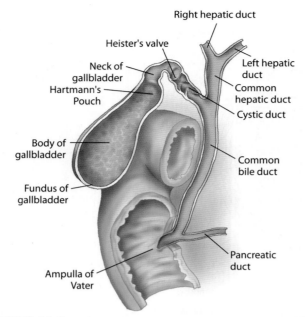

FIGURE 10-5 **Gallbladder and biliary ducts.** The first part of the duct lies in the right free edge of the lesser omentum. The second part of the duct is situated posterior to the first part of the duodenum. The third part lies in a groove on the posterior surface of the head of the pancreas. The common bile duct is joined by the main pancreatic duct, and together they open through the ampulla of Vater into the duodenal wall.

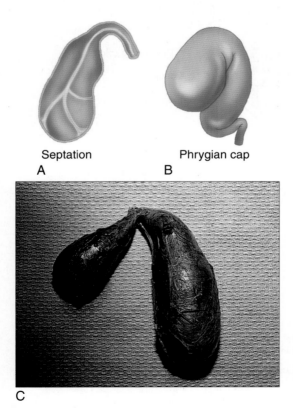

FIGURE 10-6 **A,** Septations may be found in the gallbladder. Changes in patient position will show the septation to remain in the same position in the gallbladder. **B,** The Phrygian cap is a variant in which part of the fundus of the gallbladder is bent back on itself. **C,** The double gallbladder is seen infrequently; the recognition of two distinct sacs will confirm the diagnosis.

SONOGRAPHIC EVALUATION OF THE BILIARY SYSTEM

Biliary System Protocol

Ultrasound examinations of the gallbladder and bile ducts are performed to determine cholelithiasis, changes secondary to acute and chronic cholecystitis, obstruction, and primary or metastatic tumor involvement. The examination is performed as part of a comprehensive general abdominal evaluation (Table 10-1).

1. Patient preparation: nothing by mouth (NPO) for at least 6 hours.
2. Transducer selection: broadband curvilinear or section probe 2.5 to 5 MHz.
3. Patient position: supine and decubitus (Figure 10-7).

TABLE 10-1	Abdominal Ultrasound Protocol: Gallbladder	
Organ	**Scan Plane**	**Anatomy**
GB (supine and LLD)	Long	Body/fundus
	Trv	Body/neck (measure wall) Body/neck
CBD	Trv	Portal triad
	Long	Measure duct

CBD, Common bile duct; *GB,* gallbladder; *LLD,* left lateral decubitus; *Long,* longitudinal; *Trv,* transverse.

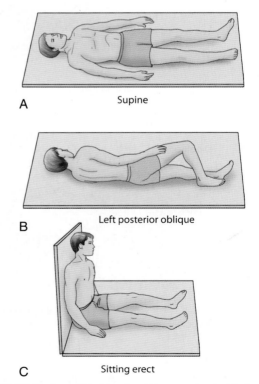

FIGURE 10-7 The gallbladder should be examined with the patient in the supine **(A),** left posterior oblique **(B),** and sometimes upright positions **(C).**

4. Images and observations should include the following (Figure 10-8).
   - The fundus, body, and neck should be surveyed.
   - Gallbladder wall thickness (normal is less than 3 mm) should be recorded. If thickened, the wall should be measured in the transverse plane at the anterior wall with the transducer perpendicular to the anterior wall.
   - The presence of echogenic foci (e.g., stones, polyps) within the gallbladder lumen should be evaluated. If echogenic foci are present, the sonographer should attempt to demonstrate acoustic shadowing and mobility with change in patient position.
   - The common bile duct should be imaged in at least the oblique long-axis plane as it lies anterior to the main portal vein before coursing posterior to the head of the pancreas.
   - The transverse scan of the porta hepatis may help delineate the portal vein from the common duct (anterior and to the right) and hepatic artery (anterior and to the left).

   - Visualization of the intrahepatic ducts may be difficult unless dilation is present. Ductal dilation may be seen as the liver is scanned, demonstrating right and left branches of the portal vein as the hepatic ducts follow a parallel course.
   - To examine gallstones, the focal point of the transducer is placed at the region of the posterior gallbladder wall, and the gain reduced. This facilitates demonstration of acoustic shadowing.

Gallbladder

To ensure maximum dilation of the gallbladder, the patient should be given nothing to eat for at least 6 hours before the ultrasound examination. The patient is initially examined in the supine position in full inspiration. Transverse, sagittal, and oblique scans are made over the upper abdomen to identify the gallbladder, biliary system, liver, right kidney, and head of the pancreas (Figure 10-9, *A*). The oblique scans are

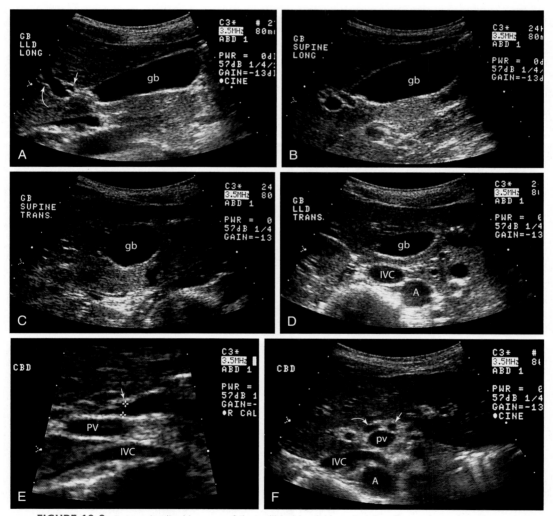

FIGURE 10-8 A, Longitudinal images of the gallbladder *(gb),* main lobar fissure *(arrow),* and portal vein *(curved arrow).* **B,** Longitudinal image of gallbladder, including the neck. **C,** Transverse image of gallbladder. **D,** Transverse image of gallbladder, inferior vena cava *(IVC),* and aorta *(A).* **E,** Longitudinal image of common bile duct *(arrow)* anterior to portal vein *(PV)* that lies anterior to the inferior vena cava. **F,** Transverse image of portal tried in the center of the image: portal vein with common bile duct *(curved arrow)* anterior and lateral; hepatic artery *(arrow)* anterior and medial; inferior vena cava and aorta.

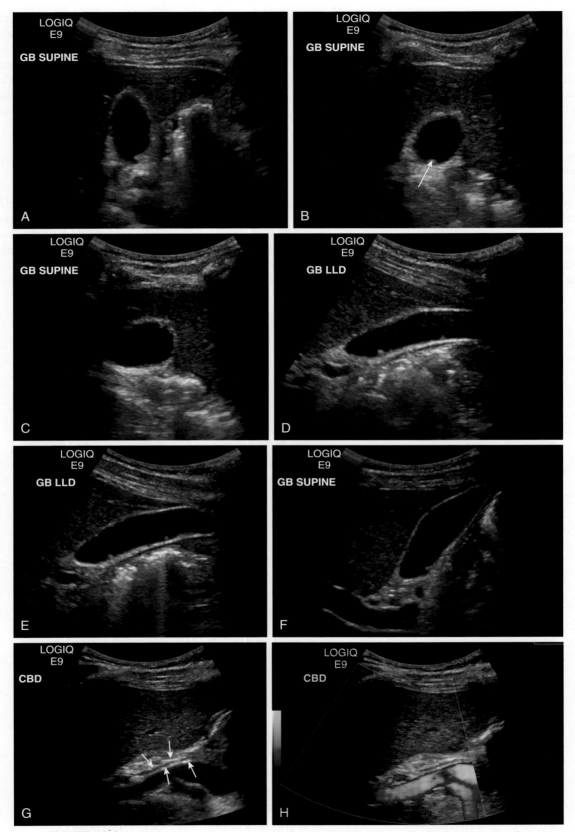

FIGURE 10-9 A–C, Supine transverse images of the gallbladder. Note the small echogenic adenoma attached to the posterior wall *(arrow)*. This does not move with alterations in patient position. **D–E,** Left lateral decubitus images of the long axis of the gallbladder. **F–H,** Supine longitudinal images of the gallbladder and common bile duct *(arrows)*.

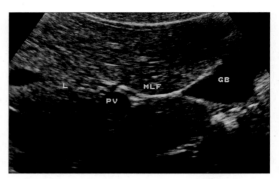

FIGURE 10-10 The main lobar fissure *(MLF)* is seen as an echogenic linear echo within the liver *(L)* connecting the right portal vein *(PV)* to the neck of the gallbladder *(GB)*.

made with the transducer in the subcostal position with a slight cephalic angulation. The probe sweep is aligned between the right shoulder and left hip of the patient. If stones or polyps are suspected, the patient should also be rolled into a steep decubitus or upright position (to ensure there are no stones within the gallbladder) in an attempt to separate small stones from the gallbladder wall or cystic duct.

The gallbladder may be identified as a sonolucent oblong structure located anterior to the right kidney, lateral to the head of the pancreas and duodenum. The gallbladder fossa causes a slight indentation on the posterior surface of the medial aspect of the right lobe of the liver (see Figure 10-9). The sagittal scans show the right kidney posterior to the gallbladder. The fundus is generally oriented slightly more anterior and, on sagittal scans, often reaches the anterior abdominal wall. Box 10-1 lists the sonographic characteristics of the normal gallbladder.

The middle hepatic vein lies in the same anatomic plane and may prove to be a useful landmark in locating the gallbladder. A sweep from cephalad to caudad shows the interlobar fissure (a structure that separates the right and left hepatic lobes) as a bright linear echo within the liver connecting the gallbladder fossa and the right portal vein (Figure 10-10). The neck of the gallbladder usually comes into contact with the main segment of the portal vein near the origin of the left portal vein. The gallbladder commonly resides in a fossa on the medial aspect of the liver. Because of fat or fibrous tissue within the main lobar fissure of the liver (which lies between the gallbladder and the right portal vein), this bright linear

reflector is a reliable indicator of the location of the gallbladder. The gallbladder lies in the posterior and caudal aspect of the fissure. The caudal aspect of the linear echo "points" directly to the gallbladder. If the gallbladder has been removed, the fossa appears as an echogenic line as a result of the remaining connective tissues.

A small echogenic fold has been reported to occur along the posterior wall of the gallbladder at the junction of the body/neck. It may be very small (3 to 5 mm) but may give rise to an acoustic shadow in the supine position. It is not duplicated in the oblique position. The cause for such a **junctional fold** is the indentation between the body/neck or Heister's valve, which is a spiral fold beginning in the neck of the gallbladder and lining the cystic duct (see Figure 10-5).

A prominent gallbladder may be normal in some individuals secondary to their fasting state (Figure 10-11). A large gallbladder has also been detected in patients with diabetes, patients bedridden with protracted illness or pancreatitis, and patients taking anticholinergic drugs. A large gallbladder may even fail to contract after a fatty meal or intravenous **cholecystokinin;** other studies may be needed before making a diagnosis of obstruction.

If a gallbladder appears abnormally enlarged, a fatty meal may be administered and further sonographic evaluation made to detect whether the enlargement is abnormal or

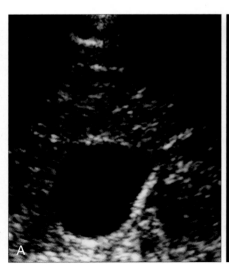

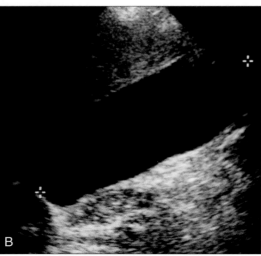

FIGURE 10-11 A, Transverse and **B,** longitudinal scans of the distended gallbladder. The gallbladder size may be quite variable from patient to patient. A good rule of thumb is to compare the size of the gallbladder with the transverse view of the right kidney. The width should always be smaller, ≤4 cm.

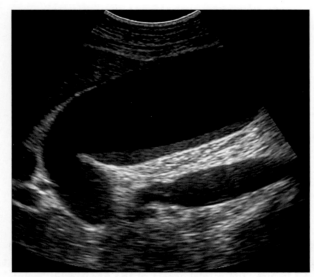

FIGURE 10-12 Distention (hydrops) of the gallbladder may be found in patients who have been on intravenous fluids for several days or may be secondary to a mass or enlarged lymph nodes compressing the common bile duct.

normal. If the gallbladder fails to contract during the examination, the pancreatic area should be investigated further. Courvoisier's sign indicates an extrahepatic mass compressing the common bile duct, which can produce an enlarged gallbladder (Figure 10-12). In addition, the liver should be carefully examined for the presence of dilated bile ducts.

In a well-contracted gallbladder, the wall changes from a single to a double concentric structure with the following three components: (1) a strongly reflective outer contour, (2) a poorly reflective inner contour, and (3) a sonolucent area between both reflecting structures.

Bile Ducts

Sonographically, the common duct lies anterior and to the right of the portal vein in the region of the porta hepatis and gastrohepatic ligament. The hepatic artery lies anterior and to the left of the portal vein. On a transverse scan, the common duct, hepatic artery, and portal vein have been referred to as the portal triad or "Mickey Mouse sign" (Figure 10-13). The portal vein serves as Mickey's face, with the right ear the common duct and the left ear the hepatic artery. To obtain such a cross section, the transducer must be directed in a slightly oblique path from the left shoulder to the right hip.

On sagittal scans, the right branch of the hepatic artery usually passes anterior to the common duct (Figures 10-14 and 10-15). The common duct is seen just anterior to the portal vein before it dips posteriorly to enter the head of the pancreas. The patient may be rotated into a slight (45-degree) or steep (90-degree) right anterior oblique position, with the beam directed posteromedially to visualize the duct. This enables the examiner to avoid cumbersome bowel gas and to use the liver as an acoustic window.

When the right subcostal approach is used, the main portal vein may be seen as it bifurcates into the right and left branches.

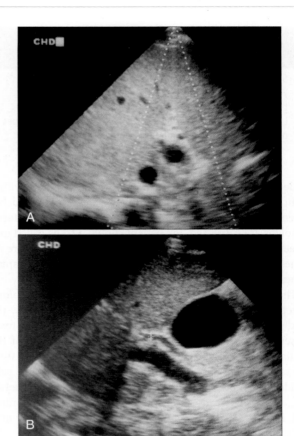

FIGURE 10-13 Transverse **(A)** and sagittal **(B)** views of the common bile duct. The transverse view shows the portal triad with the portal vein posterior, the common duct anterior and lateral, and the hepatic artery anterior and medial. The sagittal view shows the common duct anterior to the main portal vein.

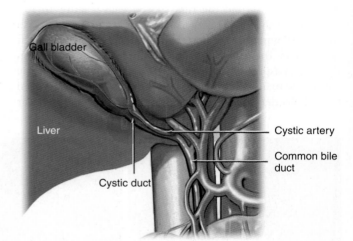

FIGURE 10-14 Anatomic relationship of the cystic duct, cystic artery, and common bile duct. The right branch of the hepatic artery usually passes anterior to the common duct. The common duct is seen just anterior to the portal vein.

As the right branch continues into the right lobe of the liver, it can be followed laterally in a longitudinal plane. The portal vein appears as an almond-shaped sonolucent structure anterior to the inferior vena cava. The common hepatic duct is seen as a tubular structure anterior to the portal vein. The right branch of

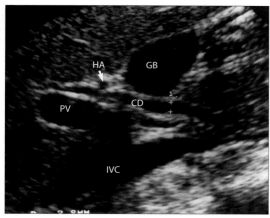

FIGURE 10-15 On this sagittal image, the hepatic artery *(HA)* is shown anterior to the common duct *(CD)*. The portal vein *(PV)* is anterior to the inferior vena cava *(IVC)*. GB, Gallbladder.

the hepatic artery can be seen between the duct and the portal vein as a small circular structure.

The small cystic duct is generally not identified. Because this landmark is necessary to distinguish the common hepatic duct from the common bile duct, the more general term *common duct* is used to refer to these structures (Figure 10-16).

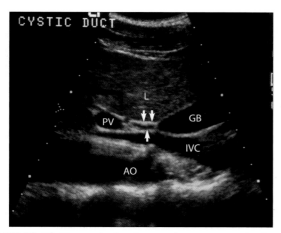

FIGURE 10-16 The cystic duct is sometimes seen to arise from the neck of the gallbladder *(arrows)*. This coronal decubitus view shows the aorta *(AO)*, inferior vena cava *(IVC)*, gallbladder *(GB)*, portal vein *(PV)*, and liver *(L)*.

PATHOLOGY OF THE GALLBLADDER AND BILIARY SYSTEM

See Table 10-2 for clinical findings, sonographic findings, and differential considerations for gallbladder and biliary diseases and conditions.

Clinical Symptoms of Gallbladder Disease

Pain. The most classic symptom of gallbladder disease is right-upper-quadrant abdominal pain, usually occurring after ingestion of greasy foods. Nausea and vomiting sometimes occur and may indicate the presence of a stone in the common bile duct. A gallbladder attack may cause referred pain to the right shoulder, with inflammation of the gallbladder often causing referred pain in the right shoulder blade.

Jaundice. Jaundice is characterized by the presence of bile in the tissues with resulting yellow-green color of the skin. It may develop when a tiny gallstone blocks the bile ducts between the gallbladder and the intestines, producing pressure on the liver and forcing bile into the blood.

Sludge. Sludge, or thickened bile, frequently occurs from bile stasis. This may be seen in patients with prolonged fasting, hyperalimentation therapy, or with obstruction of the gallbladder. Some gallbladders may be so packed with this thickened bile that the gallbladder is isoechoic and difficult to distinguish from the liver parenchyma. Occasionally sludge is also found in the common duct. Sludge is gravity dependent; therefore with alterations in the patient's position, the sonographer may be able to separate sludge from occasional artifactual echoes found in the gallbladder. Sludge will slowly resettle as the patient changes position. Sludge should be considered an abnormal finding because either a functional or a pathologic abnormality exists when calcium bilirubin or cholesterol precipitates in bile. Complications of biliary sludge are stone formation, biliary colic, acalculous cholecystitis, and pancreatitis.

Sonographic Findings. Occasionally a patient presents sonographically with a prominent gallbladder containing amorphous, low-level internal echoes without acoustic shadowing, which may be attributed to thick or inspissated bile. The source of echoes in biliary sludge is thought to be particulate matter (predominantly pigment granules with

TABLE 10-2	The Gallbladder and the Biliary System	
Clinical Findings	**Sonographic Findings**	**Differential Considerations**
Sludge		
May be asymptomatic	Low-level internal echoes layering in dependent part of GB	Pseudosludge
	Prominent gallbladder size	Empyema of GB
	Changes with patient position	Hemobilia
		Neoplasm
Acute Cholecystitis		
↑ Serum amylase	Dilation and rounding of GB	Chronic cholecystitis
Abnormal LFTs	+ Murphy's sign	Nonfasting GB
	Thick GB wall with irregular wall (edema)	Acute pancreatitis
	Stones	GB carcinoma
	Pericholecystic fluid	

Continued

TABLE 10-2	The Gallbladder and the Biliary System—cont'd	
Clinical Findings	**Sonographic Findings**	**Differential Considerations**
Chronic Cholecystitis		
↑ Serum amylase	Contraction of GB	Cholelithiasis
Abnormal LFTs	Stones	Nonfasting GB
RUQ pain—transient	WES sign	Acute pancreatitis
		GB carcinoma
Acalculous Cholecystitis		
↑ Serum amylase	Dilation of GB	Chronic cholecystitis
Abnormal LFTs	+ Murphy's sign	Nonfasting GB
	Thick GB wall with irregular wall (edema)	Acute pancreatitis
	Sludge	GB carcinoma
	Pericholecystic fluid	
	Subserosal edema	
Emphysematous Cholecystitis		
Gas-forming bacteria in GB	Bright echo in area of GB with ring-down or comet-tail artifact	Chronic cholecystitis
Abnormal LFTs	May appear as WES	GB carcinoma
Gangrenous Cholecystitis		
Abnormal LFTs	Medium to coarse echogenic densities that fill GB lumen in absence of duct obstruction	GB carcinoma
	No shadow	
	Not gravity dependent	
	Does not layer	
Cholelithiasis		
Check bilirubin levels	Dilated GB with thick wall	Duodenal gas
Acute ↑ amylase	Hyperechoic intraluminal echoes with posterior acoustic shadowing	Porcelain GB
Abnormal LFTs	WES sign	Sludge
(increased alkaline phosphatase);	Gravity-dependent calcifications in GB	
AST and ALT may be normal		
Choledochal Cysts		
Jaundice	True cysts in RUQ with or without communication with biliary system	Hepatic cyst
Possibly increased bilirubin	Classified by anatomy:	Hepatic artery aneurysm
	1. Localized dilated cystic CBD	Pancreatic pseudocyst
	2. Diverticulum of CBD	
	3. Invagination of CBD into duodenum	
	4. Dilated CBD and CHD	
Adenoma of the Gallbladder		
	Occurs as flat elevations located in the body of the GB, almost always near the fundus	Adenomyomatosis
	Does not change with position	
	No shadow produced	
Adenomyomatosis of the Gallbladder		
	Papillomas may occur singly or in groups and may be scattered over a large part of the mucosal surface of the GB	Adenoma
	Does not move with position changes.	
	Comet-tail artifact	
Porcelain Gallbladder		
Female predominance	Gallbladder wall is thickly calcified with shadowing	Gallstones with emphysematous cholecystitis
Found in patients over 60		
Choledocholithiasis		
Increased direct bilirubin	Echogenic structure in extrahepatic duct	Surgical clips
Abnormal liver enzymes	Dilated biliary tree	Artifact from right hepatic artery
Leukocytosis		Cystic duct remnant
Increased alkaline phosphatase		

ALT, alanine aminotransferase; *AST,* aspartate aminotransferase; *CBD,* common bile duct; *CHD,* common hepatic duct; *GB,* gallbladder; *LFTs,* liver function tests; *RUQ,* right upper quadrant; *WES,* wall, echo, shadow.

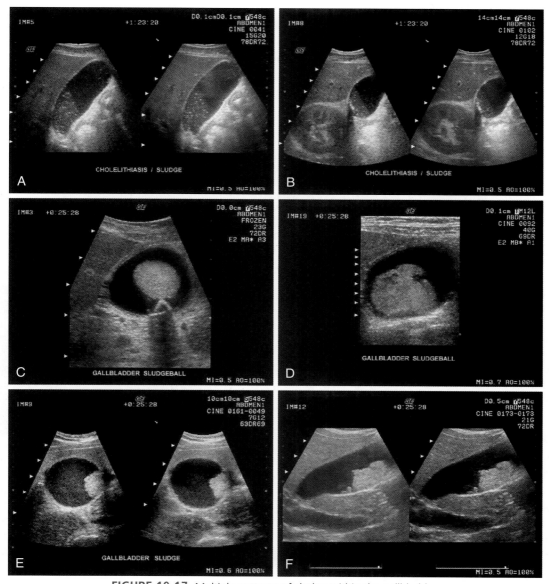

FIGURE 10-17 Multiple patterns of sludge within the gallbladder.

lesser amounts of cholesterol crystals). The viscosity does not appear to be important in the generation of internal echoes in fluids. The particles can be small and still produce perceptible echoes (Figure 10-17). Sludge may mimic polypoid tumors (tumefactive sludge). Sludge will not present with gallbladder wall thickening or internal vascularity as tumor would. Sludge may also be seen in combination with cholelithiasis, cholecystitis, and other biliary diseases.

Wall Thickness

The normal wall thickness of the gallbladder is less than 3 mm. Biliary causes of gallbladder wall thickening include cholecystitis, adenomyomatosis, cancer, acquired immunodeficiency syndrome (AIDS), cholangiopathy, severe hypoalbuminemic state, and sclerosing cholangitis (Box 10-2). Nonbiliary causes include diffuse liver disease (cirrhosis and hepatitis),

BOX 10-2	Common Causes of Thickening of the Gallbladder Wall (≥3 mm)
Intrinsic	**Extrinsic**
Cholecystitis	Hepatitis/cirrhosis
Gallbladder perforation	Hypoalbuminemia
Sepsis	Renal failure
Hyperplastic cholecystosis	Right-sided heart failure
Gallbladder carcinoma	Ascites
AIDS cholangiography	Multiple myeloma
Sclerosing cholangitis	Portal node lymphatic obstruction

pancreatitis, portal hypertension, and heart failure. A thickened wall is a nonspecific sign and is not necessarily related to gallbladder disease.

Sonographic Findings. The gallbladder wall thickness should be measured when the transducer is perpendicular to

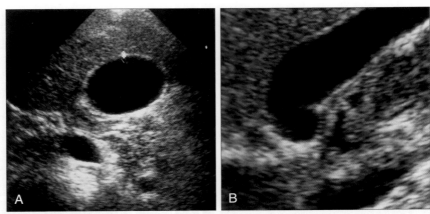

FIGURE 10-18 A, The gallbladder wall should be measured on the transverse image at the anterior wall that is perpendicular to the transducer (see markings). **B,** The sagittal image of the gallbladder is often at an angle to the transducer and may be used to measure the wall thickness when the sonographer can achieve a perpendicular angle.

the anterior gallbladder wall. This is usually done in the transverse plane, but in some cases the longitudinal plane allows a better alignment. The gain should be reduced and the focal zone aligned to the gallbladder area to clearly demarcate the anterior wall. The anterior wall is measured from outer to outer margins. Sonographically the gallbladder wall may be underestimated when the wall has extensive fibrosis or is surrounded by fat (Figure 10-18).

Cholecystitis

Cholecystitis is an inflammation of the gallbladder that may have one of several forms: acute or chronic, acalculous, emphysematous, or gangrenous (Box 10-3).

Acute Cholecystitis. The most common cause of acute cholecystitis occurs from persistent obstruction of the cystic duct or gallbladder neck by an impacted gallstone. When stones become impacted in the cystic duct or in the neck of the gallbladder (Hartmann's pouch), it results in obstruction with distention of the lumen, ischemia, and infection (cholecystitis) with eventual necrosis of the gallbladder (Figure 10-19). If the impacted stone does not spontaneously disimpact the gallbladder may become necrotic and perforate. Even though it may be difficult to visualize the actual stone that is causing the obstruction, other gallstones may be seen.

Acute cholecystitis is found three times more frequently in females than in males over 50, but it has a similar incidence at higher age-groups. Clinically the patient with acute

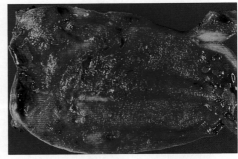

FIGURE 10-19 Gross pathology of acute cholecystitis. The gallbladder contained stones. The gallbladder wall was thick and swollen.

cholecystitis presents with acute right-upper-quadrant pain (positive **Murphy's sign**—inspiratory arrest on palpation of the gallbladder area; may be false positive in a small percentage of patients), fever, and leukocytosis; increased serum bilirubin and alkaline phosphatase levels may be present.

Cholecystectomy surgery is the treatment of choice. Antibiotics may be administered to reduce the inflammation before surgery. Complications of acute cholecystitis may be serious and include empyema, emphysematous or gangrenous cholecystitis, and perforation.

Sonographic Findings. Acute cholecystitis has very specific findings on sonography. The patient will have a positive Murphy's sign making the area of the gallbladder extremely sensitive to touch. There is a thickened gallbladder wall greater than 3 mm. This should be measured at the anterior wall with the wall parallel to the transducer (Figure 10-20). A distended gallbladder lumen greater than 4 cm is present. Gallstones are usually present and the sonographer should search for an impacted stone in Hartmann's pouch or cystic duct. Increased color Doppler flow will be present secondary to the inflammation of the gallbladder wall. There may be the presence of pericholecystic fluid collection around the gallbladder bed.

The sonographic appearance of acute cholecystitis is identified as a gallbladder with an irregular outline of a thickened wall (Figure 10-21). A sonolucent area probably caused by edema has been found within the thickened wall. If the irregular

BOX 10-3	Sonographic Findings in Cholecystitis

- Thickened gallbladder wall >3 mm
- Distended gallbladder lumen >4 cm
- Gallstones
- Impacted stone in Hartmann's pouch or cystic duct
- Positive Murphy's sign
- Increased color Doppler flow
- Pericholecystic fluid collection

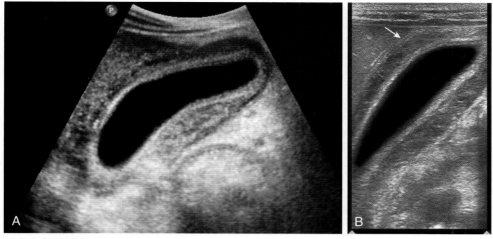

FIGURE 10-20 Acute cholecystitis. Inflammation of the gallbladder wall greater than 3 mm. This should be measured at the anterior wall with the wall parallel to the transducer.

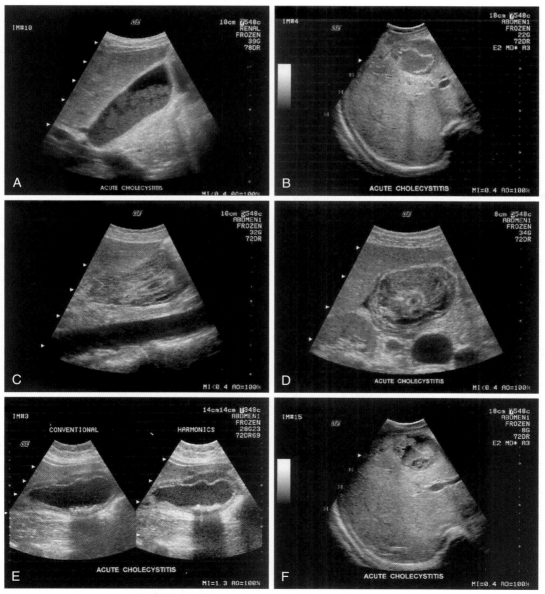

FIGURE 10-21 Multiple patterns of acute cholecystitis.

gallbladder wall shows striated sonolucencies a more advanced case of cholecystitis may be present. Some walls will be thicker because of a pericholecystic abscess. Occasionally a thickened gallbladder wall is seen in normal individuals; this is related to the degree of contraction of a normal gallbladder (Figure 10-22). Enlargement of the gallbladder is another important sign of acute cholecystitis with the width dimension more relevant that the length.

The sonographic Murphy's sign is positive when tenderness is demonstrated over the area of the gallbladder when the sonographer touches the right upper quadrant with the transducer and gentle compression is applied. When the patient takes in a deep breath, the gallbladder is displaced below the protective costal margin. This positive sign may not be present if the patient has been given analgesics before the study or if the condition has been prolonged with resultant gangrenous cholecystitis.

Color Doppler velocities (with low PRF setting) is increased in the cystic artery, which encompasses the inflamed gallbladder wall. Power Doppler may better demonstrate this increased flow because the transducer does not need to be parallel to flow as it does with color Doppler.

The sonographer should assess the presence or absence of pericholecystic fluid (Figure 10-23). The wall may become inflamed and edematous with subsequent leakage into the pericholecystic space surrounding the gallbladder.

If the thickened wall is localized and irregular, an abscess, cholecystosis, or carcinoma of the gallbladder should be considered.

Complications of Acute Cholecystitis

Emphysematous Cholecystitis. Emphysematous cholecystitis is a rare complication of acute cholecystitis that occurs more frequently in elderly men. It occurs more in diabetic patients, and often gallstones may not be present. This disease is associated with the presence of gas-forming bacteria in the gallbladder wall and/or lumen with extension into the biliary ducts. Perforation of the gallbladder is more likely to occur with emphysematous cholecystitis than with gallstone-induced cholecystitis. This condition is a surgical emergency.

▌***Sonographic Findings.*** The sonographic appearance will depend on the amount of gas within the wall of the gallbladder. If the gas is intraluminal, the sonographer should look for a prominent bright echo along the anterior wall with ring-down or comet-tail artifact directly posterior to the echogenic structure (Figure 10-24). If a large amount of gas is present, the appearance may simulate a packed bag or wall, echo, shadow (WES) sign with a curvilinear echogenic area with complete posterior fuzzy shadowing.

Gangrenous Cholecystitis.

Another serious painful complication of acute cholecystitis that may lead to perforation is gangrenous cholecystitis. This process may occur after a prolonged infection, which causes the gallbladder to undergo necrosis. The gallbladder wall may be thickened and edematous, with focal areas of exudate, hemorrhage, and necrosis. In addition, there may be ulcerations and perforations resulting

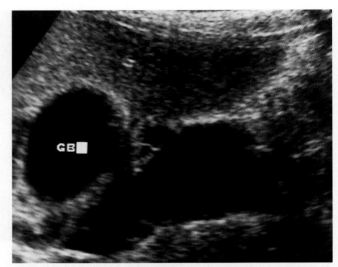

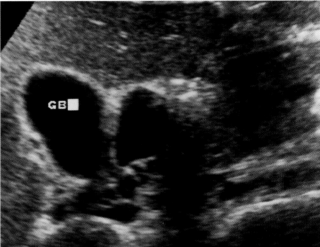

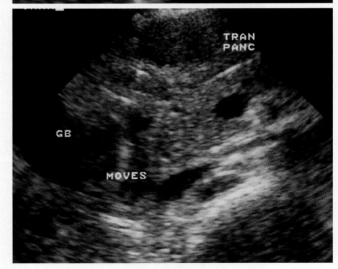

FIGURE 10-22 The sonographer should observe other fluid collections in the right upper quadrant for signs of change, or peristalsis, as illustrated in these images. The large collection of fluid was in the antrum and duodenum; with time, the fluid collection changed shape and distinct peristaltic movement could be seen with real-time imaging. *GB,* Gallbladder.

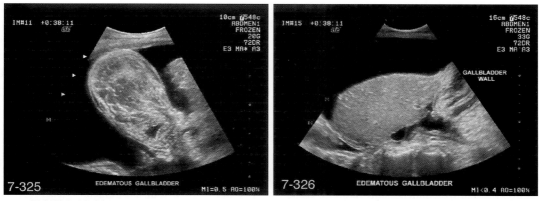

FIGURE 10-23 Swollen, edematous gallbladder was found in this middle-aged male with cirrhosis and ascites.

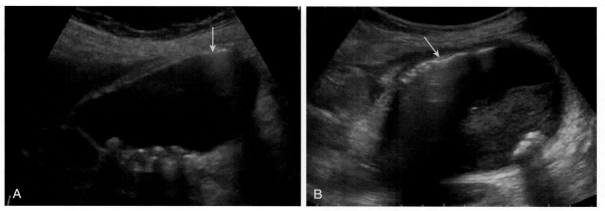

FIGURE 10-24 **Emphysematous cholecystitis.** If the gas is intraluminal, the sonographer should look for a prominent bright echo along the anterior wall with ring-down or comet-tail artifact directly posterior to the echogenic structure *(arrow)*.

in pericholecystic abscesses or peritonitis. Gallstones or fine gravel occur in 80% to 95% of patients.

Sonographic Findings. The common echo features of gangrene are the presence of diffuse medium to coarse echogenic densities filling the gallbladder lumen in the absence of bile duct obstruction. This echogenic material has the

following three characteristics: (1) it does not cause shadowing, (2) it is not gravity dependent, and (3) it does not show a layering effect (Figure 10-25). The lack of layering is attributed to increased viscosity of the bile. In addition, the gallbladder wall becomes irregular, with edematous pockets within the wall representing hemorrhage or abscess collections. The wall

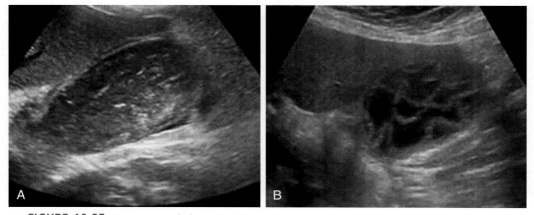

FIGURE 10-25 **Gangrenous cholecystitis.** The common echo features of gangrene are the presence of diffuse medium to coarse echogenic densities filling the gallbladder lumen in the absence of bile duct obstruction.

may become so inflamed with hemorrhage that a hemorrhagic cholecystitis develops. Pericholecystic fluid may be present in the area surrounding the gallbladder bed.

Acalculous Cholecystitis. This uncommon condition is an acute inflammation of the gallbladder in the absence of acute cholecystitis. It may develop secondary to gallbladder wall infection, ischemia, chemical toxicity to the gallbladder wall, and cystic duct obstruction. It is most likely caused by decreased blood flow through the cystic artery. Conditions that produce depressed motility (trauma, burns, postoperative patients, human immunodeficiency virus infection, etc.) may prelude the development of acalculous cholecystitis. Extrinsic compression of the cystic duct by a mass or lymphadenopathy may also cause this condition. Clinically the patient has a positive Murphy's sign.

Sonographic Findings. The gallbladder wall is extremely thickened (greater than 4 to 5 mm), and echogenic sludge is seen within a dilated gallbladder. Look for the presence of pericholecystic fluid within ascites or subserosal edema (Figure 10-26).

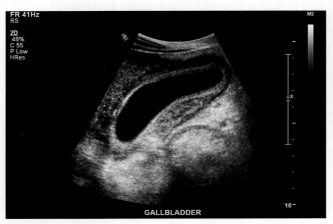

FIGURE 10-26 Acalculous cholecystitis with thickening of the gallbladder wall secondary to edema and inflammation.

Chronic Cholecystitis. Chronic cholecystitis is the most common form of gallbladder inflammation. This is the result of numerous attacks of acute cholecystitis with subsequent fibrosis of the gallbladder wall. Clinically the patients may have some transient right-upper-quadrant pain, but not the tenderness as experienced with acute cholecystitis.

Torsion of the Gallbladder

Torsion of the gallbladder is a rare condition that is found more in elderly females and is associated with a mobile gallbladder with a long suspensory mesentery. Symptoms are typical of acute cholecystitis.

Sonographic Findings. The gallbladder becomes massively inflamed and distended. The cystic artery and cystic duct may also become twisted. If the gallbladder becomes twisted more than 180 degrees, the risk of gangrene may develop. Surgical intervention is the treatment for this condition.

Cholelithiasis. Cholelithiasis, or gallstones in the gallbladder, is frequently found in a contracted gallbladder with coarse gallbladder wall thickening. The **wall, echo, shadow (WES) sign** is described as a contracted bright gallbladder with posterior shadowing caused by a packed bag of stones (Figure 10-27). When the gallbladder is completely packed full of stones, the sonographer will only be able to image the anterior border of the gallbladder, with the stones casting a distinct acoustic shadow (the WES sign). The WES sign consists of three arc-shaped lines followed by a shadow. The first line is echogenic and represents the pericholecystic fat, as well as the interface between the gallbladder wall and the liver. The second line is hypoechoic and represents the gallbladder. The third line is echogenic, reflecting the packed bag of stones within the gallbladder. The acoustic shadow is seen posterior to this third line.

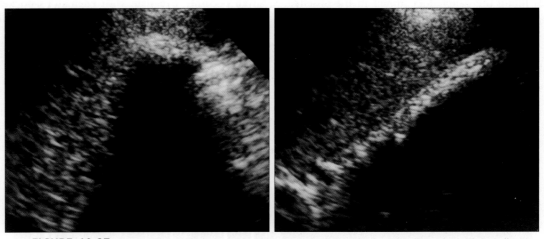

FIGURE 10-27 A 45-year-old female with right-upper-quadrant pain and distention. The wall, echo, shadow (WES) sign was visualized and indicated that the gallbladder was a packed bag. Note the sharp posterior shadow. This appearance is different from that of the porcelain gallbladder because the anterior wall is not as bright or echogenic.

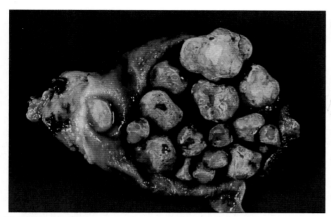

FIGURE 10-28 Gross pathology of multiple gallstones within the gallbladder.

Cholelithiasis is the most common disease of the gallbladder. In cholelithiasis there may be a single large gallstone or hundreds of tiny ones (Figure 10-28). The tiny stones are the most dangerous because they can enter the bile ducts and obstruct the outflow of bile. After a fatty meal, the gallbladder contracts to release bile; if gallstones block the outflow tract, pain results. As the bile is being stored in the gallbladder, small crystals of bile salts precipitate and may form gallstones varying from pinhead size to the size of the organ itself.

The "five F" risk factors for the patient with cholelithiasis are *fat, female, forty, fertile,* and *fair.* In addition, many other factors lead to the development of gallstones that include pregnancy, diabetes, oral contraceptive use, hemolytic diseases, diet-induced weight loss, and total parenteral nutrition. Patients may be asymptomatic until a stone lodges in the cystic or common duct, which causes biliary colic. Acute right-upper-quadrant or epigastric pain with radiation to the shoulder after a high-fat meal, nausea, and vomiting is a typical presentation for cholelithiasis. This pain may last for up to 6 hours and only ends when the stone disimpacts from the gallbladder neck or passes completely through the cystic duct.

Sonographic Findings. The evaluation of gallstones with sonography has proven to be an extremely useful procedure in patients who show symptoms of cholelithiasis. The gallbladder is evaluated for increased wall thickness, presence of internal reflections within the lumen with posterior acoustic shadowing (Figure 10-29). Gallstones appear as mobile, echogenic intraluminal structures that cast acoustic shadows. Frequently, patients with gallstones have an enlarged gallbladder lumen. Stones that are less than 1 to 2 mm may be difficult to separate from one another by ultrasound evaluation (Figure 10-30). A high-frequency transducer should be used to better delineate the stones and their shadowing characteristics. The curved array probe will allow a broader view of the near field to image the gallbladder completely. The focal zone should be adjusted to the level of the gallstone.

The patient's position should be shifted during the procedure to demonstrate the presence of movement of the stones. Patients should be scanned in the left decubitus, right lateral, or upright position. The stones should shift to the most dependent area of the gallbladder. In some cases, the bile has a thick consistency and the stones remain near the top of the gallbladder. Thus the density of the stones and the posterior shadow will be the sonographic evidence for stones.

With regard to acoustic shadowing, scattered reflections do not affect shadowing as much as specular reflections. The factors that produce a shadow are attributed to acoustic impedance of the gallstones; refraction through them or diffraction around them; their size, central or peripheral location, and position in relation to the focus of the beam; and the intensity of the beam (Figure 10-31).

All stones cast acoustic shadows regardless of the specific properties of the stones. The size of the stone is important. Stones greater than 3 mm always cast a shadow. It has been shown that any stone scanned two or more times with the same transducer and machine settings may or may not generate a shadow even when the scans are made within seconds of each other. The shadow is highly dependent on the relationship between the stone and the acoustic beam. If the central beam is aligned on the stone, a shadow can be seen. Thus some critical ratio between the stone diameter and the beam width must be achieved before shadowing is seen.

Some stones are seen to float ("floating gallstones") when contrast material from an oral cholecystogram is present because the contrast material has a higher specific gravity than the bile and indicates the floating stones are composed of cholesterol. The gallstones seek a level at which their specific gravity equals that of the mixture of bile and contrast material (Figure 10-32).

Differential diagnoses of cholelithiasis include gallbladder polyps and sludge balls. Polyps are tiny soft tissue structures that adhere to the gallbladder wall. They do not move or shadow. Sludge balls are larger than most gallstones and move, although they do not produce an acoustic shadow.

Porcelain Gallbladder

A **porcelain gallbladder** is a rare occurrence that is defined as calcium incrustation of the gallbladder wall. It is associated with gallstones in the majority of patients and may represent a form of chronic cholecystitis and inflammation. It occurs more often in the elderly female patients. The patient is generally asymptomatic and the diagnosis is generally made as an incidental finding or when a mass is found on physical examination. The clinical significance of a porcelain gallbladder is the increased risk of gallbladder carcinoma.

Sonographic Findings. On sonography, a bright echogenic echo is seen in the region of the gallbladder with

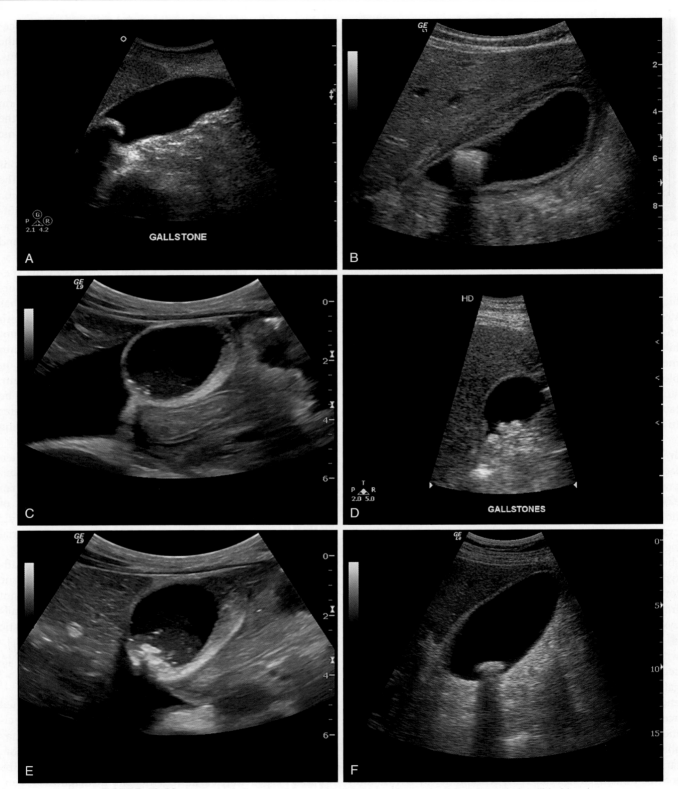

FIGURE 10-29 A, A single large gallstone is lodged into the neck of the distended gallbladder. Note the sharply defined shadow. **B,** A single large gallstone near the neck of the gallbladder. Note the thickening of the gallbladder wall. **C,** Tiny gallstones are seen within the sludge layered along the posterior margin of the gallbladder. **D,** Several medium-sized stones (without a shadow) are seen along the posterior margin of the gallbladder. The patient should be rolled into a decubitus position to watch the movement of these stones. **E,** Multiple stones with posterior shadow. **F,** Solitary stone with posterior shadow.

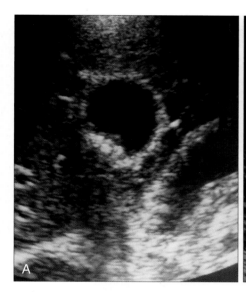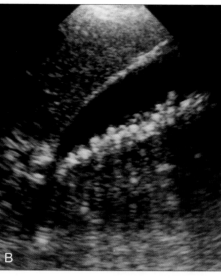

FIGURE 10-30 A, Multiple small stones are layered along the posterior wall of the gallbladder. These bright echogenic foci give acoustic shadowing beyond. **B,** A higher-frequency transducer would outline the stones and the shadowing even more clearly.

shadowing posterior (Figure 10-33). The differential will include a packed bag or WES sign. The entire gallbladder wall may not be completely calcified; thus the appearance will vary with the amount of calcification present.

Hyperplastic Cholecystosis

Hyperplastic cholecystosis is represented by a variety of degenerative and proliferative changes of the gallbladder characterized by hyperconcentration, hyperexcitability, and hyperexcretion. Cholesterolosis and adenomyomatosis of the gallbladder are two types of this condition.

Cholesterolosis. **Cholesterolosis** is a condition in which cholesterol is deposited within the lamina propria of the gallbladder. The disease process is often associated with cholesterol stones. It is often referred to as a "strawberry gallbladder" because the mucosa resembles the surface of a strawberry.

Most patients with cholesterolosis do not show thickening of the gallbladder wall on imaging studies; a small percentage of patients with this condition will show cholesterol polyps, which may be detected with ultrasound. **Polyps of the gallbladder** are small, well-defined soft tissue projections from the gallbladder wall. The cholesterol polyp is a small structure covered with a single layer of epithelium and is attached to the gallbladder with a delicate stalk. These polyps usually are found in the middle third of the gallbladder and are less than 10 mm in diameter. Cholesterol polyps are the most common pseudotumor of the gallbladder. Other masses that occur are mucosal hyperplasia, inflammatory polyps, mucous cysts, and granulomata (resulting from parasitic infections).

Sonographic Findings. Cholesterol polyps are small, smooth, ovoid wall projections seen to arise from the gallbladder wall (Figure 10-34). The polyps usually are multiple, do not shadow, and remain fixed to the wall with changes in patient position. The comet-tail artifact may be present, emanating from the cholesterol polyps, and this may be indistinguishable from adenomyomatosis.

Adenomyomatosis. **Adenomyomatosis** is a benign condition that demonstrates a hyperplastic change in the gallbladder wall. This is caused by exaggeration of the normal invaginations of the luminal epithelium (Rokitansky-Aschoff sinuses) with associated smooth muscle proliferation. The cholesterol crystals may settle within these sinus pockets. This condition is characterized by mucosal hyperplasia and thickening of the muscular layer of the gallbladder wall. Papillomas may occur alone or in groups and may be scattered over a large part of the mucosal surface of the gallbladder. These papillomas are not precursors to cancer.

Sonographic Findings. Benign tumors appear as small elevations in the gallbladder lumen. The affected areas show thickening of the gallbladder wall with internal cystic spaces. The adenomyomatosis may be focal or diffuse. Commonly small echogenic foci are seen in the gallbladder wall that create a very specific comet-tail artifact. Various patient positions and compression show the lesion to be immobile within the gallbladder. No acoustic shadow is seen posterior to this papillomatous elevation (Figure 10-35).

Adenoma. Adenomas are benign neoplasms of the gallbladder with a premalignant potential much lower than colonic adenomas. This condition usually occurs as a solitary lesion. The smaller lesions are pedunculated, whereas the larger lesions may contain foci of malignant transformation. The adenomas tend to be homogeneously hyperechoic but become more heterogeneous as they grow. If the gallbladder wall is thickened adjacent to the adenoma, malignancy should be suspected.

Gallbladder Carcinoma

Primary carcinoma of the gallbladder is rare and is nearly always a rapidly progressive disease, with a mortality rate approaching 100%. It is associated with cholelithiasis in about 80% to 90% of cases (although there is no direct proof that gallstones are the carcinogenic agent). It is twice as common as cancer of the bile ducts and occurs most frequently in women 60 years of age and older. The tumor arises in the body of the gallbladder or rarely in the cystic duct (Figure 10-36).

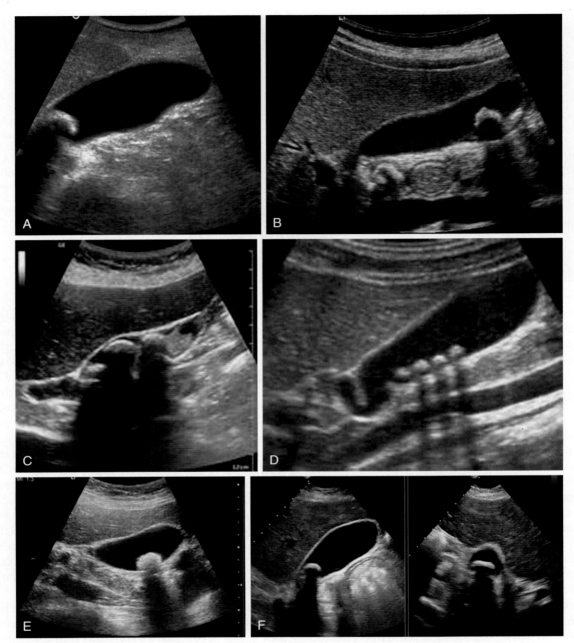

FIGURE 10-31 Multiple images of gallstones. The factors that produce a shadow are attributed to acoustic impedance of the gallstones; refraction through them or diffraction around them; their size, central or peripheral location, and position in relation to the focus of the beam; and the intensity of the beam.

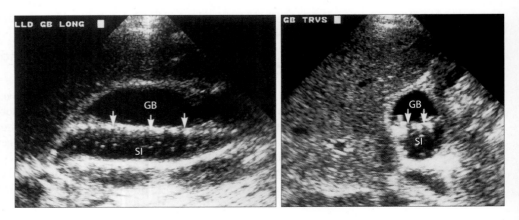

FIGURE 10-32 Longitudinal and transverse scans of the gallbladder *(GB)*, with a layer of stones "floating" *(arrows)* along the thick bile layer of sludge *(SI)*.

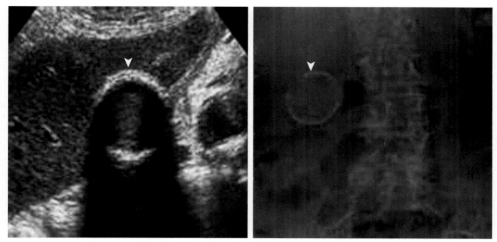

FIGURE 10-33 Porcelain gallbladder. On sonography, a bright echogenic echo *(arrow)* is seen in the region of the gallbladder with shadowing posterior.

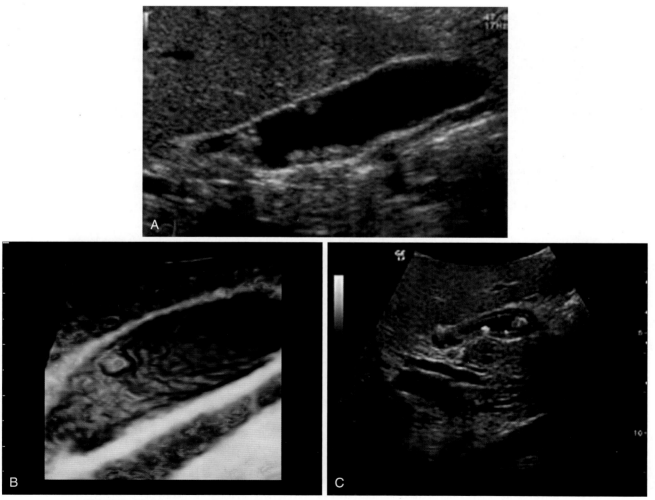

FIGURE 10-34 Polyps of the gallbladder. A, Cholesterol polyps are small, smooth ovoid wall projections seen to arise from the gallbladder wall. **B** and **C,** Cholesterol polyps do not alter their position with changes in body movement.

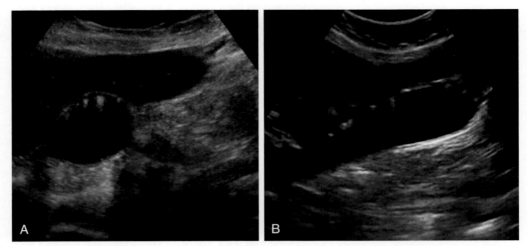

FIGURE 10-35 Adenomyomatosis. The adenomyomatosis may be focal or diffuse small echogenic foci in the gallbladder wall that create a very specific comet-tail artifact.

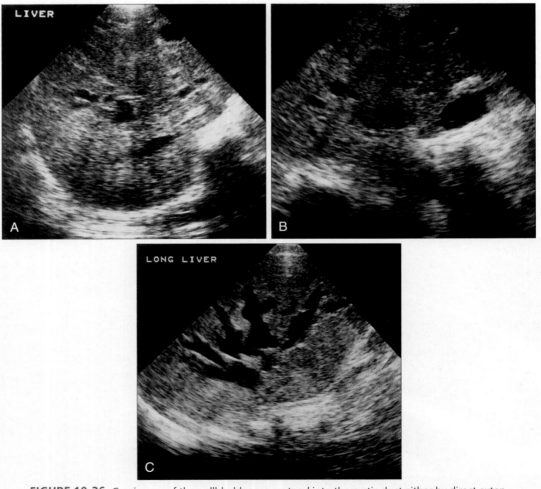

FIGURE 10-36 Carcinoma of the gallbladder may extend into the cystic duct either by direct extension of the tumor or by extrinsic compression by the involved lymph nodes. **A,** Transverse scan of the liver shows dilated ducts with an inhomogeneous liver parenchyma. **B,** Transverse scan of the inhomogeneous liver parenchyma. **C,** Transverse scan of the dilated ducts within the liver.

The tumor infiltrates the gallbladder locally or diffusely and causes thickening and rigidity of the wall. The adjacent liver is often invaded by direct continuity extending through tissue spaces, the ducts of Luschka, the lymph channels, or some combination of these. Obstruction of the cystic duct results from direct extension of the tumor or extrinsic compression by involved lymph nodes (this obstruction occurs early).

The gallbladder tumor is usually columnar cell adenocarcinoma, sometimes mucinous in type (Figure 10-37). Squamous cell carcinoma occurs but is unusual. Metastatic carcinoma in the gallbladder may occur secondary to melanoma. It usually is accompanied by liver metastases. Most patients have no symptoms that relate to the gallbladder unless there is complicating acute cholecystitis.

Sonographic Findings. The most common sonographic appearance of the soft tissue mass is a heterogeneous solid or semisolid echo texture. The mass is centered in the gallbladder fossa that completely or partially obliterates the lumen. The gallbladder wall is markedly abnormal and thickened. This thickening may be focal or diffuse, but is usually irregular and asymmetric. The identification of gallstones within the area helps to identify the mass as part of the gallbladder (Figure 10-38). The adjacent liver tissue, in the hilar area, is often heterogeneous because of direct tumoral spread. There may be dilated biliary ducts within the liver parenchyma, causing the "shotgun" sign (a "double-barrel" appearance of portal veins and dilated ducts).

Carcinoma of the gallbladder is almost never detected at a resectable stage. Obstruction of the cystic duct by the tumor or lymph nodes occurs early in the course of the disease and causes nonvisualization of the gallbladder on oral cholecystogram. Differential diagnosis for gallbladder masses included tumefactive sludge, inflammatory wall thickening, polyps, metastases, and focal adenomyomatosis.

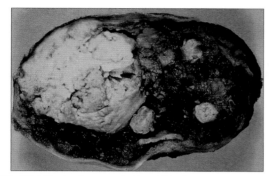

FIGURE 10-37 Carcinoma of the gallbladder shows the gallbladder partially filled and infiltrated with neoplastic tissue.

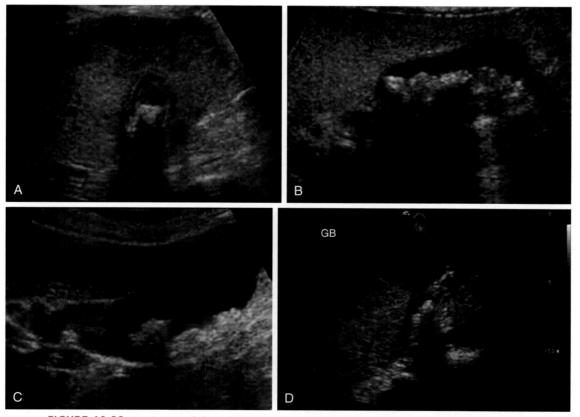

FIGURE 10-38 Carcinoma of the gallbladder. The most common sonographic appearance of the soft tissue mass is a heterogeneous solid or semisolid echo texture. The gallbladder wall is usually irregular and asymmetric and markedly abnormal and thickened.

PATHOLOGY OF THE BILIARY TREE

Choledochal Cysts

Choledochal cysts are an unusual, diverse group of diseases that may manifest as congenital, focal, or diffuse cystic dilation of the biliary tree. The choledochal cyst may be the result of pancreatic juices refluxing into the bile duct because of an anomalous junction of the pancreatic duct into the distal common bile duct, causing duct wall abnormality, weakness, and outpouching of the ductal walls. These cysts are rare; the incidence is more common in females than males (4:1), with an increased incidence in infants (the condition may occur in less than 20% of adults). Choledochal cysts may be associated with gallstones, pancreatitis, or cirrhosis. The patient presents with an abdominal mass, pain, fever, or jaundice. The diagnosis may be confirmed with a nuclear medicine hepatobiliary scan. The majority of cases are thought to be congenital and result from bile reflux. The mass presents as a cystic dilation of the biliary system.

The classification of choledochal cysts is divided into five types. Type I is a fusiform dilation of the common bile duct. Type II cysts are true diverticular outpouching of the bile ducts. Type III cysts (choledochoceles) are a dilation of the distal mural portion of the common bile duct that protrudes into the duodenum. Type IV cysts are multifocal biliary dilations of the intrahepatic and extrahepatic ducts. Type V cysts have been classified as Caroli's disease.

◢ *Sonographic Findings.* Choledochal cysts appear as true cysts in the right upper quadrant with or without an apparent communication with the biliary system (Figures 10-39 and 10-40). The cystic structure may contain internal sludge, stones, or solid neoplasm. If the cyst is very large, the connection to the bile duct may be difficult to distinguish on sonography.

Caroli's Disease. Caroli's disease is a rare congenital abnormality that is most likely inherited in an autosomal recessive fashion. This condition is a communicating cavernous ectasia of intrahepatic ducts characterized by congenital segmental saccular cystic dilation of major intrahepatic bile ducts. It is usually found in the young adult or pediatric population and may be associated with renal disease or congenital hepatic fibrosis. Patient symptoms include recurrent cramplike upper abdominal pain secondary to biliary stasis, ductal stones, cholangitis, and hepatic fibrosis. Cystic disease of the kidney (medullary sponge kidney) is strongly associated with Caroli's disease. Renal failure may be a dominant feature. There are two types of Caroli's disease: the simple classic form and the more common form that is associated with periportal hepatic fibrosis.

◢ *Sonographic Findings.* On sonographic examination, multiple cystic structures in the area of the ductal system converge toward the porta hepatis (Figure 10-41). These masses may be seen as localized or diffusely scattered cysts that communicate with the bile ducts. The differential will include cystic liver disease or biliary obstruction. In addition to the abnormality in the porta hepatis, the ducts may show a beaded appearance as they extend into the periphery of the liver. Ectasia of the extrahepatic and common bile ducts may be present. In addition, sludge or calculi may reside in the dilated ducts. Secondary signs of portal hypertension may occur. The "central dot" sign is classic for Caroli's disease and is caused by the dilated duct surrounding the adjacent hepatic artery and portal vein.

Dilated Biliary Ducts

The small size of the peripheral intrahepatic bile ducts (normally less than 2 mm) implies that sonography cannot image the ducts routinely until their size dilates to greater than 4 mm. Evaluation of the portal structures will allow the sonographer to search for the dilated ducts as they parallel the course of the portal veins. The common hepatic duct has an internal diameter of less than 4 mm. A duct diameter of 5 mm is borderline, and one of 6 mm requires further investigation. A patient may have a normal-size hepatic duct and still have distal obstruction. The distal duct is often obscured by gas in the duodenal loop. The common bile duct has an

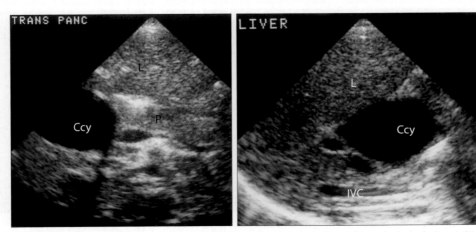

FIGURE 10-39 Transverse and longitudinal scans of a young patient with a choledochal cyst *(Ccy)* in the right upper quadrant. *IVC,* Inferior vena cava; *L,* liver; *P,* pancreas.

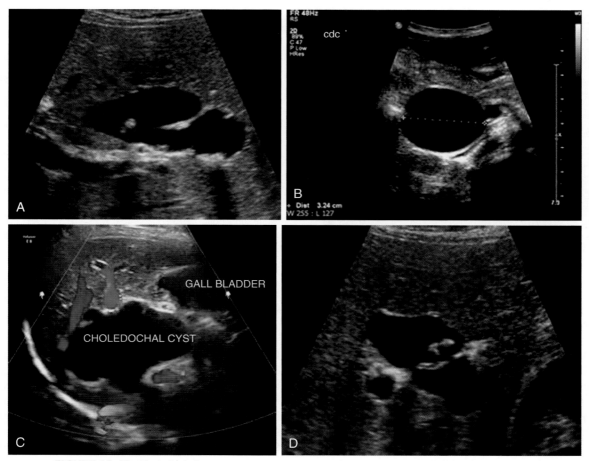

FIGURE 10-40 Choledochal cysts appear as true cysts in the right upper quadrant with or without an apparent communication with the biliary system; the cystic structure may contain internal sludge, stones, or solid neoplasm.

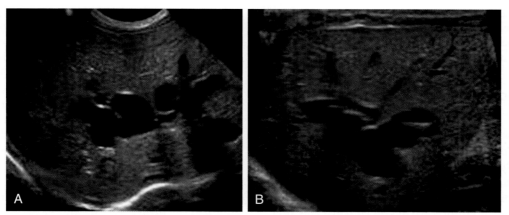

FIGURE 10-41 **Caroli's disease.** Multiple cystic structures in the area of the ductal system converge toward the porta hepatis; masses may be localized or diffusely scattered cysts that communicate with the bile ducts.

internal diameter slightly greater than that of the hepatic duct. Generally a duct more than 6 mm in diameter is considered borderline and more than 10 mm is dilated (Figure 10-42). The dilated duct is distinguished from the portal vein by its tortuosity, increased through transmission and central stellate configuration.

Biliary Obstruction

The most common cause of biliary ductal system obstruction is the presence of a tumor or thrombus within the ductal system. The process may be found in the extrahepatic or intrahepatic ductal pathway. Obstruction of the biliary ductal

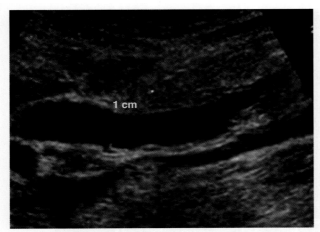

FIGURE 10-42 Longitudinal image of a dilated common bile duct measuring 1.0 cm.

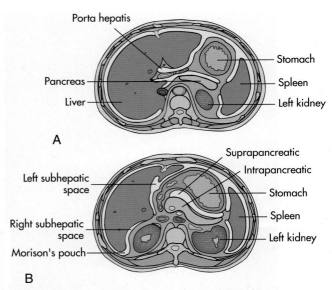

FIGURE 10-43 Levels of obstruction. **A,** Porta hepatic. **B,** Intrapancreatic and suprapancreatic.

system is diagnosed by ultrasound when the sonographer finds the presence of ductal dilation. This finding has been termed on sonography as "too many tubes" or "shotgun" sign when intrahepatic ducts are dilated. These dilated intrahepatic ducts can be seen as parallel channels adjacent to the portal veins. The normal intrahepatic ducts should not be more than 40% of the diameter of the adjacent portal vein. Likewise, the peripheral ducts should not be more than 2 mm in diameter.

Bile ducts expand centrifugally from the point of obstruction. Therefore extrahepatic dilation occurs before intrahepatic dilation. In patients with obstructive jaundice, isolated dilation of the extrahepatic duct may be present. Fibrosed or infiltrative disease of the liver may prevent intrahepatic dilation because of lack of compliance of the hepatic parenchyma.

Clinically the elevation of cholestatic liver parameters may present as jaundice. Painful jaundice is seen with acute obstruction or infection that may invade the biliary tree.

Extrahepatic Biliary Obstruction

The job of the sonographer is to localize the level and cause of the obstruction. The least restrictive segment of the bile duct is the midsegment between the right hepatic artery and the pancreas, so this segment dilates first in obstruction. Dilation is present when the duct is more than 7 mm in diameter. The sonographer should keep in mind that the duct does increase in size with age and after cholecystectomy.

Another assessment of extrahepatic ductal dilation is to measure the proximal duct at the point it crosses the right hepatic artery. A duct more than 4 mm is abnormal at this intersection. This segment may not dilate as early as the midduct. Also, there may be partial or intermittent obstruction of the duct.

There are three primary areas for obstruction to occur: (1) intrapancreatic, (2) suprapancreatic, and (3) porta hepatic (Figure 10-43).

Intrapancreatic Obstruction. There are three important conditions that cause the majority of biliary obstruction at the level of the distal duct and cause the extrahepatic duct to be entirely dilated: (1) pancreatic carcinoma, (2) choledocholithiasis, and (3) chronic pancreatitis with stricture formation (Figure 10-44, *A*).

Suprapancreatic Obstruction. This obstruction originates between the pancreas and the porta hepatis. The head of the pancreas, the intrapancreatic duct, and pancreatic duct are normal with ultrasound. The most common cause for this obstruction is malignancy or adenopathy at this level.

Porta Hepatic Obstruction. This area of obstruction is usually due to a neoplasm. In patients with obstruction at the level of the porta hepatis, ultrasound will show intrahepatic ductal dilation and a normal common duct (Figure 10-44, *B*). Hydrops of the gallbladder may be present.

Mirizzi syndrome is an uncommon cause for extrahepatic biliary obstruction resulting from an impacted stone in the cystic duct or gallbladder neck, which creates extrinsic mechanical compression of the common hepatic duct (Figure 10-44, *C*). The patient presents with painful jaundice. This stone may penetrate into the common hepatic duct or the gut, which results in a cholecystobiliary or cholecystenteric fistula. In this case the cystic duct inserts unusually low into the common hepatic duct, and thus the two ducts have parallel alignment, which allows for the development of this syndrome. Using sonography, an intrahepatic ductal dilation is seen with a normal-size common duct and a large stone in the neck of the gallbladder or cystic duct.

▶ *Sonographic Findings.* Minimal dilation may be seen in nonjaundiced patients with gallstones or pancreatitis or in jaundiced patients with a common duct stone or tumor (Figures 10-45 and 10-46). However, a diameter

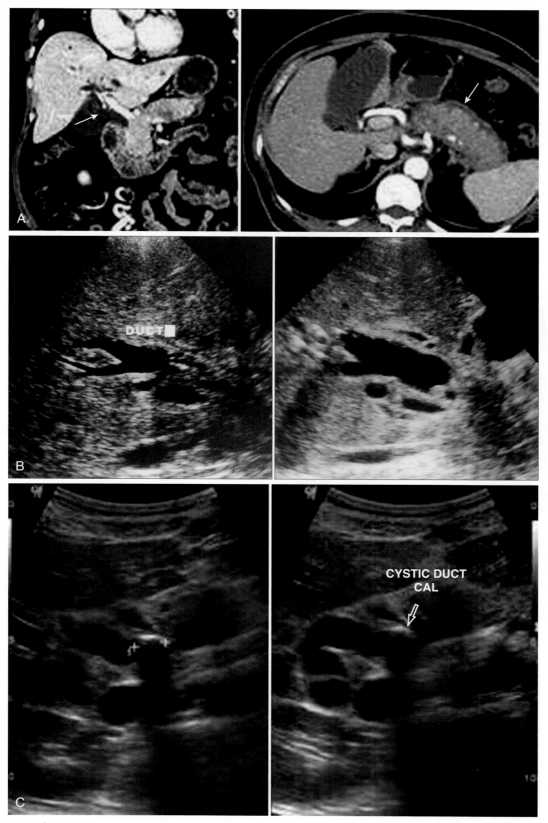

FIGURE 10-44 **Intrapancreatic obstruction. A,** Pancreatic carcinoma causing obstruction to the distal duct. **B,** Dilated intrahepatic ducts secondary to a mass in the area of the porta hepatis. **C,** Stone lodged in the cystic duct.

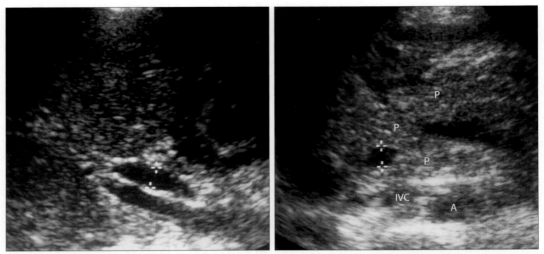

FIGURE 10-45 Inflammation of the pancreas may cause the common duct to dilate. This patient had acute pancreatitis *(P)* and dilation of the common duct *(crossbars)*. *A*, Aorta; *IVC*, inferior vena cava.

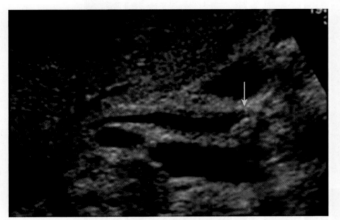

FIGURE 10-46 Arrow denotes the stone in the distal common duct.

of more than 11 mm suggests obstruction by stone or tumor of the duct or pancreas or some other source (Figure 10-47).

Dilated ducts may also be found in the absence of jaundice. The patient may have biliary obstruction involving one hepatic duct, an early obstruction secondary to carcinoma, or gallstones causing intermittent obstruction resulting from a ball-valve effect (Figure 10-48).

Choledocholithiasis

Choledocholithiasis is classified into primary and secondary forms. Primary choledocholithiasis is the de novo formation of calcium stones in the bile duct. These stones may result from disease causing strictures or dilation of the bile ducts leading to stasis, as seen in sclerosing cholangitis, Caroli's disease, parasitic infections, chronic hemolytic diseases, and prior biliary surgery. The secondary form denotes that the majority of stones in the common bile duct have migrated from the gallbladder. Common duct stones are usually associated with calculous cholecystitis.

▎ *Sonographic Findings.* Stones tend to become impacted in the distal portion of the intrahepatic duct of the ampulla of Vater and may project into the duodenum (Figure 10-49). This is the reason it is important for the surgeons to check the common bile duct when removing the gallbladder. The sonographer should look for a dilated duct with a ductal stone that appears hyperechoic and casts

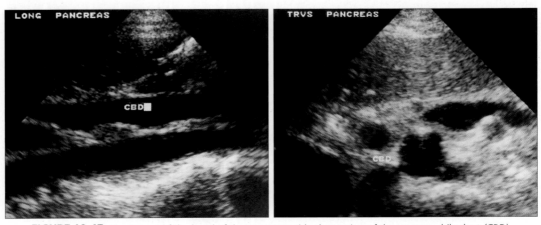

FIGURE 10-47 Carcinoma of the head of the pancreas with obstruction of the common bile duct *(CBD)*.

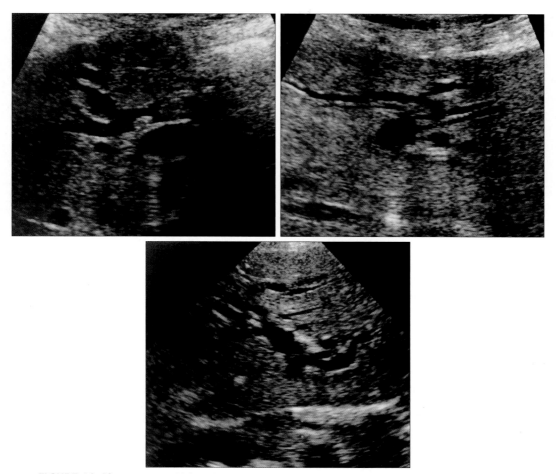

FIGURE 10-48 A 60-year-old female with a history of cholecystectomy several years previously. The patient was known to have had previous hepatic calculi and now has right-upper-quadrant pain. Moderate diffuse dilation of the right and left intrahepatic ducts is present. Echogenic ovoid structures seen in the distal right hepatic and left hepatic ducts represent calculi or sludge balls. The intrahepatic duct was minimally dilated.

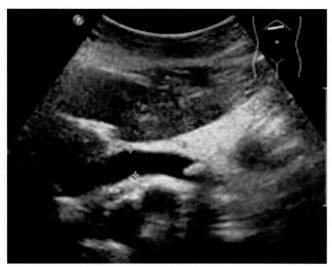

FIGURE 10-49 **Choledocholithiasis.** Stones tend to become impacted in the distal portion of the intrahepatic duct of the ampulla of Vater and may project into the duodenum.

a posterior shadow. Not all ductal stones may shadow, nor will they show mobility. Alterations in the patient position ranging from the right posterior oblique to upright scanning may help distinguish the impacted ductal stone from the duodenum.

Other Causes of Shadowing. The sonographer should be aware that structures or conditions other than stones may lead to attenuation of the ultrasound beam or shadowing. Calcifications in the hepatic artery and pancreatic head may cause shadowing to occur in the area of the gallbladder and be misinterpreted as stones. Air or gas within the duodenum may also give rise to a dirty shadow in the right upper quadrant. Intrabiliary gas is sometimes difficult to separate from stones, although the gas usually produces a brighter reflection with a ring-down artifact and dirtier shadow versus the clean sharp shadow from a stone (Figure 10-50). Another cause of shadowing in the right upper quadrant is gas in the biliary tree. This is a spontaneous occurrence resulting from the formation of a biliary enteric fistula in chronic gallbladder disease.

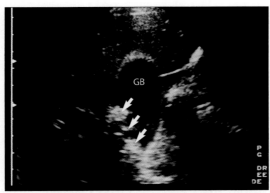

FIGURE 10-50 Gas in the right upper quadrant may cause shadowing in the area of the gallbladder (*GB, arrows*).

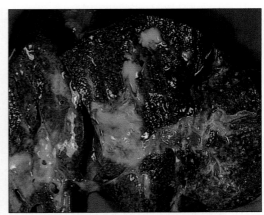

FIGURE 10-51 Gross pathology of bacterial cholangitis with pus in the bile ducts.

Intrahepatic duct stones are less common than common bile duct stones. The intrahepatic duct stones tend to form primarily in the bile ducts and typically are a complication of another biliary tract abnormality.

Hemobilia

Biliary trauma secondary to percutaneous biliary procedures or liver biopsies accounts for the majority of hemobilia cases. Other causes include cholangitis, cholecystitis, vascular malformations, abdominal trauma, and malignancies. The usual clinical findings are pain, bleeding, and jaundice. The sonographic appearance of blood in the biliary tree will depend on the length of time the blood has been present. Acute hemorrhage will appear as fluid with low-level internal echoes. Look for blood clots that may move in the duct with extension into the gallbladder.

Pneumobilia

Pneumobilia is air within the biliary tree secondary to biliary intervention, biliary-enteric anastomoses, or common bile duct stents. In the patient with an acute abdomen, pneumobilia may be caused by emphysematous cholecystitis, inflammation from an impacted stone in the common bile duct, or prolonged acute cholecystitis, which may lead to erosion of the bowel. On sonography, the air in the bile ducts presents as bright, echogenic linear structures that follow the portal triads. The posterior dirty shadow and reverberating artifact is seen. The sonographer should look for the movement of tiny air bubbles with a change in the patient's position.

Cholangitis: Bile Duct Wall Thickening

Cholangitis is an inflammation of the bile ducts (Figure 10-51). It may present as acute bacterial cholangitis, recurrent pyogenic cholangitis, or primary sclerosing cholangitis. The cause of cholangitis is dependent on the type of disease, but the obstruction may include ductal strictures, parasitic infestation, bacterial infection, stones, choledochal cysts, or neoplasm.

Cholangitis may be identified as *oriental sclerosing cholangitis* (seen more frequently in the United States with immigration). Other forms of cholangitis include AIDS cholangitis and acute obstructive suppurative cholangitis. Clinically the patient presents with malaise and fever, followed by sweating and shivering. There may be right-upper-quadrant pain and jaundice. In severe cases, the patient is lethargic, prostrate, and in shock. Elevated laboratory values show leukocytosis, as well as elevation of serum alkaline phosphatase and bilirubin.

Cholangitis is a medical emergency as it develops increasing pressure in the biliary tree with pus accumulation. Decompression of the common bile duct is necessary. More than half of the patients with sclerosing cholangitis have ulcerative colitis. Both sclerosing and AIDS cholangitis can have intrahepatic biliary changes that are nearly identical on ultrasound.

Sonographic Findings. The sonographer needs to determine the cause and level of obstruction, as well as exclude other diseases such as cholecystitis or hepatitis. The biliary tree is dilated and the common bile duct wall may show a smooth or irregular thickening (Figure 10-52). There may be choledocholithiasis with sludge. The ductal wall may be so thickened that it is difficult to recognize on sonography without careful evaluation. Cholangitis usually involves the bile duct in a more generalized manner. Careful evaluation of the liver parenchyma should also be made to look for hepatic abscesses.

The subcostal oblique imaging of the porta hepatis to image the portal venous system is the landmark to find the biliary tree. The common bile duct may or may not be enlarged, but the walls may become slightly irregular and thickened. The stones are usually lodged in the distal common bile duct or must be mobile to cause intermittent obstruction.

In patients with oriental cholangitis, the lateral segment of the left lobe of the liver is most often involved. In the acute septic phase, the patient may need urgent percutaneous biliary decompression or surgery. Atrophy of the affected duct develops with chronic stasis and inflammation followed

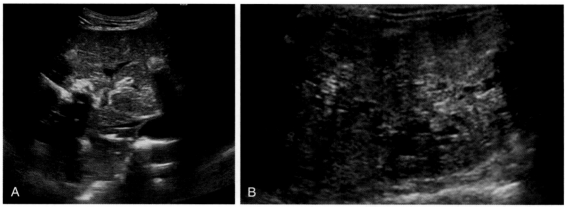

FIGURE 10-52 Cholangitis. The biliary tree is dilated and the common bile duct wall may show a smooth or irregular thickening.

by biliary cirrhosis and cholangiocarcinoma. Ultrasound is excellent for following these patients. As the biliary tree dilates, the internal lumen may be hypoechoic or echogenic with stones; these stones may not shadow, especially if they are tiny.

Ascariasis

This is a parasitic roundworm *(Ascaris lumbricoides)* that uses a fecal-oral route of transmission. The worm may be 20 to 30 cm long and 6 cm in diameter. It grows in the small bowel before entering the biliary tree through the ampulla of Vater. These worms cause acute biliary obstruction and are dramatic when seen on sonography. Clinically the patient may be asymptomatic or present with biliary colic, pancreatitis, or biliary symptoms.

Sonographic Findings. On sonography the sonographer may denote an enlarged duct with a moving "tube" or parallel echogenic lines within the biliary ducts. As the transducer is rotated into the transverse position, the worm is surrounded by the duct wall and gives a target appearance. If the transducer is held in place over the area, small discrete movements may be seen on the image. The worm may fold over itself, or there may be multiple worms that present as an amorphous echogenic filling defect in the right upper quadrant (Figure 10-53).

Intrahepatic Biliary Neoplasms

Changes in the intrahepatic biliary ducts occur secondary to extrahepatic bile duct obstruction in most cases. Occasionally intrahepatic lesions are responsible for the changes in the duct. Intrahepatic biliary tumors are rare and are primarily limited to cystadenoma and cystadenocarcinoma. The tumors are more frequently found in middle-aged women who clinically present with abdominal pain or mass or jaundice (if the mass is near the porta hepatis). The sonographic appearance is a cystic mass with multiple septa and papillary excrescences. The mass may show variations in this pattern and present as unilocular, calcified,

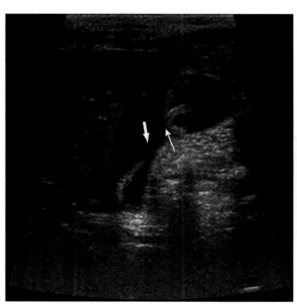

FIGURE 10-53 Ascariasis. On sonography the sonographer may denote an enlarged duct with a moving "tube" or parallel echogenic lines within the biliary ducts.

or multiple. The lesion may be associated with dilation of the intrahepatic ducts. The differential includes a hemorrhagic cyst or infection, echinococcal cyst, abscess, or cystic metastasis.

Cholangiocarcinoma

Cholangiocarcinoma is a rare malignancy that originates within the larger bile ducts, which is usually the common duct or common hepatic duct (Figure 10-54). The incidence is uncommon and the frequency increases with age. The most common risk factor in the Western world is primary sclerosing cholangitis. The classification of the tumor is based on the anatomic location: intrahepatic (peripheral), hilar (Klatskin's), and distal (Figure 10-55). Most cholangiocarcinomas are adenocarcinomas, followed by squamous

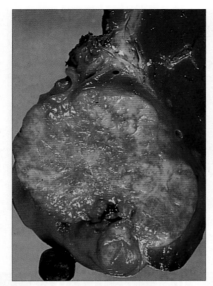

FIGURE 10-54 Gross pathology of cholangiocellular carcinoma.

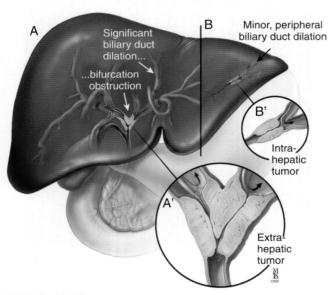

FIGURE 10-55 Cholangiocarcinoma is a rare malignancy that originates within the larger bile ducts, which is usually the common duct or common hepatic duct. *(Department of Art as Applied to Medicine/The Johns Hopkins University School of Medicine © JHU/AAAM 2000. Used with permission.)*

carcinomas. The tumors are further divided into subtypes: sclerosing, nodular, and papillary. Nodular sclerosing tumors are the most common. Hilar cholangiocarcinoma is a nodular sclerosing tumor, a firm mass surrounding and narrowing the affected duct with a nodular intraductal component. Papillary cholangiocarcinomas are found in the distal common bile duct.

Intrahepatic Cholangiocarcinoma. Although this is the least common location for cholangiocarcinomas, it represents the second most common primary malignancy of the liver. An increased incidence of this tumor has risen

over the past two decades secondary to an increasing number of patients with liver cirrhosis and hepatitis C infection. These tumors are often unresectable, with a poor prognosis.

▌ *Sonographic Findings.* On sonography, a large hepatic mass may be seen. The appearance is varied, from hypoechoic to hyperechoic. There may be a heterogeneous texture or hypovascular solid mass. Biliary ductal dilation is associated with these obstructive masses in one third of cases (Figure 10-56, *A* and *B*). Uncommonly, an intrahepatic cholangiocarcinoma presents as one or more polypoid intraductal masses. Another uncommon form may present as a solid mass within a cystic structure that represents a tumor within a very dilated duct that does not communicate with the biliary tree.

Hilar Cholangiocarcinoma. A **Klatskin's tumor** is a specific type of cholangiocarcinoma that can occur at the bifurcation of the common hepatic duct, with involvement of both the central left and right duct. The most suggestive sonographic feature to indicate cholangiocarcinoma is isolated intrahepatic duct dilation. Even though the obstructing mass may not be imaged, a nonunion of the right and left ducts is characteristic for a Klatskin's tumor (Figure 10-56, *C* and *D*).

This tumor is challenging for most imaging modalities. The patient clinically presents with jaundice, pruritus, and elevated cholestatic liver parameters. This disease usually begins in the right or left bile duct and then extends into the proximal duct and distally into the common hepatic duct and contralateral bile ducts. The tumor may extend outside the ducts to involve the adjacent portal vein and arteries. Chronic obstruction leads to atrophy of the involved lobe. The nodal disease originates in the porta hepatis and extends to the celiac axis with subsequent metastases to the liver. Although surgical resection is utilized, the majority of patients die within a year of diagnosis.

With sonography, careful attention is directed to the porta hepatis region. The sonographer should assess the level of the obstruction, the presence of a mass, lobar atrophy, and the patency of main, right, and left portal veins; the sonographer should also evaluate the encasement of the hepatic artery and look for local and distant adenopathy and metastases.

If the ducts are dilated, the sonographer should follow their course centrally toward the hepatic hilum to determine which order of branching is involved with the tumor. Resection is precluded once the tumor extension is found in the segmental ducts.

Evaluation of the portal system is critical. The narrowing of the right or left portal vein leads to compensatory increased flow in the hepatic artery. Tumor narrowing or encasing that obliterates the main portal vein or proper hepatic artery makes the tumor unresectable.

Distal Cholangiocarcinoma. This tumor is difficult to distinguish from hilar cholangiocarcinoma, although progressive jaundice is seen in the majority of patients. The

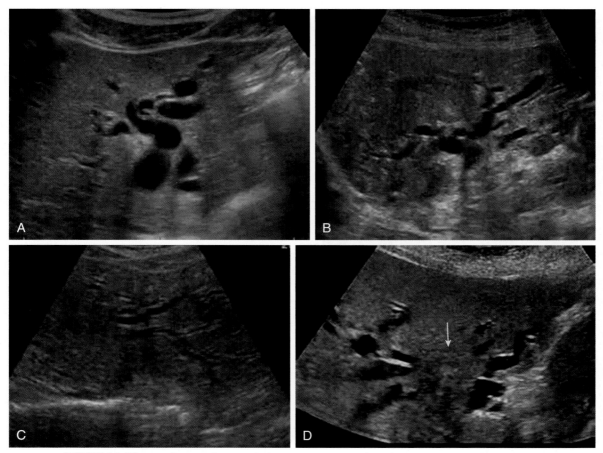

FIGURE 10-56 **A** and **B,** Intrahepatic cholangiocarcinoma. A large heterogeneous or hypovascular solid hepatic mass may be seen with a variable texture that ranges from hypoechoic to hyperechoic. Biliary ductal dilation may also be associated with these obstructive masses. **C** and **D,** Klatskin's tumor is a specific type of cholangiocarcinoma that can occur at the bifurcation of the common hepatic duct, with involvement of both the central left and right duct. The most suggestive sonographic feature to indicate cholangiocarcinoma is isolated intrahepatic duct dilation.

tumor mass may be sclerosing or polypoid. Evaluation of tumor spread in the superior ductal system and extrahepatic area should be carefully evaluated. The tumor may extend into the adjacent lymph nodes.

Sonographic Findings. On sonography, the sclerosing tumor is nodular with focal irregular ductal constriction and wall thickening (Figure 10-57). The tumor is hypoechoic and hypovascular with poorly defined margins. The more common polypoid tumor is seen as a hypovascular well-defined mass found within the distal ductal system.

Metastases to the Biliary Tree. The most common tumor sites that can spread to the biliary system are from the breast, colon, or melanoma. These metastases can affect the intrahepatic and extrahepatic ductal system. On sonography, the appearance of metastases is similar to that of cholangiocarcinoma with the tumor presenting as hyperechoic or hypoechoic and hypovascular with poorly defined margins (Figure 10-58).

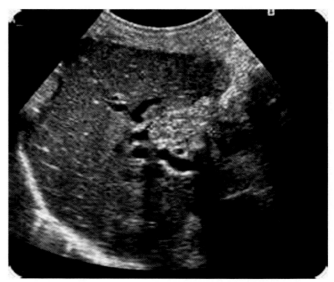

FIGURE 10-57 Distal cholangiocarcinoma on sonography shows a sclerosing tumor as nodular with focal irregular ductal constriction and wall thickening.

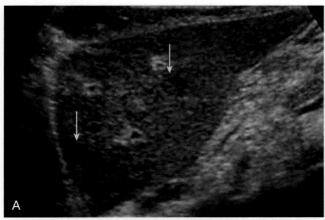

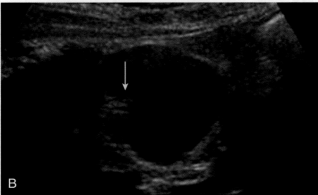

FIGURE 10-58 Metastases to the biliary tree. A, Diffuse isoechoic metastases are seen throughout the liver parenchyma. **B,** Irregular mass *(arrow)* protruding into the gallbladder lumen.

Key Pearls

- The biliary apparatus consists of the right and left hepatic ducts, the common hepatic duct, the common bile duct, the pear-shaped gallbladder, and the cystic duct.
- The bile ducts are divided into intrahepatic and extrahepatic segments. The intrahepatic ducts run in the portal triads along with the portal veins and hepatic arteries. The peripheral intrahepatic ducts run parallel and adjacent to the hepatic arteries and portal veins.
- The extrahepatic portion of the bile ducts includes the common hepatic duct, common bile duct, and a portion of the central right and left ducts.
- The right and left hepatic ducts emerge from the right lobe of the liver in the porta hepatis and unite to form the common hepatic duct, which then passes caudally and medially.
- The common bile duct is joined by the main pancreatic duct, and together they open through a small ampulla (the ampulla of Vater) into the duodenal wall.
- The middle hepatic vein is in alignment with the gallbladder fossa. The interlobar fissure extends from the right portal vein to the gallbladder fossa.
- The gallbladder is divided into the *fundus, body,* and *neck.*

- The primary functions of the extrahepatic biliary tract are (1) the transportation of bile from the liver to the intestine and (2) the regulation of its flow.
- The common duct lies anterior and to the right of the portal vein in the region of the porta hepatis and gastrohepatic ligament. The hepatic artery lies anterior and to the left of the portal vein.
- The most classic symptom of gallbladder disease is right-upper-quadrant abdominal pain, usually occurring after ingestion of greasy foods.
- Jaundice is characterized by the presence of bile in the tissues with resulting yellow-green color of the skin.
- Sludge, or thickened bile, frequently occurs from bile stasis.
- Biliary causes of gallbladder wall thickening include cholecystitis, adenomyomatosis, cancer, AIDS, cholangiopathy, severe hypoalbuminemic state, and sclerosing cholangitis.
- Nonbiliary causes of gallbladder wall thickening include diffuse liver disease (cirrhosis and hepatitis), pancreatitis, portal hypertension, and heart failure.
- Cholecystitis is an inflammation of the gallbladder that may have one of several forms: acute or chronic, acalculous, emphysematous, or gangrenous.
- The patient with acute cholecystitis presents with acute right-upper-quadrant pain (positive Murphy's sign—inspiratory arrest on palpitation of the gallbladder area), fever, and leukocytosis.
- Chronic cholecystitis is the result of numerous attacks of acute cholecystitis with subsequent fibrosis of the gallbladder wall.
- When the gallbladder is completely packed full of stones, the sonographer will only be able to image the anterior border of the gallbladder, with the stones casting a distinct acoustic shadow known as the wall, echo, shadow (WES) sign.
- Cholelithiasis is the most common disease of the gallbladder.
- A porcelain gallbladder is associated with gallstones in the majority of patients and may represent a form of chronic cholecystitis and inflammation.
- Cholesterolosis is a condition in which cholesterol is deposited within the lamina propria of the gallbladder and is often associated with cholesterol stones.
- Polyps of the gallbladder are small, well-defined soft tissue projections from the gallbladder wall.
- Adenomyomatosis is a benign condition that demonstrates a hyperplastic change in the gallbladder wall.
- Adenomas are benign neoplasms of the gallbladder with a premalignant potential much lower than colonic adenomas.
- Primary carcinoma of the gallbladder is rare and is nearly always a rapidly progressive disease and is associated with cholelithiasis.
- Choledochal cysts are an unusual, diverse group of diseases that may manifest as congenital, focal, or diffuse cystic dilation of the biliary tree.

- The most common cause of biliary ductal system obstruction is the presence of a tumor or thrombus within the ductal system.
- There are three primary areas for obstruction to occur: (1) intrapancreatic, (2) suprapancreatic, and (3) porta hepatic.
- Cholangitis is an inflammation of the bile ducts that may present as acute bacterial cholangitis, recurrent pyogenic cholangitis, or primary sclerosing cholangitis.
- Cholangiocarcinoma is a rare malignancy that originates within the larger bile ducts, which is usually the common duct or common hepatic duct.
- A Klatskin's tumor is a specific type of cholangiocarcinoma that can occur at the bifurcation of the common hepatic duct, with involvement of both the central left and right duct.

BIBLIOGRAPHY

Ahrendt AS, Nakeeb A, Pitt HA: Cholangiocarcinoma, *Clin Liver Dis* 5:191-218, 2001.

Bachar GN, Cohen M, Belenky A, et al: Effect of aging on the adult entrahepatic bile duct: a sonographic study, *J Ultrasound Med* 22:879-882, 2003.

Buljevac M, Busic Z, Cabrijan Z: Sonographic diagnosis of gallstone ileus, *J Ultrasound Med* 23:1395-1398, 2004.

Collett JA: Gallbladder polyps: prospective study, *J Ultrasound Med* 17:207, 1998.

Dobbins JM, Rao PM, Novelline RA: Posttraumatic hemobilia, *Emerg Radiol* 4:180, 1997.

Frezza EE, Mezghebe H: Gallbladder carcinoma: a 28 year experience, *Int Surg* 82:295, 1997.

Gates J, Kane RA, Hartnell GG: Primary biliary tract malignant melanoma, *Abdom Imaging* 21:453, 1996.

Ghersin E, Soudack M, Galtini D: Twinkling artifact in gallbladder adenomyomatosis, *J Ultrasound Med* 22:229-231, 2003.

Gore RM, Yaghmai V, Newmark GM, et al: Imaging benign and malignant disease of the gallbladder, *Radiol Clin North Am* 40:1307-1323, 2002.

Gremmels JM, Kruskal JB, Parangi S, Kane RA: Hemorrhagic cholecystitis simulating gallbladder carcinoma, *J Ultrasound Med* 23:993-995, 2004.

Hann LE: Cholangiocarcinoma at the hepatic hilus: sonographic findings, *Am J Roentgenol* 168:985, 1997.

Henningsen C: *Clinical guide to ultrasonography*, St Louis, 2005, Mosby.

Indar AA, Beckingham IJ: Acute cholecystitis, *BMJ* 325:639-643, 2002.

Kao EY, Desser TS, Jeffrey RB: Sonographic diagnosis of traumatic gallbladder rupture, *J Ultrasound Med* 21:1295-1297, 2002.

Kim HC, Yang DM, Jin W, et al: Large fibrous polyps of the gallbladder simulating gallbladder carcinoma, *J Ultrasound Med* 28:537-540, 2009.

Klatskin G: Adenocarcinoma of the hepatic duct at its bifurcation within the porta hepatis: an unusual tumor with distinctive clinical and pathologic features, *Am J Med* 38:241, 1965.

Kurtz AB, Middleton WD: *The gallbladder in ultrasound: the requisites*, St Louis, 2004, Mosby.

Laing FC: Sonographic appearances in the gallbladder and biliary tree with emphasis on intracholecystic blood, *J Ultrasound Med* 16:537, 1997.

Lee HJ, Choi BI, Han JK, et al: Three-dimensional ultrasound using the minimum transparent mode in obstructive biliary diseases: early experience, *J Ultrasound Med* 21:443-453, 2002.

Lim JH: Anatomic relationship of intrahepatic bile ducts to portal veins, *J Ultrasound Med* 9:137, 1990.

Markhardi BK, Rubens DJ, Huang J, Doogra VS: Sonographic features of biliary hamartomas with histopathologic correlation, *J Ultrasound Med* 25:1631-1633, 2006.

Mittelstaedt CA: Ultrasound of the bile ducts, *Semin Roentgenol* 32:161, 1997.

Pandey M: Carcinoma of the gallbladder: role of sonography in the diagnosis and staging, *J Clin Ultrasound* 28:227-232, 2000.

Rao AV, Champine JG, Forte TB, Brewington CC: Three-dimensional sonographic evaluation of the common bile duct, *J Ultrasound Med* 22:939-944, 2003.

Rumack CM, Wilson SR, Charboneau JW, Johnson J: *Diagnostic ultrasound*, ed 3, vol 1, St Louis, 2005, Mosby.

Simmons MZ: Pitfalls in ultrasound of the gallbladder and biliary tract, *Ultrasound Q* 14:2, 1998.

Ueno N, Togo S: Bleeding from the gallbladder: novel ultrasonographic features, *J Ultrasound Med* 25:111-113, 2006.

Watanabe Y: Usefulness of intraductal ultrasonography in gallbladder disease, *J Ultrasound Med* 17:33, 1998.

Spleen

Sandra L. Hagen-Ansert

The spleen is the largest single mass of lymphoid tissue in the body. It is part of the **reticuloendothelial** system and has a role in the synthesis of blood proteins. The spleen is active in blood formation (**hematopoiesis**) during the initial part of fetal life. This function decreases gradually by the fifth or sixth month, when the spleen assumes its adult characteristics and discontinues its hematopoietic (blood-producing) activities. The spleen plays an important role in the defense of the body. Although it is often affected by systemic disease processes, the spleen is rarely the primary site of disease.

The left upper quadrant may be rapidly assessed with sonography in patients with palpable splenomegaly or trauma to the left upper quadrant. The normal texture of the spleen is homogeneous, being slightly more echogenic than the texture of the liver; therefore pathology or blood collection secondary to a splenic rupture is usually easily identified.

ANATOMY OF THE SPLEEN

Normal Anatomy

The spleen is an **intraperitoneal** organ covered with peritoneum over its entire extent, except for a small area at its hilum, where the vascular structures and lymph nodes are located. The spleen lies in the posterior left hypochondrium between the fundus of the stomach and the diaphragm. The splenic axis is along the shaft of the eight to tenth ribs with the lower pole extending forward as far as the midaxillary

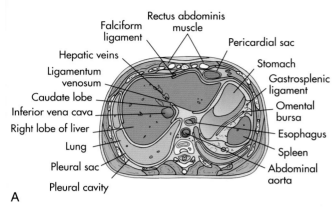

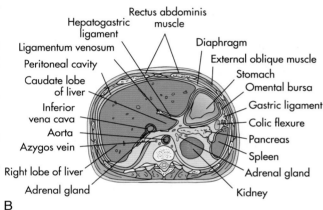

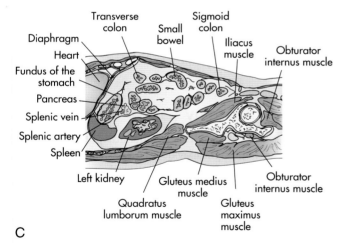

FIGURE 11-1 **A,** Transverse plane of the upper abdomen shows the posterior position of the spleen in the left upper quadrant. **B,** Transverse plane of the spleen. **C,** Sagittal plane of the spleen and left kidney.

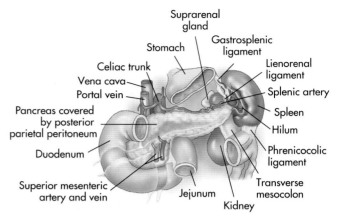

FIGURE 11-2 Anterior view of the spleen as it lies in the left hypochondrium. Note the relational anatomy, ligament attachments, and vascular landmarks.

of the dorsal mesentery that separate the lesser sac posteriorly from the greater sac anteriorly. A protective capsule covers the spleen with peritoneum. In most adults, a portion of the splenic capsule is firmly adherent to the fused dorsal mesentery anterior to the upper pole of the left kidney, which produces a "bare area" of the spleen. This bare area can be helpful in distinguishing intraperitoneal from pleural fluid collections.

Size

The spleen is of variable size and shape (e.g., "orange segment," tetrahedral, triangular) but generally is considered to be ovoid with smooth, even borders and a convex superior and concave inferior surface (see Figure 11-4). The spleen is normally measured with ultrasound on a longitudinal image from the upper margin (near the diaphragm) to the inferior margin at the long axis (Figure 11-3). Normal measurements for the average adult should be 8 to 13 cm in length, 7 cm in width, and 3 to 4 cm in thickness. The spleen decreases slightly in size with advancing age. The size of the spleen may vary in size in accordance with the nutritional status of the body.

Vascular Supply

Blood is supplied to the spleen by the tortuous **splenic artery** that travels horizontally along the superior border of the pancreas (Figure 11-4). On entering the **splenic hilum,** the splenic artery immediately branches into six smaller arteries to supply the organ with oxygenated blood to profuse the splenic parenchyma. Color Doppler imaging allows the sonographer to image the vascularity of the spleen; gray-scale imaging will show small echogenic lines throughout the spleen that represent the arterial system. The splenic arteries are subject to **infarction** because adequate anastomoses between the vessels are lacking.

The **splenic vein** is formed by multiple branches within the spleen and leaves the hilum in a horizontal direction to

line (Figure 11-1). The inferomedial surface of the spleen comes into contact with the stomach, left kidney, pancreas, and splenic flexure of the colon (Figure 11-2). The peritoneal ligament that attaches the spleen to the stomach and the kidney is called the *splenorenal ligament.* This ligament is in contact with the posterior peritoneal wall, the *phrenicocolic ligament,* and the *gastrosplenic ligament.* The **gastrosplenic ligament** is significant in that it is composed of the two layers

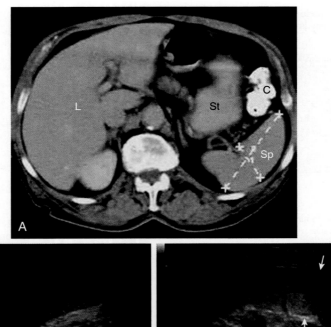

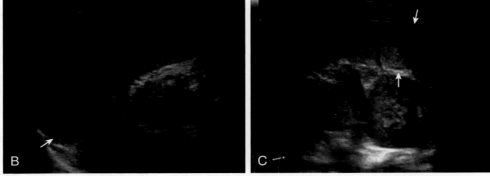

FIGURE 11-3   A, Transverse CT image of the upper left quadrant demonstrates the posterior position of the spleen. *Sp,* spleen; *L,* liver; *St,* stomach; and *C,* colon. Transverse image **(B)** and longitudinal image **(C)** of the spleen with measurements.

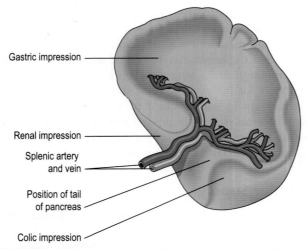

FIGURE 11-4 The spleen is variable in size and shape. The tortuous splenic artery provides the arterial supply to the spleen.

join the superior mesenteric vein. The superior mesenteric vein returns unoxygenated blood from the bowel to form the main portal vein (Figure 11-5). The splenic vein usually travels along the posteromedial border of the pancreas.

The **lymph** vessels emerge from the splenic hilum, pass through other lymph nodes along the course of the splenic artery, and drain into the celiac nodes. The nerves to the

spleen accompany the splenic artery and are derived from the celiac plexus.

Relational Anatomy

The spleen lies between the left hemidiaphragm and the stomach. The diaphragm may be seen as a bright, curvilinear, echogenic structure close to the proximal superolateral surface of the spleen. Posteriorly, the diaphragm, left pleura, left

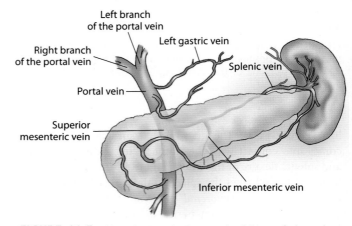

FIGURE 11-5 The splenic vein leaves the hilum of the spleen to join the main portal vein posterior to the head of the pancreas.

lung, and ribs are in contact with the spleen. The medial surface is related to the stomach and lesser sac (Figure 11-6). The fundus of the stomach may contain gas or fluid, which may cause confusion in the left upper quadrant during attempts to demonstrate the spleen. Alteration in the patient position or ingestion of fluids may help to separate stomach from splenic tissue. The tail of the pancreas lies posterior to the stomach and lesser sac as it approaches the hilum of the spleen and splenic vessels. The spleen may serve as a good acoustic window to image the tail of the pancreas. The left kidney lies inferior and medial to the spleen.

Displacement of the Spleen

The spleen is held in place by the lienorenal, gastrosplenic, and phrenocolic ligaments (see Figure 15-2). These ligaments are derived from the layers of peritoneum that form the greater and lesser sacs. A mass in the left upper quadrant may displace the spleen inferiorly. Caudal displacement may occur secondary to a subclavian abscess, splenic cyst, or left pleural effusion. Cephalic displacement may result from volume loss in the left lung, left lobe pneumonia, paralysis of the left hemidiaphragm, or a large intraabdominal mass. A normal spleen with medial lobulation between the pancreatic tail and the left kidney may be confused with a cystic mass in the tail of the pancreas.

The term **"wandering" spleen** describes a spleen that has migrated from its normal location in the left upper quadrant. It is the result of an embryologic anomaly of the dorsal mesentery that fails to fuse with the posterior peritoneum without supporting ligaments of the spleen. The patient may present with an abdominal or pelvic mass, intermittent

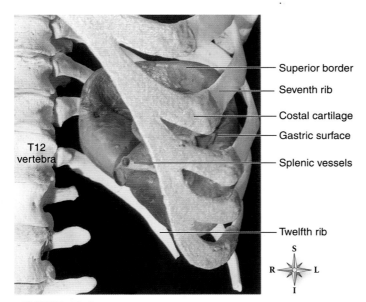

FIGURE 11-6 The spleen lies between the left hemidiaphragm and the stomach. Posteriorly, the diaphragm, left pleura, left lung, and ribs are in contact with the spleen. The medial surface is related to the stomach and lesser sac. The tail of the pancreas lies posterior to the stomach and lesser sac as it approaches the hilum of the spleen and splenic vessels. The left kidney lies inferior and medial to the spleen.

pain, and volvulus, that is, splenic torsion. The sonographer should use color Doppler to map the vascularity within the spleen. When torsion is complete, the vascular pattern shows decreased velocity.

Congenital Anomalies

Splenic Agenesis. Complete absence of the spleen (asplenia), or **splenic agenesis,** is rare and by itself causes no difficulties. However, it may occur as part of a major congenital abnormality. Visceral heterotaxy is the common name that consists of a spectrum of anomalies. Asplenic or **polysplenia** syndromes are associated with complex cardiac malformations, bronchopulmonary abnormalities, or visceral heterotaxis (anomalous placement of organs or major blood vessels, including a horizontal liver, malrotation of the gut, and interruption of the inferior vena cava with azygos continuation). The normal arrangement of asymmetric body parts is called *situs solitus.* The mirror image condition is called *situs inversus.* The term *situs ambiguous* is used when the anatomy falls in between these two conditions.

Patients with polysplenia may have bilateral left-sidedness (two morphologic left lungs, left-sided azygous continuation of an interrupted inferior vena cava, biliary atresia, absence of the gallbladder, gastrointestinal malrotation, and cardiovascular abnormalities). On the other hand, patients with asplenia may have bilateral right-sidedness (two morphologic right lungs, midline location of the liver, reversed position of the abdominal aorta and inferior vena cava, anomalous pulmonary venous return, and horseshoe kidneys). Patients with agenesis of the spleen have major problems with serious infection, as their immune response is absent.

Splenic agenesis may be ruled out by demonstrating a spleen on ultrasound. The sonographer should be careful not to confuse the spleen with the bowel, which may lie in the area normally occupied by the spleen. Color Doppler helps determine the splenic vascular pattern and thus helps to separate it from the colon.

Accessory Spleen. An **accessory spleen,** or *splenunculus,* is a more common congenital anomaly that may be found in up to 30% of patients (Figure 11-7). The accessory spleen may be difficult to demonstrate by sonography if it is very small. However, when it is seen, it appears as a homogeneous pattern similar to that of the spleen. It usually is found near the hilum or inferior border of the spleen but has been reported elsewhere in the abdominal cavity. Lesions affecting the normal spleen would also affect the accessory spleen. An accessory spleen results from failure of fusion of separate splenic masses forming on the dorsal mesogastrium; it is most commonly located in the splenic hilum or along the splenic vessels or associated ligaments. The location of the accessory spleen has been reported anywhere from the diaphragm to the scrotum, and it is usually solitary. It usually remains small and does not present as a clinical problem. The accessory spleen may simulate enlarged lymph nodes in the area of the spleen, or a tumor of the pancreatic, suprarenal, or retroperitoneal structures. As the spleen enlarges, so does the accessory spleen.

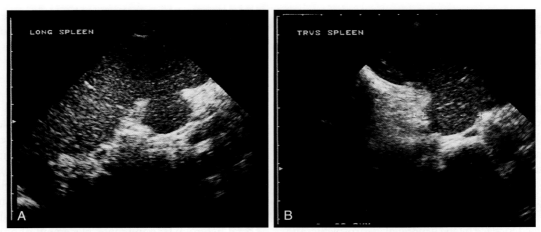

FIGURE 11-7 Accessory spleen. Long **(A)** and transverse **(B)** images of the small accessory spleen as it projects from the hilum of the spleen.

PHYSIOLOGY AND LABORATORY DATA OF THE SPLEEN

The spleen is part of the reticuloendothelial system and is rarely the site of primary disease. It is commonly involved in metabolic, hematopoietic, and infectious disorders. Blunt abdominal trauma to the spleen may result in splenic laceration and rupture. The spleen is active in the body's defense against disease; its major function is to filter the peripheral blood.

The spleen is a soft organ with elastic properties that allow it to distend as blood fills the venous sinuses. These characteristics are related to the function of the spleen as a blood reservoir. Within the lobules of the spleen are tissues called *pulp*. Two components are found within the spleen: red pulp and white pulp (Figure 11-8). *White pulp* is distributed throughout the spleen in tiny islands. This tissue consists of splenic nodules, which are similar to those found in lymph nodes and contain large numbers of lymphocytes. *Red pulp* fills the remaining spaces of the lobules and surrounds the venous sinuses. The pulp contains relatively large numbers of red blood cells, which are responsible for its color, along with many lymphocytes and macrophages.

The **red pulp** of the spleen consists of *splenic sinuses* alternating with splenic cords. The blood capillaries within the red

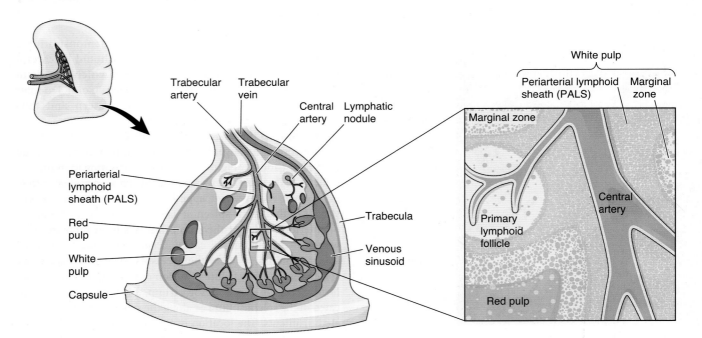

FIGURE 11-8 Within the lobules of the spleen are tissues called *pulp:* red pulp and white pulp. *White pulp* is distributed throughout the spleen in tiny islands. This tissue consists of splenic nodules, which are similar to those found in lymph nodes and contain large numbers of lymphocytes. *Red pulp* fills the remaining spaces of the lobules and surrounds the venous sinuses. The pulp contains relatively large numbers of red blood cells, which are responsible for its color, along with many lymphocytes and macrophages.

pulp are quite permeable. Red blood cells can squeeze through the pores in these capillary walls and enter the venous sinuses. The older, more fragile red blood cells may rupture as they make this passage, and the resulting cellular debris is removed by phagocytic macrophages located within the splenic sinuses. The macrophages engulf and destroy foreign particles, such as bacteria, that may be carried in the blood as it flows through the sinuses. The lymphocytes of the spleen help to defend the body against infection. The blood that leaves the splenic sinuses to enter the reticular cords passes through a complex filter. The venous drainage of the sinuses and cords is not well defined, but it is assumed that tributaries of the splenic vein connect with sinuses of the red pulp.

The **white pulp** of the spleen consists of the *malpighian corpuscles,* small nodular masses of lymphoid tissue attached to the smaller arterial branches. Extending from the splenic capsule inward are the trabeculae, which contain blood vessels and lymphatics. The lymphoid tissue or malpighian corpuscles have the same structure as the follicles in the lymph nodes; however, they differ in that the splenic follicles surround arteries, so that on cross section, each contains a central artery. These follicles are scattered throughout the organ and are not confined to the peripheral layer or cortex, as are lymph nodes.

As part of the reticuloendothelial system, the spleen plays an important role in the defense mechanisms of the body and is also implicated in pigment and lipid metabolism. It is not essential to life and can be removed with no ill effects. The functions of the spleen may be classified under two general headings: those that reflect the functions of the reticuloendothelial system and those that are characteristic of the organ itself (Box 11-1). The role of the spleen as an immunologic organ involves the production of cells capable of making antibodies (lymphocytes and plasma cells); however, antibodies are also produced at other sites.

Phagocytosis of **erythrocytes** and the breakdown of **hemoglobin** occur throughout the entire reticuloendothelial system, but roughly half the catabolic activity is localized in the normal spleen. In splenomegaly, the major portion of hemoglobin breakdown occurs in the spleen. The iron that is liberated is stored in the splenic phagocytes. In anomalies such as the hemolytic anemias, the splenic phagocytes become engorged with hemosiderin when erythrocyte destruction is accelerated. In addition to storing iron, the spleen is subject to storage diseases such as Gaucher's disease and Niemann-Pick disease. Abnormal lipid metabolites accumulate in all phagocytic reticuloendothelial cells but may also involve the phagocytes in the spleen, producing gross splenomegaly.

Functions of the spleen that are characteristic of the organ relate primarily to the circulation of erythrocytes through it. In a normal individual, the spleen contains only about 20 to 30 ml of erythrocytes. In splenomegaly the reservoir function is greatly increased, and the abnormally enlarged spleen contains many times this volume of red blood cells. Transit time is lengthened, and the erythrocytes are subject to destructive effects for a long time. In part, ptosis causes consumption of glucose, on which the erythrocyte depends to maintain normal metabolism, and the erythrocyte is destroyed. Selective destruction of abnormal erythrocytes is also accelerated by splenic pooling.

As erythrocytes pass through the spleen, the organ inspects them for imperfections and destroys those it recognizes as abnormal or senescent. **Pitting** is the process of removing the nuclei from the red blood cells. **Culling** is the process by which the spleen removes abnormal red blood cells. The normal function of the spleen keeps the number of circulating erythrocytes with inclusions at a minimum.

The spleen also pools platelets in large numbers. Entry of platelets into the splenic pool and their return to the circulation are extensive. In splenomegaly, the splenic pool may be so large that it produces thrombocytopenia. Sequestration of leukocytes in the enlarged spleen may produce **leukopenia.**

Laboratory data include the following:
- *Hematocrit.* The hematocrit indicates the percentage of red blood cells per volume of blood. Abnormally low readings indicate hemorrhage or internal bleeding within the body.
- *Bacteremia.* The test for bacteremia indicates the presence of bacteria within the body. The term *sepsis* indicates bacteria in the bloodstream. Typical symptoms of fever and chills, along with other medical conditions, may indicate the presence of an infection.
- *Leukocytosis.* An increase in the number of white cells present in the blood is usually a typical finding in infection. This finding may also occur after surgery, in malignancies, or in the presence of leukemia.
- *Leukopenia.* Abnormal decrease in white blood corpuscles may be secondary to certain medications or bone marrow disorder.
- *Thrombocytopenia.* Thrombocytopenia is an abnormal decrease in platelets, which may be due to internal hemorrhage.

SONOGRAPHIC EVALUATION OF THE SPLEEN

Spleen Protocol

Ultrasound examinations are performed to assess overall splenic architecture, to examine or detect intrasplenic masses,

---

BOX 11-1 | Functions of the Spleen

Functions of the Spleen as an Organ of the Reticuloendothelial System
Production of lymphocytes and plasma cells
Production of antibodies
Storage of iron
Storage of other metabolites

Functions Characteristic of the Spleen
Maturation of the surface of erythrocytes
Reservoir
Culling
Pitting function
Disposal of senescent or abnormal erythrocytes
Functions related to platelet and leukocyte life span

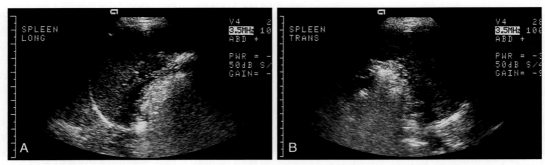

FIGURE 11-9 Normal spleen. Long **(A)** and transverse **(B)** images of the normal spleen with measurements. The parenchyma is homogeneous throughout except for the area of the hilum where the vascular structures enter and leave the spleen.

TABLE 11-1	Abdominal Protocol: Spleen
Scan Plane Anatomy	
Long spleen/left kidney; measure length; color Doppler	
Transverse splenic hilum; measure width; color Doppler	

to examine the splenic hilum and vasculature, and to determine splenic size (Figure 11-9 and Table 11-1).

1. Patient preparation: nothing by mouth (NPO) for at least 6 hours.
2. Transducer selection: broadband (2.5 to 4 MHz) curvilinear or sector.
3. Patient position: supine; or steep left lateral if echo bed with a drop-leaf component is available.
4. Images and observations include the following:
   - Coronal scans of the long axis of the spleen should be performed.
   - The left hemidiaphragm, splenic hilus, and upper and lower borders of the spleen should be demonstrated.
   - The splenic length should be measured.
   - The texture of the spleen should be compared with that of the liver. The splenic parenchyma should be homogeneous with the liver.
   - Transverse scans of the spleen at the level of the splenic hilus should be performed. The sonographer should look for increased vascularity or splenic nodes with a sweep from the superior to inferior borders.

Normal Texture and Patterns

Sonographically, the splenic parenchyma should have a fine uniform homogeneous mid- to low-level echo pattern, and slightly more echogenic than the liver parenchyma (Figure 11-10). As the spleen enlarges, echogenicity further increases. The shape of the spleen has considerable variation. The spleen has two components joined at the hilum: a superomedial component and an inferolateral component. On transverse scans, it has a "crescent" inverted comma appearance, usually with a large medial component and a thin component extending anteriorly. This part of the spleen may be seen to indent the fundus of the stomach. Moving inferiorly, only the lateral component is imaged. On longitudinal scans, the superior component extends more medially than the inferior component. The superomedial component or the inferolateral component may enlarge independently. The irregularity of these components makes it difficult to assess mild splenomegaly accurately. The length of the spleen usually measures greater than the length of the kidney.

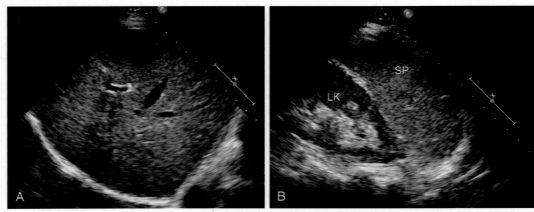

FIGURE 11-10 The splenic parenchyma should have a fine uniform homogeneous mid- to low-level echo pattern, which is slightly more echogenic than the liver. **A,** Liver and **B,** spleen. *LK,* Left kidney; *SP,* spleen.

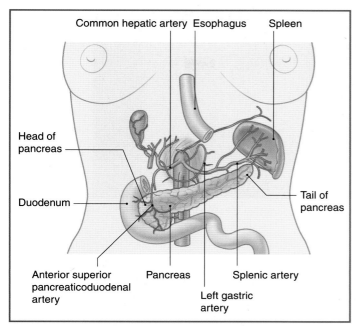

FIGURE 11-11 The spleen lies in an oblique pathway in the posterior left upper quadrant.

Splenomegaly is diagnosed when the spleen measures more than 13 cm in the adult patient, or more than normal length in the child.

Patient Position and Technique

The left upper quadrant may be imaged as the sonographer carefully manipulates the transducer between intercostal margins to image the left kidney, spleen, and diaphragm. The sector transducer may fit between the intercostal margins better than the larger curved-array transducer. The spleen generally lies in an oblique pathway in the posterior left upper quadrant (Figure 11-11); therefore with the patient supine, the transducer should be placed in the superior left upper quadrant intercostal margin and slowly sweep anterior to posterior along the long

axis of the spleen. The transducer must be positioned superior and posterior enough to image the spleen (Figure 11-12). A deep inspiration may help to bring the spleen farther into the field of view from the subcostal approach. Variations in patient respiration may also facilitate imaging of the spleen; deep inspiration causes the lungs to expand with air and displaces the diaphragm; the lungs may expand so fully that the costophrenic angle is obscured and visualization of the spleen is impeded. The sonographer should observe the patient's breathing pattern and modify the amount of inspiration to adequately image the spleen without interference from the air-filled lungs.

When the patient is lying supine, the problem of overlying air-filled stomach or bowel anterior to the spleen may interfere with adequate visualization. The steep right decubitus position with the intercostal approach is not recommended as this causes the spleen to fall away from the abdominal wall and allows aerated lung to migrate inferiorly and obscure the acoustic window. If the ultrasound laboratory has an echo bed with a drop-leaf component, the patient should be rolled onto his or her left side and the transducer directed along the left intercostal margin to image the spleen. Excellent visualization is achieved because the spleen will lie flush against the patient's abdominal wall.

In a routine abdominal examination, the spleen should be surveyed to ensure that the parenchyma is uniform with a homogeneous texture, except for the splenic hilum, which shows normal tubular vascular structures. At least two images of the spleen should be recorded in the longitudinal and transverse planes (see Figure 11-10). The longitudinal plane should demonstrate the left hemidiaphragm, the superior and inferior margins of the spleen, and the upper pole of the left kidney. The sonographer should look at the left pleural space superior to the diaphragm to see if fluid is present in the lower costal margin. The long axis of the spleen is measured from its superior-to-inferior border.

After the longitudinal oblique scan is completed, the transducer is rotated 90 degrees to survey the spleen in a transverse plane. The sonographer should obtain at least one transverse image at the hilum of the spleen. The sonographer should observe the flow of the splenic artery and

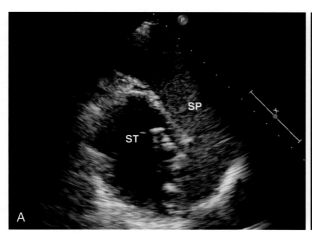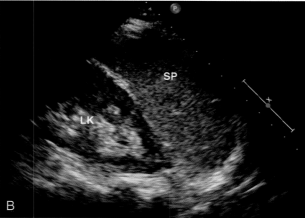

FIGURE 11-12 Normal images of the spleen. **A,** Transverse image of the spleen *(SP)* and fluid-filled stomach *(ST)*. **B,** Longitudinal image of the spleen *(SP)* and left kidney *(LK)*.

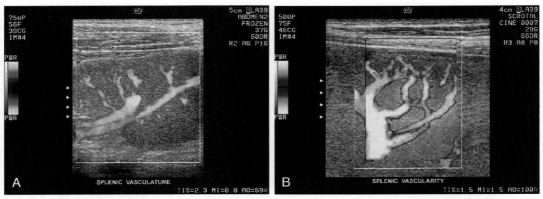

FIGURE 11-13 A, Color Doppler shows the splenic arterial system within the spleen. **B,** The splenic venous system is well demarcated with color Doppler.

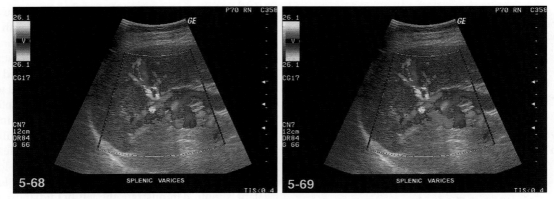

FIGURE 11-14 Color Doppler shows the dilated splenic vessels that may be seen with portal hypertension and varices.

vein with color Doppler. Forward (positive to the baseline) arterial flow should be seen entering the main splenic artery as it bifurcates into multiple branches to supply the splenic parenchyma (Figure 11-13, *A*). Conversely, returning flow (negative to the baseline) from the multiple splenic venous branches enters into the splenic vein. The splenic vein leaves the hilum of the spleen to transverse horizontally across the abdomen before joining the superior mesenteric vein, which leads into the main portal vein anterior to the inferior vena cava (Figure 11-13, *B*).

Increased hypoechoic structures in the area of the splenic hilum may indicate portal hypertension with collateral vessels or enlarged lymph nodes. A correlation has been noted between the caliber of splenic arteries and the size of the spleen in cirrhotic patients with esophageal varices. The splenic artery is larger in patients with splenomegaly (patients with cirrhosis with esophageal varices and patients with hematologic malignancies). The use of color Doppler imaging will help the sonographer determine whether the structures are vascular or nonvascular in composition (Figure 11-14).

Care should be taken when hepatomegaly is present with a prominent left lobe of the liver. The homogeneous texture of the liver may be confused as spleen, especially if the left lobe extends to the left upper quadrant. The sonographer should evaluate the patient in multiple planes in an effort to separate the splenic tissue from the hepatic structures.

Nonvisualization of the Spleen

The inability to image the spleen in its normal location may be a result of one of several conditions (e.g., asplenia syndrome, polysplenia syndrome, traumatic fragmentation of the spleen, wandering spleen).

Atrophy. Atrophy of the spleen may be found in normal individuals. It may also occur in wasting diseases. Chronic hemolytic anemias, particularly sickle cell anemia, involve excessive loss of pulp, increasing fibrosis, scarring from multiple infarcts, and encrustation with iron and calcium deposits. In the final stages of atrophy, the spleen may be so small that it is hardly recognizable. Advanced atrophy is sometimes referred to as autosplenectomy.

PATHOLOGY OF THE SPLEEN

Table 11-2 and Box 11-2 lists the clinical findings, sonographic findings, and differential considerations for selected splenic diseases and conditions to include: splenomegaly, infection, infarction, trauma, cystic disease, and primary tumors. The sonographic appearance of splenic disorders is found in Table 11-3.

TABLE 11-2	Splenic Findings	
Clinical Findings	**Sonographic Findings**	**Differential Considerations**
Splenomegaly		
Depends on cause	Long axis ≥13 cm Look for liver anomalies (e.g., cirrhosis, diffuse disease)	
Splenic Abscess		
Fever Leukocytosis	Splenomegaly Irregular, ill-defined borders May have internal septa	Hematoma Necrotic neoplasm Lymphoma Leukemia
Splenic Infarction		
Related to primary diagnosis	Acute: wedge-shaped, hypoechoic area Chronic: wedge-shaped, echogenic area (base points to periphery) Look for splenic atrophy	Infection Hemorrhage Neoplasm Lymphoma
Splenic Trauma		
↓ Hematocrit	Spleen may appear enlarged Hematoma may form later along subcapsular area or internally	
Splenic Cysts		
Asymptomatic	Solitary Anechoic ↑ Transmission Well-defined walls Look for tissue compression	Hematoma Lymphangioma Echinococcal cyst
Primary Tumors		
Depends on primary	Splenomegaly May be diffuse, single, or multiple Hypoechoic to hyperechoic	Infection

BOX 11-2	Pathologic Classification of Splenic Disorders

Hematopoiesis
Granulocytopoiesis
    Reactive hyperplasia to acute and chronic infection (low sonodensity)
Noncaseous granulomatous inflammation
Myeloproliferative syndromes (normal)
Chronic myelogenous leukemia
Acute myelogenous leukemia
Lymphopoiesis (low sonodensity or focal sonolucent)
Chronic lymphocytic leukemia
    Lymphoma
    Hodgkin's disease
Erythropoiesis (normal)
Sickle cell disease
    Hereditary spherocytosis
    Hemolytic anemia
    Chronic anemia
    Myeloproliferative syndrome
Other
    Multiple myeloma (low sonodensity)

Reticuloendothelial Hyperactivity (Normal)
Still's disease
Wilson's disease
Felty's syndrome
Reticulum cell sarcoma

Congestion (Normal or Low Sonodensity)
Hepatocellular disease

Nonspecific
Neoplasm-metastasis (focal sonodense)
Cyst (focal sonolucent)
Abscess (focal sonolucent)
Malignant neoplasm (focal sonolucent)
    Hodgkin's disease
    Lymphoma
Benign neoplasm (focal sonolucent)
    Lymphangiomatosis
Hematoma (perisplenic)

TABLE 11-3	Sonographic-Pathologic Classification of Splenic Disorders			
Uniform Splenic Sonodensity			**Focal Defects**	
Normal Sonodensity	**Low Sonodensity**	**Sonodense**	**Sonolucent**	**Perisplenic Defects**
Erythropoiesis (including myeloproliferative disorders) Reticuloendothelial Congestion Hyperactivity	Granulocytopoiesis (excluding myeloproliferative disorders) Lymphopoiesis Other (multiple myeloma) Congestion	Nonspecific (metastasis)	Nonspecific (benign primary neoplasm, cyst, abscess, malignant neoplasm [lymphopoietic])	Nonspecific (hematoma)

From Mittelstaedt CA, Partain CL: *Radiology* 134:697, 1980.

Splenomegaly

As the largest unit of the reticuloendothelial system, the spleen is involved in all systemic inflammations and generalized hematopoietic disorders and many metabolic disturbances (Box 11-3). Whenever the spleen is involved in systemic disease, splenic enlargement, or **splenomegaly,** usually develops (Figure 11-15).

Obvious gross splenomegaly is easily defined with sonography. If mild splenomegaly is present, sonographic findings may be more difficult to obtain. Volume measurements of the

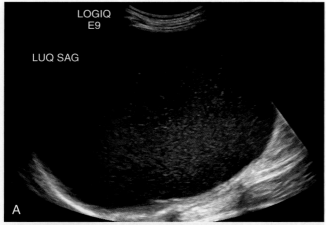

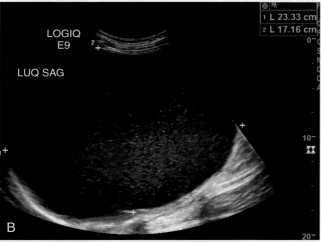

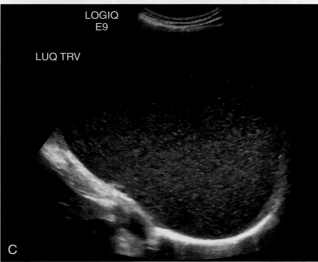

FIGURE 11-15 A and **B,** The enlarged spleen consumes the left upper quadrant in this patient with splenomegaly. **C,** Transverse image of the enlarged spleen.

spleen are necessary to determine the exact size. Although splenomegaly is the most common disease process encountered by the sonographer when evaluating this organ, careful evaluation of splenic contour and homogeneity should be undertaken to determine whether a disease process involves the spleen. Evaluation of the splenic parenchyma and vascular patterns may demonstrate changes in the size, texture, and vascularity of the organ, which could be helpful in the patient's clinical evaluation to rule out the presence of a diffuse disease process or focal lesion. The spleen may grow to enormous size with extension into the iliac fossa. The medial segment may cross the midline of the abdomen to mimic a mass inferior to the left lobe of the liver. Splenomegaly has multiple causes as noted in Box 11-4. Table 11-4 lists possible causes, depending on the degree of enlargement.

Clinical signs of splenomegaly may include left-upper-quadrant pain (secondary to stretching of the splenic capsule or ligaments) or fullness. Enlargement of the spleen may encroach on surrounding organs, such as the left kidney, pancreas, stomach, and intestines.

Congestion of the Spleen

Two types of splenic congestion are known: acute and chronic. In acute congestion, active hyperemia accompanies the reaction in the moderately enlarged spleen. In chronic venous congestion, diffuse enlargement of the spleen occurs. The venous congestion may be of systemic origin, caused by intrahepatic obstruction to portal venous drainage or by obstructive venous disorders in the portal or splenic veins. Systemic venous congestion is found in cardiac decompensation involving the right side of the heart. It is particularly severe in tricuspid or pulmonary valvular disease and in chronic cor pulmonale. The most common causes of striking

BOX 11-4	Causes of Congestive Splenomegaly
Heart failure	Generalized infections
Portal hypertension, portal or splenic vein thrombosis	Hemolytic anemias
	Glycogen storage disease
Leukemia	Malaria
Lymphoma	Myelofibrosis
Mononucleosis	

TABLE 11-4	Causes of Splenomegaly
Degree of Splenomegaly	**Possible Causes**
Mild to moderate	Infection
	Portal hypertension
	AIDS
Moderate	Leukemia
	Lymphoma
	Infectious mononucleosis
Massive	Myelofibrosis
Focal lesions	Lymphomatous involvement
	Metastatic disease
	Hematomas

congestive splenomegaly are the various forms of cirrhosis of the liver. It is also caused by obstruction to the extrahepatic portal or splenic vein (e.g., spontaneous portal vein thrombosis) (see Box 11-4).

Storage Disease

Amyloidosis. In systemic diseases leading to **amyloidosis,** the spleen is the most frequently involved organ. Two types of involvement are seen: nodular and diffuse. In the nodular type, amyloid is found in the walls of the sheathed arteries and within the follicles, but not in the red pulp (Figure 11-16). In the diffuse type, the follicles are not involved, the red pulp is prominently involved, and the spleen is usually greatly enlarged and firm. On sonography, the spleen may be of normal size or decidedly enlarged, depending on the amount and distribution of amyloid.

Gaucher's Disease. All age-groups can be affected by **Gaucher's disease.** About 50% of patients are younger than 8 years of age, and 17% are younger than 1 year of age. Clinical features follow a chronic course, with bone pain and changes in skin pigmentation. Sonographic findings show splenomegaly, diffuse inhomogeneity, and multiple splenic nodules (well-defined hypoechoic lesions). These nodules may be irregular, hyperechoic, or mixed. They represent focal areas of Gaucher's cells associated with fibrosis and infarction.

Niemann-Pick Disease. Niemann-Pick disease is a rapidly progressing fatal disease that predominantly affects female infants. Clinical features consist of hepatomegaly, digestive disturbances, and lymphadenopathy.

Diffuse Disease

Erythropoietic abnormalities include the following: sickle cell, hereditary spherocytosis, hemolytic anemia, chronic anemia, polycythemia vera, thalassemia, and myeloproliferative disorders.

Sickle Cell Anemia. In the earlier stage of **sickle cell anemia,** as seen in infants and children, the spleen is enlarged with marked congestion of the red pulp. Later, the spleen undergoes progressive infarction and fibrosis and decreases in size until, in adults, only a small mass of fibrous tissue may be found (autosplenectomy). It is generally believed that these changes result when sickle cells plug the vasculature of the splenic substance, effectively producing ischemic destruction of the spleen. Sonographic findings for sickle cell disease have different sonographic appearances, depending on its disease state (Figure 11-17). An acute **sickle cell crisis** commonly occurs in children with homozygous sickle cell disease with splenomegaly and a sudden decrease in hematocrit. In addition, these patients may develop a subacute hemorrhage that appears as a hypoechoic area in the periphery of the spleen.

Congenital Spherocytosis. In congenital or hereditary **spherocytosis,** an intrinsic abnormality of the red cells gives rise to erythrocytes that are small and spheroid rather than normal, flattened, biconcave disks (Figure 11-18).

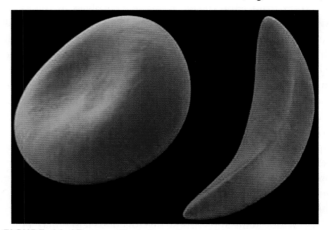

FIGURE 11-17 Magnified view of a red blood cell in a patient with sickle cell anemia (on the right) compared with the normal cell (on the left).

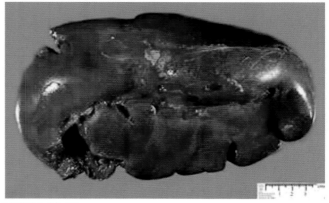

FIGURE 11-18 Gross pathology of the enlarged spleen in a patient with congenital spherocytosis.

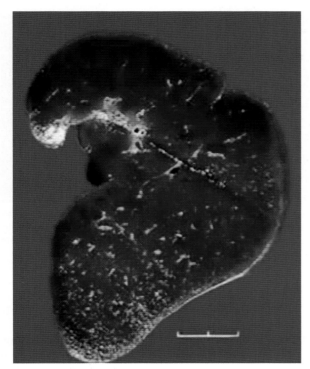

FIGURE 11-16 Gross pathology of the enlarged spleen in a patient with amyloidosis; note the diffuse involvement of the red pulp.

The two results of this disease are production by the bone marrow of spherocytic erythrocytes and increased destruction of these cells in the spleen. The spleen destroys spherocytes selectively. On sonography, splenomegaly may be seen.

Hemolytic Anemia. **Hemolytic anemia** is the general term applied to anemia linked to decreased life of the erythrocytes. When the rate of destruction is greater than what the bone marrow can compensate for, anemia results.

Autoimmune Hemolytic Anemia. **Autoimmune hemolytic anemia** can occur in its primary form without underlying disease, or it may be seen as a secondary disorder in patients already suffering from some disorder of the reticuloendothelial or hematopoietic system, such as lymphoma, leukemia, or infectious **mononucleosis.** Splenomegaly may be present.

Polycythemia Vera. **Polycythemia** is an excess of red blood cells. **Polycythemia vera** is a chronic disease of unknown cause that involves all bone marrow elements. It is characterized by an increase in red blood cell mass and hemoglobin concentration. Clinical symptoms include weakness, fatigue, vertigo, tinnitus, irritability, splenomegaly, flushing of the face, redness and pain in the extremities, and blue-and-black spots. Splenomegaly is present. Infarcts and thromboses are common in polycythemia vera (Figure 11-19).

Thalassemia. The spleen is severely involved in **thalassemia.** This hemoglobinopathy differs from the others in that an abnormal molecular form of hemoglobin is not present. Instead, suppression of synthesis of beta or alpha polypeptide chains occurs, resulting in deficient synthesis of normal hemoglobin. Not only are the erythrocytes deficient in normal hemoglobin, they are also abnormal in shape; many are target cells, whereas others vary considerably in size and shape. Their life span is short because they are destroyed by the spleen in large numbers. The disease ranges from mild to severe. Changes in the spleen are greatest in thalassemia major (Figure 11-20). Splenomegaly is present, often filling the entire abdominal cavity.

Myeloproliferative Disorders. Myeloproliferative disorders include acute and chronic myelogenous leukemias, polycythemia vera, myelofibrosis, megakaryocytic leukemia, and erythroleukemia (Figure 11-21). An isoechoic sonographic pattern is seen in this condition because the parenchyma is hypoechoic compared with the liver.

Granulocytopoietic Abnormalities. Granulocytopoietic abnormalities include reactive hyperplasia resulting from acute or chronic infection (e.g., splenitis sarcoid, tuberculosis). On sonographic examination, splenomegaly is seen with a diffusely hypoechoic pattern (less dense than the liver). Patients who have had a previous granulomatous infection may have bright echogenic lesions on sonography, with or without shadowing (Figure 11-22). Histoplasmosis and tuberculosis are the most common causes; sarcoidosis is rare. The sonographer may also find calcium in the splenic artery.

Reticuloendotheliosis. Diseases characterized by reticuloendothelial hyperactivity and varying degrees of lipid

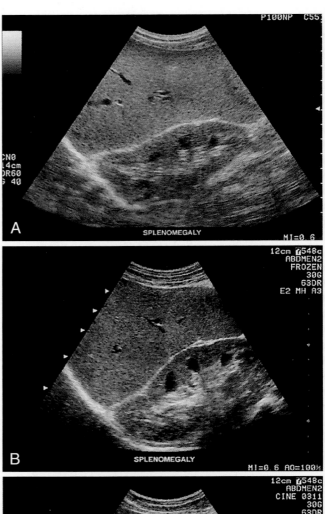

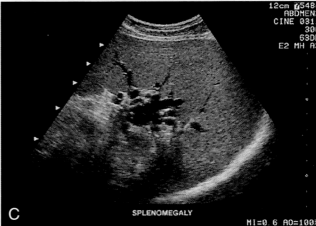

FIGURE 11-19 Patterns of splenomegaly. **A** and **B,** The tip of the enlarged spleen covers the lower pole of the kidney. **C,** The dilated splenic hilum is secondary to portal hypertension; with hepatosplenomegaly.

storage in phagocytes are included in the category of reticuloendotheliosis. On ultrasound, the spleen appears isoechoic.

Letterer-Siwe Disease. In Letterer-Siwe disease, sometimes called *nonlipid reticuloendotheliosis,* proliferation of reticuloendothelial cells occurs in all tissues, but particularly in the splenic lymph nodes and bone marrow. This disease is

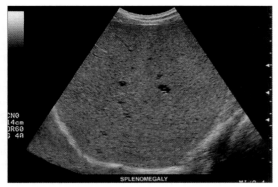

FIGURE 11-20 A patient with thalassemia major shows a huge spleen extending into the lower abdominal cavity.

generally found in children younger than 2 years of age. Clinical features include hepatosplenomegaly, fever, and pulmonary involvement. It is rapidly fatal. Usually, the spleen is only moderately enlarged, although the change may be more severe in affected older infants.

Hand-Schüller-Christian Disease. Hand-Schüller-Christian disease is benign and chronic, in spite of many features similar to those of Letterer-Siwe disease. It usually affects children older than 2 years of age. Clinical features include a chronic course, diabetes, and moderate hepatosplenomegaly.

Splenic Abscess and Infection

Splenic Abscess. The phagocytic activity of the spleen's efficient reticuloendothelial system and leukocytes help to prevent abscess formation within the spleen. However, the spleen may be infected by the following: subacute bacterial endocarditis, septicemia, decreased immunologic states, drug abuse, splenic trauma, and infarcts. In the majority of patients, the infection is spread from distant foci in the abdomen, or an inflammatory process extends directly from adjacent organs. Extrinsic processes (i.e., perinephric or subphrenic abscess, perforated gastric or colonic lesions, or pancreatic abscess) may invade the splenic parenchyma.

The abscess formations may be typical pyogenic, atypical pyogenic, or microabscess collections. The typical pyogenic abscess is a focal collection of pus within the splenic parenchyma. The appearance is hypoechoic with internal septations with low level echoes representing pus or debris. Decreased acoustic enhancement may be present. The atypical pyogenic abscess demonstrates reverberation artifacts from gas, therefore the image is echogenic. The microabscess formation demonstrates a target or bull's-eye appearance on sonography, similar to that seen in the liver.

Clinical findings may be subtle and may include fever, left-upper-quadrant tenderness, and splenomegaly. Laboratory results would demonstrate positive blood cultures and leukocytosis, depending on the type of infection present.

Sonographic Findings. Sonography may demonstrate a simple cystic pattern to mixed echo pattern (Figure 11-23). The lesion may be hypoechoic, often with hyperechoic foci that represent debris or gas. Other findings include the following: thick or shaggy walls, anechoic (without echoes

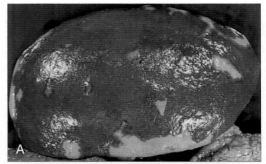

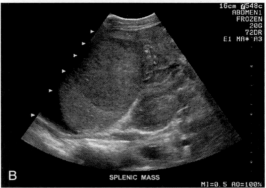

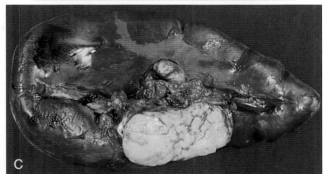

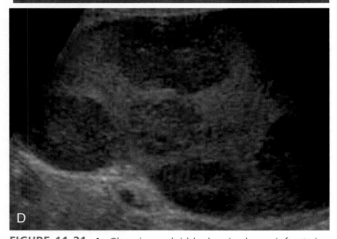

FIGURE 11-21 A, Chronic myeloid leukemia shows infarcts in a gross specimen with splenomegaly. **B,** Patient with acute myelogenous leukemia shows a large mass within the splenic parenchyma and enlarged nodes in the hilum. **C,** Lymphoblastic lymphoma. Tumor cells form a discrete mass in the spleen. **D,** On sonography, an enlarged spleen is seen with an inhomogeneous texture in this patient with lymphoma.

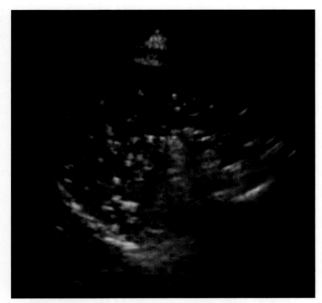

FIGURE 11-22 Patient with granulomatous infection may have bright echogenic lesions on sonography.

within a mass) appearance, poor definition of the lesion, and increased to decreased transmission (depending on the presence of gas). An abscess may be difficult to distinguish from an infarct, neoplasm, or hematoma, and clinical correlation is necessary.

Splenic Infection. Many infections can affect the spleen. The most prominent feature is splenomegaly. Many immunocompromised patients also have multiple nodules within the spleen.

Hepatosplenic candidiasis on ultrasound may show irregular masses within the spleen, the "wheels-within-wheels" pattern, with the outer wheel representing the ring of fibrosis surrounding the inner echogenic wheel of inflammatory cells, and a central hypoechoic area. Other patterns seen include bull's-eye pattern (hypoechoic rim with an echogenic central core), hypoechoic nodule, or hyperechoic nodule (Figure 11-24).

Patients with mycobacterial infections show tiny, diffuse echogenic foci throughout the spleen. Active tuberculosis shows echo-poor or cystic masses, representing abscess

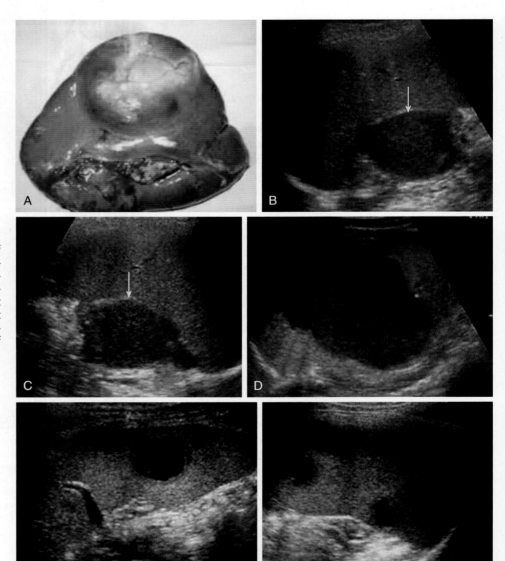

FIGURE 11-23 **A,** Gross pathology of a large splenic abscess. **B** and **C,** Transverse and longitudinal images of a patient with a splenic abscess. **D,** Sonography of a patient with a large splenic abscess. **E,** Sonography of a small splenic abscess with debris within. **F,** Sonography of the spleen with multiple areas of abscess formation.

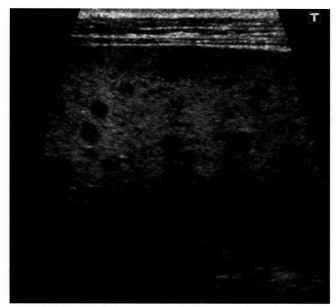

FIGURE 11-24 Sonography of an enlarged spleen with diffuse areas of hypoechoic lesions throughout in a patient with a splenic abscess.

lesions (Figure 11-25). These small punctate areas may show increased echogenity with calcification.

In patients with acquired immunodeficiency syndrome (AIDS), the most common finding is splenomegaly. There can be multiorgan involvement (i.e., liver, spleen, and kidneys). Focal lesions include *Candida, Pneumocystis jiroveci* pneumonia, *Mycobacterium,* disseminated *Pneumocystis,* Kaposi's sarcoma, and lymphoma. Sonographic findings may demonstrate focal splenic lesions displaying small, round lesions that may be multiple, hypoechoic, and well defined. Many of these lesions are caused by disseminated *Mycobacterium tuberculosis* infection, *Candida, Pneumocystis jiroveci,* or *Mycobacterium avium.* In addition, hepatomegaly with focal lesions, retroperitoneal lymphadenopathy, and ascites may be seen.

Splenic Infarction. Splenic infarction is the most common cause of focal splenic lesions resulting from occlusion of the major splenic artery or any of its branches. They are almost always the result of emboli that arise in the heart, produced from mural thrombi or from vegetation on the valves of the left side of the heart. Other causes include septic emboli and local thrombosis in patients with pancreatitis, leukemia, lymphomatous disorders, sickle cell anemia, sarcoidosis, or polyarteritis nodosa.

Sonographic Findings. Splenomegaly is not present with a splenic infarction. Sonography may show a localized hypoechoic area, depending on the time of onset. Fresh hemorrhage has a hypoechoic appearance; healed infarctions appear as echogenic, peripheral wedge-shaped lesions with their base toward the subcapsular surface of the spleen (Figure 11-26). The infarction may become nodular or hyperechoic with time. The entire spleen or focal segmental areas may be affected. The infarcted segment will be avascular.

Splenic Trauma. The spleen is most commonly injured as a result of blunt abdominal trauma. If the patient has severe left-upper-quadrant pain secondary to trauma, a splenic hematoma or subcapsular hematoma should be considered. The tear may result in linear or stellate lacerations or capsular tears, puncture wounds from foreign bodies or rib fractures, or subcapsular hematomas. Blunt trauma has two outcomes. If the capsule is intact, the outcome may be intraparenchymal or subcapsular hematoma; if the capsule ruptures, a focal or free intraperitoneal hematoma may form (Figure 11-27). In delayed rupture, a subcapsular hematoma may develop with subsequent rupture. Quick assessment of free fluid that may surround the splenic capsule in blunt abdominal trauma can lead to a life-saving diagnosis for the patient.

Sonographic Findings. Sonography is a sensitive and specific test used to examine trauma patients for abdominal injury requiring surgery (Figure 11-28). Routine abdominal ultrasound examination can be performed at the bedside in the trauma center. The use of screening ultrasound can improve clinical decision making for the use of emergency laparotomy.

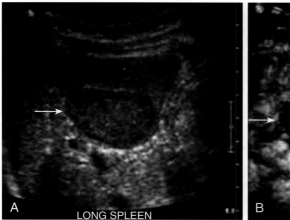
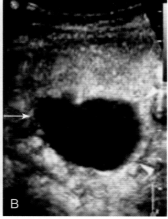

FIGURE 11-25 Sonography of a tuberculous abscess of the spleen; these collections may show echo-poor or cystic masses.

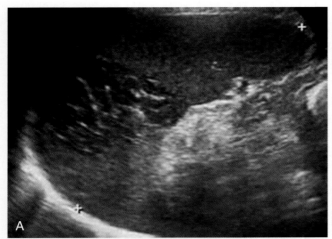

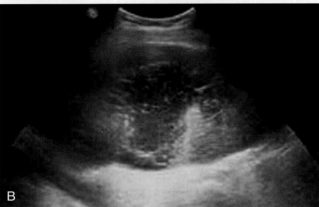

FIGURE 11-26 A, Sonography of a patient with a splenic infarct demonstrates an inhomogeneous texture in the midsplenic parenchyma. **B,** Splenic infarcts may present as wedge-shaped abnormalities within the splenic parenchyma.

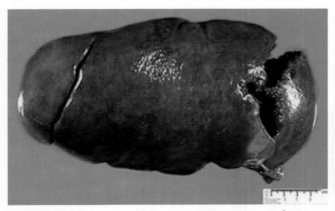

FIGURE 11-27 Gross pathology that demonstrates a large tear in the splenic parenchyma from blunt trauma.

The patient typically presents with left-upper-quadrant pain, left shoulder pain, left flank pain, or dizziness. On clinical evaluation, the patient may have tenderness over the left upper quadrant, hypotension, and decreased hemoglobin, indicating a bleed. A timely response to this emergent situation may save the patient undergoing peritoneal lavage

or exploratory surgery. The sonographer should quickly examine the four abdominopelvic quadrants: the area surrounding the kidneys (Morison's pouch), the subdiaphragmatic areas, the liver and splenic capsule, and the bladder and anterior rectal area to determine whether free fluid is present. The patient's bladder may be filled retrograde to help serve as a window in the pelvic cavity. The entire screening examination should take less than 5 minutes and may be recorded on videotape.

If the spleen has been lacerated and blood is contained within the splenic capsule, the most prominent ultrasound finding is splenomegaly, with progressive enlargement as the bleeding continues. In addition, an irregular splenic border, hematoma, contusion (splenic inhomogeneity), subcapsular and pericapsular fluid collections, free intraperitoneal blood, or left pleural effusion may be present.

Focal hematomas may have intrasplenic fluid collections. Perisplenic fluid is seen in patients with subcapsular hematomas. The sonographer should be aware that blood exhibits various echo patterns, depending on the time that has passed since the trauma. Fresh hemorrhage may appear hypoechoic and may be difficult to distinguish from normal splenic tissue. The sonographer should look for a double-contour sign depicting the hematoma as separate from the spleen. As the protein and cells resorb the hematoma, the fluid becomes organized, hyperechoic, and similar to splenic tissue. In focal areas, tiny splenic lacerations give rise to small collections of blood interspersed with disrupted splenic pulp (contusion). Over time, the hematoma becomes more fluid or appears lucent.

The echo-free, intraperitoneal fluid is probably blood mixed with peritoneal transudate. Healing of the lesion often takes months. The free fluid disappears more quickly because the fluid is moved across the pleural and peritoneal membranes rapidly (2 to 4 weeks). Intrasplenic hematomas and contusions take longer because the fluid, protein, and necrotic debris must be resorbed from within a solid organ in which the blood supply has already been focally disrupted. When the spleen returns to normal, small irregular foci may remain, or the parenchyma may be normal.

Splenic Cysts. Cystic masses do not commonly occur in the spleen. Splenic cysts may be classified as congenital or acquired in origin. The congenital cyst has an endothelial lining present. These cysts present on ultrasound as an anechoic, smooth bordered mass without septations or nodules (Figure 11-29). If they are complicated cysts there may be septations with internal echoes, a thickened wall, and usually no calcifications. Simple congenital cysts can have internal echoes at increased gain. Hemorrhage within the cyst may produce a fluid level.

The acquired cyst is considered "posttraumatic" or a "pseudocyst" as the inner cellular wall is absent, but a fibrous wall is present. Most acquired cysts are considered secondary cysts caused by trauma, infection, or infarction. These acquired cysts on sonography appear as small anechoic or mixed homogeneity. The wall may be echogenic (calcified). *Echinococcus* is the only parasite that forms

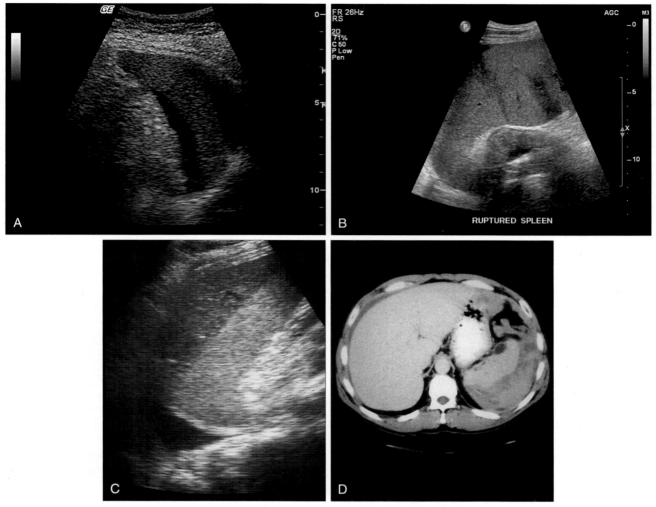

FIGURE 11-28 Splenic hematoma. **A,** Small hypoechoic separation medial to the splenic capsule represents a splenic hematoma. **B,** Inhomogeneity of the splenic texture represents a laceration in the spleen. **C,** Separation of the splenic capsule from the spleen secondary to a large hematoma resulting from an automobile accident. **D,** Computed tomography demonstrates the splenic hematoma along the posterolateral wall of the abdomen.

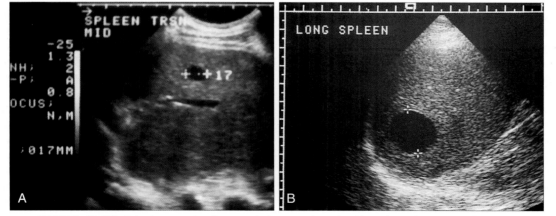

FIGURE 11-29 Splenic cyst. **A,** Tiny anechoic mass found within the splenic parenchyma as an incidental finding. **B,** Well-defined anechoic mass found within an asymptomatic young female.

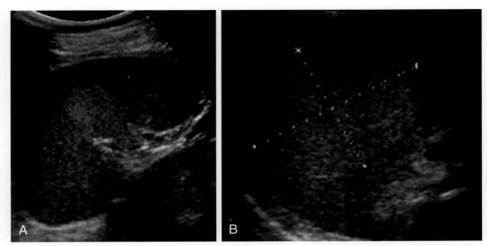

FIGURE 11-30 A, Sonography of the spleen denotes a small mass in the upper margin in a patient with a hemangioma. **B,** A large hemangioma is more echogenic than the splenic parenchyma.

splenic cysts; it is uncommon in the United States. Parasitic cysts appear as anechoic lesions with possible daughter cysts and calcification, or as solid masses with fine internal echoes and poor distal enhancement. Infectious cysts of *Echinococcus* and hydatid cysts may show calcifications within their walls. Posttraumatic cysts that have no cellular lining are called pseudocysts. These cysts may develop calcifications in their walls.

Benign Primary Neoplasms. Generally speaking, primary tumors of the spleen are rare. The tumors may be divided into two groups: benign and malignant. With benign primary tumors, splenomegaly is the first indication of an abnormality. The tumor appearance may be solid or cystic and they may be solitary or multiple. Most of these tumors appear isoechoic compared with the normal splenic parenchyma. Benign primary tumors include hemangioma, hamartoma, and lymphangioma.

Hemangioma. The hemangioma is the most common benign tumor of the spleen. It usually is found as an isolated inhomogeneous echogenic mass with multiple small hypoechoic areas (Figure 11-30). The patient displays no symptoms and becomes symptomatic only when the size of the spleen increases and it compresses other organs. Complications occur when the tumor increases in size to cause a splenic rupture with peritoneal symptoms. The sonographic appearance is variable, from a well-defined echogenic appearance to a complex mixed pattern; infarction with coagulated blood or fibrin in the cavities may be seen, but is nonspecific. Hydatid cyst, abscess, dermoid cyst, and metastasis should be considered in the differential diagnosis.

Hamartoma. The patient with a rare hamartoma is asymptomatic. The tumor may be solitary or multiple and is considered well defined but not encapsulated. The hamartoma consists of lymphoid tissue or a combination of sinuses and structures equivalent to pulp cords of normal splenic tissue. Symptomatic splenic hamartomas are rare in the pediatric age group. The hamartoma has both solid and cystic

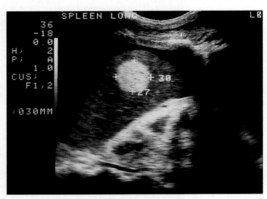

FIGURE 11-31 Hamartoma of the spleen. Small, solitary hyperechoic lesion within the spleen was seen in a young patient with ascites.

components and is generally hyperechoic on sonography (Figure 11-31).

Lymphangioma. Lymphangioma is a rare benign malformation of lymphatics, consisting of endothelium-lined cystic spaces that vary in size. If the cysts are large enough they may appear anechoic; however, if the cysts are multiple and grouped closely together they may appear as a solid lesion. This condition may involve multiple organ systems or may be confined to solitary organs, such as the liver, spleen, kidney, or colon. Cystic lymphangioma appears as a mass with extensive cystic replacement of splenic parenchyma.

Malignant Primary Neoplasms. Malignant tumors of the spleen are uncommon. Primary tumors found in the spleen include lymphoma and hemangiosarcoma. Very rare splenic tumors include malignant fibrous histiocytoma, leiomyosarcoma, and fibrosarcoma.

Lymphoma. The spleen is commonly involved in lymphoma. The lesions may be focal or diffuse. Splenomegaly may or may not be present. The most common malignant tumor is Hodgkin's and non-Hodgkin's lymphoma. It may be difficult to detect splenic lymphoma by sonography. When

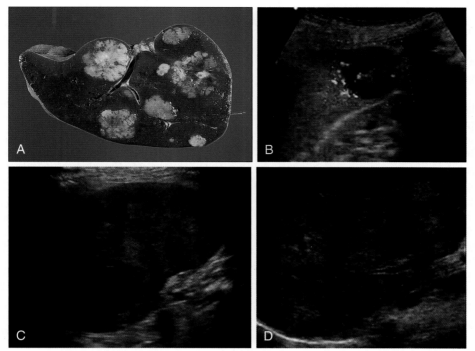

FIGURE 11-32 Metastases in the spleen with various sonographic patterns. **A,** Gross specimen of splenic metastases. **B,** Inhomogeneous vascular mass. **C,** Large complex lesion with hypoechoic central core. **D,** Diffuse isoechoic lesions with halo effect.

it is seen, however, it appears to be typically hypoechoic. Four different sonographic patterns have been reported in patients with malignant lymphoma: (1) diffuse involvement, (2) focal small nodular lesions, (3) focal large nodular lesions, and (4) bulky disease. The diffuse or small nodular pattern was seen predominantly in low-grade lymphomas and in Hodgkin's disease.

AIDS lymphoma shows a uniform decreased echogenicity or focal hypoechoic lesions in the spleen.

Hemangiosarcoma. Hemangiosarcoma is a very rare malignant neoplasm arising from the vascular endothelium of the spleen. The mixed cystic sonographic pattern of hemangiosarcoma resembles that of a cavernous hemangioma, but the tumor can also be hyperechoic.

Metastases. Metastases are the result of a hematogenous spread from another primary site. The spleen is the tenth most common site of metastases, which may originate from the breast, lung, ovary, stomach, colon, kidney, or prostate, or from melanoma. The metastatic tumors may be microscopic, causing no symptoms. The tumor may be multiple, solitary, nodular, or diffuse.

Sonographic Findings. The splenic parenchyma should be carefully examined by the sonographer to detect abnormalities of the splenic parenchyma. The tumors are usually well-defined lesions that may appear isoechoic, hypoechoic, hyperechoic, target lesions, or halo lesions (Figure 11-32). The larger lesions appear more complex. *Melanoma* deposits appear hypoechoic, but are of higher echo amplitude than lymphoma; some are echodense.

 Key Pearls

- The spleen, as part of the reticuloendothelial system, is the largest single mass of lymphoid tissue in the body.
- Splenic functions include hematopoiesis and the body's defense against disease.
- The normal texture of the spleen is homogeneous, being slightly more echogenic than the texture of the liver.
- The spleen is of variable size and shape (e.g., "orange segment," tetrahedral, triangular) but generally is considered to be ovoid with smooth, even borders and a convex superior and concave inferior surface.
- The splenic hilum contains both the splenic artery and vein.
- Variations of the spleen include "wandering" spleen, agenesis, accessory spleen, asplenia, and polysplenia.
- Significant laboratory data related to the spleen include hematocrit, bacteremia, leukocytosis, and leukopenia.
- On sonography, the spleen should be evaluated with longitudinal, transverse, and coronal views from the supine or decubitus position.
- Splenic enlargement, or splenomegaly, usually develops whenever the spleen is involved in systemic disease.
- Splenic congestion: (1) In acute congestion, active hyperemia accompanies the reaction in the moderately enlarged spleen; (2) in chronic venous congestion, diffuse enlargement of the spleen occurs.

Continued

- Storage diseases include amyloidosis, Gaucher's disease, and Niemann-Pick disease.
- Erythropoietic abnormalities include the following: sickle cell, hereditary spherocytosis, hemolytic anemia, chronic anemia, polycythemia vera, thalassemia, and myeloproliferative disorders.
- The spleen may be infected by the following: subacute bacterial endocarditis, septicemia, decreased immunologic states, drug abuse, splenic trauma, and infarcts.
- The spleen is most commonly injured as a result of blunt abdominal trauma; the tear may result in linear or stellate lacerations or capsular tears, puncture wounds from foreign bodies or rib fractures, or subcapsular hematomas.
- Cystic masses do not commonly occur in the spleen; splenic cysts may be classified as congenital or acquired in origin.
- Primary tumors of the spleen are rare; they include hemangioma, hamartoma, and lymphangioma.
- Malignant tumors of the spleen are uncommon; primary tumors found in the spleen include lymphoma and hemangiosarcoma, and very rare splenic tumors include malignant fibrous histiocytoma, leiomyosarcoma, and fibrosarcoma.

BIBLIOGRAPHY

Akhan O, Koroglu M: Hydatid disease of the spleen, *Semin Ultrasound CT, MR* 28:28-34, 2007.

Al-Salem AH, Qaisaruddin S, Al-Jams A, et al: Splenic abscess and sickle cell disease, *Am J Hematol* 58:2-8, 1998.

Aytac S, Fitoz S, Atasoy C, et al: Multimodality demonstration of primary splenic angiosarcoma, *J Clin Ultrasound* 27:92-95, 1999.

Changchien CS: Sonographic patterns of splenic abscess: an analysis of 34 proven cases, *Abdom Imaging* 27:739-745, 2002.

Danaci M, Belet U, Yalin T, et al: Power Doppler sonographic diagnosis of torsion in a wandering spleen, *J Clin Ultrasound* 28:246-248, 2000.

Elstein D, Hadas-Halpern I, Azuri Y, et al: Accuracy of ultrasonography in assessing spleen and liver size in patients with Gaucher disease: comparison to computed tomographic measurements, *J Ultrasound Med* 16:209-211, 1997.

Fitoz S, Atasoy C, Düsünceli E, et al: Post-traumatic intrasplenic pseudoaneurysms with delayed rupture: color Doppler sonographic and CT findings, *J Clin Ultrasound* 29:102-104, 2001.

Franquet T, Montes M, Lecumberri FJ, et al: Hydatid disease of the spleen: imaging findings in nine patients, *Am J Roentgenol* 154:525, 1990.

Gamblin TC, Wall Jr CE, Royer GM, et al: Delayed splenic rupture: case reports and review of the literature, *J Trauma* 59:1231-1234, 2005.

Goldberg BB, McGahan JP: *Atlas of ultrasound measurements*, St Louis, 2006, Mosby.

Gorg C, Weide R, Schwek W: Malignant splenic lymphoma: sonographic patterns, diagnosis and follow-up, *Clin Radiol* 52:7-12, 1997.

Gorg X, Zugmaier G: Chronic recurring infarction of the spleen: sonographic patterns and complications, *Ultraschall Med* 24:245-249, 2003.

Herneth AM, Pokleser P, Phillipp MO, et al: Role of Doppler sonography in the evaluation of accessory spleens after splenectomy, *J Ultrasound Med* 20:1347-1351, 2001.

Ishida H, Konno K, Ishida J, et al: Isolated splenic metastases, *J Ultrasound Med* 16:11-15, 1997.

Kamaya A, Weinstein S, Desser TS: Multiple lesions of the spleen: differential diagnosis of cystic and solid lesions, *Semin Ultrasound CT MR* 27:389-403, 2006.

Kessler A, Miller E, Keidar S, et al: Mass at the splenic hilum: a clue to torsion of a wandering spleen located in a normal left upper quadrant position, *J Ultrasound Med* 22:527-530, 2003.

Lamb PM, Lund A, Kanagasaby RR, et al: Spleen size: how well do linear ultrasound measurements correlate with 3D CT volume assessments? *Br J Radiol* 75:573-577, 2002.

McKenney MG, McKenney KL, Compton RP, et al: Can surgeons evaluate emergency ultrasound scans for blunt abdominal trauma? *J Trauma Infect Crit Care* 44:4-8, 1998.

Middleton WB, Kurtz AB, Hertzberg BS: *Ultrasound: the requisites*, ed 2, St Louis, 2004, Mosby.

Perez Fontan FJ, Soler R, Santos M, et al: Accessory spleen torsion: US, CT and MR findings, *Eur Radiol* 11:509-512, 2001.

Thibodeau GA, Patton KT: *The human body in health and disease*, St Louis, 1997, Mosby.

Warshauer DM, Hall HL: Solitary splenic lesions, *Semin Ultrasound CT MR* 27:370-388, 2006.

Wilcox TM, Speer RW, Schlinkert RT, et al: Hemangioma of the spleen: presentation, diagnosis, and management, *J Gastrointest Surg* 4:611-613, 2000.

Pancreas

Sandra L. Hagen-Ansert

OBJECTIVES

On completion of this chapter, you should be able to:
- Describe the normal anatomy and relational landmarks of the pancreas
- Name the exocrine and endocrine functions of the pancreas
- Describe the laboratory tests used to detect pancreatic disease
- Describe the sonographic technique and patterns of the normal pancreas

- Define the clinical signs and symptoms of pancreatic disease
- Name the congenital anomalies of the pancreas
- List the sonographic findings and differential diagnoses of the following diseases: pancreatitis, pancreatic cyst, and pancreatic tumor

OUTLINE

KEY TERMS

Acini cells
Amylase
Body of the pancreas
Caudal pancreatic artery
C-loop of the duodenum
Common hepatic artery
Courvoisier's sign
Dorsal pancreatic artery
Duct of Santorini
Duct of Wirsung

Endocrine
Exocrine
Glucagon
Head of the pancreas
Hypercalcemia
Hyperlipidemia
Ileus
Insulin
Islets of Langerhans
Lipase

Lymphomas
Neck of the pancreas
Pancreatic ascites
Pancreatitis
Pseudocyst
Serum amylase
Tail of the pancreas
Uncinate process

The pancreas continues to be a technical challenge for the sonographer because this gland is located in the retroperitoneal cavity posterior to the stomach, duodenum, and proximal jejunum of the small bowel. In addition, the transverse colon may obstruct visualization of the pancreas as it runs horizontally across the abdominal cavity.

Other noninvasive procedures were unsuccessful in visualization of the pancreas before the development of computed tomography (CT), magnetic resonance imaging (MRI), and ultrasound. Plain film of the abdomen may lead to a diagnosis of pancreatitis if calcification is visible in the pancreatic area, but calcification does not occur in all cases. Localized **ileus,** dilated loops of bowel without peristalsis ("paralyzed gut") caused by gas and fluid accumulation near the area of inflammation, may be shown on the plain radiograph in patients with pancreatitis. The upper gastrointestinal test series provides indirect information about the pancreas when the widened duodenal loops are visualized.

CT and MRI have become the primary modalities to image the patient with pancreatic disease because of their improved resolution of the retroperitoneal structures. However, the normal pancreas can be visualized in the majority of gas-free patients with sonography by using the neighboring organs and vascular landmarks to aid in localization. The gland appears sonographically isoechoic to more hyperechoic than the hepatic parenchyma. Variations in patient positioning or ingestion of water to fill the stomach (that serves as a window to image the pancreas) are used routinely in many laboratories to further aid in visualizing the entire gland. In addition, clinicians performing the endoscopic retrograde cholangiopancreatography (ERCP) examination of the pancreatic duct are incorporating endoscopic ultrasound as an aid in visualizing the detailed anatomy of the pancreatic area.

Sonography is readily accessible and less expensive than the other imaging modalities. The primary task of the sonographer is to distinguish the normal gland from an abnormal process, to image the ductal system, and to separate inflammation of the gland from malignancies. Sonography may also aid in percutaneous fine-needle aspiration when a lesion is found.

ANATOMY OF THE PANCREAS

Normal Anatomy

The pancreas lies anterior to the first and second lumbar bodies located deep in the epigastrium and left hypochondrium, behind the lesser omental sac (Figure 12-1). The major posterior vascular landmarks of the pancreas are the aorta and inferior vena cava. The pancreas most commonly extends in a horizontal oblique lie extending from the second portion of the duodenum to the splenic hilum. Other variations in the lie of the pancreas include transverse, horseshoe, sigmoid, L-shaped, and inverted V. When this occurs, it may be more difficult to obtain a single image of the pancreatic gland, as the tail will be in a different plane than the body and the head.

It may be surprising that the majority of the pancreas lies within the retroperitoneal cavity, with the exception of a small portion of the head that is surrounded by peritoneum. Posterior to the pancreas are the connective prevertebral tissues, the portal-splenic confluence, the superior mesenteric vessels, the aorta, the inferior vena cava, and the lower border of the diaphragm. The stomach, duodenum, and transverse colon form the superior and lateral borders of the pancreas, which makes visualization of the pancreas by ultrasound difficult (air and gas interference).

The pancreas is divided into the following four areas: head, neck, body, and tail (Figure 12-2). Each area is discussed as it relates to its surrounding anatomy. The reader is referred to the multiple cross-sectional drawings (Figures 12-3 and 12-4) to gain a relational understanding of the adjacent anatomy to the pancreas.

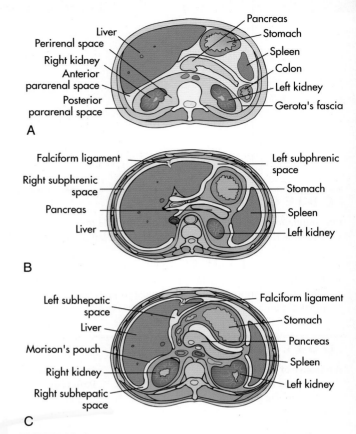

FIGURE 12-1 A, The pancreas lies in the anterior pararenal space. **B,** The stomach is anterior to the body and tail of the gland, whereas the aorta and inferior vena cava, superior mesenteric artery, and vein lie posterior to the gland. **C,** The head of the pancreas lies in the lap of the duodenum.

Head. The **head of the pancreas** is the most inferior portion of the gland. It lies anterior to the inferior vena cava, to the right of the portal-splenic confluence, inferior to the main portal vein and caudate lobe of the liver, and medial to the duodenum as it "lies in the lap" of the **C-loop of the duodenum** (see Figure 12-2). The splenic vein forms the posterior medial border of the pancreas, where it is joined by the superior mesenteric vein to form the main portal vein, thus forming the portal-splenic confluence (Figure 12-5). The superior mesenteric vein crosses anterior to the uncinate process of the head of the gland and posterior to the neck and body of the pancreas. The **uncinate process** is the small, curved tip at the end of the head of the pancreas. It lies anterior to the inferior vena cava and posterior to the superior mesenteric vein. As Figure 12-6 shows, the common bile duct passes posterior to the first part of the duodenum and courses through a groove posterior to the pancreatic head, whereas the gastroduodenal artery forms the anterolateral border.

Neck. The **neck of the pancreas** is located between the pancreatic head and body, and often it is included as "part of the body" of the gland. It is found directly anterior to the portal-splenic confluence/superior mesenteric vein (see Figure 12-5).

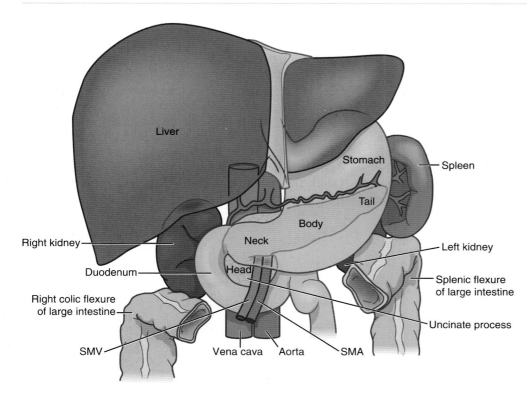

FIGURE 12-2 The aorta and inferior vena cava are the posterior landmarks of the pancreas; the stomach is the anterior border. The tail of the pancreas is directed toward the upper pole of the left kidney and hilum of the spleen. The body and head lie anterior to the prevertebral vessels. The four major areas of the pancreas are the head (with the uncinate process), the neck, the body, and the tail. The superior mesenteric vein *(SMV)* is anterior to the uncinate process. The superior mesenteric artery *(SMA)* is posterior to the neck/body.

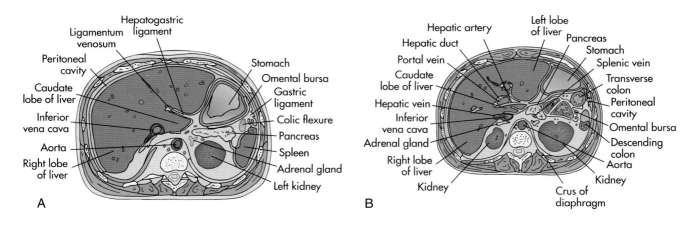

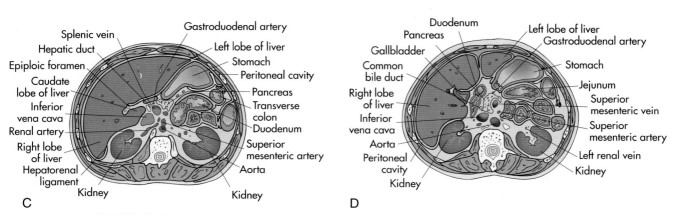

FIGURE 12-3 Transverse planes of the pancreas. **A,** Note the relationship of the tail of the pancreas to the spleen, left kidney and adrenal gland, stomach, and colic flexure. **B,** The body of the pancreas is adjacent to the left lobe of the liver, the stomach, the omental bursa, and the left kidney. **C,** The size of the left lobe of the liver helps to push the stomach away from the pancreatic area for better visualization. **D,** The head of the pancreas is adjacent to the duodenum, superior mesenteric vessels, inferior vena cava, and aorta.

Body. The **body of the pancreas** is the largest section of the pancreas. It lies anterior to the aorta and celiac axis, left renal vein, adrenal gland, and kidney. The tortuous splenic artery is the superior border of the gland (see Figure 12-5). The anterior border is the posterior wall of the antrum of the stomach. The neck of the pancreas forms the right lateral border.

Tail. The **tail of the pancreas** is more difficult to image because it lies anterior to the left kidney and posterior to the left colic flexure and transverse colon. The tail begins to the left of the lateral border of the aorta and extends toward the splenic hilum (see Figure 12-5). The splenic vein is the posterior border of the body and tail. The splenic artery forms the superior border of the tail, whereas the stomach is the anterior border.

Pancreatic Ducts. Two ducts are seen within the pancreas, the duct of Wirsung and the duct of Santorini. To aid in the transport of pancreatic fluid, the ducts have smooth muscle surrounding them. The **duct of Wirsung** is a primary duct extending the entire length of the gland (see Figure 12-6). It receives tributaries from lobules at right angles and enters the medial second part of the duodenum with the common bile duct at the ampulla of Vater (guarded by the sphincter of Oddi). The **duct of Santorini** is a secondary duct that drains the upper anterior head. It enters the duodenum at the minor

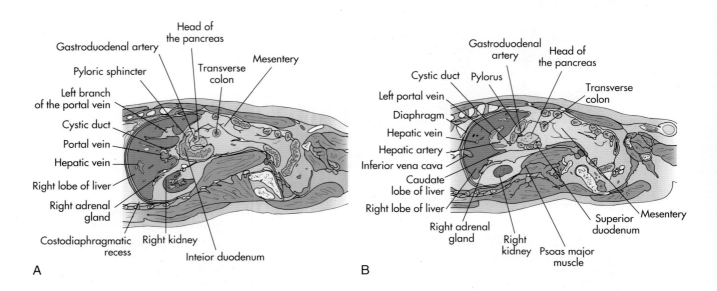

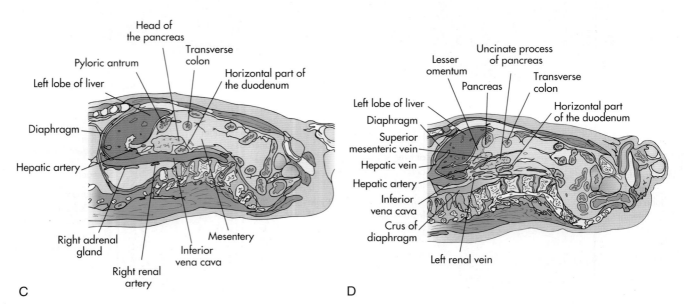

FIGURE 12-4 Sagittal planes of the pancreas. **A,** The head of the pancreas lies in the lap of the duodenum. The gastroduodenal artery is the anterior lateral border of the head. **B,** The head of the pancreas may be obscured by mesenteric fat and air in the duodenum. **C,** The head of the pancreas lies anterior to the inferior vena cava and inferior to the portal vein. **D,** Note the adjacent relationship of the lesser omentum to the pancreas. The superior mesenteric vein is posterior to the neck and anterior to the uncinate process.

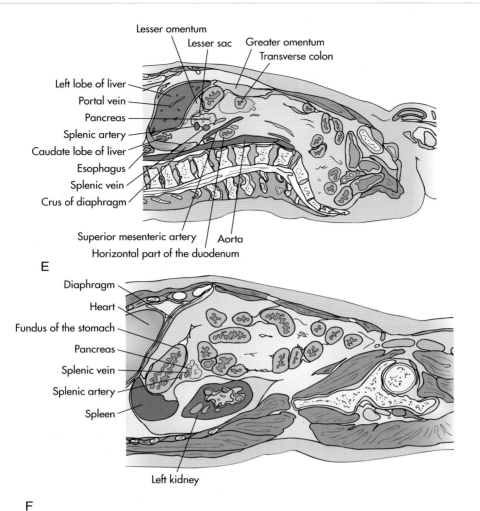

Lesser omentum
Lesser sac
Greater omentum
Transverse colon
Left lobe of liver
Portal vein
Pancreas
Splenic artery
Caudate lobe of liver
Esophagus
Splenic vein
Crus of diaphragm
Superior mesenteric artery
Aorta
Horizontal part of the duodenum

E

Diaphragm
Heart
Fundus of the stomach
Pancreas
Splenic vein
Splenic artery
Spleen
Left kidney

F

FIGURE 12-4, cont'd E, Note the intimate relationship of the splenic vein and artery, superior mesenteric artery, aorta, and left lobe of the liver to the pancreas. **F,** The tail of the pancreas is more difficult to image on the sagittal plane secondary to the adjacent colon and small bowel. Occasionally a fluid-filled stomach, prominent spleen, or left kidney may help to localize the tail of the pancreas.

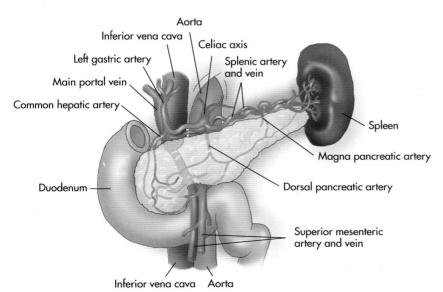

Aorta
Inferior vena cava
Celiac axis
Left gastric artery
Splenic artery and vein
Main portal vein
Common hepatic artery
Spleen
Magna pancreatic artery
Dorsal pancreatic artery
Duodenum
Superior mesenteric artery and vein
Inferior vena cava   Aorta

FIGURE 12-5 The portal venous system is the posterior border of the pancreas. The splenic vein lies along the posterior border, the superior mesenteric vein crosses anterior to the uncinate process and posterior to the neck, and the main portal vein is the posterior border to the head of the pancreas. The tortuous splenic artery is the superior border to the body and tail of the pancreas. The hepatic artery gives rise to the gastroduodenal artery, which serves as the anterolateral border to the head of the pancreas. The splenic artery branches into the magna pancreatic artery and dorsal pancreatic artery. The celiac axis rises from the anterior abdominal aorta just below the diaphragm and serves as the superior border of the pancreas.

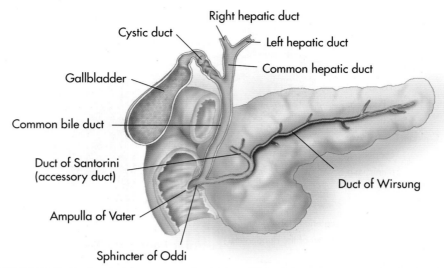

Right hepatic duct
Cystic duct
Left hepatic duct
Gallbladder
Common hepatic duct
Common bile duct
Duct of Santorini
(accessory duct)
Duct of Wirsung
Ampulla of Vater
Sphincter of Oddi

FIGURE 12-6 The head of the pancreas lies in the C-loop of the duodenum. The common bile duct passes posterior to the first part of the duodenum and courses through a groove posterior to the pancreatic head, where it meets the pancreatic duct to enter the duodenum through the ampulla of Vater. This opening is guarded by the sphincter of Oddi.

papilla about 2 cm proximal to the ampulla of Vater. The duct of Wirsung is easier to visualize on ultrasound as it courses through the midline of the body of the gland. It appears as an echogenic line or lucency bordered by two echogenic lines. The duct should measure less than 2 mm, with tapering as it reaches the tail. Color Doppler imaging may help distinguish the dilated pancreatic duct from the vascular structures (splenic vein and artery) in the area.

Common Bile Duct. The common bile duct runs inferiorly in the free edge of the lesser omentum to the level of the duodenum. Then it travels posterior to the first portion of the duodenum and the head of the pancreas to the right of the main pancreatic duct. The common bile duct opens into the duodenum after forming a common trunk with the pancreatic duct.

Size of the Pancreas

The normal length of the pancreas (head to tail) is about 15 cm, with the range extending between 12 and 18 cm. The head is the thickest part of the gland, measuring 2 to 3 cm in its anterior-to-posterior dimension. The neck measures 1.5 to 2.5 cm, the body measures 2 to 2.5 cm, and the tail measures 1 to 2 cm. The sonographer should evaluate the total size, contour, and texture of the gland to determine enlargement. The gland appears larger or thicker in children than in adults and decreases in size with advancing age.

Vascular Supply

The blood supply for the pancreas is the splenic artery and pancreaticoduodenal arteries (Figure 12-7). The anterior and inferior pancreaticoduodenal arteries supply the head and part of the duodenum. The splenic artery supplies the body and tail of the pancreas through four smaller branches: (1) suprapancreatic (rises from the celiac axis/splenic artery), (2) pancreatic, (3) prepancreatic (before leaving the pancreas), and (4) prehilar (before leaving the spleen) and hepatic artery (gastroduodenal artery). The **dorsal pancreatic artery** rises from the suprapancreatic section, the pancreatica magna artery rises from the pancreatic section, and the **caudal pancreatic artery** rises from the prepancreatic or prehilar section. Venous drainage is through tributaries of the splenic and superior mesenteric veins.

Vascular and Ductal Landmarks to the Pancreas

Celiac Axis and Branches. The celiac axis originates from the anterior abdominal aorta and serves as the superior border of the pancreas. It gives rise to three branches: the left gastric, common hepatic, and splenic arteries (see Figure 12-7).

Splenic Artery. The splenic artery follows a tortuous course along the superior border of the pancreatic body and tail as it crosses horizontally toward the splenic hilum.

Common Hepatic Artery. The **common hepatic artery** rises from the celiac axis and courses along the superior margin of the first portion of the duodenum to divide into the proper hepatic artery and gastroduodenal artery, usually when it crosses anterior to the portal vein. The common hepatic artery forms the right superior border of the body and head of the gland and gives rise to the gastroduodenal artery. In some patients the right hepatic artery rises from the superior mesenteric artery and courses posterior to the medial portion of the splenic vein.

Gastroduodenal Artery. The gastroduodenal artery is seen along the anterolateral border of the pancreas as it

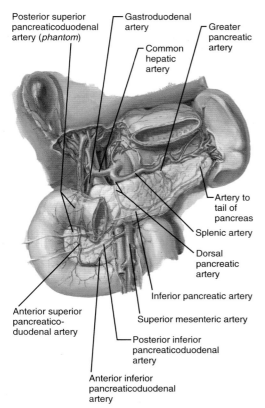

Posterior superior pancreaticoduodenal artery (*phantom*)

Gastroduodenal artery

Common hepatic artery

Greater pancreatic artery

Artery to tail of pancreas

Splenic artery

Dorsal pancreatic artery

Inferior pancreatic artery

Superior mesenteric artery

Posterior inferior pancreaticoduodenal artery

Anterior inferior pancreaticoduodenal artery

Anterior superior pancreatico-duodenal artery

FIGURE 12-7 The blood supply for the pancreas is the splenic artery and pancreaticoduodenal arteries. *(Copyright 2017 Elsevier Inc. All rights reserved. www.netterimages.com.)*

travels a short distance along the anterior aspect of the pancreatic head just to the right of the neck before it divides into the superior pancreaticoduodenal branches; they join with the inferior pancreaticoduodenal branches, which rise from the superior mesenteric artery (see Figure 12-7).

Superior Mesenteric Artery. The superior mesenteric artery rises from the aorta inferior to the celiac axis and posterior to the lower portion of the pancreatic body and courses anterior to the third portion of the duodenum to enter the small bowel mesentery (see Figure 12-7).

Portal Vein and Tributaries. The main portal vein is formed posterior to the neck of the pancreas by the junction of the superior mesenteric vein and splenic vein (see Figure 12-5). The splenic vein runs from the splenic hilum along the posterior aspect of the pancreas. The superior mesenteric vein runs posterior to the neck of the pancreas and anterior to the uncinate process, which forms the small, curved tip of the pancreatic head.

Common Bile Duct. The common bile duct crosses the anterior aspect of the portal vein to the right of the proper hepatic artery. The portal vein is anterior to the inferior vena cava. The duct passes along the anterior border of the portal vein and travels posterior to the first portion of the duodenum to course inferior and somewhat posterior in the parenchyma of the head of the pancreas (see Figure 12-6). It joins the pancreatic duct close to the ampulla of Vater.

Congenital Anomalies

Congenital abnormalities of the pancreas are uncommon. The following abnormalities are presented: agenesis, pancreas divisum, ectopic pancreatic tissue, and annular pancreas.

Agenesis. Agenesis of the body and tail, with hypertrophy of the pancreatic head, is a congenital defect.

Pancreas Divisum. This rare condition is caused by the lack of fusion of the dorsal and ventral pancreatic buds. The drainage of the dorsal pancreas is through the minor papilla, with the ventral part draining through the major papilla. On sonography, this diagnosis is challenging. A persistent dorsal pancreatic duct in the head may be identified, but communication with the ventral duct is difficult to ascertain with sonography (Figure 12-8, *A*).

Ectopic Pancreatic Tissue. Ectopic pancreatic tissue is the most common pancreatic anomaly, usually in the form of intramural nodules. The ectopic tissue may be found in various places in the gastrointestinal tract. Frequent sites are the stomach, duodenum, small bowel, and large bowel. On palpation these lesions may seem polypoid, and they characteristically have a central dimple. They consist of elements of the pancreas, usually the acinar and ductal structures and less frequently the islets of Langerhans. They are generally small (0.5 to 2 cm), and acute pancreatitis or tumor may occur within these elements.

Annular Pancreas. Annular pancreas is a rare anomaly in which the head of the pancreas surrounds the second portion of the duodenum (Figure 12-8, *B* and *C*). It is more common in males than in females, and all grades (from an overlapping of the posterior duodenal wall to a complete ring) may be found. It may be associated with complete or partial atresia of the duodenum and is susceptible to any of the diseases of the pancreas.

PHYSIOLOGY AND LABORATORY DATA OF THE PANCREAS

Physiology

The pancreas is both a digestive (**exocrine**) and hormonal (**endocrine**) gland. The primary exocrine function is to produce pancreatic juice, which enters the duodenum together with bile. The exocrine secretions of the pancreas and those of the liver, which are delivered into the duodenum through duct systems, are essential for normal intestinal digestion and absorption of food. Pancreatic secretion is under the control of the vagus nerve and two hormonal agents, secretin and pancreozymin, that are released when food enters the duodenum. The endocrine function controls the secretion of glucagons and insulin into the blood. Failure of the pancreas to furnish sufficient insulin leads to diabetes mellitus.

Exocrine Function. Exocrine function is performed by **acini cells** of the pancreas, which can produce up to 2 L of pancreatic juice per day. These cells are arranged in saclike clusters (acini) connected by small intercalated ducts to larger excretory ducts. The excretory ducts converge into

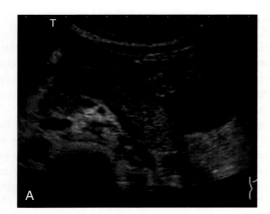

A

Annular
pancreas
constricting
duodenum

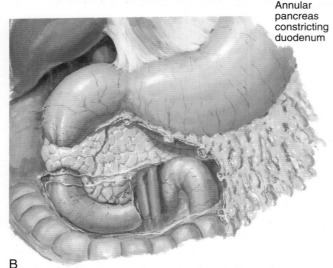

B

Annular pancreas occurs when the ventral bud fails to rotate
with the duodenum and instead surrounds it. This may resutlt
in duodenal obstruction.

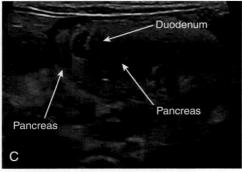

Duodenum

Pancreas

Pancreas

C

FIGURE 12-8 A, Pancreas divisum. This rare condition is caused by
the lack of fusion of the dorsal and ventral pancreatic buds.
B and **C,** Annular pancreas. A rare anomaly in which the head of the
pancreas surrounds the second portion of the duodenum. *(Copyright
2017 Elsevier Inc. All rights reserved. www.netterimages.com.)*

one or two main ducts, which deliver the exocrine secretion of the pancreas into the duodenum. The enzymes of
the pancreatic juice that aid in digestion include **lipase,**
which digests fats; **amylase,** which digests carbohydrates;
carboxypeptidase, trypsin, and chymotrypsinogen, which
digest proteins; and nucleases, which digest nucleic acids
(Table 12-1).

TABLE 12-1	Pancreatic Exocrine Function
Enzymes of Pancreatic Juice	**Digestive Action**
Lipase	Fats
Amylase	Carbohydrates
Trypsin, chymotrypsinogen, carboxypeptidase	Proteins
Nucleases	Nucleic acids

Pancreatic juice is the most versatile and active of the
digestive secretions. Its enzymes are capable of nearly com-
pleting the digestion of food in the absence of all other digestive secretions. Because the digestive enzymes that are
secreted into the lumen of the small intestine require an almost neutral pH for best activity, the acidity of the contents
entering the duodenum must be reduced. Thus the pancreatic
juice contains a relatively high concentration of sodium bicarbonate, and this alkaline salt is largely responsible for the
neutralization of gastric acid.

The nervous secretion of pancreatic juice is thick and rich
in enzymes and proteins. The chemical secretion, resulting
from pancreozymin activity, also is thick, watery, and rich in
enzymes. Pancreatic juice is alkaline and becomes more so
with increasing rates of secretion. This is because of a simultaneous increase in bicarbonates and decrease in chloride
concentration.

The proteolytic enzyme trypsin may hydrolyze protein
molecules to polypeptides. Chymotrypsinogen is activated by trypsin. Amylase causes hydrolysis of starch with
the production of maltose, which is further hydrolyzed to
glucose. Lipase is capable of hydrolyzing some fats to monoglycerides and some to glycerol and fatty acids. Although
lipases are also secreted by the small intestine, what is
secreted by the pancreas accounts for 80% of all fat digestion.
Thus impaired fat digestion is an important indicator of pancreatic dysfunction.

Partially digested food, or chyme, in the duodenum stimulates the release of hormones that act on pancreatic juice
formation. These hormones include gastrin, cholecystokinin,
acetylcholine (all digestive enzymes), and secretin (stimulates
production of sodium bicarbonate).

The pancreatic juice enters the duodenum through the
duct of Wirsung. This duct joins the common bile duct as it
drains bile from the liver and both enter the duodenum
through the ampulla of Vater. The sphincter of Oddi is a
muscle surrounding the ampulla of Vater that relaxes to allow
pancreatic juice and bile to empty into the duodenum.

Endocrine Function. The endocrine function is located
in the **islets of Langerhans** in the pancreas. Specialized
cells within the islets are called *alpha, beta,* and *delta* cells.
The beta cells are most prevalent and produce **insulin,** a
hormone that causes glycogen formation from glucose in
the liver. It also enables cells within insulin receptors to
take up glucose (to decrease blood sugar). Alpha cells produce **glucagon,** a hormone that causes the cells to release
glucose to meet the energy needs of the body. Glucagon

TABLE 12-2	Pancreatic Endocrine Function	
Pancreatic Hormone	**Cell Type**	**Action**
Insulin	Beta	Glucose to glycogen
Glucagon	Alpha	Glycogen to glucose
Somatostatin	Delta	Alpha and beta inhibitor

stimulates the liver to convert glycogen to glucose to increase sugar levels. Delta cells are the smallest composition of endocrine tissue and produce somatostatin. This hormone inhibits the production of both insulin and glucagon. All the hormones are released into the bloodstream (Table 12-2).

Laboratory Tests

There are specific enzymes of the pancreas that may become altered in pancreatic disease, namely amylase and lipase. Increased glucose levels may indicate abnormalities of the pancreas (Table 12-3).

Amylase. Amylase is a digestive enzyme for carbohydrates. It is secreted by the pancreas, parotid glands, gynecologic system, and bowel. In certain types of pancreatic disease, the digestive enzymes of the pancreas escape into the surrounding tissue, producing necrosis with severe pain and inflammation. Under these circumstances there is an increase in **serum amylase.** A serum amylase level of twice normal usually indicates acute pancreatitis.

Other conditions that may cause an increase in amylase include chronic pancreatitis, obstruction of the pancreatic duct, perforated peptic ulcer, acute cholecystitis, and alcohol poisoning. Less common conditions include mumps, ischemic bowel disease, and pelvic inflammatory disease.

TABLE 12-3	Laboratory Values for Pancreatic Disease
Condition	**Amylase Level**
Acute pancreatitis	Twice normal
Chronic pancreatitis	No change
Mumps, ischemic bowel disease, pelvic inflammatory disease	↑
Condition	**Lipase Level**
Acute pancreatitis	↑
Carcinoma of the pancreas	↑
Condition	**Blood Glucose Level**
Severe diabetes	↑
Chronic liver disease	↑
Overactive endocrine glands	↑
Tumor in islet of Langerhans	↓

↑, Increased; ↓, decreased.

Urine Amylase. Urine amylase may be elevated in pancreatitis. Diseases not affecting the pancreas may cause the elevation of serum amylase without elevation of urine amylase.

Lipase. Lipase is an enzyme that is excreted specifically by the pancreas and that parallels the elevation in amylase levels. The lipase test is performed to assess damage to the pancreas. The pancreas secretes lipase, and small amounts pass into the blood. The lipase level rises in acute pancreatitis and in carcinoma of the pancreas. Both amylase and lipase rise at the same rate, but the elevation in lipase concentration persists for a longer period. Lipase may also be elevated with obstruction of the pancreatic duct, pancreatic carcinoma, and acute cholecystitis.

Glucose. Glucose controls the blood sugar level in the body. The glucose tolerance test is performed to discover whether there is a disorder of glucose metabolism. An increased blood glucose level is found in severe diabetes, chronic liver disease, and overactivity of several of the endocrine glands. There may be a decreased blood sugar level in tumors of the islets of Langerhans in the pancreas.

SONOGRAPHIC EVALUATION OF THE PANCREAS

The pancreas is one of the most difficult abdominal organs to image with sonography because it lies posterior to the stomach and sometimes the transverse colon. To help visualize the pancreas, the patient should fast 6 to 8 hours; this decreases the amount of air and fluid in the stomach and colon that may impede visualization. It also promotes dilation of the gallbladder and ducts. If fluid is administered to better visualize the gland, real-time visualization of peristaltic movement of food particles within the duodenum and stomach can be a useful landmark to help outline the head, body, and tail of the pancreas. This will be discussed in more detail later in the chapter.

Pancreas Protocol

The pancreas is examined as part of a comprehensive general abdominal study (Figure 12-9 and Table 12-4). Specific indications for pancreatic scanning include abdominal pain, clinically manifested acute or chronic pancreatitis, abnormal laboratory values, cholecystitis, or obstructive jaundice. The examination determines the presence of cystic and solid masses, biliary and ductal dilation, and the presence of extrapancreatic masses and fluid collections.

1. Patient preparation: nothing by mouth for at least 6 hours; may need to give water to fill the stomach as a window to image the pancreas.
2. Transducer selection: broadband 2.5 to 5 MHz curvilinear.
3. Patient position: supine, decubitus, or upright.
4. Images and observations should include the following:
   - The head, neck/body, and tail should be well delineated once the celiac axis, superior mesenteric artery and vein, aorta, and inferior vena cava are identified. (Often the lie of the pancreas makes it difficult to image the

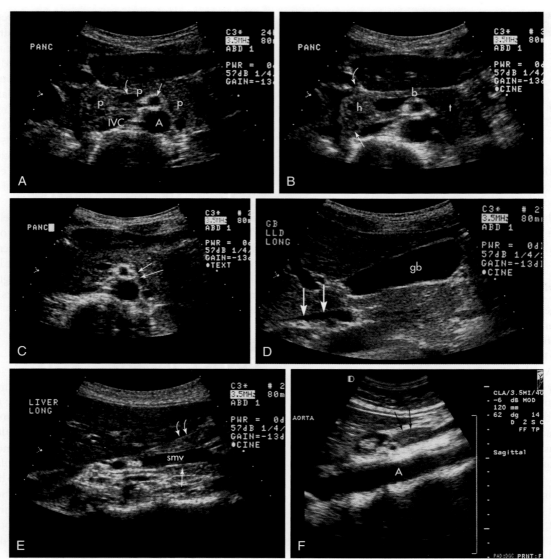

FIGURE 12-9 A, Transverse image of pancreas *(p)* as it lies anterior to superior mesenteric artery *(arrow)* and vein *(curved arrow)*. The aorta *(A)* and inferior vena cava *(IVC)* are anterior to the horseshoe shape of the spine. **B,** Transverse image of head *(h)*, body *(b)*, and tail *(t)* of the pancreas. The gastroduodenal artery *(curved arrow)* is the anterolateral border of the head; the common bile duct *(arrow)* is the posterolateral border of the head. **C,** Transverse image of the pancreas; a sliver of splenic vein *(arrows)* lies posterior to the body and tail. **D,** Longitudinal image of the pancreas (posterior to the gallbladder) with the common bile duct *(arrows)* beginning to move posterior to join the pancreatic duct. **E,** Longitudinal image of the superior mesenteric vein *(smv)* as it flows anterior to the uncinate process *(arrow)* and posterior to the head of the pancreas *(curved arrows)*. **F,** Longitudinal image of the body of the pancreas *(arrows)* anterior to the aorta *(A)*.

TABLE 12-4	Abdominal Ultrasound Protocol: Pancreas	
Organ	**Scan Plane**	**Anatomy**
Pancreas (Figures 8-58–8-63)	Trv	Head/IVC/SMV
		Body and tail/SMV/SMA
	Long	Head/portal vein/IVC
		Body and tail/aorta

IVC, Inferior vena cava; *Long,* longitudinal; *SMA,* superior mesenteric artery; *SMV,* superior mesenteric vein; *Trv,* transverse.

gland in one plane; the tail may be seen on an image that is more superior than the head of the gland.)

- Transverse scans along the region of the splenic vein should be performed to demonstrate the body and tail of the pancreas.
- The pancreatic duct may be seen on the transverse scan as it courses through the body of the gland.
- The longitudinal view of the pancreatic head lies anterior to the inferior vena cava and inferior to the portal vein.

- The superior mesenteric vein may be seen to course anterior to the uncinate process of the head and posterior to the body.
- The pancreatic tail may be seen as gentle but firm pressure is applied to the abdomen to displace overlying gas in the antrum of the stomach or transverse colon. The tail may also be seen with the patient in a right decubitus position as the transducer is angled through the spleen and left kidney; the pancreatic tail is anterior to the left kidney.
- The presence of dilated pancreatic or biliary ducts should be assessed and their size measured.
- The presence of cystic or solid masses should be assessed.
- The presence of peripancreatic nodes should be assessed.
- The presence of peripancreatic fluid collections (e.g., pseudocysts) should be assessed.
- The presence of any pancreatic calcifications detected should be recorded.

Normal Pancreatic Texture

The echogenicity of the pancreas is discussed in terms of how it relates to the liver's homogeneous soft echo pattern. The normal pancreas has an echo pattern that is slightly more hyperechoic and finer in texture than that of the surrounding retroperitoneum. The echo intensity of the pancreas is usually slightly less than that of surrounding soft tissue and slightly greater than that of the liver.

The parenchymal texture of the pancreas depends on the amount of fat between the lobules and to a lesser extent on the interlobular fibrous tissue. The internal echoes of the pancreas consist of closely spaced elements of the same intensity with uniform distribution throughout the gland. Fat is strongly echogenic, and the extensive fatty infiltrations of the pancreas are difficult to visualize by ultrasound because the pancreas blends in with the surrounding retroperitoneal fat. A lesser degree of fatty infiltration may not render the pancreas invisible but may raise the amplitude of returning pancreatic echoes, resulting in the clinical observation that the pancreas returns stronger echoes than the liver. Fibrous tissue may also account for the portion of increased echogenicity. Box 12-1 lists the sonographic characteristics of the normal pancreas.

Sonographic Scan Technique

The patient is usually examined in the supine, oblique, and sometimes upright positions. Sonographic techniques vary according to the patient's body habitus. For adult patients, use a low-frequency broadband transducer with a midfocal zone; for pediatric patients, use at least a 5- to 7.5-MHz transducer. The curved array transducer allows for a better near field of view than the sector transducer allows. The time gain compensation and overall gain should be adjusted so that the pancreatic tissue has the same echo brightness or slightly greater than the normal liver. The texture of the pancreas will appear coarser than the liver depending on the amount of fibrous/fatty tissue interfaces within the gland. The younger pediatric patients tend to have less echogenicity of the pancreas than the older patients do (i.e., more fatty interfaces in the gland of the older patient). The diabetic patient may be challenging to image through the fatty liver texture; therefore a lower-frequency transducer may be useful. With the patient in deep inspiration, gentle pressure on the abdomen with the transducer allows the sonographer to get as close as possible to the pancreatic tissue to improve visualization.

Box 12-2 summarizes the normal pancreatic landmarks. The sonographer should identify the head, neck, body, and tail in the transverse and longitudinal planes (Figures 12-10 and 12-11). The sonographer should evaluate the shape, contour, lie, and texture of the pancreas (compared with the liver parenchyma). The oblique or upright position of the patient may improve visualization of the pancreas and peripancreatic region. The following surrounding structures should be identified: superior mesenteric artery and vein, portal and splenic veins, aorta and inferior vena cava, common bile duct, gastroduodenal artery, left renal vein, duodenal bulb, posterior wall of the stomach, and pancreatic duct.

Windows for Visualization. Difficulties in visualization of the pancreas may result from bowel gas, a transverse stomach obscuring the anatomy, or a small left lobe of the liver. A left lobe measuring at least 2 to 2.5 cm makes an excellent sonic window for imaging the pancreatic area. The subcostal view can be used with a slight caudal angle of the transducer (15 to 20 degrees) as the transducer is directed from the midabdomen (at the level of the xiphoid process), through the left lobe of the liver, and angled through the pancreatic area with the prevertebral vessels demarcating its posterior border.

BOX 12-1 Normal Characteristics of the Pancreas

Size: Head ≤3 cm; neck ≤2.5 cm; body ≤2.5 cm; tail ≤2 cm
Echogenicity: >liver </>spleen (depends on fatty/fibrous texture)
Echotexture: Homogeneous
Surface: Smooth to slightly lobular (islets of Langerhans)

BOX 12-2 Normal Pancreatic Landmarks

Head: Anterior to inferior vena cava, lateral to duodenum; gastroduodenal artery is anterolateral border; common bile duct is posterior medial border. On sagittal plane, portal vein is superior to head of the pancreas.
Uncinate process: Anterior to inferior vena cava, posterior to superior mesenteric vein.
Body: Anterior to superior mesenteric artery and vein, aorta, splenic vein; posterior to stomach, inferior to splenic artery.
Tail: Medial to hilum of spleen; superior to left kidney.
Pancreatic duct: Runs through middle portion of body of pancreas.

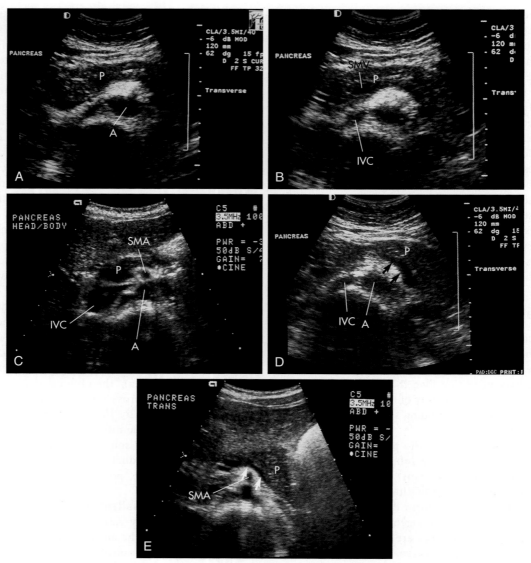

FIGURE 12-10 Transverse images of the pancreas *(P)*. **A,** Body and tail of the pancreas drape anterior to the aorta *(A)*. **B,** Head, body, and tail of the pancreas shown anterior to the aorta, superior mesenteric vein *(SMV)*, and inferior vena cava *(IVC)*. **C,** The superior mesenteric artery *(SMA)*, aorta *(A)*, and inferior vena cava *(IVC)* are posterior borders to the pancreas. **D,** The splenic vein outlines the posterior border of the tail of the pancreas *(arrows)*. **E,** The SMA and splenic vein *(arrows)* outline the posterior border of the tail of the pancreas.

The patient should be in full inspiration to image the pancreas well. This causes the liver to be inferiorly displaced and provides a better scanning window. If the patient has a concave abdomen, ask the patient to take in a deep breath and push out the abdomen to provide a better scanning window.

If the sonographer is unable to image the pancreas, the water ingestion technique may be an effective window to image the gland. The initial scans of the biliary system should be made before asking the patient to drink 32 to 300 ml of fluid through a straw (to prevent swallowing of air) in the erect or right lateral decubitus position. In the upright position, the stomach can be used as an acoustic window; if the patient is unable to sit up, the examination can be done in the right lateral decubitus position. This water method fills the body and antrum of the stomach initially to help outline the body and tail of the pancreas (Figure 12-12). The fluid then fills the duodenal cap to outline the lateral margin of the head of the pancreas. The upright position allows the air to move from the gastric antrum to the fundus of the stomach and causes the upper viscera to move downward for a better sonic window. The upright position also results in distention of the venous structures, which further aids in the localization of the pancreas (see Box 12-2).

Transverse Plane. Generally the pancreas is imaged first in the transverse plane. The patient should be in full inspiration to distend the venous structures that serve as posterior landmarks to visualize the pancreas. As previously mentioned, the sonographer should use the left lobe of the liver at the level of

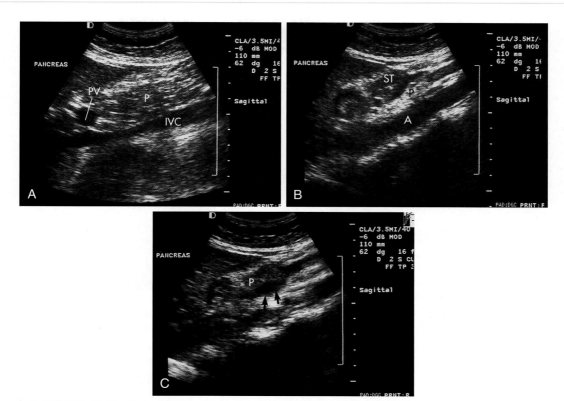

FIGURE 12-11 Sagittal images of the pancreas *(P)*. **A,** The pancreas lies inferior to the portal vein *(PV)* and anterior to the inferior vena cava *(IVC)*. **B,** The stomach *(ST)* is anterior to the pancreas. The aorta *(A)* is the posterior border. **C,** A small segment of the superior mesenteric vein *(arrows)* is seen along the posterior border of the neck of the pancreas.

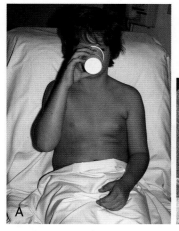

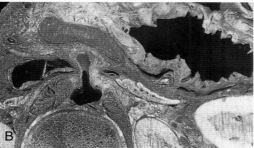

FIGURE 12-12 A, To better visualize the pancreas, the patient should drink more than 16 ounces of water and be imaged in the semiupright position. **B,** Gross anatomy of the midepigastrium at the level of the superior mesenteric artery. The body of the pancreas is clearly seen anterior to the superior mesenteric artery and posterior to the stomach.

the xiphoid and angle the transducer slightly toward the feet to image the aorta and celiac axis. This is near the superior border of the pancreas (remember that the tortuous splenic artery may be seen rising from the celiac axis to demarcate the superior border of the pancreas) (Figure 12-13). The body and tail of the gland should be imaged as the transducer is slowly angled inferiorly from the celiac axis. Visualization of the superior mesenteric vessels, left renal vein, and inferior vena cava also helps delineate the borders of the body of the pancreas (Figure 12-14). The stomach may be seen as the walls are collapsed because it lies anterior to the pancreas (Figure 12-15).

The duodenum, gastroduodenal artery, and common bile duct are useful landmarks in identifying the lateral margin of the pancreatic head (Figure 12-16). The sonographer may watch for peristalsis or fluid to pass through the second part of the duodenum as it forms the C-loop around the lateral border of the head.

Sagittal Plane. The initial scan should be made slightly to the right of midline with the patient in full inspiration. The dilated inferior vena cava is seen as the posterior border (Figure 12-17). The main portal vein or right branch of the portal vein is the next landmark seen anterior to the cava.

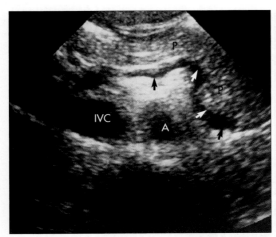

FIGURE 12-13 The tortuous splenic artery *(arrows)* rises from the celiac axis. The pancreas is usually inferior to the splenic artery; however, in this patient the gland is shown anterior to the vessel. *A,* Aorta; *IVC,* inferior vena cava; *P,* pancreas.

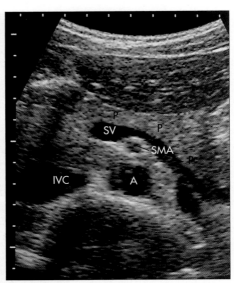

FIGURE 12-14 Transverse scan of the normal pancreas and its vascular landmarks. *A,* Aorta; *IVC,* inferior vena cava; *P,* pancreas; *SMA,* superior mesenteric artery; *SV,* splenic vein.

FIGURE 12-15 A, The collapsed wall of the stomach *(arrows)* may be seen as two parallel lines anterior to the body of the pancreas. **B,** The fluid-filled duodenum *(Du)* marks the lateral border of the head of the pancreas *(P). A,* Aorta; *IVC,* inferior vena cava.

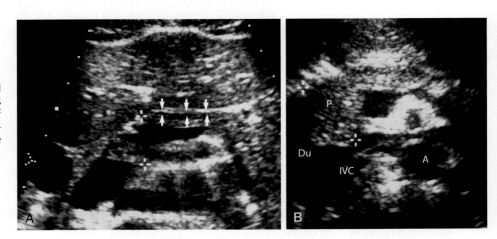

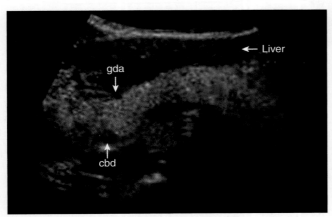

FIGURE 12-16 The small gastroduodenal artery *(gda)* is the anterolateral border of the head of the pancreas. *A,* Aorta.

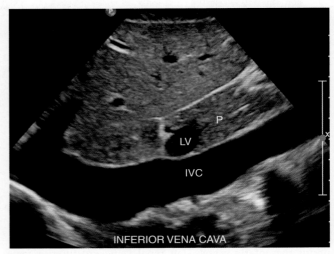

FIGURE 12-17 Sagittal image of the dilated inferior vena cava *(IVC)* as it demarcates the posterior border of the pancreas *(P).* The portal vein *(pv)* is seen anterior to the inferior vena cava and cephalad to the pancreas.

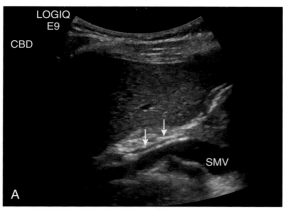
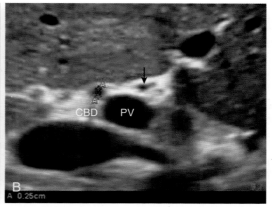

FIGURE 12-18 **A,** Sagittal scan of the common bile duct *(arrows)* and its surrounding vascular landmarks. *SMV/PV,* Superior mesenteric/portal vein confluence. **B,** The common bile duct *(open arrows)* is seen anterior and lateral to the portal vein *(PV)* while the hepatic artery *(arrow)* is anterior medial. The patient is in a decubitus position.

The pancreas lies just inferior to the portal vein and anterior to the inferior vena cava. As the pancreas enlarges, a slight indentation is apparent on the anterior border of the cava. This view is also good for visualizing the common bile duct because it lies anterior to the portal vein before dropping posterior to enter the head of the pancreas (Figure 12-18). The hepatic artery is sometimes visible as a circular tube when the common duct is seen. The use of color Doppler may help the sonographer separate the hepatic artery from the common duct.

Subsequent scans are made slightly to the left of the midline to image the aorta and superior mesenteric artery and vein because they form the posterior border of the body of the pancreas. The superior mesenteric vein flows cephalad to join the portal vein and may be seen as a long, tubular structure posterior to the neck of the pancreas and anterior to the uncinate process (Figure 12-19). The tail of the pancreas is more difficult to see, but it may be imaged as the sonographer angles slightly to the left of the aorta. The patient may be rolled into a steep right decubitus position to image the tail of the gland as it lies in the hilum of the spleen near the left kidney.

The antrum of the stomach appears as a collapsed bull's-eye and may be identified anterior and slightly caudal to the body of the pancreas (Figure 12-20, *A*). The splenic vein is a circular sonolucent structure posterior to the cephalic portion of the gland (Figure 12-20, *B*). The left renal vein is a slitlike

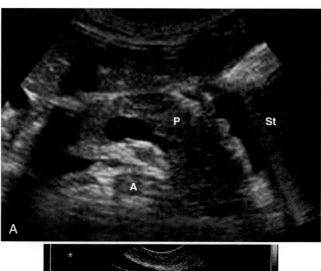

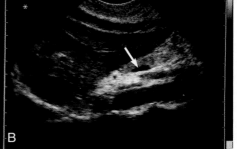

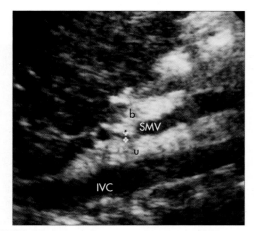

FIGURE 12-19 Sagittal scan of the right upper quadrant shows the superior mesenteric vein *(SMV)* as it flows anterior to the uncinate process *(u)* and posterior to the body *(b)* of the pancreas. *IVC,* Inferior vena cava.

FIGURE 12-20 **A,** The collapsed antrum of the stomach *(ST)* is seen as a target lesion anterior to the body of the pancreas. **B,** The splenic vein is seen as a circle on the sagittal plane as it flows along the posteromedial border of the pancreas *(arrow).*

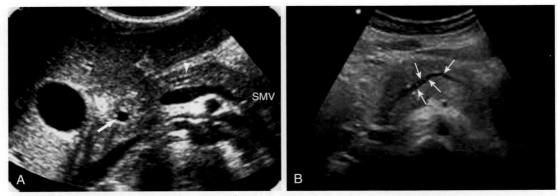

FIGURE 12-21 A, Normal pancreatic duct *(closed arrow)* within the midbody of the pancreas; gastroduodenal artery *(arrow)* marks the anterolateral border of the pancreatic head. **B,** Dilated pancreatic duct *(arrows).*

sonolucency between the aorta and the superior mesenteric artery.

Pancreatic Duct. The main pancreatic duct may be visualized best on the transverse image as it courses through the body of the gland (Figure 12-21). The sonographer should be sure to identify pancreatic tissue on both sides of the duct so as not to confuse it with vascular structures that may lie near it. The splenic vein is usually too posterior and the hepatic artery too anterior to be confused with the duct. Color Doppler may be used to help distinguish a dilated duct from vascular structures. The duct appears as an echo-free area sharply marginated by two parallel echogenic lines. A thin strip of retroperitoneal fat may underlie the anterior aspect of the pancreas. This sonolucent linear pattern should not be mistaken for duct. On transverse scans, the posterior wall of the antrum can be seen overlying the pancreas. Care should be taken to distinguish the antrum of the collapsed stomach from the small pancreatic duct.

PATHOLOGY OF THE PANCREAS

Pancreatitis

Pancreatitis is inflammation of the pancreas; this condition may be chronic or acute. Pancreatitis occurs when the pancreas becomes damaged and malfunctions as a result of increased secretion and blockage of ducts. When this occurs, the pancreatic tissue may be digested by its own enzymes. Pancreatitis may be classified as acute or chronic with a further subdescription of mild to severe. In patients with acute pancreatitis, ultrasound may not always be the first imaging performed because often ileus is associated with this condition. Therefore the optimal imaging procedure is the dynamic intravenous and oral contrast-enhanced computed tomography. See Table 12-4 for clinical findings, sonographic findings, and differential considerations for pancreatitis.

Acute Pancreatitis. Acute pancreatitis is an inflammation of the pancreas caused by the inflamed acini releasing pancreatic enzymes into the surrounding pancreatic tissue. Normally these enzymes do not become active until they

reach the duodenum, where they enable the breakdown of food in the system. The classification of acute pancreatitis is further divided into the following three categories: (1) mild acute pancreatitis, characterized by the absence of organ failure and local or systemic complications; (2) moderately severe acute pancreatitis, characterized by transient organ failure and/or local or systemic complications without persistent organ failure; and (3) severe acute pancreatitis, characterized by persistent organ failure that may involve one or multiple organs.

The clinical features of acute pancreatitis usually do not last more than several days. Most patients present with acute onset of persistent, severe epigastric pain accompanied by nausea and vomiting. In patients with gallstone pancreatitis, the pain is well localized and the onset of pain is rapid, reaching maximum intensity in 10 to 20 minutes. In contrast, in patients with pancreatitis secondary to alcohol, metabolic, or hereditary causes, the pain is usually not as abrupt and is poorly localized. The pain may radiate to the back, persisting for several hours to days. The patient may be at risk for abscess and hemorrhage secondary to the pancreatitis (Figure 12-22).

An acute attack of pancreatitis is commonly related to biliary tract disease and alcoholism. The most common cause

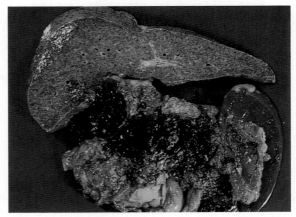

FIGURE 12-22 Gross pathology of acute hemorrhagic pancreatitis. The pancreas has been completely obliterated by blood.

of pancreatitis in the United States is biliary tract disease. Gallstones are present in 40% to 60% of patients, and 5% of patients with gallstones have acute pancreatitis. Gallstone pancreatitis causes a relatively sudden onset of constant biliary pain. As the pancreatic parenchyma is further damaged, the pain becomes more severe and the abdomen becomes rigid and tender.

Alcohol abuse is the second most common cause of pancreatitis. Other less common causes include trauma, inflammation from adjacent peptic ulcer or abdominal infection, pregnancy, mumps, tumors, congenital causes, vascular thrombosis or embolism, and drugs.

The laboratory analysis of pancreatic enzymes is the key to pancreatic destruction (see Table 12-4). Serum amylase rises within 6 to 12 hours of the onset of acute pancreatitis. Amylase has a short half-life of approximately 10 hours and in uncomplicated attacks returns to normal within 3 to 5 days. Serum lipase rises within 4 to 8 hours of the onset of symptoms, peaks at 24 hours, and returns to normal within 8 to 14 days. Lipase elevations occur earlier and last longer compared with elevations in amylase and are therefore especially useful in patients who seek treatment more than 24 hours after the onset of pain. Serum lipase is also more sensitive compared with amylase in patients with pancreatitis secondary to alcohol abuse.

Acute pancreatitis may be mild to severe (Figure 12-23). Damage to the acinar tissue and ductal system results either in exudation of pancreatic juice into the gland's interstitium, leakage of secretions into the peripancreatic tissues, or both. After the acini or duct disrupts, the secretions migrate to the surface of the gland. The common course is for fluid to break through the pancreatic connective tissue layer and thin posterior layer of the peritoneum and enter the lesser sac. The mild form of pancreatitis demonstrates interstitial edema within the gland with little or no peripancreatic inflammation. There may be small areas of acinar cell necrosis within the pancreas. As the process becomes more severe, fat necrosis, parenchymal necrosis, and necrosis of the blood vessels develops with subsequent hemorrhage and peripancreatic inflammation within 1 to 2 days. With time, this necrotic tissue is replaced by diffuse or focal fibrosis,

calcifications, and irregular ductal dilations. The formation of a pseudocyst may develop secondary to acute pancreatitis.

The pancreatic juice enters the anterior pararenal space by breaking through the thin layer of the fibrous connective tissue, or the fluid may migrate to the surface of the gland and remain within the confines of the fibrous connective tissue layer.

Collections of fluid in the peripancreatic area generally retain communication with the pancreas. A dynamic equilibrium is established so that fluid is continuously absorbed from the collection and replaced by additional pancreatic secretions. The drainage of juices may cease as the pancreatic inflammatory response subsides and the rate of pancreatic secretions returns to normal. The collections of extrapancreatic fluid should be reabsorbed or, if drained, should not recur with recovery of proper drainage through the duct.

Sonographic Findings. The sonographic description of acute pancreatitis may be defined by distribution (focal or diffuse) and by severity (mild, moderate, or severe). In the early stages of acute pancreatitis the gland may not show swelling on sonography (Figure 12-24). When swelling does occur, the gland is hypoechoic to anechoic and is less echogenic than the liver because of the increased prominence of lobulations and congested vessels (Figure 12-25). The borders may be somewhat indistinct but smooth. On a longitudinal scan, the anterior compression of the inferior vena cava by the swollen head of the pancreas may be apparent. Thus pancreatic enlargement and decreased pancreatic echogenicity are sonographic landmarks for acute pancreatitis.

If localized enlargement is present, it may be difficult to separate from neoplastic involvement of the gland (Figure 12-26). Analysis of patient history and laboratory values should enable the clinician to make the distinction. If the serum amylase level is normal and the patient is asymptomatic, the mass is likely to represent a neoplasm. However, if the patient has severe abdominal pain, tender to the touch, this focal hypoechogenicity is more likely caused by pancreatitis than by a neoplastic growth. If the mass has calcification within an enlarged ductal system, a neoplasm is more likely suspected. The evaluation by ERCP may

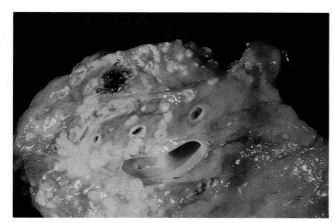

FIGURE 12-23 Gross pathology of acute pancreatitis. The foci of fat necrosis appear as white opaque patches.

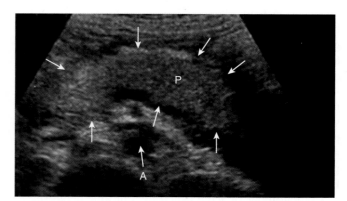

FIGURE 12-24 A middle-aged male presented with midepigastric pain, elevated amylase and lipase levels, and tenderness. The pancreas is diffusely enlarged representing acute pancreatitis. Transverse scans over the upper abdomen show the inflamed pancreatic tissue. *A,* Aorta; *P,* pancreas *(arrows).*

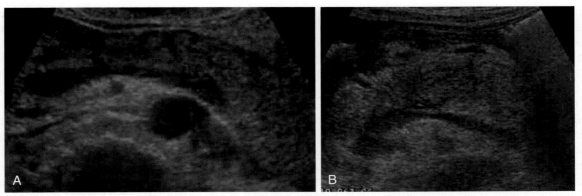

FIGURE 12-25 In acute pancreatitis, the gland is hypoechoic to anechoic and is less echogenic than the liver because of the increased prominence of lobulations and congested vessels.

provide better resolution of the pancreatic head and ductal system to further delineate neoplastic growth from pancreatitis.

The pancreatic duct may be obstructed in acute pancreatitis as a result of inflammation, spasm, edema, swelling of the papilla, or pseudocyst formation. The detection of biliary obstruction is important as so many of the patients have coexisting liver disease. Obstruction of the biliary system may be due to stricture in the distal common duct or to compression of the common bile duct by a pseudocyst or inflammation of the head of the pancreas.

The alteration in the size and echogenic texture of the pancreas may be subtle; therefore the diagnosis of pancreatitis may be based on the visualization of peripancreatic fluid collections in a patient with abnormal pancreatic enzymes and clinical history suggestive of pancreatitis. Fluid collections around the pancreatic bed, along the pararenal spaces, within Morison's pouch, and around the duodenum may be present in a patient with acute pancreatitis.

In diffuse pancreatitis, the pancreas enlarges and the texture becomes hypoechogenic compared with the "normal" liver texture. Because alcohol is a frequent cause of pancreatitis, the development of a hyperechoic diffuse fatty liver makes this comparison invalid. As the disease progresses, the decreased echogenicity and enlargement are readily seen secondary to increased fluid content in the interstitium caused by the inflammation. The pancreas may be diffusely inhomogeneous. The pancreatic duct may be either compressed by the edema or dilated (from the focal pancreatic inflammation or obstruction of the stone or tumor).

Sonography is not as effective as CT in the early stages of pancreatitis, as CT is more specific in its ability to demonstrate the detail of the pancreas and the retroperitoneal structures, regardless of bowel interference. CT can detect necrosis and acute fracture of the pancreas. Sonographic detection of pancreatitis is effective when ileus is not present to obstruct the visualization of the pancreatic area.

Complications of acute pancreatitis include hemorrhage, pseudocyst formation, inflammatory mass, and intrapancreatic and extrapancreatic fluid collections. Sonography may directly guide the interventionalist for needle aspiration to help differentiate between an infected and noninfected inflammatory mass and pseudocyst collection.

Extrapancreatic Fluid Collections and Edema. The findings of fluid collections and edema are frequent in patients with severe acute pancreatitis. The most common sites for fluid collection are found in the lesser sac, anterior pararenal spaces, mesocolon, perirenal spaces, and peripancreatic soft tissue spaces. For the sonographer, the fluid in the lesser sac that is found between the stomach and the pancreas is easily imaged. Fluid in the superior recess of the lesser sac is seen to surround the caudate lobe with visualization of the gastrohepatic ligament. Fluid that lies in the perirenal space may also be demonstrated on sonography. As fluid collects in the anterior pararenal space, it is best demonstrated on the sagittal sonographic image. The fluid may be anechoic or contain fine linear lines within that represent septations secondary to infection or hemorrhage. The more solid composition of the retroperitoneal or intraperitoneal fluid collections is most difficult to image with sonography because of bowel interference. These extrapancreatic fluid collections occur within 4 weeks from the acute onset of the pancreatitis and may resolve spontaneously. The formation of a pseudocyst occurs when the fluid collection develops into a well-defined, walled-off fluid collection of amylase. Other sonographic findings may include ascites, thickened wall of the gallbladder, and thickening of the adjacent gastrointestinal tract.

Chronic Pancreatitis. Chronic pancreatitis results from recurrent attacks of acute pancreatitis and causes continuing destruction of the pancreatic parenchyma that result in permanent structural damage, which can lead to impairment of exocrine and endocrine function (see Table 12-4). There are several features to distinguish chronic from acute pancreatitis. Patients with chronic pancreatitis may be asymptomatic over long periods of time, may present with a fibrotic mass, or may have symptoms of pancreatic insufficiency without pain. Acute pancreatitis is most always associated with epigastric pain. The laboratory values of serum amylase and lipase are usually normal in chronic pancreatitis, but almost always elevated in patients with acute disease. Characteristically, chronic pancreatitis presents with patchy focal fibrotic disease, whereas acute pancreatitis usually involves the entire gland.

Clinical findings in patients with chronic pancreatitis include abdominal pain and pancreatic insufficiency. The abdominal pain is epigastric, radiating to the back, and may be associated with nausea and vomiting. Patients with severe pancreatic exocrine dysfunction cannot properly digest complex foods or absorb partially digested breakdown products. Glucose intolerance may develop in patients with chronic pancreatitis.

Chronic pancreatitis is generally associated with chronic alcoholism or biliary disease, although patients with **hypercalcemia** (elevated calcium levels) and **hyperlipidemia** (elevated fat levels) are more predisposed to chronic pancreatitis. In chronic alcoholic pancreatitis, the alcoholic intake causes increased pancreatic protein secretion with subsequent ductal obstruction resulting in chronic calcifying pancreatitis. The fibrous connective tissue rapidly grows around the ducts and between the lobules with resultant scarring that leads to a nodular, irregular surface of the pancreas. The pancreatic ducts become obstructed with a buildup of protein plugs with resultant calcifications along the duct. The less common type is chronic obstructive pancreatitis with a nonlobular distribution, less ductal epithelial damage, and rarely calcified stones. This form is usually caused by stenosis of the sphincter of Oddi by cholelithiasis or pancreatic tumor.

Patients with chronic pancreatitis may develop pseudocysts, a dilated common bile duct, or thrombosis of the splenic vein with extension into the portal vein. Patients with chronic pancreatitis have an increased risk of developing pancreatic cancer.

On pathologic examination, the pancreas shows an increase in the interlobular fibrous tissue and chronic inflammatory infiltration changes. Stones of calcium carbonate may be found inside the ductal system, and pseudocysts are common (Figure 12-27). There is calcification of the gland in 20% to 40% of the patients.

Sonographic Findings. Chronic pancreatitis appears as a mixed pattern. The tissue affected may appear as a diffuse or localized involvement of the gland (Figure 12-28). Echogenicity of the pancreas is usually increased beyond normal because of fibrotic and fatty changes, with a mixture of hypoechoic (from inflammation) and hyperechoic foci. The size of the gland is reduced and the borders are irregular, and the pancreatic duct may be irregular and dilated

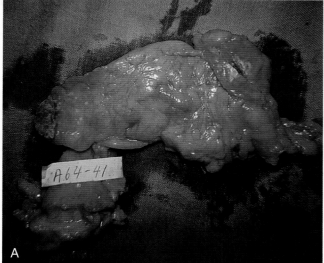
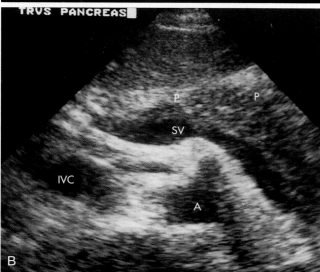
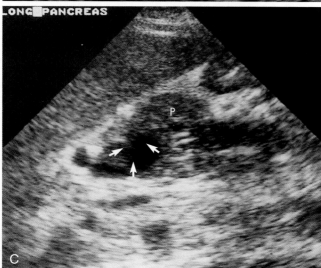

FIGURE 12-26 **A,** Gross specimen of an inflamed pancreas. **B,** A 37-year-old male patient with AIDS presented with pancreatitis, hepatosplenomegaly, and peripancreatic adenopathy. The pancreas is enlarged and slightly hypoechoic. *A,* Aorta; *IVC,* inferior vena cava; *P,* pancreas; *SV,* splenic vein. **C,** Sagittal scan of the enlarged pancreas *(P)* with adenopathy *(arrows).*

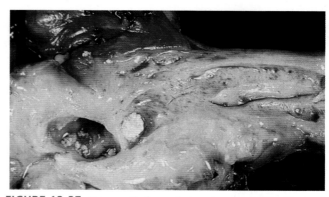

FIGURE 12-27 Gross pathology of chronic pancreatitis. The main pancreatic duct is dilated and contains calculi. The pancreatic acini have been replaced by fibrous tissue.

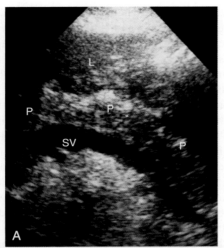

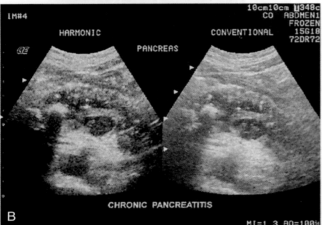

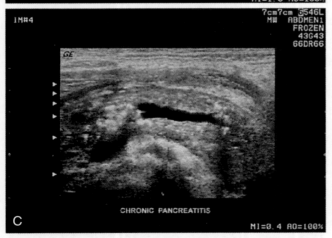

FIGURE 12-28 Ultrasound patterns in chronic pancreatitis. **A,** Calcifications are seen along the body of the pancreas *(P). L,* Liver; *SV,* splenic vein. **B,** The pancreas is shrunken in size. **C,** The pancreatic duct is enlarged.

secondary to stricture or as the result of an extrinsic stone moving from a smaller pancreatic duct into a major duct. The classic sonographic finding is calcifications. With pancreatic ductal lithiasis, shadowing may be present, with the most common site of obstruction at the papilla. Generally speaking, chronic pancreatitis is more highly suspected

when the duct contains calcification and no obstructing mass lesion is seen, whereas carcinoma is suggested when a parenchymal mass lesion is identified at the site of obstruction of the pancreatic duct.

A focal mass or enlargement may be seen in the pancreas secondary to perilobular scarring with edema and inflammation. The presence of calcification is useful to differentiate such focal enlargements from neoplasms. Pseudocysts over 5 cm in size that persist beyond 6 weeks require decompression with significant risk of complications. Decompression may also be required in smaller pseudocysts that compress adjacent structures to cause persistent symptoms or if significant complications arise such as infection, hemorrhage, or perforation.

Complications of Pancreatitis

Pancreatitis may be associated with a variety of complications. These include walled-off pancreatic fluid collections, bile duct or duodenal obstruction, pancreatic ascites or pleural effusion, splenic vein thrombosis, pseudoaneurysms, and pancreatic cancer. Pancreatic and parapancreatic fluid collections are the most common complications of pancreatitis.

Walled-off Pancreatic Fluid Collections. The inflammatory pancreatic fluid collections include acute peripancreatic fluid collections, pseudocysts, acute necrotic collections, and walled-off pancreatic necrosis. The acute peripancreatic fluid collections occur in the setting of acute interstitial pancreatitis within 4 weeks of the onset of pancreatitis. They typically are extrapancreatic and do not have a definable wall. The fluid contains no solid material, and no pancreatic necrosis is present. The pseudocyst represents a more mature fluid collection, is located outside the pancreas, has a well-defined wall, and has no solid internal material or necrosis. Acute necrotic collections occur in necrotizing pancreatitis, may be adjacent to or involve the pancreas, have no definable wall, and may contain liquid and solid material. The walled-off pancreatic necrosis is a mature mass that may be intrapancreatic or extrapancreatic with an encapsulated collection of necrosis with liquid and solid components. Walled-off pancreatic fluid collections include pseudocysts and walled-off pancreatic necrosis. Most walled-off pancreatic fluid collections are now classified as walled-off pancreatic necrosis rather than pseudocysts.

Although many of these walled-off pancreatic fluid collections resolve without intervention, a variety of clinical problems may develop depending on the location and extent of the fluid collection and if the collection becomes infected. The expansion of the fluid collection may produce abdominal pain, duodenal or biliary obstruction, vascular occlusion, or fistula formation into adjacent viscera, the pleural space, or pericardium. If an adjacent vessel is digested by the pancreatic enzymes, a pseudoaneurysm can develop, which can produce sudden, painful expansion of the cyst or gastrointestinal bleeding due to the bleeding into the pancreatic duct. Pancreatic ascites or pleural effusion may result from

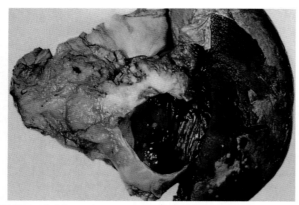

FIGURE 12-29 Gross pathology of pancreatic pseudocyst filled with hemorrhagic fluid in the tail with extension into the hilum of the spleen.

disruption of the pancreatic duct with fistulization to the abdomen or chest.

The walled-off pancreatic fluid collection known as the **pseudocyst** may be defined as a collection of fluid that arises from the loculation of inflammatory processes, necrosis, trauma, or hemorrhage (Figure 12-29). Pseudocysts are always acquired; they result from trauma to the gland or acute or chronic pancreatitis (see Table 12-4). In approximately 10% to 20% of patients with acute pancreatitis, a pseudocyst develops over 4 to 6 weeks after the onset of pancreatitis. This collection is formed when pancreatic enzymes escape from the gland and break down tissue to form a sterile abscess somewhere in the abdomen. Its walls are not true cyst walls, hence the name *pseudo-*, or false, cyst. Pseudocysts generally take on the contour of the available space around them and therefore are not always spherical, as are normal cysts. There may be more than one pseudocyst, so the sonographer should search for daughter collections.

The patient does not experience symptoms as a result of the pseudocyst until it becomes large enough to cause pressure on the surrounding organs. Pseudocysts usually develop through the lesser omentum, displacing the stomach or widening the duodenal loop. Although the most common association of pseudocyst development is in patients with alcoholic or biliary disease, it may also develop after blunt trauma or secondary to pancreatic malignancy. Clinically the patient may present with a history of pancreatitis, persistent pain, and elevated amylase levels.

Locations of a Pseudocyst.
The most common location of a pseudocyst is in the lesser sac anterior to the pancreas and posterior to the stomach. The second most common location is in the anterior pararenal space (posterior to the lesser sac, bounded by Gerota's fascia). The spleen is the lateral border of the anterior pararenal space on the left. Fluid occurs more commonly in the left pararenal space than the right. Sometimes the posterior pararenal space is fluid filled; fluid spreads from the anterior pararenal space to the posterior pararenal space on the same side. Fluid may enter the peritoneal cavity via the foramen of Winslow or by disrupting the peritoneum in the anterior surface of the lesser sac. It may extend into the mediastinum by extending through the esophageal or aortic hiatus, or it may extend into small bowel mesentery or down into the retroperitoneum into the pelvis and groin.

Sonographically, the walled-off pseudocyst usually appears as a well-defined mass with essentially sonolucent, echo-free interior. Debris seen within the collection may occur from complications of infection or hemorrhage; scattered echoes may be seen at the bottom of the cysts, and increased through-transmission is present (Figure 12-30). The borders are very echogenic, and the cysts usually are thicker than other simple cysts. Calcification may develop within the walls of the pseudocyst. When a suspected pseudocyst is located near the stomach, the stomach should be drained so the cyst is not mistaken for a fluid-filled stomach. If the patient has been on continual drainage before the ultrasound examination, this problem is eliminated. Spontaneous rupture is the most common complication of a pancreatic pseudocyst, occurring in 5% of patients. In 3% of these patients, drainage is directly into the peritoneal cavity. Clinical symptoms are sudden shock and peritonitis. The mortality rate is 50%.

Walled-off Necrotic Intrapancreatic or Extrapancreatic Fluid Collections.
The walled-off necrotic intrapancreatic or extrapancreatic fluid collection appears as a heterogeneous collection with liquid and solid components with varying degrees of loculation. This necrosis is well defined and completely encapsulates the fluid collection.

Pancreatic ascites occurs when the pancreatic pseudocyst ruptures into the abdomen. Pancreatic ascites that develops as a consequence of spontaneous rupture may be differentiated from pancreatic ascites associated with cirrhosis in patients who have known rupture of a pseudocyst by analysis of the fluid for elevated amylase and protein content (Figure 12-31). In 2% of patients, the rupture is into the gastrointestinal tract. Such patients may present a confusing picture sonographically. The initial scan shows a typical pattern for a pseudocyst formation, but the patient may have intense pain develop secondary to the rupture, and consequent examination shows the disappearance of the mass.

Hemorrhagic Pancreatitis.
Hemorrhagic pancreatitis is a rapid progression of acute pancreatitis with rupture of pancreatic vessels and subsequent hemorrhage (see Table 12-4). In hemorrhagic pancreatitis, there is diffuse enzymatic destruction of the pancreatic substance caused by a sudden escape of active pancreatic enzymes into the glandular parenchyma (Figure 12-32). These enzymes cause focal areas of fat necrosis in and around the pancreas, which leads to rupture of pancreatic vessels and hemorrhage. Nearly half of these patients have sudden necrotizing destruction of the pancreas after an alcoholic binge or an excessively large meal.

Specific sonographic findings depend on the age of the hemorrhage. A well-defined homogeneous mass in the area of the pancreas may be seen with areas of fresh necrosis. Foci of extravasated blood and fat necrosis are also seen. Further necrosis of the blood vessels results in the development of hemorrhagic areas referred to as Grey Turner's sign (discoloration of the flanks). At 1 week, the mass may appear cystic with solid elements or septation. After several weeks the hemorrhage may appear cystic.

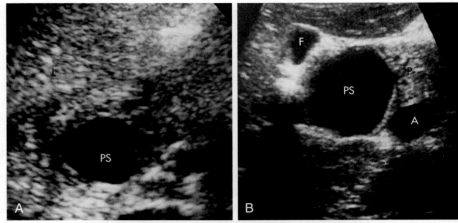

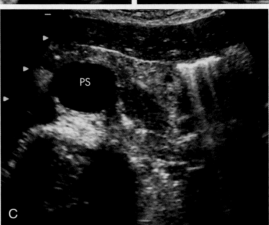

FIGURE 12-30 Ultrasound patterns of a typical pancreatic pseudocyst. *A,* Aorta; *F,* fluid; *L,* liver; *P,* pancreas; *PS,* pseudocyst.

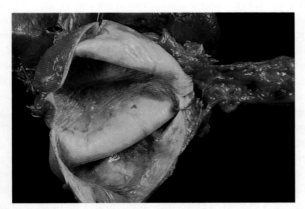

FIGURE 12-31 Gross pathology of a pancreatic pseudocyst rupture.

Phlegmonous Pancreatitis. A phlegmon is an inflammatory process that spreads along fascial pathways, causing localized areas of diffuse inflammatory edema of soft tissue that may proceed to necrosis and suppuration. Extension outside the gland occurs in 18% to 20% of patients with acute pancreatitis. The phlegmonous tissue appears on ultrasound as hypoechoic texture with good through-transmission (Figure 12-33). The phlegmon usually involves the lesser sac, left anterior pararenal space, and transverse mesocolon. Less commonly, it involves the small bowel mesentery, lower retroperitoneum, and pelvis. See Table 12-4 for sonographic

findings and differential considerations for phlegmonous pancreatitis.

Pancreatic Abscess. Pancreatic abscess has a low incidence, although it is a serious complication of pancreatitis; the condition is related to the degree of tissue necrosis (see Table 12-4). The majority of patients develop abscess secondary to pancreatitis that develops from postoperative procedures. A very high mortality rate is associated with this condition if left untreated. An abscess may rise from a neighboring infection, such as a perforated peptic ulcer, acute appendicitis, or acute cholecystitis. A pancreatic abscess may be unilocular or multilocular and can spread superiorly into the mediastinum, inferiorly into the transverse mesocolon, or down the retroperitoneum into the pelvis. Acute peritonitis may develop as the pseudocyst ruptures into the peritoneal cavity.

Sonographic Findings. A pancreatic abscess is imaged with sonography as a poorly defined hypoechoic mass with smooth or irregular thick walls, causing few internal echoes; it may be echo-free to echodense (Figure 12-34). The sonographic appearance depends on the amount of debris present. If air bubbles are present, an echogenic region with a shadow posterior is imaged. A pseudocyst that forms during acute necrotizing pancreatitis has a higher likelihood of spontaneous regression, whereas a pseudocyst that forms secondary to chronic pancreatitis and develops calcification in its walls usually does not resolve on its own.

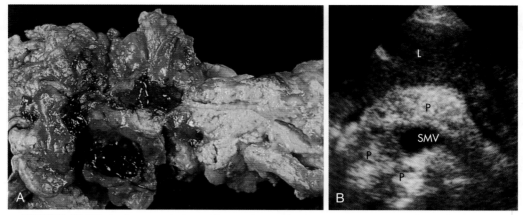

FIGURE 12-32 **A,** Gross pathology of acute hemorrhagic pancreatitis. Hemorrhagic fat necrosis and a pseudocyst filled with blood are seen on cross section. **B,** Pancreatitis with hemorrhage. The gland is enlarged and echogenic secondary to freshly clotted blood. *L,* Liver; *P,* pancreas; *SMV,* superior mesenteric vein.

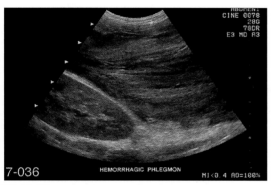

FIGURE 12-33 Hemorrhagic phlegmon is a complication of pancreatitis. The phlegmon is ill defined as it lies anterior to the kidney.

Benign Cystic Lesions of the Pancreas

A wide variety of cystic lesions of the pancreas may be seen on imaging studies of the abdomen. Pancreatic cysts may be neoplastic or nonneoplastic. Ultrasound, CT, MRI, and ERCP are imaging modalities that are used to help narrow the differential diagnosis to aid the clinician in arriving at a diagnosis when correlated with clinical, pathologic, and laboratory findings. See Table 12-5 for clinical findings, sonographic findings, and differential considerations for pancreatic cysts.

Multiple Pancreatic Cysts (Table 12-6)

Autosomal Dominant Polycystic Disease. This disease is characterized by the presence of multiple small cysts in the kidney and liver, with rare extension into the pancreas. These cysts vary from microscopic to several centimeters in diameter and with increasing size may destroy the normal pancreatic tissue.

Von Hippel–Lindau Syndrome. Von Hippel–Lindau syndrome is an inherited disorder characterized by the formation of tumors and fluid-filled sacs (cysts) in many different parts of the body (Figure 12-35). The tumors may be either noncancerous or cancerous and most frequently appear during young adulthood; however, the signs and symptoms of von Hippel–Lindau syndrome can occur

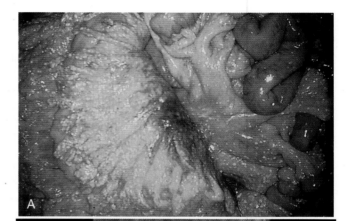
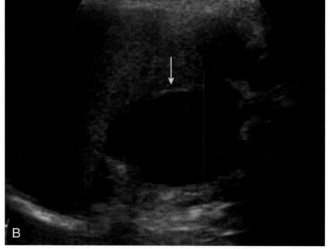

FIGURE 12-34 **A,** Gross pathology of peritonitis complicating acute pancreatitis. The mesentery shows foci of fat necrosis and hemorrhage. Bloody ascites has already been removed. **B,** A pancreatic abscess is imaged with sonography as a poorly defined hypoechoic mass with smooth or irregular thick walls, causing few internal echoes; it may be echo-free to echodense.

TABLE 12-5 Pancreatitis Findings

Clinical Findings	Sonographic Findings	Differential Considerations
Acute Pancreatitis		
Sudden onset of moderate to severe abdominal pain with radiation to back	Ranges from normal size to focal/diffuse enlargement	Hemorrhagic pancreatitis
Nausea and vomiting	Hypoechoic texture (edema)	Lymphoma
History of gallstones (localized) or alcoholism	Borders distinct but irregular	Retroperitoneal neoplasm
Mild fever	Enlargement of head causes depression on inferior vena cava	
↑ Pancreatic enzymes in blood (amylase, lipase)	40%–60% have gallstones Pancreatic duct may be enlarged	
Leukocytosis (↑ white blood cells)	Parapancreatic fluid collections	
Abdominal distention		
Hemorrhagic Pancreatitis		
↓ Hematocrit and serum calcium level	Depends on age of hemorrhage	Chronic hemorrhage
Intense, severe pain radiating to back, with subsequent shock and ileus	Well-defined homogeneous mass in area of pancreas	
Hypotension despite volume replacement, with metabolic acidosis and adult respiratory distress syndrome		
Phlegmonous Pancreatitis		
See *Acute pancreatitis*	Hypoechoic, ill-defined mass	Chronic hemorrhage
Pancreatic Abscess		
Fever, chills	Hypoechoic mass with smooth borders	Acute pancreatitis
↑ Leukocytosis	Thick walls	Chronic pancreatitis
Hypotension	Echo-free to echogenic	
Tender abdomen		
Chronic Pancreatitis		
Severe abdominal pain radiating to back	Gland is small and fibrotic	Acute pancreatitis
Malabsorption	Irregular borders	Thrombosis of portal system
Fatty stools	Mixed echogenicity	Pancreatic pseudocyst
Signs of diabetes Weight loss	Dilated pancreatic duct (string of pearls sign with dilated duct)	Dilated common bile duct
Jaundice	Look for calculi within duct	
↑ Amylase and lipase		
Pancreatic Pseudocyst		
Asymptomatic unless large enough to put pressure on other organs	Well-defined mass, usually in area of pancreas	True cyst Fluid-filled cystadenoma
↑ Amylase and lipase	↑ Through-transmission	
↑ Alkaline phosphatase if obstruction develops	Variable size (round or oval) May have debris at bottom	

throughout life. Tumors called *hemangioblastomas* are characteristic of von Hippel–Lindau syndrome. These growths are made of newly formed blood vessels. Although they are typically noncancerous, they can cause serious or life-threatening complications. People with von Hippel–Lindau syndrome commonly develop cysts in the kidneys, pancreas, and genital tract. They are also at an increased risk of developing a type of pancreatic cancer called a *pancreatic neuroendocrine tumor.*

Cystic Fibrosis. Cystic fibrosis is a hereditary disease that causes excessive production of thick mucus by the endocrine glands. The most common pancreatic abnormality found is fatty replacement of the pancreas, sometimes with calcifications. The cysts develop from inspissated mucin that obstructs the pancreatic ducts. The cysts are either single or multiple. Most are microscopic, but they can also be several centimeters in diameter.

Cystic Pancreatic Neoplasms

There are four subtypes of pancreatic cystic neoplasms that have varying malignant potential: serous cystic tumors, mucinous cystic neoplasms, intraductal papillary mucinous neoplasms, and solid pseudopapillary neoplasms. The cystic neoplasms of the pancreas account for between 10% and 15% of all pancreatic cysts and less than 1% of all pancreatic malignancies.

TABLE 12-6	Congenital Pancreatic Lesions		
Clinical Findings	**Sonographic Findings**		**Differential Considerations**
Autosomal Dominant Polycystic Kidney Diseases			
Asymptomatic, often found in patients with polycystic renal disease	Well-defined mass with serous fluid Size varies from microscopic to several centimeters		Pseudocyst Other cystic lesions of the pancreas
Von Hippel–Lindau Disease Asymptomatic Patients may have central nervous system and retinal hemangioblastomas, visceral cysts, pheochromocytomas, and renal cell carcinoma	Well-defined mass with thick fluid; calcifications Single or multiple Size varies from microscopic to several centimeters		Pseudocyst Other cystic lesions of the pancreas
Cystic Fibrosis Asymptomatic	Well-defined mass with serous fluid Size varies from microscopic to several centimeters		Pseudocyst Other cystic lesions of the pancreas
True Pancreatic Cysts Asymptomatic, often found in infants	Well-defined mass with serous fluid Unilocular or multilocular		Pseudocyst Other cystic lesions of the pancreas

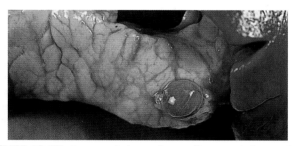

FIGURE 12-35 Gross pathology of a small congenital cyst of the pancreas.

Serous Cystic Tumors. Serous cystadenoma is a rare, benign, well-circumscribed tumor with multiple tiny cysts found more often in elderly females (Figure 12-36). This lesion is the least likely to develop malignant potential. The sonographic appearance depends on the number and size of the cysts. The lesions may appear cystic, solid, or even echogenic if the cysts are very small and more numerous along the periphery. The coarsely lobulated cystic tumors sometimes present sonographically with cyst walls thicker than the membranes between

multilocular cysts (Figure 12-37). A minority of the cysts have an echogenic central stellate scar that may have calcification. The pseudocapsule and septa of the mass tends to be hypervascular and seen well with color Doppler. The mass usually does not cause obstruction of the pancreatic duct. It is difficult to differentiate a serous cystadenoma from a malignant mucinous cystic tumor without pathologic confirmation.

Mucinous Cystic Neoplasms. Mucinous cystadenoma/cystadenocarcinoma is an uncommon, slow-growing tumor that rises from the ducts as a cystic neoplasm. The tumor may be either malignant or benign with a significant "malignant potential." It occurs predominantly in middle-aged and elderly females, usually in the body or tail. Clinically patients present with epigastric pain or a palpable mass, weight loss, abdominal mass, or jaundice. Many patients have concurrent diseases: diabetes, calculous disease of the biliary tract, or arterial hypertension.

This lesion presents as well-circumscribed, smooth-surfaced, thin- or thick-walled, unilocular or multilocular cystic lesions of variable sizes (usually more than 20 mm in diameter and less than six in number) on sonography. The tumor is typically

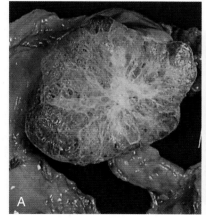
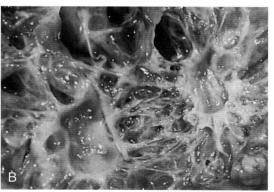

FIGURE 12-36 Gross pathology of serous cystadenoma. **A,** Well-circumscribed tumor. **B,** Tumor appears microcystic.

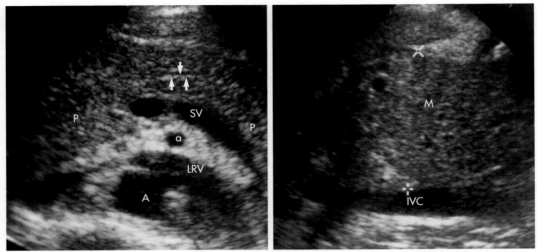

FIGURE 12-37 A 65-year-old patient with cystadenoma in the head of the pancreas that is not causing obstruction of the pancreatic duct. **A,** Transverse image of the pancreas (P), pancreatic duct (arrows), splenic vein (SV), superior mesenteric artery (a), left renal vein (LRV), and aorta (A). **B,** Large mass (M) in the head of the pancreas seen compressing the inferior vena cava (IVC).

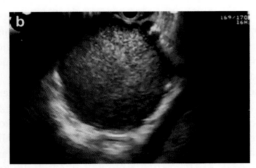

FIGURE 12-38 Mucinous cystadenoma. This lesion presents as well-circumscribed, smooth-surfaced, thin- or thick-walled, unilocular or multilocular cystic lesions of variable sizes comprised of well-defined cysts containing thick mucinous fluid, internal septations, or mural nodules.

comprised of well-defined cysts containing thick mucinous fluid, internal septations, or mural nodules (Figure 12-38). The large cyst (greater than 5 cm) with or without septations, irregular wall, and calcification of the cyst wall has a significant malignant potential; compared with adenocarcinoma of the pancreas, the survival is better with cystadenocarcinoma if the lesion is intact. Frequently, foci of calcification may be seen within the pancreas.

Intraductal Papillary Mucinous Neoplasms. The intraductal papillary mucinous tumor is a form of mucinous cystic neoplasm. The tumor originates from the main pancreatic duct or its branches. This slow-growing lesion affects both elderly men and women. The histology ranges from benign to malignant. Many patients with intraductal papillary mucinous neoplasms are asymptomatic. However, some patients have a recurrent history of acute pancreatitis or symptoms suggestive of chronic pancreatitis, which result from intermittent obstruction of the pancreatic duct with mucous plugs. The presence of back pain, jaundice, weight loss, anorexia, steatorrhea, and diabetes may be precursors to malignancy.

The ductal tumors demonstrate specific patterns on abdominal imaging. The main pancreatic duct type presents as segmental or diffuse dilation of the duct with or without side branch dilation. The branch type shows a single or multicystic mass with a microcystic or macrocystic appearance (Figure 12-39). Careful demonstration of the mass should show communication with the pancreatic duct, usually best seen with ERCP. The tumors may present as nonvascular nodules within the dilated ducts. The presence of vascular nodules and a thick wall differentiates the mass benign from malignant.

Solid Pseudopapillary neoplasms. The finding of a heterogeneous sonographic pattern with solid and cystic components in a young woman is suggestive of a solid pseudopapillary neoplasm. This tumor has a lower incidence of malignancy. Patients with pseudopapillary neoplasm are

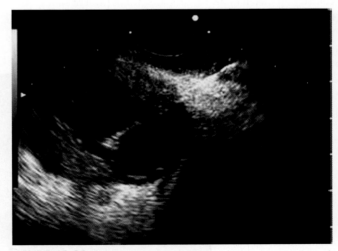

FIGURE 12-39 The intraductal papillary mucinous tumor branch type shows a single or multicystic mass with a microcystic or macrocystic appearance. (Biopsy needle is noted.)

TABLE 12-7	Pancreatic Tumor Findings	
Clinical Findings	**Sonographic Findings**	**Differential Considerations**
Adenocarcinoma		
Depends on size and location of tumor (symptoms occur late if located in body or tail) Weight loss	Loss of normal pancreatic parenchyma Hypoechoic poorly defined mass Focal mass with irregular border Enlargement of pancreas	Pseudocyst Cystadenoma Lymphoma
Decreased appetite Nausea, vomiting Stool changes	If mass is located in head of pancreas, look for hydrops, compression of inferior vena cava, and dilated ducts	
Pain radiating to back Painless jaundice if tumor is located in the head (hydrops of GB—Courvoisier's sign) Metastasizes to lymph nodes, liver, lungs, bone, duodenum, peritoneum, and adrenal glands		
Cystadenoma		
↑ Amylase	Anechoic mass with posterior enhancement May have internal septa Thick walls Small size of tumor makes it difficult to image Single or multiple Occur in body and tail Hypoechoic	Pseudocyst Metastases
Cystadenocarcinoma		
Epigastric pain or palpable mass Abdominal pain	Irregular lobulated cystic tumor Thick walls Hypoechoic mass	Pseudocyst Cystadenoma Adenocarcinoma Islet-cell tumor

usually symptomatic with abdominal pain, nausea, vomiting, and weight loss. Additional symptoms of abdominal mass, gastrointestinal obstruction, anemia, jaundice, and pancreatitis may also be present. These tumors are usually smaller in size and thus MRI is more specific.

Endocrine Pancreatic Neoplasms

The endocrine tumors rise from the islet cells of the pancreas. There are several types of islet-cell tumors; they may be functional or nonfunctional and may be classified as benign adenomas or malignant tumors. Nonfunctioning islet-cell tumors comprise one third of all islet-cell tumors, with the majority (85%) classified as adenocarcinoma (see Table 12-7).

Functional Endocrine Pancreatic Neoplasm. The most common functioning islet-cell tumor is insulinoma (60%) followed by gastrinoma (18%). The tumor size is small (1 to 2 cm), and it is well encapsulated with a good vascular supply (Figure 12-40). A large percentage of insulinoma tumors occur in patients with hyperinsulinism and hypoglycemia. Most gastrinomas are malignant, with up to 40% appearing with metastatic disease at the time of diagnosis.

Insulinoma (B-Cell Tumor). Insulinoma is the most common functioning islet-cell tumor. The clinical triad is found in patients in their fourth to sixth decades of life with hypoglycemic symptoms with immediate relief of symptoms

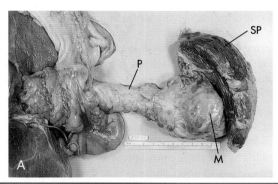

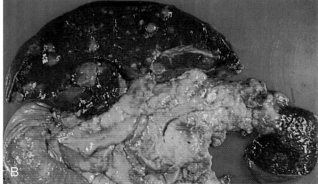

FIGURE 12-40 A, Gross specimen of a pancreatic mass *(M)* in the tail of the gland. *P,* Pancreas; *SP,* spleen. **B,** Carcinoma of the body of the pancreas. The tumor has metastasized to the liver.

after the administration of intravenous glucose. Clinical symptoms include palpitations, headache, confusion, pallor, sweating, slurred speech, and coma. This tumor is usually benign. A small percent of insulinomas are multiple, 10% are malignant, and 10% of patients have hyperplasia rather than neoplasia. Most of the insulinomas are small, well encapsulated, and hypervascular. Some of the lesions contain calcification.

Gastrinoma (G-Cell Tumor). Gastrinoma is the second most common functioning islet-cell tumor and produces the Zollinger-Ellison syndrome. This condition is caused by non–insulin-secreting pancreatic tumors, which secrete excessive amounts of gastrin. This stimulates the stomach to secrete great amounts of hydrochloric acid and pepsin, which in turn leads to peptic ulceration of the stomach and small intestine. These lesions usually affect young adults who have peptic ulcer disease (when ulcers are recurrent, intractable, multiple, or in unusual locations). Diarrhea is common because of the increased gastrin on the small bowel. Gastrinomas are frequently multiple, extrapancreatic, and difficult to locate, and 60% are malignant. Total gastrectomy and local excision of the pancreatic tumor may be performed if metastases have not appeared. Most gastrinomas are found in the pancreas with a small amount (10% to 15%) arising in the duodenum.

Nonfunctioning Islet-Cell Tumors. These tumors comprise 33% of all islet-cell neoplasms. These tumors have a tendency to present as large tumors in the head of the pancreas with a high incidence of malignancy. Adenocarcinoma is the most common malignant tumor.

Adenocarcinoma. The most common primary neoplasm of the pancreas is adenocarcinoma. This fatal tumor involves the exocrine portion of the gland (ductal epithelium) and accounts for greater than 90% of all malignant pancreatic tumors (see Figure 12-40). Pancreatic carcinoma accounts for approximately 5% of all cancer deaths and is the fourth most common cause of cancer-related mortality, after lung, breast, and colon cancers. Carcinoma of the pancreas is rare before age 40; the majority of patients present after age 60. The prognosis is poor with a median survival time of 2 to 3 months and a 1-year survival of only 8%.

Clinical symptoms depend on the location of the tumor. Tumors in the pancreatic head present symptoms early, causing obstruction of the common bile duct with subsequent jaundice and hydrops of the gallbladder (**Courvoisier's sign**). A palpable, nontender gallbladder accompanied by jaundice is present in 25% of patients with pancreatic carcinoma. Tumors in the body and tail of the gland present with less specific symptoms, most commonly weight loss, pain, jaundice, and vomiting as the gastrointestinal tract becomes invaded by tumor. The tumors in the body and tail are more frequently larger in size and tend to invade the adjacent organs such as the stomach, transverse colon, spleen, and adrenal gland. These organs tend to present with metastases more often than tumors in the head. Metastases to the liver, regional lymph nodes, lungs, peritoneum, and adrenal glands have been reported. Peripancreatic, gastric, mesenteric, omental, and portohepatic nodes have been identified with adenocarcinoma.

On pathology, nearly all adenocarcinomas of the pancreas originate in the ductal epithelium, with less than 1% arising in the acini. The tumor may be either mucinous or nonmucinous. The most frequent site of occurrence is in the head of the gland (60% to 70%), with 20% to 30% in the body and 5% to 10% in the tail. One fifth of the tumors are diffuse.

Sonographic Findings. The sonographic appearance of adenocarcinoma is the loss of the normal pancreatic parenchymal pattern (Figure 12-41). The most common finding

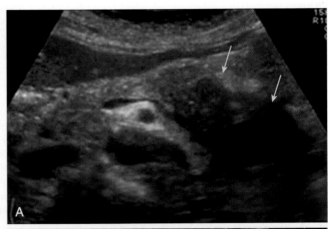
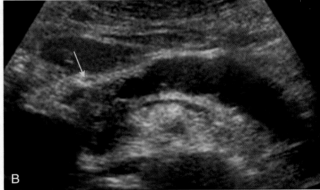
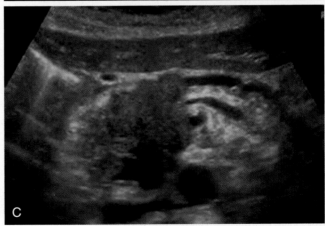

FIGURE 12-41 Adenocarcinoma of the pancreas. A, Transverse images of the pancreas demonstrate a large heterogeneous irregular lesion within the tail of the gland. **B,** Moderate heterogeneous lesion *(arrows)* in the head of the gland, causing obstruction of the common bile duct. **C,** Large irregular heterogenous lesion in the head of the pancreas with pancreatic ductal enlargement.

on sonography is a poorly defined mass in the region of the pancreas. The lesion represents localized change in the echogenicity of the pancreas texture. The echo pattern is hypoechoic or isoechoic, with a texture less dense than the pancreas or liver. (The hypoechoic or isoechoic ill-defined tumor is better identified when the pancreatic texture is more echogenic.) Rarely, necrosis will be seen as a cystic area within the mass. The borders of the gland become irregular and the pancreas may be enlarged. There may be secondary enlargement of the common duct resulting from edema or tumor invasion of the pancreatic head. If the mass causes obstruction of the duct, look for dilation of the pancreatic duct (greater than 2 to 3 mm). If the tumor is located within the head, look for biliary duct dilation. Remember the level of the obstruction may be in the head, above the head, or in the porta hepatis, depending on the size of the lesion. The distinction of echogenic sludge within the common bile duct may be difficult to separate from tumor extension. Dilation of both the pancreatic and common bile duct may be seen in chronic pancreatitis, as well as pancreatic adenocarcinoma.

There may be expansion or compression of the adjacent structures. The formation of a pseudocyst secondary to associated pancreatitis may be seen adjacent to the carcinoma. A diffuse spread of the tumor throughout the pancreas may appear as edematous pancreatitis. The sonographer should carefully evaluate the gland for the vague appearance of a lobulated mass and correlate with clinical symptoms.

The sonographer should look for metastatic spread into the liver, lymph nodes (abnormal displacement of the superior mesenteric artery), or portal venous system. The superior mesenteric vessels may be displaced posteriorly by the pancreatic mass; anterior displacement is present when the carcinoma is in the uncinate process, and posterior displacement is present when the tumor is in the head or body. A soft tissue thickening caused by neoplastic infiltration of perivascular lymphatics may be seen surrounding the celiac axis or superior mesenteric artery may be seen more with carcinoma of the body and tail.

Many patients with a mass in the head of the gland will have obstructive jaundice and anterior wall compression of the inferior vena cava. A tumor in the tail may compress the splenic vein, producing secondary splenic enlargement. A tumor may displace or invade the splenic or portal vein or produce thrombosis. Atrophy of the gland proximal to an obstructing mass in the head may appear hypoechoic or hyperechoic.

Doppler patterns feature characteristics of other malignant lesions with increased velocity and diminished flow impedance. The increased velocity is most likely from arteriovenous shunting and the diminished impedance to vascular spaces that lack muscular walls.

Significance of Sonography in Staging Pancreatic Tumors. Sonography may play an important screening role not only in identifying the pancreatic tumor mass but also in assessing the possibility of tumor resection. Surgery remains the treatment of choice in carcinomas that are considered resectable, but it comes with a high rate of mortality and morbidity. The ability to identify the extension of the carcinoma beyond the border of the pancreas—including invasion of the carcinoma into the

lymph nodes, surrounding venous structures and organs, retroperitoneal fat, and liver metastases—precludes the feasibility of surgery. This abdominal/pelvic imaging survey has been more effective with CT evaluation. The demonstration of anatomic structures by sonography will be determined by the adequate image quality. The retroperitoneal structures are often precluded by bowel gas interference and thus inadequate image quality results. However, if the pancreas can be adequately imaged in its entirety and has a normal appearance, pancreatic carcinoma can be excluded with a high degree of certainty.

The sonographer should strive to carefully evaluate the vascular structures surrounding the pancreas. The gland lies in the middle of a significant vascular highway, the celiac plexus, and if a mass is present in the pancreas it may easily travel to adjacent organs. It may be difficult to distinguish compression and invasion of the venous structures. Secondary signs should be noted, such as interruption of a vein, organomegaly, or collateral formation in the peripancreatic and periportal region and along the stomach wall. Enlargement of the lymph nodes in the pancreatic area may lead to encasement of the celiac axis or superior mesenteric artery.

Differential Diagnosis for Pancreatic Carcinoma. The primary differential diagnosis of pancreatic carcinoma is focal pancreatitis or a focal mass associated with chronic pancreatitis. Calcification may be seen in patients with pancreatitis to help delineate the gland. However, it is possible to have concurrent neoplastic growth in the presence of pancreatitis. Comparative imaging with CT and ERCP may be necessary to evaluate the texture of the gland and retroperitoneal area and to further assess the pancreatic duct.

Enlarged lymph nodes in the peripancreatic area may be differentiated from pancreatic cancer by identifying the echogenic septa between each of the hypoechoic nodes. The absence of jaundice in the presence of a mass near the head of the pancreas favors the presence of lymphadenopathy over pancreatic carcinoma.

Ampullary adenocarcinomas have a better prognosis than pancreatic adenocarcinoma when lesions are less than 2 cm. Endoscopic ultrasound has allowed the visualization of the pancreatic duct to stage this neoplastic growth. Dilation of the pancreatic and common duct is common with the ampullary tumor.

Metastatic Disease to the Pancreas

Generally speaking, metastasis to the pancreas is uncommon but has been reported to be found in 10% of patients with cancer. Primary tumors that can metastasize to the pancreas include melanomas, breast tumors, gastrointestinal tumors, and lung tumors.

Parapancreatic Neoplasms

Lymphomas are malignant neoplasms that rise from the lymphoid tissues. They are the most frequent parapancreatic neoplasm. It may be difficult to separate a parapancreatic lymphadenopathy from a primary lesion in the pancreas. An

FIGURE 12-42 A, An intraabdominal lymphoma may appear as a hypoechoic mass or with necrosis, a cystic mass in the pancreas. **B,** Sagittal sonogram of the midabdomen demonstrates multiple enlarged homogeneous lymph nodes *(arrows)* surrounding the inferior vena cava *(IVC).*

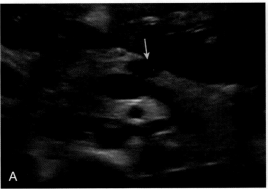

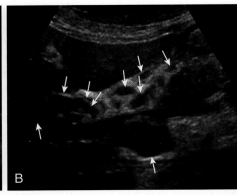

intraabdominal lymphoma may appear as a hypoechoic mass or with necrosis, a cystic mass in the pancreas (Figure 12-42). The superior mesenteric vessels may be displaced anterior instead of posterior as seen with a primary pancreatic mass. Multiple nodes are seen along the pancreas, duodenum, porta hepatis, and superior mesenteric vessels; they may be difficult to distinguish from a pancreatic mass. The enlarged nodes appear hypoechoic and well defined.

Other types of retroperitoneal neoplasms that may appear as a cystic lesion near the area of the pancreas include lymphangiomas, paragangliomas, cystic teratomas, and metastases. The lymphangiomas are most often thin-walled, homogeneous, small cysts, but they have also been seen to have septa, thick walls, calcification, and internal debris. The paragangliomas are usually found near the inferior mesenteric artery or near the kidney. The cystic teratomas are found more frequently in children and young adults. Their appearance is a mixed sonographic pattern of cystic, solid, fat, and calcifications.

 Key Pearls

- The pancreas lies anterior to the first and second lumbar bodies located deep in the epigastrium and left hypochondrium, behind the lesser omental sac.
- The majority of the pancreas lies within the retroperitoneal cavity, with the exception of a small portion of the head that is surrounded by peritoneum.
- The pancreas is divided into the following four areas: head, neck, body, and tail.
- Two ducts are seen within the pancreas, the duct of Wirsung and the duct of Santorini.
- The blood supply for the pancreas is the splenic artery and pancreaticoduodenal arteries.
- The splenic artery supplies the body and tail of the pancreas through four smaller branches: (1) suprapancreatic (rises from the celiac axis/splenic artery), (2) pancreatic, (3) prepancreatic (before leaving the pancreas), and (4) prehilar (before leaving the spleen) and hepatic artery (gastroduodenal artery).
- The gastroduodenal artery is seen along the anterolateral border of the pancreas as it travels a short distance along the anterior aspect of the pancreatic head just to the right of the neck before it divides into the superior pancreaticoduodenal branches.

- Annular pancreas is a rare anomaly in which the head of the pancreas surrounds the second portion of the duodenum.
- The pancreas is both a digestive (exocrine) and hormonal (endocrine) gland.
- The primary exocrine function is to produce pancreatic juice, which enters the duodenum together with bile.
- Exocrine function is performed by acini cells of the pancreas, which can produce up to 2 L of pancreatic juice per day.
- The endocrine function controls the secretion of glucagons and insulin into the blood.
- The endocrine function is located in the islets of Langerhans in the pancreas.
- There are specific enzymes of the pancreas that may become altered in pancreatic disease, namely amylase and lipase.
- Lipase is an enzyme that is excreted specifically by the pancreas and that parallels the elevation in amylase levels.
- Glucose controls the blood sugar level in the body.
- The normal pancreas has an echo pattern that is slightly more hyperechoic and finer in texture than that of the surrounding retroperitoneum.
- The echo intensity of the pancreas is usually slightly less than that of surrounding soft tissue and slightly greater than that of the liver.
- Pancreatitis is inflammation of the pancreas; this condition may be chronic or acute.
- Pancreatitis occurs when the pancreas becomes damaged and malfunctions as a result of increased secretion and blockage of ducts.
- Acute pancreatitis is an inflammation of the pancreas caused by the inflamed acini releasing pancreatic enzymes into the surrounding pancreatic tissue.
- An acute attack of pancreatitis is commonly related to biliary tract disease and alcoholism.
- Collections of fluid in the peripancreatic area generally retain communication with the pancreas.
- The pancreatic duct may be obstructed in acute pancreatitis as a result of inflammation, spasm, edema, swelling of the papilla, or pseudocyst formation.
- The alteration in the size and echogenic texture of the pancreas may be subtle; therefore the diagnosis of pancreatitis may be based on the visualization of peripancreatic fluid collections in a patient with abnormal pancreatic enzymes and clinical history suggestive of pancreatitis.

- Complications of acute pancreatitis include hemorrhage, pseudocyst formation, inflammatory mass, and intrapancreatic and extrapancreatic fluid collections.
- Complications of acute pancreatitis include hemorrhage, pseudocyst formation, inflammatory mass, and intrapancreatic and extrapancreatic fluid collections.
- Chronic pancreatitis results from recurrent attacks of acute pancreatitis and causes continuing destruction of the pancreatic parenchyma that result in permanent structural damage, which can lead to impairment of exocrine and endocrine function.
- Chronic pancreatitis is generally associated with chronic alcoholism or biliary disease, although patients with hypercalcemia (elevated calcium levels) and hyperlipidemia (elevated fat levels) are more predisposed to chronic pancreatitis.
- The most common location of a pseudocyst is in the lesser sac anterior to the pancreas and posterior to the stomach.
- A phlegmon is an inflammatory process that spreads along fascial pathways, causing localized areas of diffuse inflammatory edema of soft tissue that may proceed to necrosis and suppuration.
- Benign cystic lesions of the pancreas include autosomal dominant polycystic disease, von Hippel–Lindau syndrome, and cystic fibrosis.
- There are four subtypes of pancreatic cystic neoplasms that have varying malignant potential: serous cystic tumors, mucinous cystic neoplasms, intraductal papillary mucinous neoplasms, and solid pseudopapillary neoplasms.
- The endocrine tumors rise from the islet cells of the pancreas.
- There are several types of islet-cell tumors; they may be functional or nonfunctional and may be classified as benign adenomas or malignant tumors.
- The most common functioning islet-cell tumor is insulinoma followed by gastrinoma.
- The most common primary neoplasm of the pancreas is adenocarcinoma.
- Many patients with a mass in the head of the gland will have obstructive jaundice and anterior wall compression of the inferior vena cava.
- Primary tumors that can metastasize to the pancreas include melanomas, breast tumors, gastrointestinal tumors, and lung tumors.
- Lymphomas are malignant neoplasms that rise from the lymphoid tissues; they are the most frequent parapancreatic neoplasm.
- Other types of retroperitoneal neoplasms that may appear as a cystic lesion near the area of the pancreas include lymphangiomas, paragangliomas, cystic teratomas, and metastases.

BIBLIOGRAPHY

Bang UC, Benfield T, Hyldstrup L, et al: Mortality, cancer, and comorbidities associated with chronic pancreatitis: a Danish nationwide matched-cohort study, *Gastroenterology* 146:989, 2014.

Banks PA, Bollen TL, Dervenis C, et al: Classification of acute pancreatitis—2012; revision of the Atlanta classification and definitions by international consensus, *Gut* 62:102, 2013.

Barge JU, Lopera JE: Vascular complications of pancreatitis: role of interventional therapy, *Korean J Radiol* 13(Suppl 1):S45, 2012.

Bergman S, Melvin WS: Operative and nonoperative management of pancreatic pseudocysts, *Surg Clin North Am* 87:1447, 2007.

Carpenter SL, Scheiman JM: Pancreatic imaging, *Curr Opin Gastroenterol* 12:442, 1996.

Demos TC, Posniak HV, Harmath C, et al: Cystic lesions of the pancreas, *Am J Roentgenol* 179:1375-1388, 2002.

Dietrich CF, Chichakli M, Hirche TO, et al: Sonographic findings of the hepatobiliary-pancreatic system in adult patients with cystic fibrosis, *J Ultrasound Med* 21:409-416, 2002.

Goodman M, Willmann JK, Jeffrey RB: Incidentally discovered solid pancreatic masses: imaging and clinical observations, *Abdom Imaging* 37:91, 2012.

Grogan JR, Saeian K, Taylor AJ, et al: Making sense of mucin-producing pancreatic tumors, *Am J Roentgenol* 176:921-929, 2001.

Grube J: Epigastric pain. In Henningsen C, editor: *Clinical guide to ultrasonography*, St Louis, 2004, Mosby.

Gumaste VV, Pitchumoni CS: Pancreatic pseudocyst, *Gastroenterologist* 4:33, 1996.

Jung-Hee Y, Han SS, Cha SS, Lee SJ: Color Doppler ultrasonography of a pancreatic arteriovenous malformation, *J Ultrasound Med* 24:113-117, 2005.

Khalid A, Brugge W: ACG practice guidelines for the diagnosis and management of neoplastic pancreatic cysts, *Am J Gastroenterol* 102:2339, 2007.

Lim JH, Lee G, Oh YL: Radiologic spectrum of intraductal papillary mucinous tumor of the pancreas, *RadioGraphics* 21:323-337, 2001.

Lundstedt C, Dawiskiba S: Serous and mucinous cystadenomas/cystadenocarcinomas of the pancreas, *Abdom Imaging* 25:201-206, 2000.

Megibow AJ, Lavelle MT, Rofsky NM: Cystic tumors of the pancreas: the radiologist, *Surg Clin North Am* 81:489-495, 2001.

Middleton WD, Kurtz AB, Hertzberg BS: *Ultrasound: the requisites*, ed 2, St Louis, 2004, Mosby.

Morgan DE, Baron TH: Practical imaging in acute pancreatitis, *Semin Gastrointest Dis* 9:41, 1998.

Neumyer MM: Ultrasonographic assessment of renal and pancreatic transplants, *J Vasc Technol* 19:321, 1995.

Nicolau C, Torra R, Bianchi L, et al: Abdominal sonographic study of autosomal dominant polycystic disease, *J Clin Ultrasound* 28:277-282, 2000.

Ocampo C, Oria A, Zandalazini H, et al: Treatment of acute pancreatic pseudocysts after severe acute pancreatitis, *J Gastrointest Surg* 11:357, 2007.

Porta M, Fabregat X, Malats N, et al: Exocrine pancreatic cancer: symptoms at presentation and their relation to tumour site and stage, *Clin Transl Oncol* 7:189, 2005.

Rumack CM, Wilson SR, Charboneau JW, Johnson J: *Diagnostic ultrasound*, ed 3, St Louis, 2005, Mosby.

Ryan DP, Hong TS, Bardeesy N: Pancreatic adenocarcinoma, *N Engl J Med* 371:1039, 2014.

Scott J, Martin I, Redhead D: Mucinous cystic neoplasm of the pancreas: imaging features and diagnostic difficulties, *Clin Radiol* 55:187-192, 2000.

Sharma A: Tumors of the pancreas. In Greenberger NJ, Blumberg RS, Burakoff R, editors: *Current diagnosis and treatment: gastroenterology, hepatology and endoscopy*, New York, 2009, McGraw-Hill, p 318.

Siegel RL, Miller KD, Jemal A: Cancer statistics, 2015, *CA Cancer J Clin* 65:5, 2015.

Tseng JF, Warshaw AL, Sahani DV, et al: Serous cystadenoma of the pancreas: tumor growth rates and recommendations for treatment, *Ann Surg* 242:413, 2005.

Yoon SH, Lee JM, Cho JY, et al: Small (<20 mm) pancreatic adenocarcinomas: analysis of enhancement patterns and secondary signs with multiphasic multidetector CT, *Radiology* 259:442, 2011.

CHAPTER

13

Gastrointestinal Tract

Sandra L. Hagen-Ansert

OBJECTIVES

On completion of this chapter, you should be able to:
- Describe the anatomy and relational landmarks of the gastrointestinal system
- Discuss the size of wall thickness and diameters of the gastrointestinal tract
- Describe the sonographic technique used to image the gastrointestinal tract and appendix
- Differentiate the sonographic appearances of the pathologies covered in this chapter

OUTLINE

Anatomy of the Gastrointestinal Tract
  Normal Anatomy
  Vascular Anatomy
Physiology and Laboratory Data of the Gastrointestinal Tract

Sonographic Evaluation of the Gastrointestinal Tract
  Stomach
  Duodenum
  Small Bowel

Appendix
Colon
Pathology of the Gastrointestinal Tract
  Upper Gastrointestinal Tract
  Lower Gastrointestinal Tract

KEY TERMS

Abscess
Absorption
Alimentary tract
Appendicolith
Ascites
Cardiac orifice
Cholecystokinin
Crohn's disease
Digestive system
Diverticulum
Duodenal bulb
Fecalith
Gastrin
Gastrohepatic ligament

Gastrointestinal tract
Gastrophrenic ligament
Gastrosplenic ligament
Greater omentum
Haustra
Hemorrhage
Hepatic flexure
Lesser omentum
Lienorenal ligament
McBurney's point
McBurney's sign
Meckel's diverticulum
Mesentery
Mesothelium

Mucosa
Muscularis
Paralytic ileus
Peristalsis
Polyp
Pyloric canal
Rugae
Secretin
Serosa
Splenic flexure
Submucosa
Target sign
Valvulae conniventes
Villi

Sonography is not the primary imaging tool to investigate the gastrointestinal system due to the limited visualization of many structures. However, there are patients who have non-specific complaints related to the gastrointestinal tract that sonography may be able to help direct the further workup of the patient. The gastrointestinal tract may be difficult to image with ultrasound in most patients unless they ingest fluids or some other acoustic transmittable contrast agent. Many laboratories have begun to investigate various contrast agents in pursuit of the ideal medium for imaging the stomach, duodenum, small bowel, and colon. The retrograde infusion of

water can also be used to distend the colon to evaluate for abnormalities.

ANATOMY OF THE GASTROINTESTINAL TRACT

Normal Anatomy

The digestive tract, also known as the **alimentary tract,** is a tube about 8 m long extending from the mouth to the anus (Figure 13-1). The **gastrointestinal tract** is that part of the

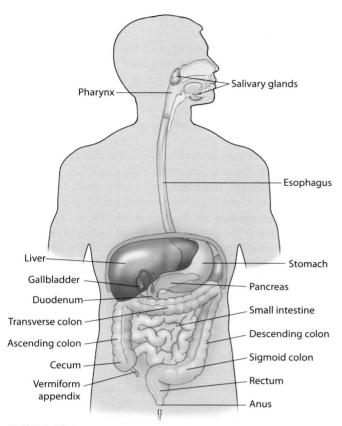

FIGURE 13-1 The digestive system includes the mouth, pharynx, esophagus, stomach, small intestine, large intestine, rectum, and anus.

digestive system below the diaphragm. Together, the digestive tract and gastrointestinal tract comprise the **digestive system.** The sequential parts of the digestive system include the mouth, pharynx, esophagus, stomach, small intestine, and large intestine. Three types of accessory digestive glands—the salivary glands, liver, and pancreas—secrete digestive juices into the digestive system.

Esophagus. The esophagus extends from the pharynx through the thoracic cavity, then passes through the diaphragm and empties into the stomach (see Figure 13-1). The lower end of the esophagus is a circular muscle that acts as a sphincter, constricting the tube so that the entrance to the stomach, at the **cardiac orifice,** is generally closed. This helps to prevent gastric acid from moving up into the esophagus.

Stomach. The stomach is a large, smooth, muscular organ that has two surfaces: the lesser curvature and the greater curvature (Figure 13-2). The stomach is divided into three parts: The *fundus* is found in the superior aspect, the *body* makes up the major central axis, and the *pylorus* is the lower aspect. The pylorus is further subdivided into the antrum, the pyloric canal, and the pyloric sphincter. The **pyloric canal** is a muscle that connects the stomach to the proximal duodenum.

Supporting ligaments of the greater curvature of the stomach include the **greater omentum,** the **gastrophrenic ligament,** the **gastrosplenic ligament,** and the **lienorenal ligament.** Ligaments that support the lesser curvature of the stomach include the **gastrohepatic ligament** of the **lesser omentum.** Folds of the **mucosa** and **submucosa** are called **rugae.**

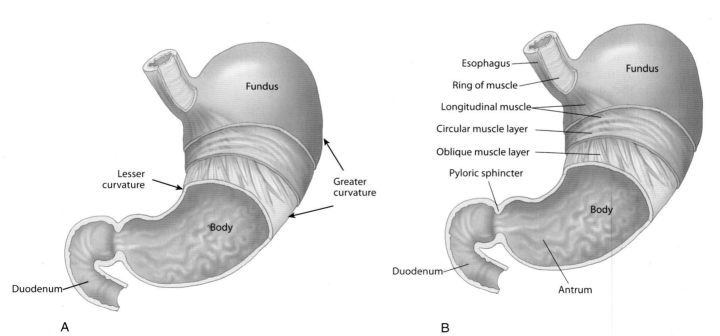

A   B

FIGURE 13-2 A, Lesser curvature and greater curvature of the stomach. **B,** Food enters the stomach after leaving the esophagus through the gastroesophageal junction at the level of the diaphragm. The three parts of the stomach (fundus, body, and antrum) are shown. Food leaves the stomach through the pylorus and pyloric sphincter to enter the duodenum.

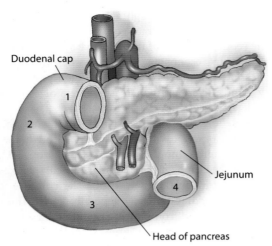

FIGURE 13-3 The duodenal cap is an excellent landmark for the head of the pancreas. The duodenum is divided into four sections. See text for explanation. (The fourth part of the duodenum is posterior to the jejunum.)

Small Intestine. The small intestine is a long, coiled tube about 5 m long by 4 cm in diameter (see Figure 13-1). The first 22 cm is the duodenum, which is curved like the letter C. The duodenum is subdivided into four segments: (1) superior, (2) descending, (3) transverse, and (4) ascending (Figure 13-3). The first part of the duodenum is not attached to the mesentery; the remainder of the small intestine, including the rest of the duodenum, is attached to the mesentery. The **mesentery** projects from the parietal peritoneum and attaches to the small intestine to anchor it to the posterior abdominal wall.

The first part of the duodenum, the **duodenal bulb,** begins at the pylorus and terminates at the neck of the gallbladder, posterior to the left lobe of the liver and medial to the gallbladder. The duodenal bulb is peritoneal, supported by the hepatoduodenal ligament, and passes anterior to the common bile duct, gastroduodenal artery, common hepatic artery, hepatic portal vein, and head of the pancreas. This is an important point for sonographers to recognize: if there is air in the duodenal bulb, it will be more difficult to image the common bile duct and smaller vessels that help to define the head of the pancreas. This is avoided by changing patient position (decubitus or upright) or giving the patient water to fill the duodenal loop and serve as an acoustic window to image these structures.

The second part (descending) of the duodenum is retroperitoneal and runs parallel, posterior, and to the right of the spine. The transverse colon crosses anterior to the middle third of the descending duodenum. The pancreatic head is medial to the duodenum at this point. The common bile duct joins the pancreatic duct to enter the ampulla of Vater.

The third part (transverse) of the duodenum begins at the right of the fourth lumbar vertebra and passes anterior to the aorta, inferior vena cava, and crura of the diaphragm. The superior mesenteric vessels course anterior to the duodenum.

The fourth part (ascending) of the duodenum ascends superiorly to the left of the spine and aorta to the second lumbar vertebra, where it joins the proximal jejunum (duodenojejunal flexure). This portion lies on the left crus of the diaphragm. It is held in place by the ligament of Treitz (which courses from the left toward the right crus of the diaphragm).

As the duodenum turns downward, it is called the *jejunum* (Figure 13-4). The jejunum extends for about 2 m before becoming the ileum. The inner wall of the small intestine is marked by circular folds of the mucous membrane, **villi.** The **valvulae conniventes** are large folds of mucous membrane that project into the lumen of the bowel and help retard the passage of food to provide greater absorption. The lower part of the small intestine is the ileum. The ileocecal orifice marks the entry into the large intestine and prevents food from reentering the small intestine.

Large Intestine. This is the last part of the digestive system. The large intestine is larger in diameter and shorter in length than the small intestine. The cecum and vermiform appendix, ascending colon, transverse colon, and descending colon, sigmoid colon, and rectum all make up the large intestine (Figure 13-5). The **haustra** (singular *haustrum*) of the colon are the small pouches caused by sacculation, which give the colon its segmented appearance (Figure 13-6). The ascending colon extends from the cecum vertically to the lower part of the liver. It turns horizontally at the **hepatic flexure** and moves to become the transverse colon. On the left side of the abdomen, at the **splenic flexure,** it then descends vertically to become the descending colon and eventually the sigmoid colon, which empties into the rectum. The rectum is 12 cm long, terminating at the anus. The mucosa of the large intestine lacks villi and produces no digestive enzymes. The surface epithelium consists of cells specialized for absorption and goblet cells that secrete mucus.

Vascular Anatomy

Esophagus. The arteries that supply the esophagus rise from the high, middle, and lower sections of this muscular tube. The inferior thyroid branch of the subclavian artery supplies the upper esophagus, the descending thoracic aorta supplies the middle of the esophagus, and the gastric branch of the celiac axis and the left inferior phrenic artery of the abdominal aorta supply the lower end of the esophagus. Varices may be seen to rise from the gastroesophageal arteries (Figure 13-7).

Stomach. The vascular supply to the stomach is provided by the right gastric arterial branch, pyloric and right gastroepiploic branches of the hepatic artery, left gastroepiploic branch and vasa brevia of the splenic artery, and left gastric artery (see Figure 13-6). The venous system of the stomach is parallel to the arterial vessels, which drain into the portal venous system.

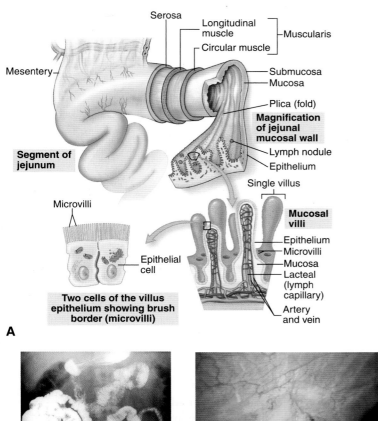

Serosa
Longitudinal muscle
Circular muscle
Muscularis
Mesentery
Submucosa
Mucosa
Plica (fold)
Magnification of jejunal mucosal wall
Lymph nodule
Epithelium
Segment of jejunum
Single villus
Microvilli
Mucosal villi
Epithelium
Microvilli
Mucosa
Lacteal (lymph capillary)
Artery and vein
Epithelial cell
Two cells of the villus epithelium showing brush border (microvilli)

A

FIGURE 13-4 The small intestine. A, The folds of mucosa are covered with villi; each villus is covered with epithelium, which increases the surface area for absorption of food. **B,** Anteroposterior (AP) X-ray image obtained during a contrast (barium-enhanced) study of the small intestine. The individual is lying supine on the x ray table. **C,** Laparoscopic view of the small intestine.

B   **C**

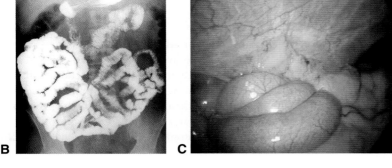

Transverse colon
Aorta
Splenic vein
Splenic (left side) Flexure
Inferior vena cava
Superior transverse artery
Hepatic (right colic) flexure
Interior transverse artery and vein
Ascending colon
Descending colon
Right colic artery
Mesentery
Ileocecal valve
Sigmoid artery and vein
Cecum
Sigmoid colon
Ileum
Vermiform appendix
Rectum
Superior rectal artery and vein

FIGURE 13-5 Divisions of the large intestine.

Small Intestine. The mesentery outlines the small intestine and contains superior mesenteric vessels, nerves, lymphatic glands, and fat between its two layers. The celiac axis supplies the duodenum through its right gastric, gastroduodenal, and superior pancreaticoduodenal branches (Figure 13-8). The superior mesenteric artery has multiple branches to the small bowel, which include the inferior pancreaticoduodenal, jejunal, and ileal arteries. The venous system parallels the arterial system and empties into the portal venous system.

Large Intestine. The celiac, superior mesenteric, and inferior mesenteric arteries supply both the small and the large intestine. The superior mesenteric arterial branches include the ileocolic, right colic, and middle colic arteries (Figure 13-9). The inferior mesenteric artery supplies the intestine from the left border of the transverse colon to the rectum, rising from the anterior surface of the abdominal aorta at the level of the third lumbar vertebra and descending retroperitoneally. Branches of the inferior mesenteric artery include the left colic, sigmoid, and superior rectal arteries. The venous system parallels the arterial system and empties into the portal venous system.

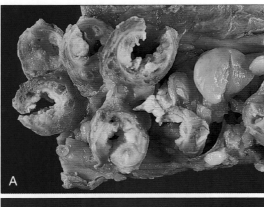

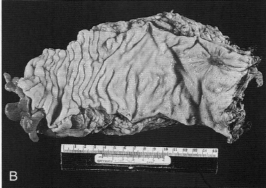

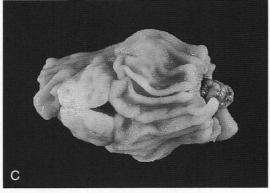

FIGURE 13-6 A, Gross specimen of the small intestine. **B** and **C,** Gross specimens of the large intestine.

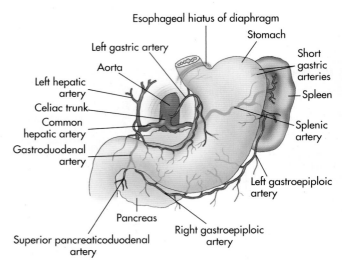

FIGURE 13-7 Vascular supply to the stomach is received from the branches of the celiac axis. The left gastric artery supplies the lower third of the esophagus and the upper right part of the stomach. The right gastric artery supplies the lower right part of the stomach. The short gastric arteries supply the fundus. The left gastroepiploic artery supplies the upper part of the greater curvature of the stomach, and the right gastroepiploic artery supplies the lower part of the greater curvature of the stomach.

PHYSIOLOGY AND LABORATORY DATA OF THE GASTROINTESTINAL TRACT

Digestion and absorption are the primary functions of the gastrointestinal tract. Food is ingested through the mouth, chewed, and swallowed. The molecules of food must be further digested, or mechanically broken down, and chemically split into small molecules. The chemical digestion of food breaks down long-chain organic molecules (i.e., polysaccharides or proteins). Each reaction is carried on with the help of a specific enzyme produced by cells of the digestive tract or its accessory glands. When these particles are small enough, nutrient molecules pass through the wall of the intestine into the blood or lymph system by **absorption.**

Nutrients are transported to the liver after they are absorbed by the blood; the liver processes and stores nutrients. Remaining nutrients in the blood are transported to cells throughout the body. Undigested and unabsorbed food is eliminated from the digestive tract by the process of defecation.

When food enters the stomach, the rugae gradually smooth out, causing the stomach to stretch and increase its capacity for food intake. Contractions of the stomach help to mix the food. The three layers of smooth muscle in the wall enable the stomach to mash and churn food and move it along through **peristalsis.** Large amounts of mucus are secreted in the stomach. Gastric glands secrete gastric juice containing hydrochloric acid and enzymes. Over a 3- to 4-hour period, food is converted into chyme. This soupy mixture is moved toward the pylorus and into the small intestine. Small quantities of water, salts, and lipid-soluble substances, such as alcohol, are absorbed through the stomach mucosa. The pyloric sphincter is a strong band of muscle that relaxes at the time necessary to release the food.

Villi within the small intestine increase its surface area for digestion and absorption of nutrients. If the villi were not present, food would move quickly through the intestine without time for absorption. The intestinal glands are found between the villi and secrete large amounts of fluid that serve as a medium for digestion and absorption of nutrients. The hormone **gastrin,** which is released by the stomach mucosa, stimulates the gastric glands to secrete. Most digestion occurs within the duodenum. Bile and enzymes from the liver and pancreas are secreted into the duodenum to act on the chyme and break down the food particles for absorption. The intestinal glands are stimulated to release their fluid mainly by local

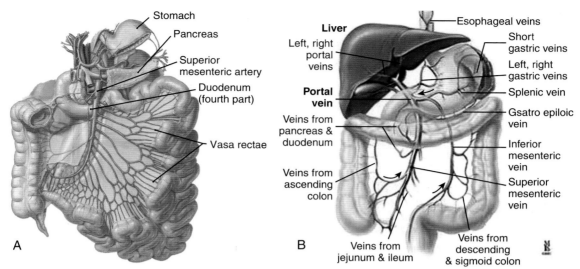

FIGURE 13-8 **A,** Arterial supply for the small intestine. **B,** Venous supply for the gastrointestinal system. *(Department of Art as Applied to Medicine/The Johns Hopkins University School of Medicine © JHU/AAAM 2000. Used with permission.)*

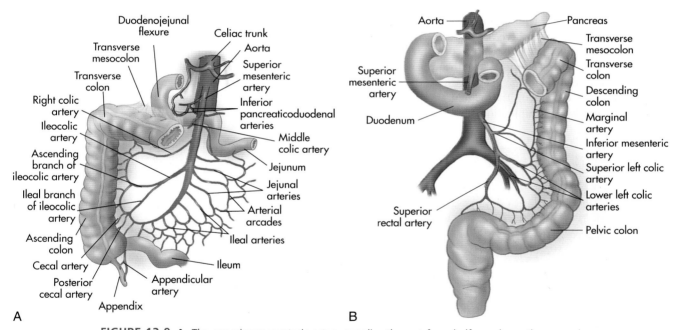

FIGURE 13-9 **A,** The superior mesenteric artery supplies the gut from halfway down the second part of the duodenum to the distal third of the transverse colon. **B,** The inferior mesenteric artery supplies the large bowel from the distal third of the transverse colon to halfway down the anal canal. It forms an anastomosis with the middle colic branch of the superior mesenteric artery.

reflexes initiated when the small intestine is distended by chyme.

Other gastrointestinal hormones include **cholecystokinin** and **secretin.** Cholecystokinin is released by the presence of fat in the intestine and regulates gallbladder contraction and gastric emptying. Secretin is released from the small bowel to stimulate the secretion of bicarbonate to decrease the acid content of the intestine.

A period of 1 to 3 days or longer may be required for the journey through the large intestine. Within the large intestine, undigestible chime becomes stool as most of the remaining sodium and water are reabsorbed. Some of the undigestible remains of the chime are devoured by gut bacteria. Most of the absorption process of sodium and water occurs in the cecum.

The most common laboratory data the sonographer may come across in a patient with gastrointestinal disease relate to the presence of blood in the stool. If chronic, this blood loss can lead to anemia. Blood in the stool indicates the presence of a bleed somewhere in the gastrointestinal system. Infection would show elevation of the white blood count. An increase in the carcinoembryonic antigen is found in patients with inflammatory bowel disease.

Clinical signs and symptoms of nausea, vomiting, and diarrhea are common with gastrointestinal problems. Abdominal pain and fever may also be present with gastrointestinal conditions, such as colitis, bowel abscess, acute diverticulitis, and appendicitis.

SONOGRAPHIC EVALUATION OF THE GASTROINTESTINAL TRACT

Visualization of the gastrointestinal tract with ultrasound may be difficult because intraluminal air produces an echogenic shadow, which prevents the sound beam from penetrating structures posteriorly. The scattering and reflection effect of gas in the gastrointestinal tract often produces an incomplete or mottled distal acoustic shadow. The rim of lucency represents the wall (i.e., intima, media, and serosa), and its periserosal fat produces the outer echogenic border of the tract wall.

The bowel wall consists of five layers (Box 13-1). The odd-numbered walls (first, third, and fifth) are echogenic, and the even-numbered walls (second and fourth) are hypoechoic, with an average total thickness of 3 mm if distended and 5 mm if undistended.

The technique used to observe the upper gastrointestinal tract is for the patient to drink 10 to 40 oz of water through a straw after a baseline ultrasound study of the upper abdomen is completed. The straw helps prevent ingestion of excess air when the water is consumed. The patient should be in an upright position for the examination; this causes air in the

stomach to rise to the fundus of the stomach and not interfere with the ultrasound beam (Figure 13-10). The lower gastrointestinal tract requires no preparation. When imaging the lower colon, it may be useful to give the patient a water enema to better delineate the colon.

Stomach

The gastroesophageal junction is seen on the sagittal scan to the left of the midline as a bull's-eye or target-shaped structure anterior to the aorta, posterior to the left lobe of the liver, and inferior to the hemidiaphragm (Figure 13-11). The left lobe of the patient's liver must be large enough to allow imaging of the gastroesophageal junction. The gastric antrum can be seen as a target shape in the midline (Figure 13-12). The remainder of the stomach usually is not visualized well unless dilated with fluid (Figure 13-13).

BOX 13-1	Layers of Bowel

1. **Mucosa:** directly contacts the intraluminal contents; lined with epithelial folds; echogenic
2. **Submucosa:** contains blood vessels and lymph channels
3. **Muscularis:** contains circular and longitudinal bands of fiber
4. **Serosa:** thin, loose layer of connective tissue
5. **Mesothelium:** covers intraperitoneal bowel loops

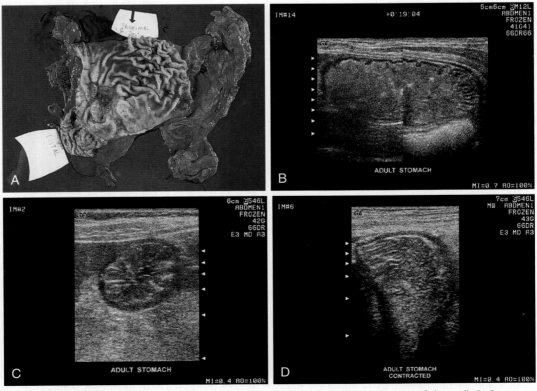

FIGURE 13-10 A, Gross specimen of the stomach showing the internal rugae of the wall. **B,** Sagittal image of the fluid-filled stomach. Rugae may be seen along the peripheral margins of the wall. **C,** Transverse image of the prominent stomach and rugae. **D,** Contracted stomach after fluid has passed through the pylorus.

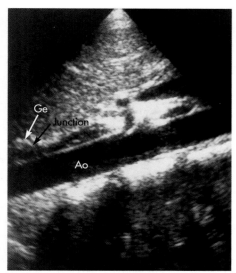

FIGURE 13-11 Sagittal image of the gastroesophageal *(Ge)* junction, which is shown as a small bull's-eye shape anterior to the aorta *(Ao)* and posterior to the left lobe of the liver, inferior to the hemidiaphragm.

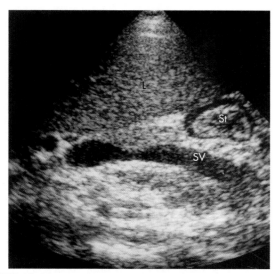

FIGURE 13-12 Transverse view of the left lobe of the liver *(L)*. The antrum of the stomach *(St)* is seen posterior to the liver and anterior to the splenic vein *(SV)*.

When pathology is present, the serosal layer of the normal gastric wall is seen running toward the serous side of a tumor, which allows differentiation of intramural from extraserosal tumors. If a serosal bridging layer (three layers are seen on the mucosal side of the tumor, and at least two of them are continuous with the first and second layers of normal gastric wall) is present, the tumor lies within the gastric wall. If mucosal bridging is continuous with the mucosal layers of the normal gastric wall, is intramucosal, or is deeply infiltrated, carcinoma can be excluded. The sonographer should orient the transducer vertical to the area of transition between the lesion and the stomach wall to show their relationship.

Cystic Mass in the Left Upper Quadrant. If a patient has a cystic mass in the left upper quadrant, several measurements can be taken to determine whether the mass is the fluid-filled stomach or another mass arising from adjacent organs. The sonographer may give the patient a carbonated drink to see bubbles in the stomach, ask the clinician to place a nasogastric tube for drainage, watch for a change in the shape or size of the "stomach" mass with ingestion of fluids, alter the patient's position by scanning in an upright or left or right lateral decubitus position, watch for peristalsis, or ask the patient to drink water to see the swirling effect.

Duodenum

Usually, only the gas-filled duodenal cap is seen to the right of the pancreas. As discussed previously, the duodenum is divided into the following four segments:

1. A superior portion that courses anteroposteriorly from the pylorus to the level of the neck of the gallbladder
2. A sharp bend in the duodenum into the descending portion that runs along the inferior vena cava at the level of L4
3. A transverse portion that passes right to left with a slight inclination upward in front of the great vessels and crura
4. An ascending portion that rises to the right of the aorta and reaches the upper border at L2, where at the duodenojejunal flexure, it turns forward to become the jejunum (usually not seen with ultrasound)

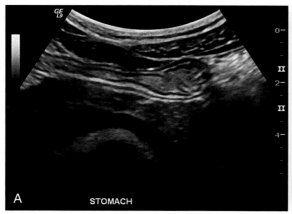

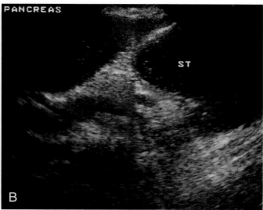

FIGURE 13-13 A, Transverse image of the collapsed empty stomach anterior to the pancreas and splenic vein. **B,** Transverse view of the fluid-filled stomach. Real-time imaging shows movement throughout the stomach *(ST)*.

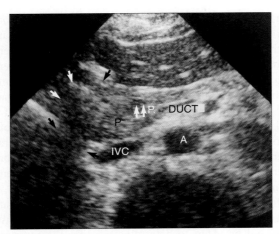

FIGURE 13-14 The duodenum, when filled with a small amount of fluid *(arrows)*, serves as an excellent landmark for the head of the pancreas *(P)*. *A,* Aorta; *IVC,* inferior vena cava.

The duodenum can be outlined easily with water ingestion or a change in position (Figure 13-14). Generally, the right lateral decubitus position allows the fluid to drain from the antrum of the stomach into the duodenum. Observation of peristalsis is useful to delineate the duodenum.

Small Bowel

The sonographer usually cannot see the small bowel with sonography; the valvulae conniventes may be seen as linear echo densities spaced 3 to 5 mm apart (Figure 13-15). This is called the "keyboard sign" and can be seen in the duodenum and jejunum. The ileum is smooth walled, and the small bowel wall is less than 3 mm thick. The small bowel is more difficult to image unless contrast or fluid is present. When fluid is present in the bowel loops, the sonographer may be able to look for peristalsis, air movement, or movement of intraluminal fluid contents to rule out obstruction.

Appendix

The vermiform appendix is a remnant of what was originally the apex of the cecum. It is a long, tubular structure extending from the cecum in one of several directions; it may lie superiorly behind the cecum, medially behind the ileum and mesentery, or downward and medial into the true pelvis (see Figure 13-5). The appendix is located on the abdominal wall under McBurney's point. **McBurney's point** is located by drawing a line from the right anterosuperior iliac spine to the umbilicus. At approximately the midpoint of this line lies the root of the appendix.

The appendix varies from 2 to 20 cm in length, averaging 9 cm, with an average diameter of 7 to 8 mm. It is retained in position by a fold of the peritoneum that forms a mesentery for the appendix. This triangular structure covers two thirds of the appendix, leaving the distal one third completely uncovered by peritoneum. A branch of the ileocolic

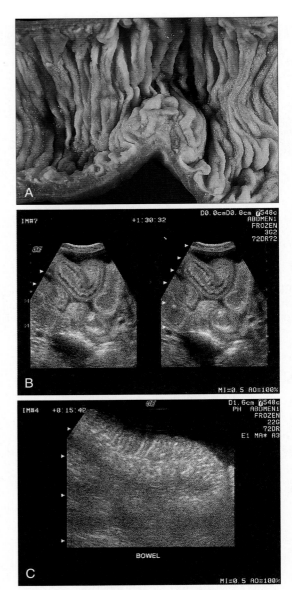

FIGURE 13-15 A, Gross specimen showing the valvulae conniventes within the small bowel lumen. **B** and **C,** Ultrasound images of prominent small bowel with valvulae conniventes.

artery, the artery of the appendix, lies between the layers of this mesentery. This artery runs the entire length of the appendix.

The small canal of the appendix communicates with the cecum by an orifice that is below and behind the ileocecal opening. The cellular layers that make up the appendix are the serosa or adventitia, muscularis propria, submucosa, and mucosa—the same layers as in the intestine. An abundant amount of retiform tissue is found in the mucosa layer, especially in younger ages. The appendix has no known physiologic significance.

Colon

A prominent fluid-filled colon may present as a mass (Figure 13-16). The water enema technique should be used

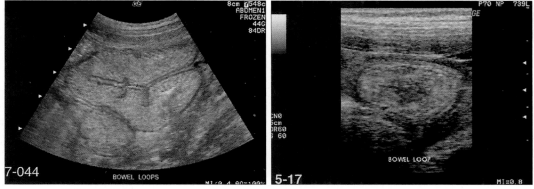

FIGURE 13-16 Target or bull's-eye sign. Ultrasound images of the prominent colon.

to help delineate if the mass is within the colon, separate from the colon, or just the colon itself. The patient should have a full bladder when scanned to help push the small bowel out of the pelvis. The water in the enema should be lukewarm and the patient rolled into the left lateral decubitus position. Only a small amount of water needs to be given as the sonographer follows the rectum and rectosigmoid colon with the endoluminal probe. The normal wall thickness measures 4 mm. The colon consists of five layers: From innermost to outermost, the first two layers are mucosa, the third is submucosa, the fourth is muscularis propria, and the fifth is subserosal fatty tissue. If the colon is dilated, the sonographer should measure from the fluid to the outside of the wall. Distention is considered adequate if the lower bowel is larger than 5 cm; the entire halo should measure less than 2 cm (target sign).

PATHOLOGY OF THE GASTROINTESTINAL TRACT

Upper Gastrointestinal Tract

Table 13-1 lists the clinical findings, sonographic findings, and differential considerations for upper gastrointestinal tract diseases and conditions.

Duplication Cyst. Duplication cysts are embryologic mistakes. They may cause symptoms, depending on their size, location, and histology (see Table 13-1). The criteria for a duplication cyst are as follows: (1) The cyst is lined with alimentary tract epithelium, (2) the cyst has a well-developed muscular wall, and (3) the cyst is contiguous with the stomach. These cysts may come from the pancreas or duodenum and occur more often in females than in males. They usually are found on the greater curvature of the stomach. Clinical symptoms include high intestinal obstruction-distention, vomiting, and abdominal pain; **hemorrhage** and fistula formation may also occur. Differential considerations include mesenteric or omental cyst, pancreatic cyst or pseudocyst, enteric cyst, renal cyst, splenic cyst, congenital cyst of the left lobe of the liver, and gastric distention.

Sonographic Findings. On ultrasound examination, duplication cysts appear anechoic with a thin inner echogenic rim (mucosa) and a wider outer hypoechoic rim (muscle layer).

Gastric Bezoar. A gastric bezoar is an intragastric mass composed of accumulated ingested material. Bezoars are divided into the following three categories: (1) trichobezoars—hair balls in young women, (2) phytobezoars—vegetable matter (e.g., unripe persimmons), and (3) concretions—inorganic materials (e.g., sand, asphalt, shellac). Gastric bezoars are movable intraluminal masses of congealed ingested materials that are seen on upper gastrointestinal radiographs. Clinically, patients may present with nausea, vomiting, crampy epigastric pain, or signs of bowel obstruction (see Table 13-1). Differential diagnosis would include gastric carcinoma, postprandial food, or intramural mass.

Sonographic Findings. Radiography (Figure 13-17) or computed tomography is the imaging modality of choice; however, with sonographic evaluation, a complex mass is seen with internal mobile echogenic components. In the fasting patient, the sonographer would see a broad band of high-amplitude echoes or a hyperechoic curvilinear dense strip at the anterior margin.

Benign Tumors

Polyp. A **polyp** is a protruding, space-occupying, epithelial lesion within the stomach. A gastric polyp is an outgrowth of tissue from the gastric wall (Figure 13-18). Patients are asymptomatic when the polyp is small. As the polyp grows, abdominal pain may be present. See Table 13-1 for clinical findings, sonographic findings, and differential considerations for upper gastrointestinal tract polyps.

Sonographic Findings. Polyps may be seen as an incidental finding with fluid distention of the stomach and appear as solid masses that adhere to the gastric wall. The polyp has variable echogenicity. A large polyp may be inhomogeneous; its contours may be sharply defined, depending on the nature of the surface; a pedicle may be detected.

Intramural Benign Gastric Tumors. These tumors are defined as a benign mass composed of one or more tissue elements of the gastric wall. There are many different types of benign tumors, such as gastrointestinal stromal tumor,

TABLE 13-1	Upper Gastrointestinal Tract Findings	
Clinical Findings	Sonographic Findings	Differential Considerations
Duplication Cysts		
↓ Hematocrit with hemorrhage	Anechoic mass with thin inner echogenic rim Wide outer hypoechoic rim	Mesenteric or omental cyst Pancreatic cyst Enteric cyst Renal cyst Splenic cysts Hepatic cyst in LLL
Gastric Bezoar		
Nausea Vomiting Pain	Complex mass with internal mobile components Hyperechoic curvilinear dense strip at anterior margin	Tumor Cyst
Polyps		
Abdominal pain	Echogenic Heterogeneous	Leiomyoma
Leiomyomas		
N/A	Hypoechoic and contiguous with muscular layer of stomach Solid with cystic areas (necrosis)	Carcinoma Polyp
Gastric Carcinoma		
↑ LFTs Abdominal pain	Target or pseudokidney sign Gastric wall thickening	Leiomyoma Lymphoma Metastatic disease
Lymphoma		
Nausea, vomiting Weight loss	Large, hypoechoic mass Thickened gastric walls Spoke-wheel pattern	Gastric carcinoma Leiomyosarcoma Metastatic disease
Leiomyosarcoma		
N/A	Target lesion with variable pattern Irregular echoes Cystic cavity	Lymphoma Gastric carcinoma Metastatic disease
Metastatic Disease		
Secondary to other cancers	Target pattern Circumscribed thickening Uniform widening of wall without layering	Lymphoma Gastric carcinoma Leiomyosarcoma

LFTs, Liver function tests; *LLL,* left lobe of the liver; *N/A,* not applicable.

leiomyoma, leiomyoblastoma, schwannoma, neurofibroma, lipoma, hemangioma, and lymphangioma.

Leiomyoma is the most common tumor of the stomach. Leiomyoma is seen as a small mass similar to carcinoma. Clinically the patient is asymptomatic (see Table 13-1). Differential diagnosis includes gastric carcinoma, gastric metastases and lymphoma, ectopic pancreatic tissues, and gastric or duodenal ulcer.

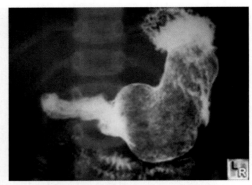

FIGURE 13-17 Radiograph of a patient with a large gastric bezoar.

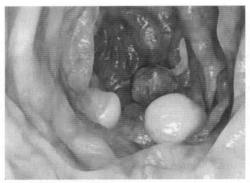

FIGURE 13-18 Endoscopic view of a polyp in the gastrointestinal tract.

Sonographic Findings. On sonography, the mass is seen as hypoechoic and continuous with the muscular layer of the stomach (Figure 13-19). It may also be seen as a circular or oval space-occupying lesion with a homogeneous echo pattern and hemispheric bulging into the lumen, frequently separated from the lumen by two or three layers continuous with those of normal wall. The mass may appear as a solid with cystic areas that represent necrosis.

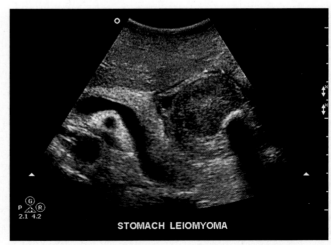

FIGURE 13-19 Transverse image of the left upper quadrant demonstrates a complex tumor in the region of the stomach, which was diagnosed as a leiomyoma.

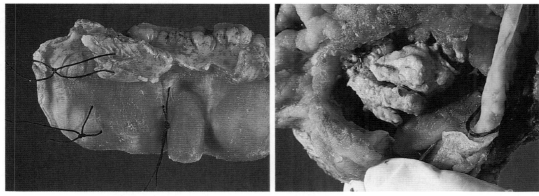

FIGURE 13-20 Gross specimen of adenocarcinoma of the stomach.

Malignant Tumors

Gastric Carcinoma. Stomach cancer or gastric cancer develops from the lining of the stomach. Gastric carcinoma is the fifth leading cause of cancer and the third leading cause of death from cancer; it occurs twice as often in males than in females and is more common in Eastern Asia and Eastern Europe. Clinical symptoms range from asymptomatic to non-specific. Patients may experience indigestion or a burning sensation, loss of appetite, and abdominal discomfort. One half of these tumors occur in the pylorus, and one fourth occur in the body and fundus of the stomach. The lesions may be ulcerated, diffuse, polypoid, superficial, or some combination of these (see Table 13-1) (Figure 13-20).

Sonographic Findings. The sonographer should look for the target or pseudokidney sign; the patient may have gastric wall thickening. The mass will be polypoid or circumferential with no peristalsis through the lesion. The poylpoid cancer can be lobulated or fungating (Figure 13-21). Gastric outlet obstruction may be present secondary to the mass.

Lymphoma. Lymphoma can occur as a primary tumor of the gastrointestinal tract with 3% comprising stomach tumors. In patients with disseminated lymphoma, a primary tumor occurs as a multifocal lesion in the gastrointestinal tract. The stomach has enlarged and thickened mucosal folds, multiple submucosal nodules, ulceration, and a large extraluminal mass. Clinical symptoms include nausea and vomiting with weight loss (see Table 13-1).

Sonographic Findings. The sonographer will note a large and poorly echogenic (hypoechoic) mass, thickening of the gastric walls, and a spoke-wheel or bull's-eye pattern within the mass (Figure 13-22).

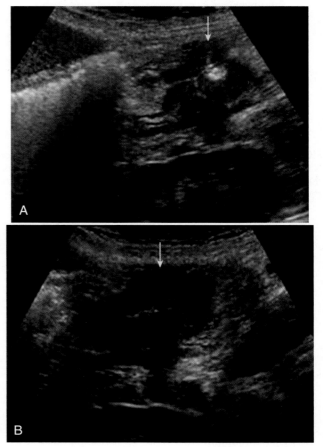

FIGURE 13-22 Lymphoma. On sonography, a large and poorly echogenic (hypoechoic) mass, thickening of the gastric walls, and a spoke-wheel or bull's-eye pattern may be noted within the mass.

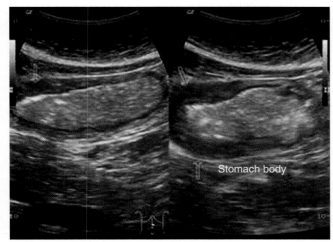

FIGURE 13-21 Sonographic images of a large heterogeneous cancerous mass within the stomach.

Leiomyosarcoma. The second most common malignant tumor is the leiomyosarcoma gastric sarcoma comprising 1% to 5% of tumors. The mass is generally globular or irregular; it may become huge, outstripping its blood supply, with central necrosis leading to cystic degeneration and cavitation (see Table 13-1).

Sonographic Findings. A target-shaped hypoechoic lesion is visible on sonography. Although the pattern is variable, hemorrhage and necrosis may occur, causing irregular echoes or a cystic cavity (Figure 13-23).

Metastatic Disease. Metastatic disease to the stomach is rare; it may result from a melanoma or lung or breast cancer. The tumor is found in the submucosal layer, forming circumscribed nodules or plaques (see Table 13-1).

Sonographic Findings. A target pattern with circumscribed thickening or uniform widening of the stomach wall without layering is visible (Figure 13-24).

Lower Gastrointestinal Tract

Table 13-2 lists the clinical findings, sonographic findings, and differential diagnoses for lower gastrointestinal tract diseases and conditions.

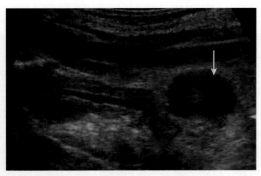

FIGURE 13-23 **Leiomyosarcoma.** A target-shaped hypoechoic lesion is visible on sonography. Although the pattern is variable, hemorrhage and necrosis may occur, causing irregular echoes or a cystic cavity.

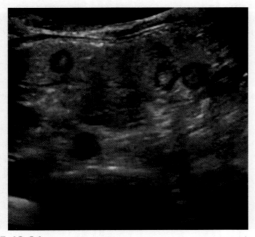

FIGURE 13-24 **Metastatic disease.** A target pattern with circumscribed thickening or uniform widening of the stomach wall without layering is visible.

TABLE 13-2	Lower Gastrointestinal Tract Findings	
Clinical Findings	Sonographic Findings	Differential Considerations
Obstruction and/or Dilation		
Epigastric pain	Tubular, round, echo-free lesion Compressibility of bowel	Appendicitis
Acute Appendicitis		
Pain rebound tenderness over McBurney's point Diarrhea Fever Nausea, vomiting	Thickened muscular wall and ↑ appendiceal diameter (6 mm) Lack of peristalsis Not compressible ↑ Blood flow (Doppler)	Ruptured ectopic pregnancy Fluid-filled colon Inflammation of Meckel's diverticulum
Mucocele		
↑ Leukocytes RLQ pain Asymptomatic	Variable: anechoic, hypoechoic, complex	Appendicitis
Meckel's Diverticulitis		
Rectal bleeding Tenderness	Loop pattern	Acute appendicitis
Crohn's Disease		
Diarrhea Fever RLQ pain	Symmetrically swollen bowel Target pattern with preserved parietal layers around stenotic and hyperdense lumen ↑ Wall thickening Rigidity to pressure Peristalsis absent or sluggish	Appendicitis Meckel's diverticulum Diverticulitis
Lymphoma		
Abdominal pain Palpable mass Weight loss Blood loss	Large, discrete mass Exoenteric pattern	Pseudokidney Leiomyosarcoma
Leiomyosarcoma		
Abdominal pain Palpable mass	Large, solid mass Contained in necrotic areas	Lymphoma

RLQ, Right lower quadrant.

Obstruction and Dilation. A small-bowel obstruction is associated with dilation of the bowel loops proximal to the site of obstruction (Figure 13-25). In 6% of cases, the dilated loops are fluid filled and can be mistaken for a soft tissue mass on x-ray examination (see Table 13-2).

Sonographic Findings. The dilated loops have a tubular or round echo-free appearance. In adynamic ileus, the dilated bowel has normal to somewhat increased peristaltic activity and less distention than in dynamic ileus. In dynamic ileus, the loops are round, with minimal deformity at the interfaces with adjacent loops of distended bowel; valvulae

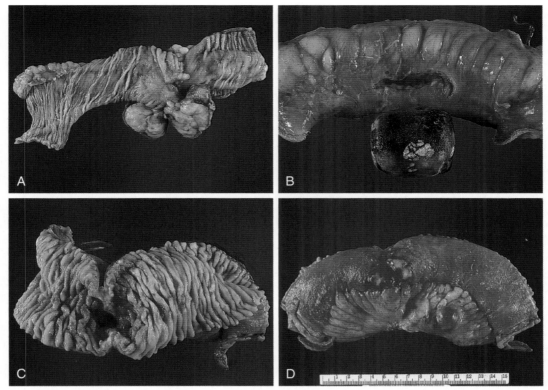

FIGURE 13-25 **A,** Gross specimen example of small-bowel obstruction. **B,** Small-bowel obstruction secondary to gallstones. **C** and **D,** Small-bowel adenocarcinoma. The tumor may cause obstruction of the small bowel.

conniventes and peristalsis are seen. The fluid loops are not always associated with obstruction; they can occur with gastroenteritis and **paralytic ileus,** or in dilated, fluid-filled bowel loops without peristalsis. The sonographer should demonstrate pliability and compressibility of the bowel wall (Figure 13-26). With volvulus (closed-loop obstruction), the involved loop is doubled back on itself abruptly, so that a U-shaped appearance is seen on sagittal scan, and a C-shaped anechoic area with a dense center is seen on transverse scan. The dense center represents medial bowel wall and mesentery.

Abnormalities of the Appendix

Acute Appendicitis. Acute appendicitis is the result of luminal obstruction and inflammation, leading to ischemia of the vermiform appendix (Figure 13-27). This may produce necrosis, perforation, and subsequent abscess formation and peritonitis. The appendix lumen may be obstructed by fecal material, a foreign body, carcinoma of the cecum, stenosis, inflammation, kinking of the organ, or even lymphatic hypertrophy resulting from systemic infection. Obstruction results in edema, which can compromise the vascular supply to the appendix. Subsequently, the permeability of the mucosa increases, and bacterial invasion of the wall of the appendix results in infection and inflammation. Increased intraluminal pressure may cause occlusion of the appendicular end artery. If the condition persists, the appendix may necrose, leading to gangrene, rupture, and subsequent local or generalized peritonitis.

Periappendiceal abscess or peritonitis does not necessarily mean perforation; the organism may permeate the wall in the absence of perforation to cause these extra-appendiceal complications.

The symptoms of acute appendicitis are pain and rebound tenderness, which is usually localized over the right lower quadrant (**McBurney's sign**). Typically, the pain is followed by nausea and vomiting, diarrhea, and systemic signs of inflammation, such as leukocytosis and fever (see Table 13-2). Acute appendicitis can occur at any age but is more prevalent at younger ages.

Progression of acute appendicitis to frank perforation is more rapid in the younger child, sometimes occurring within 6 to 12 hours. The rate of perforation in the preschool child can be as high as 70% compared with the overall figure of 30% for children and 21% to 22% for adults. Women age 20 to 40 years are at high risk for misdiagnosis of the condition on initial physical examination.

Diagnosis of even the classic case of appendicitis is complicated by the fact that many disorders present with a similar clinical picture of an acute condition in the abdomen. Differential diagnosis may include the following: (1) acute gastroenteritis, (2) mesenteric lymphadenitis in children, (3) ruptured ectopic pregnancy, (4) mittelschmerz, (5) inflammation of Meckel's diverticulum, (6) regional enteritis, and (7) right ovarian torsion.

Sonographic Findings. The normal appendix occasionally can be visualized with gradual compression sonography.

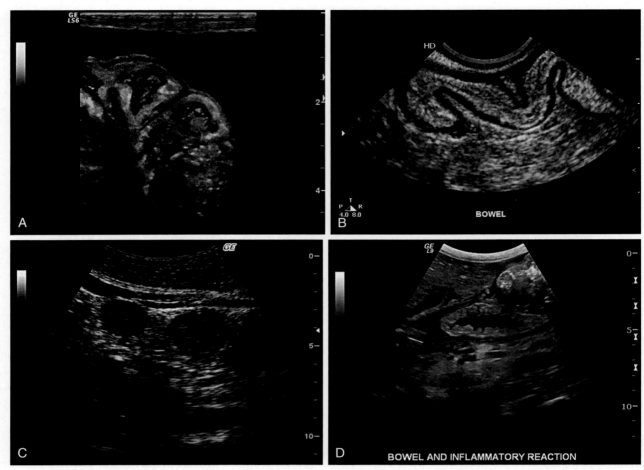

FIGURE 13-26 A, Transverse image of prominent fluid-filled bowel loops. **B,** The bowel is surrounded by ascitic fluid. **C,** Inflammation of the bowel demonstrates prominent dilated loops of bowel shown as circular bull's-eye or target structures in the lower abdomen. **D,** Inflammatory reaction of the bowel.

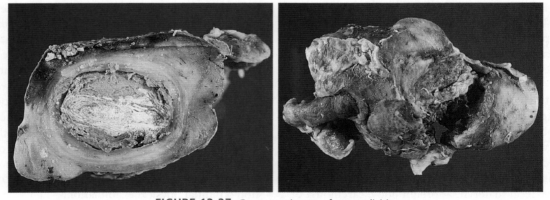

FIGURE 13-27 Gross specimens of appendicitis.

The maximal outer diameters of the normal appendix can measure up to 6 mm. The inflamed appendix will show edema of the wall measuring greater than 2 mm thick; perforation may be present when asymmetric wall thickening is seen. In inflamed specimens, both the integrity and the stratification of wall layers are altered. The distinction of layers is impaired, and each layer is sonographically inhomogeneous.

Wall appearance should not be the only criterion for confirmation of appendicitis. The ultrasound pattern of acute appendicitis is characterized by a target-shaped appearance of the appendix in transverse view. Views of the appendix in the transverse plane should demonstrate a thickened muscular wall and increased appendiceal diameter (Figure 13-28). The typical target-shaped lesion consists of a hypoechoic, fluid-distended lumen, a hyperechoic

Retrocecal appendicitis is seen in approximately 28% of pediatric appendicitis patients and is easy to diagnose by ultrasound. No bowel loops are interposed between the appendix and the lateral wall of the abdomen. The inflamed appendix is identified on cross section as a **target sign** underneath the abdominis muscle. The incidence of complex masses is greater in retrocecal appendicitis, reflecting a higher incidence of perforation. The sonographic appearance of an appendiceal abscess is a complex mass. Sometimes the sonographer can recognize the appendix inside the mass. The omentum wrapping the appendix is seen as an echogenic band and bowel loops.

The initial inflammatory changes in appendicitis are more pronounced in the distal half of the appendix and may be focally confined to the appendiceal tip. Ulcerations and necrosis may cause loss of the echogenic submucosal layer in the tip of the appendix. The appendix should be compressed to the tip and visualized longitudinally and transversely to its blind termination. **Appendicoliths** are **fecaliths** or calculi in the appendix. They are seen as intraluminal foci of high-amplitude echoes with acoustic shadowing.

In infancy and childhood, the appendix frequently becomes decompressed after perforation, and the inflammatory process may not wall off or form a well-defined abscess, as is typically seen in adults. With perforation and decompression and an abnormally thickened wall, a collapsed appendix may still be identified. In some patients, however, no appendix may be found, and only questionable remnants remain. Supplemental findings, such as free abdominal fluid with debris or thickening of the adjacent abdominal wall, may suggest the diagnosis. However, the possibility of appendicitis cannot be ruled out even in a patient who lacks an abnormal appendix or a well-defined abscess. Radiographic contrast studies may help diagnosis.

Gas collections within the appendix may be a pitfall in ultrasound evaluation. Gas within the appendix is diagnosed on the basis of sonographic findings of high-amplitude echogenic foci, causing distal reverberation artifacts (i.e., "comet tails" or "dirty" acoustic shadowing). Although this is a relatively rare finding, its importance lies in the fact that it may be misconstrued as a normal bowel loop or a gas-forming appendiceal abscess. Gas collections from within the bowel loops should be distinguished from an inflamed appendix. The inflamed appendix is noncompressible and demonstrates other specific anatomic features.

Graded compression ultrasound is an alternative technique for diagnosing appendicitis; it has a sensitivity of 88% and a specificity of 96%. Color Doppler ultrasound imaging can be used to detect increased flow, demonstrating hyperperfusion associated with inflammation. Vessels can be seen coursing through the periphery of the dilated appendix. Addition of color Doppler alone does not increase the sensitivity for detecting appendicitis compared with ultrasound alone. Color Doppler is a simple means of confirming gray-scale sonographic findings.

Mucocele. Mucocele of the appendix is a rare pathologic entity. This term designates gross enlargement of the appendix

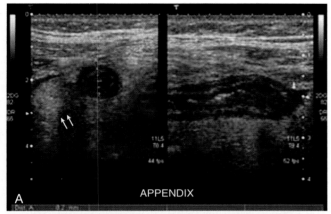

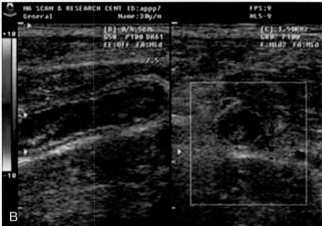

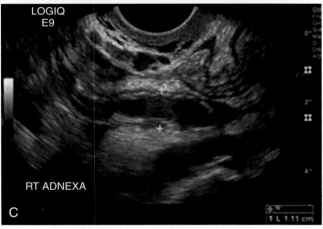

FIGURE 13-28 Acute appendicitis. A, The appendix in the transverse plane should demonstrate a thickened muscular wall and increased appendiceal diameter. **B,** Color Doppler will show the increased velocity secondary to the inflamed appendix. **C,** Transvaginal imaging allows the sonographer to image the inflamed appendix without bowel interference.

inner ring representing mainly the mucosa and the submucosa, and an outer hypoechoic ring representing the **muscularis** externa. The inflamed appendix is further characterized by lack of peristalsis and compressibility, and by demonstration of its "blind end tip." It is important to carefully survey the entire length of the appendix to prevent a false-negative examination.

from accumulation of mucoid substance within the lumen. Scarring or fecalith after an appendectomy is the most common cause of mucocele, although proximal obstruction of the lumen by inflammatory fibrosis, cecal carcinoma, carcinoid polyp, and even endometriosis has been reported. Mucoceles have been classified into three distinct entities: mucosal hyperplasia (an innocuous hyperplastic process), mucinous cystadenoma (a benign neoplasm), and mucinous cystadenocarcinoma (a malignant tumor).

Several classifications of mucoceles are known. If the tumor remains encapsulated and no malignant cells are present, this lesion is called a *mucocele.* If the mucus spreads through the abdominal cavity without evidence of malignant cells, this condition is called *pseudomyxoma peritonei.* Pseudomyxoma assumes a malignant potential only when epithelial cells occur within the gelatinous peritoneal fluid in association with carcinoma.

Appendiceal mucoceles reportedly show a female-to-male predominance of 4:1, with an average age at presentation of 55 years. The most common clinical complaint is right lower quadrant pain (see Table 13-2). About 25% of cases are asymptomatic. Other symptoms include right iliac fossa mass, sepsis, and urinary symptoms. Bloating of the abdomen is specific to patients with pseudomyxoma peritonei. Laboratory values show an increased erythrocyte sedimentation rate and an elevated leukocyte count. Also, elevated levels of carcinoembryonic antigen have been reported. Pseudomyxoma peritonei significantly decreases survival of patients with appendiceal cystadenocarcinomas.

Sonographic Findings. The sonographer should locate the appendix in the right lower quadrant, referencing the psoas muscle and iliac vessels. The image varies according to the content of the mucocele, which may be anechoic when mucoid material is more fluid. The following patterns have been defined: (1) a purely cystic lesion with anechoic fluid; (2) a hypoechoic mass containing fine internal echoes; and (3) a complex mass with high-level echoes (Figure 13-29). As it enlarges, inspissation of the mucoid material creates this internal echo pattern. This mass has an irregular inner wall

caused by mucinous debris with varying degrees of epithelial hyperplasia. Calcification of the rim can produce acoustic shadowing. Internal, thin septations have been seen along with variable degrees of mucosal atrophy and ulceration.

Pseudomyxoma peritonei is a clinical condition caused by cancerous cells (mucinous adenocarcinoma) that produce abundant mucin or gelatinous ascites. The tumors cause fibrosis of tissues and impede digestion or organ function, and if left untreated, the tumors and mucin they produce will fill the abdominal cavity. This will result in compression of organs and will destroy the function of colon, small intestine, stomach, or other organs. Prognosis with treatment in many cases is optimistic, but the disease is lethal if untreated, with death by cachexia, bowel obstruction, or other types of complications.

This disease is most commonly caused by an appendiceal primary cancer (cancer of the appendix); mucinous tumors of the ovary have also been implicated, although in most cases ovarian involvement is favored to be a metastasis from an appendiceal or other gastrointestinal source. Disease is typically classified as low- or high-grade disease (with signet ring cells). When disease presents with low-grade histologic features the cancer rarely spreads through the lymphatic system or through the bloodstream.

With sonography, the disease is seen as septated **ascites** (fluid in the abdomen) with numerous suspended echoes that do not mobilize as the patient changes position. When combined with ultrasound, paracentesis may accurately establish the diagnosis of gelatinous ascites.

Meckel's Diverticulitis. A **diverticulum** is a pouchlike herniation through the muscular wall of a tubular organ that occurs in the stomach, the small intestine, or, most commonly, the colon. **Meckel's diverticulum** is located in the distal ileum, usually within 60 to 100 cm of the ileocecal valve. This blind segment or small pouch is about 3 to 6 cm long and may have a greater lumen diameter than that of the ileum. It runs antimesenterically and has its own blood supply. It is a remnant of the connection from the yolk sac to the small intestine present during embryonic development. It is a

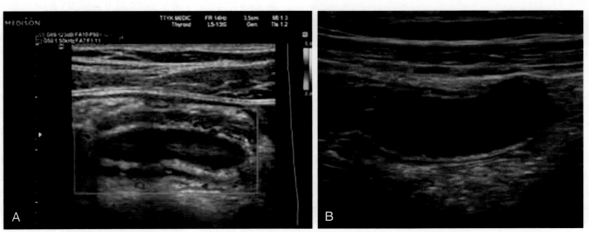

FIGURE 13-29 Mucocele. The image varies according to the content of the mucocele, which may be anechoic when mucoid material is more fluid.

true diverticulum, consisting of all three layers of the bowel wall (mucosa, submucosa, and muscularis propria).

As the vitelline duct is made up of pluripotent cell lining, Meckel's diverticulum may harbor abnormal tissues, containing embryonic remnants of other tissue types. Jejunal, duodenal mucosa, and Brunner's tissue were each found in 2% of ectopic cases. Heterotopic rests of gastric mucosa and pancreatic tissue are seen in 60% and 6% of cases, respectively. Heterotopic means the displacement of an organ from its normal anatomic location. Inflammation of Meckel's diverticulum may mimic appendicitis. Therefore during appendectomy the ileum should be checked for the presence of Meckel's diverticulum, and if it is found to be present it should be removed along with appendix.

In Meckel's diverticulitis, adults may present with intestinal obstruction, rectal bleeding, or diverticular inflammation (see Table 13-2). Acute appendicitis and acute Meckel's diverticulitis may not be distinguished clinically.

Sonographic Findings. The wall of Meckel's diverticulum consists of mucosal, muscular, and serosal layers. Noncompressibility of the obstructed, inflamed diverticulum indicates that intraluminal fluid is trapped (Figure 13-30). The area of maximal tenderness is evaluated along with its distance from the cecum.

Crohn's Disease. **Crohn's disease** is regional enteritis, a recurrent granulomatous inflammatory disease that affects the terminal ileum, colon, or both at any level (Figure 13-31). The reaction involves the entire thickness of the bowel wall. Clinical symptoms include diarrhea, fever, and right lower quadrant pain (see Table 13-2).

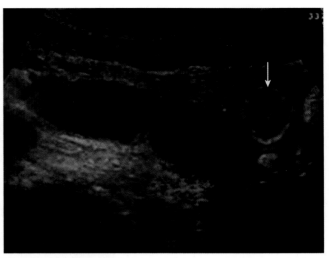

FIGURE 13-30 **Meckel's diverticulitis.** The wall of Meckel's diverticulum consists of mucosal, muscular, and serosal layers. Noncompressibility of the obstructed, inflamed diverticulum indicates that intraluminal fluid is trapped.

Sonographic Findings. A symmetrically swollen bowel target pattern with preserved parietal layers around the stenotic and echogenic lumen is seen on sonography (Figure 13-32). Findings are most prominent in ileocolonic disease, with uniformly increased wall thickness involving all layers, especially the mucosa and submucosa. A matted-loop pattern is found in late stages. Patients with Crohn's disease show rigidity to pressure exerted with the transducer. Peristalsis is absent or sluggish.

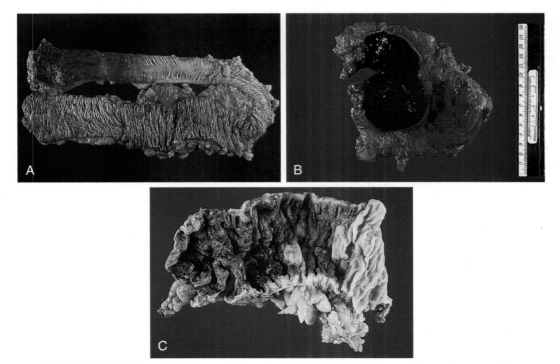

FIGURE 13-31 **A,** Gross specimen of ulcerative colitis. **B** and **C,** Gross specimens show complications of colitis: hematoma in the colon **(B)** and gangrenous colon **(C)**.

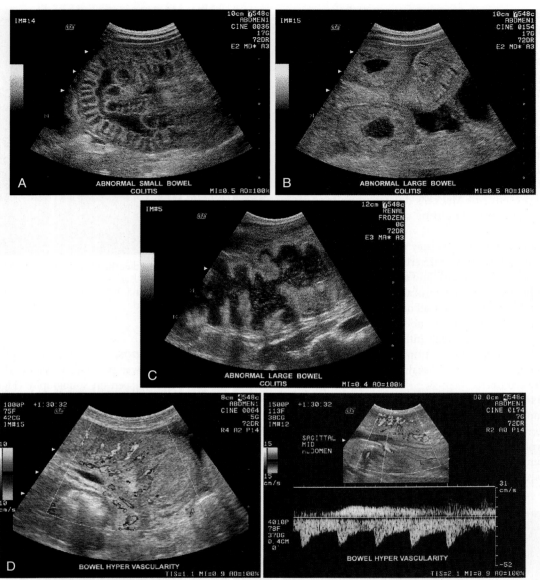

FIGURE 13-32 Ulcerative colitis. A, Small-bowel colitis. **B** and **C,** Dilated colon with colitis. **D,** Prominent colon with increased vascularity.

Tumors of the Colon

Lymphoma. Lymphoma is a tumor that usually occurs late in life, near the sixth decade; it is also the most common tumor of the gastrointestinal tract in children younger than 10 years of age. Intraperitoneal masses frequently involve the mesenteric vessels that encase them. Clinical signs include intestinal blood loss, weight loss, anorexia, and abdominal pain (see Table 13-2). The patient may have an intestinal obstruction or a palpable mass.

Sonographic Findings. The sonographer may see a large, discrete mass with a target pattern, an exoenteric pattern with a large mass on the mesenteric surface of bowel, and a small anechoic mass representing subserosal nodes or mesenteric nodal involvement (Figure 13-33).

Lymphomatous involvement of the intestinal wall may lead to pseudokidney or hydronephrotic pseudokidney. The lumen may be dilated with fluid and may demonstrate lack of peristalsis. The bowel wall is uniformly thickened, with homogeneous low echogenicity between the well-defined mucosal and serosal surfaces that contain a persistent, echo-free, wide, and long lumen.

Leiomyosarcoma. Leiomyosarcoma is a rare, malignant (cancerous) smooth muscle tumor. It must not be confused with leiomyoma, which is a benign tumor originating from the same tissue. Leiomyosarcomas can be very unpredictable. They can remain dormant for long periods of time and recur after years. It is a resistant cancer, meaning generally not very responsive to chemotherapy or radiation. The best outcomes occur when it can be removed surgically with wide margins early, while small and still in situ.

Smooth muscle cells make up the involuntary muscles, which are found in most parts of the body, including the

Understanding the structure

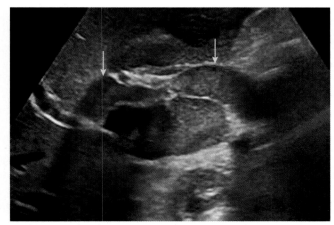

FIGURE 13-33 **Lymphoma.** A large, discrete mass with a target pattern, an exoenteric pattern with a large mass on the mesenteric surface of bowel, and a small anechoic mass representing subserosal nodes or mesenteric nodal involvement may be seen in a patient with lymphoma.

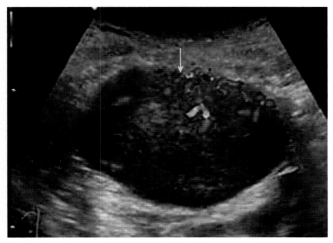

FIGURE 13-34 **Metastatic disease.** A large solid mass containing necrotic areas anterior to solid viscus may be found; color Doppler with demonstrate a low-velocity flow within the mass.

uterus, the stomach and intestines, the walls of all blood vessels, and the skin. It is therefore possible for leiomyosarcomas to appear at any site in the body (including the breasts); they are most commonly found in the uterus, stomach, small intestine, and retroperitoneum. This tumor can have a primary site of origin anywhere in the body where there is a blood vessel. Leiomyosarcoma represents 10% of primary small-bowel tumors. Approximately 10% to 30% of these occur in the duodenum, 30% to 45% in the jejunum, and 35% to 55% in the ileum. Patients are in their fifth to sixth decade of life.

Sonographic Findings. A large solid mass containing necrotic areas anterior to solid viscus may be found. Color Doppler with demonstrate a low-velocity flow within the mass (Figure 13-34).

Key Pearls

- The digestive tract and gastrointestinal tract comprise the digestive system.
- The stomach is divided into three parts: The *fundus* is found in the superior aspect, the *body* makes up the major central axis, and the *pylorus* is the lower aspect.
- The duodenum is subdivided into four segments: (1) superior, (2) descending, (3) transverse, and (4) ascending.
- The valvulae conniventes of the small intestine are large folds of mucous membrane that project into the lumen of the bowel and help retard the passage of food to provide greater absorption.
- The haustra of the colon are the small pouches caused by sacculation, which give the colon its segmented appearance.
- The arteries that supply the esophagus rise from the high, middle, and lower sections of this muscular tube.
- Varices may be seen to rise from the gastroesophageal arteries.
- The celiac axis supplies the duodenum through its right gastric, gastroduodenal, and superior pancreaticoduodenal branches.
- The celiac, superior mesenteric, and inferior mesenteric arteries supply both the small and the large intestine.
- Digestion and absorption are the primary functions of the gastrointestinal tract.
- Visualization of the gastrointestinal tract with ultrasound may be difficult because intraluminal air produces an echogenic shadow, which prevents the sound beam from penetrating structures posteriorly.
- The bowel wall consists of five layers: the odd-numbered walls (first, third, and fifth) are echogenic, and the even-numbered walls (second and fourth) are hypoechoic, with an average total thickness of 3 mm if distended and 5 mm if undistended.
- The gastroesophageal junction is seen on the sagittal scan to the left of the midline as a bull's-eye or target-shaped structure anterior to the aorta, posterior to the left lobe of the liver, and inferior to the hemidiaphragm.
- The duodenum can be outlined easily with water ingestion or a change in position.
- The sonographer usually cannot see the small bowel with sonography; the valvulae conniventes may be seen as linear echo densities spaced 3 to 5 mm apart.
- The vermiform appendix is a remnant of what was originally the apex of the cecum.
- The appendix is located on the abdominal wall under McBurney's point, located by drawing a line from the right anterosuperior iliac spine to the umbilicus: the appendix lies at the midpoint of this line.
- The criteria for a duplication cyst are as follows: (1) The cyst is lined with alimentary tract epithelium, (2) the cyst

Continued

has a well-developed muscular wall, and (3) the cyst is contiguous with the stomach.

- A gastric bezoar is an intragastric mass composed of accumulated ingested material.
- A polyp is a protruding, space-occupying, epithelial lesion within the stomach.
- Leiomyoma is the most common tumor of the stomach.
- Gastric carcinoma is the fifth leading cause of cancer and the third leading cause of death from cancer.
- A small-bowel obstruction is associated with dilation of the bowel loops proximal to the site of obstruction.
- Acute appendicitis is the result of luminal obstruction and inflammation, leading to ischemia of the vermiform appendix.
- The symptoms of acute appendicitis are pain and rebound tenderness, which is usually localized over the right lower quadrant.
- The inflamed appendix will show edema of the wall measuring greater than 2 mm thick; perforation may be present when asymmetric wall thickening is seen.
- Mucocele of the appendix is a gross enlargement of the appendix from accumulation of mucoid substance within the lumen.
- Meckel's diverticulum is a pouchlike herniation through the muscular wall of a tubular organ that occurs in the stomach, the small intestine, or, most commonly, the colon.
- Crohn's disease is regional enteritis, a recurrent granulomatous inflammatory disease that affects the terminal ileum, colon, or both at any level.
- Lymphomatous involvement of the intestinal wall may lead to pseudokidney or hydronephrotic pseudokidney.

BIBLIOGRAPHY

Birnbaum BA, Jeffrey RB Jr: CT and sonographic evaluation of acute right lower quadrant abdominal pain, *Am J Roentgenol* 170:361-371, 1998.

Chaubal N, Manjiri D, Shah M, Chaubal J: Sonography of the gastrointestinal tract, *J Ultrasound Med* 25:87-97, 2006.

Curry R, Tempkin B, editors: *Sonography: introduction to normal anatomy and structure*, ed 3, Philadelphia, 2010, Saunders.

Eisen K: Gastrointestinal imaging. In Henningsen C, editor: Clinical guide to ultrasonography, St Louis, 2004, Mosby.

Khaja M, Kilani R, Jacobson W, Hiett AK: Gastrointestinal stromal tumor presenting as a mass on pelvic sonography, *J Ultrasound Med* 26:117-120, 2007.

Landen S, Bertrand C, Maddern GJ, et al: Appendiceal mucoceles and pseudomyxoma peritonei, *Surg Gynecol Obstet* 175:401, 1992.

Limberg B: Sonographic features of colonic Crohn's disease: comparison of in vivo and in vitro studies, *J Clin Ultrasound* 18:161, 1990.

Liu JB, Miller LS, Bagley DH, Goldberg BB: Endoluminal sonography of the genitourinary and gastrointestinal tracts, *J Ultrasound Med* 21:323-337, 2002.

Lorentzen T, Nolsoe CP, Khattar SC, et al: Gastric and duodenal wall thickening on abdominal ultrasonography: positive predictive value, *J Ultrasound Med* 12:633-637, 1993.

Quillin SP, Siegel MJ: Appendicitis: efficacy of color Doppler sonography, *Radiology* 191:557, 1994.

Rapp CL, Stavros AT, Meyers PR: Ultrasound of the normal appendix: the how and why, *J Diagn Med Sonogr* 14:195, 1998.

Rumack C, Wilson S, Charboneau W, Johnson J: *Diagnostic ultrasound*, ed 3, St Louis, 2005, Mosby.

Stavros AT, Rapp CL, Thickman D: Sonography of inflammatory conditions, *Ultrasound Q* 13:1, 1995.

Tarantino L, Nocera V, Perrotta M, et al: Primary small-bowel melanoma: color Doppler ultrasonographic, computed tomographic, and radiological findings with pathologic correlations, *J Ultrasound Med* 26:121-127, 2007.

Wilson SR, Toi A: The value of sonography in the diagnosis of acute diverticulitis of the colon, *Am J Roentgenol* 154:1199, 1990.

Worrell JA, Drolshagen LF, Kelly TC, et al: Graded compression ultrasound in the diagnosis of appendicitis: a comparison of diagnostic criteria, *J Ultrasound Med* 9:145, 1990.

Yacoe ME, Jeffrey RB Jr: Sonography of appendicitis and diverticulitis, *Radiol Clin North Am* 32:899-912, 1994.

Peritoneal Cavity and Abdominal Wall

Sandra L. Hagen-Ansert

OBJECTIVES

On completion of this chapter, you should be able to:
- Describe the normal anatomy of the abdominal wall
- List the peritoneal and retroperitoneal organs
- Compare and contrast the different locations of fluid and their sonographic appearances

- Discuss the pathology and sonographic findings of the peritoneal cavity, mesentery, omentum, peritoneum, and abdominal wall

OUTLINE

KEY TERMS

Abscess

Ascites

Gutters

Hemorrhage

Leukocytosis

Mesentery

Morison's pouch

Omentum

Peritonitis

Pyogenic

Sandwich sign

Sepsis

Septicemia

Subhepatic

Subphrenic

Urinoma

ANATOMY AND SONOGRAPHIC EVALUATION OF THE PERITONEAL CAVITY AND ABDOMINAL WALL

Peritoneal Cavity

The peritoneal cavity is made up of multiple peritoneal ligaments and folds that connect the viscera to each other and to the abdominopelvic walls. Within the cavity are the lesser and greater omentum, the mesenteries, the ligaments, and multiple fluid spaces (lesser sac, perihepatic space, and subphrenic space). The peritoneum is a smooth membrane that lines the entire abdominal cavity and is reflected over the contained organs. The section that lines the walls of the cavity is the parietal peritoneum, and the part covering the abdominal organs to a greater or lesser extent is the visceral peritoneum (Figure 14-1). In the male, the peritoneum forms a closed cavity; in the female, there is a "communication" outside the peritoneum through the uterine tubes, uterus, and vagina. In reality, however, the complex linings of the uterus and fallopian tubes tend to close off any potential space and prohibit the entrance of air into the peritoneal cavity.

The relationship of the peritoneum to the abdominal structures may be understood with the visualization of an inflated balloon (the peritoneum) within an empty box (the abdominal cavity) (Figure 14-2). If one were to place objects within the box, yet outside the balloon, these objects might impinge

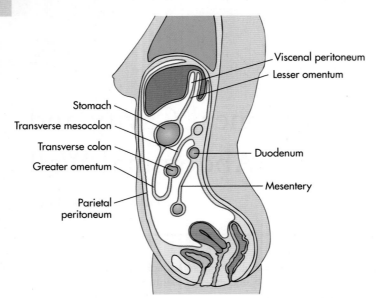

FIGURE 14-1 The peritoneum that lines the walls of the cavity is the parietal peritoneum, and the part covering the abdominal organs to a greater or lesser extent is the visceral peritoneum.

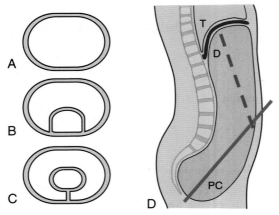

FIGURE 14-2 A, The "abdominal cavity" containing a "balloon" (peritoneum). **B,** An organ inside the abdomen and partly covered by peritoneum, such as the kidney, which is said to be in the retroperitoneal cavity. **C,** An organ suspended from the abdominal wall by a fold of peritoneum, such as the small intestine suspended by its mesentery. **D,** When supine, the backward tilt of the pelvis makes it the lowest part of the peritoneal cavity. Long axis of abdomen *(dotted line);* long axis of pelvis *(solid line); PC,* pelvic part of peritoneal cavity; *D,* diaphragm; *T,* thorax.

on the balloon shape. This is the same condition that the kidneys and the ascending and descending colon have on the peritoneal cavity. Because these structures lie along the posterior surface of the peritoneal cavity, they are considered "retroperitoneal," and they are overlaid by visceral peritoneum. If an object bulges so far into the balloon that it loses contact with the box, the object would become surrounded by a fold of the balloon. This is the situation with the small intestine, transverse colon, and the sigmoid colon; they are suspended from the posterior abdominal wall by a double fold of peritoneum called the **mesentery**. Thus the peritoneal cavity

is really empty of abdominal organs, as they bulge into or are covered by the cavity, but are not located within the cavity.

The general peritoneal cavity is known as the greater sac of the peritoneum. With the development of the stomach and the spleen, a smaller sac, called the lesser sac (omental bursa), is the peritoneal recess posterior to the stomach (Figure 14-3). This sac communicates with the greater sac through a small vertical opening known as the epiploic foramen. The epiploic foramen is just inferior to the liver and superior to the first part of the duodenum; the inferior vena cava is posterior, and the portal vein is anterior (Figure 14-4).

The attachments of the peritoneum to the abdominal walls and organs help determine the way abnormal collections of fluid within the peritoneal cavity can collect or move (Figure 14-5). When the patient is lying supine, the lowest part of the body is the pelvis. On a transverse view, the flanks are lower than the midabdomen. Fluid will accumulate in the lowest parts of the body; therefore the pelvis and lateral flanks (**gutters**) should be carefully examined for pathologic collections of fluid.

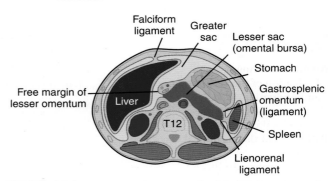

FIGURE 14-3 The general peritoneal cavity is known as the greater sac of the peritoneum. With the development of the stomach and the spleen, a smaller sac, called the lesser sac (omental bursa), is the peritoneal recess posterior to the stomach.

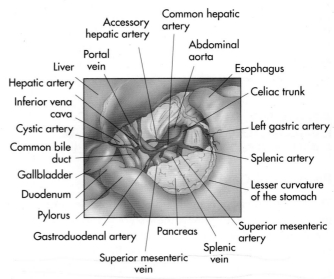

FIGURE 14-4 Upper abdominal dissection, with part of the left lobe of the liver and the lesser omentum removed to show the celiac trunk, portal vein, bile duct, and related structures.

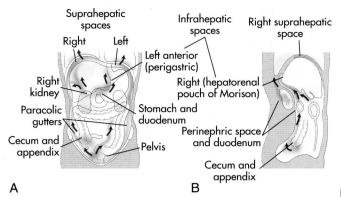

FIGURE 14-5 A, Anterior view of the collection of fluid in the abdominal and pelvic cavities. **B,** Sagittal view of the right abdomen shows how the fluid collects in the most dependent areas of the abdomen and pelvis.

The lesser omentum is a double layer of peritoneum, extending from the liver to the lesser curvature of the stomach. This structure acts as a sling for the stomach, suspending it from the liver (Figure 14-6).

The greater omentum is an apron-like fold of peritoneum that hangs from the greater curvature of the stomach (Figure 14-7). The omentum lies freely over the intestine

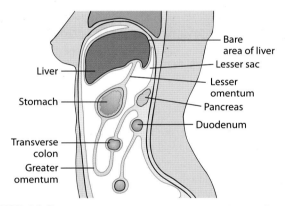

FIGURE 14-6 The lesser omentum is a double layer of peritoneum, extending from the liver to the lesser curvature of the stomach; this structure acts as a sling for the stomach, suspending it from the liver.

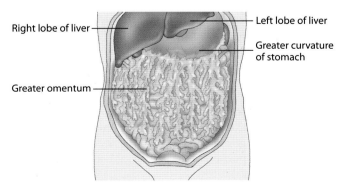

FIGURE 14-7 The greater omentum is an apron-like fold of peritoneum that hangs from the greater curvature of the stomach

except for the upper part, which is fused with the transverse colon and mesocolon. The greater omentum is able to adhere to diseased organs, which in turn helps prevent further spread of infected fluid by essentially "walling it off" from the rest of the body. The greater omentum is profusely supplied with blood vessels by the epiploic branches of the gastroepiploic vessels and thus can bring masses of blood phagocytes to the areas it adheres to, which in turn helps combat infection.

Determination of Intraperitoneal Location. The determination of intraperitoneal fluid from pleural, subdiaphragmatic, subscapular, or retroperitoneal fluid is necessary to determine a differential diagnosis or to locate a fluid pocket for aspiration or a biopsy.

Pleural versus Subdiaphragmatic. Because of the coronary ligament attachments, collections in the right posterior subphrenic space cannot extend between the bare area of the liver and the diaphragm. On the other hand, because the right pleural space extends medially to the attachment of the right superior coronary ligament, pleural collections may appear apposed to the bare area of the liver (Figure 14-8). Unless it is loculated, the pleural fluid tends to distribute posteromedially in the chest (Figure 14-9).

Subcapsular versus Intraperitoneal. Subcapsular liver and splenic collections are seen when they are inferior to the diaphragm unilaterally, and they conform to the shape of an organ capsule (Figure 14-10). They may extend medially to the attachment of the superior coronary ligament.

Retroperitoneal versus Intraperitoneal. A mass is confirmed to be within the retroperitoneal cavity when anterior renal displacement or anterior displacement of the dilated ureters can be documented (Figure 14-11). The mass interposed anteriorly or superiorly to kidneys can be located either intraperitoneally or retroperitoneally.

Fatty and collagenous connective tissues in the perirenal or anterior pararenal space produce echoes that are best

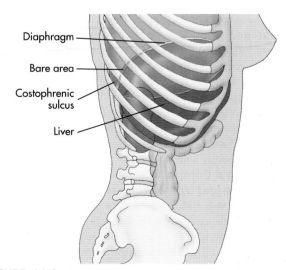

FIGURE 14-8 Sagittal plane of the body shows the diaphragm and liver with the highlighted "bare" area of the liver. The costophrenic sulcus forms the sharp border posterior to the liver and may be identified when fluid is present.

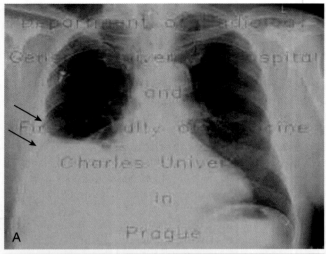

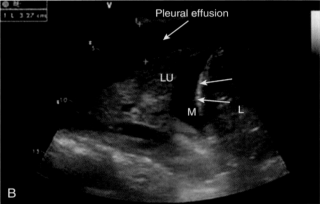

FIGURE 14-9 **A,** Chest radiography demonstrating a large right pleural effusion with blunting of the costophrenic sulcus *(arrows)*. **B,** Sonogram of the right pleural space demonstrating a large right pleural effusion. Diaphragm *(D, curved arrows)*, lung *(Lu)*, liver *(L)*.

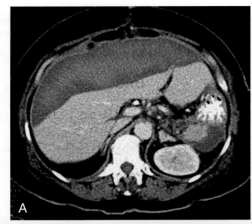

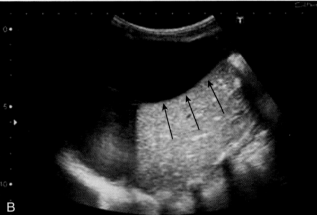

FIGURE 14-10 **A,** Computed tomography image of a patient with a large subcapsular hematoma *(arrows)*. **B,** Ultrasound image of the subcapsular hematoma *(arrows)*.

demonstrated on sagittal scans. Retroperitoneal lesions displace echoes ventrally and cranially; hepatic and **subhepatic** lesions produce inferior and posterior displacement.

The anterior displacement of the superior mesenteric vessels, splenic vein, renal vein, and inferior vena cava excludes an intraperitoneal location. A large, right-sided retroperitoneal mass rotates the intrahepatic portal veins to the left. This causes the left portal vein to show reversed flow. Right posterior hepatic masses of similar dimensions may produce minor displacement of the intrahepatic portal vein. Primary liver masses should move simultaneously with the liver.

Intraperitoneal Compartments

Perihepatic and Upper Abdominal Compartments. Ligaments on the right side of the liver form the subphrenic and subhepatic spaces (Figure 14-12). The falciform ligament divides the subphrenic space into right and left components. The ligamentum teres hepatis ascends from the umbilicus to the umbilical notch of the liver within the free margin of the falciform ligament before coursing within the liver.

The *bare area* is delineated by the right superior and inferior coronary ligaments, which separate the posterior

subphrenic space from the right superior subhepatic space **(Morison's pouch).** Lateral to the bare area and right triangular ligament, the posterior subphrenic and subhepatic spaces are continuous.

A single large and irregular perihepatic space surrounds the superior and lateral aspects of the left lobe of the liver, with the left coronary ligaments anatomically separating the subphrenic space into anterior and posterior compartments. The left subhepatic space is divided into an anterior compartment (the gastrohepatic recess) and a posterior compartment (the lesser sac) by the lesser omentum and stomach (Figure 14-13). The lesser sac lies anterior to the pancreas and posterior to the stomach. With fluid in the lesser and greater omental cavities, the lesser omentum may be seen as a linear, undulating echodensity extending from the stomach to the porta hepatis.

Gastrosplenic Ligament. The gastrosplenic ligament is the left lateral extension of the greater omentum that connects the gastric greater curvature to the superior splenic hilum and forms a portion of the left lateral border of the lesser sac (see Figure 14-12, *C*).

Splenorenal Ligament. The splenorenal ligament is formed by the posterior reflection of the peritoneum of the spleen and passes inferiorly to overlie the left kidney

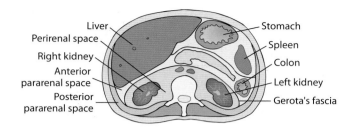

A

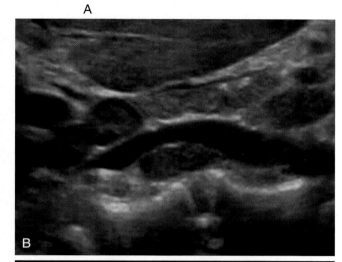

B

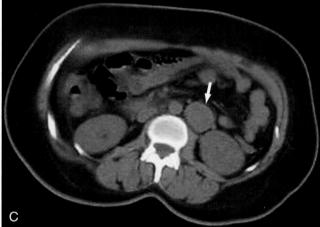

C

FIGURE 14-11 **A,** Transverse view of the retroperitoneal space. **B,** Enlarged lymph nodes surrounding the inferior vena cava. **C,** Computed tomography presentation of an enlarged node *(arrow).*

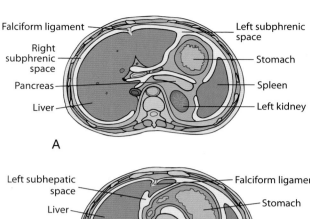

A

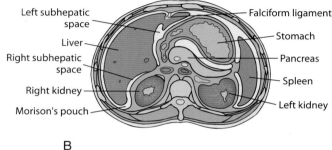

B

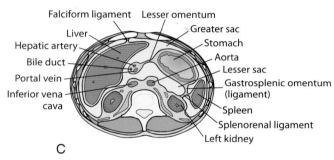

C

FIGURE 14-12 **A,** Transverse view of the subphrenic spaces. **B,** Transverse view of the subhepatic spaces and Morison's pouch. **C,** Transverse view of the abdomen showing the greater and lesser sac, the falciform ligament, the gastrosplenic ligament, and the splenorenal ligament.

(see Figure 14-12, *C*). It forms the posterior portion of the left lateral border of the lesser sac and separates the lesser sac from the renosplenic recess.

The Lesser Omental Bursa. The lesser omental bursa is subdivided into a larger lateroinferior and a smaller mediosuperior recess by the gastropancreatic folds, which are produced by the left gastric and hepatic arteries (Figure 14-14). The lesser sac extends to the diaphragm. The superior recess of the bursa surrounds the anterior, medial, and posterior surfaces of the caudate lobe, making the caudate a lesser sac structure. The lesser sac collections may extend a considerable distance below the plane of the pancreas by inferiorly displacing the transverse mesocolon or extending into the inferior recess of the greater omentum.

Lower Abdominal and Pelvic Compartments. The supravesical space and the medial and lateral inguinal fossae represent intraperitoneal paravesical spaces formed by indentation of the anterior parietal peritoneum by the bladder, obliterated umbilical arteries, and inferior epigastric vessels. The retrovesical space is divided by the uterus into an anterior vesicouterine recess and a posterior rectouterine sac (pouch of Douglas) (see Figure 14-14). The peritoneal reflection over the dome of the bladder may have an inferior recess extending anterior to the bladder. Ascites displaces the distended urinary bladder inferiorly but not posteriorly. Intraperitoneal fluid compresses the bladder from its lateral aspect in cases of loculation. Fluid in the extraperitoneal prevesical space has a "dumbbell" configuration, displacing the bladder posteriorly and compressing it from the sides along its entire length (Figure 14-15).

Abdominal Wall

The paired rectus abdominis muscles are delineated medially in the midline of the body by the linea alba (Figure 14-16). Laterally the aponeuroses of external oblique, internal oblique, and transversus abdominis muscles unite to form a bandlike

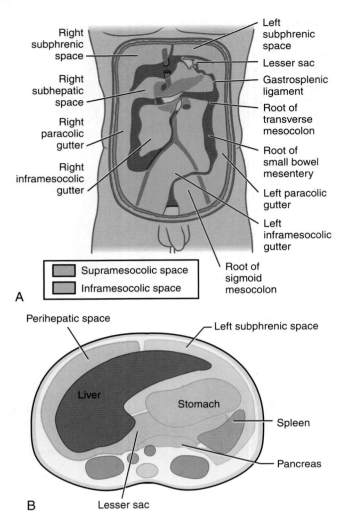

Right subphrenic space

Right subhepatic space

Right paracolic gutter

Right inframesocolic gutter

Left subphrenic space

Lesser sac

Gastrosplenic ligament

Root of transverse mesocolon

Root of small bowel mesentery

Left paracolic gutter

Left inframesocolic gutter

Root of sigmoid mesocolon

Supramesocolic space
Inframesocolic space

A

Perihepatic space

Left subphrenic space

Liver

Stomach

Spleen

Pancreas

Lesser sac

B

FIGURE 14-13 A, The left subhepatic space is divided into an anterior compartment (the gastrohepatic recess) and a posterior compartment (the lesser sac) by the lesser omentum and stomach. **B,** The lesser sac lies anterior to the pancreas and posterior to the stomach.

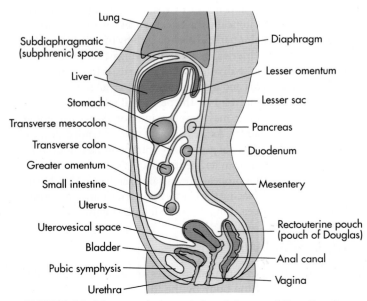

Lung

Subdiaphragmatic (subphrenic) space

Liver

Stomach

Transverse mesocolon

Transverse colon

Greater omentum

Small intestine

Uterus

Uterovesical space

Bladder

Pubic symphysis

Urethra

Diaphragm

Lesser omentum

Lesser sac

Pancreas

Duodenum

Mesentery

Rectouterine pouch (pouch of Douglas)

Anal canal

Vagina

FIGURE 14-14 Sagittal view of the abdomen delineating the peritoneal cavity.

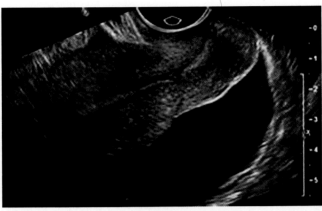

FIGURE 14-15 Transvaginal image of fluid in the extraperitoneal prevesical space displacing the uterus anteriorly.

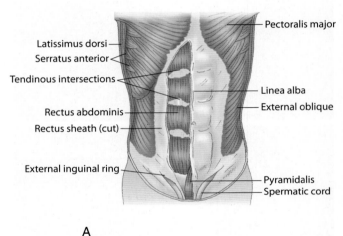

Latissimus dorsi

Serratus anterior

Tendinous intersections

Rectus abdominis

Rectus sheath (cut)

External inguinal ring

Pectoralis major

Linea alba

External oblique

Pyramidalis

Spermatic cord

A

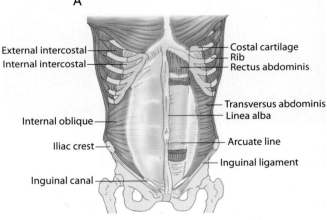

External intercostal

Internal intercostal

Internal oblique

Iliac crest

Inguinal canal

Costal cartilage

Rib

Rectus abdominis

Transversus abdominis

Linea alba

Arcuate line

Inguinal ligament

B

FIGURE 14-16 A, The rectus abdominis muscle rises from the front of the symphysis pubis and the pubic crest. **B,** The muscles of the anterior and lateral abdominal walls include the external oblique, internal oblique, transversus, rectus abdominis, and pyramidalis.

vertical fibrous groove called the linea semilunaris or spigelian fascia. The sheath of the three anterolateral abdominal muscles invests the rectus both anteriorly and posteriorly. Midway between the umbilicus and symphysis pubis, the aponeurotic sheath passes anteriorly to the rectus.

Below the peritoneal line, the rectus muscle is separated from the intraabdominal contents only by the transversalis fascia and the peritoneum. The rectus muscles are seen as a biconvex muscle group delineated by the linea alba and linea semilunaris. The peritoneal line is seen as a discrete linear echogenicity in the deepest layer of the abdominal wall.

PATHOLOGY OF THE PERITONEAL CAVITY

Ascites

Ascites is the accumulation of serous fluid in the peritoneal cavity. The amount of intraperitoneal fluid depends on the location, volume, and patient position. Factors other than fluid volume that affect the distribution of intraperitoneal fluid include peritoneal pressure, the area from which fluid originates, rapidity of fluid accumulation, presence or absence of adhesions, density of fluid with respect to other abdominal organs, and degree of bladder fullness.

Sonographic Findings. Serous ascites appears as echo-free fluid regions indented and shaped by the organs and viscera it surrounds or between where it is interposed (Figure 14-17). The fluid first fills the pouch of Douglas, then the lateral paravesical recesses, before it ascends to both paracolic gutters. The major flow from the pelvis is via the right paracolic gutter. Small volumes of fluid in the supine patient first appear around the

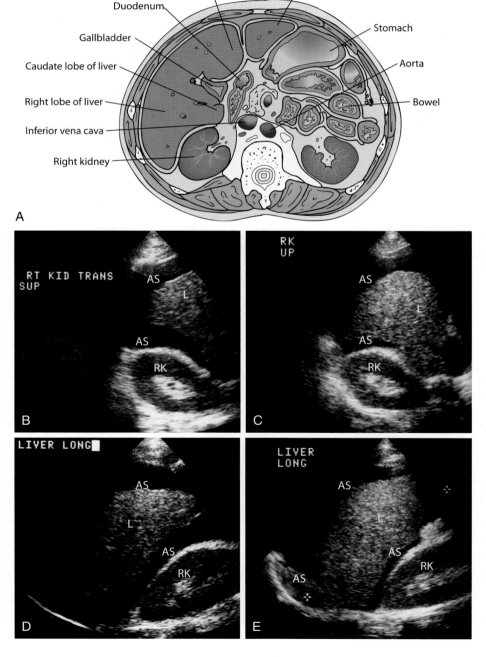

FIGURE 14-17 **A,** Transverse view of the posterior pararenal space. This space is located between the posterior renal fascia and the transversalis fascia. It communicates with the peritoneal fat, lateral to the lateroconal fascia. The space merges inferiorly with the anterior pararenal space and retroperitoneal tissue of the iliac fossa. Ascites may fill the peritoneal cavity. Small volumes of fluid in the supine position first appear around the inferior tip of the right lobe of the superior portion of the right flank. **B,** Transverse view. *AS,* ascites; *L,* liver; *RK,* right kidney. **C,** Transverse view. **D,** Longitudinal view with fluid in Morison's pouch. **E,** Longitudinal view.

inferior tip of the right lobe in the superior portion of the right flank and in the pelvic cul-de-sac, then in the paracolic gutters, before moving lateral and anterior to the liver (Figure 14-18).

The small bowel loops, sinks, or floats in the surrounding ascitic fluid, depending on relative gas content and amount of fat in the mesentery (Figure 14-19). The middle portion of the transverse colon usually floats on top of fluid because of its gas content, whereas the ascending portions of the colon, which are fixed retroperitoneally, remain in their normal location with or without gas.

Floating loops of small bowel, anchored posteriorly by the mesentery and with fluid between the mesenteric folds, have a characteristic anterior convex fan shape or arcuate appearance. An overdistended bladder may mask small quantities of fluid.

Inflammatory or Malignant Ascites. The sonographer should look for findings within the ascitic fluid that may suggest an inflammatory or malignant process. In searching for inflammatory or malignant ascites, the sonographer should look for fine or coarse internal echoes; loculation; unusual distribution, matting, or clumping of bowel loops; and thickening of interfaces between the fluid and neighboring structures (Figure 14-20).

Hepatorenal Recess. Generalized ascites, inflammatory fluid from acute cholecystitis, fluid resulting from pancreatic

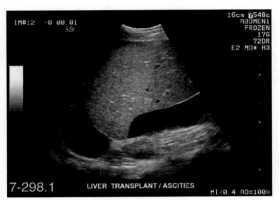

FIGURE 14-18 Ascites secondary to liver transplant is shown in this sagittal image.

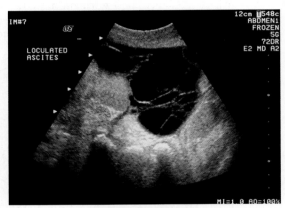

FIGURE 14-19 Loculated ascites with matted bowel.

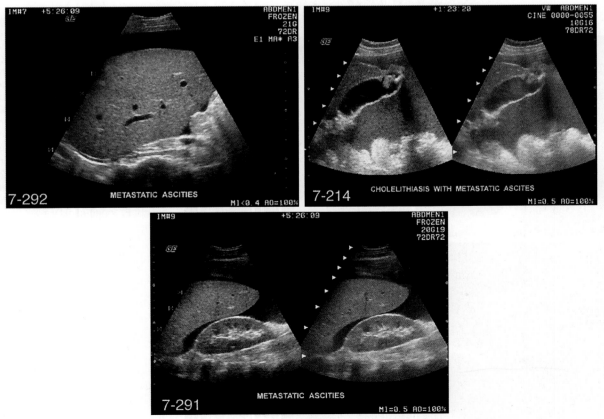

FIGURE 14-20 Malignant ascites. Fine internal echoes are seen in these images of malignant ascites.

autolysis, or blood from a ruptured hepatic neoplasm or ectopic gestation may contribute to the formation of hepatorenal fluid collections. Abdominal fluid collections do not persist 1 week after abdominal surgery as a normal part of the healing process.

Sonographic Findings. Loculated ascites tends to be more irregular in outline, shows less mass effect, and may change shape slightly with positional variation (Figure 14-21).

Abscess Formation and Pockets in the Abdomen and Pelvis

An **abscess** is a cavity formed by necrosis within a solid tissue or a circumscribed collection of purulent material. The sonographer is frequently asked to evaluate a patient to rule out an abscess formation. The patient may present with a fever of unknown origin or with tenderness and swelling from a postoperative procedure. Other clinical signs include chills, weakness, malaise, and pain at the localized site of infection. Laboratory findings include normal liver function values, increased white blood cell count (**leukocytosis**), generalized **sepsis,** and bacterial cultures (if superficial).

Sonographic Findings. Abscess collections can appear quite varied in their texture depending on the length of time the abscess has been forming and the space available for the abscess to localize. Therefore many collections appear predominantly fluid filled with irregular borders; they can also be complex, with debris floating within the cystic mass, or they may show a more solid pattern (Figure 14-22). If the collection is in the pelvis, careful analysis of bowel patterns and peristalsis should be made in an attempt to separate the bowel from the abscess collection.

Classically an abscess appears as an elliptical sonolucent mass with thick and irregular margins. The margins tend to be under tension and displace surrounding structures. A septated appearance may result from previous or developing adhesions. Necrotic debris produces low-level internal echoes that may be seen to float within the abscess. Fluid levels are secondary to layering, probably because of the settling of debris.

Gas-Containing Abscess. Scattered air reflectors may be the sonographer's clue in a gas- or air-filled abscess collection.

Sonographic Findings. Gas-containing abscesses have varying echo patterns. Generally, they appear as a densely echogenic mass with or without acoustic shadowing and otherwise increased through-transmission (Figure 14-23). A teratoma may mimic the pattern of a gas-containing abscess, but clinical history and x-rays exclude this tumor from the diagnosis. A gas-containing abscess may be confused with a solid lesion because it can be difficult to determine the presence of through-transmission.

Peritonitis. **Peritonitis** and the resultant abscess formation may be a generalized or localized process. Multiloculated abscesses or multiple collections should be recorded and their size determined as accurately as possible to help plan drainage and improve accuracy in follow-up studies.

Lesser-Sac Abscess. The small slitlike epiploic foramen usually seals off the lesser sac from inflammatory processes extrinsic to it. If the process begins within the lesser sac, such as with a pancreatic abscess, the sac may be involved along with other secondarily affected peritoneal and retroperitoneal

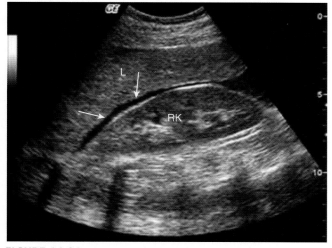

FIGURE 14-21 Fluid in Morison's pouch seen anterior to the right kidney in this sagittal view. *Arrows,* fluid; *L,* liver; *RK,* right kidney.

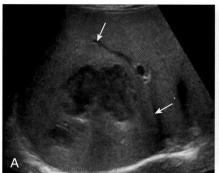
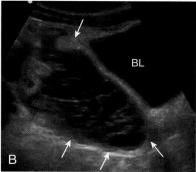
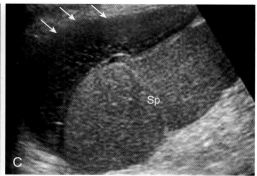

FIGURE 14-22 Abscess collections can appear quite varied in their texture: irregular borders, complex, or debris floating within cystic mass. **A,** Liver abscess *(arrows)* in right lobe displacing the vascular structures. **B,** Pelvic abscess *(arrows)* superior to the bladder (Bl). **C,** Splenic abscess *(arrows)*. *Sp,* spleen.

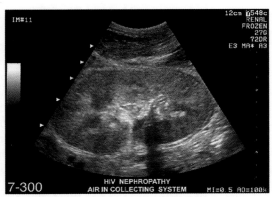

FIGURE 14-23 Patient with human immunodeficiency virus *(HIV)* nephropathy showed air with shadowing in the renal collecting system.

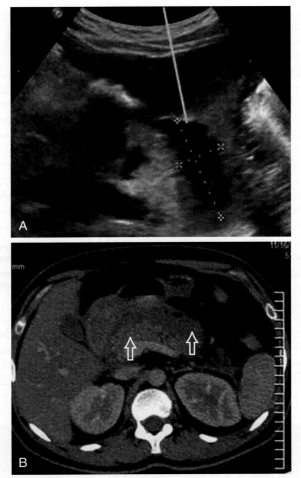

FIGURE 14-24 If the process begins within the lesser sac, such as with a pancreatic abscess, the sac may be involved along with other secondarily affected peritoneal and retroperitoneal spaces. **A,** Small localized collection of complex fluid in the lesser sac. **B,** Computed tomography of the upper abdomen that shows a complex fluid in the lesser sac *(arrows)* near the pancreas.

may alter the patient's position to a right lateral decubitus position to scan along the coronal plane of the body, or prone, to use the spleen as a window. A sonographer must decide if the fluid collection is above or below the diaphragm. With the patient in a right lateral decubitus position, the probe is placed at the midaxilla line over the dome of the liver. As the patient takes in a breath, the diaphragm moves and the distinction of the fluid collection may be seen either below the diaphragm, or above the diaphragm, extending into the costal phrenic sulcus (Figure 14-25). The sonographer may also perform the scan with the patient upright to better demonstrate the pleural and subdiaphragmatic areas.

Subcapsular Collections. Intraabdominal fluid may be differentiated by its smooth border and its tendency to conform

spaces (Figure 14-24). Differential diagnosis should include pseudocyst, pancreatic abscess, gastric outlet obstruction, and fluid-filled stomach.

Subphrenic Abscess. The left upper quadrant may be difficult to examine because of the air interference. The sonographer

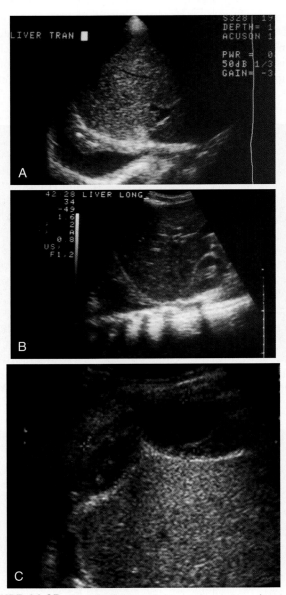

FIGURE 14-25 Pleural effusion. A, Transverse image shows the pleural effusion posterior to the liver as the transducer is angled in a cephalic direction. **B,** Sagittal images of a patient with a moderate pleural effusion shown superior to the liver. **C,** Subphrenic abscess seen in the anterior pocket of the right upper quadrant.

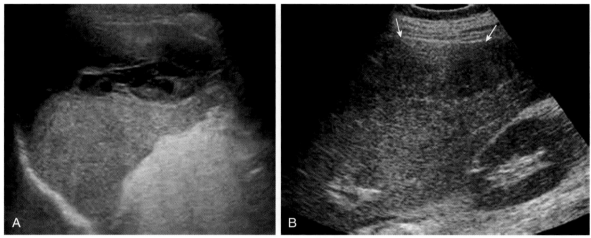

FIGURE 14-26 Subcapsular collections of fluid within the liver can mimic loculated subphrenic fluid. **A,** Sonogram of a moderate size subcapsular heterogeneous collection in the right upper quadrant. **B,** Isoechoic subcapsular hematoma of the liver *(arrows)*.

to the contour of the liver. It displaces the liver medially, rather than indenting the border locally, as subcapsular fluid might. A tense subphrenic abscess can displace the liver. The subcapsular fluid collections may be the result of a traumatic injury or other abscess formation. The sonographic pattern is usually heterogeneous (Figure 14-26).

It may be difficult to distinguish a subphrenic abscess from ascites. To do so, the sonographer can look at the margins of the fluid collection or look for other collections of fluid (in the pelvis) to distinguish ascites from abscess. Preperitoneal fat anterior to the liver may mimic a localized fluid collection. An abscess collects in the most dependent area of the body; therefore all the gutters should be examined, including the "pockets" and "pouches" and the spaces above and around the various organs (Box 14-1).

Biloma Abscess. Bilomas are extrahepatic loculated collections of bile that may develop because of iatrogenic, traumatic, or spontaneous rupture of the biliary tree. On sonography, a biloma abscess may appear cystic with weak internal echoes or a fluid-fluid level if clots or debris are not present (Figure 14-27). They usually have sharp margins. The extrahepatic bilomas are usually crescentic, surrounding and compressing structures with which they come in contact.

General Abdominal Abscess. A high percentage of abdominal and pelvic abscesses appear after surgery or trauma. The hepatic recesses and perihepatic spaces are the most

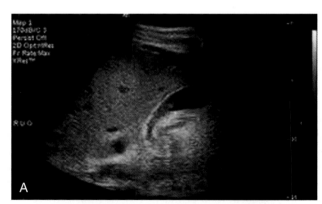

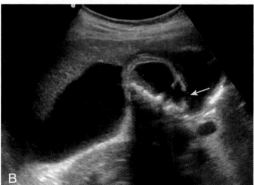

FIGURE 14-27 On sonography, a biloma abscess may appear cystic with weak internal echoes or a fluid-fluid level if clots or debris are not present.

BOX 14-1	**Sonography of Abscesses**

If an abscess is suspected (e.g., the patient has a fever of unknown origin), the sonographer should evaluate the following areas:
- Subdiaphragmatic area (liver and spleen)
- Splenic recess and borders
- Hepatic recess and borders
- Pericolic gutters
- Lesser omentum
- Transverse mesocolon
- Morison's pouch
- Gastrocolic ligament
- Phrenicosplenic ligament
- Recesses between intestinal loops and colon
- Extrahepatic falciform ligament
- Pouch of Douglas
- Broad ligaments (female)
- The area anterior to the urinary bladder

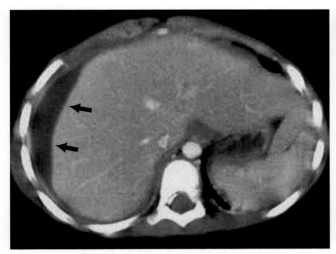

FIGURE 14-28 The hepatic recesses and perihepatic spaces are the most common sites for abscess formation. Computed tomography images of the upper abdomen show a fluid collection along the right lateral margin of the liver.

common sites for abscess formation (Figure 14-28). The pelvis is another common site. (Free fluid below the transverse mesocolon often flows into the pouch of Douglas and perivesical spaces.) An abscess may form in the right subhepatic space. The fluid ascends the right pericolic gutter into Morison's pouch. When the fluid fills Morison's pouch, it spreads past the coronary ligament over the dome of the liver. The presence of a right subhepatic abscess generally implies previous contamination of the right subhepatic space.

PATHOLOGY OF THE MESENTERY, OMENTUM, AND PERITONEUM

A mass or lesion within the mesentery and omentum may have solid or cystic characteristics, whereas a mass within the peritoneum may show an infiltrative pattern (Table 14-1). With an omental mass, at least one third of these lesions are malignant, and secondary neoplasms are more frequent than primary. In the mesentery, a benign primary tumor is more common than a malignant tumor, and secondary neoplasms are more frequent than primary. A cystic mass is more common than a solid mass. Malignant solid tumors are more likely found near the root of the mesentery, whereas benign solid tumors are found in the periphery near the bowel.

Cysts

Abdominal cysts may have (1) embryologic, (2) traumatic or acquired, (3) neoplastic, or (4) infective and degenerative origins. It is important to determine the organ of origin of the mass. If the mass is adherent to the mesentery or small intestine, it may be difficult for ultrasound to distinguish the anatomic landmarks necessary to determine the point of origin; therefore many patients will have a computed tomography scan or magnetic resonance imaging of the abdomen to better define these borders. **Hemorrhage** into omental or

TABLE 14-1	Description of Peritoneal, Omental, and Mesenteric Masses	
Solid	**Cystic**	**Infiltrative**
Peritoneal Mass		
Peritoneal mesothelioma	Cystic mesothelioma	Peritoneal mesothelioma
Peritoneal carcinomatosis	Pseudomyxoma peritonei Bacterial/ mycobacterial infection	
Solid	**Cystic**	**Infiltrative**
Omental Mass		
Benign: leiomyoma, lipoma, neurofibroma Malignant: leiomyosarcoma, liposarcoma, fibrosarcoma, lymphoma, peritoneal mesothelioma, hemangiopericytoma, metastases Infection: tuberculosis	Hematoma	
Round	**Loculated Cystic**	**Ill-Defined/ Stellate**
Mesenteric Mass		
Metastases, especially from colon, ovary Lymphoma Leiomyosarcoma Neural tumor Lipoma, lipomatosis, liposarcoma Fibrous histiocytoma Hemangioma	Cystic lymphangioma Pseudomyxoma Peritonei Cystic mesothelioma Mesenteric cyst Mesenteric hematoma Benign cystic teratoma Cystic spindle cell tumor	Metastases (ovary) Lymphoma Fibromatosis Fibrosing mesenteritis Lipodystrophy Mesenteric panniculitis Stellate: peritoneal mesothelioma, retractile mesenteritis, fibrosis reaction of carcinoid, desmoid tumor, tuberculous peritonitis, metastases, diverticulitis, pancreatitis

mesenteric cysts may cause rapid distention and clinically mimic ascites. Peritoneal inclusion cysts are considered in the differential diagnosis when large adnexal cystic structures are identified in a young woman. Fungal infections present as peritoneal cystic lesions.

▶ ***Sonographic Findings.*** Mesenteric and omental cysts may be uniloculated or multiloculated with smooth walls and thin internal septations (Figure 14-29). The internal echoes are correlated with fat globules, debris, superimposed hemorrhage, or infection. They may follow the contour of the

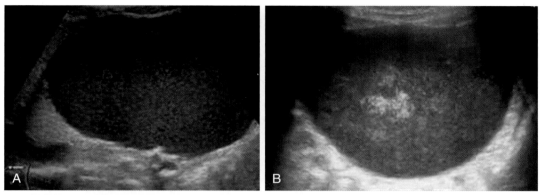

FIGURE 14-29 Mesenteric and omental cysts may be uniloculated or multiloculated with smooth walls and thin internal septations.

underlying bowel and conform to the anterior abdominal wall rather than produce distention.

Urachal Cyst. A urachal cyst is an incomplete regression of the urachus during development. The apex of the bladder is continuous with the allantois, which becomes obliterated and forms a fibrous core, the urachus. The urachus persists throughout life as a ligament that runs from the apex of the bladder to the umbilicus and is called the median umbilical ligament.

Sonographic Findings. On sonography, the sonographer may see a cystic mass between the umbilicus and the bladder (Figure 14-30). The mass may be small or giant, multiseptated, and extend into the upper abdomen.

Urinoma

A **urinoma,** an encapsulated collection of urine, may result from a closed renal injury or surgical intervention or may develop spontaneously secondary to an obstructing lesion. The extraperitoneal extravasation may be subcapsular or perirenal; the latter collections are sometimes termed *uriniferous pseudocysts*. The extravasation may leak around the ureter, where the perinephric fascia is weakest, or into adjoining fascial planes and peritoneal cavity.

Sonographic Findings. Cystic masses are most often oriented inferomedially, with upward and lateral displacement

of the lower pole of the kidney along with medial displacement of the ureter. They usually present on ultrasound as anechoic or contain low-level echoes (Figure 14-31).

Peritoneal Metastases

Peritoneal metastases develop from cellular implantation across the peritoneal cavity. The most common primary sites are the ovaries, stomach, and colon. Other less common sites are the pancreas, biliary tract, kidneys, testicles, and uterus. Metastases may arise from tumors, such as sarcomas, melanomas, teratomas, or embryonic tumors.

Sonographic Findings. The metastases form a nodular, sheetlike, irregular configuration. Multiple small nodules are seen along the peritoneal line. The larger masses obliterate the line and cause adhesion to bowel loops (Figure 14-32).

Lymphomas of the Omentum and Mesentery

Lymphoma presents as a uniformly thick, hypoechoic, band-shaped structure that follows the convexity of the anterior and lateral abdominal wall, creating the omental band.

Sonographic Findings. On ultrasound examination, omental and mesenteric lymphomas present as a lobulated, confluent, hypoechoic mass surrounding a centrally positioned

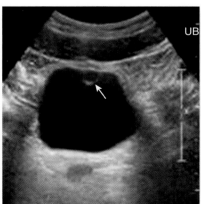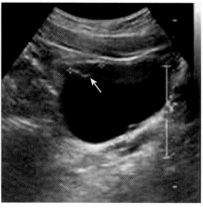

FIGURE 14-30 Urachal cyst. The sonographer may see a cystic mass between the umbilicus and the bladder.

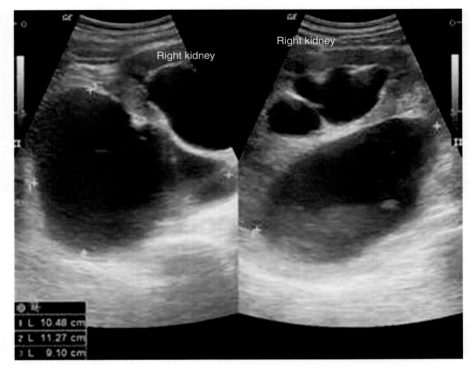

FIGURE 14-31 A urinoma may result from a closed renal injury or surgical intervention or may develop spontaneously secondary to an obstructing lesion. Patient with a recent renal transplant developed a urinoma adjacent to the kidney.

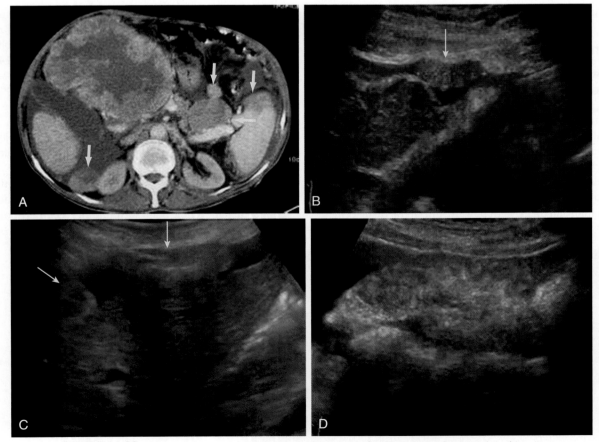

FIGURE 14-32 Computed tomography **(A)** and sonographic **(B–D)** images of omental "caking."

echogenic area. The **sandwich sign** represents a mass infiltrating the mesenteric leaves and encasing the superior mesenteric artery (Figure 14-33).

Tumors of the Peritoneum, Omentum, and Mesentery

Secondary tumors and lymphoma are neoplasms that most commonly involve the peritoneum and mesentery. Peritoneal and omental mesotheliomas most often occur in middle-aged men as the result of exposure to asbestos. The common symptoms are abdominal pain, weight loss, and ascites.

Sonographic Findings. The tumor may present as a large mass with discrete smaller nodes scattered over large areas of the visceral and parietal peritoneum, or it may present as diffuse nodes and plaques that coat the abdominal cavity and envelope and mat together in the abdominal viscera (Figure 14-34).

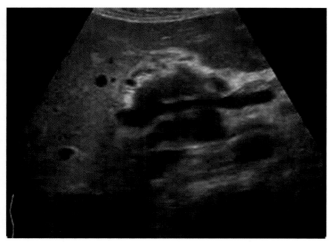

FIGURE 14-33 The "sandwich sign" of lymphoma or enlarged nodes represents a mass infiltrating the mesenteric leaves and encasing the superior mesenteric artery.

PATHOLOGY OF THE ABDOMINAL WALL

Abdominal Wall Masses

Lesions found within the superficial abdominal wall include inflammatory lesions, hematomas, neoplasms, hernias, and postsurgical lesions. Symmetry of the rectus sheath muscles is a key factor in determining whether an abdominal wall mass is present. The higher-resolution transducers may help the sonographer distinguish between the amount of fat and muscle present and an abnormal lesion.

Lymphoceles. A lymphocele is a collection of fluid that occurs after surgery in the pelvis, retroperitoneum, or recess cavities. Lymphoceles generally look like loculated, simple fluid collections, although they may have a more complex, usually septated, morphology (Figure 14-35). Differentiation from loculated ascites is usually possible because the mass effect of a lymphocele that is under tension displaces the surrounding organs. Differentiation from other fluid collections is mainly made by aspiration.

Extraperitoneal Hematoma

Extraperitoneal rectus sheath hematomas are acute or chronic collections of blood lying either within the rectus muscle or between the muscle and its sheath. They occur as the result of direct trauma, pregnancy, cardiovascular and degenerative muscle diseases, surgical injury, anticoagulation therapy, steroids, or extreme exercise. Clinically the patient may present with acute, sharp, persistent nonradiating pain.

Hematomas are caused by surgical injury to tissue or by blunt trauma to the abdomen. Laboratory values may show a decrease in hematocrit and red blood cell count; the patient may go into shock.

Sonographic Findings. On ultrasound examination, the sonographer notices an asymmetry between the rectus sheath muscles. The hematoma may appear as an anechoic mass

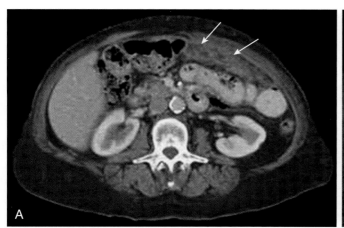
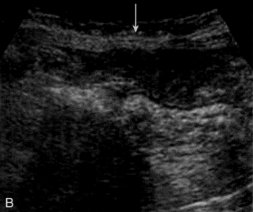

FIGURE 14-34 The secondary tumor may present as a large mass with discrete smaller nodes scattered over large areas of the visceral and parietal peritoneum, or it may present as diffuse nodes and plaques that coat the abdominal cavity and envelope and mat together in the abdominal viscera.

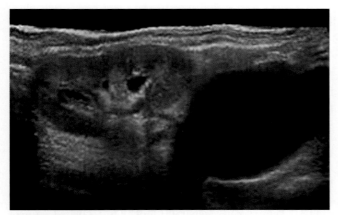

FIGURE 14-35 Lymphoceles generally look like loculated, simple fluid collections, although they may have a more complex, usually septated, morphology.

with scattered internal echoes (Figure 14-36). The sonographic appearance depends on the stage of the bleed. Acute bleeds are primarily cystic, with some debris and blood clots; as the blood begins to organize and clot, the mass becomes more solid in appearance. Newly formed clots may be very homogeneous. Hematomas can become infected and at any stage may be sonographically indistinguishable from abscesses. They may mimic subphrenic fluid.

Bladder-Flap Hematoma. A bladder-flap hematoma is a collection of blood between the bladder and lower-uterine segment, resulting from a lower-uterine transverse cesarean section and bleeding from the uterine vessels.

Subfascial Hematoma. A subfascial hematoma is found in the prevesicular space and is caused by a disruption of the inferior epigastric vessels or their branches during a cesarean section.

Inflammatory Lesion (Abscess)

An abscess or inflammation in the abdominal wall may occur after surgery. The sonogram may show cystic, complex, or solid characteristics. Generally the masses are superficial and are easy to locate and needle aspirate with ultrasound guidance if necessary. A high-frequency, linear array transducer should be used to image the superficial area. The patient may present with leukocytosis, **septicemia,** or a previous history of **pyogenic** infection.

▶ *Sonographic Findings.* An abdominal wall abscess presents as an anechoic or echoic mass with internal echoes from debris. The mass usually has irregular margins and shape (Figure 14-37). It may have gas bubbles within that show shadowing on the ultrasound image.

Neoplasm or Peritoneal Thickening

Neoplasms of the abdominal wall include lipomas, desmoid tumors, or metastases. The desmoid tumor is a benign fibrous neoplasm of aponeurotic structures. It most commonly occurs in relation to the rectus abdominis and its sheath (Figure 14-38). The tumor may present as hypoechoic to cystic (except lipomas).

▶ *Sonographic Findings.* A desmoid tumor presents as anechoic to hypoechoic, with smooth and sharply defined walls (Figure 14-39). The peritoneal lining is not seen as a distinct structure during sonography unless it is thickened. This is usually secondary to metastatic implants or to direct extension of the tumor from the viscera or mesentery. Primary mesotheliomas occur rarely.

Hernia

An abdominal hernia is the protrusion of a peritoneal-lined sac through a defect in the weakened abdominal wall (Figure 14-40). The viscera beneath the weakened tissue may protrude, resulting in a hernia. The most common areas of weakness are the umbilical area and the femoral and inguinal rings. (The inguinal hernia is discussed in Chapter 23.) An incarcerated hernia is one that cannot be "reduced" or pushed back into the abdominal cavity. Complications may arise if edema develops or if the opening constricts so much that the protrusion cannot be placed back into position. Strangulation (interruption of the blood supply) of the bowel can also occur in an incarcerated hernia that is not surgically repaired in a timely manner. This bowel can become necrotic and require resection.

The abdominal wall hernia consists of three parts: the sac, the contents of the sac, and the covering of the sac. Common locations for hernias are umbilical (congenital or acquired), epigastric, inguinal, femoral, and at the separation of the

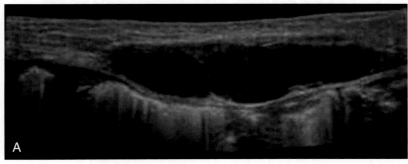
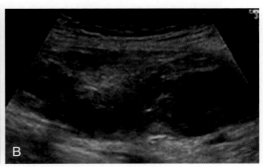

FIGURE 14-36 The rectus sheath hematoma may appear as an anechoic mass with scattered internal echoes.

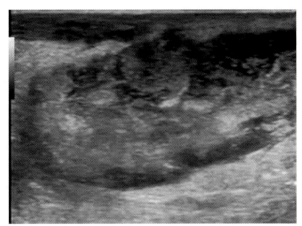

FIGURE 14-37 An abdominal wall abscess presents as an anechoic or echoic mass with internal echoes from debris.

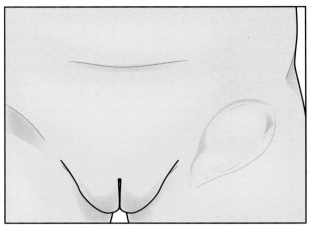

FIGURE 14-40 Femoral hernia causing a bulging enlargement of the femoral canal.

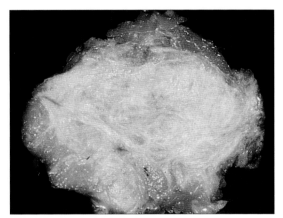

FIGURE 14-38 Gross pathology of a desmoid tumor of the abdominal wall.

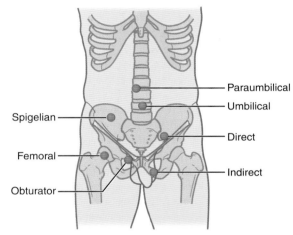

FIGURE 14-41 Common locations of hernias in the abdominal and pelvic cavities.

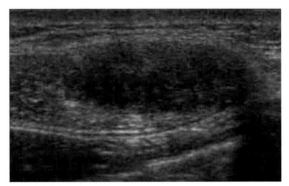

FIGURE 14-39 A desmoid tumor presents as anechoic to hypoechoic, with smooth and sharply defined walls.

rectus abdominis (Figure 14-41). The hernia may involve the omentum only or it may mimic other masses. The hernia commonly originates near the junction of the linea semilunaris and arcuate line in the paraumbilical area.

Epigastric hernias are found in the widest part of the linea alba between the xiphoid process and the umbilicus. This hernia is usually filled with fat, which over the years may carry a piece of omentum along with it.

A spigelian hernia is a variant of the ventral hernia, which is found more laterally in the abdominal wall.

Sonographic Findings. Many hernias are palpable and do not require sonographic evaluation. However, if the mass is not well defined on physical examination, ultrasound evaluation may be helpful. If a hernia is present, the sonographer will note an interruption of the peritoneal line separating the muscles and abdominal contents (Figure 14-42).

Sonography may outline the contents of the mass where it is fluid filled or contains peristaltic bowel or mesenteric fat. The sonographer should look for a peristalsing bowel within the mass, although the peristalsis may be absent with incarceration. If the hernia is not readily apparent, the patient may be asked to lift the head or to strain (Valsalva maneuver) to see if the mass moves or changes shape. The sonographic criteria for a hernia include (1) demonstration of an abdominal wall defect, (2) presence of bowel loops or mesenteric fat within a lesion, (3) exaggeration of the lesion with strain (Valsalva), and (4) reducibility of the lesion by gentle pressure.

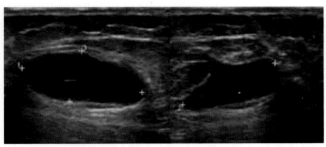

FIGURE 14-42 If a hernia is present, the sonographer will note an interruption of the peritoneal line separating the muscles and abdominal contents.

Key Pearls

- The peritoneal cavity is made up of multiple peritoneal ligaments and folds that connect the viscera to each other and to the abdominopelvic walls.
- Within the cavity are the lesser and greater omentum, the mesenteries, the ligaments, and multiple fluid spaces (lesser sac, perihepatic space, and subphrenic space).
- The section that lines the walls of the cavity is the parietal peritoneum, and the part covering the abdominal organs to a greater or lesser extent is the visceral peritoneum.
- The general peritoneal cavity is known as the greater sac of the peritoneum. With the development of the stomach and the spleen, a smaller sac, called the lesser sac (omental bursa), is the peritoneal recess posterior to the stomach.
- The attachments of the peritoneum to the abdominal walls and organs help determine the way abnormal collections of fluid within the peritoneal cavity can collect or move.
- Because of the coronary ligament attachments, collections in the right posterior subphrenic space cannot extend between the bare area of the liver and the diaphragm.
- Ligaments on the right side of the liver form the subphrenic and subhepatic spaces.
- The bare area is delineated by the right superior and inferior coronary ligaments, which separate the posterior subphrenic space from the right superior subhepatic space (Morison's pouch).
- A single large and irregular perihepatic space surrounds the superior and lateral aspects of the left lobe of the liver, with the left coronary ligaments anatomically separating the subphrenic space into anterior and posterior compartments.
- The retrovesical space is divided by the uterus into an anterior vesicouterine recess and a posterior rectouterine sac (pouch of Douglas).
- Ascites is the accumulation of serous fluid in the peritoneal cavity.
- An abscess is a cavity formed by necrosis within a solid tissue or a circumscribed collection of purulent material.
- A mass or lesion within the mesentery and omentum may have solid or cystic characteristics, whereas a mass within the peritoneum may show an infiltrative pattern.

- With an omental mass, at least one third of these lesions are malignant, and secondary neoplasms are more frequent than primary.
- In the mesentery, a benign primary tumor is more common than a malignant tumor, and secondary neoplasms are more frequent than primary.
- A cystic mass is more common than a solid mass in the mesentery.
- A urachal cyst is an incomplete regression of the urachus during development.
- A urinoma, an encapsulated collection of urine, may result from a closed renal injury or surgical intervention or may develop spontaneously secondary to an obstructing lesion.
- Lymphoma presents as a uniformly thick, hypoechoic, band-shaped structure that follows the convexity of the anterior and lateral abdominal wall, creating the omental band.
- Secondary tumors and lymphoma are neoplasms that most commonly involve the peritoneum and mesentery.
- Lesions found within the superficial abdominal wall include inflammatory lesions, hematomas, neoplasms, hernias, and postsurgical lesions.
- A lymphocele is a collection of fluid that occurs after surgery in the pelvis, retroperitoneum, or recess cavities.
- Extraperitoneal rectus sheath hematomas are acute or chronic collections of blood lying either within the rectus muscle or between the muscle and its sheath.
- Neoplasms of the abdominal wall include lipomas, desmoid tumors, and metastases.
- An abdominal hernia is the protrusion of a peritoneal-lined sac through a defect in the weakened abdominal wall.

BIBLIOGRAPHY

Abrahams PH, Boon J, Spratt JD: *McMinn's clinical atlas of human anatomy with DVD*, ed 6, St Louis, 2008, Mosby.

Damjanov I: *Pathology for the health professions*, ed 3, Philadelphia, 2006, Saunders.

Damjanov I, Linder J: *Pathology: a color atlas*, St Louis, 2000, Mosby.

Fakuda T, Sakamoto I, Kohzaki S, et al: Spontaneous rectus sheath hematomas: clinical and radiologic features, *Abdom Imaging* 21:58-61, 1996.

Gould BE, Dyer R: *Pathophysiology for the health professions*, ed 4, Philadelphia, 2011, Saunders.

Hamrick-Turner JE, Chichi MV, Abbitt PL, et al: Neoplastic and inflammatory processes of the peritoneum, omentum, and mesentery: diagnosis with CT. *RadioGraphics* 12:1051-1068, 1992.

Jamadar DA, Jacobson JA, Girish G, et al: Abdominal wall hernia mesh repair: sonography of mesh and common complications, *J Ultrasound Med* 27:907-917, 2008.

Musoles FB, Machado LE, Bailas LA, et al: Abdominal wall defects: two-versus three-dimensional ultrasonographic diagnosis, *J Ultrasound Med* 20:379-389, 2001.

Spencer JA, Swift SE, Wilkinson N, et al: Peritoneal carcinomatosis: image-guided peritoneal core biopsy for tumor type and patient care, *Radiology* 221:173, 2001.

Sudheer G: Sonography in identification of abdominal wall lesions presenting as palpable masses, *J Ultrasound Med* 25:1199-1209, 2006.

Yeh HC, Halton KP, Gray CE: Anatomic variations and abnormalities in the diaphragm seen with ultrasound, *RadioGraphics* 10:1019, 1990.

Yeh HC: Ultrasonography of peritoneal tumors, *Radiology* 133:419-424, 1979.

Urinary System

Kerry Weinberg, Shpetim Telegrafi, and Mariana Kozirovsky

OBJECTIVES

On completion of this chapter, you should be able to:

- Discuss normal anatomic location, function, and sonographic appearance of urinary system organs
- Discuss normal physiology of the urinary system
- Describe the sonographic scanning technique to image the urinary system
- Define and discuss the pathologies discussed in this chapter

- Identify and define the sonographic appearance of pathologies included in this chapter
- Discuss the role and limitations of sonography in post–renal transplant patients
- Describe the clinical signs and symptoms of urinary tract problems and the laboratory tests that are used to evaluate them

OUTLINE

Anatomy of the Urinary System
   Normal Anatomy
   Vascular Supply
Physiology and Laboratory Data of the Urinary System
   Excretion
   Laboratory Tests for Renal Disease
Sonographic Evaluation of the Urinary System
   Kidneys

Renal Variants
Renal Anomalies
Evaluation of a Renal Mass
Aspiration of Renal Masses
Lower Urinary Tract
Bladder
Pathology of the Urinary System
   Renal Cystic Disease
   Renal Neoplasms
   Renal Disease
   Renal Failure

Hydronephrosis
Renal Infections
Urinary Tract Calcifications
Renal Artery Stenosis
Renal Infarction
Arteriovenous Fistulas and
   Pseudoaneurysm
Kidney Stone (Urolithiasis)
Bladder Diverticulum
Bladder Inflammation (Cystitis)
Bladder Tumors

KEY TERMS

Afferent arteriole
Arcuate arteries
Blood urea nitrogen (BUN)
Bowman's capsule
Calyx
Columns of Bertin
Cortex
Creatinine (Cr)
Dromedary hump
Ectopic kidney
Efferent arteriole
Gerota's fascia
Glomerulus

Hilus
Homeostasis
Horseshoe kidney
Hydronephrosis
Loop of Henle
Major calyces
Medulla
Minor calyces
Morison's pouch
Nephron
Renal agenesis
Renal capsule
Renal corpuscle

Renal ectopia
Renal hilum
Renal hypoplasia
Renal pelvis
Renal pyramids
Renal sinus
Retroperitoneum
Specific gravity
Ureter
Urethra
Urinary bladder
Urolithiasis

The urinary system has two principal functions: excreting wastes and regulating the composition of blood. Blood composition must not be allowed to vary beyond tolerable limits, or the conditions in tissue necessary for cellular life will be lost. Regulating blood composition involves not only removing harmful wastes but also conserving water and metabolites in the body.

ANATOMY OF THE URINARY SYSTEM

Normal Anatomy

Kidneys. The urinary system is located posterior to the peritoneum lining the abdominal cavity in an area called the

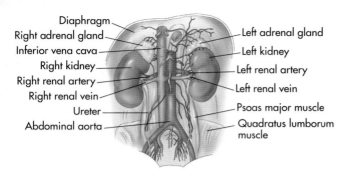

FIGURE 15-1 Relationships of the kidneys, suprarenal glands (adrenal), and vascular structures to one another.

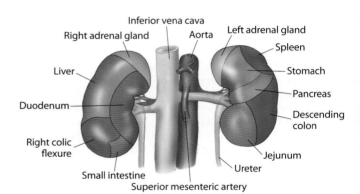

FIGURE 15-2 The kidney cut longitudinally to show the internal structure.

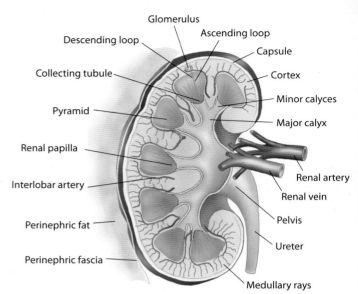

FIGURE 15-3 Anatomic structures related to the anterior surfaces of the kidneys.

retroperitoneum. The kidneys lie in the retroperitoneal cavity near the posterior body wall, just below the diaphragm (Figure 15-1). The lower ribs protect both kidneys. The right kidney lies slightly inferior to the left kidney because the large right lobe of the liver pushes it inferiorly. The kidneys move readily with respiration; on deep inspiration, both kidneys move downward approximately 1 inch.

The kidneys are dark red, bean-shaped organs that measure 9 to 12 cm long, 5 cm wide, and 2.5 cm thick. The outer **cortex** of the kidney is darker than the inner **medulla** because of the increased perfusion of blood. The inner surface of the medulla is folded into projections called **renal pyramids,** which empty into the renal pelvis. The **arcuate arteries** are located at the base of the pyramids and separate the medulla from the cortex. Numerous collecting tubules bring the urine from its sites of formation in the cortex to the pyramids. The renal tubules, or **nephrons,** are the functional units of the kidney.

On the medial surface of each kidney is a vertical indentation called the **renal hilum,** where the renal vessels and ureter enter and exit. Within the **hilus** of the kidney are other vascular structures, a ureter, and the lymphatics. The renal artery is posterior and superior to the renal veins. The two branches of the renal vein are anterior to the renal artery (Figure 15-2). The ureter is located slightly inferior to the renal artery. When present, the third branch of the renal artery may be seen to arise from the hilus. The lymph vessels and sympathetic fibers also are found within the renal hilus.

Three layers of tissue surround and protect the kidneys. The inner layer that surrounds the kidney is a fibrous capsule called the true capsule. Outside of this fibrous capsule is a covering of perinephric fat. The perinephric fascia surrounds the perinephric fat and encloses the kidneys and adrenal glands. The perinephric fascia is a condensation of areolar tissue that is continuous laterally with the fascia transversalis. The renal fascia, known as **Gerota's fascia,** surrounds the true capsule and perinephric fat.

Anterior to the right kidney are the right adrenal gland, liver, **Morison's pouch,** second part of the duodenum, and right colic flexure (Figure 15-3). Anterior to the left kidney are the left adrenal gland, spleen, stomach, pancreas, left colic flexure, and coils of jejunum.

Posterior to the right kidney are the diaphragm, costodiaphragmatic recess of the pleura, twelfth rib, psoas muscle, quadratus lumborum, and transversus abdominis muscles. The subcostal (T12), iliohypogastric, and ilioinguinal (L1) nerves run downward and laterally. Posterior to the left kidney are the diaphragm, costodiaphragmatic recess of the pleura, eleventh and twelve ribs, psoas muscle, quadratus lumborum, and transversus abdominis muscles. The same nerves are seen near the left kidney as in the right.

Within the kidney, the upper expanded end of the ureter, known as the **renal pelvis** of the ureter, divides into two or three **major calyces,** each of which divides further into two or three **minor calyces** (see Figure 15-2). The apex of a medullary pyramid, called the renal papilla, indents each minor **calyx.** The kidney consists of an internal medullary portion and an external cortical substance. The medullary substance consists of a series of striated conical masses, called the renal pyramids. The pyramids vary from 8 to 18 in number, and their bases are directed toward the outer circumference of the kidney. Their apices converge toward the **renal sinus,** where their prominent papillae project into the lumina of the minor calyces. Spirally arranged muscles surround the calyces and may exert a milking action on these tubes, aiding in the flow of urine into the renal pelvis. As the pelvis leaves the renal sinus, it rapidly becomes smaller and ultimately merges with the ureter.

Nephron. The nephrons are located in the renal parenchyma and consists of two main structures—a renal corpuscle and a renal tubule. Nephrons filter the blood and produce urine. Blood is filtered in the renal corpuscle. The filtered fluid passes through the renal tubule. As the filtrate moves through the tubule, substances needed by the body are returned to the blood. Waste products, excess water, and other substances not needed by the body pass into the collecting ducts as urine.

The **renal corpuscle** consists of a network of capillaries called the **glomerulus,** which is surrounded by a cuplike structure known as **Bowman's capsule.** Blood flows into the glomerulus through a small **afferent arteriole** and leaves the glomerulus through an **efferent arteriole.** This arteriole conducts blood to a second set of capillaries, the peritubular capillaries, which surround the renal tubule.

Filtrate passes into the renal tubule through an opening in the bottom of Bowman's capsule. The first part of the renal tubule is the coiled proximal convoluted tubule. After passing through the proximal convoluted tubule, filtrate flows into the **loop of Henle** and then into the distal convoluted tubule. Urine from the distal convoluted tubules of several nephrons drains into a collecting duct. A portion of the distal convoluted tubule curves upward and contacts the afferent and efferent arterioles. Some cells of the distal convoluted tubule and some cells of the afferent arteriole are modified to form the juxtaglomerular apparatus, a structure that helps regulate blood pressure in the kidney.

The renal corpuscle, the proximal convoluted tubule, and the distal convoluted tubule of each nephron are located within the renal cortex. The loops of Henle dip down into the medulla.

Ureter. The **ureter** is a 25-cm tubular structure whose proximal end is expanded and continuous with the funnel shape of the renal pelvis. The renal pelvis lies within the hilus of the kidney and receives major calyces. The ureter emerges from the hilus of the kidney and runs vertically downward behind the parietal peritoneum along the psoas muscle, which separates it from the tips of the transverse processes of the lumbar vertebrae. It enters the pelvis by crossing the bifurcation of the common iliac artery anterior to the sacroiliac joint. The ureter courses along the lateral wall of the pelvis to the region of the ischial spine and turns forward to enter the lateral angle of the bladder. The ureter from the ureteropelvic junction to the bladder is not routinely visualized on a sonogram. The ureters are located in the retroperitoneal cavity with the superior and distal ends of the ureters more readily visualized than the midsection due to overlying bowel gas.

Three constrictions occur along the ureter's course: (1) where the ureter leaves the renal pelvis, (2) where it is kinked as it crosses the pelvic brim, and (3) where it pierces the bladder wall.

Urinary Bladder. The **urinary bladder** is a large muscular bag located above and behind the pubic bone. It has a posterior and lateral opening for the ureters and an anterior opening for the urethra. The interior of the bladder is lined with highly elastic transitional epithelium. When the bladder is full, the lining is smooth and stretched; when it is empty, the lining is a series of folds. In the middle layer, a series of smooth muscle coats distend as urine collects and contract to expel urine through the urethra. Urine is produced almost continuously and accumulates in the bladder until the increased pressure stimulates the organ's nervous receptors to relax the urethra's sphincter and urine is released from the urinary bladder. The urinary bladder is visualized sonographically when it is distended with fluid.

Urethra. The **urethra** is a membranous tube that passes from the anterior part of the urinary bladder to the outside of the body. It includes two sphincters: the internal sphincter and the external sphincter. The urethra is not routinely visualized sonographically.

Vascular Supply

The main renal artery supplies blood to the kidney. When a person is at rest, approximately 1.2 liters of blood per minute is pumped to the kidneys. The renal arteries are lateral branches of the aorta that are located just inferior to the superior mesenteric artery (Figure 15-4). The branches of the renal artery may vary in size and number. In most cases, the renal artery is divided into two primary branches: a larger anterior and a smaller posterior. These arteries break down into smaller segmental arteries, then into interlobar arteries, and finally into tiny arcuate arteries.

Five to six veins join to form the main renal vein. This vein emerges from the renal hilus anterior to the renal artery. The renal vein drains into the lateral walls of the inferior vena cava (see Figure 15-4). The left renal vein courses transversely across the body going anterior to the aorta and posterior to the superior mesenteric artery.

The lymphatic vessels follow the renal artery to the lateral aortic lymph nodes near the origin of the renal artery.

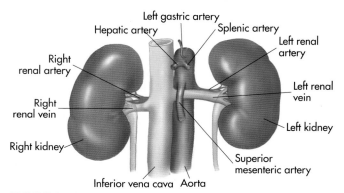

FIGURE 15-4 Vascular relationships of the great vessels and their tributaries to the kidneys.

Nerves originate in the renal sympathetic plexus and are distributed along the branches of the renal vessels.

Blood supply to nephrons begins at the renal artery. The artery subdivides within the kidneys. A small vessel (afferent arteriole) enters Bowman's capsule, where it forms a tuft of capillaries, the glomerulus, which entirely fills the concavity of the capsule. Blood leaves the glomerulus via the efferent arteriole, which subdivides into a network of capillaries that surround the proximal and distal tubules and eventually unite as veins, which become the renal vein.

The renal vein returns the cleansed blood to the general circulation. Movements of substances between the nephron and the capillaries of the tubules change the composition of the blood filtrate moving along in the tubules. From the nephrons, the fluid moves to collecting tubules and into the ureter, leading to the bladder, where urine is stored.

The arterial supply to the ureter is provided by the following three sources: the renal artery, the testicular or ovarian artery, and the superior vesical artery.

PHYSIOLOGY AND LABORATORY DATA OF THE URINARY SYSTEM

The urinary system consists of two kidneys, which remove wastes from the blood and produce urine, and two ureters, which act as tubal ducts leading from the hilus of the kidneys and drain into the urinary bladder. The bladder collects and stores urine, which is eventually discharged through the urethra. The urinary system is located posterior to the peritoneum lining the abdominal cavity in an area called the retroperitoneum.

The function of the kidneys is to excrete urine. More than any other organ, the kidneys regulate the amounts of water and electrolytes leaving the body so that these equal the amounts of substances entering the body. The formation of urine involves the following three processes: glomerular filtration, tubular reabsorption, and tubular secretion.

Excretion

Cells in the body continually carry on metabolic activities that produce waste products. If permitted to accumulate, metabolic wastes eventually reach toxic concentrations and threaten **homeostasis.** To prevent this, metabolic wastes must be quickly excreted. The process of excretion entails separating and removing substances harmful to the body. The skin, lungs, liver, large intestine, and kidneys carry out excretion.

The principal metabolic waste products are water, carbon dioxide, and nitrogenous wastes, including urea, uric acid, and **creatinine (Cr).** Nitrogen is derived from amino acids and nucleic acids. Amino acids break down in the liver, and the nitrogen-containing amino group is removed. The amino group is then converted to ammonia, which is chemically converted to urea. Uric acid is formed from the breakdown of nucleic acids. Both urea and uric acid are carried away from the liver into the kidneys by the vascular system. Creatinine is nitrogenous waste produced from phosphocreatine in the muscles.

Laboratory Tests for Renal Disease

The clinical symptoms of a patient with specific renal pathology may be nonspecific. Therefore a patient with symptoms of renal infection, renal insufficiency, or disease may undergo a number of laboratory tests to help the clinician determine the cause of the problem.

A patient's history of infection, previous urinary tract problems (renal stones), or hypertension or family history of renal cystic disease is useful information. A patient with a renal infection or disease process may have any of the following symptoms: flank pain, hematuria, polyuria, oliguria, fever, urgency, weight loss, or general edema.

Urinalysis. Urinalysis is essential to detect urinary tract disorders in patients whose renal function is impaired or absent. Most renal inflammatory processes introduce a characteristic exudate for a specific type of inflammation into the urine. The presence of an acute infection causes *hematuria,* or red blood cells in the urine; *pyuria* is pus in the urine.

Urine pH. Urine pH is very important in managing diseases such as bacteriuria and renal calculi. The pH refers to the strength of the urine as a partly acidic or alkaline solution. The abundance of hydrogen ions in a solution is called pH. If urine contains an increased concentration of hydrogen ions, the urine is acidic. The formation of renal calculi depends in part on the pH of urine. Other conditions, such as renal tubular acidosis and chronic renal failure, are associated with alkaline urine.

Specific Gravity. The **specific gravity** is the measurement of the kidney's ability to concentrate urine. The concentration factor depends on the quantity of dissolved waste products. Excessive intake of fluids or decreased perspiration may cause a large output of urine and a decrease in the specific gravity. Low fluid intake, excessive perspiration, or diarrhea can cause the output of urine to be low and the specific gravity to increase. The specific gravity is especially low in cases of renal failure, glomerular nephritis, and pyelonephritis. These diseases cause renal tubular damage, which affects the ability of the kidneys to concentrate urine.

Blood. Hematuria is the appearance of blood cells in the urine; it can be associated with early renal disease. An abundance of red blood cells in the urine may suggest renal trauma, neoplasm, calculi, pyelonephritis, or glomerular or vascular inflammatory processes, such as acute glomerulonephritis and renal infarction.

Leukocytes may be present whenever inflammation, infection, or tissue necrosis originates from anywhere in the urinary tract.

Hematocrit. The hematocrit is the relative ratio of plasma to packed cell volume in the blood. Decreased hematocrit occurs with acute hemorrhagic processes secondary to disease or blunt trauma.

Hemoglobin. Hemoglobin is present in urine whenever extensive damage or destruction of the functioning erythrocytes occurs. This condition injures the kidney and can cause acute renal failure.

Protein. When glomerular damage is evident, albumin and other plasma proteins may be filtered in excess, allowing the overflow to enter the urine, which lowers the blood serum albumin concentration. Albuminuria is commonly found with benign and malignant neoplasms, calculi, chronic infection, and pyelonephritis.

Creatinine Clearance. Specific measurements of creatinine concentrations in urine and blood serum are considered an accurate index for determining the glomerular filtration rate. Creatinine is a by-product of muscle energy metabolism; it is normally produced at a constant rate as long as the body muscle mass remains relatively constant. Creatinine normally goes through complete glomerular filtration without being reabsorbed by the renal tubules. Decreased urinary creatinine clearance indicates renal dysfunction because creatinine blood levels are constant, and only decreased renal function prevents the normal excretion of creatinine.

Blood Urea Nitrogen. The **blood urea nitrogen (BUN)** is the concentration of urea nitrogen in blood and is the end product of cellular metabolism. Urea is formed in the liver and is carried to the kidneys through the blood to be excreted in urine. Impairment of renal function and increased protein catabolism result in BUN elevation that is relative to the degree of renal impairment and the rate of urea nitrogen excretion by the kidneys.

Serum Creatinine. Renal dysfunction also results in serum creatinine elevation. Blood serum creatinine levels are said to be more specific and more sensitive in determining renal impairment than BUN.

SONOGRAPHIC EVALUATION OF THE URINARY SYSTEM

Kidneys

Sonographic evaluation of the kidneys is a noninvasive, relatively inexpensive, reproducible diagnostic test used to evaluate renal anatomy and pathology. In patients with renal colic without a history of renal stones, a noncontrast computed tomography (NCCT) is typically performed. NCCT requires no patient preparation and is not operator or patient dependent. The main disadvantages of NCCT are cost and the use of ionizing radiation. Patients with a history of renal stones require a plain film x-ray, and a renal sonogram with Doppler is usually the first diagnostic test performed.

Magnetic resonance imaging (MRI) using magnetic resonance urography (MRU) is currently being investigated for diagnosing renal disease. MRU can assess renal function, in addition to diagnosing obstructive uropathy. MRI can assess other abdominal organs for disease.

A renal sonogram is able to identify the presence and location of both kidneys, image renal congenital anomalies, determine renal size, show parenchymal detail, and delineate an abnormal lie of a kidney resulting from an extrarenal mass. In addition, sonography can demonstrate the acoustic properties of a mass, or determine whether hydronephrosis is secondary to renal stones. Sonography can also define perirenal

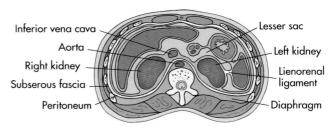

FIGURE 15-5 Transverse section of the abdominal cavity through the epiploic foramen.

fluid collections, such as a hematoma or an abscess, and detect dilated ureters and **hydronephrosis.**

Normal Texture and Patterns. The kidneys are imaged by sonography as organs with smooth, thin outer contours surrounded by reflected echoes of perirenal fat. The renal parenchyma surrounds the fatty central renal sinus, which contains the calyces, infundibula, pelvis, vessels, and lymphatics (Figure 15-5). Because of the fat interface, the renal sinus is imaged as an area of intense echoes with variable contours. If two separate collections of renal sinus fat are identified, a double collecting system should be suspected.

Generally, patients are given nothing by mouth before a sonogram or other imaging examinations are performed. This state of dehydration causes the infundibula and renal pelvis to be collapsed and thus indistinguishable from the echo-dense renal sinus fat. If, on the other hand, the bladder is distended from rehydration, the intrarenal collecting system also will become distended. An extrarenal pelvis may be seen as a fluid-filled structure medial to the kidney on transverse scans. The normal variant from obstruction is differentiated by noting the absence of a distended intrasinus portion of the renal pelvis and infundibula. Dilation of the collecting system has also been noted in pregnant patients. (The right kidney is generally involved with a mild degree of hydronephrosis. This distention returns to normal shortly after delivery.)

Patient Position and Technique. The patient should be in a supine and/or decubitus position using the liver as a window to image the right kidney (Figures 15-6 and 15-7) or through the spleen for the left kidney (Figure 15-8). Several alternative scanning windows can be used to image the kidney. These include the right posterior oblique, right lateral decubitus, and left lateral decubitus views. Having the patient take in a deep breath will move the liver and spleen distally, which may create a better window to enhance visualization of the kidneys. A subcostal or intercostal transducer approach may be used for visualization of the upper and lower poles of the kidneys.

Proper adjustment of time gain compensation (TGC) with adequate sensitivity settings allows a uniform acoustic pattern throughout the image. The renal cortical echo amplitude should be compared with the normal liver parenchymal echo amplitude at the same depth to effectively set the TGC and sensitivity.

If the patient has a substantial amount of perirenal fat, a high-frequency transducer may not provide the penetration

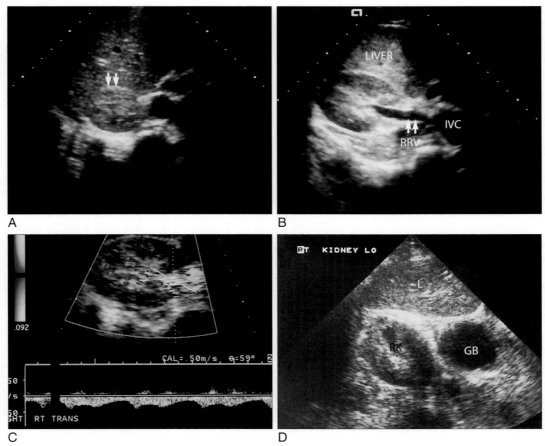

A

B

C

D

FIGURE 15-6 A and **B,** Transverse scan of the normal upper pole of the right kidney imaged through the homogeneous liver. Scans are made from the upper pole, from the mid pole to include the right renal vein (RRV), and from the inferior vena cava (IVC) to the lower pole. **C,** Normal blood flow is seen through the right renal vein to the IVC. **D,** A slight decubitus position allows the liver (L) to roll anterior to the right kidney (RK) and gallbladder (GB) for better visualization.

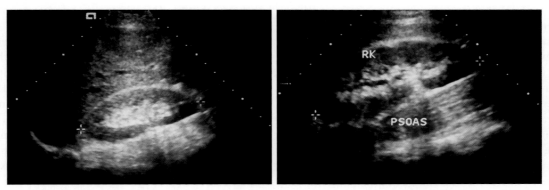

FIGURE 15-7 Longitudinal scans through the long axis of the right kidney (RK) and psoas muscle. Measurements are made along the maximum length of the right kidney from upper pole to lower pole.

necessary to optimally visualize the area. The deeper areas of the kidney may appear hypoechoic. Renal detail may also be obscured if the patient has hepatocellular disease, gallstones, rib interference (Figures 15-9 and 15-10), or other abnormal collections between the liver and kidney. The use of harmonic imaging or tissue contrast enhancement

technology (Figure 15-11) may help to optimize visualization of the kidneys.

Renal Parenchyma. The parenchyma is the area from the renal sinus to the outer renal surface (Figure 15-12). The arcuate arteries and interlobar vessels are found within and are best demonstrated as intense specular echoes in

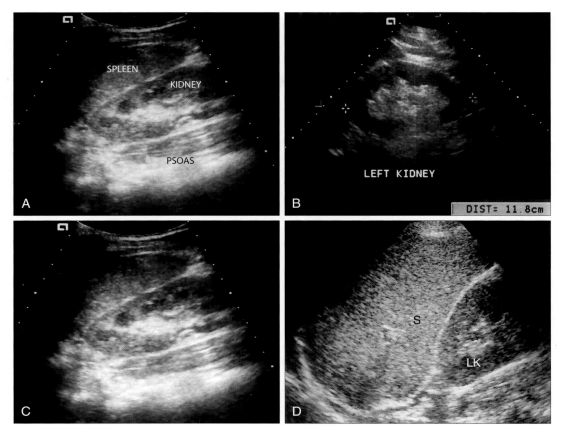

FIGURE 15-8 A, Longitudinal scan of the normal left kidney as imaged through the homogeneous spleen. The psoas muscle is the posterior medial border of the kidney. **B,** Measurements are made along the maximum length of the kidney from the upper pole to the lower pole. **C,** The patient may be rolled into a right lateral decubitus position for better visualization of the renal medullary pyramids and parenchyma. **D,** Splenomegaly *(S)* aids in visualization of the upper pole of the left kidney.

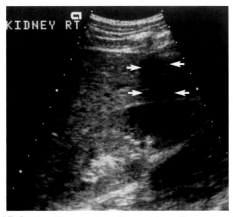

FIGURE 15-9 The ribs may interfere with uniform visualization of the kidney. Variations in respiration help the sonographer find the best window through which to image the renal parenchyma without rib interference.

cross section or oblique section at the corticomedullary junction.

The cortex generally is mid-level echo producing (Figure 15-13) (although its echoes are less echogenic than those from normal liver), whereas the medullary pyramids are hypoechoic (Figure 15-14). The two are separated

from each other by bands of cortical tissue, called columns of Bertin, which extend inward to the renal sinus.

Diseases of the renal parenchyma are those that accentuate cortical echoes but preserve or exaggerate the corticomedullary junction (type I) and those that distort the normal anatomy, obliterating the corticomedullary differentiation in a focal or diffuse manner (type II).

Criteria for type I changes include the following: (1) The echo intensity in the cortex must be equal to or greater than that in the adjacent liver or spleen, and (2) the echo intensity in the cortex must be equal to that in the adjacent renal sinus. Minor signs would include the loss of identifiable arcuate vessels and the accentuation of corticomedullary definition.

Type II changes can be seen in focal disruption of normal anatomy with any mass lesion, including cysts, tumors, abscesses, and hematomas.

Renal Vessels. The arteries are best seen with the supine and left lateral decubitus views (right side up). The right renal artery extends from the lateral wall of the aorta to enter the central renal sinus (Figure 15-15). On the longitudinal scan, the right renal artery can be seen as a round anechoic structure posterior to the inferior vena cava (Figure 15-16). The right renal vein extends from the central renal sinus directly into the inferior vena cava

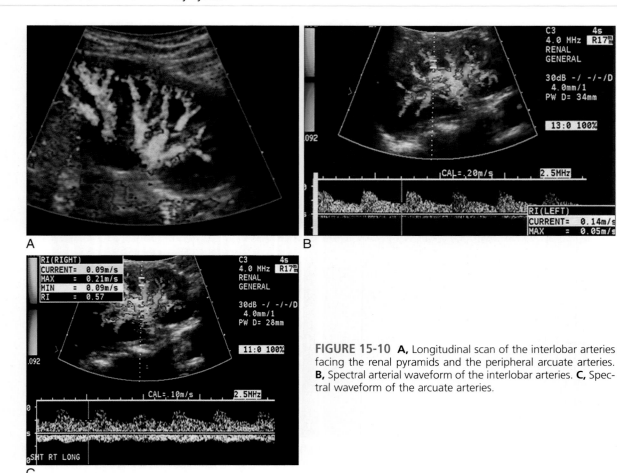

FIGURE 15-10 **A,** Longitudinal scan of the interlobar arteries facing the renal pyramids and the peripheral arcuate arteries. **B,** Spectral arterial waveform of the interlobar arteries. **C,** Spectral waveform of the arcuate arteries.

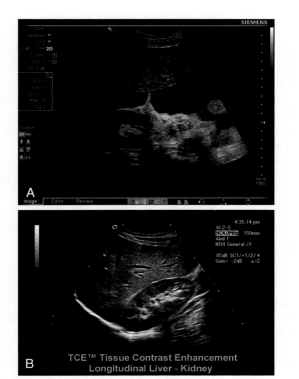

FIGURE 15-11 **A,** Transverse view of right kidney with ascites in Morison's pouch. **B,** Sagittal view of normal liver/kidney using tissue contrast enhancement technology (TCE). *(Courtesy Siemens Medical Solutions USA, Inc.)*

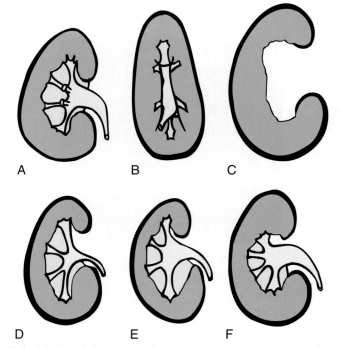

FIGURE 15-12 Thickness of the renal substance. **A,** Maximal in the polar regions, medium in the middle zone. **B,** Medial plane showing the pelvis emerging through the hilum and minimal thickness anteriorly and posteriorly. **C,** Hypertrophy. **D,** Normal adult proportions of the renal substance. **E,** Senile atrophy. **F,** Normal appearance in a 2-year-old child.

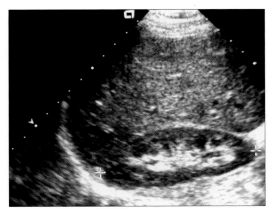

FIGURE 15-13 Sagittal scan of the normal kidney. The cortex is the brightest of the echoes within the renal parenchyma. The medullary pyramids are echo free. The pyramids are separated from the cortex by bands of cortical tissue and the columns of Bertin that extend inward to the renal sinus.

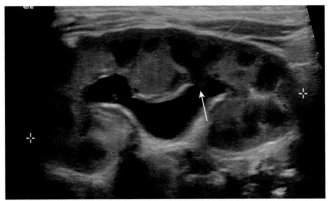

FIGURE 15-14 Longitudinal image of a neonatal left kidney using a 18 MHz transducer with white arrow pointing to normal hypoechoic renal pyramids.

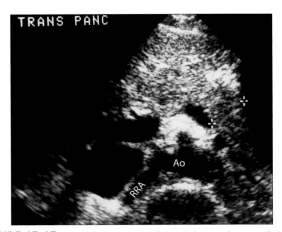

FIGURE 15-15 Transverse image of the right renal artery (RRA) as it extends from the posterior lateral wall of the aorta (Ao) to enter the central renal sinus.

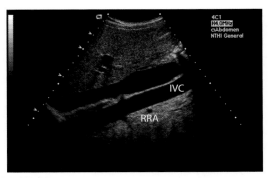

FIGURE 15-16 On longitudinal scan of the IVC and aorta at renal bifurcation, the right renal artery (RRA) can be seen as a circular structure posterior to the inferior vena cava (IVC).

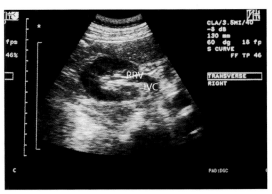

FIGURE 15-17 The right renal vein (RRV) extends from the central renal sinus directly into the inferior vena cava (IVC).

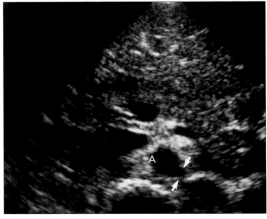

FIGURE 15-18 The left renal artery (arrows) flows from the posterior lateral wall of the aorta (A) to the central renal sinus.

(Figure 15-17). Both vessels appear as tubular structures in the transverse plane.

The renal arteries have an echo-free central lumen with highly echogenic borders that consist of a vessel wall and surrounding retroperitoneal fat and connective tissue. They lie posterior to the veins and can be demonstrated with certainty if their junction with the aorta is seen.

The left renal artery flows from the lateral wall of the aorta to the central renal sinus (Figure 15-18). The left renal vein flows from the central renal sinus, anterior to the aorta and posterior to the superior mesenteric artery, to join the inferior vena cava (Figure 15-19). It is seen as a tubular structure on the transverse scan.

The diaphragmatic crura run transversely in the para-aortic region. The crura lie posterior to the renal arteries and

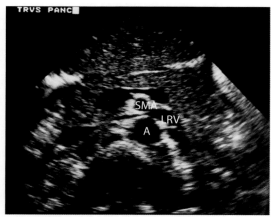

FIGURE 15-19 The left renal vein *(LRV)* flows from the central renal sinus, anterior to the aorta *(A)* and posterior to the superior mesenteric artery *(SMA)*, to join the inferior vena cava.

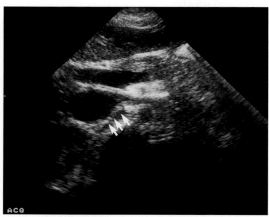

FIGURE 15-20 The crura of the diaphragm lie posterior to the renal arteries and should be identified by their lack of pulsations and lack of Doppler flow *(arrows)*.

should be identified by their lack of pulsations and absence of Doppler flow (Figure 15-20). They vary in echogenicity, depending on the amount of surrounding retroperitoneal fat. They may appear hypoechoic, as lymph nodes do.

Renal Medulla. The renal medulla consists of hypoechoic pyramids dispersed in a uniform distribution, separated by bands of intervening parenchyma that extend toward the renal sinus. The pyramids are uniform in size, shape (triangular), and distribution. The apex of the pyramid points toward the sinus, and the base lies adjacent to the renal cortex. The interlobar arteries lie alongside the pyramids, and arcuate vessels lie at the base of the pyramids (see Figures 15-2 and 15-10).

Renal Variants

Renal variants include slight alterations in anatomy that may lead the sonographer to suspect an abnormality is present when it really is a normal variation. See Table 15-1 for a description of renal variants and anomalies.

TABLE 15-1   Renal Anomalies and Variants

Type	Location	Sonographic Appearance	Differential Considerations	Distinguishing Characteristics
Column of Bertin	Medulla	Indentation of the renal sinus	Renal mass effect	Similar to renal parenchyma; contiguous with cortex
Dromedary hump	Lateral border of the kidney	Identical to the renal cortex	Mass effect	Usually seen on the left kidney
Junctional parenchymal defect	Upper pole of renal parenchyma	Echogenic triangular area	Mass effect	Best seen on sagittal scans
Fetal lobulation	Surface of the kidney	Indentations between the calyces	Mass effect	Best seen on sagittal scans
Lobar dysmorphism	Middle and upper calyces	Elongation of upper and middle calyces	Column of Bertin	Best seen on sagittal scans
Duplex collecting (complete) system	Central renal sinus	Two echogenic regions separated by moderately echogenic parenchymal tissue	Mass effect	"Faceless"; no echogenic renal pelvis seen on transverse view at the level of the midpole
Bifid renal pelvis (incomplete duplication)	Central renal sinus	Middle calyces, two echogenic regions	Pseudomass effect	One ureter entering the bladder on each side of the bladder
Extrarenal pelvis	Long renal pelvis that extends outside the renal border	Central cystic region that extends beyond the medial renal border	Renal aneurysm, dilated proximal ureter	Best seen on a transverse view at the level of the midpole
Horseshoe kidney	Kidneys seen more medial and anterior to the spine	Fusion of the polar region, usually the lower poles	Inferior poles lie more medial, associated with pyelocaliectasis, anomalous extrarenal pelvis, urinary calculi	

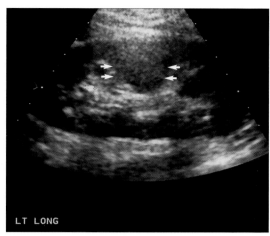

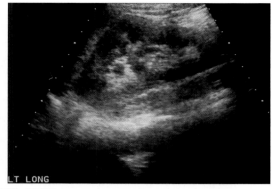

FIGURE 15-22 Coronal view of the left kidney. The dromedary hump is a cortical bulge that occurs on the lateral border of the kidney, typically on the left more than on the right.

FIGURE 15-21 Longitudinal scan of the kidney with prominent column of Bertin.

Columns of Bertin. The **columns of Bertin** are prominent invaginations of the cortex located at varying depths within the medullary substance of the kidneys. Hypertrophied columns of Bertin contain renal pyramids and may be difficult to differentiate from an avascular renal neoplasm. The columns are most exaggerated in patients with complete or partial duplication (Figure 15-21).

Sonographic Findings. Sonographic features of a renal mass effect produced by a hypertrophied column of Bertin include the following: a lateral indentation of the renal sinus, a clear definition from the renal sinus, or a maximum dimension that does not exceed 3 cm. Contiguity with the renal cortex is evident, and overall echogenicity is similar to that of the renal parenchyma.

Dromedary Hump. A **dromedary hump** is a bulge of cortical tissue on the lateral surface of a kidney (usually the left), resembling the hump of a dromedary camel. It is seen in persons whose spleen or liver presses down. It is a normal variant but may resemble a renal neoplasm.

Sonographic Findings. On sonography, the echogenicity is identical to the rest of the renal cortex, and a renal pseudotumor needs to be considered (Figure 15-22).

Junctional Parenchymal Defect. A junctional parenchymal defect is a triangular, echogenic area typically located anteriorly and superiorly. It is a result of partial fusion of two embryonic parenchymal masses called renunculi during normal development (Figure 15-23).

Sonographic Findings. Junctional parenchymal defects are best demonstrated on sagittal scans and must not be confused with pathologic processes such as parenchymal renal scars and angiomyolipoma. A lobar dysmorphism is a lobar fusion variant in which malrotation of the renal lobe occurs. The middle and upper calyces may be splayed and displaced, and the lower calyx is deviated posteriorly. The dysmorphic lobe may resemble a mass or prominent column of Bertin on a sonogram (Figure 15-24).

Fetal Lobulation. Fetal lobulation is developmental variation that is usually present in children up to 5 years old, and may be persistent in up to 51% of adults. The surfaces of the kidneys are generally indented in between the calyces, giving the kidneys a slightly lobulated appearance (Figure 15-25).

Sinus Lipomatosis. Sinus lipomatosis is a condition characterized by deposition of a moderate amount of fat in the renal sinus with parenchymal atrophy (Figure 15-26). In sinus lipomatosis, the abundant fibrous tissue may cause enlargement of the sinus region with increased echogenicity and regression toward the center of the parenchymal. Occasionally, a fatty mass is localized in only one area; this is called lipomatosis circumscripta.

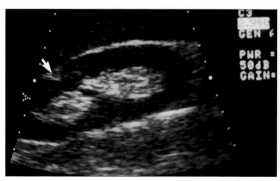

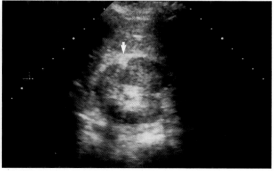

FIGURE 15-23 The junctional parenchymal defect *(arrows)* is a triangular area in the upper pole of the renal parenchyma.

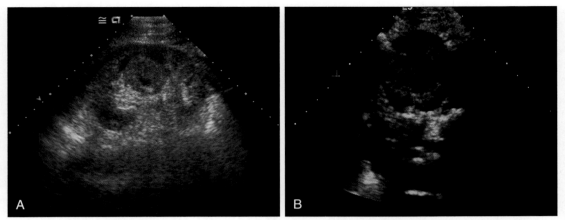

FIGURE 15-24 **A,** Longitudinal scan of lobar dysmorphism. **B,** Transverse view of lobar dysmorphism.

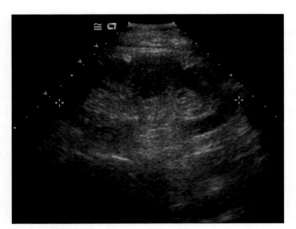

FIGURE 15-25 Remnant fetal renal lobulations (an irregularly shaped renal border).

Extrarenal Pelvis. The normal renal pelvis is a triangular structure. Its axis points inferiorly and medially. The intrarenal pelvis lies almost completely within the confines of the central renal sinus. This is usually small and foreshortened. The extrarenal pelvis tends to be larger with long major calyces.

⬛ *Sonographic Findings.* On sonography, the pelvis appears as a central cystic area that may be partially or entirely

beyond the confines of the bulk of the renal substance. Transverse views are best for viewing continuity with the renal sinus. The dilated extrarenal pelvis will usually decompress when the patient is placed in the prone position (Figure 15-27).

Renal Anomalies

Renal anomalies comprise abnormalities in number, size, position, structure, or form (Figures 15-28 and 15-29) (see Table 15-1). Anomalies in number include agenesis, dysgenesis (defective embryonic development of the kidney), and supernumerary kidney. Supernumerary kidney is an additional kidney to the number usually present, which is two. In some cases, separation of the reduplicated organ is incomplete (fused supernumerary kidney). *Bifid* means *cleft,* or *split into two parts.* Bifid renal pelvis is a common anomaly and is considered a normal variant. The renal pelvis may appear to be more prominent on sonography. A pseudotumor is an overgrowth of cortical tissue that indents the echogenic renal sinus and may be mistaken for a renal tumor on sonography.

Renal Agenesis.   **Renal agenesis** is absence of the kidney or failure of the kidney to form; it may be bilateral or unilateral. Bilateral renal agenesis is very rare and is incompatible with life. Unilateral renal agenesis results in a solitary kidney. Congenital absence of one kidney is rare, and is

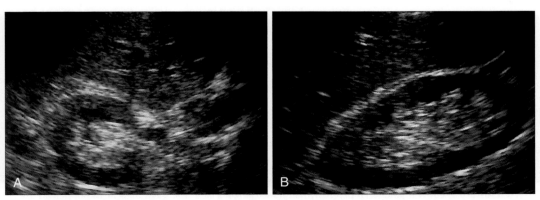

FIGURE 15-26 Transverse **(A)** and longitudinal **(B)** scans of a patient with renal sinus lipomatosis.

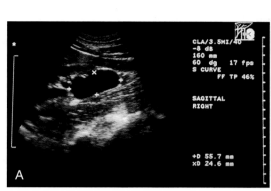

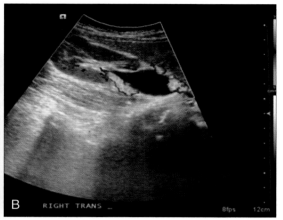

FIGURE 15-27 Extrarenal pelvis. **A,** Scan of the right kidney with an extrarenal pelvis appearing as a cystic area that extends beyond the confines of the renal borders. **B,** Color Doppler confirming the extrarenal pelvis.

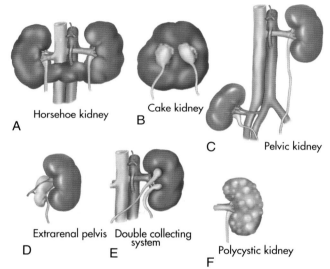

A Horseshoe kidney

B Cake kidney

C Pelvic kidney

D Extrarenal pelvis

E Double collecting system

F Polycystic kidney

FIGURE 15-28 Variations of renal anatomy, position within the retroperitoneal cavity, and pathology. **A,** Horseshoe kidney shown as two kidneys connected by an isthmus anterior to the great vessels and inferior to the inferior mesenteric artery. **B,** Cake kidney with a double collecting system. **C,** Pelvic kidney with one kidney in the normal retroperitoneal position. **D,** Extrarenal pelvis. **E,** Double collecting system in a single kidney. **F,** Polycystic kidney.

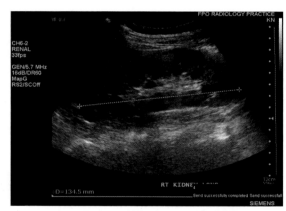

FIGURE 15-30 Enlarged solitary kidney with unilateral renal agenesis.

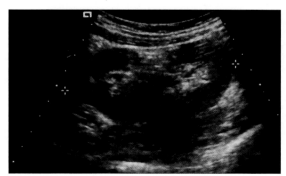

FIGURE 15-29 Longitudinal view of a malrotated right kidney, with the renal pelvis facing anteriorly.

commonly associated with other congenital anomalies such as seminal vesical cyst, vaginal agenesis, or bicorn uterus. Renal compensatory hypertrophy (enlargement) generally occurs with a solitary kidney (Figure 15-30).

Renal hypoplasia is incomplete development of the kidney, usually with fewer than five calyces. Functionally and morphologically, the kidney is normal and should be differentiated from an atrophy kidney secondary to pyelonephrosis or renal artery stenosis. Usually, the pyelonephritic kidney is scarred and echogenic, and the small kidney that results from renal artery stenosis has abnormal Doppler parameters (tardus and parvus waveform).

Bifid Renal Pelvis. A common renal anomaly with a duplication of the renal pelvis and one ureter is considered a normal variant.

Incomplete Duplication. Incomplete, or partial, duplication is the most frequently occurring congenital anomaly in the neonate. Duplication consists of two collecting systems and two ureters, with a single ureter entering into the urinary bladder. The two ureters join and form a single ureter anywhere between the kidney and the bladder.

Complete Duplication. Complete duplication is the rare condition of a duplex collecting system. This anomaly results in two separate collecting systems, each with its own ureter that enters the bladder. In cases of double ureter, the ureter from the upper pole of the kidney usually opens below and medial to the one from the lower pole (rule of Weigert-Meyer). The ureter of the lower calyx inserts into the bladder more superiorly and laterally to the normal location of the vesicoureteral orifice, with a short intramural portion. This short intramural portion of the ureter increases the chance of a prevesicoureteral reflux. The ureter from the upper pole calyx inserts into the bladder medially and distally to the normal location of the vesicoureteral orifice. The low insertion of the ureter into the bladder causes an ectopic posterior insertion of the urethra with posterior displacement of the vagina, which increases the chance of urethral obstruction by a stricture or ureterocele, vesicoureteral reflux, or both.

Sonographic Findings. The way to confirm a complete collecting system is to demonstrate two ureteral jets entering the bladder on the same side. The duplex kidney is usually enlarged with smooth margins. The central renal sinus appears as two echogenic regions separated by a cleft of moderately echogenic tissue similar in appearance to the normal renal parenchyma. On the transverse view, the area separating the renal pelvis is called "faceless" because the tissue is homogenous, with no central echogenic renal pelvis.

Hydronephrosis of the upper pole with a ureterocele, or hydronephrosis of the upper pole and lower pole calyces, may be present (Figures 15-31 and 15-32).

Renal Ectopia. **Renal ectopia,** or **ectopic kidney,** describes a kidney that is not located in its usual position, the renal fascia. It results when the kidney fails to ascend from its origin in the true pelvis or from a superiorly ascended kidney located in the thorax. Pelvic kidney, also called sacral kidney, is the most common renal ectopia and should not be misdiagnosed as a primary pelvic tumor. It is almost always malrotated; the renal pelvis faces anteriorly and is predisposed to reflux, infection, ureteropelvic junction (UPJ) obstruction, and stone formation (Figure 15-33). Pelvic kidney may be bilateral, but this is very rare. A thoracic kidney migrates through the diaphragm into the thoracic cavity. It is a rare finding and is not easily diagnosed with ultrasound. Other renal ectopias include intrathoracic kidney and abdominal (iliac crest) kidney.

Two types of crossed renal ectopia can occur: fused and nonfused. Both are associated with malrotation. Fused crossed renal ectopia occurs more frequently than nonfused and most often on the right side. In most cases of crossed renal ectopia, the ureters are not ectopic. Cystoscopy reveals a normal trigone, and the incidence of associated congenital anomalies is low. Renal calculi are the most common complication. Sonography shows both kidneys located on the same side, with most demonstrating fusion (Figure 15-34).

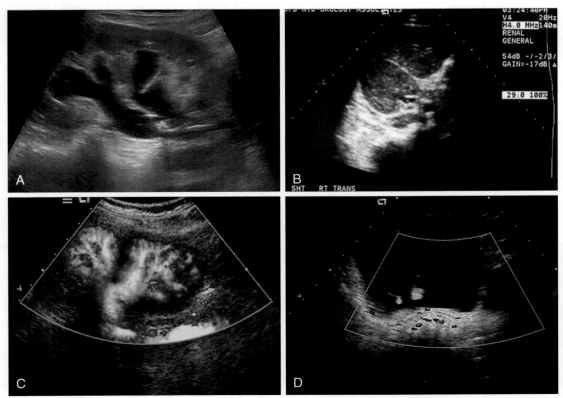

FIGURE 15-31 A, Bifid kidney. **B,** Transverse view of the echogenic tissue that separates the renal sinus ("faceless"). **C,** Power Doppler of duplex collecting system. **D,** Double right ureteral jets confirm a complete duplex collecting system.

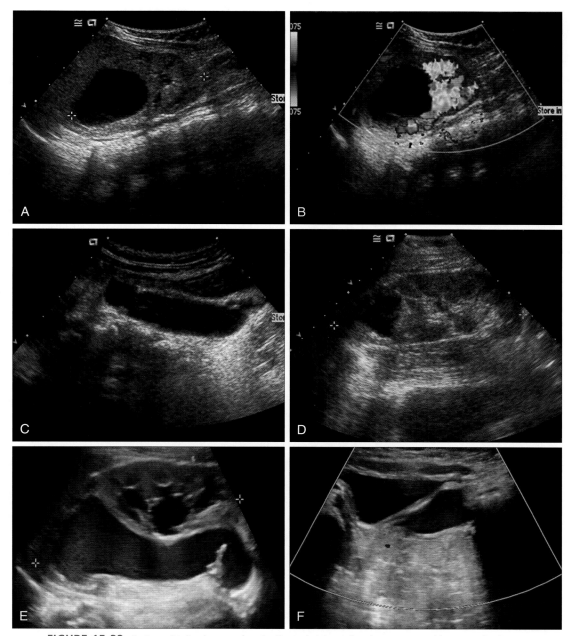

FIGURE 15-32 A, Longitudinal scan of a duplicated right collecting system with severe hydrone-phrosis of upper moiety. **B,** Ectopic right distal ureter. **C,** Longitudinal scan of a duplicated right collecting system with moderate hydronephrosis of the upper moiety. **D,** Ureterocele of the distal right ureter ("rule of Weigert-Meyer"). **E & F,** Longitudinal scan of a left collecting system with severe upper moiety, hydronephrosis, and ectopic ureter.

Horseshoe Kidney. Horseshoe kidney is the most common anomaly of renal fusion. Fusion of the lower poles occurs in 96% of cases, with ureters passing anterior to the renal parenchyma and variation of arterial land venous blood supply. The isthmus, or connecting bridge, typically consists of renal parenchymal tissue; rarely is it fibrotic tissue. The most common complications associated with horseshoe kidney are kidney malrotation, urolithiasis, UPJ obstruction, and infection. The isthmus of the kidney lies anterior to the spine and may simulate a solid pelvic mass or enlarged lymph nodes (Figure 15-35).

Evaluation of a Renal Mass

Before starting the sonographic examination for the evaluation of a renal mass, the sonographer should review the patient's chart, including the laboratory findings and previous diagnostic examinations, which may include a plain radiograph of the abdomen, computed tomography (CT), or MRI. Whenever possible, these films should be obtained before the sonogram is done, so the examination can be tailored to address the clinical problem. The sonographer should evaluate the sonographic images to determine the shape and size

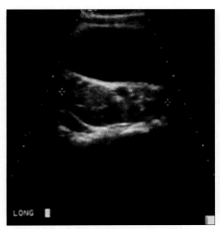

FIGURE 15-33 Ectopic kidney found in the pelvis, just posterior to the distended urinary bladder.

echoes (anechoic); and (5) increased posterior acoustic enhancement.

A solid lesion projects as a nongeometric shape with irregular borders, a poorly defined interface between the mass and the kidney, low-level internal echoes, a weak posterior border caused by increased attenuation of the mass, and poor through-transmission.

Areas of necrosis, hemorrhage, abscess, or calcification within the mass may alter the classification and cause the lesion to fall into the complex category. This means the mass shows characteristics associated with both cystic and solid lesions.

Sonography allows the sonographer to carefully evaluate the renal parenchyma in many stages of respiration. If the mass is very small, respiratory motion may cause it to move in and out of the field of view. Careful evaluation of the best respiratory phase combined with use of the cine-loop feature will allow the sonographer to adequately image most renal masses to determine their characteristic composition.

Aspiration of Renal Masses

Most renal masses that have met the criteria for a simple cystic mass do not require needle aspiration. The Bosniak classification of cysts is used to determine the appropriate workup for a cystic mass (Table 15-2). A needle aspiration

of the kidney and the location of the mass lesion, to observe distortion of the renal or ureter structure, and to look for calcium stones or gas within the kidney.

Renal masses are categorized as cystic, solid, or complex by a sonographic evaluation. A cystic mass sonographically displays several characteristic features: (1) smooth, thin, well-defined border; (2) round or oval shape; (3) sharp interface between the cyst and the renal parenchyma; (4) no internal

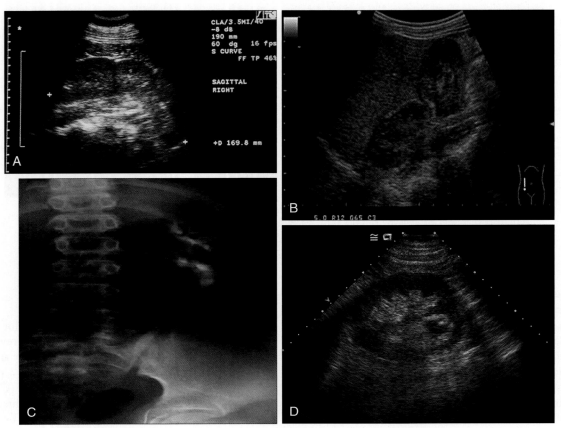

FIGURE 15-34 A, Crossed kidney on the right side of the body. Sonogram **(B)** and IVP **(C)** of the left crossed fused kidney. **D,** Cake kidney.

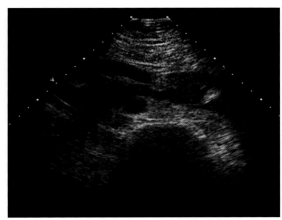

FIGURE 15-35 Transverse scan of the horseshoe kidney with isthmus connecting each pole.

TABLE 15-2	Bosniak Cyst Categories, Criteria, and Workup	
Category	**Criteria**	**Workup**
Simple cyst (I)	Thin, smooth wall, anechoic, round or oval in shape; increased through-transmission	None
Mildly complex cyst (II)	Thin septation or calcified wall	2–3 month follow-up with CT or sonogram
Mildly complex (IIF)	Atypical features; does not fall into category II	6–12 month follow-up
Indeterminate lesion (III)	Multiple septa, thickened septa, internal echoes	Biopsy or partial nephrectomy—increased risk for malignancy
Malignant lesion (IV)	Solid component, irregular walls	Nephrectomy

may be recommended to obtain fluid from the lesion to evaluate its internal composition.

The patient should be placed in a prone position with sandbags or rolled sheets under the abdomen to help push the kidneys toward the posterior abdominal wall and provide a flat scanning surface. Sterile technique is used for aspiration and biopsy procedures. The transducer must be gas sterilized. Sterile lubricant is used to couple the transducer to the patient's skin.

The renal mass should be located in the transverse and longitudinal planes, with scans performed at midinspiration. Hold the transducer lightly over the scanning surface so as not to compress the subcutaneous tissue. The depth of the mass should be noted from its posterior to anterior borders, so the exact depth can be given to aid in placement of the needle. Compression of the subcutaneous tissue results in an inaccurate depth measurement. When the area of aspiration is outlined on the patient's back, the distance is measured from the posterior surface to the middle of the lesion.

A beveled needle causes multiple echoes within the walls of the lesion. If the needle is slightly bent, many echoes

appear until the bent needle is completely out of the transducer's path. The larger the needle gauge, the stronger the reflection.

The patient's skin is painted with tincture of benzalkonium (Zephiran), and sterile drapes are applied. A local anesthetic agent is administered over the area of interest, and the sterile transducer is used to relocate the lesion. The needle is inserted into the central core of the cyst. The needle stop helps ensure that the needle does not go through the cyst. The fluid is then withdrawn according to volume calculations. The volume of the cyst may be determined by measuring the radius of the mass and using the following formula: $V = 4/3\pi r^3$.

The diameter of the mass can be applied to this formula:

$$V = d^3/2$$

Lower Urinary Tract

Ureters

Stricture. Ureteral narrowing due to fibrosis is a common form of ureteral stricture. Ureteral strictures may also result from inflammatory disease, tuberculosis, localized periureteral fibrosis, impacted ureteral stone, schistostomiasis, iatrogenic ureteral injury, or radiation therapy. Other causes include amyloidosis, adjacent malignancies, metastases, extrinsic compression due to primary retroperitoneal tumors, enlarged lymph nodes, and medial lower pole renal masses (Box 15-1).

Ureterocele. A ureterocele is a cystlike enlargement of the lower end of the ureter (Figure 15-36) caused by congenital or acquired stenosis of the distal end of the ureter. Ureteroceles are usually small and asymptomatic, although they may cause obstruction and infection of the upper urinary system. If large, a ureterocele may cause bladder outlet obstruction. Ureteroceles are found more often in adults than in children and may be unilateral or bilateral. On sonography, a *cobra head* appearance is seen in sagittal view.

Sonographic Findings. A large ureterocele may fill the urinary bladder and have the same sonographic appearance as diverticula. If the patient can partially empty the bladder, a better diagnostic-quality image will be produced, as the ureterocele will be empty. One of the advantages of ultrasound is dynamic imaging; alternate filling and emptying of the ureterocele as the result of peristalsis may be demonstrated. Calculi may also be present.

BOX 15-1	Causes of Narrowing of the Ureter
Internal causes	Radiation therapy
Fibrosis	Amyloidosis
Inflammatory disease	Extrinsic compression
Tuberculosis	Adjacent malignancies
Localized periureteral fibrosis	Metastases
Impacted ureteral stone	Primary retroperitoneal tumors
Schistosomiasis	Enlarged lymph nodes
Iatrogenic ureteral injury	Medial lower renal pole mass

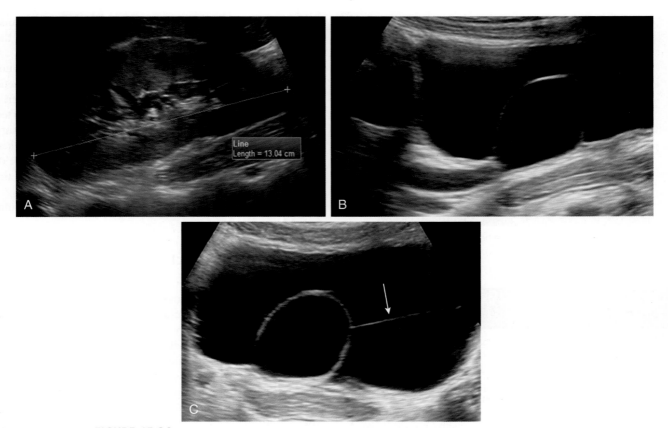

FIGURE 15-36 **A,** Normal right kidney, no hydronephrosis. **B,** Large right ureterocele protruding into urinary bladder. **C,** In gray scale the white arrow is pointing to the continuous ureteral jet known as the candle sign.

Ectopic Ureterocele. Ectopic ureteroceles are rare and are found more commonly in children and young adults, especially in females. They usually are associated with complete ureteral duplication. The ureter, which empties the upper pole, inserts low in the bladder by the bladder neck, urethra, or lower genital tract. The ectopic ureter may become stenotic and cause ureteral obstruction, which is associated with hydroureter and hydronephrosis. The ureterocele sac may obstruct the bladder outlet or may prolapse through the urethra.

Sonographic Findings. An ectopic ureterocele appears on sonography as a round, thin-walled cystic structure that may contain debris protruding into the bladder.

Bladder

Ultrasound is not the imaging modality of choice to examine the bladder. Cystoscopy is usually used to examine the bladder because of its ability to diagnose early neoplasms. Transabdominal sonography will allow visualization of most lesions greater than 5 mm. A transurethral intravesicular sonographic approach has been used to evaluate bladder tumors.

The urinary bladder should be examined at the same time as the upper urinary tract. A complete review of the patient's chart, including previous diagnostic imaging procedures, should be conducted before a sonographic examination of the bladder is begun.

A sonogram of the bladder is obtained with a distended bladder. The patient lies in a supine position. A right or left decubitus position may be used to demonstrate movement of calculi. Proper adjustment of the TGC allows for minimization of anterior wall reverberations and anechoic bladder, with posterior acoustic enhancement. The depth of the image should be set to visualize any structure that may lie posterior or caudal to the bladder. A 3.5-MHz transducer is usually used. In very thin patients, a 5-MHz transducer may be used. If evaluation of the anterior bladder wall is indicated, a high-frequency, curved linear-array transducer or linear transducer will give a larger anterior field if view.

The transducer should be placed in the middle of the filled urinary bladder and angled laterally, inferiorly, and superiorly. The bladder walls should be smooth and thin (3 to 6 mm). The bladder should be midline and should not be deviated to either side or have any irregular or asymmetric indentations.

Sonography is used to evaluate residual bladder volume in patients with outflow obstruction. The postvoid bladder is scanned in two planes: anteroposterior and transverse. Measurements are obtained in three planes: anteroposterior, transverse, and longitudinal. Images and measurements are obtained at the largest dimensions. Because bladder shape

BOX 15-2	Conditions That Cause Incomplete Emptying of Bladder

Bladder calculi	Radiation therapy
Diabetes mellitus	Rectal or vaginal fistulas
Foley catheter	Renal disease
Inflammation	Sexual intercourse
Neoplasms—benign or malignant	Trauma (blood clot)
	Tuberculosis (lower ureteric stricture)
Neurogenic bladder	
Postsurgical intervention	Urethral stricture
Pregnancy	

varies, any volume measurement can be used to approximate volume. A residue of less than 20 ml of urine is considered normal in an adult.

Ureteral jets should be identified as flashes of Doppler color entering the bladder from the lateral posterior border of the bladder and coursing superior and medial.

An enlarged prostate, enlarged uterus, pelvic mass, or filled loop of bowel may indent and displace the urinary bladder. Box 15-2 lists the conditions under which the bladder may not empty completely.

PATHOLOGY OF THE URINARY SYSTEM

See Table 15-3 for clinical findings, sonographic findings, and differential considerations for various renal diseases and conditions. Box 15-3 lists the main signs and symptoms of common renal diseases.

Renal Cystic Disease

Simple renal cystic disease encompasses a wide range of disease processes, which may be typical, complicated, or atypical. The disease may be acquired (nongenetic) or inherited (genetic) (e.g., von Hippel–Lindau disease, tuberous sclerosis). Cystic disease may occur in the renal cortex, medulla, or renal sinus (see Table 15-3).

Simple Renal Cyst. The most common renal mass lesion is a simple cortical renal cyst. Although the origin is unknown, these cysts are considered acquired lesions, probably arising from obstructed ducts or tubules. It is estimated that they occur in 50% of the population older than 50 years of age. Most patients with a simple cyst are asymptomatic, and the cyst is detected as an incidental finding in the kidney. A renal simple cyst can be solitary or multiple, involving one or both kidneys. Rarely, several simple cysts may involve only one kidney or a localized portion of a kidney. In rare cases, a large lower pole cyst may obstruct the collecting system and cause hydronephrosis and/or hypertension. Local pain and hematuria may be caused by distention of the cyst wall or spontaneous bleeding into the cyst. Occasionally, a simple cyst can be complicated by hemorrhage, infection, or calcification, which causes it to become a complex cyst. Renal cysts are unusual in children, with an overall frequency of less than 1%. A cyst in a child must be examined carefully to differentiate a benign cyst from a cystic form of nephroblastoma (Wilms' tumor).

Sonographic Findings. Sonography is the most efficient imaging modality for confirming the presence of a simple cyst that is poorly seen during CT and/or MRI. Classical sonographic criteria used to diagnose a simple renal cyst include a

TABLE 15-3	Renal Findings	
Clinical Findings	**Sonographic Findings**	**Differential Considerations**
Simple Cysts		
Usually asymptomatic Usually normal laboratory findings	Found anywhere in the kidney, but usually in cortex Round or ovoid in shape, anechoic Thin, well-defined walls No color flow or Doppler in mass	Hemorrhagic cyst, infected cyst, necrotic cyst, malignant cyst, obstruction of upper pole, calyceal diverticula, pseudoaneurysm, arteriovenous malformation
Parapelvic Cysts		
Usually asymptomatic May present with hypertension or obstruction (hilum cyst) Pain Usually normal laboratory findings	Found in the renal hilum or renal sinus Well-defined sonolucent mass with regular or irregular borders Good through-transmission Not connected to the renal collecting system	Hydronephrosis
von Hippel–Lindau Cysts		
Flank pain General discomfort Involves many body systems Usually presents in third to fifth decade Initial clinical symptoms caused by cerebellar or spinal cord hemangioblastomas, not abdominal If renal involvement occurs, there is an ↑ chance of renal carcinoma No hypertension or renal failure	Bilateral cysts and masses Other organs are affected Masses may develop within the cysts Hyperplastic linings of cysts Pancreatic cysts	Multiple cysts Renal adenoma

Continued

TABLE 15-3	Renal Findings—cont'd	
Clinical Findings	**Sonographic Findings**	**Differential Considerations**
Tuberous Sclerosis Involves several body systems Patient usually presents with mental retardation, seizures, and cutaneous lesions	Multiple cysts or angiomyolipomas Multiple organs involved Multiple angiomyolipomas that may become large	Angiomyolipomas
Acquired Cystic Disease of Dialysis Usually occurs in patients on renal dialysis for ≥3 yr Flank pain	Found in cortex Simple cysts Atypical because of hemorrhage Normal or small echogenic kidneys with ↓ in corticomedullary distinction with simple or atypical cysts	Renal cyst Adenoma Renal cell carcinoma
Adult Polycystic Kidney Disease Hypertension Renal failure Abdominal, flank pain Fever, chills (infection) Uremia Palpable mass Polycythemia Hematuria	Bilateral enlarged kidneys with multiple cysts of varied size Kidneys lose their reniform shape; in the late stages, no normal renal parenchyma may be identified Cysts may be atypical because of infection or hemorrhage Cysts may be found in liver, spleen, testes, pancreas	Cortical cysts Localized hydronephrosis Renal tuberculosis Multilocular cyst

Infantile Polycystic Kidney Disease
May be seen in utero
Renal insufficiency
Lung hypoplasia, usually fatal depending on the amount of renal function
In juvenile form:
    Portal hypertension
    Hepatic fibrosis
    GI hemorrhage
	Bilateral enlarged echogenic kidneys
	Cysts too small to be seen
	No distinction between the corticomedullary region
		In utero—ADPKD, dysplasia, glomerulocystic kidney disease

Multicystic Dysplastic Kidney Most common palpable mass in neonates Restricted growth in children Polyuria Hypertension Infection Usually unilateral; bilateral is incompatible with life	Multiple cysts of varying size No renal parenchyma surrounding the cyst Enlarged kidneys in children Small kidneys in adults Absence of renal vascularity	Hydronephrosis
Medullary Sponge Kidney Usually asymptomatic unless calculus is present, then hematuria and infections Pain Hydronephrosis Infection	Normal or small kidneys with echogenic parenchyma (cysts too small to be resolved on a sonogram) *or* Small cysts in medulla and corticomedullary region with ↑ echogenicity	Papillary necrosis Nephrocalcinosis Renal cystic disease Pyelonephritic cysts
Medullary Cystic Disease Normal renal function Anemia Salt loss Progressive azotemia Polyuria Pain Infection	Normal or small echogenic kidneys with Widening of the renal sinus after 2 cm in the medulla or corticomedullary junction	Medullary sponge kidney small cysts under 2 cm

TABLE 15-3	Renal Findings—cont'd	
Clinical Findings	**Sonographic Findings**	**Differential Considerations**
Renal Cell Carcinoma		
Hematuria	Cystic or complex mass that may have areas	Angiomyolipoma
Weight loss	of calcifications	Transitional cell carcinoma
Fatigue	May displace renal pyramids and invade renal	Lymphoma
Fever	architecture	Oncocytoma
Flank pain	Irregular margins	Column of Bertin
Palpable mass	Hypervascular	Renal vein or IVC thrombus
Hypertension	Renal vein or IVC thrombosis	
Transitional Cell Carcinoma		
Hematuria	Solid hypoechoic mass	Squamous cell tumor
Weight loss	Not well defined within the renal sinus	Renal cell carcinoma
Fatigue	May be multiple	Adenoma
Fever		Blood clot
Flank pain		Fungus ball
Squamous Cell Carcinoma		
Gross hematuria	Large bulky mass	Transitional cell carcinoma
History of chronic irritation	Invasion of the renal vein and IVC	
Palpable kidney if severe hydronephrosis is present		
Renal Lymphoma		
Not a primary site; usually caused by adjacent	Hypoechoic mass may be bilateral	Renal cell carcinoma
lymph involvement	Enlarged kidney	Cyst
More common in patients with non-Hodgkin's		
lymphoma		
Usually no renal symptoms		
Asymptomatic		
Pain		
Hematuria		
Wilms' Tumor		
Palpable abdominal mass in children	Usually unilateral, may be bilateral	Nephroblastoma
Abdominal pain	Heterogeneous	Renal cell carcinoma
Nausea and vomiting	Look for extension into renal vein and inferior	Mesoblastoma
Hematuria	vena cava	Multicystic kidney
		Retroperitoneal sarcoma
Benign Renal Tumor		
Usually asymptomatic	Well-defined mass—hyperechoic to	Angiomyolipoma
May cause painless hematuria	hypoechoic	Transitional cell carcinoma
		Oncocytoma
		Lymphoma
		Column of Bertin
Adenoma		
Asymptomatic	Well-defined mass with calcifications	Renal cell carcinoma
Angiolipoma		
Usually asymptomatic	Usually echogenic homogeneous mass with	Oncocytoma
Possible flank pain	well-defined borders	Renal cell carcinoma
Normal laboratory values	Hemorrhagic neoplasm	
Hematuria if tumor hemorrhages		
Lipoma		
Usually asymptomatic	Well-defined echogenic mass	Fibromas
Normal laboratory values		Adenoma
Oncocytoma		
Asymptomatic	Well-defined mass with spoke-wheel patterns	Renal abscess
	of enhancement and central scar	

Continued

TABLE 15-3	Renal Findings—cont'd	
Clinical Findings	**Sonographic Findings**	**Differential Considerations**
Acute Glomerulonephritis		
Nephrotic syndrome Hypertension Anemia Peripheral edema	↑ Cortical echoes	Chronic glomerulonephritis Acute tubular nephrosis AIDS Lupus nephritis Acute interstitial nephritis
Acute Interstitial Nephritis		
Uremia Hematuria Rash Fever Eosinophilia	Enlarged kidneys with ↑ cortical echoes	Acute glomerulonephritis Chronic glomerulonephritis Acute tubular necrosis AIDS Lupus nephritis
Lupus Nephritis		
Hematuria Proteinuria Renal vein thrombus Renal insufficiency	↑ Cortical echoes and renal atrophy	Acute glomerulonephritis Chronic glomerulonephritis Acute tubular necrosis AIDS Acute interstitial nephritis
Acquired Immunodeficiency Syndrome (AIDS)		
Renal dysfunction	Kidneys are normal or enlarged Echogenic parenchyma ↑ Cortical echoes	Acute glomerulonephritis Chronic glomerulonephritis Acute tubular necrosis Lupus nephritis Acute interstitial nephritis
Sickle Cell Nephropathy		

Hematuria
Renal vein thrombosis
	Varies—*patients with acute renal vein thrombosis:*
	    Enlarged kidneys with ↓ echogenicity
	Subacute:
	    Enlarged kidneys with ↑ cortical echogenicity
		Lupus nephritis

Hypertensive Nephropathy		
Uncontrolled hypertension	Small kidneys with smooth borders may have distortion of intrarenal anatomy	Hypoplasia
Papillary Necrosis		
Hematuria Flank pain Hypertension Dysuria Acute renal failure	Fluid-filled spaces at the corticomedullary junction Round or triangular Mimics calculi	Congenital megacalyces Hydronephrosis Postobstruction atrophy
Renal Atrophy		
Renal failure	Small echogenic kidneys	Renal hypoplasia Chronic renal failure
Renal Sinus Lipomatosis		
Asymptomatic	Enlarged kidneys with ↑ echogenicity of renal sinus Hyperechoic areas ↓ Renal parenchyma	Infection Atrophy Hydronephrosis
Acute Renal Failure		
Renal insufficiency ↓ Urine output	Hydronephrosis Enlarged hypoechoic kidneys Renal artery stenosis	Prerenal, renal, or postrenal causes

TABLE 15-3	Renal Findings—cont'd	
Clinical Findings	**Sonographic Findings**	**Differential Considerations**
Obstructive Hydronephrosis		
Renal insufficiency	Fluid-filled renal collecting system	Extrarenal collecting system
↓ Urine output	Thin parenchyma	Parapelvic cyst
Hypertension	Hydroureter	Reflux
	↓ or absent ureteral jets	Renal artery aneurysm
		Transient diuresis
		Congenital megacalyces
		Papillary necrosis
		Arteriovenous malformation
Renal Infarction		
Asymptomatic	Irregular triangle masses in the renal parenchyma	Renal lobulations
	Lobulated renal contour	Dromedary hump
Acute Tubular Necrosis		
Renal insufficiency	Bilaterally enlarged kidneys with hyperechoic	Nephrocalcinosis
Hematuria	pyramids	
Chronic Renal Failure		
Renal failure	Bilateral small echogenic kidneys	Multiple causes
Hypertension		AIDS
		Chronic parenchymal infection
Pyonephrosis		
Renal insufficiency	Dilated collecting system with low-level	Hydronephrosis
Hematuria	echoes or ↓ through-transmission	Hemorrhage
		Blood clot
		Uroepithelial tumors
Xanthogranulomatous Pyelonephritis		
Multiple infections	"Staghorn appearance"	Hydronephrosis
Nonfunctioning kidneys	Destruction of renal parenchyma	Renal calculi
	↑ Echogenicity	
	↑ Renal size	
	Dilated calyces	

↑, Increase; ↓, decrease; *GI*, gastrointestinal; *IVC*, inferior vena cava.

BOX 15-3	Signs and Symptoms of Renal Disease

Renal Cystic Disease
Inflammatory or necrotic cysts
- Flank pain
- Hematuria
- Proteinuria
- White blood cells in urine
- ↑ Protein

Renal subcapsular hematoma
- Hematuria
- ↓ Hematocrit

Renal Inflammatory Processes
Abscess
  Acute onset of symptoms
  Fever
  Palpable mass
  ↑ White blood cell count
  Pyuria
Acute focal bacterial nephritis
- Fever
- Flank pain

- Pyuria
- ↑ Blood urea nitrogen
- ↑ Albumin
- ↑ Total plasma proteins

Acute tubular necrosis
- Moderate to severe intermittent flank pain (caused by renal calculi)
- Vomiting (caused by renal calculi)
- Hematuria
- Infection
- Leukocytosis with infection

Chronic renal failure
- ↑ Concentration of urea in blood
- High urine protein excretion
- ↑ Creatinine
- Presence of granulocytes

Renal cell carcinoma
- Erythrocytosis may occur
- Leukocytosis
- Red blood cells in urine
- Pyuria
- ↑ Lactic acid dehydrogenase

round or oval shape, anechoic, thin walls, and posterior acoustic enhancement. If all of these sonographic findings are present, no further evaluation is required (Figure 15-37).

Complex Cyst. If a renal cyst does not meet all of the criteria for a simple cyst, it is termed *complex* and must be considered malignant until proven otherwise. Complex cysts may contain septations, thick walls, calcifications, internal echoes, and mural nodularity.

Sonographic Findings. Thick walls: Anything thicker than 1 mm is considered abnormal, and the cystic form of a renal carcinoma often presents in this manner (Figure 15-38). Most of the time, internal echoes within a cyst are the result of protein content, hemorrhage, and/or infection. Any irregularity at the base of the cyst should be considered a malignant growth (Box 15-4). Thin septations can be detected by sonography, and their presence alone does not suggest malignancy. If irregularity of septa (thicker than 1 mm) showing vascularity on color or power Doppler is seen, the lesion must be presumed malignant. Fine, thin linear calcification in the cyst wall or in a septum without associated soft tissue mass or enhancement on CT likely represents a complex cyst, rather than a malignancy.

Bosniak classification of cysts was introduced in 1986, before CT or MRI was used for diagnosing renal cystic disease. In 2005 the Bosniak classification was updated from four categories—I, II, III, and renal cyst IV—to five categories:

- **Category I** lesions are simple benign cysts: anechoic, thin walls, no calcifications or septations; no atypical features; and no further evaluation is needed.
- **Category II** lesions are cystic lesions with one or two thin (≤1 mm thick) septations, fine calcifications in the walls

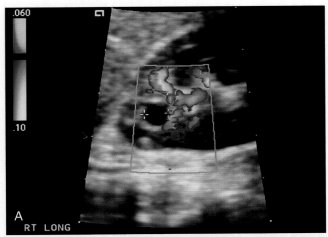
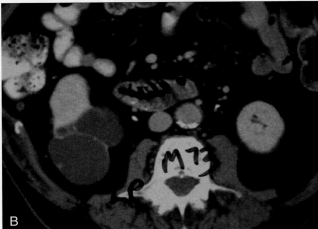
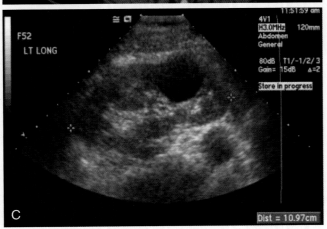

FIGURE 15-37 **A,** Upper pole renal cyst with no blood flow to the cyst. **B,** CT scan of the lower pole complicated cyst. **C,** Sagittal view of the left kidney with a cystic mass.

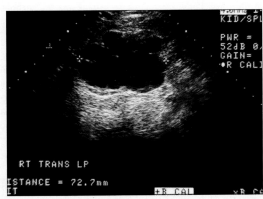

FIGURE 15-38 Transverse view of lower pole with a complex cyst.

BOX 15-4	What to Do When a Renal Mass Is Discovered

- If the renal mass is solid, it must be considered malignant, unless fat is present within the mass.
- The presence of calcifications in a renal mass is always a sign of malignancy.
- If a cystic renal mass does not meet the sonographic criteria for a simple renal cyst, it must be considered malignant.
- A renal pseudotumor needs to be considered when a renal mass is discovered.
- Metastasis rate is 10% to 15% at time of diagnosis.

Sonographic Considerations
- Evaluate the renal vein and inferior vena cava into the right atrium to look for thrombus/tumor.
- Evaluate the contralateral kidney, liver, and retroperitoneum for metastases.

or septa (wall thickening >1 mm advances the lesion into surgical category III), and hyperdense benign cysts with all features of category I cysts, except for being homogeneously hyperechoic. A benign category II lesion must be 3 cm or less in diameter, must have one quarter of its wall extending outside the kidney so the wall can be assessed, and must show no vascularity (must be nonenhancing after contrast material is administered on CT) on color Doppler.

- **Category IIF** comprises minimally complicated cysts that need follow-up. This is a group not well defined by Bosniak, but it consists of lesions that do not fall neatly into category II. These lesions have some atypical features and are most likely benign. Six months to 1 year follow-up is required.

- **Category III** consists of true indeterminate cystic masses showing uniform wall thickening, nodularity (especially in the base of the cyst), thick or irregular peripheral calcification, or a multilocular nature with multiple vascular (enhancing) septa. These cysts cannot be distinguished from malignancies and require a biopsy and/or surgery for evaluation. The distinction between some categories,

especially IIF and III, is not clear, and variability in how the cysts in these two categories are classified may occur.

- **Category IV** cysts have diffuse wall thickening and may include areas with increased vascularity, or large nodules in the wall, or clearly solid vascular components in the cystic lesion—all features that strongly suggest malignancy. The cystic masses are presumed to be renal cell carcinoma and the same treatment is followed, typically a nephrectomy.

Sonographically, it is difficult to differentiate between a septated cyst and small, adjacent cortical cysts known as "kissing" cysts (Figure 15-39). A cyst may also have a cyst or mass within it (Figure 15-40). Sometimes small sacculations or infoldings of the cystic wall produce wall irregularity; a cyst puncture or aspiration may be recommended to ascertain the pathology of the fluid within the mass.

Low-level echoes within a renal cyst may be artifacts (sensitivity too high or transducer frequency too low) or may result from infection, hemorrhage (Figures 15-41 and 15-42), or a necrotic cystic tumor, or, in rare cases, malignancy.

Renal Sinus Parapelvic Cysts. The parapelvic cyst originates from the renal sinus and is most likely lymphatic in origin.

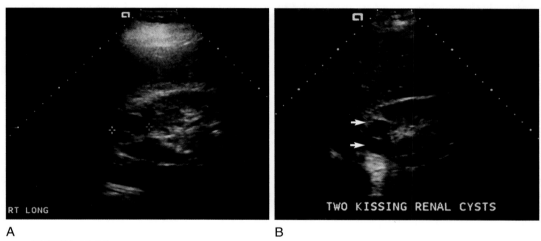

A   B

FIGURE 15-39 A, A single upper-pole cortical cyst with a thin septation. **B,** Two small adjacent renal cysts ("kissing" cysts).

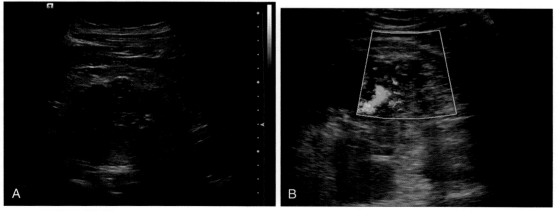

FIGURE 15-40 A, A small 15 mm mass within a cyst. **B,** Color Doppler demonstrates intratumoral vascularity.

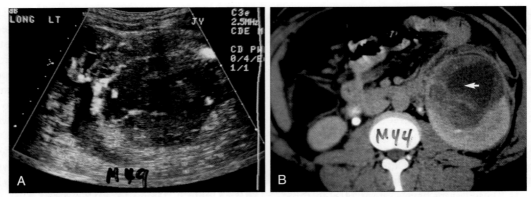

FIGURE 15-41 A, Transverse scan of a hemorrhagic cyst with no increase in blood flow. **B,** CT scan of hemorrhagic cyst.

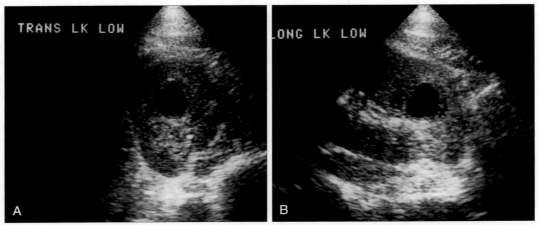

FIGURE 15-42 Transverse **(A)** and longitudinal **(B)** scans of a renal sinus cyst. Good through-transmission is noted beyond the renal parenchyma.

These small cysts do not communicate with the collecting system. Most often, patients with parapelvic cysts are asymptomatic. Clinical symptoms are infrequent, but occasionally the cyst may cause pain, hematuria, hypertension, or obstruction.

Sonographic Findings. The sonogram shows a well-defined mass with no internal septations. The cyst can have irregular borders because it may compress adjacent renal sinus structures. Parapelvic cysts (especially those located in the medial lower portion of the kidney) may cause obstruction; peripelvic cysts do not. The sonographer should be able to differentiate the parapelvic cyst from hydronephrosis by trying to connect the dilated renal pelvis centrally. A transverse view is very useful. The dilated renal pelvis may present a cauliflower-like appearance, whereas the parapelvic cyst is more spherical in appearance.

Renal Cysts Associated with Renal Neoplasms

von Hippel–Lindau. Von Hippel–Lindau disease is an autosomal dominant genetic disorder. Several areas of the body may be affected. Predominant abnormalities include retinal angiomas, cerebellar hemangioblastomas, and a variety of abdominal cysts and tumors, including renal and pancreatic cysts, renal adenomas, and frequent multiple and bilateral renal adenocarcinoma tumors. Renal cell carcinoma in patients with this disease is multifocal and bilateral. A high incidence of renal cysts is found in patients with von Hippel–Lindau disease, usually of cortical origin.

Tuberous Sclerosis. Tuberous sclerosis is an autosomal dominant genetic disorder characterized by mental retardation, seizures, and adenoma sebaceum. Associated renal lesions include multiple renal cysts or angiomyolipomas and/or cutaneous, retinal, and cerebral hamartomas. This disease may be difficult to separate from adult polycystic kidney disease.

Acquired Cystic Kidney Disease. This condition is found in native kidneys of patients with renal failure who need to undergo renal dialysis or peritoneal dialysis. Patients with this condition have been shown to have a slightly increased incidence of renal cysts, adenomas, and renal carcinoma. It is theorized that epithelial hyperplasia caused by tubular obstruction that occurs as a result of toxic substances plays a role in the development of these masses. Incidence increases with time, particularly after the first 3 years of dialysis. It increases up to 90% after 5 years of dialysis. Renal cysts can show spontaneous bleeding and hemorrhage, causing pain and flank discomfort. Solid tumors, including adenomas, oncocytomas, and renal cell carcinomas, are seen in up to 7% of patients.

Sonographic Findings. On a sonogram, the native kidneys are small and echogenic with several small cysts. In a patient with chronic renal failure, three to five cysts in each kidney are diagnostic. The incidence of hemorrhage into the renal cysts is increased; this will reveal internal echoes within the cyst or hyperechoic cysts. Renal masses with internal echoes, mural nodularities, and increased vascularity on color Doppler, with no posterior acoustic enhancement, are likely to be renal carcinoma.

Polycystic Kidney Disease. Polycystic renal disease may present in one of two forms: the infantile autosomal recessive form and the adult autosomal dominant form.

Autosomal Recessive Polycystic Kidney Disease. Autosomal recessive polycystic kidney disease (ARPKD), also called infantile polycystic disease, is a fairly rare genetic disorder. The gene that causes this disorder has been located on chromosome 6. Dilation of the renal collecting tubules causes renal failure, and in later forms of the disease, liver involvement is seen. Four forms of ARPKD are classified according to the age of the patient at the onset of clinical signs: perinatal, neonatal, infantile, and juvenile. The perinatal form is found in utero and usually progresses to renal failure, causing pulmonary hypoplasia and intrauterine demise. On the perinatal sonogram, oligohydramnios, hypoplastic lungs, and massively enlarged echogenic kidneys may be visualized.

The juvenile form may present with hypertension, renal insufficiency, nephromegaly, hepatic cysts, bile duct proliferation, and Caroli's disease, which may be associated with periportal fibrosis (which causes portal hypertension and esophageal varices). Renal function is usually decreased secondary to hepatic problems when ARPKD appears later in life. In older children, the kidneys are enlarged with an echogenic cortex and medulla and lack of corticomedullary differentiation. Microscopic or small cysts (1 to 2 mm) may be located in the medulla, often associated with hepatic fibrosis and splenomegaly.

Autosomal Dominant Polycystic Kidney Disease. Autosomal dominant polycystic kidney disease (ADPKD) (previously known as adult polycystic renal disease) is a common genetic disease that occurs in both men and women. The severity of the disease varies depending on the genotype. The most common type is ADPKD1 (located on the short arm of the sixteenth chromosome), which affects the kidneys more severely than ADPKD2 (located on the long arm of the fourth chromosome). A number of people have no known genetic disposition to ADPKD, but it may result from spontaneous mutations. It is a bilateral disease that is characterized by enlarged kidneys with multiple asymmetric cysts varying in size and location in the renal cortex and medulla. The disease is progressive and does not usually clinically manifest until the fourth or fifth decade when hypertension or hematuria develops. By age 60, approximately 50% of patients will have end-stage renal disease (ESRD). Clinical symptoms include pain (common complaint), hypertension, palpable mass, hematuria, headache, urinary tract infection, and renal insufficiency.

There is a high incidence of urolithiasis. Complications may include infection, hemorrhage, rupture of cyst, and renal obstruction.

Associated abnormalities include cysts in the liver, spleen, pancreas, thyroid, ovary, testes, or breast; cerebral berry aneurysm; and abdominal aortic aneurysm. Patients who are on renal dialysis have an increased incidence of renal cell carcinoma.

Sonographic Findings. The sonographic appearance of ADPKD is similar to the autosomal recessive form of polycystic disease. In the neonate, sonography demonstrates diffusely enlarged kidneys, due to multiple interfaces of the small cysts. This appearance is not unique to ADPKD, but further screening is warranted when noted on prenatal sonographic examination. Diagnosis is based on family history and tissue sampling.

In the adult patient, bilateral renal enlargement occurs with multiple asymmetric cysts of varying size in both cortex and medulla. In the most advanced cases, the normal renal parenchyma is replaced bilaterally with multiple cysts (Figures 15-43 and 15-44) and the kidneys lose their reniform shape. The cysts may grow large enough to obliterate the renal sinus. They may become infected or hemorrhagic, which is characterized sonographically by internal debris within the cysts or thickened walls. The walls of the cysts may be calcified, or stones may form. A complicated cyst may result in spontaneous bleeding, causing flank pain for the patient (see Table 15-3).

Multicystic Dysplastic Kidney. Multicystic dysplastic kidney (MCDK) disease is a common nonhereditary renal dysplasia that usually occurs unilaterally, with the kidney functioning poorly, if at all. MCDK is the most common form of cystic disease in neonates and is believed to be the consequence of early in utero urinary tract obstruction. Dysplastic changes usually involve the entire kidney but, rarely, may be segmental or focal. Bilateral MCDK is incompatible with life. Complications arising from a multicystic dysplastic kidney that is not removed include hypertension, hematuria, infection, and flank pain. A slightly increased risk of malignant transformation can occur if the kidney is not removed.

Sonographic Findings. In neonates and children, the kidneys are multicystic, with absence of renal parenchyma, renal sinus, and atretic renal artery. In adults, the kidneys may be small (atrophic and calcified) and echogenic. Other possible findings include ureteral atresia (failure of the ureter to develop from the calyceal system), contralateral ureteropelvic obstruction (in 30% of patients) (development of the ureter from the bladder with retrograde filling), and a nonfunctioning kidney.

Medullary Cystic Disease

Medullary Sponge Kidney. Medullary sponge kidney (MSK) is a development anomaly that occurs in the medullary pyramids and consists of cystic or fusiform dilation of the distal collecting ducts (ducts of Bellini), causing stasis of urine and stone formation. Because the medullary sponge kidney is an anatomic rather than a metabolic defect, the pathologic process may be unilateral or segmental. The cause is unknown. Many patients remain asymptomatic, but patients

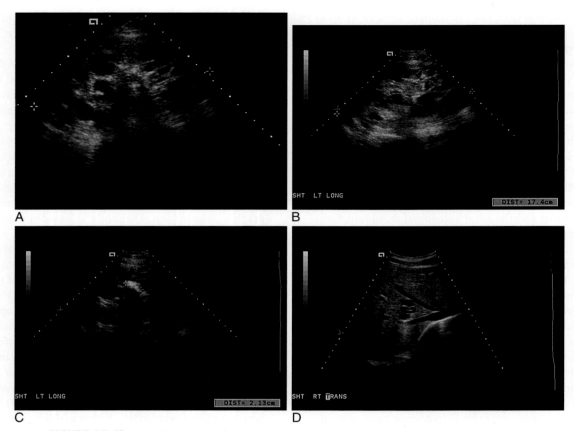

FIGURE 15-43 A and **B,** Images of a young adult male with polycystic renal disease. Longitudinal scans of both kidneys show enlarged kidneys (right kidney [RK] 15.2 cm and left kidney [LK] 17.4 cm) with a variety of cyst sizes. **C,** Polycystic kidney with stone. **D,** About one third of patients with polycystic renal disease also have cysts on the liver or other organs.

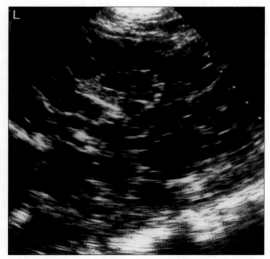

FIGURE 15-44 A 30-year-old male with a solitary left polycystic kidney and hematuria was sent to rule out obstruction. It is very difficult to rule out obstruction with so many small cysts.

with hematuria, infection, and renal stones should be evaluated for medullary sponge kidney.

MSK may be associated with a variety of other congenital and inherited disorders, including Beckwith-Wiedemann syndrome, polycystic kidney disease (PKD) (about 3% of patients

with autosomal dominant polycystic kidney disease have evidence of MSK), Caroli's disease, and congenital hepatic fibrosis.

Medullary Cystic Kidney Disease and Nephronophthisis. Nephronophthisis and medullary cystic kidney disease are inherited disorders that eventually lead to ESRD. They are grouped together because they share many features. Pathologically, they cause cysts restricted to the renal medulla or corticomedullary border, as well as a triad of tubular atrophy, tubular basement membrane disintegration, and interstitial fibrosis.

Medullary cystic kidney disease (MCKD) is very similar to the childhood disease familial juvenile nephronophthisis (NPH). Both lead to scarring of the kidney and formation of fluid-filled cavities (cysts) in the deeper parts of the kidney. In these conditions, the kidneys do not concentrate the urine enough, leading to excessive urine production and loss of sodium and other chemical changes in the blood and urine.

MCKD occurs in older patients and is inherited in an autosomal dominant pattern. NPH occurs in young children and is usually due to autosomal recessive inheritance.

Sonographic Findings. The patient presents with small echogenic kidneys, with loss of corticomedullary differentiation, and multiple small medullary cysts (smaller than 2 cm). With MCKD, sonography shows hyperechoic calyces, with or without stones (Figures 15-45 and 15-46).

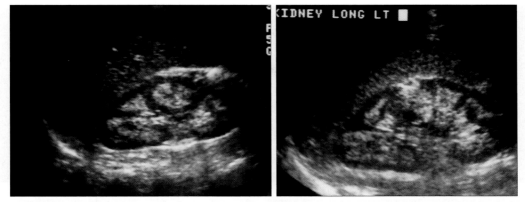

FIGURE 15-45 Longitudinal scans of a young patient with medullary sponge kidney show nephrocalcinosis and stone formation.

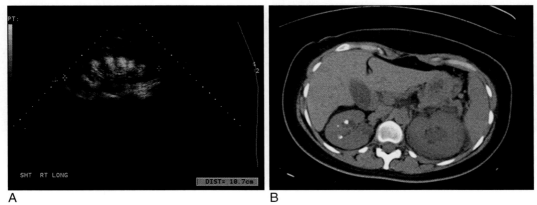

A   B

FIGURE 15-46 A, Longitudinal view of the right kidney with hyperechoic calyces and stones. **B,** Tiny medullary calculi are detected on CT.

Renal Neoplasms

Sonography is often the first imaging modality that detects renal masses. Often these masses are incidental findings. Even though ultrasound may not be as sensitive as CT or MRI in finding small masses, ultrasound is able to accurately differentiate cysts from solid masses, especially in cases where CT and MRI fail to do so. The sonographic appearance of most renal masses is nonspecific. Very often, the sonographic characteristic patterns of benign and malignant tumors cannot be differentiated from one another. In the study of the solid renal masses the role of the sonography has been focused on the differentiation of renal cell carcinoma and angiomyolipoma, the most common malignant and benign solid renal tumors.

Research in using contrast-enhanced sonography along with Doppler in identifying tumor vascularity to differentiate between a benign and malignant mass has provided encouraging results. The use of contrast agents in sonography has not, however, been approved by the Food and Drug Administration in the United States. If a solid mass is detected, renal cell carcinoma, oncocytoma, angiomyolipoma, transitional cell carcinoma, or secondary neoplasms (e.g., metastasis, lymphoma) must be considered (see Box 15-4).

Renal Cell Carcinoma. Renal cell carcinoma (RCC), also called hypernephroma, or Grawitz's tumor, is the most common

of all renal neoplasms and represents 85% of all kidney tumors. It is twice as common in males as in females, usually in the sixth to seventh decade of life. The classical clinical presentation is nonspecific; however, the patient may report hematuria, flank pain, and a palpable mass. The tumor appears bilaterally in 0.1% to 1.5% of patients, and is multifocal in 13% of cases. An association with von Hippel–Lindau disease, acquired cystic disease (dialysis patients), and tuberous sclerosis is reported. Regardless of histologic subtype, the sonographic appearance of most RCCs is solid with no predilection for left or right kidney or location in the organ. One to two percent of RCCs are predominantly cystic, and very rarely the tumor may be entirely cystic.

Sonographic Findings. Most RCCs are isoechoic, but they may also present as hyperechoic (Figure 15-47). Usually, large tumors have a heterogeneous echotexture, caused by intratumoral hemorrhage and necrosis. Small tumors (less than 3 cm in diameter) have the same hyperechoic appearance as fat-containing tumors, such as angiomyolipomas. A hypoechoic rim, which represents a vascular pseudocapsule on color Doppler, may be very helpful in making the diagnosis of RCC. The presence of intratumoral calcifications is considered specific for RCC. In cases in which renal cell carcinoma is represented as cystic, a

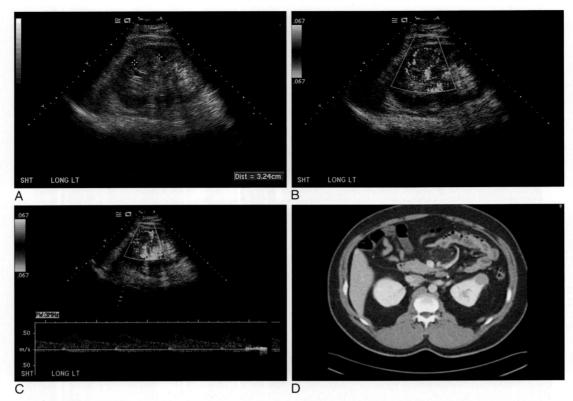

FIGURE 15-47 A, Longitudinal view of a small hyperechoic renal cell carcinoma. **B** and **C,** Color Doppler demonstrates peripheral vascularity of the tumor ("basket sign"). **D,** Contrast CT confirms a small enhancing renal tumor; pathology confirmed cell carcinoma.

variety of types, such as unilocular, multilocular, completely necrotic, and tumor originating in a cyst, may be demonstrated on sonography.

Use of color Doppler for the detection of tumor vascularity shows high sensitivity for malignant renal tumors, especially RCC. In RCC tumor vascularity can be demonstrated in up to 92% of cases, and the most common vascular patterns include a "basket sign" and/or "vessels within the tumor." High systolic and high end-diastolic arterial flow with low resistive index is the most typical flow pattern in spectral Doppler waveforms. Renal vein and inferior vena cava invasion occurs in 5% to 24% of RCCs at the time of diagnosis, and metastasis from renal malignancies is seen in lungs, mediastinum, other nodes, liver, bone, adrenal glands, and the opposite kidney. CT and MRI with contrast are the most sensitive radiographic examinations for the detection and characterization of renal masses (Figures 15-48 to 15-50). Box 15-5 summarizes the sonographic characteristics of malignant renal tumors.

Transitional Cell Carcinoma. Transitional cell carcinoma (TCC) accounts for 90% of malignancies that involve the renal pelvis, ureter, and bladder, and for up to 7% to 10% of all

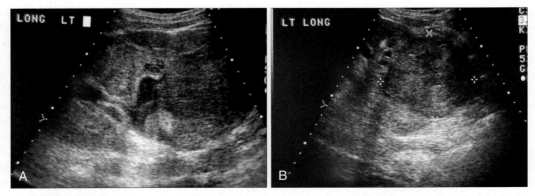

FIGURE 15-48 Stage III renal cell carcinoma with invasion into the inferior vena cava. **A,** Longitudinal scan shows lower pole mass with no normal renal parenchyma. **B,** Measurement of the lower pole mass.

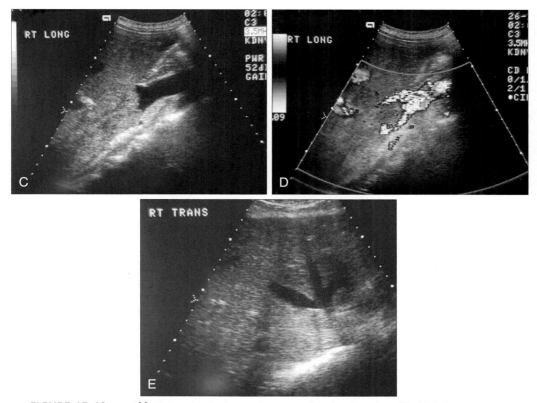

FIGURE 15-48, cont'd C, Longitudinal scan demonstrating the thrombus-filled inferior vena cava (IVC). **D,** Longitudinal scan of IVC with color flow showing obstruction. **E,** Transverse view of the dome of the liver with patent hepatic veins and nonvisualization of the IVC.

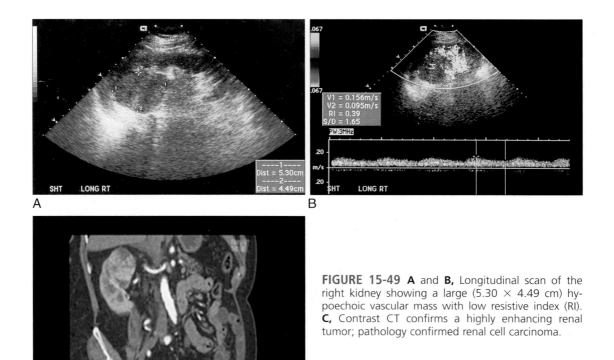

FIGURE 15-49 A and **B,** Longitudinal scan of the right kidney showing a large (5.30 × 4.49 cm) hypoechoic vascular mass with low resistive index (RI). **C,** Contrast CT confirms a highly enhancing renal tumor; pathology confirmed renal cell carcinoma.

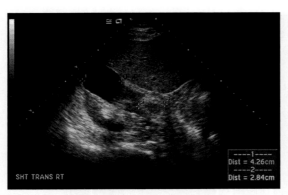

FIGURE 15-50 A transverse view of the right kidney demonstrating a cyst and a small hyperechoic mass, which is consistent with renal cell carcinoma.

BOX 15-5	Sonographic Characteristics of a Malignant Renal Tumor

- Renal cell carcinomas (RCCs) less than 2 to 3 cm in diameter are always hyperechoic.
- The bigger the tumor, the more heterogeneous is its echotexture.
- Hypoechoic rim represents a vascular pseudocapsule.
- In up to 92% of RCCs, peripheral (basket sign) and/or central (vessel within the tumor) vascularity can be demonstrated on color Doppler.
- Invasion of the renal vein and/or inferior vena cava occurs in 5% to 24% of cases.

In Cases with Cystic Appearance
- Thick wall >1 mm
- Irregularity at the base of the cyst
- Septations
- Calcifications
- Presence of vascularity in the septa and/or cystic wall

renal tumors. The tumor is often multifocal, with a 40% to 80% incidence. TCC occurs twice as often in men as in women, with a peak occurrence in the seventh decade. TCC of the renal pelvis is 2 to 3 times more common than ureteral neoplasm, and is almost 50 times less common than TCC of the urinary bladder. The TCC may be papillary or flat.

Papillary TCCs are more common, with an exophytic polypoid appearance attached to mucosa. They usually are low-grade malignancies and tend to have a more benign course. Small TCCs tend to be flat and are difficult to detect with any type of imaging. Small TCCs are generally high-grade malignancy tumors and metastasize easily to the other tissues and organs. Clinically, the patient may present with gross or microscopic hematuria and flank pain. The differential diagnosis includes other tumors of the renal pelvis, such as squamous cell tumor, adenoma, a blood clot, or a fungus ball (see Table 15-2).

Sonographic Findings. The typical appearance is that of a hypoechoic mass within the collecting system, with low vascularity on color Doppler and, extremely rarely, calcifications. TCC may invade adjacent renal parenchyma and form an infiltrating mass, which usually preserves the renal contour.

Squamous Cell Carcinoma. Squamous cell carcinoma is a rare, highly invasive tumor with a poor prognosis. Clinically, the patient usually has a history of chronic irritation and gross hematuria, with a palpable kidney secondary to severe hydronephrosis.

Sonographic Findings. The sonographic finding is usually a large mass in the renal pelvis. Obstruction from kidney stones may also be present (Figures 15-51 and 15-52).

Renal Lymphoma. Primary lymphomatous involvement of the kidneys is rare, with a 3% occurrence. The secondary form is more common. This form of lymphoma may occur as a hematogenous spread (90%) or as direct extension via the retroperitoneal lymphatic channels with a contiguous spread from the retroperitoneum (see Table 15-2). Non-Hodgkin's lymphoma is more common than Hodgkin's lymphoma. Lymphoma is more common as a bilateral invasion with multiple nodules.

Sonographic Findings. The kidneys are enlarged and hypoechoic relative to the renal parenchyma (the mass may simulate a renal cyst without posterior acoustic enhancement). The mass rarely demonstrates a sonographic halo of hypoechoic mass in the perinephric regions (Figure 15-53). The sonographer should be careful of highly hypoechoic renal tumors with poorly defined margins without posterior

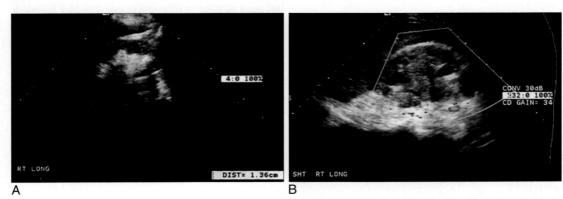

FIGURE 15-51 A, Longitudinal scan of the right kidney with a small hypoechoic mass (transitional cell carcinoma [TCC]) in the mid-upper collection system and a 1.36 cm nonobstructing stone in the lower pole. **B,** A large vascular hypoechoic mass occupying most of the collecting system and causing an obstruction *(arrows).*

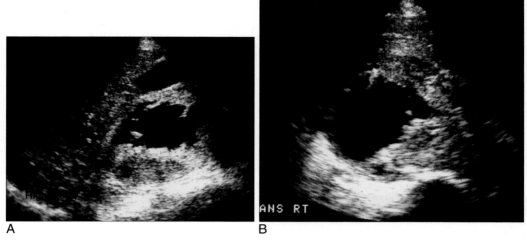

FIGURE 15-52 Sixty-year-old patient with metastatic disease. **A,** Sagittal image of right kidney shows irregularly shaped mass filling the renal sinus. **B,** Transverse image of the squamous cell carcinoma.

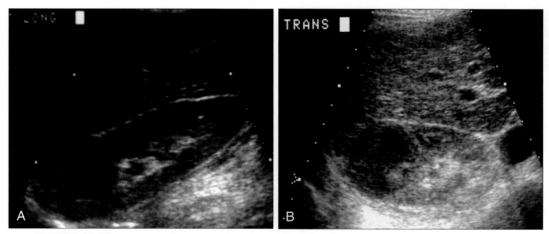

FIGURE 15-53 A and **B,** Sixty-year-old patient with bilateral renal lymphomas. **A,** Sagittal image of right kidney with hypoechoic upper pole mass. **B,** Transverse image of upper pole of right kidney with hypoechoic lymphoma.

enhancement, as they may be mistaken initially for "renal cysts."

Secondary Malignancies of the Kidneys. Metastases to the kidneys are relatively common, occurring late in the course of the disease. Secondary malignancies are bilateral in one third of cases and multiple in more than 50%. The most common primary malignancies that metastasize to the kidneys include carcinoma of the lung or breast and RCC of the contralateral kidney. On sonography, the lesion usually presents as multiple, poorly marginated hypoechoic masses. Renal enlargement without a discrete mass also may occur.

Sonographic Findings. The tumor may spread beyond the **renal capsule** and invade the renal vein. The tumor cells can extend into the inferior vena cava to the right atrium and can eventual metastasis into the lungs. The tumor may be multifocal in a small percentage of patients.

Nephroblastoma. Nephroblastoma, or Wilms' tumor, is the most common abdominal malignancy in children and the most common solid renal tumor in pediatric patients 1 to 8 years old. Peak incidence is seen at 2.5 to 3 years of age; 90% of patients are younger than 5 years old, and 70% are younger than 3 years old. Nephroblastoma is 2 to 8 times more common in patients with horseshoe kidney. Clinical signs may include abdominal flank mass, hematuria, fever, and anorexia.

Sonographic Findings. The mass varies from hypoechoic to moderately echogenic. A 5% to 10% incidence of bilateral tumors has been reported, so careful evaluation of both kidneys is crucial. Up to 40% of patients with Wilms' tumor have renal vein thrombosis and/or vena cava or atrial thrombus by the time of diagnosis. Venous obstruction may result, with findings of leg edema, varicocele, or Budd-Chiari syndrome (Figures 15-54 to 15-56).

Benign Renal Tumors. Benign renal tumors are rare. All renal tumors are treated as malignant until proven otherwise. The patient usually is asymptomatic and presents with

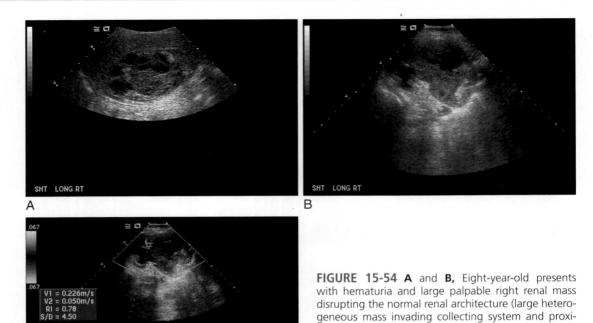

A

B

C

FIGURE 15-54 A and **B,** Eight-year-old presents with hematuria and large palpable right renal mass disrupting the normal renal architecture (large heterogeneous mass invading collecting system and proximal ureter). **C,** Color spectral Doppler shows increased vascularity of the mass.

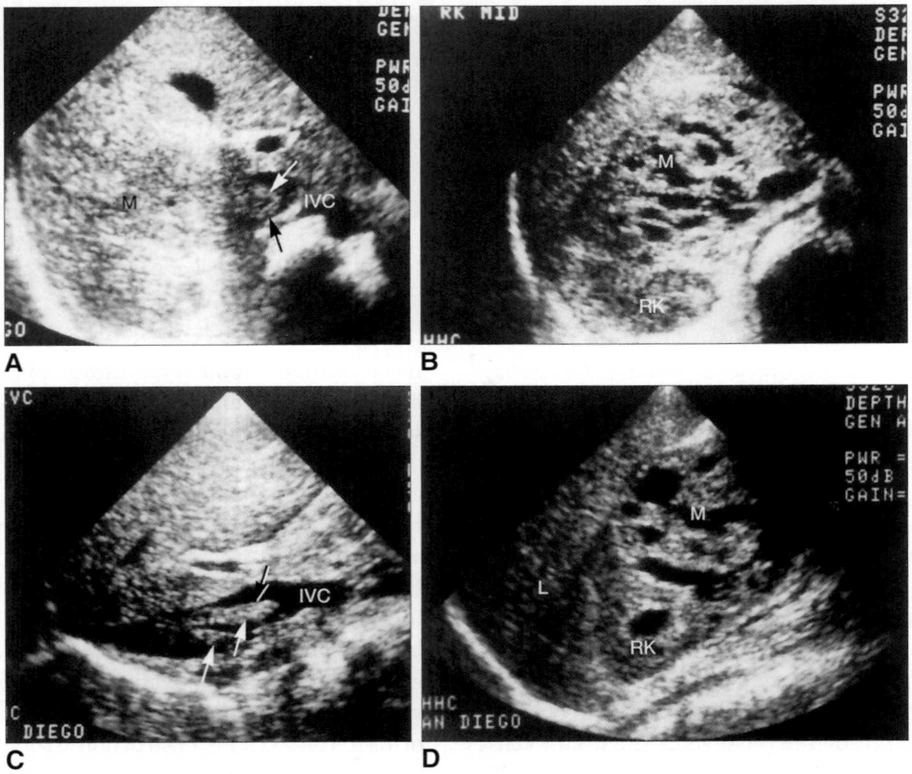

A

B

C

D

FIGURE 15-55 A, One of the complications of a Wilms' tumor *(M)* is spread beyond the renal capsule into the renal vein and inferior vena cava *(IVC)*. **B,** This 18-month-old child had a large, complex tumor with extension into the inferior vena cava *(IVC, arrows)*. *RK,* Right kidney. **C** and **D,** Longitudinal scan, showing the dilated inferior vena cava with tumor echoes along the posterior border. The tumor may extend into the right atrium of the heart. *L,* Liver; *RK,* right kidney.

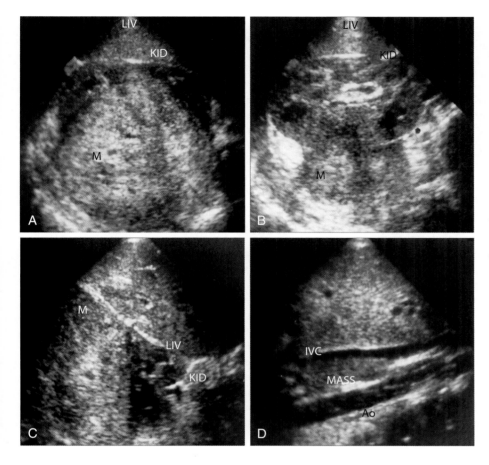

FIGURE 15-56 **A** through **D,** A 14-month-old child with a large Wilms' tumor *(M)* extending from the right kidney *(KID)* into the inferior vena cava *(IVC).* On coronal scan **(D),** the tumor mass is seen within the IVC. The patient is rolled into a slight decubitus position for better imaging of the IVC and aorta *(Ao). LIV,* Liver.

flank pain only if the mass is large or if hemorrhage from the mass occurs. Adenomas and oncocytomas are two common benign renal tumors (see Table 15-3).

Renal Angiomyolipoma. Renal angiomyolipoma (AML) is the most common benign renal tumor. It is composed of varying proportions of fat, muscle, and blood vessels. AML has an incidence of 0.07% to 0.3% in the general population; 80% of cases occur in females, and 80% in the right kidney. The tumor is found in 80% of patients with tuberous sclerosis. Tumor size varies between 1 and 20 cm and may be multifocal.

Sonographic Findings. The echo pattern of AML is usually hyperechoic, depending on the proportions of fat,

muscle, and vessels within the mass. Intratumoral hemorrhage and organ displacement are the primary complications. Differential diagnosis is made with small (less than 3 cm) renal cell carcinomas, which are also hyperechoic in echotexture and may simulate AML in up to 33% of cases. A hypoechoic rim, presented as a basket sign on color Doppler, favors renal cell carcinoma. Color Doppler shows no intratumoral vascularity. On angiography, the tumor is highly vascular; CT is determinant in the diagnosis of AML because of its sensitivity in detecting intratumoral fat (Figures 15-57 and 15-58).

Renal Adenomatous Tumors. Renal adenomatous tumors can be seen as nephrogenic adenofibroma or embryonal

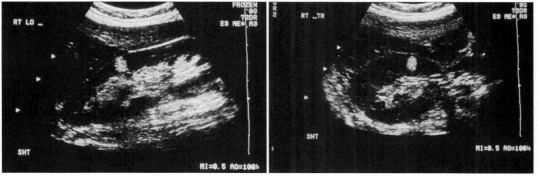

FIGURE 15-57 Angiomyolipoma appears as an echogenic focal mass in the renal parenchyma.

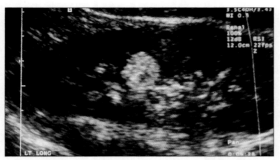

FIGURE 15-58 Angiolipomas are common benign tumors that usually appear as unilateral solitary or multiple echogenic masses in middle-aged women. Renal function is normal.

adenoma. Patients are usually asymptomatic. Incidental findings may be noted if the mass is large or if intratumoral hemorrhage occurs. In some cases, these tumors may cause hematuria.

Sonographic Findings. These tumors appear as solid masses on sonography, are hyperechoic to hypoechoic in echotexture, and are hypovascular on color Doppler (Figure 15-59). As with oncocytomas, renal adenomatous tumors may be indistinguishable from RCC.

Oncocytoma. Oncocytoma is another uncommon renal tumor that is usually benign. Incidence is increased in the middle-aged or elderly patient. This lesion represents 3.1% to 6% of all renal tumors. Tumor size varies, with an average size of 6 cm. The patient is typically asymptomatic, but the tumor may cause pain and hematuria.

Sonographic Findings. In more than 50% of cases, the mass is hypoechoic in echotexture. Oncocytomas resemble "spoke-wheel" patterns of enhancement with a central scar. It is practically impossible to differentiate them from RCC; 5% of oncocytomas are initially diagnosed as RCC (Figure 15-60).

Lipomas. A lipoma consists of fat cells and is the most common of the mesenchymal type of tumors. This tumor is found more often in females than in males. The patient is typically asymptomatic, but the tumor has been reported to cause hematuria.

Sonographic Findings. Lipomas appear as well-defined echogenic masses within the kidney (Figure 15-61).

Renal Disease

Intrinsic renal disease can be identified by examining the renal parenchyma with ultrasound. Two classifications of disease processes have been described. One group produces a generalized increase in cortical echoes, believed to result from deposition of collagen and fibrous tissue. This group includes interstitial nephritis, acute tubular necrosis, amyloidosis, diabetic nephropathy, systemic lupus erythematosus, and myeloma. The second group of diseases may cause loss of normal anatomic detail, resulting in inability to distinguish the cortex and medullary regions of the kidneys. This group of diseases includes chronic pyelonephritis, renal tubular ectasia, and acute bacterial nephritis (see Table 15-3).

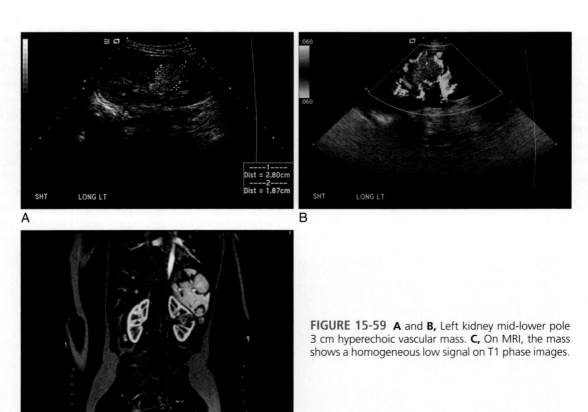

FIGURE 15-59 A and **B,** Left kidney mid-lower pole 3 cm hyperechoic vascular mass. **C,** On MRI, the mass shows a homogeneous low signal on T1 phase images.

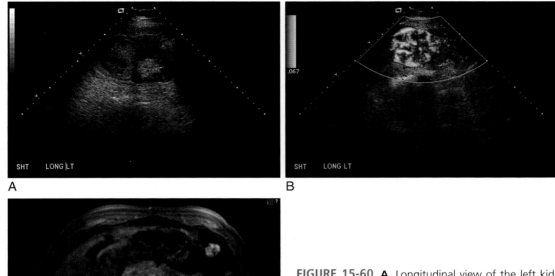

FIGURE 15-60 **A,** Longitudinal view of the left kidney shows large exophytic heterogeneous mass. **B,** Hypervascular on power Doppler. **C,** MRI transverse view of the kidneys shows enhancement of the mass *(arrow)* with a central scar. Mass proved to be oncocytoma.

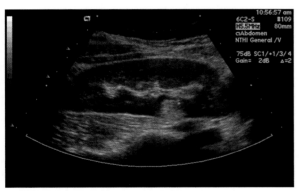

FIGURE 15-61 Sagittal view of left kidney with lipoma. *(Courtesy Siemens Medical Solutions USA, Inc.)*

The end stage of many of these disease processes is renal atrophy, which can be identified on a sonogram by measuring renal length and cortical thickness. Some acute renal disorders produce exactly the opposite findings—decreased parenchymal echogenicity and renal enlargement. Examples include acute renal vein thrombosis, acute pyelonephritis, and acute renal transplant rejection. Interstitial edema is believed to be the most likely cause of these findings.

Acute Glomerulonephritis. In acute glomerulonephritis, necrosis or proliferation of cellular elements (or both) occurs in the glomeruli. The vascular elements, tubules, and interstitium become secondarily affected; the end result is enlarged, poorly functioning kidneys.

Sonographic Findings. Different forms of glomerulonephritis, including membranous, idiopathic, membranoproliferative, rapidly progressive, and poststreptococcal, can be associated with abnormal echo patterns from the renal parenchyma on a sonogram (Figure 15-62). Increased cortical echoes probably result from changes within the glomerular, interstitial, tubular, and vascular structures. Patients have many symptoms, including nephrotic syndrome, hypertension, anemia, and peripheral edema.

Acute Interstitial Nephritis. Acute interstitial nephritis has been associated with the infectious processes of scarlet fever and diphtheria. It may be a manifestation of an allergic reaction to certain drugs. Patient signs and symptoms

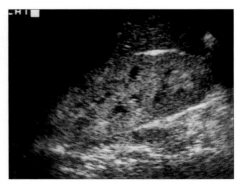

FIGURE 15-62 Acute glomerulonephritis may be suspected when the echogenicity of the renal parenchyma exceeds that of the liver.

include uremia, proteinuria, hematuria, rash, fever, and eosinophilia.

Sonographic Findings. The kidneys are enlarged and mottled. On a sonogram, renal cortical echogenicity is increased. The increase in echogenicity is greatest in cases of diffuse active disease. This increase is less apparent in diffuse scarring.

Lupus Nephritis. Systemic lupus erythematosus is a connective tissue disorder believed to result from an abnormal immune system. Females are affected more often than males, and incidence peaks between 20 and 40 years of age. The kidneys are involved in more than 50% of patients. Renal manifestations include hematuria, proteinuria, hypertension, renal vein thrombosis, and renal insufficiency.

Sonographic Findings. Sonographic appearance is increased cortical echogenicity and renal atrophy (Figure 15-63).

Acquired Immunodeficiency Syndrome. Acquired immunodeficiency syndrome (AIDS) is a highly contagious disease, spread mainly by unprotected sexual activity or infected needles. The virus destroys T cells and then replicates rapidly within the body. It affects many organs. Patients have various symptoms (see Table 15-2).

Unexplained uremia or azotemia may indicate renal dysfunction resulting from AIDS; it is usually a late finding. Causes of renal dysfunction in AIDS patients include acute

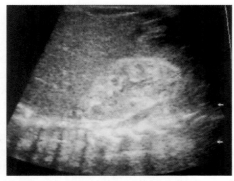

FIGURE 15-63 Patients with lupus nephritis demonstrate a highly echogenic renal parenchymal pattern compared with the liver. Renal atrophy is usually present.

tubular necrosis, nephrocalcinosis, interstitial nephritis, and focal segmental glomerulosclerosis.

Sonographic Findings. An echogenic parenchymal pattern is evident on a sonogram. Cortical echogenicity is increased. Kidneys are normal in size or enlarged (Figures 15-64 to 15-66). If AIDS-related lymphoma or Kaposi's sarcoma occurs, the kidneys appear enlarged and hypoechoic on a sonogram.

Sickle Cell Nephropathy. Renal involvement is common in patients with sickle cell disease. Abnormalities include glomerulonephritis, renal vein thrombosis, and papillary necrosis. Hematuria is common.

Sonographic Findings. The sonographic appearance depends on the type of disorder. In acute renal vein thrombosis, the kidneys are enlarged with decreased echogenicity secondary to edema. In patients with subacute cases, renal enlargement is present with increased cortical echoes.

Hypertensive Nephropathy. Uncontrolled hypertension can lead to progressive renal damage and azotemia.

Sonographic Findings. Sonographically, the kidneys are small with smooth borders. Superimposed scars of pyelonephritis or lobar infarction may distort the intrarenal anatomy. Bilateral small kidneys occur secondary to end-stage disease as a result of hypertension, inflammation, or ischemia.

Papillary Necrosis. Renal papillary necrosis (RPN) is not a pathologic entity, but rather a descriptive term for a condition—necrosis of the papillae. The renal papillae (the apex of the renal pyramid that projects into the minor calyx) are vulnerable to ischemic necrosis. Diabetes is the most frequent condition associated with RPN in adults. Other conditions that cause RPN include analgesic abuse, sickle cell disease, obstructive uropathy, renal vein thrombosis, tuberculosis, pyelonephritis, and renal transplant. Necrosis may develop within weeks or months after renal transplantation, especially in patients previously treated for rejection and those with cadaveric kidney. Ischemia is believed to have an important role in necrosis.

Symptoms depend on the etiology of RPN and most of the time complications suggest calculus or an inflammatory process. Complaints include hematuria, flank pain, dysuria,

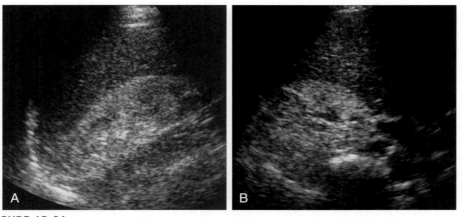

FIGURE 15-64 Longitudinal **(A)** and transverse **(B)** scans in a patient with acquired immunodeficiency syndrome (AIDS) show cortical echogenicity with normal to slightly increased renal size.

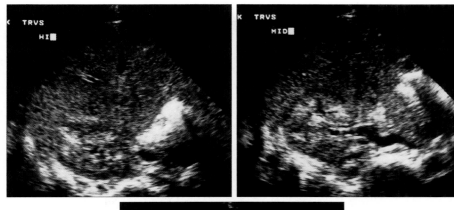

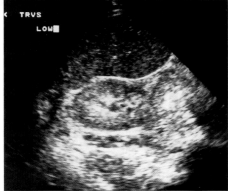

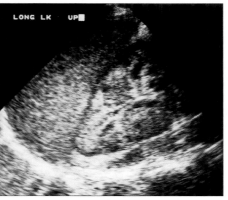

FIGURE 15-65 Transverse scans of a young male with acquired immunodeficiency syndrome (AIDS) show a mildly echogenic renal parenchyma.

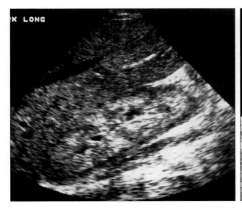

FIGURE 15-66 Longitudinal scans of a 26-year-old male with acquired immunodeficiency syndrome (AIDS).

fever, hypertension, and acute renal failure. Differential considerations include congenital megacalyces, hydronephrosis, and postobstructive atrophy.

Sonographic Findings. Sonographic findings include one or more fluid spaces at the corticomedullary junction that correspond to the distribution of the renal pyramids. The cystic spaces may be round or triangular. Sloughed papillae may appear as echogenic material within the necrotic medullary cavities. Correlation with clinical and laboratory findings help distinguish renal papillary necrosis from other renal abnormalities that have similar features on sonography and that are associated with areas of increased echogenicity (e.g., nephrocalcinosis).

Renal Atrophy. Renal atrophy results from numerous disease processes. Intrarenal anatomy is preserved with uniform loss of renal tissue. Renal sinus lipomatosis occurs secondary to renal atrophy. More severe lipomatosis results from a tremendous increase in renal sinus fat content in cases of marked renal atrophy caused by hydronephrosis and chronic calculus disease.

Sonographic Findings. The kidneys appear enlarged with a highly echogenic, enlarged renal sinus and a thin cortical rim. Renal sinus fat is easily seen on a sonogram as highly echogenic reflections (Figure 15-67).

Renal Failure

The excretory and regulatory functions of the kidneys are decreased in acute and chronic renal failure. Acute renal failure (ARF) is a common medical condition that can be caused by

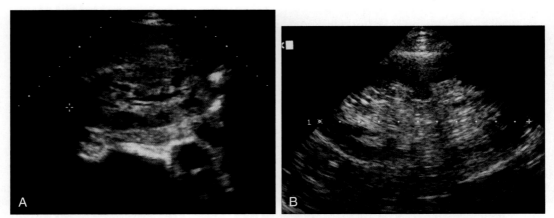

FIGURE 15-67 A, A 73-year-old man with chronic renal disease. Small echogenic kidney with inability to distinguish the medulla from the cortex region of the kidney. **B,** Renal sinus lipomatosis appears as enlarged kidneys with an echogenic, enlarged renal sinus and a thin cortical rim. Renal sinus fat is easily seen on ultrasound as highly echogenic reflections.

numerous medical diseases or pathophysiologic mechanisms. ARF is typically an abrupt transient decrease in renal function often heralded by oliguria. Pathophysiologic states that cause varying degrees of renal malfunction have been categorized as prerenal, renal, and postrenal (Box 15-6). Decreased perfusion of the kidneys can cause prerenal failure (e.g., renal vein thrombus, congestive heart failure, renal artery occlusion) and can be diagnosed by clinical and laboratory data and also by color Doppler. Renal causes of acute azotemia include parenchymal disease (e.g., acute glomerulonephritis, acute interstitial nephritis, acute tubular necrosis) and hydronephrosis. Major postrenal causes of acute renal failure include bladder, pelvic, or retroperitoneal tumor and calculi. Prompt diagnosis and treatment of postrenal failure is crucial; the condition is potentially reversible.

Chronic renal failure may be caused by obstructive nephropathies, parenchymal diseases, renovascular disorders, or any process that progressively destroys nephrons. See Table 15-3 for clinical findings, sonographic findings, and differential considerations for malfunctioning kidney conditions.

Numerous studies have previously documented that sonography is extremely sensitive in diagnosing hydronephrosis. Patients for whom laboratory test results indicate compromised

renal function should receive rule-out obstruction studies. Most agree that sonography is the initial procedure of choice in evaluating all patients with known or suspected renal failure. See Table 15-3 for clinical findings, sonographic findings, and differential considerations for renal failure.

Acute Renal Failure. ARF may occur in prerenal, renal, or postrenal failure stages (see Box 15-6). The prerenal stage is secondary to hypoperfusion of the kidney. The renal stages may be caused by parenchymal diseases (i.e., acute glomerulonephritis, acute interstitial nephritis, or acute tubular necrosis). They may also be caused by renal vein thrombosis or renal artery occlusion. In postrenal failure, radiologic imaging plays a major role. This condition is usually the result of outflow obstruction and is potentially reversible. Postrenal failure is usually increased in patients with malignancy of the bladder, prostate, uterus, ovaries, or rectum. Less frequent causes include retroperitoneal fibrosis and renal calculi.

Sonographic Findings. The cause of acute renal disease urinary outflow obstruction can be differentiated from parenchymal disease. The kidneys may appear normal in size or enlarged and may be hypoechoic with parenchymal disease. Obstruction is responsible for approximately 5% of cases of ARF. The most important issue is the presence or absence of urinary tract dilation. The degree of dilation does not necessarily reflect the presence or severity of an obstruction. A sonographer should try to determine the level of obstruction. A normal sonogram does not totally exclude urinary obstruction. In the clinical setting of acute obstruction secondary to calculi, a nondistended collecting system can be present.

Acute Tubular Necrosis. Acute tubular necrosis is the most common medical renal disease to produce acute renal failure, although it can be reversible.

Sonographic Findings. The sonogram shows bilaterally enlarged kidneys with hyperechoic pyramids; this can revert to a normal appearance. Differential considerations include nephrocalcinosis. In pediatric patients, the renal pyramids are highly echoic without shadowing. The calculi may be

BOX 15-6	Causes of Renal Failure

Prerenal
   Hypoperfusion
   Hypotension
   Congestive heart failure
Renal
   Infection
   Nephrotoxicity
   Renal artery occlusion
   Renal mass or cyst
Postrenal
   Lower urinary tract obstruction (ureter, bladder)
Retroperitoneal fibrosis

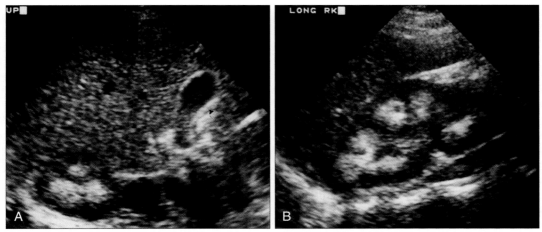

FIGURE 15-68 Transverse **(A)** and longitudinal **(B)** scans of the pediatric patient with acute tubular necrosis and nephrocalcinosis. The echogenic renal pyramids are well seen.

too small to cause dilation and shadowing of the pyramids (Figure 15-68). As renal function improves, echogenicity decreases. This can occur in the medulla or the cortex. If the condition reverses, it is probably acute tubular necrosis.

Chronic Kidney Disease. Chronic kidney disease (CKD) is the loss of renal function as a result of disease, most commonly parenchymal disease. Three primary types of chronic renal failure are known: nephron, vascular, and interstitial abnormalities. Glomerulonephritis, chronic pyelonephritis, renal vascular disease, and diabetes are a few of the diseases that lead to renal failure.

Intrarenal fibrosis is a final common pathway for all CKD, and the degree of fibrosis correlates with disease severity. Nonfocal renal biopsy is the only method in current clinical use for the evaluation of intrarenal fibrosis. However, nonfocal renal biopsy has significant disadvantages: it is invasive, with risk of major complications; it is expensive; and it is subject to sampling error, as the biopsy cores comprise a small fraction of the renal parenchyma, and highly fibrotic kidneys often have insufficient glomerular tissue on biopsy samples to permit accurate histopathologic diagnosis.

There is an increased incidence of CKD in individuals with diabetes and hypertension-related nephropathies. CKD causes end-stage renal failure with high morbidity and mortality rates. In most types of kidney diseases the progressive fibrotic processes may first involve either glomeruli (glomerulosclerosis) or the interstitial spaces (interstitial fibrosis), depending on the initial nephropathy. In renal transplantation the development of interstitial fibrosis and tubular atrophy is the major determinant of renal allograft failure.

Sonographic Findings. Chronic renal disease is a diffusely echogenic kidney with loss of normal anatomy. It is a nonspecific sonographic finding; chronic renal disease can have multiple causes (AIDS can produce echogenic kidneys). If chronic renal disease is bilateral, small kidneys are identified. This may result from hypertension, chronic inflammation, or chronic ischemia.

Shear wave elastography (SWE) is an emerging ultrasound technique that permits the noninvasive measurement of tissue stiffness. SWE uses focused acoustic energy pulses to produce microscopic tissue displacement, which induces perpendicular shear waves that are sonographically tracked as they progress through tissue. Stiffer tissues have been shown to have increased shear wave velocities. SWE may be a low-cost way to provide additional diagnostic information in CKD. Further studies are required to determine the relationship between estimated renal stiffness and renal fibrosis severity. Whereas native kidneys are quite deep within the abdomen and hardly compressible, renal transplants are much more superficial, located in the iliac fossa.

Hydronephrosis

Hydronephrosis–Urinary Tract Obstruction. Hydronephrosis is the separation of renal sinus echoes by interconnected fluid-filled calyces. Box 15-7 lists the causes of hydronephrosis.

BOX 15-7	Causes of Hydronephrosis

Acquired
Bladder tumors
Calculi
Carcinoma of the cervix
Neurogenic bladder
Normal pregnancy
Pelvic mass
Prostatic enlargement
Retroperitoneal fibrosis

Intrinsic
Bladder neck obstruction
Calculus
Congenital
Inflammation
Posterior urethral valves
Pyelonephritis
Stricture
Ureterocele
Ureteropelvic junction obstruction

Dilation of the pelvocalyceal system is called hydronephrosis. In 1988 the Society for Fetal Urology proposed the following classification of grading hydronephrosis:

- Grade 1: small fluid-filled separation of the renal pelvis
- Grade 2: dilation of some but not all of the calyces; calyx orientation still concave
- Grade 3: complete pelvocaliectasis; calyx orientation changed in convex; echogenic line separating collecting system from renal parenchyma can be demonstrated (Figure 15-69)
- Grade 4: prominent dilation of the collecting system, thinning of renal parenchyma, and no differentiation between collecting system and renal parenchyma

Urinary tract obstruction is not synonymous with dilation; in almost 35% of cases with acute urinary obstruction, no dilation is seen. Nonobstructive dilation is also seen in childhood during vesicoureteral reflux (see Box 15-7).

Sonographic Findings. Whenever the renal collecting system is dilated, the ureters and bladder are scanned to locate the level of obstruction. It is possible to identify the site of obstruction by using sonography. A congenital obstruction of the ureteropelvic junction can be seen in utero and in infants. The collecting system will be dilated without dilation of the ureter. Localized hydronephrosis occurs as a result of strictures, calculi, focal masses, or a duplex collecting system (Figures 15-70 and 15-71). Hydronephrosis with a dilated ureter indicates obstruction of the ureterovesical junction; hydroureteronephrosis with a dilated bladder indicates obstruction of the posterior urethra (posterior urethral valves).

A mildly distended collecting system can be caused by overhydration, a normal variant of extrarenal pelvis, or by a previous urinary diversion procedure (Figure 15-72). Postvoid scanning techniques are helpful in preventing these errors.

If hydronephrosis is suspected, the sonographer should examine the bladder. If it is full, a postvoid longitudinal scan of each kidney should be done to show that hydronephrosis has disappeared or remains the same. At the level of obstruction, the sonographer should sweep the transducer back and forth in two planes to see if a mass or stone can be distinguished. The sonographer must be able to

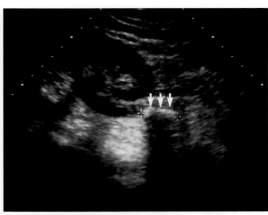

FIGURE 15-70 Slight dilatation of the collecting system is seen. A longitudinal left kidney scan with dilatation of the proximal ureter caused by a stone *(arrows)*.

rule out a parapelvic cyst (septations may be numerous) or a crossing renal vessel in the peripelvic area (color flow Doppler is extremely useful). An extrarenal pelvis would protrude outside of the renal area, and the sonographer probably would not confuse this pattern with hydronephrosis.

In evaluating the patient for hydronephrosis, the sonographer must be sure to look for a dilated ureter, an enlarged prostate, or an enlarged bladder (which may occur secondary to an enlarged prostate). Bladder carcinoma may obstruct the pathway of the urethra, causing urine to back into both ureters and renal pelvis. A ureterocele may also block urine output. This condition occurs with an anomalous insertion of the ureter into the bladder wall. The ureter can turn inside out and obstruct the orifice.

Obstructive Hydronephrosis. Dilation of the renal pelvis is just one factor present in patients with obstructive hydronephrosis. (See Table 15-3 for clinical findings, sonographic findings, and differential considerations for obstructive hydronephrosis.)

Sonographic Findings. In cases of acute urinary tract obstruction (UTO), the resistive index (RI) of the interlobar and arcuate intrarenal vessels may be greater than 0.70, starting 6 hours after acute onset and up to 72 hours (Figure 15-73). The RI returns to normal value after 120 hours of obstruction. The value of the RI may be higher than 0.70 in some normal conditions, as in neonates and infants up to 6 years old and in elderly patients, and in some pathologic conditions related to intrinsic renal disease, diabetes, and/or hypertension. Use of nonsteroidal antiinflammatory drugs may lower the value of the RI on the affected side, which decreases the sensitivity of Doppler ultrasound in identifying UTO. Level of obstruction is another important factor in elevation of the RI value. The resistive index is greater in patients with an obstruction in the proximal ureter or in the distal intramural ureteral portion.

It is very important to measure and compare the RI in both kidneys, because a ΔRI is more useful for diagnosis of UTO than a solid value for RI. No ureteral jet will be seen on the affected side if the obstruction is complete, or the jet may be noted if obstruction is partial.

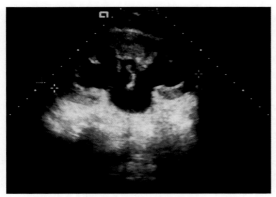

FIGURE 15-69 Hydronephrosis of the kidney. The dilated pyelocaliceal system appears as separation of the renal sinus echoes by fluid-filled areas that conform anatomically to the infundibula, calyces, and pelvis.

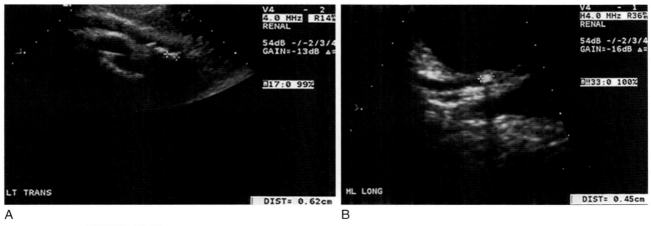

FIGURE 15-71 **A,** Three small left uretral stones at the level of the crossing iliac vessels. Mild hydronephrosis is seen. **B,** Small right distal UVJ stone causing obstruction of the ureter.

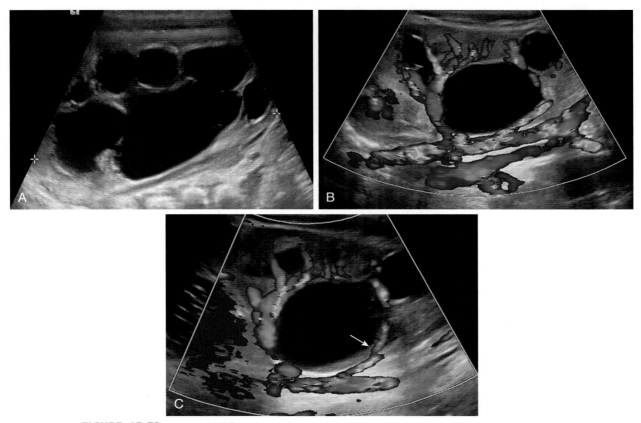

FIGURE 15-72 **A,** Severe left pelvocaliectasis. Note the absence of a dilated ureter after the ureteral pelvic junction (UPJ). **B,** Severe left pelvocaliectasis without a dilated ureter after UPJ. **C,** Color Doppler demonstrates the crossing vessel causing UPJ obstruction.

Classical sonographic findings in the diagnosis of UTO include the following: grade I or II hydronephrosis; Doppler showing elevated RI or difference of ΔRI; absence of the respective ureteral jet; and visualization of the dilated ureter and/or stone. Sonography can be normal in up to 50% of cases in the first 6 hours after acute onset, which means that the normal sonogram does not exclude acute urinary obstruction, and a noncontrast CT will be necessary.

Ureteral Jet Phenomenon. The ureteral jet phenomenon picked up by gray-scale or color Doppler is caused by the difference in density between urine in the bladder and urine coming from the ureter (kidney). The frequency and size (velocity) of the ureteral jet range from 0.2 to 1.7 m/sec. Duration of the jets is 0.6 to 4.1 seconds, with a 30-second interval jet time. The jets are directed upward and toward the contralateral side, and the shape of

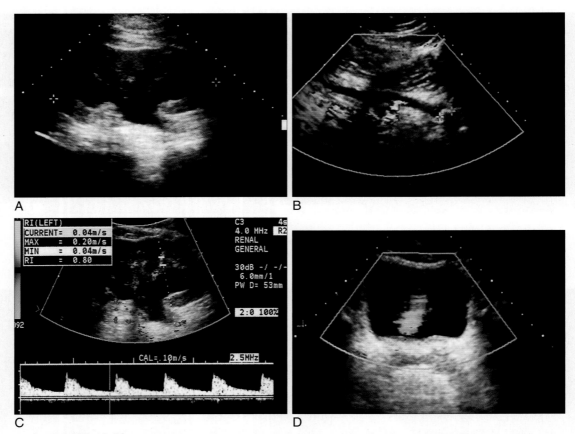

FIGURE 15-73 **A,** Grade 2 to grade 3 left uretero-hydronephrosis. **B,** 1 cm obstructing stone in the lower portion of the left ureter. **C,** High resistive index (RI = 0.80) documenting an acute urinary obstruction. **D,** Absence of the left ureteral jet.

the spectral Doppler curve varies with the amount of urine produced. Complete obstruction shows absence of the respective ureteral jet; partial obstruction may show a low-level jet on the side of obstruction and/or asymmetry of the ureteral jets.

Urine fills the bladder at a rate of up to 2 ml/min. Patients who have voided before the renal examination and are rehydrated may have a false-positive absence of ureteral jets. This occurs because the concentration of urine in the recently distended bladder is similar in density to that of urine entering

the bladder. Comparison of the two ureteral jets is necessary to confirm that nonvisualization of the symptomatic side is not related to the fact that the density of urine in the ureter is similar to that in the bladder (Figures 15-74 and 15-75).

Nonobstructive Hydronephrosis. Dilation of the renal pelvis does not always mean that obstruction is present. Several other factors, such as reflux, infection, large extrarenal pelvis, high-flow states (polyuria), distended renal bladder, atrophy after obstruction, or pregnancy dilation, may cause the renal pelvis to be dilated. (The enlarged uterus can compress the ureter; this

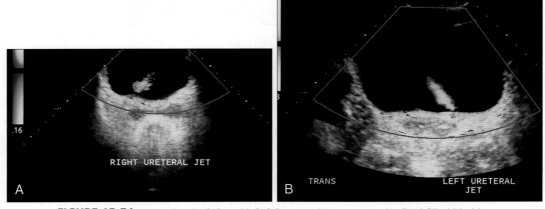

FIGURE 15-74 Normal right **(A)** and left **(B)** ureteral jets seen in the fluid-filled bladder.

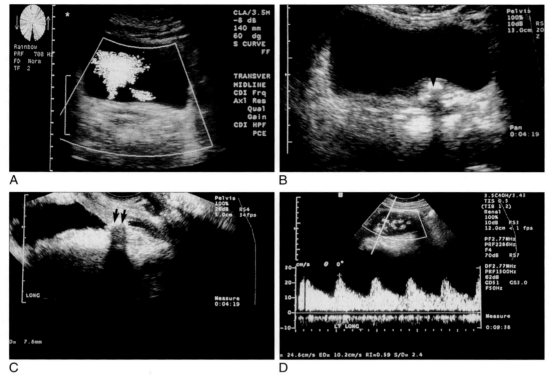

FIGURE 15-75 A, Transverse scan of a fluid-filled bladder with a normal right ureteral jet. A partially obstructed left ureter with decreased flow. **B,** Transverse scan of a partially obstructed distal left ureter. *Arrows* indicate the stone and shadowing posterior to the stone. **C,** Transvaginal scan of the dilated distal ureter with a ureteral stone. **D,** Normal resistive index (RI) of 0.59 for left kidney.

usually occurs more frequently on the right during the third trimester, causing the so-called "hydronephrosis of pregnancy" with normal RI.)

False-Positive Hydronephrosis. Many conditions may mimic hydronephrosis (Box 15-8); these include extrarenal pelvis, parapelvic cyst, reflux, multicystic kidney, central renal cyst, transient diuresis, congenital megacalyces, papillary necrosis, renal artery aneurysm (color can help distinguish that this enlargement, not the renal pelvis, is vascular), or an arteriovenous malformation (color can distinguish this abnormality).

Localized hydronephrosis may occur secondary to strictures, calculi, or focal masses (transitional). It may also be seen in a duplex system when one of the systems can be obstructed by an ectopic insertion of the ureter. In females, the ureter can insert below the external urinary sphincter, causing dribbling.

False-Negative Hydronephrosis. A dilated renal pelvis may be distinguished from other conditions by the use of other techniques. In patients with retroperitoneal fibrosis or necrosis, give liquids to see if the renal pelvis dilates. In patients with distal calculi, no obstruction can be seen unless the calculi have been there for several days. A staghorn calculus can mask an associated dilation.

The conditions of adult polycystic disease and multicystic renal disease with severe hydronephrosis may be confused. In patients with severe hydronephrosis, the image shows dilated calyces as they radiate from a larger central fluid collection in the renal pelvis. The kidney usually retains a normal shape. The sonographer sees fluid-filled sacs in a radiating pattern or cauliflower configuration. In patients with adult polycystic renal disease or multicystic renal disease, the renal cysts are randomly distributed, the contour is disturbed, and the cysts are variable in size. Once obstruction has been ruled out, consider renal medical disease, which is the leading cause of ARF.

Renal Infections

A spectrum of severity is possible in renal infection. The disease can progress from pyelonephritis to focal bacterial nephritis to an abscess. An abscess can be transmitted through the parenchyma into the blood. Most renal infections stay in

BOX 15-8	Conditions That Mimic Hydronephrosis

Arteriovenous malformation
Congenital megacalyces
Extrarenal pelvis
Papillary necrosis
Parapelvic cysts
Persistent diuresis
Reflux
Renal artery aneurysm

the kidney and are resolved with antibiotics. A perirenal abscess may occur from direct extension. (See Table 15-3 for clinical findings, sonographic findings, and differential considerations for renal infections.)

Pyonephrosis. Pyonephrosis occurs when pus is found within the collecting renal system. It is often associated with severe urosepsis and represents a true urologic emergency that requires urgent intravenous antibiotic therapy and/or percutaneous drainage. It usually occurs secondary to long-standing ureteral obstruction resulting from calculus disease, stricture, or a congenital anomaly.

Sonographic Findings. Sonographic findings include the presence of low-level echoes with a fluid-debris level (Figure 15-76). The sonographer should be aware that an anechoic dilated system may be found. (Sonographic guided aspiration or CT may be necessary.)

Emphysematous Pyelonephritis. Emphysematous pyelonephritis occurs when air is present in the parenchyma (diffuse gas-forming parenchymal infection). It may be caused by *Escherichia coli* bacteria. When this occurs in diabetic patients, they become very sick. It generally is found unilaterally and may be cause for an emergency nephrectomy.

Sonographic Findings. On a sonogram, the enlarged kidneys appear hypoechoic and inflamed (Figure 15-77).

Xanthogranulomatous Pyelonephritis. Xanthogranulomatous pyelonephritis is an uncommon renal disease associated with chronic obstruction and infection. It involves destruction of renal parenchyma and infiltration of lipid-laden histiocytes. Clinically, the patient presents with a large nonfunctioning kidney, staghorn calculus, and multiple infections (Figure 15-78). The disease is more common in females and is poorly understood. It is thought to represent an impaired host response to infection in a chronically obstructed and infected kidney.

Sonographic Findings. The sonographic appearance may show bright echogenicity from the staghorn calculus. (Peripelvic fibrosis can prevent the staghorn from shadowing.) The renal parenchyma is replaced by cystic spaces. Overall renal size is increased. The disease process may be diffuse or segmental.

Urinary Tract Calcifications

Renal Calcifications. Renal calcifications may be seen as localized parenchymal calcifications, resulting from scar

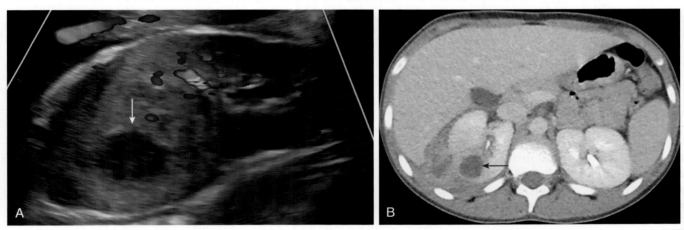

FIGURE 15-76 Renal infection. This patient presented with an elevated white blood cell count and spiking fever. **A,** Supine sagittal scan reveals a homogeneous, slightly irregular mass arising from the upper pole of the right kidney. **B,** CT confirms right renal abscess extending into posterior pararenal space.

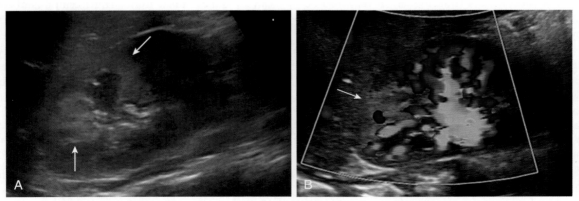

FIGURE 15-77 A, Right upper pole focal pyelonephritis. **B,** Longitudinal view right kidney shows slightly hyperechoic, avascular area consistent with focal pyelonephritis.

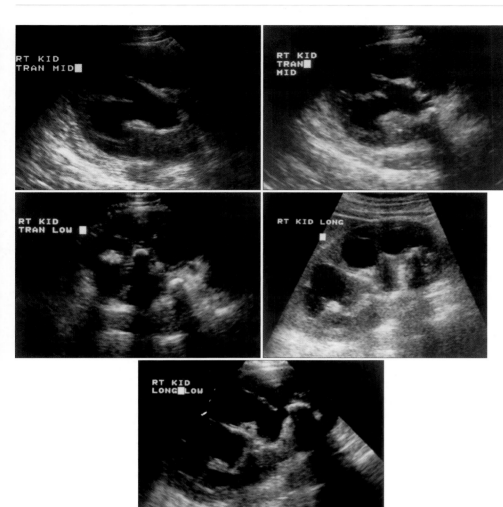

FIGURE 15-78 Patient with xanthogranulomatous pyelonephritis shows a large, nonfunctioning right kidney secondary to a stone. Multiple areas of shadowing are seen within the renal parenchyma from the renal stones.

tissue caused by bacterial infection, renal abscess, infected hematoma, urinoma, lymphocele, tuberculosis, or infarction, or post–percutaneous renal procedures. Malignant solid and/or cystic masses often demonstrate calcifications, but benign renal masses may also calcify. Linear vascular calcifications commonly are associated with renal artery atherosclerosis and/or vascular malformation.

Most of the intraluminal renal calcifications seen on sonography are renal calculi. Milk of calcium cyst and obstructed calyceal diverticulum are rare conditions with suspension of small calcified crystals and/or small stones in layers within the renal cystic structure.

Medullary Sponge Kidney. As was previously discussed, medullary sponge kidney (MSK), or intratubular renal calcification, is a developmental anomaly that occurs in the medullary pyramids and consists of cystic or fusiform dilation of the distal collecting ducts (ducts of Bellini), causing stasis of the urine and stone formation. Because MSK is an anatomic rather than a metabolic defect, the pathologic process may be unilateral or segmental. The cause is unknown. Many patients remain asymptomatic, but patients with hematuria,

infection, and renal stones should be evaluated for MSK. Sonographically, MSK appears as hyperechoic calyces, with or without stones (Figure 15-79).

Nephrocalcinosis. Nephrocalcinosis, or parenchymal calcification, involves diffuse foci of calcium deposits, which

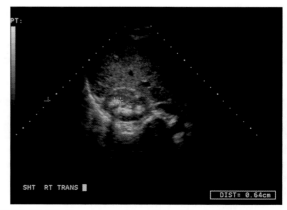

FIGURE 15-79 Transverse view of the right kidney for measuring the renal stone.

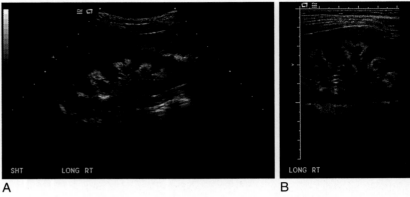

FIGURE 15-80 A and **B,** Longitudinal scans of the right kidney show hyperechoic pyramids, consistent with nephrocalcinosis.

A   B

usually are located in the medulla but infrequently can be seen in the renal cortex. Both kidneys are affected. Calcification may be dystrophic from devitalized tissues, ischemia, and/or necrosis, or from hypercalcemic states, hyperparathyroidism, renal tubular acidosis, and renal failure.

Metastatic nephrocalcinosis is based on location and is classified as cortical or medullary. Cortical nephrocalcinosis is most commonly seen with chronic glomerulonephritis, chronic hypercalcemic states, sickle cell disease, and rejected renal transplants. Medullary nephrocalcinosis occurs more often with disorders such as hyperparathyroidism (40%), renal tubular acidosis (20%), MSK, chronic pyelonephritis, hyperthyroidism, sickle cell disease, and renal papillary necrosis.

Sonographic Findings. Sonographically, cortical nephrocalcinosis appears as increased cortical echogenicity with spared pyramids (Figure 15-80). In cases of medullary nephrocalcinosis, the pyramids become more echogenic than the adjacent cortex. A combination corticomedullary form exists, which shows both renal cortex and medulla as echogenic.

Renal Artery Stenosis

Renal artery stenosis (RAS) is the most common correctable cause of hypertension. Only 1% to 5% of hypertensive patients have a renovascular origin; most patients have essential hypertension. Renovascular hypertension is renin mediated and occurs as a response to renal ischemia, and later as a response to high circulating levels of angiotensin II. The most common causes of renal artery stenosis are atherosclerosis and fibromuscular dysplasia (Box 15-9).

Atherosclerosis is associated with hypertension, which is more common in older patients, and accounts for one third

of cases of RAS. It occurs more frequently in males. Atherosclerosis usually occurs within the first 2 cm of the renal artery, and because this is a generalized process, it may be multifocal, or both renal arteries may be affected.

Fibromuscular dysplasia accounts for approximately two thirds of renal artery stenosis cases and is seen in younger patients. Fibromuscular dysplasia may involve any layer of the renal artery wall and is classified as intimal, medial, or adventitial, creating a smooth stenosis, usually in the midportion of the renal artery. Involvement of the medial layer is seen in the most common subtype of fibromuscular dysplasia, accounting for more than 90% of cases. Medial dysplasia consists of the replacement of smooth muscle by collagen, forming thick ridges and alternating with areas of small aneurysm formation, which results in the classic "string of beads" appearance on arteriography or CT angiography. Fibromuscular dysplasia is most commonly seen in young women. It is progressive and may be seen not only in renal arteries but also in cephalic, visceral, and peripheral arteries.

Sonographic Findings. Selective renal arteriography is the gold standard for visualizing renal artery stenosis. Color Doppler sonography was developed as a noninvasive alternative to detect RAS in hypertensive patients. Direct evaluation of the main renal artery and indirect evaluation via the arcuate and intralobar renal arteries are the two methods used. Accuracy rate depends on operator hand, patient body habitus, and adequacy of the technique.

The most reliable signs for diagnosing RAS using the main renal artery are (1) increased velocity through the stenotic area greater than 150 to 190 cm/sec and (2) turbulence distal to the narrowing. Use of peak systolic velocity has not proved accurate because of overestimation caused by suboptimal angles of incidence. The use of frequency ranges has been shown to be of little value because of the tortuosity of the renal artery, which causes varied frequencies throughout the vessel.

A problem that occurs when the main renal artery is used to evaluate renal blood flow is that more than one renal artery may be found. The main renal artery may have normal blood flow and a stenotic accessory renal artery, causing hypertension. Evaluating the entire course of the main renal arteries is a long and tedious study and one that sonographers and

BOX 15-9	Sonographic Characteristics of Renal Artery Stenosis

Kidney smaller than contralateral side
Absence of early systolic peak
Overall waveform shape: "tardus and parvus" waveform
Delayed systolic rise time: $\Delta T < 0.1$ sec
Peak systolic velocity: PSV > 160/180 cm/sec
Resistive index: RI = $(S - D)/S \geq 0.70$

sonologists try to avoid. Several technical factors (body habitus, tortuosity of the vessel, overlying bowel gas, respiratory motion, and underlying arteriosclerotic disease) may prohibit visualization of the entire length of the renal artery. The proximal portion of the renal arteries may be difficult to evaluate because of cardiac or aortic pulse frequencies.

Evaluating the segmental and intralobar renal vessels is an indirect method of evaluating for RAS. They are easier to see than the main renal artery with the use of convergent color or power color (Figures 15-81 to Figure 15-83). It is very

difficult to obtain a 60-degree angle of the renal vessels. Convergent color and power color are not angle dependent.

Studies have used various Doppler parameters to assist in the evaluation of RAS. The normal intrarenal Doppler signal has a rapid systolic upstroke and an early systolic peak (Figures 15-84 and 15-85). The absence of early systolic peak and a prolonged systolic upstroke or acceleration time, together with decreased peak systole and dampening of the distal waveform, are indications of RAS. The term *tardus-parvus* is used to describe the decreased acceleration time and the decreased peak (Figure 15-86).

Clinical studies with contrast agents are continuing to improve the use of sonography and Doppler for evaluation of renal vascularity. The use of three-dimensional imaging to demonstrate the renal vasculature is also being investigated (Figure 15-87).

Renal Infarction

A renal infarction occurs when part of the tissue undergoes necrosis after cessation of the blood supply, usually as a result of artery occlusion. Renal function is usually normal. This may result from a thrombus, a tumor infiltration, or obstruction, or it may be iatrogenic. (See Table 15-3 for clinical findings,

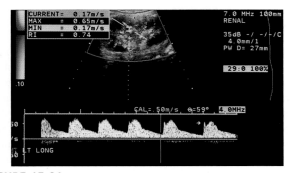

FIGURE 15-81 Normal resistive index (RI) of 0.74 in a 4-year-old female. The *arrow* indicates an early systolic peak.

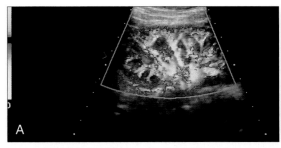 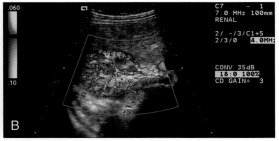

FIGURE 15-82 Longitudinal **(A)** and transverse **(B)** color Doppler of normal intrarenal vessels with vascular flow throughout the renal cortex.

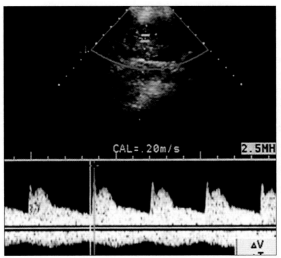

FIGURE 15-83 Normal renal spectral waveform taken at the interlobar arteries.

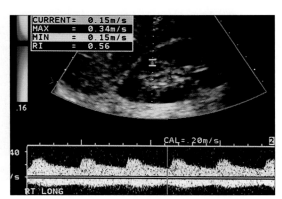

FIGURE 15-84 Normal arcuate vessel Doppler spectral signal. A rapid systolic rise with a resistive index (RI) of 0.56. A gradual decrease into diastole.

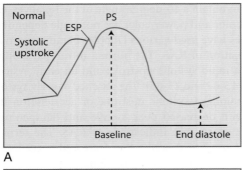

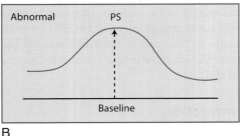

FIGURE 15-85 A, Diagram of a normal renal artery spectral waveform with early systolic peak *(ESP)* and a rapid systolic upstroke followed by peak systole *(PS)* and a gradual decrease into diastole. **B,** Diagram of an abnormal renal artery spectral waveform with absence of early systolic peak and a long systolic upstroke.

sonographic findings, and differential considerations for renal infarction.)

Sonographic Findings. Infarcts within the renal parenchyma appear as irregular areas, somewhat triangular in shape, along the periphery of the renal border. The renal contour may be somewhat "lumpy-bumpy." Remember that lobulations in the pediatric patient may be normal, except for the dromedary hump variant. In the adult patient, the renal contour should be smooth. In a patient with a renal infarct, the irregular area may be slightly more echogenic than the renal parenchyma.

Arteriovenous Fistulas and Pseudoaneurysm

Arteriovenous fistulas (AVFs) are most often acquired rather than congenital. AVFs may be due to renal biopsies, complications from partial nephrectomies, or trauma. Gray-scale sonography shows no abnormalities in the kidney, but color Doppler easily depicts the arteriovenous malformation. The diagnosis is based on detection of a perivascular artifact that reflects local tissue vibration produced by the arteriovenous shunt. Because power Doppler usually demonstrates a larger, artifactual area of uniform color signal that is more pronounced than on conventional color Doppler imaging, it has the potential to facilitate detection of small, low-flow AVF. No

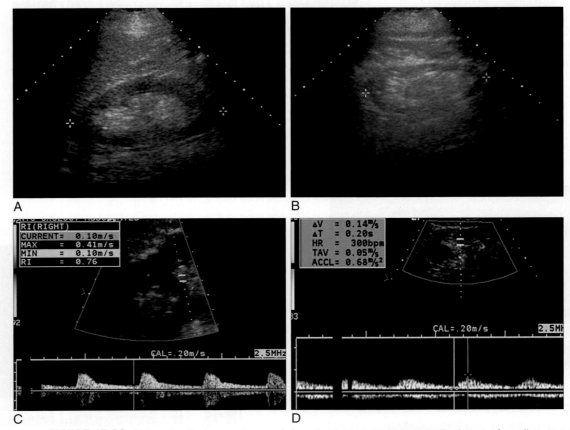

FIGURE 15-86 A, Longitudinal scan of normal size of right kidney. **B,** Longitudinal scan of small (shrunken) left kidney with cortical atrophy. **C,** Normal spectral waveform right kidney. **D,** Parvus-tardus (delayed SRT) left kidney consistent with renal artery stenosis.

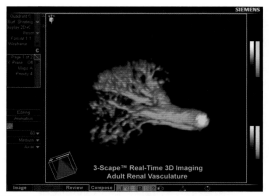

FIGURE 15-87 Adult renal vasculature demonstration using 3-Scape real-time three-dimensional imaging. *(Courtesy Siemens Medical Solutions USA, Inc.)*

abnormalities or small cystic lesions are evident on gray scale. Spectral Doppler shows increased flow velocities, decreased resistive indexes, and arterialization of the draining vein, regardless of the cause of arteriovenous malformation.

Pseudoaneurysm may develop following graft anastomosis, renal biopsy, or intratumoral hemorrhage (angiomyolipomas),

or it may occur after renal surgery (partial nephrectomies) or after trauma; as with AVF, it is very rarely congenital. Color flow Doppler sonographic patterns associated with pseudoaneurysm have been well described in the literature. Sonography shows a round hypoechoic or cystic mass in the renal parenchyma that fills with color signal on color flow Doppler imaging. Spectral analysis performed at the level of the communicating channel shows a typical pattern known as the to-and-fro sign, which signifies both systolic feeding arterial flow and diastolic draining arterial flow—in other words, bidirectional flow occurs (Figures 15-88 and 15-89).

Kidney Stone (Urolithiasis)

A stone located in the urinary system is called **urolithiasis.** Most urinary tract stones are formed in the kidney and course down the urinary tract. Stones consist of a combination of chemicals that precipitate out of urine. The most common chemical found in stones is calcium, along with oxalate or phosphate. Uric acid, cystine, and xanthine can also be found in kidney stones. Kidney stones are one of the most common kidney problems that can occur; they may cause

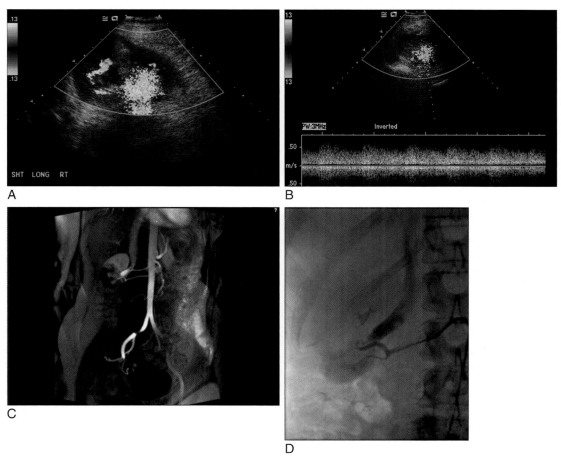

FIGURE 15-88 A, Color duplex Doppler with a pulsating vascular malformation in the right renal hilum. **B,** Arterialization of renal venous flow. **C,** MRI coronal view with simultaneous visualization of the renal artery (aorta) and the inferior vena cava (IVC) consistent with an arteriovenous (AV) fistula. **D,** Renal angiogram shows early visualization of the IVC.

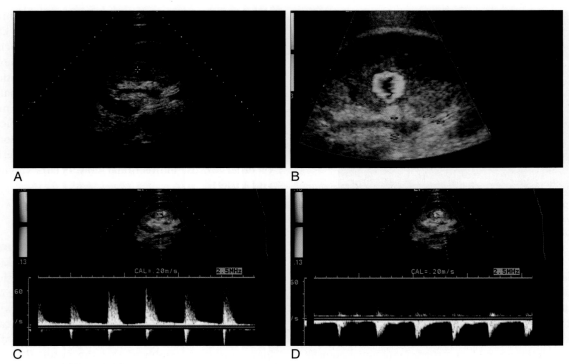

FIGURE 15-89 A, Longitudinal scan of the right kidney 1 week post-ureteroscopic laser treatment for a mid calyx stone with a perinephric fluid collection and a newly discovered 1.8 cm cystic structure. **B,** Color Doppler shows a typical "yin-yang" or swirling appearance consistent with a renal artery pseudoaneurysm. **C** and **D,** Spectral arterial waveform demonstrates clean bidirectional arterial blood flow above and below baseline, consistent with a renal pseudoaneurysm.

obstruction, and this obstruction can be extremely painful. Most kidney stones are small and can travel through the urinary system without treatment or with increased hydration. Stones that are large and fill the renal collecting system are called staghorn calculi. Kidney stones that travel down the urinary system may obstruct the ureter in constricted areas.

The number of people with kidney stones in the United States has increased in the past 20 years. Kidney stones are more common in men. Some people are more likely to form kidney stones than others, and once a kidney stone has formed, the person is at increased risk of getting stones in the future. Kidney stones are associated with renal acidosis (a rare hereditary disorder); people taking the protease inhibitor indinavir are at increased risk for developing kidney stones. The initial clinical sign of a kidney stone is extreme pain, typically followed by cramping on the side on which the stone is located; nausea and vomiting may also occur. The pain may subside while the stone is traveling down the ureter.

Treatment for stones that cause obstruction varies depending on the size and location of the stone. Treatment can include extracorporeal shockwave lithotripsy (ESWL), percutaneous nephrolithotomy, and ureteroscopic stone removal. ESWL uses ultrasound or x-ray to locate the stone, and shockwaves are used to break up the stone into smaller particles, which can readily pass through the urinary system. Percutaneous nephrolithotomy is a surgical procedure in which an opening is made in the kidney, and a nephroscope is used to remove the stone from the kidney. For mid- and lower urinary tract stones, a ureteroscope (which has a basket-like end) can be placed through the urethra and bladder and guided up to the level of the stone to capture and remove the stone. Early treatment of stones that cause obstruction is important to reverse any renal damage that the obstruction may cause.

Sonographic Findings. Renal stones are highly echogenic foci with posterior acoustic shadowing (Figure 15-90). When searching for renal stones, the sonographer should scan along the lines of renal fat; usually, stones smaller than 3 mm may not shadow with the use of traditional B-mode. Prominent renal sinus fat, mesenteric fat, and bowel have high attenuation and may appear as an indistinct echogenic focus with questionable posterior acoustic shadowing, making it difficult to differentiate from stones. The use of tissue harmonics can demonstrate the shadowing of small stones measuring millimeters in size (Figure 15-91). Color and power Doppler have increased the sensitivity of confirming the presence of stones. Color and power Doppler cause a twinkling artifact posterior to the stone. This artifact is referred to as the *twinkling sign* and is imaged as a rapidly changing mixture of red and blue colors posterior to the stone (Figure 15-92). Color and power Doppler are more sensitive when an "all-digital" processing technology is used because of its increased color sensitivity and acoustic power.

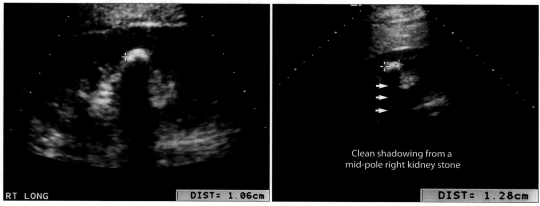

RT LONG   DIST= 1.06cm

Clean shadowing from a
mid-pole right kidney stone

DIST= 1.28cm

FIGURE 15-90   A 69-year-old male presented with right flank pain. A midpole echogenic structure with indicating posterior shadowing *(arrows)*, representative of a renal stone.

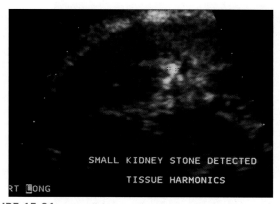

SMALL KIDNEY STONE DETECTED

TISSUE HARMONICS

RT LONG

FIGURE 15-91   A small (3.1 mm) right renal stone detected using tissue harmonics.

If the stone causes obstruction, hydronephrosis will be noted, and depending on the location of the stone, the ureter may be dilated superior to the level of obstruction (Figure 15-93). The ureter—from the ureteropelvic junction to the bladder—is not routinely visualized on a sonogram unless dilated. The superior and distal ends of the ureters are more readily visualized than the midsection. The ureters lie in the retroperitoneal cavity and are obscured by bowel gas. Stones can also be imaged when

the urinary bladder is distended with fluid (Figures 15-94 and 15-95).

Bladder Diverticulum

A bladder diverticulum is a herniation of the bladder wall. These outpouchings may be singular or multiple and are thinner than the normal bladder wall (Figure 15-96). Diverticula can be congenital or acquired. An acquired bladder diverticulum is an outpouching of bladder mucosa between muscle bundles caused by increased intravesical pressure. A diverticulum lacks a muscular layer and has a neck, which usually is narrow. Acquired diverticula are commonly associated with calculi and are more prevalent in patients with chronic bladder outlet obstruction or neurogenic bladder.

Congenital bladder diverticula are rare. They originate at the posterior angle of the bladder trigone and contain all components of the bladder wall.

Sonographic Findings.   The sonographic finding is a neck of varying size connecting the adjacent fluid-filled structure to the bladder. The diverticulum may still be filled with fluid after the patient empties the bladder. Urine stasis leads to recurrent infection and stone formation (Figure 15-97).

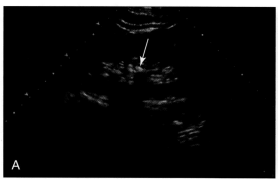
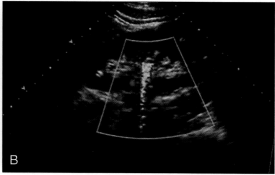

A   B

FIGURE 15-92   **A,** Small stone in the renal sinus *(arrow).* **B,** Color Doppler. A twinkle effect.

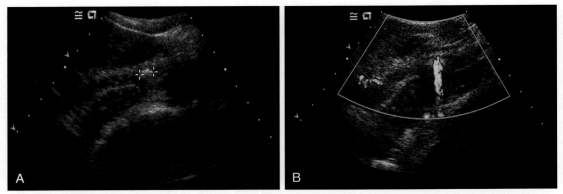

FIGURE 15-93 A, An 8 mm right midpole obstructing ureteral stone. **B,** Color Doppler shows twinkle sign.

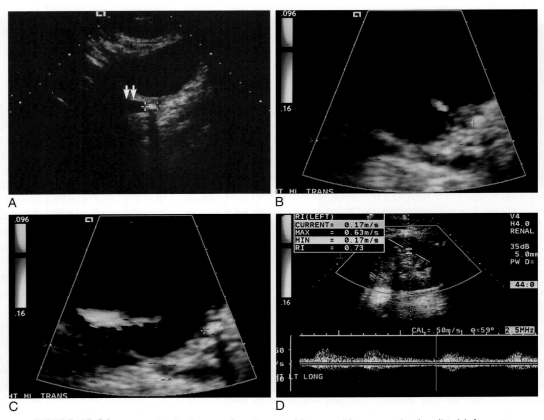

FIGURE 15-94 A, Longitudinal scan of a 65-year-old man with a stone in the distal left ureter *(arrows)*. **B,** Partial obstruction of left ureter with decreased ureteral jet. **C,** Transverse scan of bladder with left ureteral stone measuring 8 mm and normal right ureteral jet. **D,** Increased left intrarenal resistive index (RI) of 0.73.

Bladder Inflammation (Cystitis)

Inflammation of the bladder has several infectious and non-infectious causes. Cystitis is usually secondary to another condition that causes stasis of urine in the bladder. Conditions that cause incomplete emptying of the bladder include urethral stricture, benign and malignant neoplasms, bladder calculi, trauma (blood clot), tuberculosis (lower ureteric strictures), pregnancy, neurogenic bladder, and radiation therapy. Other causes of cystitis include Foley catheter, common rectal or vaginal fistulas, renal disease, sexual intercourse, poor hygiene, diabetes mellitus, and inflammation following surgical intervention.

▌ *Sonographic Findings.* Sonographically, the bladder wall may appear normal in the early stages of inflammatory disease. As the duration of inflammation increases, the smooth bladder wall will become diffuse or nondiffuse with hypoechoic thickening. As the inflammatory process progresses,

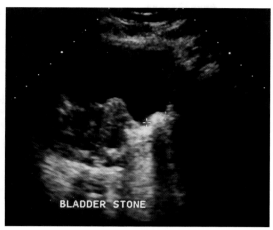

FIGURE 15-95 Transverse scan of the bladder stone with shadowing measuring 1.21 cm.

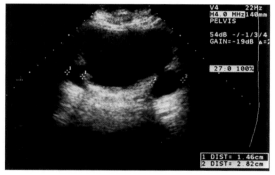

FIGURE 15-96 Transverse scan of two bladder diverticula, one on either side.

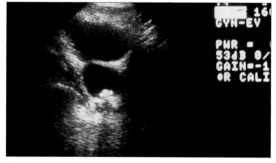

FIGURE 15-97 Transverse scan of the urinary bladder with a stone in the diverticulum.

the bladder wall will become fibrotic and scarred. The bladder wall will appear more echogenic on a sonogram.

Bladder Tumors

Most bladder tumors in adults (95%) are transitional cell carcinoma. Bladder tumors usually are not detected until they have become advanced. Patients usually present with gross hematuria and may also present with dysuria, urinary frequency, or urinary urgency. Sonography cannot distinguish between benign and malignant masses. A cystoscopy or

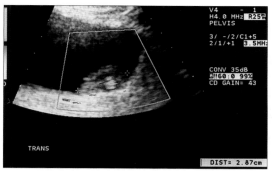

FIGURE 15-98 Carcinoma of the urinary bladder with blood flow seen within the mass.

a biopsy may allow differentiation between a benign and a malignant neoplasm. The bladder may be the secondary site of malignancy. The most common site is the prostate. Invasion of the bladder may result from colon, uterine, or ovarian carcinoma or endometriosis.

 Sonographic Findings. The sonographic appearance of bladder masses varies; they commonly appear as a focal bladder wall thickness. Sonography, CT, or MRI may be used to perform staging of bladder carcinoma. A transabdominal sonographic approach can detect intravesical lesions as small as 3 to 4 mm. Sonography is limited and is unable to detect a perivesical extension and pelvic wall involvement. A transrectal approach can be used to detect intravesicular involvement.

Benign tumors are typically hypoechoic compared with malignant bladder tumors, but they may have the same echogenicity. All primary bladder tumors—squamous cell carcinoma, adenocarcinoma, and rhabdomyosarcoma in children—have the same sonographic appearance: an irregular echogenic mass that projects into the lumen of the bladder. Color Doppler can be used to determine increased vascularity (Figure 15-98). Any bladder mass may cause outflow obstruction, and the kidneys should be evaluated for hydronephrosis.

Key Pearls

- The normal urinary system has two principal functions: excreting wastes and regulating the composition of blood.
- The urinary system is located posterior to the peritoneum lining the abdominal cavity in an area called the retroperitoneum.
- Within the kidney, the upper expanded end of the ureter, known as the renal pelvis of the ureter, divides into two or three major calyces, each of which divides further into two or three minor calyces.
- The renal corpuscle consists of a network of capillaries called the glomerulus, which is surrounded by a cuplike structure known as Bowman's capsule. Blood flows into the glomerulus through a small afferent arteriole and leaves the glomerulus through an efferent arteriole.

Continued

- Three constrictions occur along the ureter's course: (1) where the ureter leaves the renal pelvis, (2) where it is kinked as it crosses the pelvic brim, and (3) where it pierces the bladder wall.
- The renal arteries are lateral branches of the aorta that are located just inferior to the superior mesenteric artery.
- Five to six veins join to form the main renal vein. This vein emerges from the renal hilus anterior to the renal artery.
- Hematuria is the appearance of blood cells in the urine; it can be associated with early renal disease.
- Leukocytes may be present whenever inflammation, infection, or tissue necrosis originates from anywhere in the urinary tract.
- The blood urea nitrogen (BUN) is the concentration of urea nitrogen in blood and is the end product of cellular metabolism.
- The columns of Bertin are prominent invaginations of the cortex located at varying depths within the medullary substance of the kidneys.
- A dromedary hump is a bulge of cortical tissue on the lateral surface of a kidney (usually the left), resembling the hump of a dromedary camel.
- A junctional parenchymal defect is a triangular, echogenic area typically located anteriorly and superiorly.
- Sinus lipomatosis is a condition characterized by deposition of a moderate amount of fat in the renal sinus with parenchymal atrophy.
- Renal hypoplasia is incomplete development of the kidney, usually with fewer than five calyces.
- Incomplete, or partial, duplication is the most frequently occurring congenital anomaly in the neonate. Duplication consists of two collecting systems and two ureters, with a single ureter entering into the urinary bladder.
- Complete duplication is the rare condition of a duplex collecting system. This anomaly results in two separate collecting systems, each with its own ureter that enters the bladder. In cases of double ureter, the ureter from the upper pole of the kidney usually opens below and medial to the one from the lower pole (rule of Weigert-Meyer).
- Renal ectopia (ectopic kidney) describes a kidney that is not located in its usual position, the renal fascia.
- Horseshoe kidney is the most common anomaly of renal fusion. Fusion of the lower poles occurs in 96% of cases, with ureters passing anterior to the renal parenchyma and variation of arterial land venous blood supply.
- A cystic mass sonographically displays several characteristic features: (1) smooth, thin, well-defined border; (2) round or oval shape; (3) sharp interface between the cyst and the renal parenchyma; (4) no internal echoes (anechoic); and (5) increased posterior acoustic enhancement.
- Complex cysts may contain septations, thick walls, calcifications, internal echoes, and mural nodularity.
- Polycystic renal disease may present in one of two forms: the infantile autosomal recessive form and the adult autosomal dominant form.
- Autosomal recessive polycystic kidney disease, also called infantile polycystic disease, is a fairly rare genetic disorder.
- Multicystic dysplastic kidney (MCDK) disease is a common nonhereditary renal dysplasia that usually occurs unilaterally, with the kidney functioning poorly, if at all. MCDK is the most common form of cystic disease in neonates and is believed to be the consequence of early in utero urinary tract obstruction.
- Medullary sponge kidney is a development anomaly that occurs in the medullary pyramids and consists of cystic or fusiform dilation of the distal collecting ducts (ducts of Bellini), causing stasis of urine and stone formation.
- A solid lesion projects as a nongeometric shape with irregular borders, a poorly defined interface between the mass and the kidney, low-level internal echoes, a weak posterior border caused by increased attenuation of the mass, and poor through-transmission.
- Renal cell carcinoma, also called hypernephroma, or Grawitz's tumor, is the most common of all renal neoplasms and represents 85% of all kidney tumors.
- Transitional cell carcinoma accounts for 90% of malignancies that involve the renal pelvis, ureter, and bladder, and for up to 7% to 10% of all renal tumors.
- Metastases to the kidneys are relatively common, occurring late in the course of the disease. Secondary malignancies are bilateral in one third of cases and multiple in more than 50%. The most common primary malignancies that metastasize to the kidneys include carcinoma of the lung or breast and renal cell carcinoma of the contralateral kidney.
- Nephroblastoma, or Wilms' tumor, is the most common abdominal malignancy in children and the most common solid renal tumor in pediatric patients 1 to 8 years old.
- Renal angiomyolipoma is the most common benign renal tumor. It is composed of varying proportions of fat, muscle, and blood vessels.
- A ureterocele is a cystlike enlargement of the lower end of the ureter caused by congenital or acquired stenosis of the distal end of the ureter.
- Different forms of glomerulonephritis, including membranous, idiopathic, membranoproliferative, rapidly progressive, and poststreptococcal, can be associated with abnormal echo patterns from the renal parenchyma on a sonogram.
- Acute interstitial nephritis has been associated with the infectious processes of scarlet fever and diphtheria.
- Systemic lupus erythematosus is a connective tissue disorder believed to result from an abnormal immune system. Females are affected more often than males, and incidence peaks between 20 and 40 years of age.
- Renal involvement is common in patients with sickle cell disease. Abnormalities include glomerulonephritis, renal vein thrombosis, and papillary necrosis.
- Renal papillary necrosis is not a pathologic entity, but rather a descriptive term for a condition—necrosis of the

papillae. The renal papillae (the apex of the renal pyramid that projects into the minor calyx) are vulnerable to ischemic necrosis.

- The excretory and regulatory functions of the kidneys are decreased in acute and chronic renal failure.
- Acute renal failure is a common medical condition that can be caused by numerous medical diseases or pathophysiologic mechanisms.
- Acute tubular necrosis is the most common medical renal disease to produce acute renal failure, although it can be reversible.
- Chronic kidney disease is the loss of renal function as a result of disease, most commonly parenchymal disease. Three primary types of chronic renal failure are known: nephron, vascular, and interstitial abnormalities.
- Hydronephrosis is the separation of renal sinus echoes by interconnected fluid-filled calyces.
- Pyonephrosis occurs when pus is found within the collecting renal system.
- Emphysematous pyelonephritis occurs when air is present in the parenchyma (diffuse gas-forming parenchymal infection).
- Renal calcifications may be seen as localized parenchymal calcifications, resulting from scar tissue caused by bacterial infection, renal abscess, infected hematoma, urinoma, lymphocele, tuberculosis, or infarction, or post–percutaneous renal procedures.
- A renal infarction occurs when part of the tissue undergoes necrosis after cessation of the blood supply, usually as a result of artery occlusion.
- Arteriovenous fistulas (AVFs) are most often acquired rather than congenital. AVFs may be due to renal biopsies, complications from partial nephrectomies, or trauma.
- Kidney stones are one of the most common kidney problems that can occur; they may cause obstruction, and this obstruction can be extremely painful.
- Stones that are large and fill the renal collecting system are called staghorn calculi.
- A bladder diverticulum is a herniation of the bladder wall. These outpouchings may be singular or multiple and are thinner than the normal bladder wall.
- Inflammation of the bladder has several infectious and noninfectious causes. Cystitis is usually secondary to another condition that causes stasis of urine in the bladder.
- Most bladder tumors in adults (95%) are transitional cell carcinoma.

BIBLIOGRAPHY

Abed A, El-Nahas AR, Al-Kandari AM, Shokeir AA: Percutaneous nephrolithotomy (PCNL) in the treatment of stones within horseshoe kidneys and in patients with autosomal dominant polycystic kidney disease. In *Difficult cases in endourology*, London, 2013, Springer, pp. 115-121.

Bajwa ZH, Gupta S, Warfield CA, et al: Pain management in polycystic kidney disease, *Int Soc Nephrol* 60:1631-1644, 2001.

Brun M, Maugey-Laulom B, Eurin D, et al: Prenatal sonographic patterns in autosomal dominant polycystic kidney disease: a multicenter study, *Ultrasound Obstet Gynecol* 24:55-61, 2004.

Buturovic-Ponikvar J, Visnar-Perovic A: Ultrasonography in chronic renal failure, *Eur J Radiol* 46:115-122, 2003,

Cai Y, Lianfang D, Li F, Jiying G: Quantification of enhancement of renal parenchymal masses with contrast-enhanced ultrasound, *Ultrasound Med Biol* 40(7):1387-1393, 2014. doi: http://dx.doi.org/10.1016/j.ultrasmedbio.2014.02.003

Gordon D: Imaging in cystic renal disease, *Arch Dis Child* 83:533, 2000.

Hélénon O, Correas JM, Balleyguier C, et al: Ultrasound of renal tumors, *Euro Radiol* 11:1890-1901, 2001.

Hennerici M, Neuerbrug-Hensler D: *Vascular diagnosis with ultrasound*, New York, 1998, Thieme.

Henningsen C: *Clinical guide to ultrasonography*, St Louis, 2004, Mosby.

Kamaya A, Tuthill T, Rubin J: Twinkling artifact on color Doppler sonography: depending on machine parameters and underlying cause, *Am J Roentgenol* 180:215-222, 2003.

Lee HY, Grant EG: Sonography in renovascular hypertension, *J Ultrasound Med* 21:431-441, 2002.

Lee JY, Kim AH, Cho JY, et al: Color and power Doppler twinkling artifacts from urinary stones, *Am J Roentgenol* 176:1441-1445, 2001.

Lucisano G, Comi N, Pelagi E, et al: Can renal sonography be a reliable diagnostic tool in the assessment of chronic kidney disease? *J Ultrasound Med* 34(2):299-306, 2015. doi: 10.7863/ultra.34.2.299J

Mostbeck GH, Gossinger HD, Mallek R: Effect of heart rate on Doppler measurements of RI in renal arteries, *Radiology* 175:511, 1990.

Nicolau C, Torra R, Bianchi L, et al: Abdominal sonographic study of autosomal dominant polycystic kidney disease, *J Clin Ultrasound* 22:277-282, 2000.

Oei T, Hedgire S, Harisinghan M: Advanced cross-sectional imaging techniques for the detection and characterization of renal masses, *Imaging Med* 3(2):207-218, 2001.

Pepe P, Motta L, Pennisi M, et al: Functional evaluation of the urinary tract by color-Doppler ultrasonography (CDU) in 100 patients with renal colic, *Eur Radiol* 53:131-135, 2005.

Pickerwell D: Elastography: imaging of tomorrow? *J Diagn Medical Sonography*, pp 1-5, May 2010.

Redmond A, McDevitt M, Barnes S: Acute renal failure: recognition and treatment in ward patients, *Nurs Stand* 18:46-55, 2004.

Shokeir AA: Renal colic: new concepts related to pathophysiology, diagnosis and treatment, *Curr Opin Urol* 12:263-269, 2002.

Tempkin B: *Ultrasound scanning: principles and protocols*, ed 3, Philadelphia, 2009, Saunders.

Wolf SJ Jr: State of the art article evaluation and management of solid and cystic renal masses, *J Urol* 159:1120, 1998.

Retroperitoneum*

Sandra Hagen-Ansert

OBJECTIVES

On completion of this chapter, you should be able to:
- Identify the retroperitoneal anatomy
- List the adrenal gland hormones and describe the syndromes associated with hypersecretion and hyposecretion
- Describe the sonographic appearance and clinical findings of adrenal tumors, retroperitoneal fibrosis, and retroperitoneal fluid collections
- Explain the role that sonography plays in the evaluation of para-aortic nodes and describe the sonographic technique used to visualize them

OUTLINE

KEY TERMS

Addison's disease
Adenoma
Adrenocorticotropic hormone (ACTH)
Cortex

Cushing's syndrome
False pelvis
Hyperplasia
Lymphadenopathy

Lymphoma
Medulla
Neuroectodermal tissue
Pheochromocytoma

ANATOMY OF THE RETROPERITONEUM

Normal Anatomy

The retroperitoneal space is the area between the posterior portion of the parietal peritoneum and the posterior abdominal wall muscles (Figure 16-1). It extends from the diaphragm to the pelvis. Laterally, the boundaries extend to the extraperitoneal fat planes within the confines of the transversalis fascia, and medially the space encloses the great vessels. It is subdivided into the following three categories: anterior pararenal space, perirenal space, and posterior pararenal space (Box 16-1).

The perirenal space surrounds the kidney, adrenal, and perirenal fat. The anterior pararenal space includes the duodenum, pancreas, and ascending and transverse colon. The posterior pararenal space includes the iliopsoas muscle, ureter, and branches of the inferior vena cava and aorta and their lymphatics.

The retroperitoneum is protected by the spine, ribs, pelvis, and musculature and has been a difficult area to assess clinically

---

*The author would like to recognize Kerry Weinberg and Shpetim Telegrafi for their contribution to the previous edition of this chapter.

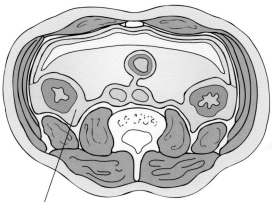

Retroperitoneal space

FIGURE 16-1 Schematic transverse section of the abdominal cavity at the level of the fourth lumbar vertebra. The retroperitoneal space is outlined in blue.

BOX 16-1	Organs in the Retroperitoneal Spaces

Anterior Pararenal Space
- Pancreas
- Duodenal sweep
- Ascending and transverse colon

Perirenal Space
- Adrenal glands
- Kidneys
- Ureter
- Great vessel

Posterior Pararenal Space
- Blood
- Lymph nodes

Iliac Fossa
- Ureter
- Major branches of great vessels
- Lymphatics

Retrofascial Space
Three Compartments
- Psoas
- Lumbar (quadratus lumborum)
- Iliacus

Pathologic processes can stretch from the anterior abdominal wall to the subdiaphragmatic space, mediastinum, and subcutaneous tissues of the back and flank. The retrofascial space, which includes the psoas, quadratus lumborum, and iliacus muscles (muscles posterior to the transversalis fascia), is often the site of extension of retroperitoneal pathologic processes.

Anterior Pararenal Space. The anterior pararenal space is bound anteriorly by the posterior parietal peritoneum and posteriorly by the anterior renal fascia. It is bound laterally by the lateroconal fascia formed by the fusion of the anterior and posterior leaves of the renal fascia. (This space merges with the bare area of the liver by the coronary ligament.) The pancreas, duodenum, and ascending and transverse colon are the structures included in the anterior pararenal space (Figure 16-2).

Perirenal Space. The perirenal space is surrounded by the anterior and posterior layers of the renal fascia (Gerota's fascia), attaching to the diaphragm superiorly. They are united loosely at their inferior margin at the iliac crest level or superior border of the **false pelvis.** Collections in the perinephric space can communicate within the iliac fossa of the retroperitoneum (Figure 16-3).

The lateroconal fascia (the lateral fusion of the renal fascia) proceeds anteriorly as the posterior peritoneum. The posterior renal fasciae fuse medially with the psoas or quadratus lumborum fascia (Figure 16-4). The anterior renal fascia fuses medially with connective tissue surrounding the great vessels. (This space contains the adrenal gland, kidney, and ureter; the great vessels, also within this space, are largely isolated within their connective tissue sheaths—see Figure 16-3.) The perirenal space contains the adrenal gland and kidney (in a variable amount of echogenic perinephric fat, the thickest portion of which is posterior and lateral to the kidney's lower pole). The kidney is anterolateral to the psoas muscle, anterior to the quadratus lumborum muscle, and posteromedial to the ascending and descending colon.

by sonography. Computed tomography (CT) imaging is better to outline the retroperitoneal cavity. Occasionally, however, the sonographer is asked to rule out fluid collection, hematoma, urinoma, or ascitic fluid in the retroperitoneal space.

The retroperitoneum is delineated anteriorly by the posterior peritoneum, posteriorly by the transversalis fascia, and laterally by the lateral borders of the quadratus lumborum muscles and peritoneal leaves of the mesentery. Proceeding from a superior to inferior direction, the retroperitoneum extends from the diaphragm to the pelvic brim. Superior to the pelvic brim the retroperitoneum can be partitioned into the lumbar and iliac fossae. The pararenal and perirenal spaces are included in the lumbar fossa.

Anterior perirenal space

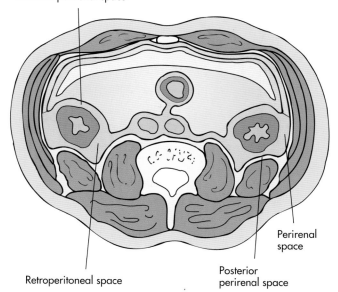

Retroperitoneal space

Posterior perirenal space

Perirenal space

FIGURE 16-2 Transverse drawing of the anterior pararenal space, perirenal space, and posterior perirenal space.

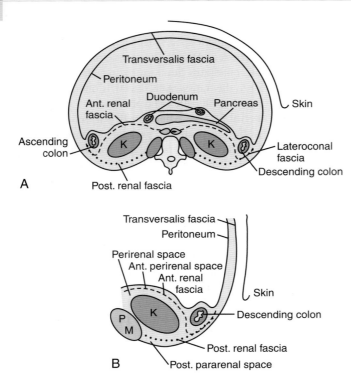

FIGURE 16-3 Retroperitoneal spaces based on the traditional concept of retroperitoneal anatomy. Anterior (dashed lines) and posterior (dotted lines) perirenal fascia join to form lateroconal fascia. These fasciae divide the retroperitoneum into (1) the anterior pararenal space, which contains the duodenum, pancreas, and right and left colon; (2) the perirenal space, which contains the kidney and adrenal gland; and (3) the posterior pararenal space, which contains fat. **A,** Axial section of the pancreas. **B,** Axial section of the left upper quadrant just caudal to the pancreatic tail. The anterior pararenal space is subtended ventrally by the posterior peritoneum and dorsolaterally by the anterior renal fascia and lateroconal fascia. The posterior pararenal space is demarcated ventrally by the posterior perirenal fascia and lateroconal fascia and dorsolaterally by transversalis fascia.

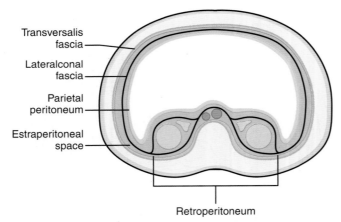

FIGURE 16-4 Illustration of the lateroconal fascia.

The second portion of the duodenum is anterior to the renal hilum on the right. On the left, the kidney is bounded by the stomach anterosuperiorly, the pancreas anteriorly, and the spleen anterolaterally.

Adrenal Glands. In the adult patient the adrenal glands are anterior, medial, and superior to the kidneys (Figure 16-5). The right adrenal is more superior to the kidney, whereas the left

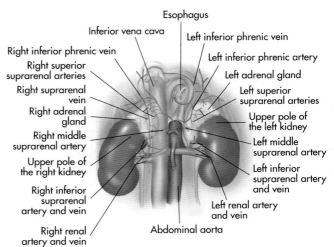

FIGURE 16-5 The adrenal glands are retroperitoneal organs that lie on the upper pole of each kidney. They are surrounded by perinephric fat. The right adrenal gland is triangular and caps the upper pole of the right kidney. It extends medially behind the inferior vena cava and rests posteriorly on the diaphragm. The left adrenal gland is semilunar and extends along the medial borders of the left kidney. It lies posterior to the pancreas, the lesser sac, and the stomach and rests posteriorly on the diaphragm.

adrenal is more medial to the kidney. The medial portion of the right adrenal gland is immediately posterior to the inferior vena cava (above the level of the portal vein and lateral to the crus). The lateral portion of the gland is posterior and medial to the right lobe of the liver and posterior to the duodenum.

The left adrenal gland is lateral or slightly posterolateral to the aorta and lateral to the crus of the diaphragm. The superior portion is posterior to the lesser omental space and posterior to the stomach. The inferior portion is posterior to the pancreas. The splenic vein and artery pass between the pancreas and the left adrenal gland.

The adrenal glands vary in size, shape, and configuration; the right adrenal is triangular and caps the upper pole of the right kidney. The left adrenal is semilunar in shape and extends along the medial border of the left kidney from the upper pole to the hilus. The internal texture is medium in consistency; the cortex and medulla are not distinguished.

The adrenal gland is a distinct hypoechoic structure; sometimes highly echogenic fat is seen surrounding the gland. The normal size is usually smaller than 3 cm.

Neonatal Adrenal. The neonatal adrenal glands are characterized by a thin echogenic core surrounded by a thick transonic zone. This thick rim of transonicity represents the hypertrophied adrenal cortex, whereas the echogenic core is the adrenal medulla. An infant adrenal gland is proportionally larger than an adult adrenal gland (one third the size of the kidney; in adults it is one thirteenth the size) (Figure 16-6).

Diaphragmatic Crura. The diaphragmatic crura begins as tendinous fibers from the lumbar vertebral bodies, disks, and transverse processes of L3 on the right and L1 on the left (Figure 16-7). The right crus is longer, larger, and more lobular and is associated with the anterior aspect of the lumbar vertebral ligament. The right renal artery crosses anterior to the crus and posterior to the inferior vena cava at the level of

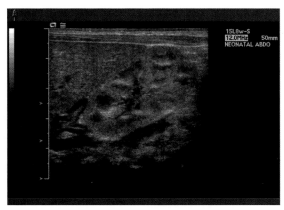

FIGURE 16-6 Neonatal right kidney and adrenal gland.

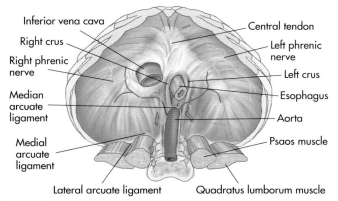

FIGURE 16-7 The crura of the diaphragm begin as tendinous fibers from the lumbar vertebral bodies, disks, and transverse processes of L3 on the right and L1 on the left.

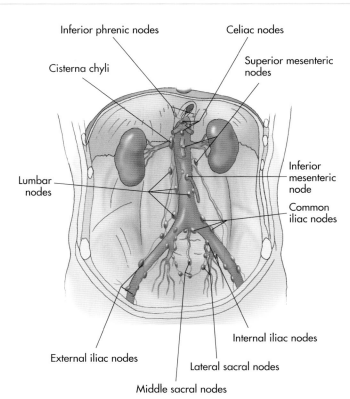

FIGURE 16-8 Lymphatic chain along the aorta and iliac artery.

the right kidney. The right crus is bounded by the inferior vena cava anterolaterally and the right adrenal and right lobe of liver posterolaterally.

The left crus courses along the anterior lumbar vertebral bodies in a superior direction and inserts into the central tendon of the diaphragm.

Para-aortic Lymph Nodes. There are two major lymph-node-bearing areas in the retroperitoneal cavity: the iliac and hypogastric nodes within the pelvis and the para-aortic group in the upper retroperitoneum. The lymphatic chain follows the course of the thoracic aorta, abdominal aorta, and iliac arteries (Figure 16-8). Common sites are the para-aortic and paracaval areas near the great vessels, peripancreatic area, renal hilar area, and mesenteric region. Normal nodes are smaller than the tip of a finger, less than 1 cm, and are not imaged on a sonogram. However, if these nodes enlarge because of infection or tumor, they can be seen on a sonogram.

Posterior Pararenal Space. The posterior pararenal space is located between the posterior renal fascia and the transversalis fascia. It communicates with the peritoneal fat, lateral to the lateroconal fascia. The posterior pararenal space merges inferiorly with the anterior pararenal space and retroperitoneal tissues of the iliac fossa (see Figure 16-4).

The psoas muscle, the fascia of which merges with the posterior transversalis fascia, makes up the medial border of this posterior space. This space is open laterally and inferiorly. The

blood and lymph nodes embedded in fat may be found in the posterior pararenal space.

Iliac Fossa. The iliac fossa is the region extending between the internal surface of the iliac wings, from the crest to the iliopectineal line. This area is known as the false pelvis and contains the ureter and major branches of the distal great vessels and their lymphatics. The transversalis fascia extends into the iliac fossa as the iliac fascia.

Retrofascial Space. The retrofascial space is made up of the posterior abdominal wall, muscles, nerves, lymphatics, and areolar tissue behind the transversalis fascia. It is divided into the following three compartments:

1. The psoas compartment: a muscle that spans from the mediastinum to the thigh (Figure 16-9). The fascia attaches to the pelvic brim.
2. The lumbar region consists of the quadratus lumborum, a muscle that originates from the iliolumbar ligament, the adjacent iliac crest, and the superior borders of the transverse process of L3 and L4, and inserts into the margin of the twelfth rib (Figure 16-10). It is adjoining and posterior to the colon, kidney, and psoas muscle.
3. The iliac area, which is made up of the iliacus and extends the length of the iliac fossa. The psoas passes through the iliac fossa medial to the iliacus and posterior to the iliac fascia (see Figure 16-9). These two muscles merge as they extend into the true pelvis. The iliopsoas takes on a more anterior location caudally to lie along the lateral pelvic side wall.

Pelvic Retroperitoneum. The pelvic retroperitoneum lies between the sacrum and pubis from back to front, between the pelvic peritoneal reflection above and pelvic diaphragm (coccygeus and levator ani muscles) below, and between the

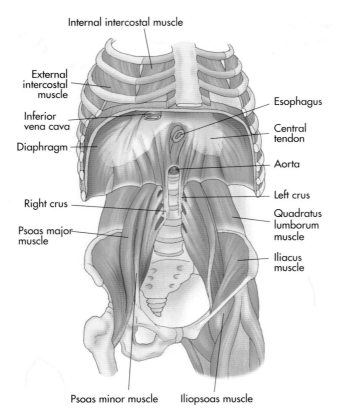

FIGURE 16-9 The psoas muscle extends from the mediastinum to the thigh.

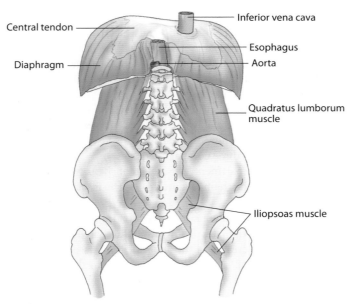

FIGURE 16-10 The quadratus lumborum muscle originates from the iliolumbar ligament, the adjacent iliac crest, and the superior borders of the transverse process of L3 and L4 and inserts into the margins of the twelfth rib.

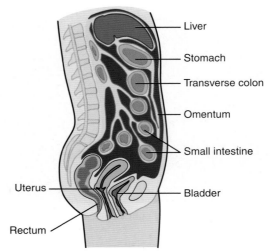

FIGURE 16-11 The pelvic retroperitoneum lies between the sacrum and pubis from back to front, between the pelvic peritoneal reflection above and pelvic diaphragm (coccygeus and levator ani muscles) below, and between the obturator internus and piriformis muscles.

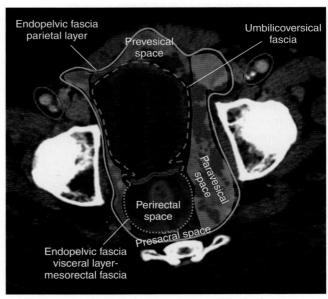

FIGURE 16-12 The prevesical space extends from the pubis to the anterior margin of the bladder. It is bordered by the obturator fascia on its lateral margins. The space between the bladder and rectum is the rectovesical space.

obturator internus and piriformis muscles (Figure 16-11). There are four subdivisions: (1) prevesical, (2) rectovesical, (3) presacral, and (4) bilateral pararectal (and paravesical) spaces.

Prevesical and Rectovesical Spaces. The prevesical space spans from the pubis to the anterior margin of the bladder. It is bordered laterally by the obturator fascia. The connective tissue covering the bladder, seminal vesicles, and prostate is continuous with the fascial lamina within this space. The space is an extension of the retroperitoneal space of the anterior abdominal wall deep to the rectus sheath, which is continuous with the transversalis fascia. The space between the bladder and rectum is the rectovesical space (Figure 16-12).

Presacral Space. The presacral space lies between the rectum and fascia covering the sacrum and posterior pelvic floor musculature.

Bilateral Pararectal Space. The pararectal space is bounded laterally by the piriformis and levator ani fascia and medially by the rectum. It extends anteriorly from the bladder, medially to

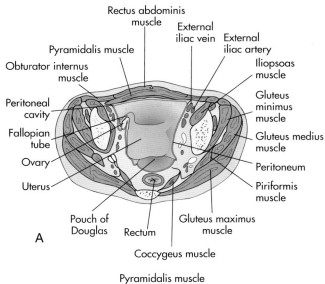

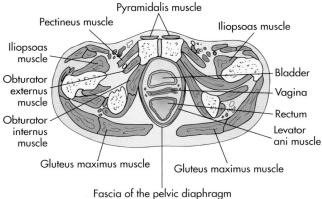

FIGURE 16-13 A, The pararectal space is bounded laterally by the piriformis and levator ani fascia and medially by the rectum. **B,** The pararectal space extends anteriorly from the bladder, medially to the obturator internus, and laterally to the external iliac vessels.

the obturator internus, and laterally to the external iliac vessels (Figure 16-13).

The paravesical and pararectal spaces are traversed by the two ureters. The pelvic wall muscles, iliac vessels, ureter, bladder, prostate, seminal vesicles, and cervix are retroperitoneal structures within the true pelvis. The obturator internus muscle lines the lateral aspect of the pelvis. Posteriorly the piriformis muscle is seen extending anterolaterally from the region of the sacrum.

Vascular Supply

Aorta. The aorta enters the abdomen posterior to the diaphragm at the level of L1 and passes posterior to the left lobe of the liver. The aorta has a straight horizontal course to the level of L4, where it bifurcates into the common iliac arteries. A slight anterior curve of the aorta is the result of lumbar lordosis.
Inferior Vena Cava. The inferior vena cava extends from the junction of the two common iliac veins to the right of L5 and travels cephalad. Unlike the aorta, it curves anterior toward its termination into the right atrial cavity.

Adrenal Glands. Three arteries supply each adrenal gland: the suprarenal branch of the inferior phrenic artery, the suprarenal branch of the aorta, and the suprarenal branch of the renal artery. A single vein from the hilum of each gland drains into the inferior vena cava on the right, and on the left the vein drains into the left renal vein.

PHYSIOLOGY AND LABORATORY DATA OF THE RETROPERITONEUM

Each adrenal gland is made up of two endocrine glands. The **cortex,** or outer part, secretes a range of steroid hormones; the **medulla,** or core, secretes epinephrine and norepinephrine.

Cortex

The steroids secreted by the adrenal cortex fall into the following three main categories: mineralocorticoids, glucocorticoids, and sex hormones (androgen and estrogen).
Mineralocorticoids. Mineralocorticoids regulate electrolyte metabolism. Aldosterone is the principal mineralocorticoid. It has a regulatory effect on the relative concentrations of mineral ions in the body fluids and therefore on the water content of tissue. An insufficiency of this steroid leads to increased excretion of sodium and chloride ions, and water into the urine. This is accompanied by a fall in sodium, chloride, and bicarbonate concentrations in the blood, resulting in a lowered pH or acidosis.
Glucocorticoids. Glucocorticoids play a principal role in carbohydrate metabolism. They promote deposition of liver glycogen from proteins and inhibit use of glucose by the cells, thus increasing blood sugar level. Cortisone and hydrocortisone are the primary glucocorticoids. They diminish allergic response, especially the more serious inflammatory types (rheumatoid arthritis and rheumatic fever).
Sex Hormones. Androgens are the male sex hormones, and estrogens are the female sex hormones. The adrenal gland secretes both types of hormones regardless of the patient's gender. Normally these are secreted in minute quantities and have almost insignificant effects. With oversecretion, however, a marked effect is seen. Adrenal tumors in women can promote secondary masculine characteristics. Hypersecretion of the hormone in prepubertal boys accelerates adult masculine development and the growth of pubic hair. The adrenal cortex is controlled by **adrenocorticotropic hormone (ACTH)** from the pituitary. A diminished glucocorticoid blood concentration stimulates the secretion of ACTH. Consequent increase in adrenal cortex activity inhibits further ACTH secretion.

Hypofunction of the adrenal cortex in humans is called **Addison's disease.** Symptoms and signs include hypotension, general weakness, fatigue, loss of appetite and weight, and a characteristic bronzing of the skin (hyperpigmentation).

Oversecretion of the adrenal cortex may be caused by an overproduction of ACTH resulting from a pituitary tumor, **hyperplasia,** or a tumor in the cortex itself. Hypersecretion of the cortical hormones produces distinct syndromes. The features of the syndromes often overlap and can be either acquired or congenital. Adrenal hyperfunction can cause Cushing's syndrome, Conn's syndrome, or adrenogenital syndrome (see Adrenal Pathology).

Medulla

The adrenal medulla makes up the core of the gland in which groups of irregular cells are located amid veins that collect blood from the sinusoids. The adrenal medulla produces epinephrine and norepinephrine. Both of these hormones are amines, sometimes referred to as catecholamines. They elevate the blood pressure, the former working as an accelerator of the heart rate and the latter as a vasoconstrictor. The two hormones together promote glycogenolysis, the breakdown of liver glycogen to glucose, which causes an increase in blood sugar concentration.

The adrenal medulla is not essential for life and can be removed surgically without causing untreatable damage. An increase in the production of the medulla hormones may be caused by a **pheochromocytoma.**

SONOGRAPHIC EVALUATION OF THE RETROPERITONEUM

No specific patient preparation is necessary to image the retroperitoneal cavity, although 6 to 8 hours of fasting may help to eliminate bowel gas. To image the retroperitoneum, scans should be made in the longitudinal and transverse planes from the diaphragm to the iliac crest, with the patient in a supine, decubitus, or prone position, and from the crest to the symphysis, with the patient in a supine position and having a full bladder. The upper abdomen may also be scanned with the patient in a decubitus position. All scans should include the kidneys and retroperitoneal muscles.

Adrenal Glands

Although sonography has proven useful in evaluating soft tissue structures within the abdominal cavity, visualization of the adrenal glands has been difficult because of their small size, medial location, and surrounding perirenal fat. Sonography is not the imaging modality of choice for evaluation of an adrenal mass. If the adrenal gland becomes enlarged secondary to disease, it is easier to image and separate from the upper pole of the kidney.

Visualization of the adrenal area depends on several factors: the size of the patient and the amount of perirenal fat surrounding the adrenal area, the presence of bowel gas, and the ability to move the patient into multiple positions.

With the patient in the decubitus position, the sonographer should attempt to align the kidney and ipsilateral paravertebral vessels (inferior vena cava or aorta). The right adrenal gland has a "comma" or triangular shape in the transaxial plane (Figure 16-14). The best visualization is obtained by a transverse scan with the patient in a left lateral decubitus position. When the patient assumes this position, the inferior vena cava moves forward, and the aorta rolls over the crus of the diaphragm, offering a good window to image the upper pole of the right kidney and adrenal gland. If the patient is obese, it may be difficult to recognize the triangular- or crescent-shaped adrenal gland. The adrenal should not appear rounded; if it does, the finding suggests a pathologic process.

The longitudinal scan is made through the right lobe of the liver, perpendicular to the linear right crus of the diaphragm. The retroperitoneal fat must be recognized as separate from the liver, crus of the diaphragm, adrenal gland, and great vessel (Figure 16-15).

The left adrenal gland is closely related to the left crus of the diaphragm and the anterior-superior-medial aspect of the upper pole of the left kidney. It may be more difficult to image the left adrenal gland because of the stomach gas interference. The patient should be placed in a right lateral decubitus position and transverse scans made in an attempt to align the left kidney and the aorta. The left adrenal gland is seen by scanning along the posterior axillary line (Figure 16-16). The patient should be in deep inspiration in an effort to bring the adrenal and renal area into better view.

Sonography Pitfalls

- Right crus of the diaphragm
- Second portion of the duodenum

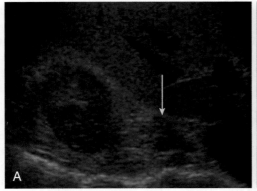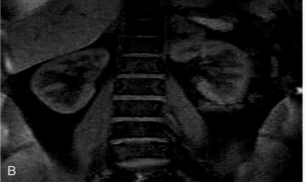

FIGURE 16-14 A, The right adrenal gland has a "comma" or triangular shape in the transaxial plane. **B,** CT coronal image of the left adrenal gland.

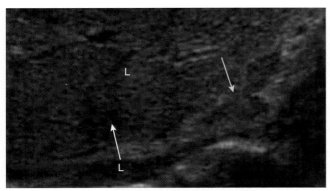

FIGURE 16-15 Longitudinal scan of the right adrenal gland is made through the right lobe of the liver *(L)*, adrenal gland *(arrow)*.

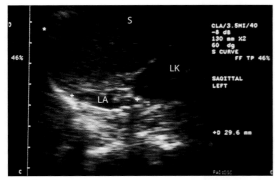

FIGURE 16-16 Longitudinal scan of the left adrenal gland *(LA)* and the anterior superior aspect of the upper pole of the left kidney *(LK)* and spleen *(S)*.

- Gastroesophageal junction (cephalad to the left adrenal gland)
- Medial lobulations of the spleen
- Splenic vasculature
- Body-tail region of the pancreas
- Fourth portion of the duodenum

The normal right adrenal gland can be visualized in more than 90% of patients, and the left is seen in 80% of patients.

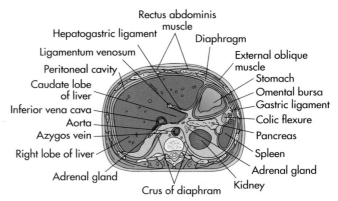

FIGURE 16-17 The right crus of the diaphragm passes posterior to the inferior vena cava, and the left crus passes anterior to the aorta.

Diaphragmatic Crura

The crus of the diaphragm may be imaged in the transverse or longitudinal coronal plane. The right crus is seen in a plane that passes through the right lobe of the liver, kidney, and adrenal gland (Figure 16-17). The left crus is seen using the spleen and left kidney as a window, with the crus to the left of the aorta.

Para-aortic Lymph Nodes

Sonography patterns associated with nodes include rounded, focal, echo-poor lesions (1 to 3 cm in size and larger), and confluent, echo-poor masses, which often displace the kidney laterally. The sonographer may also detect a "mantle" of nodes in the paraspinal location, a "floating" or anteriorly displaced aorta secondary to the enlarged nodes, or the mesenteric "sandwich" sign representing the anterior and posterior node masses surrounding mesenteric vessels (Figures 16-18 to 16-21).

The lymph nodes lie along the lateral and anterior margins of the aorta and inferior vena cava (Figure 16-22); thus the best scanning is done with the patient in the supine or decubitus position. A left coronal view using the left kidney as a window may be used to discover para-aortic nodes. It is always important to examine the patient in two planes because

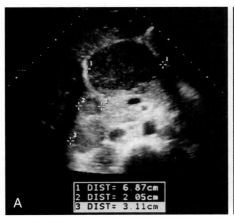

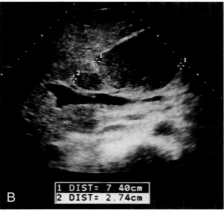

FIGURE 16-18 **A,** A 39-year-old female with lymphoma. Three nodes were seen peripancreatic *(crossbars): 1,* anterior to the pancreas; *2,* lateral to the pancreas head; and *3,* paracaval. **B,** Two nodes paraportal *(crossbars): 1,* anterior and compressing the main portal vein; and *2,* a smaller, sonolucent homogeneous node.

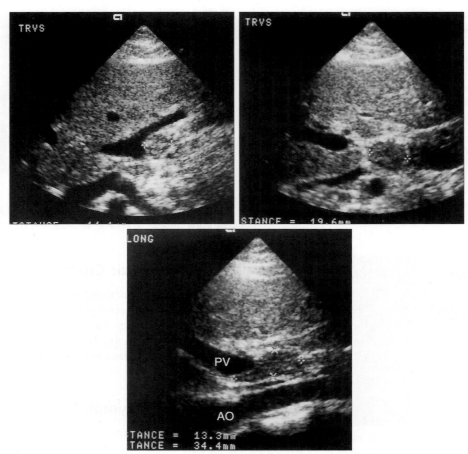

FIGURE 16-19 A 32-year-old female with right upper quadrant pain and fever. Two paracaval nodes were seen anterior to the aorta *(AO)* and inferior to the portal vein *(PV)*.

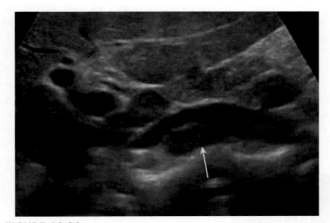

FIGURE 16-20 Longitudinal view of the aorta *(Ao)* surrounded by prominent lymph nodes.

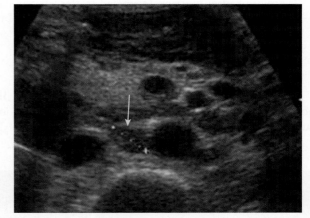

FIGURE 16-21 Transverse view of the great vessels and enlarged lymph node *(arrow)*.

in only one plane the enlarged nodes may mimic an aortic aneurysm or tumor.

Longitudinal scans may be made first to outline the aorta and to search for enlarged lymph nodes. The aorta provides an excellent background for the hypoechoic nodes. Scans should begin at the midline, and the transducer should be angled both to the left and right at small angles to image the anterior and lateral borders of the aorta and inferior vena cava.

Transverse scans are made from the level of the xiphoid to the symphysis. Careful identification of the great vessels, organ structures, and muscles is important. Patterns of a fluid-filled duodenum or bowel may make it difficult to outline the great vessels or may cause confusion in diagnosing **lymphadenopathy.**

Scans below the umbilicus are more difficult because of interference from the small bowel. Careful attention should be given to the psoas and iliacus muscles within the pelvis

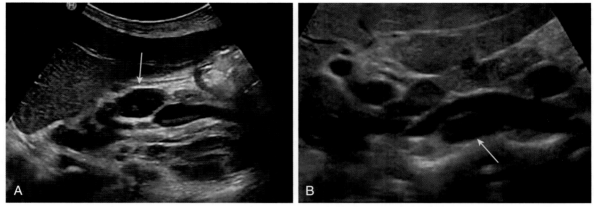

FIGURE 16-22 A, Transverse view of the enlarged lymph node *(arrow)* adjacent to the splenic vein. **B,** Longitudinal view of the lymph nodes lifting the abdominal aorta.

where the iliac arteries run along their medial border. Both muscles serve as a hypoechoic marker along the pelvic side wall. Enlarged lymph nodes can be identified anterior and medial to these margins. A smooth sharp border of the muscle indicates no nodal involvement. The bladder should be filled to help push the small bowel out of the pelvis and to serve as an acoustic window to better image the vascular structures. Color Doppler may be used to help delineate the vascular structures.

Splenomegaly should also be evaluated in patients with lymphadenopathy. As the sonographer moves caudal from the xiphoid, attention should be on the splenic size and great vessel area to detect nodal involvement near the hilus of the spleen (Figure 16-23 and 16-24).

Lymph nodes remain as consistent patterns, whereas bowel and the duodenum display changing peristaltic patterns when imaged with a sonogram. As gentle pressure is applied with the transducer in an effort to displace the bowel, the lymph nodes remain constant in shape. The echo pattern posterior to each structure is different. Lymph nodes are homogeneous and thus transmit sound easily; the bowel presents a more complex pattern with dense central echoes

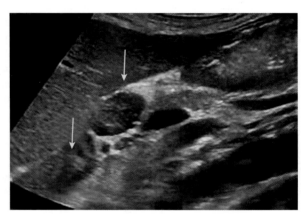

FIGURE 16-23 Transverse view of the aorta with large para-aortic nodes.

from its mucosal pattern. Often the duodenum has air within its walls, causing a shadow posteriorly. Enlarged lymph nodes should be reproducible on a sonogram in two projections. After the abdomen is completely scanned, repeat sections over the enlarged nodes should demonstrate the same pattern as on the earlier scan.

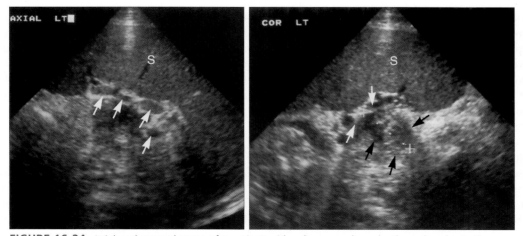

FIGURE 16-24 Axial and coronal scans of a patient with splenomegaly and enlarged nodes in the area of the splenic hilus. Color flow imaging should be used to document that the lesions are nodes and not dilated vascular structures. *Arrows,* nodes; *S,* spleen.

PATHOLOGY OF THE RETROPERITONEUM

Adrenal Cortical Syndromes

The cortical syndromes that the sonographer may encounter while scanning for an adrenal mass are as follows:

- *Addison's disease (adrenocortical insufficiency).* Affects males and females equally and can be diagnosed in any age-group. It is characterized by atrophy of the adrenal cortex with decreased production of cortisol and sometimes aldosterone. Usually the majority of the cortical tissue is destroyed before adrenal insufficiency is diagnosed. Primary causes of reduced adrenal cortical tissue include an autoimmune process, tuberculosis, an inflammatory process, a primary neoplasm, or metastases. Secondary adrenal insufficiencies are caused by pituitary dysfunction and a decrease in production of the pituitary hormone ACTH. The clinical signs and symptoms usually manifest during metabolic stress or trauma. Symptoms include increased sodium retention, which leads to tissue edema; increased plasma volume; increased potassium excretion; hyperpigmentation; and a mild alkalosis. Fatigue and muscle and bone weakness are common. Prognosis is good with steroid replacement therapy.
- *Adrenogenital syndrome (adrenal virilism).* Results from the excessive secretion of the sex hormones and adrenal androgens. It is caused either by an adrenal tumor or by hyperplasia. The symptoms and clinical signs vary depending on the age and sex of the person. In a newborn there may be ambiguous genitalia with or without adrenal hyperplasia. (Things other than adrenal hyperplasia can also cause ambiguous genitalia.) Adrenal virilism has masculinizing effects on adult women. The clinical signs and symptoms in a female adult include hirsutism, baldness, and acne; deepening of the voice; atrophy of the uterus; decreased breast size; clitoral hypertrophy; and increased muscularity. Prepubescent males will have signs of masculine development, deepening voice, and an increase in body hair. The imaging modalities of choice to confirm the presence or absence of an adrenal tumor are CT and magnetic resonance imaging (MRI).
- *Conn's syndrome (aldosteronism).* Conn's syndrome occurs in 0.5% of patients with sustained hypertension and is caused by excessive secretion of aldosterone, usually because of a cortical **adenoma** of the glomerulosa cells or less frequent causes, including adrenal hyperplasia or adrenal carcinoma. Hyperplasia is more common in males and adrenal adenomas are more common in females. Adenomas measure 0.5 to 3 cm in diameter and contralateral adrenal atrophy is identified. Clinical signs and symptoms include muscle weakness, hypertension, and abnormal electrocardiogram. If an adenoma is causing the hyperaldosteronism, removal of the adenoma is performed. In rare cases a bilateral adrenalectomy is necessary. In cases of secondary aldosteronism, the hypertension may be caused by renal artery disease.
- *Cushing's syndrome.* **Cushing's syndrome** is caused by excessive secretion of cortisol resulting from adrenal hyperplasia, cortical adenoma, adrenal carcinoma, or elevated ACTH resulting from a pituitary adenoma. Cushing's syndrome symptoms include truncal obesity, "pencil-thin" extremities, "buffalo hump," "moon face," hypertension, renal stones, irregular menses in females, and psychiatric disturbances. If an adrenal tumor is present, the secretion of androgens may increase and cause masculinizing effects in women. Cushing's syndrome can also be caused by an anterior pituitary tumor. Treatment to decrease the production of cortisol varies depending on the cause of the hypersecretion. If an adrenalectomy is performed, the patient will require replacement steroids for life. Functioning adrenal adenomas are usually small (2 to 5 cm) and hypoechoic. They typically are associated with contralateral adrenal atrophy.
- *Waterhouse-Friderichsen syndrome.* With Waterhouse-Friderichsen syndrome there is a fulminant bacterial sepsis, shock, and necropsy with evidence of bilateral adrenal hemorrhage that is complicated with acute adrenocortical insufficiency in up to 25% of severely traumatized patients. Adrenal hemorrhage may occur 20% bilateral, which most often is caused by severe meningococcal infection. It is characterized by acute adrenal gland insufficiency, which is fatal if not treated immediately. With sonography, depending on the stage of hemorrhage, the echo pattern can range from a hyperechoic to an anechoic suprarenal mass. Subsequently, over a period of time, the mass may shrink, and calcifications may appear as focal hyperechoic areas with acoustic shadowing (Table 16-1).

Adrenal Cysts

Adrenal cysts are uncommon lesions that produce no clinical symptoms when the lesion is small. The cysts affect females more often than males (3:1). Adrenal cysts are usually unilateral and tend to be found incidentally. They may vary in size and can be unilocular or multilocular.

Sonographic Findings. Sonographically, adrenal cysts present a typical cystic pattern, with a strong posterior wall, no internal echoes, and good through-transmission. Adrenal cysts have the tendency to become calcified, which gives them the sonographic appearance of a somewhat sonolucent solid mass appearing with a sharp posterior border and poor through-transmission (Figure 16-25). Hemorrhage within the cyst would appear as a complex mass with multiple internal echoes and good through-transmission.

Adrenal Hemorrhage

Adrenal hemorrhage in adults is rare and is usually caused by severe trauma or infection. Posttraumatic hemorrhage is usually unilateral and does not cause any major clinical problems. A bilateral hemorrhage may cause adrenal insufficiency. Adrenal hemorrhages are more common in neonates who experienced a traumatic delivery with stress, asphyxia, and

TABLE 16-1	Adrenal Pathology	
Adrenal Diseases	Hormone Secreted	Distinguishing Characteristics
Addison's disease	Hyposecretion of cortisol, aldosterone	Increases when there is stress or trauma Hypotension, general weakness, loss of appetite, hyperpigmentation (bronzing of skin), may have renal failure
Adrenogenital syndrome	Excessive secretion of androgens (male) Excessive secretion of estrogen (female)	Prepubertal males accelerate adult masculine development and growth of pubic hair Female: masculine characteristics
Conn's syndrome	Excessive secretion of aldosterone	Cortical adenoma, carcinoma
Cushing's syndrome	Excessive secretion of glucocorticoids	Hyperplasia, benign tumor, carcinoma
Waterhouse-Friderichsen syndrome		Bilateral hemorrhage into adrenal glands
Medulla tumor Pheochromocytoma	Excessive secretion of epinephrine and norepinephrine	Intermittent hypertension; large tumor with varied sonographic pattern (cystic, solid, calcified components)

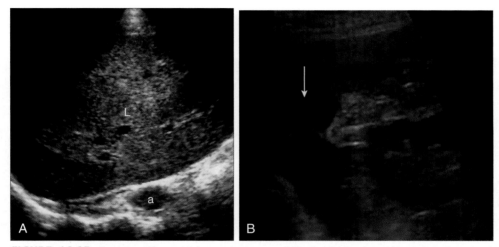

FIGURE 16-25 **A,** Adrenal cysts *(a)* may become calcified, which gives them the ultrasound appearance of a "solid" mass with decreased transmission. *L,* liver. **B,** Small adrenal cyst *(arrow)* adjacent to the kidney.

septicemia. The adrenal glands in a neonate are very vascular and the glands are proportionally larger than in an adult. Clinical signs and symptoms include abdominal mass, anemia, and hyperbilirubinemia.

Sonographic Findings. The sonographic appearance of an adrenal hemorrhage will vary depending on the age of the hemorrhage. The adrenal gland will appear as a solid mass initially, and over time the mass will have a more cystic or complex appearance. As the hemorrhage resolves, the mass will decrease in size. The adrenal gland may go back to a normal size with focal areas of calcification (Figure 16-26).

Adrenal Tumors

Sonography can detect 90% of known adrenal masses that were first detected by CT. Sonography is used to characterize a known adrenal mass as cystic or solid, evaluate the position and patency of the inferior vena cava and draining veins, evaluate tumor invasion into adjacent structures, and determine the origin of a large retroperitoneal mass. Sonography is also used to follow an adrenal mass that is not surgically removed.

Adrenal Adenoma. Benign nonfunctioning adenoma is the most common primary adrenal tumor. Adrenal nodules are usually less than 2.5 cm. There is a high incidence of adrenal adenomas in older patients with diabetes or hypertension. A significant percentage of the malignant adrenal adenomas may be due to metastases.

Sonographic Findings. In nonfunctioning adenomas, sonographic findings demonstrate a well-defined, round, slightly hypoechoic homogeneous mass (Figure 16-27). Almost always the mass is detected as an incidental finding. On rare occasions the mass may be so large that it may compress the adjacent structures.

Further pathology of the adrenal glands is related to the tumors arising within them and their hyposecretion or hypersecretion of hormones. Rare nonfunctional adrenal tumors include myelolipomas, hemangiomas, teratomas, lipomas, and fibromas. These tumors are typically not seen on a sonogram and are more frequently imaged with CT or MRI.

Adrenal Malignant Tumors. Primary adrenal carcinomas are rare and may be hyperfunctional or nonfunctional. Hyperfunctional malignant tumors are more common in females.

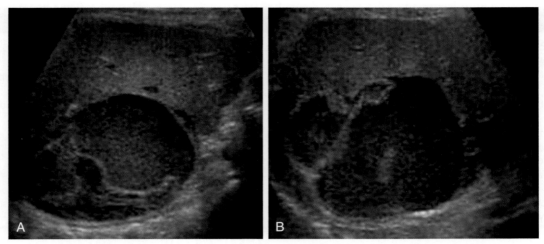

FIGURE 16-26 The sonographic appearance of an adrenal hemorrhage will vary depending on the age of the hemorrhage. The adrenal gland will appear as a solid mass initially, and over time the mass will have a more cystic or complex appearance.

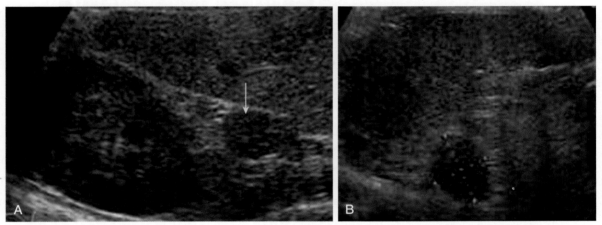

FIGURE 16-27 In nonfunctioning adenomas, sonographic findings demonstrate a well-defined, round, slightly hypoechoic homogeneous mass.

Adrenal malignant tumors may be a cause of Cushing's syndrome, Conn's syndrome, or adrenogenital syndrome. The origin of the tumor should be clearly defined. Functional tumors tend to be smaller than nonfunctional tumors because they are typically diagnosed earlier. The tumors are homogeneous with the same echogenicity as the renal cortex. The larger neoplasms tend to be nonfunctional and heterogeneous, with a central area of necrosis and hemorrhage.

Sonographic Findings. If the mass is small (2 to 6 cm), it is well defined and homogeneous. If the mass is larger, it tends to have necrosis with central hemorrhage and often calcifies. In color Doppler, the tumor is hypervascular with a high incidence of invasion of the adrenal or renal vein, inferior vena cava, hepatic veins, and lymph nodes (Figure 16-28). The sonographic appearance of a mass cannot be used to differentiate between a benign or malignant tumor, as this is a histologic diagnosis.

Metastasis. Adrenals glands are the fourth most common site in the body for metastasis, after the lungs, the liver, and the bones. Primarily there are metastases from

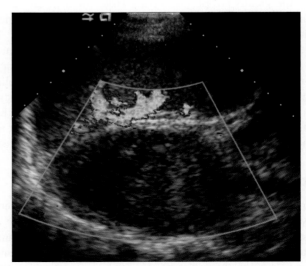

FIGURE 16-28 A coronal scan through the spleen with a large left malignant adrenal mass compressing the splenic hilum. *(Courtesy Robert DeJong, RDMS, RVT, FSDMS.)*

lung in 33% and breast carcinomas in 30%, followed by melanoma, gastric carcinoma, colon, kidney, and thyroid. Bilateral involvement is seen in more than half of the patients. Metastases to the adrenal gland typically cause adrenal insufficiency.

Sonographic Findings. Adrenal glands vary in size and echogenicity. Metastatic lesions have a nonspecific appearance. Large masses may contain areas of necrosis and hemorrhage. Sometimes differentiation of a common benign adenoma from a metastatic lesion is difficult when there is no other evidence of metastatic disease and the adrenal mass is unilateral (Figure 16-29). Often central necrosis causes sonolucent areas within the tumor.

Adrenal Medulla Tumors

Pheochromocytoma. The pheochromocytes of the adrenal medulla may produce a tumor called a pheochromocytoma, which secretes epinephrine and norepinephrine in excessive quantities. A small percentage of patients will have ectopic adrenal pheochromocytomas rising from the **neuroectodermal tissue**; these tumors tend to be malignant. The clinical symptoms include intermittent hypertension, severe headaches, heart palpitations, and excess perspiration. Treatment usually is removal of the tumor.

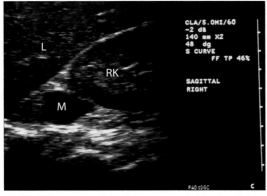

FIGURE 16-29 Patient with a large mass *(M)* in the right adrenal gland representing metastases from a melanoma. *L,* liver; *M,* mass; *RK,* right kidney.

Sonographic Findings. The tumor has a homogeneous pattern that can be differentiated from a cyst by its weak posterior wall and poor through-transmission (Figure 16-30). Pheochromocytomas are usually unilateral and may be large, bulky tumors with a variety of sonographic patterns, including cystic, solid, and calcified components.

Adrenal Neuroblastoma. The adrenal neuroblastoma is the most common malignancy of the adrenal glands in childhood and the most common tumor of infancy, representing 30% of all neonatal tumors. Neuroblastoma is a well-encapsulated tumor that usually displaces the kidney inferiorly and laterally and elevates the levels of vanillylmandelic acid and homovanillic acid. More than 90% of fetal neuroblastomas are located in the adrenal glands, and 50% of these have cystic components. Generally, the tumor develops within the adrenal medulla. Although children are usually asymptomatic, some do present with a palpable abdominal mass that must be differentiated from a neonatal hemorrhage and hydronephrosis. It is known to be one of the most common tumors of childhood. Spontaneous regression is common before age 1. Otherwise it has a poor prognosis and is not responsive to either irradiation or chemotherapy.

Sonographic Findings Lesions generally are heterogeneously echogenic with poorly defined margins. A small percentage of neuroblastomas demonstrate internal calcifications with anechoic "cystic" areas. The "ultrasound lobule" (an area of increased echogenicity in the tumor) seems to be characteristic for neuroblastomas. The use of color Doppler may be helpful in demonstrating capsular flow and low-resistance arterial waveforms (Figure 16-31). Evaluation of the surrounding retroperitoneum and liver should be made to rule out metastases. When a large, solid, upper abdominal mass is identified in an infant or young child, the differential diagnosis should include neuroblastoma, Wilms' tumor (nephroblastoma), and hepatoblastoma.

Retroperitoneal Fat

The anatomic origin of the right upper quadrant mass may be difficult to determine. The reflection produced by the retroperitoneal fat is displaced in a characteristic manner by masses originating from this area. This pattern of displacement helps

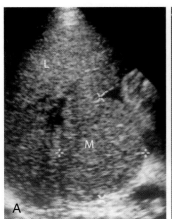
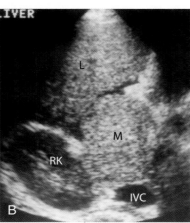

FIGURE 16-30 The pheochromocytoma is a homogeneous tumor that has a weak posterior wall and decreased through-transmission. This tumor can grow quite large. **A,** Longitudinal view. *L,* liver; *M,* mass. **B,** Transverse view. *IVC,* inferior vena cava; *M,* mass; *RK,* right kidney.

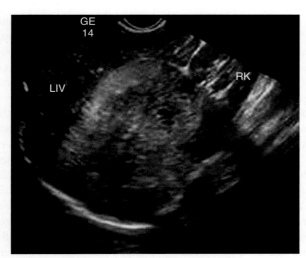

FIGURE 16-31 A small percentage of neuroblastomas demonstrate internal calcifications with anechoic "cystic" areas. The "ultrasound lobule" (an area of increased echogenicity in the tumor) seems to be characteristic for neuroblastomas.

to localize the origin of the mass. Retroperitoneal lesions cause ventral and often cranial displacement of the lesion.

Sonographic Findings The lesions in the liver or in Morison's pouch displace the echoes posterior and inferior, whereas renal and adrenal lesions cause anterior displacement of structures. An extrahepatic mass may shift the inferior vena cava anteromedially (anterior displacement of right kidney).

Primary Retroperitoneal Tumors

A primary retroperitoneal tumor (PRT) is one that originates independently within the retroperitoneal space. Primary malignancies are more common than benign neoplasms, but both are rare.

Lymphoma is the most common PRT. Sonographic evaluation for abdominal lymphoma is performed to determine the presence or absence of lymphadenopathy and the primary areas to be evaluated include the hepatic and splenic hilum, origin of celiac and superior mesenteric artery (peripancreatic, mesenteric), para-aortic, and renal hilar areas. Accuracy of sonographic detection is close to 90% when the lymph nodes are larger than 2 cm in diameter. The sonographic appearance varies from round, hypoechoic masses to anechoic masses with good posterior enhancement. Color Doppler shows increased intranodal vascularity. The primary criteria for differentiating a malignant from a benign lymph node are size greater than 2 cm; shape, round; and resistive index (RI) greater than 0.70 (Figure 16-32).

The other PRT can develop anywhere, with most tumors proving to be malignant. The tumor is derived either from mesenchymal or neurogenic tissues. Mesenchymal tumors develop within connective tissues of the retroperitoneum, and most fat-containing tumors are liposarcomas, which is the third most common malignant tumor of soft tissues. More than one third of the tumors originate from perirenal fat, including malignant fibrous histiocytomas, fibrosarcomas, and desmoid tumors. All of these tumors are nonspecific by sonography.

Neurogenic tumors are usually encountered in the paravertebral region, where they rise from nerve roots or sympathetic chain ganglia. They extend into the retroperitoneum and may be classified as benign or malignant tumors. The sonographic patterns of neurogenic tumors are quite variable.

Tumors of Muscle Origin. Leiomyosarcoma is the second most common PRT. This tumor may originate from smooth muscles of small blood vessels or within the gastrointestinal tract and extend into the retroperitoneum. On sonography leiomyosarcomas generally present as a large complex mass with areas of necrosis and cystic degeneration.

Fibrosarcomas and rhabdomyosarcomas may be quite invasive and may infiltrate widely into muscles and adjoining soft tissue. They often extend across the midline and appear similar to lymphomas. Sonographically, they are highly reflective tumors.

Germ Cell Tumors. Germ cell tumors can be either benign or malignant and the retroperitoneal space is the fourth most

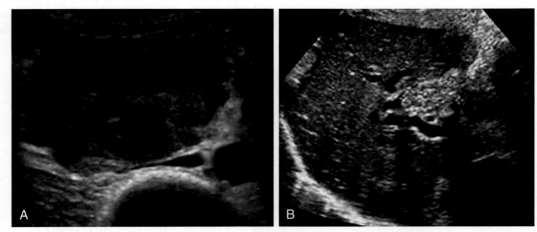

FIGURE 16-32 Sonographic evaluation for abdominal lymphoma is performed to determine the presence or absence of lymphadenopathy. The primary areas to be evaluated include the hepatic and splenic hilum, origin of celiac and superior mesenteric artery (peripancreatic, mesenteric), para-aortic, and renal hilar areas.

frequent site (ovaries, testes, anterior mediastinum, retro-peritoneum, and sacrococcygeal region). Teratomatous tumors may arise within the upper retroperitoneum and the pelvis. They may contain calcified echoes from bones, cartilage, teeth, and soft tissue elements (Figure 16-33).

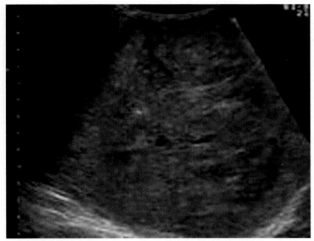

FIGURE 16-33 Teratomatous tumors may arise within the upper retroperitoneum and the pelvis. They may contain calcified echoes from bones, cartilage, teeth, and soft tissue elements.

Teratomas are seen more commonly in childhood and are usually located in the upper pole of the left kidney. Sonographically they are heterogeneous tumors with solid areas, calcifications, and cystic spaces.

Secondary Retroperitoneal Tumors

Metastatic disease may occur anywhere in the retroperitoneum, secondary to hematogenous or lymphatic spread, or by direct extension. The most common primary malignancies that spread into the retroperitoneum are from the breast, lung, testis, or the recurrence of previously resected urologic or gynecologic tumor.

Ascitic fluid, along with a retroperitoneal tumor, usually indicates seeding or invasion of the peritoneal surface. Evaluation of the para-aortic region should be made for extension to the lymph nodes (Figure 16-34). The liver should also be evaluated for metastatic involvement.

Retroperitoneal Fluid Collections

Urinoma. A urinoma is a walled-off collection of extravasated urine that develops spontaneously after trauma, surgery, or a subacute or chronic urinary obstruction.

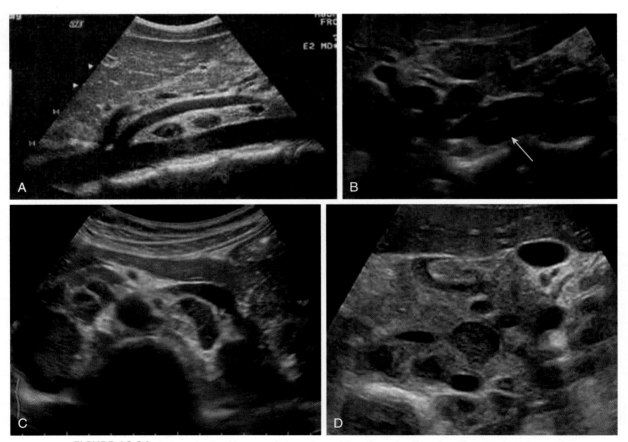

FIGURE 16-34 A, Longitudinal image of the enlarged lymph nodes elevating the superior mesenteric artery. **B,** Longitudinal image of the "sandwich sign" or mantle sign as the enlarged nodes surround the aorta, elevating its position away from the spine. **C** and **D,** Transverse images of the enlarged nodes surrounding the great vessels.

Urinomas usually collect around the kidney or upper ureter in the perinephric space. Occasionally urinomas dissect into the pelvis and compress the bladder.

■ *Sonographic Findings.* Generally the sonographic pattern of urinomas is sonolucent unless they become infected.

Hemorrhage. A retroperitoneal hemorrhage may occur in a variety of conditions, including trauma, vasculitis, bleeding diathesis, a leaking aortic aneurysm, or a bleeding neoplasm.

■ *Sonographic Findings.* Sonographically the hemorrhage may be well localized and produce displacement of other organs, or it may present as a poorly defined infiltrative process. Fresh hematomas present as sonolucent areas, whereas an organized thrombus with clot formation shows echo densities within the mass (Figure 16-35). Calcification may be seen in long-standing hematomas.

Abscess. Abscess formation may result from surgery, trauma, or perforation of the bowel or duodenum.

■ *Sonographic Findings.* Sonographically the abscess usually has a complex pattern with debris. Gas within the abscess causes a "reflective" pattern on sonography and casts an acoustic shadow. The sonographer should be careful not to mistake a gas-containing abscess for "bowel" patterns. The radiograph should be evaluated in this case. The abscess frequently extends along or within the muscle planes, is of an irregular shape, and lies in the most dependent portion of the retroperitoneal space.

Retroperitoneal Fibrosis (Ormond's Disease)

Retroperitoneal fibrosis (RPF) is an idiopathic condition characterized by thick sheets of fibrous tissue in the retroperitoneal cavity. The fibrosis may encase and obstruct the ureters and vena cava, with resultant hydronephrosis. RPF can be also associated with infiltrating neoplasms, acute immune diseases (e.g., Crohn's disease), ulcerative colitis, sclerosing cholangitis, and so on. Clinically the patient may present with abdominal pain, hypertension, and oligo-anuria. Radiographically an intravenous pyelogram shows medial displacement and bilateral (one third are

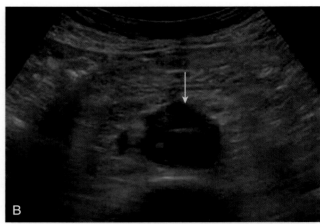

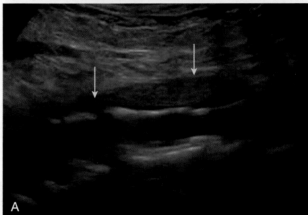

FIGURE 16-36 Retroperitoneal fibrosis is an idiopathic condition characterized by thick sheets of fibrous tissue in the retroperitoneal cavity. Sonography may demonstrate abnormal hypoechoic tissue surrounding the anterolateral aspect of the aorta or inferior vena cava.

unilateral) hydronephrosis. Sonography may demonstrate abnormal hypoechoic tissue surrounding the anterolateral aspect of the aorta or inferior vena cava (Figure 16-36). Sonography may also be useful to evaluate the kidneys, as well as fibrosis regression in response to steroids. Further imaging with CT may be necessary to establish whether there is a benign or malignant disease process.

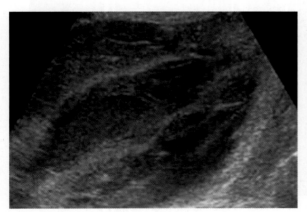

FIGURE 16-35 Fresh hematomas present as sonolucent areas, whereas an organized thrombus with clot formation shows echo densities within the mass.

Key Pearls

- The retroperitoneal space is the area between the posterior portion of the parietal peritoneum and the posterior abdominal wall muscles. It extends from the diaphragm to the pelvis.
- Laterally, the boundaries extend to the extraperitoneal fat planes within the confines of the transversalis fascia, and medially the space encloses the great vessels.
- It is subdivided into the following three categories: anterior pararenal space, perirenal space, and posterior pararenal space.

- The perirenal space surrounds the kidney, adrenal, and perirenal fat.
- The anterior pararenal space includes the duodenum, pancreas, and ascending and transverse colon.
- The posterior pararenal space includes the iliopsoas muscle, ureter, and branches of the inferior vena cava and aorta and their lymphatics.
- The right adrenal is more superior to the kidney, whereas the left adrenal is more medial to the kidney.
- There are two major lymph-node-bearing areas in the retroperitoneal cavity: the iliac and hypogastric nodes within the pelvis and the para-aortic group in the upper retroperitoneum.
- The retrofascial space is made up of the posterior abdominal wall, muscles, nerves, lymphatics, and areolar tissue behind the transversalis fascia.
- The pelvic retroperitoneum lies between the sacrum and pubis from back to front, between the pelvic peritoneal reflection above and pelvic diaphragm (coccygeus and levator ani muscles) below, and between the obturator internus and piriformis muscles.
- The prevesical space spans from the pubis to the anterior margin of the bladder. It is bordered laterally by the obturator fascia.
- The presacral space lies between the rectum and fascia covering the sacrum and posterior pelvic floor musculature.
- The pararectal space is bounded laterally by the piriformis and levator ani fascia and medially by the rectum. It extends anteriorly from the bladder, medially to the obturator internus, and laterally to the external iliac vessels.
- Sonography patterns associated with nodes include rounded, focal, echo-poor lesions (1 to 3 cm in size and larger), and confluent, echo-poor masses, which often displace the kidney laterally.
- The sonographer may also detect a "mantle" of nodes in the paraspinal location, a "floating" or anteriorly displaced aorta secondary to the enlarged nodes, or the mesenteric "sandwich" sign representing the anterior and posterior node masses surrounding mesenteric vessels.
- Adrenal hemorrhages are more common in neonates who experienced a traumatic delivery with stress, asphyxia, and septicemia.
- Benign nonfunctioning adenoma is the most common primary adrenal tumor.
- Adrenals glands are the fourth most common site in the body for metastasis, after the lungs, the liver, and the bones.
- The pheochromocytes of the adrenal medulla may produce a tumor called a pheochromocytoma, which secretes epinephrine and norepinephrine in excessive quantities.
- The adrenal neuroblastoma is the most common malignancy of the adrenal glands in childhood and the most common tumor of infancy, representing 30% of all neonatal tumors.
- Lymphoma is the most common primary retroperitoneal tumor.
- Metastatic disease may occur anywhere in the retroperitoneum, secondary to hematogenous or lymphatic spread, or by direct extension.
- A urinoma is a walled-off collection of extravasated urine that develops spontaneously after trauma, surgery, or a subacute or chronic urinary obstruction.
- A retroperitoneal hemorrhage may occur in a variety of conditions, including trauma, vasculitis, bleeding diathesis, a leaking aortic aneurysm, or a bleeding neoplasm.
- Retroperitoneal fibrosis is an idiopathic condition characterized by thick sheets of fibrous tissue in the retroperitoneal cavity.

BIBLIOGRAPHY

Abdu A, KrissV, Bada H: Adrenal hemorrhage in a newborn, *Am J Perinatal* 26:553-557, 2009.

Beer MH, Berkow R: *The Merck manual,* ed 17, Whitehouse Station, NJ, 1999, Merck Research Laboratories.

Choyke PL, Glenn G, Walther M: Von Hippel-Lindau disease: genetic, clinical and imaging features, *Radiology* 194:629, 1996.

Dalrymple NC, John R, Leyendecker JR, Oliphant M: *Problem solving in abdominal imaging,* St Louis, 2009, Mosby Elsevier, pp. 464-566.

Dunnick NR, Korobkin M, Francis I: Adrenal radiology: distinguishing benign from malignant adrenal masses, *Am J Roentgenol* 167:861, 1996.

Heinz-Peer G, Memarsadeght M, Niederle B: Imaging of adrenal masses, *Curr Opin Urol* 17:32-38, 2007.

Henningsen C: *Clinical guide to ultrasonography,* St Louis, 2004, Mosby.

Hsu CW, Ho C, Sheu W: Adrenal insufficiency caused by primary aggressive non-Hodgkin's lymphoma of bilateral adrenal glands: report of a case and literature review, *Ann Hematol* 78:151, 1999.

Krebs C, Rawls K: Techniques for successful scanning: positioning strategy for optimal visualization of a left adrenal mass, *J Diag Med Sonogr* 5:286, 1990.

Little AF: Adrenal gland and renal sonography, *World J Surg* 24:171, 2000.

Mittelstaedt CA: *General ultrasound,* New York, 1992, Churchill Livingstone.

Rosenblatt GS, Takesita K, Fuch G, et al: Adrenal metastasis with inferior vena cava tumor thrombus through adrenal vein, *Clin Urol* 74:290-291, 2009.

Rumack CM, Wilson SR, Charbonneau JW, et al: *Diagnostic ultrasound,* ed 3, vol 1, St Louis, 2005, Mosby, pp 425-489.

Sivit CJ, Hung W, Taylor G: Sonography in neonatal congenital adrenal hyperplasia, *Am J Roentgenol* 156:141, 1991.

Suzuki Y, Sasagawa S, Suzuki H, et al: The role of ultrasonography in the detection of adrenal masses: comparison with computed tomography and magnetic resonance imaging, *Int Urol Nephrol* 32:303-306, 2001.

Udelsman R, Fishman EK: Radiology of the adrenal, *Endocrinol Metab Clin North Am* 29(1):27-42, viii, 2000.

Abdominal Applications of Ultrasound Contrast Agents

Daniel A. Merton

OBJECTIVES

On completion of this chapter, you should be able to:
- List the current limitations of ultrasound imaging that may be overcome by the use of ultrasound contrast agents
- Describe the properties that an ultrasound contrast agent must have to be clinically accepted
- Describe the difference between tissue-specific ultrasound contrast agents and vascular agents
- Describe how contrast harmonic imaging improves the clinical capabilities of ultrasound contrast agents
- Describe the hepatic applications of contrast agents

OUTLINE

Types of Ultrasound Contrast Agents
　　Vascular Ultrasound Contrast Agents
　　Tissue-Specific Ultrasound Contrast Agents

Ultrasound Equipment Modifications
Clinical Applications
　　Hepatic Applications
　　Renal Applications
　　Splenic Applications

Pancreatic Applications
Organ Transplants
Other Applications
Conclusion

KEY TERMS

Acoustic emission
Contrast-enhanced sonography (CES)
Harmonic imaging (HI)
Induced acoustic emission

Mechanical index (MI)
Molecular imaging agents
Tissue-specific ultrasound contrast agent

Ultrasound contrast agents (UCAs)
Vascular ultrasound contrast agents

Since the 1980s, a significant amount of research has been conducted toward the development of **ultrasound contrast agents (UCAs)**.[61] Most of the work has centered on developing agents that can be administered intravenously to evaluate blood vessels, blood flow, tumors, and solid organs.

The clinical utilization of **contrast-enhanced sonography (CES)** has been shown to reduce or eliminate some of the current limitations of ultrasound (US) imaging and Doppler blood flow detection. These include limitations of spatial and contrast resolution on gray-scale US and the detection of low-velocity blood flow and flow in very small vessels using Doppler flow detection modes, including color flow imaging and pulsed-wave Doppler with spectral analysis. Advances in US equipment technology following the development of UCAs have resulted in contrast-specific imaging modes, including gray-scale US methods that allow detection and display of blood flow without the limitations of Doppler US. The use of CES is growing

around the world and there are published clinical guidelines describe the most appropriate use of CES for a variety of abdominal, retroperitoneal, and other applications.[30] Ultrasound contrast agents are increasingly being used to improve the sensitivity and specificity of US diagnoses and are expanding sonography's already broad range of clinical applications.

TYPES OF ULTRASOUND CONTRAST AGENTS

Vascular Ultrasound Contrast Agents

Sonographic detection of blood flow is limited by factors including the depth and size of a vessel, the attenuation properties of intervening tissue, or low-velocity flow. Limitations of US equipment sensitivity and the operator dependence of Doppler US are also factors that may affect the results of a vascular examination. Vascular or blood-pool UCAs enhance Doppler (color and spectral) flow signals by adding more and better acoustic scatterers to the bloodstream (Figures 17-1 and 17-2). The use of these UCAs improves the color flow imaging detection of blood flow from vessels that are often difficult to assess without their use, such as the renal arteries, intracranial vessels, and small capillaries within organs (i.e., tissue perfusion) (Figure 17-3). In addition to enhancing Doppler signals, **vascular ultrasound contrast agents** also improve gray-scale US visualization of flowing blood and demonstrate changes to the gray-scale echogenicity of tissues with the use of contrast-specific imaging software such as contrast harmonic imaging (CHI).

The concept of a UCA was first introduced by Gramiak and Shah in 1968, who, in their initial work, injected agitated saline directly into the ascending aorta and cardiac chambers during echocardiographic examinations.[27] The microbubbles formed by agitation resulted in strong reflections arising

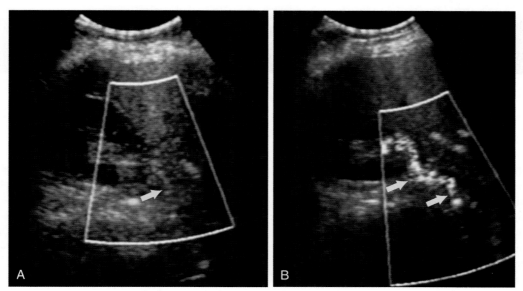

FIGURE 17-1 Color Doppler imaging of a patient's right renal artery before **(A)** and after **(B)** administration of a vascular UCA. Note the increased visualization of flow in the renal artery *(arrows)* after intravenous injection of contrast. In this case no vascular abnormality was detected.

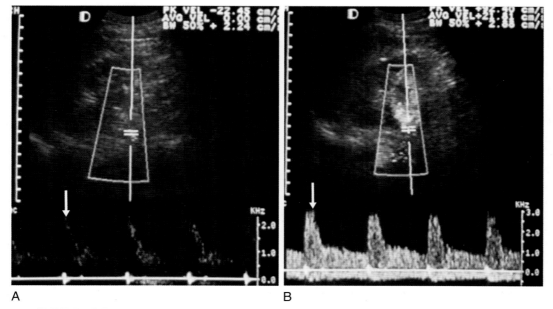

FIGURE 17-2 Color flow imaging and spectral Doppler analysis of renal artery flow. **A,** Before contrast, the spectral waveforms are weak and there is minimal color flow information. **B,** After intravenous administration of a contrast, the spectral wave forms have a higher signal intensity and additional color flow information is provided.

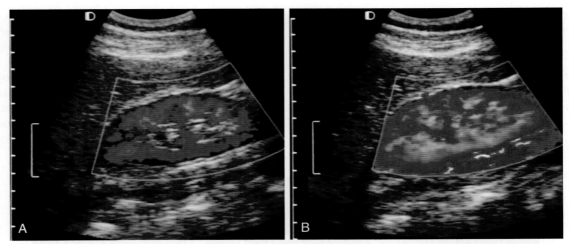

FIGURE 17-3 Power Doppler imaging of a normal right kidney before **(A)** and after **(B)** injection of a vascular UCA. Note the improved demonstration of flow in the renal parenchyma after intravenous injection of contrast.

from within the normally echo-free lumen of the aorta and chambers of the heart. Eventually other solutions were discovered that could produce similar effects. However, microbubbles produced by simple agitation are nonuniform in size, relatively large, and unstable, which makes them unsuitable for sonographic evaluations of the left side of the heart and systemic circulation, because the microbubbles do not persist through passage of the pulmonary and cardiac circulations. Furthermore, to provide contrast enhancement, agitated saline required direct injection into the vessel under evaluation (e.g., the aorta) and a more clinically practicable administration method, such as intravenous (IV) injection, was desired.

For a UCA to be clinically useful, it should be nontoxic, have microbubbles or microparticles that are small enough to traverse the pulmonary capillary beds (i.e., less than 8 microns in size), and be stable enough to provide multiple recirculations. Furthermore, the contrast agent should be administered via IV injection and provide enhancement of ultrasound signals. A number of agents possess these desirable traits, and presently several microbubble-based UCAs are commercially available worldwide (Tables 17-1 and 17-2).

The specific type of gas contained within a UCA microbubble and its shell composition influence the microbubble's acoustic behavior (e.g., reflectivity and elasticity), method of metabolism, and stability within the blood pool.[10,95] In 1998, Optison (FSO 69) was approved by the U.S. Food and Drug Administration (FDA) for cardiac applications in the United States. The microbubbles of Optison are composed of a shell of 5% sonicated human serum albumen that contains a high-molecular-weight gas (perfluoropropane), which extends the stability and plasma longevity of the agent. Optison has shown potential for use with gray-scale CHI and Doppler modes for echocardiography, as well as systemic vascular, tumor characterization, and abdominal applications.[19,21,42,97]

TABLE 17-1	Ultrasound Contrast Agents That Are Commercially Available in the United States and Their Food and Drug Administration–Approved Indications*
Agent Name, Manufacturer	**Approved Indications**
Optison, GE Healthcare, Princeton, NJ	LVO/EBD
Definity, Lantheus Medical Imaging, N. Billerica, MA	LVO/EBD
Imagent, IMCOR Pharmaceuticals, Inc., San Diego, CA (Imagent is not currently being marketed)	LVO/EBD
Lumason Bracco International, Milan, Italy	LVO/EBD and characterization of focal hepatic tumors in adult and pediatric patients.

EBD, Endocardial border definition; *LVO,* left ventricular opacification.
*This information is considered accurate as of June 2016. The status of UCAs is subject to change.

SonoVue (BR-1) is an aqueous suspension of phospholipid-stabilized sulfur hexafluoride (SF-6) microbubbles having a low solubility in blood.[29] SonoVue enhances the echogenicity of blood and provides opacification of the cardiac chambers resulting in improved left ventricular endocardial border definition. In clinical trials it has been shown to increase US's accuracy in detection or exclusion of abnormalities in intracranial, extracranial carotid, and peripheral arteries. SonoVue also increases the quality of Doppler flow signals and the duration of clinically useful signal enhancement in portal vein assessments. SonoVue improves the detection of liver and breast lesion vascularity resulting in more specific lesion characterization.[82,83] SonoVue has been approved for use in Europe for echocardiography and macrovascular applications.

TABLE 17-2	Ultrasound Contrast Agents That Are Commercially Available Outside the United States and Their Approved Indications*		
Agent Name, Manufacturer	**Countries**		**Approved Indications**
Definity, Lantheus Medical Imaging, London, U.K. (Marketed as Luminity in some countries)	Canada, Mexico, Israel, New Zealand, India, Australia †European Union, Korea, Singapore, United Arab Emirates		LVO/EBD, liver, kidney
Optison, GE Healthcare, Chalfont St. Giles, U.K.	European Union		LVO/EBD
Sonazoid, Daiichi Pharmaceutical Co., LTD, Tokyo, Japan (Manufactured and distributed in partnership with GE Healthcare)	Japan		Focal liver lesions Focal breast lesions
SonoVue, Bracco International, Milan, Italy	European Union, Norway, Switzerland, China, Singapore, Hong Kong, S. Korea, Iceland, India ‡Canada		LVO/EBD, breast, liver, portal vein, extracranial carotid, peripheral arteries (macrovascular and microvascular)

EBD, endocardial border definition; *LVO*, left ventricular opacification.
*This information is considered accurate as of June 2016. The status of UCAs around the world is subject to change.
†Approved in these countries only for LVO/EBD.
‡Approved in Canada for LVO/EBD and diagnostic assessment of vessels.

In the United States SonoVue is marketed as Lumason, and it received FDA approval for echocardiography applications in 2014.[29] Lumason has also been studied for liver lesion characterization,[72,75] and in April 2016 it became the first UCA to gain FDA approval for a non-cardiac indication. It is FDA approved for characterization of focal liver lesion in adult and pediatric patients.[96]

Tissue-Specific Ultrasound Contrast Agents

The kinetics of UCA microbubbles following IV injection is complex, and each agent has its own unique characteristics.[6] In general, after IV administration, blood-pool UCAs are contained exclusively in the body's vascular spaces. Once a vascular agent's microbubbles are ruptured or otherwise destroyed, the microbubble shell products are metabolized or eliminated by the body, and the gas is exhaled.[95]

Tissue-specific ultrasound contrast agents differ from vascular agents in that the microbubbles of these agents are removed from the blood pool and taken up by, or have an affinity toward, specific tissues, for example, the reticuloendothelial system (RES) in the liver and spleen, or thrombi in blood vessels. Over time the presence of contrast microbubbles within or attached to the target tissue changes its sonographic appearance. By changing the signal impedance (or other acoustic characteristics) of normal and abnormal tissues, these agents improve the detectability of abnormalities and permit more specific sonographic diagnoses. Tissue-specific UCAs are typically administered by IV injection. Some tissue-specific UCAs also enhance the sonographic detection of blood flow and are therefore potentially multipurpose. Because tissue-specific UCAs target specific types of tissues and their behavior is predictable, they can be considered in the category of **molecular imaging agents.**[55]

Sonazoid is a tissue-specific UCA that contains microbubbles of perfluorobutane gas in a stable lipid shell.[40] Sonazoid is currently approved for use in Japan.[87] After being injected intravenously, Sonazoid behaves as a vascular agent (i.e., enhances the detection of flowing blood) and, over time, the microbubbles are phagocytosed by the RES (macrophage Kupffer cells) of the liver and spleen.[6] The intact microbubbles may remain stationary in the tissue for several hours. When insonated after uptake, the stationary contrast microbubbles increase the reflectivity of the contrast-containing tissue. If an appropriate level of acoustic energy is applied to the tissue, the microbubbles first oscillate (emitting harmonic signals that can be detected with gray-scale CHI) and then rupture. The rupture of the microbubbles results in random Doppler shifts appearing as a transient mosaic of colors on a color Doppler display (Figure 17-4). This effect has been termed **induced acoustic emission** (IAE), *stimulated acoustic emission* (SAE), or simply **acoustic emission** (AE).[25,28] By exploiting the color Doppler–depicted AE phenomenon, masses that have destroyed or replaced the normal Kupffer cells will be displayed as color-free areas and thus become more sonographically conspicuous. These same AE effects can also be demonstrated using gray-scale CHI (see the CHI discussion that follows) (Figure 17-5).[20,28] Improvements in contrast-specific US technologies have obviated the use of Doppler modes with UCAs for the majority of applications.[28]

It is important to remember that the AE effects are independent of contrast motion. In other words, the AE effect can result from oscillation and eventual rupture of stationary contrast microbubbles, and agents that demonstrate the AE phenomenon also can be utilized for nonvascular applications where there is little or no movement of the microbubbles.

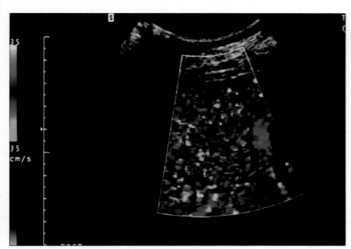

FIGURE 17-4 Color Doppler imaging display of acoustic emission after IV injection of a tissue-specific UCA. The rupture of contrast microbubbles present within the RES cells of the liver results in the characteristic random color display.

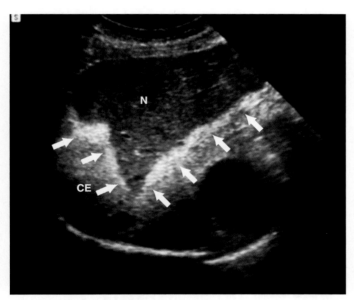

FIGURE 17-5 Gray-scale contrast harmonic imaging display of the acoustic emission effect after IV injection of a tissue-specific UCA. As the acoustic energy traverses through the liver parenchyma, it causes the contrast microbubbles to rupture, resulting in a characteristic wave of intense echoes *(arrows)*. The normal echogenicity of the liver parenchyma in the near field *(N)* is restored after the microbubbles have ruptured, whereas deep to the AE wave the contrast-enhanced tissue *(CE)* remains echogenic because of the presence of intact microbubbles. This effect is dramatic when visualized in real time.

Currently, tissue-specific agents that are taken up by the RES appear to be most useful in the assessment of patients with suspected liver abnormalities, including the ability to both detect and characterize liver tumors using CES. Other target- or tissue-specific agents are being developed to enhance the detection of thrombus and tumors.

ULTRASOUND EQUIPMENT MODIFICATIONS

Microbubble-based UCAs enhance the detection of blood flow when used with conventional ultrasound imaging techniques, including gray-scale US, and Doppler techniques (i.e., color flow imaging and pulsed-wave Doppler with spectral analysis). However, research and experience have led to a better understanding of the complex interactions between acoustic energy (i.e., the US beam) and UCA microbubbles, which in turn has led to contrast-specific US imaging modes that greatly improve the clinical utility of CES.[70]

Harmonic imaging (HI) uses the same broadband transducers used for conventional US, but in HI mode the US system is configured to receive only echoes at the second harmonic frequency, which is twice the transmit frequency (e.g., 7.0 MHz for a 3.5-MHz transducer).[17,43] When using a microbubble-based UCA, the microbubbles oscillate (i.e., they get larger and smaller) when subjected to the acoustic energy present in the US field. The reflected echoes from the oscillating microbubbles contain energy components at the fundamental frequency and at the higher and lower harmonics (i.e., subharmonics). Contrast harmonic imaging (CHI) allows detection of contrast-enhancement of blood flow and organs with B-mode US. The use of CHI for CES avoids many of the limitations and artifacts encountered when using Doppler US techniques and UCAs, such as angle dependence and "color blooming" artifacts.[18] In CHI mode the echoes from the oscillating microbubbles have a higher signal-to-noise ratio than would be provided by using conventional US, so that regions with microbubbles (e.g., blood vessels and organ parenchyma) are more easily appreciated visually. Advanced CHI technology (e.g., wideband HI, phase-inversion HI, and pulse-inversion HI) employ image processing algorithms to subtract echoes arising from body tissues while echoes arising from contrast microbubbles are preferentially displayed.[43] Thus CHI provides a way to better differentiate areas with and without contrast and has the potential to demonstrate real-time B-mode blood-pool imaging (i.e., "perfusion imaging"). The benefits of using CHI for CES (e.g., higher frame rates, improved contrast resolution, reduced artifacts) are so great that conventional (non-HI) color flow imaging is neither necessary nor advised.

When using microbubble-based UCAs, the energy present within the acoustic field can have a detrimental effect on the contrast microbubbles.[10] A significant number of the microbubbles can be destroyed by the acoustic pressure even though the actual pressure contained within the US field is relatively low. Once the microbubble is destroyed, contrast enhancement is no longer provided, which reduces the clinical utility and duration of contrast enhancement. Several approaches have been used to minimize this problem. One relatively easy technique is to use a low acoustic output power as defined by the **mechanical index (MI)**.[69] However, reducing the MI also limits tissue penetration, so this is not always an adequate solution. Furthermore, the MI may be an imprecise predictor of the effect of acoustic energy on contrast microbubbles.[22,28]

Equipment manufacturers have incorporated *intermittent imaging* (also referred to as *interval delay imaging*) capabilities on their systems to provide an additional option to the user seeking to reduce microbubble destruction during contrast-enhanced examinations.[43,53,69,80] In this mode the system is gated to only transmit and receive data at predetermined intervals. The gating may be triggered on a specific portion of the electrocardiogram (e.g., the r-wave) or a time interval such as once or twice per second. Intermittent imaging reduces the exposure of contrast microbubbles to the acoustic energy and allows additional microbubbles to enter the field between signal transmissions. The additional microbubbles then contribute to an even greater increase in reflectivity of the contrast-containing blood or tissue than would be possible by continuous real-time imaging. A disadvantage to intermittent imaging is its lack of a real-time display of data, but advances in instrumentation such as "flash echocardiography" address this weakness.[65] Intermittent imaging is commonly combined with CHI to further improve the clinical utility of CES.

Moriyasu and colleagues[57] used intermittent imaging for CES of hepatic tumors. This study showed that the signal intensity is dependent on an interscan delay time during which the acoustic power is lowered under the threshold for passive cavitation of the microbubbles. A study by Sirlin and colleagues[80] demonstrated that intermittent imaging improved image contrast resolution and a 1-frame-per-second rate provided greater contrast resolution than that provided by continuous real-time imaging.

Other contrast-specific technologies include advanced three-dimensional (3D) and four-dimensional (4D) imaging (Figures 17-6 and 17-7). Furthermore, a number of

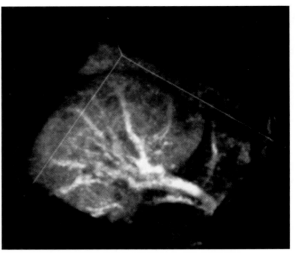

FIGURE 17-7 The combination of 3D gray-scale harmonic imaging and administration of a vascular UCA results in an "ultrasound angiogram."

contrast-specific measurements and calculations can be performed, including onboard video densitometry, calculation of the integrated backscatter from contrast, measurement of the transit time of contrast-containing blood through normal and diseased tissue, estimations of blood volume, and assessment of tissue perfusion differences in solid organs.[5,38,93] Systems have been developed that allow onboard calculation of the unique data provided by the use of UCAs (Figure 17-8).

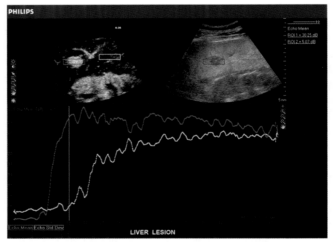

FIGURE 17-8 Contrast-specific quantification of changes in signal intensity within a liver tumor compared with the normal liver. Time-intensity curves generated after IV administration of contrast from regions of interest placed over the tumor (red box) and the normal liver (yellow box). The graphic displays time on the x-axis and signal intensity on the y-axis. Note that the signal intensity on the tumor (red tracing) demonstrates more rapid up-take of contrast and higher signal intensity as compared to the normal liver (yellow tracing). Contrast enhancement can also be seen in the right kidney deep to the liver. *(Courtesy of Philips Healthcare, Bothell, WA)*

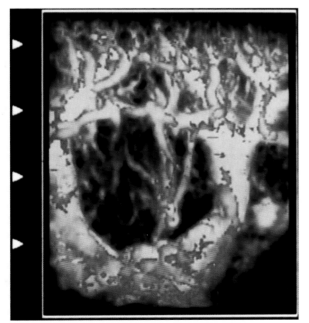

FIGURE 17-6 Contrast-enhanced 3D power Doppler imaging of a kidney in an animal model. Note the fine detail of the renal vasculature.

CLINICAL APPLICATIONS

Hepatic Applications

There are limitations to the sonographic evaluation of hepatic lesions and other hepatic abnormalities. Although US is usually sensitive for the detection of medium to large hepatic lesions, it is limited in its ability to detect small (less than 10 mm), isoechoic, or peripherally located lesions, particularly in obese patients or patients with diffuse liver disease. Furthermore, sonography is not as effective as computed tomography (CT) or magnetic resonance imaging (MRI) for characterization of hepatic tumors.

Hepatic US blood flow studies are limited by low-velocity blood flow (e.g., in cases of portal hypertension) or for the detection of flow in the intrahepatic artery branches. Ultrasound contrast agents have shown the potential to improve the accuracy of hepatic sonography, including enhanced detection and characterization of hepatic masses and improved detection of intrahepatic and extrahepatic blood flow.

Hepatic Blood Flow. Vascular UCAs have been shown to improve the assessment of hepatic blood flow in normal subjects, as well as in patients with liver disease and portal hypertension (PHT).[1,11,37,45,77]

Most sonographic examinations for PHT include qualitative assessment of blood flow with color flow imaging to identify the presence and direction of flow in the splenic and superior mesenteric veins, as well as the main portal vein and the intrahepatic portal and hepatic veins. When scanning patients with PHT, slow-moving portal flow can be difficult to detect using conventional Doppler techniques. Studies have found that the increased reflectivity of contrast-containing blood allows the detection of abnormal blood flow in the portal and hepatic veins, as well as in portal-systemic collaterals.[33,71,77]

Contrast-enhanced sonography has also been used effectively in the assessment of flow through transjugular intrahepatic portosystemic shunts (TIPS).[54,91]

Uggowitzer and colleagues[91] found that Levovist provided Doppler signal enhancement lasting from 30 seconds to 7 minutes, and Levovist-enhanced scans improved the diagnosis of stent stenosis compared with conventional US examinations.

Published reports have described CES-detectable alterations in blood flow transit time through the livers of patients with diffuse hepatic disease compared with normal controls.[1,46,77] In cases of cirrhosis there is often reduced portal venous flow and a compensatory increase in hepatic artery flow. Zhou and colleagues[100] examined blood flow in the hepatic arteries and hepatic veins of 52 patients with metastases and 23 normal control subjects after bolus injections of SonoVue. The parameters that were evaluated included contrast arrival time, time to peak enhancement, and peak intensity values in the vessels. Additionally, the difference between the arrival times in the hepatic artery and the hepatic veins was calculated. The arrival times and transit times in the patient group were significantly shorter than those of the control group, and the peak intensity values in the patient group were significantly higher than those of the control

group. The results of this study suggest that CES assessment of changes in the hemodynamic parameters of the hepatic artery and vein can be used to improve diagnosis of liver metastases possibly before sonographic detection of focal lesions.

Hepatic Tumors. Many patients who have hepatic tumors first identified sonographically eventually require a CT or MRI examination to better determine the extent of disease and to more accurately characterize the lesions. Using CES, it is possible to distinguish the various phases of blood flow to and within the liver. In normal situations after IV administration of a UCA, contrast-enhanced flow in the hepatic artery is identified first (arterial phase), followed by enhanced portal venous flow (portal venous phase). Detection of flow in the hepatic capillaries is identified later (late phase) as a parenchymal blush (Figure 17-9). If an RES-specific agent is used, identification of the delayed enhancement phase representing the enhancement from the stationary microbubbles that have been phagocytosed by the RES is possible.[87]

Diagnostic criteria used for contrast-enhanced CT or MRI, including the evaluation of the phase, degree, and pattern of vascularity in and around hepatic tumors, is also used for CES[32,47] (Table 17-3). In fact, CES, because of its ability to image dynamic events in real time, may prove to be better than CT or MRI in the evaluation of hemodynamics that occur in the various hepatic vascular phases. Numerous published reports suggest that CES can improve the detection and characterization of liver lesions.*

Strobel and colleagues[85,86] evaluated the diagnostic accuracy of CES for diagnosis of liver tumors in 1349 patients who had hepatic tumors that could not be definitively diagnosed with conventional sonography. Low-MI CHI was utilized to assess contrast enhancement patterns in the focal lesions during the arterial, portal, and late phases, and CES results were compared with histology, CT, or MRI. The diagnostic accuracy of CES was 83% for all benign lesions (82% for hemangiomas and 87% for focal nodular hyperplasia lesions) and 96% for all malignant lesions (91% for metastases and 85% for hepatocellular carcinomas). Late-phase hypoenhancement was seen in 95% of all liver metastases.

Cavernous hemangiomas are common benign solid neoplasms of the liver and are frequently detected during hepatic US examinations. Not all hemangiomas have the classic US appearance of a rounded, homogeneously hyperechoic mass that has well-defined margins, nor can they be accurately characterized sonographically (Figure 17-10). Several reports have suggested that CES can improve the assessment of hemangiomas.[83,85,94]

SonoVue was used in a study of atypical hemangiomas reported by Solbiati and colleagues.[83] Seven atypical hemangiomas (1.5 to 6.5 cm) were evaluated with CHI before and after bolus administration of contrast. Four lesions appeared hypoechoic or anechoic; the other three were isoechoic and "almost undistinguishable" on baseline (unenhanced) US. Arterial, portal, and late vascular phase imaging was performed following contrast administration. In the arterial phase,

---

*References 15, 19, 20, 32, 39, 41, 42, 46, 47, 82, 83, 86, 87, 88, 92, 97, and 100.

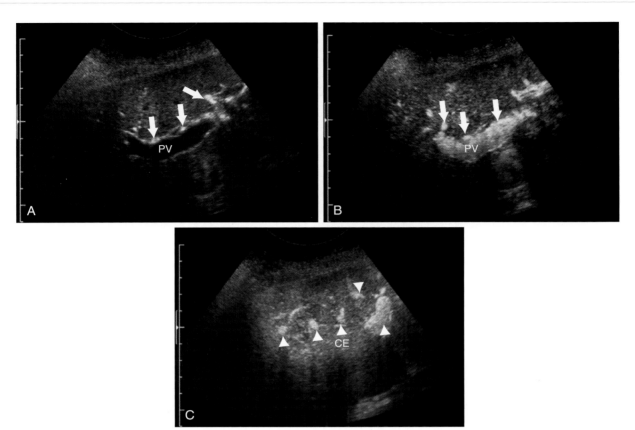

FIGURE 17-9 Contrast-enhanced demonstration of the various phases of hepatic blood flow. **A,** Twenty-five seconds after IV injection of an UCA, the first vessels to demonstrate contrast enhancement in the liver are the hepatic arteries *(arrows)*, whereas the portal vein *(PV)* remains anechoic in the arterial phase. **B,** In this patient, the portal venous phase occurred 37 seconds after injection with contrast seen in the portal vein. **C,** In the late vascular phase at 71 seconds after injection, the liver parenchyma is becoming echogenic (i.e., contrast-enhanced; *CE*) and there is persistent enhancement of the major hepatic vessels *(arrowheads)*.

TABLE 17-3	Typical Contrast-Enhancement Patterns of Benign and Malignant Focal Hepatic Tumors as Compared with Surrounding Liver Parenchyma		
Tumor Type	**Arterial Phase**	**Portal Venous Phase**	**Late Phase**
Hemangioma	Peripheral nodular enhancement Small lesions may show rapid centripetal enhancement	Gradual partial to complete centripetal filling	Complete enhancement May have nonenhancing areas
Focal nodular hyperplasia	Rapid, complete enhancement from center May demonstrate spoke-wheel pattern	Hyperenhanced	Hyperenhanced or isoenhanced, may demonstrate central scar
Focal fatty sparing	Isoenhanced	Isoenhanced	Isoenhanced
Focal fatty infiltration	Isoenhanced	Isoenhanced	Isoenhanced
Hepatocellular carcinoma	Hyperenhanced throughout, may have nonenhanced areas, may demonstrate chaotic vessels	Isoenhanced, may have nonenhanced areas	Hypoenhanced, may have nonenhanced areas
Hypovascular metastases	Peripheral enhancement, may have complete enhancement or nonenhanced areas	Hypoenhanced	Hypoenhanced, may have nonenhanced areas
Hypervascular metastases	Hyperenhanced, may demonstrate chaotic vessels	Hypoenhanced	Hypoenhanced, may have nonenhanced areas

all lesions demonstrated only peripheral enhancement. In the portal phase, and even more so in the late vascular phase, progressive centripetal filling lasting from 5 to 7 minutes was observed in all lesions. The lesions got progressively more echogenic over time, which permitted a confident diagnosis. The authors concluded that multiphase sonography was necessary for accurate diagnosis of atypical hemangiomas and that CES has the potential to obviate the need for CT scans.

Several reports have described the CES appearance of hepatocellular carcinoma (HCC) as having intense enhancement in the early arterial phase and relatively rapid wash-out of contrast in the portal venous phase (Figure 17-11).[36,82,97]

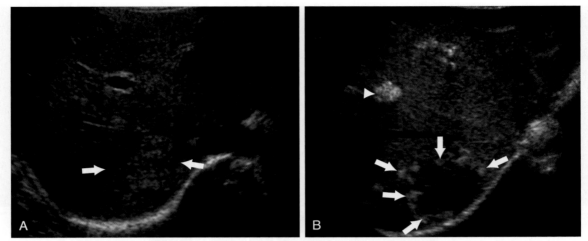

FIGURE 17-10 Improved detection and characterization of a liver hemangioma. **A,** A conventional ultrasound examination identified a poorly demarcated mass *(arrows)* in the right posterior lobe of the liver. **B,** After contrast administration using CHI there is pooling of contrast-containing blood at the periphery of the lesion and increased echogenicity of the normal liver parenchyma. This pattern is characteristic for hemangiomas.

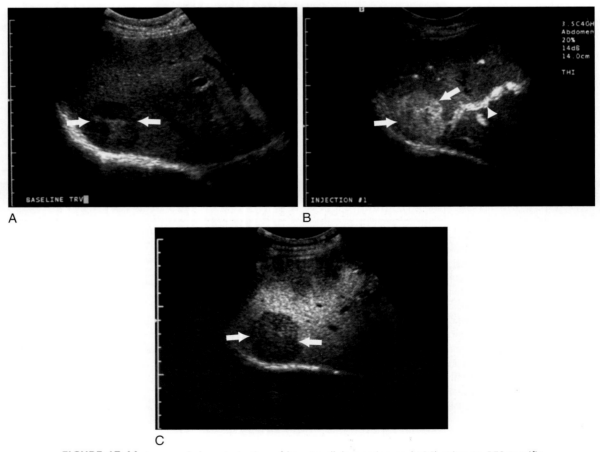

FIGURE 17-11 Improved characterization of hepatocellular carcinoma (HCC) using an RES-specific UCA. **A,** A conventional US examination identified a mass *(arrows)* in the right posterior lobe of the liver having mixed echogenicity. **B,** After contrast administration using CHI, the hepatic artery and portal veins filled with contrast *(arrowheads)* and the mass became brightly echogenic compared with the surrounding liver tissue in the arterial and portal venous phases. **C,** On delayed imaging the lesion was hypoechoic compared with the surrounding liver tissue. This CES pattern is characteristic for HCC.

When using an RES-specific agent, HCC lesions can have a similar appearance to focal nodular hyperplasia (FNH) in the early arterial phase. However, on delayed phase imaging the HCC tumor will be hypoechoic relative to the surrounding normal liver tissue (because of the lack of Kupffer cells within the tumor), whereas FNH tumors, because they contain abundant amounts of Kupffer cells, will be isoechoic to the surrounding normal liver tissue (Figure 17-12). The central feeding artery and spoke-wheel radiating branches that are characteristic of FNH on dynamic CT angiography can also be depicted by CES, and can be used to differentiate HCC from FNH.[36,85,90,92]

Contrast-enhanced sonography has been shown to improve the detection and delineation of liver metastases (Figure 17-13).[87,90,100] However, accurate characterization of metastatic liver tumors with CES can be problematic because the degree of vascularity in these lesions is related to the primary cancer.[97] Therefore some metastatic liver lesions will be hypervascular, whereas others are hypovascular. One imaging characteristic of liver metastases that has been identified during delayed phase imaging using an RES-specific UCA is an echogenic rim around the tumor.[47] The echogenic rim is thought to reflect the higher concentration of Kupffer cells around metastases or a higher degree of contrast, which results from compression of the normal liver parenchyma around the metastases.[47]

A 2009 report described the results of a multicenter study that compared CES to CT or MRI for characterization of focal liver lesions.[90] The study included 134 patients with one focal liver lesion detected in baseline ultrasound imaging. The lesions were classified as malignant, benign, or indeterminate based on imaging findings. Compared with unenhanced US, CES markedly improved sensitivity and specificity for differentiating malignant from benign liver lesions. The authors concluded that CES was the most sensitive, most specific, and most accurate imaging modality for the characterization of focal liver lesions.

By providing a means to detect and differentiate the various vascular enhancement patterns (e.g., degree, architecture, and phasicity) in and around hepatic lesions in real time, CES has been proven to improve characterization of liver lesions, including HCC, FNH, metastases, and hemangiomas. Numerous published reports have confirmed the clinical utility and

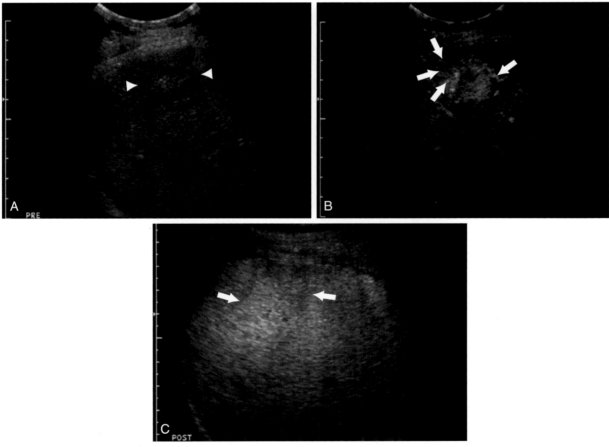

FIGURE 17-12 Improved characterization of focal nodular hyperplasia (FNH) using an RES-specific UCA. **A,** A conventional US examination identified a hypoechoic mass *(arrowheads)* in the right anterior lobe of the liver. **B,** After contrast administration using CHI, the mass became brightly echogenic and intratumoral vessels having a radiating spoke-like pattern could be identified *(arrows)*. A central hypoechoic area within the mass that did not enhance represents a scar. **C,** On delayed imaging the lesion was isoechoic compared with the surrounding liver tissue. This CES pattern is characteristic for FNH.

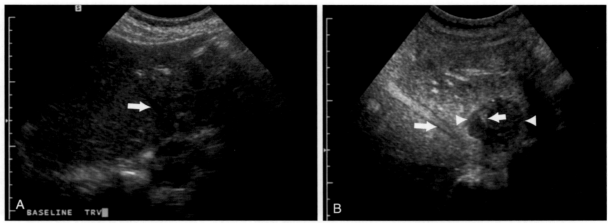

FIGURE 17-13 Improved detection and delineation of a colorectal carcinoma liver metastasis. **A,** A transverse conventional US image at the level of the middle hepatic vein *(arrow)* did not identify the mass, which had been detected on a prior CT examination. **B,** After UCA administration using CHI in the portal venous phase, there was increased echogenicity of the surrounding liver parenchyma that resulted in improved delineation of the tumor *(arrowheads).* Contrast-enhanced blood flow could also be identified in the hepatic vein *(arrow)* and small vessels within the mass *(short arrow).* In this case the patient was being evaluated for possible US-guided radiofrequency ablation of this nonresectable tumor, and the CES results enhanced the ability to identify the location of the tumor, as well as its size and margins.

diagnostic accuracy of CES for liver lesion characterization. Liver lesion characterization is recognized around the world as one of the most important applications of CES. CES has established itself as an important diagnostic tool for the evaluation of patients with focal liver lesions of unknown origin and has the potential to reduce the use of competing imaging modalities for this application.

Renal Applications

Published reports have described the use of UCAs in a variety of renal applications, including the evaluation of suspected renal masses and renal artery stenosis.* These reports provide an indication as to what may be expected once vascular UCAs become available for widespread clinical use in the United States.

Renal Artery Stenosis. The sonographic evaluation of the main and intrarenal renal arteries in patients with suspected renal artery stenosis (RAS) is fraught with problems. Because the main renal arteries are retroperitoneal in location, these vessels are typically difficult to evaluate sonographically, particularly in the obese patient. A significant number of patients will have anatomic variations of the renal vasculature, including duplicate or accessory renal arteries, and these variations can be difficult to identify using conventional US. Furthermore, US examinations for RAS are often time consuming and are extremely operator dependent. These factors likely contribute to the wide variability reported in the accuracy of US when used for RAS examinations.[4,64] Although not a common clinical application of

CES, it has been investigated as a salvage tool employed when conventional US RAS examinations are nondiagnostic (Figure 17-14).[56,60]

Renal Masses. Diagnostic sonography has been a reliable method of evaluating patients with renal masses, particularly in the differentiation of cystic from solid lesions. Sonography is usually accurate in its ability to identify large (greater than 2 cm) renal cell carcinomas and to identify tumor thrombus in the renal veins or inferior vena cava. However, in a small percentage of cases sonography cannot identify small neoplasms or differentiate solid hypoechoic renal lesions from hemorrhagic cysts or other benign processes (Figure 17-15). Furthermore, normal anatomic variations such as a prominent column of Bertin or persistent fetal lobulation may mimic renal tumors. In these cases other imaging studies such as CT or MRI or needle biopsy may be indicated for a definitive diagnosis. The use of an UCA and CHI allows detection of normal renal blood flow using a non-Doppler mode (Figure 17-16).

The use of CES improves the ability to identify the normal renal vasculature and detect the presence of lesions that distort the vascular architecture (Figure 17-17).[67]

Splenic Applications

Several reports have described the clinical value of CES for the evaluation of the spleen.[8,9,51,63,68] Picardi and colleagues[68] compared CES to CT and fluorodeoxyglucose positron emission tomography (PET) for the detection of nodular infiltration in the spleen of 100 patients with newly diagnosed Hodgkin's lymphoma. Malignant nodules were detected with CT in 13 patients, with PET in 13 patients,

---

*References 12, 14, 44, 48, 56, 59, 67, 74, and 93.

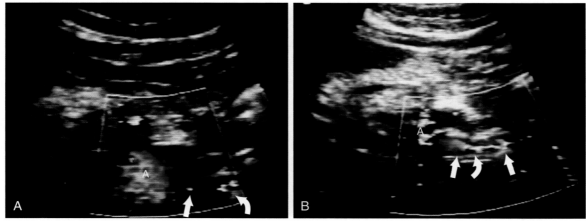

FIGURE 17-14 Transverse color Doppler images of the abdominal aorta and proximal left renal artery in a patient with suspected renal artery stenosis. **A,** Before intravenous administration of contrast, flow in the aorta *(A)* and proximal most renal artery *(arrow)* are visualized and there is aliasing of the color flow display *(curved arrow)*. **B,** After injection of contrast, the stenotic vessel lumen *(arrows)* can be clearly visualized. Advances in contrast imaging modes have obviated the use of color flow imaging modes when performing contrast-enhanced examinations.

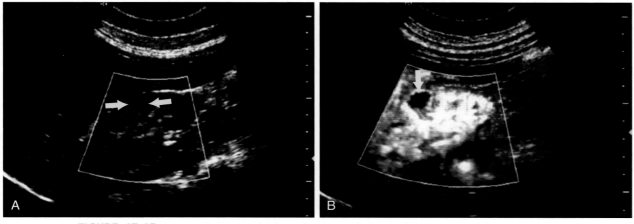

FIGURE 17-15 Improved characterization of a hypoechoic renal mass. **A,** On the precontrast power Doppler image, a hypoechoic mass *(arrows)* is visualized in the midpole of the right kidney. **B,** After injection of a vascular UCA, blood flow is demonstrated with PDI within the normal renal parenchyma but no flow was detected from within the mass *(arrow)*. The mass was later determined to represent a benign hemorrhagic cyst.

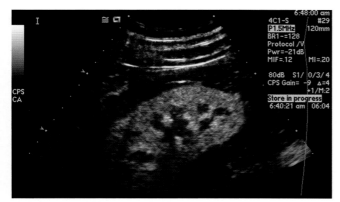

FIGURE 17-16 Contrast harmonic imaging after IV administration of contrast demonstrates a uniform increase in the signal intensity within a normal kidney parenchyma.

and with CES in 30 patients. The authors concluded that CES provides a higher sensitivity than does CT or PET in the detection of splenic involvement by Hodgkin's lymphoma.

Catalano and colleagues[9] studied 55 patients with a variety of suspected splenic abnormalities including traumatic injuries and tumors. The CES results were compared with baseline (noncontrast) US, CT, or MRI. In this series, parenchymal injuries were detected with a sensitivity of 63% on baseline US, whereas the sensitivity improved to 89% after CES. Parenchymal injuries included posttraumatic infarctions that were not identified on baseline US but were identified with CES. CES also identified 35 of 39 proven focal lesions in patients with Hodgkin's disease, whereas baseline US detected only 23 lesions.

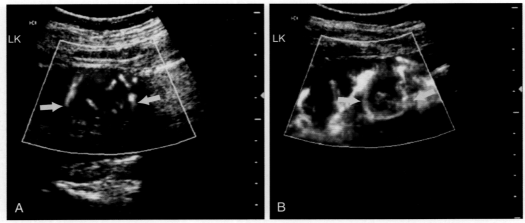

FIGURE 17-17 Power Doppler imaging (PDI) of a suspicious renal mass before and after IV administration of contrast. **A,** On the precontrast image a subtle hypoechoic mass was identified near the lower pole of the left kidney but PDI only demonstrates flow around the mass. **B,** After injection of contrast there are significantly more flow signals detected including intratumoral flow. This was later confirmed to represent a renal cell carcinoma.

Pancreatic Applications

Visualization of the pancreas using transabdominal US is often hampered by the gland's deep location within the retroperitoneum and the presence of overlying bowel. Advances in US technology (e.g., endoscopic US), combined with UCAs, has led to a significant improvement in the diagnostic potential of US for a range of pancreatic disorders.[52] Several published reports describe the ability of UCAs to improve pancreatic US evaluations.[7,16,34,35,52,58,60,73]

Kersting and colleagues[35] evaluated the value of transabdominal CES for differential diagnosis of pancreatic ductal adenocarcinoma (PDAC) and focal inflammatory masses resulting from chronic pancreatitis. Time-intensity curves were obtained in two regions of interest within the lesion and within the normal pancreatic tissue, and CES data were evaluated using quantification software. Of the 60 patients examined, histology revealed 45 PDACs and 15 inflammatory masses. The time-dependent parameters (arrival time and time-to-peak) were significantly longer in PDACs compared with focal masses. The authors concluded that PDAC and focal inflammatory masses exhibit different perfusion patterns that can be visualized with CES. Additionally, the contrast quantification software provided objective criteria that could be used to facilitate pancreatic lesion diagnoses.

Organ Transplants

Sonography is routinely used to evaluate kidney, liver, and pancreas transplants. The modality is often employed as a first-line examination tool in the immediate postsurgical period, as well as for serial studies to confirm organ viability. After organ transplantation, sonography is used to detect postsurgical fluid collections, to identify urinary or bile obstructions, and to assess blood flow to and from the transplanted organ. Conventional sonography is also useful in the evaluation of blood flow within the organ, but it does not have an adequate level of sensitivity to detect flow at the microvascular level (i.e., tissue perfusion). When a vascular abnormality is suspected, angiography or contrast-enhanced CT can provide a definitive diagnosis. However, angiography is invasive, CT requires ionizing radiation, and administration of contrast media required for these examinations may be contraindicated.

The enhanced detection of blood flow provided by CES improves the assessment of blood flow in the arteries and veins that supply the transplanted organ and the vessels to which these vessels are anastomosed. CES has also been found to improve the ability to detect the lack of flow within transplanted organs (i.e., ischemic regions) within renal and pancreatic grafts.[3,7,16,34,41]

Reports also suggest that CES is useful for the evaluation of liver transplant recipients.[3,41,49,78,79]

For renal transplants, CES can permit better differentiation of regions that have decreased perfusion from true vascular defects resulting from a renal artery branch occlusion or acute rejection.[13] The use of CES has also been investigated as a means to detect early organ rejection.[76]

Contrast-enhanced sonography has also been found to be superior to conventional sonography for differentiating parenchymal abnormalities in renal transplants, such as acute tubular necrosis (ATN), from other abnormalities.[3,99]

Benozzi and colleagues[3] performed serial CES and power Doppler imaging (PDI) of 39 kidney recipients within 30 days of transplantation and compared the imaging results with clinical findings and functional assessments. Both CES and PDI identified grafts with early dysfunction, but only some CES-derived parameters distinguished ATN from acute rejection episodes. The authors concluded that the use of CES in the early postoperative period provided important prognostic information about renal transplants.[49,50,79]

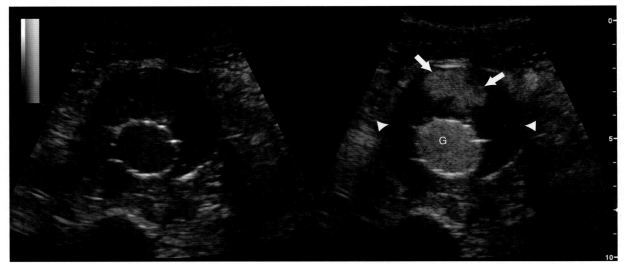

FIGURE 17-18 CES detection of an endovascular aortic aneurysm graft leak. This transverse CHI image using a dual display (*A;* the contrast-specific imaging mode is on the right and a conventional gray-scale US image is on the left) demonstrates the aneurismal sack *(arrowheads)* and contrast-enhanced blood flow in the graft *(G).* Contrast-containing blood *(arrows)* is identified in the aneurismal sack consistent with an endoleak. *(Courtesy of Dirk Clevert, MD, University of Munich, Munich, Germany).*

Other Applications

Other common abdominal/retroperitoneal applications of US include assessment of flow in the mesenteric arteries (for mesenteric ischemia), as well as the aorta and iliac arteries for aneurysms, stenoses, endovascular leaks, or dissections. Often these examinations are limited by the presence of overlying bowel and bowel gas, or the effects of signal attenuation resulting from the deep location of the vessels. Vascular UCAs have been used with success to improve the assessment of the abdominal vasculature and blood flow.[24,31,62,66]

A promising application for CES is for surveillance of patients after endovascular aneurysm repair (EVAR) of abdominal aortas (Figure 17-18).[24,98] Postsurgical surveillance of these patients is required to detect endoleaks, and patients commonly are followed for months or even years after EVAR. Administration of a UCA provides several minutes of contrast enhancement, thereby allowing time to assess the graft for both fast-flowing and slow-flowing endoleaks. This is an advantage over CT, as the CE-CT scans may only use one or a few phases (to limit ionizing radiation exposure). CES has been found to allow assessment of the precise location of the endoleak, as well as differentiate between type I and type II endoleaks.

Finally, contrast has been used successfully to diagnose and monitor treatment of patients with focal tumors who are going to have or have had chemotherapy, radiofrequency, ethanol, or other focal tumor ablation techniques[26,84,89] (see Figure 17-12). Ultrasound contrast agents used during the planning stage of a US-guided ablation can provide a means to better define tumor size and delineate tumor margins, which would help ensure that the entire tumor is ablated while normal tissue is preserved. Patients that have had a tumor ablation procedure receive serial imaging examinations to check for residual viable tumor at the ablation site and to screen for tumor recurrence. Currently, CT and MRI are most commonly used for these serial studies. However, the use of CES has been investigated as an alternative method for the follow-up examinations.[2,23]

CONCLUSION

Several UCAs are currently marketed in the United States, but they are FDA approved only for echocardiographic applications. In the future, additional agents or clinical applications of existing agents are likely to become available. Many published reports on the efficacy and clinical utility of CES are coming from European and Asian investigators because of the greater availability and utilization of UCAs in those regions of the world. Vascular agents have been shown to improve the detection of blood flow in small and deep vessels throughout the body. Reports have also described the ability of UCAs to improve the sonographic detection and characterization of tumors and other abnormalities within the abdomen.

The enhancement capabilities of UCAs have been shown to have the ability to salvage nondiagnostic US examinations and render them diagnostic. The use of UCAs has also resulted in new US evaluations (e.g., the assessment of contrast transit time and phasicity of blood flow in and around liver tumors) that were not possible without their use. Improvements in US technology designed to exploit the acoustic behavior of contrast microbubbles are complementing the use of UCAs. Advances in both US instrumentation and the development of UCAs will continue to have a positive impact on the future of diagnostic sonography.

Key Pearls

- The clinical utilization of contrast-enhanced sonography (CES) has been shown to reduce or eliminate some of the current limitations of ultrasound (US) imaging and Doppler blood flow detection.
- Sonographic detection of blood flow is limited by factors including the depth and size of a vessel, the attenuation properties of intervening tissue, or low-velocity flow.
- The use of UCAs improves the detection of blood flow from vessels that are often difficult to assess without their use, such as the renal arteries, intracranial vessels, and small capillaries within organs (i.e., tissue perfusion).
- For a UCA to be clinically useful, it should be nontoxic, have microbubbles or microparticles that are small enough to traverse the pulmonary capillary beds (i.e., less than 8 microns in size), and be stable enough to provide multiple recirculations.
- The specific type of gas contained within a UCA microbubble and its shell composition influence the microbubble's acoustic behavior (e.g., reflectivity and elasticity), method of metabolism, and stability within the blood pool.
- Once a vascular agent's microbubbles are ruptured or otherwise destroyed, the microbubble shell products are metabolized or eliminated by the body, and the gas is exhaled.
- Tissue-specific ultrasound contrast agents differ from vascular agents in that the microbubbles of these agents are removed from the blood pool and taken up by, or have an affinity toward, specific tissues, for example, the reticuloendothelial system in the liver and spleen, or thrombi in blood vessels.
- Harmonic imaging (HI) uses the same broadband transducers used for conventional US, but in HI mode the US system is configured to receive only echoes at the second harmonic frequency, which is twice the transmit frequency.

REFERENCES

1. Albrecht T, Blomley MJ, Cosgrove DO, et al: Non-invasive diagnosis of hepatic cirrhosis by transit-time analysis of an ultrasound contrast agent, *Lancet* 353:1579-1583, 1999.
2. Allard CB, Coret A, Dason S, et al: Contrast-enhanced ultrasound for surveillance of radiofrequency-ablated renal tumors: a prospective, radiologist-blinded pilot study, *Urology* 86(6):1174-1178, 2015.
3. Benozzi L, Cappelli G, Granito M, et al: Contrast-enhanced sonography in early kidney graft dysfunction, *Transplant Proc* 41(4):1214-1215, 2009.
4. Berland LL, Koslin DB, Routh WD, Keller FS: Renal artery stenosis: prospective evaluation of diagnosis with color duplex US compared with angiography, *Radiology* 174:421-423, 1990.
5. Blomley MJ, Lim AK, Harvey CJ, et al: Liver microbubble transit time compared with histology and Child-Pugh score in diffuse liver disease: a cross sectional study, *Gut* 52(8):1188-1193, 2003.
6. Blomley MJK, Harvey CJ, Eckersley RJ, Cosgrove DO: Contrast kinetics and Doppler intensitometry. In Goldberg BB, Raichlen JR, Forsberg F, editors: *Ultrasound contrast agents: basic principles and clinical applications,* ed 2, London, 2001, Martin Dunitz, pp 81-89.
7. Boggi U, Morelli L, Amorese G, et al: Contribution of contrast-enhanced ultrasonography to nonoperative management of segmental ischemia of the head of a pancreas graft, *Am J Transplant* 9(2):413-418, 2009.
8. Catalano O, Aiani L, Barozzi L, et al: CEUS in abdominal trauma: multi-center study, *Abdom Imaging* 34(2):225-234, 2009.
9. Catalano O, Lobianco R, Sandomenico F, et al: Realtime contrast-enhanced ultrasound of the spleen: examination technique and preliminary clinical experience, *Radiol Med* 106(4):338-356, 2003.
10. Chomas JE, Dayton PA, Allen J, Ferrara KW: Optical and acoustical observation of contrast-agent destruction. In Goldberg BB, Raichlen JS, Forsberg F, editors: *Ultrasound contrast agents,* ed 2, London, 2001, Martin Dunitz, pp 259-266.
11. Cocciolillo S, Parruti G, Marzio L: CEUS and Fibroscan in non-alcoholic fatty liver disease and non-alcoholic steatohepatitis, *World J Hepatol* 6(7):496-503, 2014.
12. Correas J, Claudon M, Tranquart F, Helenon O: Contrast-enhanced ultrasonography: renal applications, *J Radiol* 84:2041-2054, 2003.
13. Correas J, Helenon O, Moreau JF: Contrast-enhanced ultrasonography of native and transplanted kidney diseases, *Eur Radiol* 9(Suppl 3):S394-S400, 1999.
14. Dowling RJ, House MK, King PM, et al: Contrast-enhanced Doppler ultrasound for renal artery stenosis, *Australas Radiol* 43(2):206-209, 1999.
15. Ernst H, Hahn EG, Balzer T, et al: Color Doppler ultrasound of liver lesions: signal enhancement after intravenous injection of the ultrasound contrast agent Levovist, *J Clin Ultrasound* 24:31-35, 1996.
16. Faccioli N, Crippa S, Bassi C, D'Onofrio M: Contrast-enhanced ultrasonography of the pancreas, *Pancreatology* 9(5):560-566, 2009.
17. Forsberg F, Goldberg BB, Liu JB, et al: On the feasibility of real-time, in vivo harmonic imaging with proteinaceous microspheres, *J Ultrasound Med* 15:853-860, 1996.
18. Forsberg F, Liu JB, Burns PN, Merton DA, Goldberg BB: Artifacts in ultrasound contrast agent studies, *J Ultrasound Med* 13:357-365, 1994.
19. Forsberg F, Liu JB, Merton DA, et al: Tumor detection using an ultrasound contrast agent, *J Ultrasound Med* 4:S8, 1995.
20. Forsberg F, Liu JB, Merton DA, et al: Gray scale second harmonic imaging of acoustic emission signals improves detection of liver tumors in rabbits, *J Ultrasound Med* 19:557-563, 2000.
21. Forsberg F, Liu JB, Rawool NM, et al: Gray-scale and color Doppler flow harmonic imaging with proteinaceous microspheres, *Radiology* 197(2):403, 1995.
22. Forsberg F, Shi WT, Merritt CRB, et al: Does the Mechanical Index predict destruction rates of contrast microbubbles? *J Ultrasound Med* 20:S12, 2001.
23. Gao Y, Zheng DY, Cui Z, et al: Predictive value of quantitative contrast-enhanced ultrasound in hepatocellular carcinoma recurrence after ablation, *World J Gastroenterol* 21(36):10418-10426, 2015.
24. Giannoni MF, Palombo G, Sbarigia E, et al: Contrast-enhanced ultrasound for aortic stent-graft surveillance, *J Endovasc Ther* 10(2):208-217, 2003.
25. Goldberg BB, Forsberg F, Fitzsch T, et al: Induced acoustic emission as a contrast mechanism for detection of hepatic abnormalities, *J Ultrasound Med* 14:S7, 1995.
26. Goldberg BB, Liu JB, Merton DA, et al: The role of contrast-enhanced US for RF ablation of liver tumor, *Radiology* 217(2):607, 2000.
27. Gramiak R, Shah PM: Echocardiography of the aortic root, *Invest Radiol* 3:356-366, 1968.
28. Harvey CJ, Blomley MJK, Cosgrove DO: Acoustic emission imaging. In Goldberg BB, Raichlen JS, Forsberg F, editors: *Ultrasound contrast agents,* ed 2, London, 2001, Martin Dunitz, pp 71-80.
29. http://imaging.bracco.com/us-en/bracco-diagnostics-inc-receives-us-fda-approval-new-ultrasound-contrast-agent-0. Accessed Nov 13, 2015.

30. http://www.efsumb.org/guidelines/guidelines01.asp. Accessed Nov 13, 2015.
31. Iezzi R, Cotroneo AR, Basilico R, et al: Endoleaks after endovascular repair of abdominal aortic aneurysm: value of CEUS, *Abdom Imaging* 35(1):106-114, 2010.
32. Isozaki T, Numata K, Kiba T, et al: Differential diagnosis of hepatic tumors by using contrast enhancement patters at US, *Radiology* 229(3):798-805, 2003.
33. Jeong WK, Kim TY, Sohn JH, et al: Severe portal hypertension in cirrhosis: evaluation of perfusion parameters with contrast-enhanced ultrasonography, *PLoS One* 10(3):e0121601, 2015.
34. Karamehic J, Scoutt LM, Tabakovic M, Heljic B: Ultrasonography in organ transplantation, *Med Arh* 58(1 Suppl 2):107-108, 2004.
35. Kersting S, Konopke R, Kersting F, et al: Quantitative perfusion analysis of transabdominal contrast-enhanced ultrasound of pancreatic masses and carcinomas, *Gastroenterology* 137(6):1903-1911, 2009.
36. Kim EA, Yoon KH, Lee YH, et al: Focal hepatic lesions: contrast-enhancement patterns at pulse-inversion harmonic US using a microbubble contrast agent, *Korean J Radiol* 4:224-233, 2003.
37. Kim MY, Suk KT, Baik SK, et al: Hepatic vein arrival time as assessed by contrast-enhanced ultrasonography is useful for the assessment of portal hypertension in compensated cirrhosis, *Hepatology* 56(3):1053-1062, 2012.
38. Kishimoto N, Mori Y, Nishiue T, et al: Renal blood flow measurement with contrast-enhanced harmonic ultrasonography: evaluation of dopamine-induced changes in renal cortical perfusion in humans, *Clin Nephrol* 59(6):423-428, 2003.
39. Kitamura H, Miyagawa Y, Yokoyama T, et al: Kupffer cell imaging with ultrasound contrast agent for diagnosis of histological grade of hepatocellular carcinoma, *J Ultrasound Med* 20:S10, 2001.
40. Klein HG: Ultrasound contrast agents: A commercial perspective. In Goldberg BB, Raichlen JS, Forsberg F, editors: *Ultrasound contrast agents,* ed 2, London, 2001, Martin Dunitz, pp 387-405.
41. Koda M, Matsunaga Y, Ueki M, et al: Qualitative assessment of tumor vascularity in hepatocellular carcinoma by contrast-enhanced coded ultrasound: comparison with arterial phase of dynamic CT and conventional color/power Doppler ultrasound, *Eur Radiol* 14(6):1100-1108, 2004.
42. Kono Y, Mattrey RF, Pinnell SP, et al: Contrast-enhanced B-mode harmonic imaging for the evaluation of HCC viability after therapy in cirrhotic patients, *J Ultrasound Med* 20:S10, 2001.
43. Kono Y, Mattrey RT: Harmonic imaging with contrast microbubbles. In Goldberg BB, Raichlen JS, Forsberg F, editors: *Ultrasound contrast agents,* ed 2, London, 2001, Martin Dunitz, pp 37-46.
44. Lacourciere Y, Levesque J, Onrot JM, et al: Impact of Levovist ultrasonographic contrast agent on the diagnosis and management of hypertensive patients with suspected renal artery stenosis: a Canadian multicentre pilot study, *Can Assoc Radiol J* 53(4):219-227, 2002.
45. Lee KH, Choi BI, Kim KW, et al: Contrast-enhanced dynamic ultrasonography of the liver: optimization of hepatic arterial phase in normal volunteers, *Adbom Imaging* 28(5):652-656, 2003.
46. Leen E, Anderson WG, Cooke TG, McArdle CS: Contrast enhanced Doppler perfusion index: detection of colorectal liver metastases, *Radiology* 209(1):292, 1998.
47. Leen E: Radiological applications of contrast agents in the hepatobiliary system. In Goldberg BB, Raichlen JS, Forsberg F, editors: *Ultrasound contrast agents,* ed 2, London, 2001, Martin Dunitz, pp 278-288.
48. Lencioni R, Pinto S, Cioni D, Bartolozzi C: Contrast-enhanced Doppler ultrasound of renal artery stenosis: prologue to a promising future, *Echocardiography* 16(7, Pt 2):767-773, 1999.
49. Leutoff UC, Scharf J, Richter GM, et al: Use of ultrasound contrast medium Levovist in after-care of liver transplant patients: improved vascular imaging in color Doppler ultrasound, *Radiology* 38:399-404, 1998.
50. Lyu SQ, Ren J, Zheng RQ, et al: Contrast-enhanced sonography for diagnosing collateral transformation of the hepatic artery after liver transplantation, *J Ultrasound Med* 34(9):1591-1598, 2015.
51. Manetta R, Pistoia ML, Bultrini C, et al: Ultrasound enhanced with sulphur-hexafluoride-filled microbubbles agent (SonoVue) in the follow-up of mild liver and spleen trauma, *Radiol Med* 114(5):771-779, 2009.
52. Martínez-Noguera A, Montserrat E, Torrubia S, et al: Ultrasound of the pancreas: update and controversies, *Eur Radiol* 11(9):1594-1606, 2001.
53. Merton DA: An easily implemented method to improve detection of ultrasound contrast in body tissues: frame one imaging, *J Diag Med Sonography* 16(1):14-20, 2000.
54. Micol C, Marsot J, Boublay N, et al: Contrast-enhanced ultrasound: a new method for TIPS follow-up, *Abdom Imaging* 37(2):252-260, 2012.
55. Postema M, Gilja OH: Contrast-enhanced and targeted ultrasound, *World J Gastroenterol* 17(1):28-41, 2011.
56. Missouris CG, Allen CM, Balen FG, et al: Non-invasive screening for renal artery stenosis with ultrasound contrast enhancement, *J Hypertens* 14(4):519-524, 1996.
57. Moriyasu F, Kono Y, Nada T, et al: Flash echo (passive cavitation) imaging of the liver by using US contrast agents and intermittent scanning sequence, *Radiology* 201(1):196, 1996.
58. Nagase M, Furuse J, Ishii H, Yoshino M: Evaluation of contrast enhancement patters in pancreatic tumors by coded harmonic sonographic imaging with a microbubble contrast agent, *J Ultrasound Med* 22(8):789-795, 2003.
59. Needleman L: Review of a new ultrasound contrast agent—EchoGen emulsion, *Appl Rad* 26(S):8-12, 1997.
60. Numata K, Yutaka O, Noritoshi K, et al: Contrast-enhanced sonography of autoimmune pancreatitis: comparison with pathologic findings, *J Ultrasound Med* 23(2):199-206, 2004.
61. Ophir J, Gobuty A, McWhirt RE, Maklad NF: Ultrasonic backscatter from contrast producing collagen microspheres, *Ultrasound Imaging* 2:67-77, 1980.
62. Oka MA, Rubens DJ, Strang JG: Ultrasound contrast agent in evaluation of abdominal vessels, *J Ultrasound Med* 20:S84, 2001.
63. Oldenburg A, Hohmann J, Skrok J, Albrecht T: Imaging of paediatric splenic injury with contrast-enhanced ultrasonography, *Pediatr Radiol* 34(4):351-354, 2004.
64. Olin JW, Piedmonte MR, Young JR, et al: The utility of duplex ultrasound scanning of the renal arteries for diagnosing significant renal artery stenosis, *Ann Intern Med* 122:833-838, 1995.
65. Pelberg RA, Wei K, Kamiyama N, et al: Potential advantage of flash echocardiography for digital subtraction of B-mode images acquired during myocardial contrast echocardiography, *J Am Soc Echocardiogr* 12:85-93, 1999.
66. Pfister K, Rennert J, Uller W, et al: Contrast harmonic imaging ultrasound and perfusion imaging for surveillance after endovascular abdominal aneurysm repair regarding detection and characterization of suspected endoleaks, *Clin Hemorheol Microcirc* 43(1):119-128, 2009.
67. Peterson CL, Barr RG: Contrast-enhanced sonography in patients with renal pathology, *J Diag Med Sonography* 16(2):53-56, 2000.
68. Picardi M, Soricelli A, Pane F, et al: Contrast-enhanced harmonic compound US of the spleen to increase staging accuracy in patients with Hodgkin lymphoma: a prospective study, *Radiology* 251(2):574-582, 2009.
69. Porter TR, Xie F: Accelerated intermittent harmonic imaging. In Goldberg BB, Raichlen JS, Forsberg F, editors: *Ultrasound contrast agents,* ed 2, London, 2001, Martin Dunitz, pp 67-70.
70. Porter TR, Xie F: Contrast echocardiography: latest developments and clinical utility, *Curr Cardiol Rep* 17(3):569, 2015.
71. Qu EZ, Zhang YC, Li ZY, et al: Contrast-enhanced sonography for quantitative assessment of portal hypertension in patients with liver cirrhosis, *J Ultrasound Med* 33(11):1971-1977, 2014.
72. Quaia E, De Paoli L, Angileri R, et al: Indeterminate solid hepatic lesions identified on non-diagnostic contrast-enhanced computed tomography: assessment of the additional diagnostic value of contrast-enhanced ultrasound in the non-cirrhotic liver, *Eur J Radiol* 83(3):456-462, 2014.

73. Rickes S, Unkrodt K, Neye H, et al: Differentiation of pancreatic tumours by conventional ultrasound, unenhanced and echo-enhanced power Doppler sonography, *Scand J Gastroenterol* 37(11): 1313-1320, 2002.

74. Robbin ML, Lockhart ME, Barr RG: Renal imaging with ultrasound contrast: current status, *Radiol Clin North Am* 41(5):963-978, 2003.

75. Ryu SW, Bok GH, Jang JY, et al: Clinically useful diagnostic tool of contrast enhanced ultrasonography for focal liver masses: comparison to computed tomography and magnetic resonance imaging, *Gut Liver* 8(3):292-297, 2014.

76. Schwenger V, Hankel V, Seckinger J, et al: Contrast-enhanced ultrasonography in the early period after kidney transplantation predicts long-term allograft function, *Transplant Proc* 46(10):3352-3357, 2014.

77. Sellars ME, Sidhu PS, Heneghan M, et al: Infusions of microbubbles are more cost-effective than bolus injections in Doppler studies of the portal vein: a quantitative comparison of normal volunteers and patients with cirrhosis, *Radiology* 217(2):396, 2000.

78. Sidhu PS, Marshall MM, Ryan SM, et al: Clinical use of Levovist, an ultrasound contrast agent, in the imaging of liver transplantation: assessment of the pre- and post-transplant patient, *Eur Radiol* 10(7):1114-1126, 2000.

79. Sidhu PS, Shaw AS, Ellis SM, et al: Microbubble ultrasound contrast in the assessment of hepatic artery patency following liver transplantation: role in reducing frequency of heaptic artery arteriography, *Eur Radiol* 14(1):21-30, 2004.

80. Sirlin CB, Girard MS, Baker K, et al: Effect of gated US acquisition on liver and portal vein contrast enhancement, *Radiology* 201(1):158, 1996.

81. Skjoldbye B, Weislander S, Struckmann J, et al: Doppler ultrasound assessment of TIPS patency and function-the need for echo enhancers, *Acta Radiol* 39:675-679, 1998.

82. Solbiati L, Cova L, Ierace T, et al: Characterization of focal lesions in patients with liver cirrhosis using second generation contrast-enhanced (CE) wideband harmonic sonography (WBHS) in different enhancement phases, *J Ultrasound Med* 20:S10, 2001.

83. Solbiati L, Cova L, Ierace T, et al: Diagnosis of atypical hemangioma using contrast-enhanced wideband harmonic sonography (CE-WBHS), *J Ultrasound Med* 20:S9, 2001.

84. Solbiati L, Goldberg SN, Ierace T, et al: Radio-frequency ablation of hepatic metastases: post procedural assessment with a US microbubble contrast agent: early experience, *Radiology* 211:643-649, 1999.

85. Strobel D, Seitz K, Blank W, et al: Tumor-specific vascularization pattern of liver metastasis, hepatocellular carcinoma, hemangioma and focal nodular hyperplasia in the differential diagnosis of 1,349 liver lesions in contrast-enhanced ultrasound (CEUS), *Ultraschall Med* 30(4):376-382, 2009.

86. Strobel D, Krodel U, Martus P, et al: Clinical evaluation of contrast-enhanced color Doppler sonography in the differential diagnosis of liver tumors, *J Clin Ultrasound* 28:1-13, 2000.

87. Sugimoto K, Shiraishi J, Moriyasu F, et al: Improved detection of hepatic metastases with contrast-enhanced low mechanical-index pulse inversion ultrasonography during the liver-specific phase of Sonazoid: observer performance study with JAFROC analysis, *Acad Radiol* 16(7):798-809, 2009.

88. Tanaka S, Kitamra T, Yoshioka F, et al: Effectiveness of galactose-based intravenous contrast medium on color Doppler sonography of deeply located hepatocellular carcinoma, *Ultrasound in Med Biol* 21:157-160, 1995.

89. Tawada K, Yamaguchi T, Kobayashi A, et al: Changes in tumor vascularity depicted by contrast-enhanced ultrasonography as a predictor of chemotherapeutic effect in patients with unresectable pancreatic cancer, *Pancreas* 38(1):30-35, 2009.

90. Trillaud H, Bruel JM, Valette PJ, et al: Characterization of focal liver lesions with SonoVue® enhanced sonography: International multicenter-study in comparison to CT and MRI, *World J Gastroenterol* 15(30):3748-3756, 2009.

91. Uggowitzer MM, Hausegger KA, Machan L, et al: Echo-enhanced Doppler sonography in the evaluation of transjugular intraheptic portosystemic shunts: clinical applications of a new transpulmonary US contrast agent, *Radiology* 201(1,3):266, 748, 1996.

92. von Herbay A, Vogt C, Haussinger D: Pulse inversion sonography in the early phase of the sonographic contrast agent Levovist: differentiation between benign and malignant focal liver lesions, *J Ultrasound Med* 21:1191-1200, 2002.

93. Wei K, Le E, Bin JP, et al: Quantification of renal blood flow with contrast-enhanced ultrasound, *J Am Coll Cardiol* 37(4):1135-1140, 2001.

94. Weskott HP: Contrast-enhanced reperfusion imaging in atypical hepatic hemangiomas, *J Ultrasound Med* 20:S9, 2001.

95. Wheatley MA: Composition of contrast microbubbles: basic chemistry of encapsulated and surfactant-coated bubbles. In Goldberg BB, Raichlen JS, Forsberg F, editors: *Ultrasound contrast agents,* ed 2, London, 2001, Martin Dunitz, pp 3-13.

96. Bracco Diagnostic Inc: *First approval by U.S. Food and Drug Administration for contrast enhanced ultrasonography of the liver received by Bracco Diagnostics Inc. for LUMASON® (sulfur hexafluoride lipid-type A microspheres) for injectable suspension, for intravenous use* (website). http://imaging.bracco.com/us-en/first-approval-us-food-and-drug-administration-contrast-enhanced-ultrasonography-liver-received. Accessed June 17, 2016.

97. Wilson SR, Burns PN, Muradali D, et al: Harmonic hepatic US with microbubble contrast agent: initial experience showing improved characterization of hemangioma, hepatocellular carcinoma, and metastasis, *Radiology* 215:153-161, 2000.

98. Yang X, Chen YX, Zhang B, et al: Contrast-enhanced ultrasound in detecting endoleaks with failed computed tomography angiography diagnosis after endovascular abdominal aortic aneurysm repair, *Chin Med J (Engl)* 128(18):2491-2497, 2015.

99. Zeisbrich M, Kihm LP, Drüschler F, et al: When is contrast-enhanced sonography preferable over conventional ultrasound combined with Doppler imaging in renal transplantation? *Clin Kidney J* 8(5):606-614, 2015.

100. Zhou JH, Li AH, Cao LH, et al: Haemodynamic parameters of the hepatic artery and vein can detect liver metastases: assessment using contrast-enhanced ultrasound, *Br J Radiol* 81(962):113-119, 2008.

Ultrasound-Guided Interventional Techniques

M. Robert DeJong

Ultrasound has been used to assist in interventional procedures since the 1970s by means of specially designed A-mode and B-mode transducers. The use of ultrasound as a primary imaging modality to guide interventional examinations continues to grow. Multiple factors contribute to this growth: increased system resolution, new developments in transducer designs, new technology developments such as compound imaging and fusion technologies, and the development of more versatile transducer needle guide attachments, which offer multiple angles. Another important factor is economics, as ultrasound-guided procedures are less costly than other imaging modalities. One of the economic benefits of

interventional examinations is that performing a biopsy under ultrasound allows improved patient throughput to continue through the computed tomography (CT) scanner. Performing a biopsy under CT would mean a decrease of four to five patients per hour in the CT scanner as opposed to one less patient in the ultrasound room. Ultrasound is now being used to perform a variety of invasive procedures on various organs and masses located in the neck, chest, abdomen, retroperitoneum, musculoskeletal system, and pelvis, as well as to drain various fluid and abscess collections. There has been an increase in the number of nonimaging physicians who use ultrasound for the placement of peripherally inserted central catheter lines, subclavian and jugular lines, and even to assist in starting intravenous (IV) lines.

ULTRASOUND-GUIDED PROCEDURES

In recent years, there has been a movement to perform more and more procedures under ultrasound guidance. Retroperitoneal masses, pleural-based masses, deep masses in the liver, and musculoskeletal masses that were once typically biopsied under CT guidance or in open surgical biopsies are now being successfully performed using ultrasound guidance (Figure 18-1).

Ultrasound can be used to do the following:
- Biopsy malignant or benign masses.
- Biopsy organs for parenchymal disease or transplant rejection.
- Drain fluid collections, such as cysts, ascites, or pleural fluid.
- Drain or obtain samples of abscesses to determine the type of organism, especially on patients who are not responding to antibiotic therapy.
- Assist in placement of drainage tubes or catheters.
- Assist in placement of catheters in arteries and veins.
- Mark spots for fluid taps to be performed without direct sonographic guidance.

The main advantage of using ultrasound for guidance is to have continuous real-time visualization of the biopsy needle, which allows adjustment of the needle as needed during the procedure. As the biopsy specimen is being obtained, the needle tip can be watched in real-time to ensure that it does not slip outside the mass. This is especially important for small masses or if the patient has trouble holding his or her breath. Ultrasound also has the advantage of allowing different patient positions and approaches to be considered. The patient may be turned into a decubitus or oblique position to allow safe access to the mass (Figure 18-2). Subcostal approaches can allow the use of steep angles with the needle directed cephalic in liver masses. This can reduce the risk of

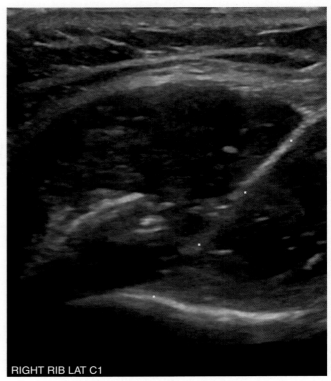

RIGHT RIB LAT C1

FIGURE 18-1 Chondrosarcoma of the rib.

a **pneumothorax** or bleeding from an injury to an intercostal artery when using intercostal techniques. Using ultrasound the patient can be placed in a comfortable position and not be made to lie supine or prone. For example, the patient's head may be slightly elevated or the patient can move slightly between passes to relieve back or joint pain. Another benefit is the ability to comfort and reassure the patient as the sonologist, sonographer, and nurse are all with the patient during the procedure. Even the most anxious patients can be coached to cooperate when the team is by their side and not constantly in and out of the room. Other advantages include the ability to

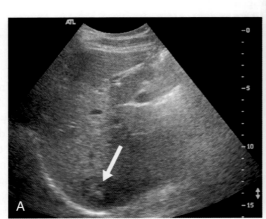
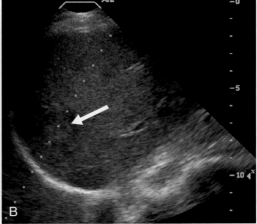

FIGURE 18-2 **A,** With the patient supine, the liver mass *(arrow)* is 15 cm deep. **B,** The patient is now in the left lateral decubitus position, the liver has fallen forward, and the same mass *(arrow)* is now only 7 cm deep. An easy, successful biopsy showed metastatic disease from a pancreas primary.

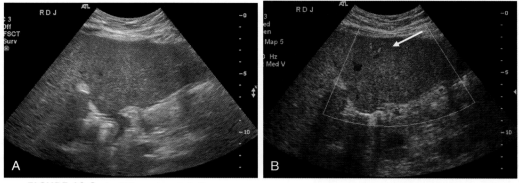

FIGURE 18-3 A, Although a definite mass was seen on a contrast magnetic resonance imaging (MRI), it was not appreciated by ultrasound. **B,** Using the MRI as a guide and color Doppler to assess for areas of abnormal flow, a successful biopsy was performed on this patient with infiltrative hepatocellular carcinoma *(arrow)*.

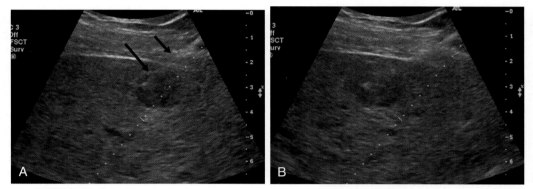

FIGURE 18-4 A, The needle *(arrows)* deviated from the projected path of the guide *(dotted line)*. **B,** Because of the constant deviation of the needle from the projected path, the sonographer had to compensate by moving the transducer laterally so that the needle would pass through the center of the mass. Note that the projected path does not even go through the mass. A diagnosis of hepatocellular carcinoma was obtained.

perform the biopsy in a single breath hold, portability, lack of radiation, and shorter procedure times.

Despite all its benefits, ultrasound guidance does have some limitations. Not all masses can be visualized with ultrasound, as the mass may be isoechoic to the normal tissue. The sonographer should look for indirect signs of the presence of a mass, such as displaced vessels, capsule bulges, or the presence of tumor vessels (Figure 18-3). Abdominal masses may also be obscured by bowel gas. Sometimes the sonographer can press the gas out of the way with the transducer, allowing for a successful biopsy. Gas may move during the procedure, causing difficulty in seeing the mass, which can delay the biopsy until the gas moves or even in some cases canceling the biopsy under ultrasound and finishing it under CT. The needle tip may be difficult to see if it deviates from the projected path because of bending or deflection of the needle. This can call on the sonographer's scanning skills to maneuver the transducer to find the needle tip or to correct for needle deviation (Figure 18-4). Other disadvantages may include sonographer inexperience, the comfort level of the radiologist with performing biopsies under CT, and having to use fixed angles when using needle guides.

INDICATIONS FOR A BIOPSY

The most common indication for a biopsy is to confirm malignancy of a mass. The mass may be a primary tumor in a patient with an undiagnosed malignancy or a metastatic mass in a patient with a known primary malignancy. Other indications include the need to differentiate between a metastatic and a second primary mass, to determine the cause of metastases in a patient with multiple primaries, to differentiate recurrent tumor from postoperative or therapy scarring, to differentiate malignancy from inflammatory or infectious disease, to determine metastatic lymph adenopathy from lymphoma, and to characterize a benign mass. Other common reasons for a biopsy are to obtain a sample of the parenchyma in an organ to determine the severity or progression of a disease process such as hepatitis or renal failure or to determine the cause of rejection in a transplanted organ (Figure 18-5).

CONTRAINDICATIONS FOR A BIOPSY

Contraindications of ultrasound-guided procedures are few because of the procedure's minimally invasive nature. However, contraindications do include an uncorrectable bleeding

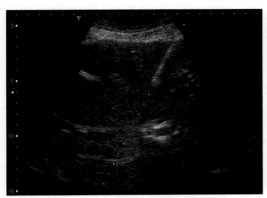

FIGURE 18-5 Liver core biopsy in a patient with hepatitis C.

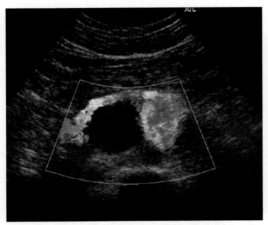

FIGURE 18-6 This retroperitoneal lymph node could not be biopsied under ultrasound because of the vessels that surrounded it.

disorder, the lack of a safe needle path (Figure 18-6), or an uncooperative patient. Patient cooperation is needed so that the mass may be biopsied safely. If the patient will not hold still, is jumpy, or cannot control his or her breathing, the risk of a complication for the patient increases significantly, as does the risk to the sonographer or sonologist of being stuck by a contaminated needle.

LABORATORY TESTS

With the exception of bleeding times, blood or urine tests typically are not requested before an ultrasound-guided procedure. Usually, an abnormal laboratory value will be part of the patient's workup that led to the biopsy. Some abnormal values that may trigger a request for a biopsy or aspiration include elevated **alpha-fetoprotein (AFP)** in the presence of a liver lesion, elevated **prostate-specific antigen (PSA)** to evaluate for prostate cancer, changes in thyroglobulin levels in a patient with a history of thyroid cancer, increased white blood cell count (leukocytosis) when an abscess is suspected, and hematuria along with a renal mass.

Laboratory tests that should be reviewed before most procedures are the patient's bleeding times. These tests measure the time it takes the blood to form a clot. This is especially true for patients who are on blood thinners such as warfarin

(Coumadin), heparin, or aspirin therapy. Because vitamin K is essential in the blood clotting process, patients with liver disease are at risk for prolonged bleeding and the formation of hematomas. To eliminate patient rescheduling or cancellation, test results should be obtained as close to the date of the procedure as possible, although results may be acceptable up to 3 to 4 weeks before the scheduled procedure. These simple blood tests can also be performed the morning of the procedure as results can usually be obtained in 2 to 3 hours.

At least a dozen factors are needed to form a blood clot to stop bleeding; they all interact through a complex series of reactions called the coagulation cascade. There are three pathways in the blood clotting process: intrinsic, extrinsic, and common. To evaluate all three pathways, both **prothrombin time (PT)** and **partial thromboplastin time (PTT)** are evaluated. PTT can be used to evaluate the effects of heparin, aspirin, and antihistamines on the blood-clotting process. PTT evaluates factors found in the intrinsic and common pathways. PTT values may vary depending on the method and activators used, with normal values typically between 60 and 70 seconds. PT is used to evaluate factors found in the extrinsic pathway, which may be affected by patients on Coumadin. Normal values are typically between 10 and 13 seconds.

Because of the variability of PT results between laboratories, a method of standardization was developed called the **international normalized ratio (INR).** The INR was created in 1983 by the World Health Organization to account for the various thromboplastin reagents used to determine PT, which caused fluctuations in normal values. The INR is a calculation that adjusts for the variations in PT processing and values so that test results from different laboratories can be compared. The INR is expressed as a number. Values of less than 1.4 are needed to ensure a safe procedure. The INR/PT is not used on patients with liver disease or on heparin. It is evaluated on patients taking anticoagulants, especially Coumadin.

PT, PTT, and platelet count are required before most procedures. Some departments may not require a hemostatic evaluation for fluid aspirations and superficial or low-risk biopsies such as of the thyroid, neck nodes, or prostate. Anticoagulants should be discontinued before the biopsy to reduce the risk of postprocedural bleeding. Patients should be off their blood thinners before the procedure as follows: 4 to 6 hours for heparin, 3 to 4 days for Coumadin, and 5 to 7 days for aspirin, although these values can be different for different hospitals or imaging centers. Patients should also be informed to stop taking supplements that can prolong bleeding times such as omega-3, fish oils, and flaxseed oil. Patients with a defect in their blood-clotting mechanism (**coagulopathy**) will need to have a platelet transfusion just before and during the procedure to ensure that they do not have excessive bleeding.

TYPES OF PROCEDURES

Biopsies are used to confirm if a mass is benign, malignant, or infectious. Most biopsies are easily and safely performed as an outpatient procedure. Biopsy success rates have been reported to have sensitivities of greater than 85% and specificities of greater than 95%. Cell type is often needed to determine treatment type and options, as specific tumors respond better to certain types of chemotherapy or to radiation therapy.

Fine-needle aspiration (FNA), or cytologic aspiration, uses thin-gauge needles to obtain cells from within the mass. FNAs are performed using a 20- to 25-gauge needle with a cutting tip, such as a Franseen, Chiba, or spinal needle (Figure 18-7). These types of needles have the least risk associated with their use, allowing multiple passes as needed. The number of the gauge corresponds to the diameter of the needle: the higher the number, the smaller the diameter. Needles are described by their length and gauge. For example, if the physician asks for a 20, 15, or 20 × 15, he or she wants a 20-gauge needle that is 15 cm in length. If different types of needles are available, the

physician might ask for a Franseen 20, 15. A word of caution: Seeing the length of the needle may cause a patient to become quite apprehensive. The sonographer should explain to the patient that *most of the needle will be inside the needle guide.* The specimen is obtained by using a capillary action technique. This involves a steady, quick up-and-down motion of the needle (after the stylet is removed), which obtains the needed cells through a scraping or cutting action. As the needle is removed from the body, the physician will place his or her thumb over the open hub so that the cells are not sucked back into the body. An FNA technique reduces the trauma to the cells and decreases the amount of background blood. If the sample is scant, suction techniques can be used. Suction technique involves using a syringe and tubing attached to the needle. As the needle is being moved up and down, suction is applied to draw up the cells into the needle. Once the needle is removed, the physician will place the tip of the needle over the slide to deposit the cells so that they can be smeared for staining and evaluation. The physician may also express the cells into a container holding special fluid to preserve the cells. Because of its thin size, the needle can safely go through the large or small bowel and near vascular structures. FNA in conjunction with onsite cytopathology can help ensure that the procedure is diagnostic and minimize the number of passes.

A core biopsy utilizes an automated, spring-loaded device, termed a *biopsy gun,* to obtain a core of tissue for histologic analysis. The biopsy device is cocked and the needle tip is placed just inside the mass, on the outside edge of the mass or inside the organ itself. The button is then pushed and the cutting needle is thrown, obtaining a core of tissue, which is deposited into a slot on the inner needle (Figure 18-8). Various throw

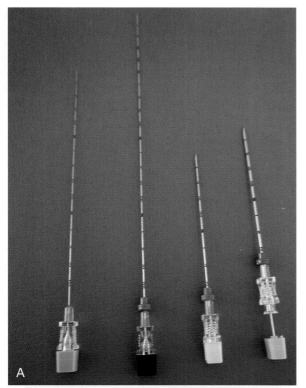

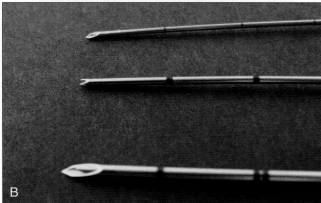

FIGURE 18-7 **A,** Different types of needles and gauges used for FNA biopsies. Blue: 25 gauge × 15 cm, black: 22 gauge × 20 cm, yellow: 20 gauge × 9 cm, pink: 18 gauge × 9 cm. **B,** Example of different types of needle tips. From top: Chiba, Franseen, Spinal.

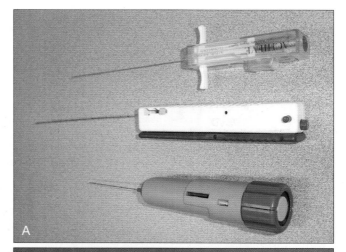

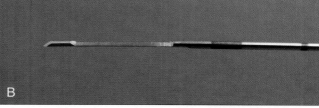

FIGURE 18-8 Different types of biopsy devices used for core biopsies. **B,** Close-up of a core needle where the specimen is deposited.

lengths are available, ranging from 10 to 23 mm, which will also correspond to the length of specimen that is obtained. The throw length is the distance that the needle will advance when fired. The proper throw distance needs to be determined so that the needle does not go through the back wall of the mass and damage underlying structures or vessels (Figure 18-9). The snapping sound that the device makes can be startling to the patient, and it is advised to let the patient hear the sound before obtaining the specimen. This also ensures that the device is not defective. Core biopsy needles are larger in diameter and range in size from 14 to 20 gauge. A core biopsy can be used in conjunction with FNA techniques, especially if a definitive diagnosis could not be determined from just the FNA or if the cytopathologist requires more tissue for a more accurate diagnosis or special stains. Core biopsies are used to diagnose diffuse parenchymal disease of the liver or kidney, in transplanted organs, masses in the breast, and in prostate biopsies.

Ultrasound is routinely used to guide needle placement to drain or obtain samples from ascites or pleural effusions. Usually, these procedures are performed without the use of a needle guide unless the fluid is multiloculated, is only a small amount, or is unsafe to drain by free-hand techniques. If a small amount of fluid is needed, a 22- or 20-gauge needle may be used. If the fluid is viscous, an 18- or 16-gauge needle may be required. If the goal is to drain as much fluid as possible, a special needle called a centesis catheter is used (Figure 18-10).

After the needle is properly placed, the stylet is removed, leaving a catheter with side holes to safely drain the fluid. For large volume drainage, 1-liter vacuum bottles are used to remove the fluid. Ultrasound can be used to periodically check the amount of fluid remaining or to help reposition the catheter to free it from bowel that may be sucked against the wall of the catheter (Figure 18-11). The sonographer can usually scan outside the sterile field. In a patient with massive ascites, a large volume of fluid may be drained for patient comfort. It is usually recommended that no more than 5 liters be drained because more than that can place the patient at risk for electrolyte imbalance, hypovolemia, hypotension, and hepatorenal syndrome. If more than 5 liters are to be removed, the patient is usually given IV albumin to decrease the chance of these complications.

Fluid or abscess collections are usually performed using a needle guide. Abscess or fluid collections may be located in or around the liver; in the peripancreatic, perinephric, intraabdominal, pelvic, or intramuscular regions; or in the prostate gland. Ultrasound can also be used to provide guidance to drain the gallbladder in patients who have cholecystitis, especially acalculous cholecystitis, or in patients too sick for

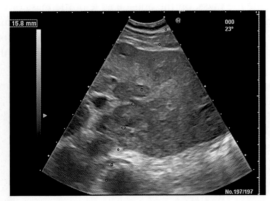

FIGURE 18-9 The sonographer measured the lesion (calipers) to determine the size of the core needle to be used. The diameter of the lesion along the needle path is 15.8 mm, so a 15-mm throw is needed to stay within the lesion.

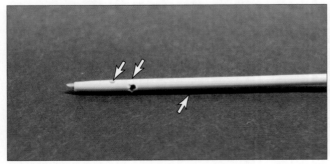

FIGURE 18-10 A centesis catheter. The arrows are pointing to the side holes.

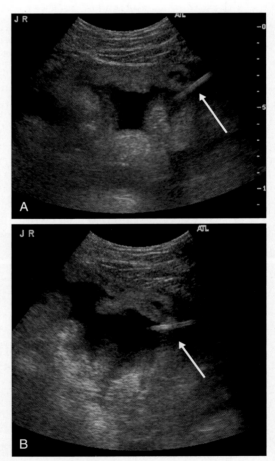

FIGURE 18-11 A, Bowel has been sucked up against the catheter (*arrow*), obstructing the flow of fluid. **B,** By having the patient roll into an oblique position, the fluid collected to the dependent portion and the bowel loop floated away from the catheter (*arrow*), allowing drainage to continue.

surgery. The needle gauge used to drain the abscess depends on the thickness of the fluid. For pelvic collections, depending on their location, an endovaginal approach should be considered in women, and endorectal approaches in both men and women. For prostatic abscess drainage, an endorectal technique is used. Fluid is obtained to determine the type of organism present, so that the correct antibiotics can be administered to the patient. For a larger abscess, catheters may be left in place to drain the collection. Patients may have follow-ups to monitor that the cavity is getting smaller and to check that the catheter is still in the correct position. These follow-up examinations are usually performed under fluoroscopy in a procedure called a sinogram, although ultrasound can also be used.

Ultrasound is currently being used to guide placements of catheters and lines in various vessels including the subclavian, jugular, brachial, and femoral vessels; to assist in transjugular intrahepatic portosystemic shunt (TIPS) procedures; and to place nephrostomy tubes in obstructed kidneys. There are even dedicated ultrasound units available to help with image-guided peripheral IV insertion.

ULTRASOUND GUIDANCE METHODS

There are two methods in performing ultrasound-guided procedures: free-hand techniques and the use of needle guides. The free-hand technique is performed without the use of a needle guide on the transducer. The transducer is placed in a sterile cover, and the radiologist or physician that performs the biopsy will hold the transducer in one hand and the needle in the other hand. Care must be taken to align the needle with the transducer and the sound beam or else the needle tip will not be seen. If the needle tip disappears while advancing the needle on the image, the transducer should be repositioned in alignment with the needle path to bring the needle tip back into view. The free-hand technique allows more flexibility in choosing the needle path, but it is more technically challenging, especially on deep lesions (Figure 18-12). A variation of this technique allows the sonographer to scan outside the sterile field while the physician performs the biopsy (Figure 18-13). Again, it is important to remember that to see the needle tip, the transducer must be aligned to the needle path. If the needle is not going to the area of interest, then either the transducer must be realigned to the needle path to find the needle or the needle must be removed and reinserted toward the transducer. If there is a light or color mark on the transducer, the sonographer can tell the physician to go toward the light. Free-hand techniques are typically used to drain ascites (Figure 18-14), pleural fluid, and in superficial lesions. Some physicians prefer using free-hand techniques for thyroid, native renal, and renal transplant biopsies.

The second method involves using a needle guide that is attached to the transducer (Figure 18-15). The predicted

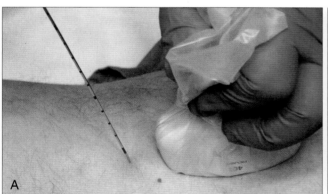

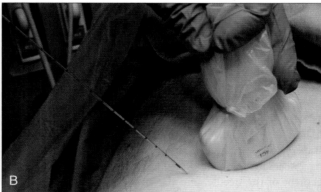

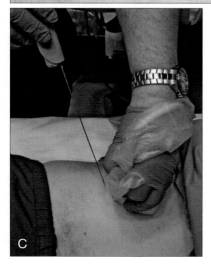

FIGURE 18-12 One-person free-hand technique. **A,** The needle is in plane with the transducer. **B,** Notice that the needle is not in plane with the transducer. **C,** This is the same patient and position as B, with the transducer now moved to be in line with the needle.

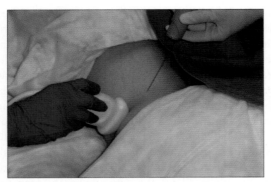

FIGURE 18-13 Two-person free-hand technique with the sonographer scanning outside the sterile field.

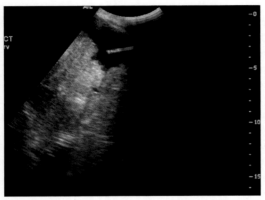

FIGURE 18-14 This paracentesis was performed without the use of a guide, as the fluid was superficial.

needle path is displayed on the screen either as a single line or as two parallel lines. The mass is then lined up along the path, either on the single line or between the two lines. Some transducers offer a choice of angles, usually a steep angle and a shallow angle (Figure 18-16). This gives some flexibility around vessels or other structures. There are many benefits to using a needle guide, including a faster learning curve, faster placement of the needle, and the ability to keep the needle going through the anesthetized area when multiple passes are required (Figure 18-17). The use of needle guides has expanded the role of ultrasound-guided procedures by allowing biopsies of pleural-based lung lesions, deep retroperitoneal lesions, small masses, and musculoskeletal masses. When the sonographer attaches the needle guide to the transducer, it is important to attach it correctly and set the angle on the guide the same as the angle on the screen. The needle guides are precision-made devices and need to be handled with care and attached properly. If another angle is set on the transducer, the needle will appear to deviate, as it is not following the projected path on the screen; if the guide is put on backward, the needle will come in from the opposite side of the guide (Figure 18-18).

Both methods have their pros and cons, and the physician performing the biopsy or procedure will decide which technique—free-hand or needle-guided—to use.

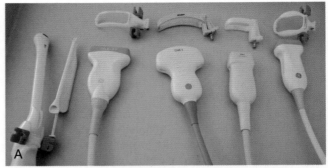

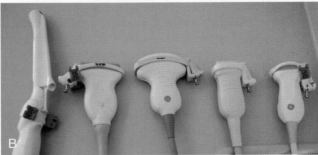

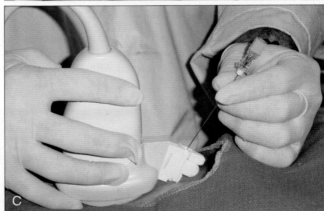

FIGURE 18-15 A, Various types of transducers and their guides. **B,** Same transducers with their guides attached. **C,** Biopsy using a needle guide.

CYTOPATHOLOGY

Some ultrasound departments collaborate with the cytopathology department by having the cytopathology team present during the procedure. Usually, one to three passes are made, placed on the sterile slides, and stained in the ultrasound room. The cytopathologist looks at the slides to determine if the material is diagnostic. This can ensure that enough diagnostic material is obtained and help to minimize the number of passes. The cytopathologist may request additional material for special stains and flow cytometry. (Flow cytometry may be needed when lymphoma is suspected.) The cytopathologist may also request that a core sample be obtained to enhance the chances of obtaining a diagnosis for the patient. It typically takes 3 to 5 minutes to stain and evaluate the slides per pass or group of passes. The benefit of having cytopathology onsite is that it increases

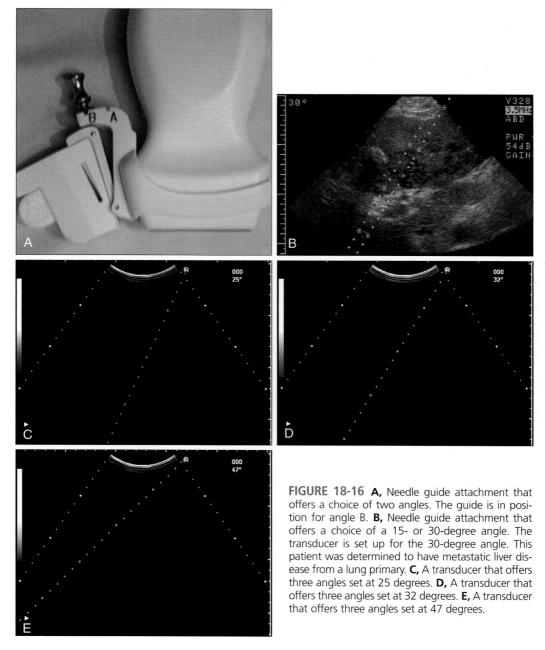

FIGURE 18-16 **A,** Needle guide attachment that offers a choice of two angles. The guide is in position for angle B. **B,** Needle guide attachment that offers a choice of a 15- or 30-degree angle. The transducer is set up for the 30-degree angle. This patient was determined to have metastatic liver disease from a lung primary. **C,** A transducer that offers three angles set at 25 degrees. **D,** A transducer that offers three angles set at 32 degrees. **E,** A transducer that offers three angles set at 47 degrees.

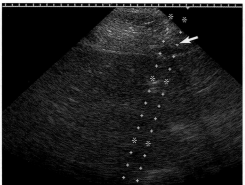

FIGURE 18-17 The arrow is pointing to a hypoechoic area, which is the lidocaine that was injected adjacent to the liver capsule. It is important for the sonographer to keep the transducer in this position so that the biopsy needle goes through the anesthetized area.

the percentage of successful biopsies, helps to minimize the number of passes, and possibly reduces overall procedure time.

Inconclusive Specimens

Unfortunately, not all biopsies yield sufficient material to provide a diagnosis. There are multiple reasons that lead to an inconclusive result, including insufficient material, necrotic lesion, and not biopsying the area of malignancy. If this occurs, a repeat biopsy may be required. This possibility should have been explained to the patient during the consent process. To increase the success of the repeat biopsy, a cytopathologist should be present.

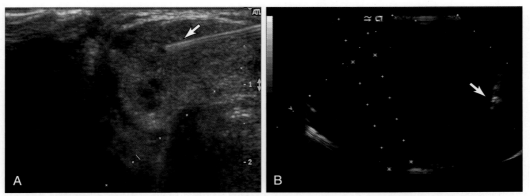

FIGURE 18-18 **A,** The arrow is pointing to the needle, which appears to be deviating. What is actually happening is that the guide on the transducer is set for angle A, but the biopsy line displayed on the screen is set for angle B. **B,** The transducer was attached backward. When the needle is inserted *(arrow),* it appears from the opposite side of the screen.

BIOPSY COMPLICATIONS

Complications from an ultrasound-guided biopsy are usually minor and may include postprocedural pain or discomfort, vasovagal reactions, and hematomas. Serious complications, although rare, include bleeding, hemorrhage, pneumothorax, pancreatitis, biliary leakage, peritonitis, infection, and possibly death. Seeding of the needle track by malignant cells is rare, with an estimated occurrence of 1 in 20,000 patients. These potential complications must be explained to the patient during the consent process. It is important for the sonographer to look for signs of a complication both by observing the patient and with ultrasound. The sonographer should scan after every pass to look for any sonographic sign of a complication using both gray scale and color Doppler (Figure 18-19). The sonographer should also help in observing the patient for any indications of a vasovagal reaction, pain, or bleeding from the biopsy site. Any visual or sonographic signs of a complication should be reported to the physician immediately. Applying pressure with the transducer over the area of bleeding can treat both internal and external bleeding. For bleeding from the skin at the biopsy site, cover the puncture site with a sterile 4 × 4 or other sterile material and press with the transducer. The sterile

4 × 4 will absorb the blood so that it does not drip down the patient's side and lend stability to the transducer so that it is not slippery. **Vasovagal** patient symptoms include profuse sweating, complaining of feeling faint or lightheaded, and nausea. Patients who experience any or all of these symptoms should be placed in a Trendelenburg position or have their feet elevated with a stack of sheets. A cold cloth or compress can also be placed on the forehead. After these feelings pass, the biopsy may continue.

FUSION TECHNOLOGY

Newer technologies have improved the percentage of procedures that can be performed using ultrasound guidance. Harmonic imaging and compound imaging have improved resolution by improving visualization of subtler lesions as well as of the needle tip. However, there are still a small percentage of lesions that cannot be seen by ultrasound. These are typically isoechoic lesions, especially in the liver. These lesions may also only be seen on a contrast-enhanced CT, thus making it difficult to perform the biopsy under CT guidance. Recently some ultrasound companies have developed ultrasound equipment that can import the patient's CT or magnetic resonance

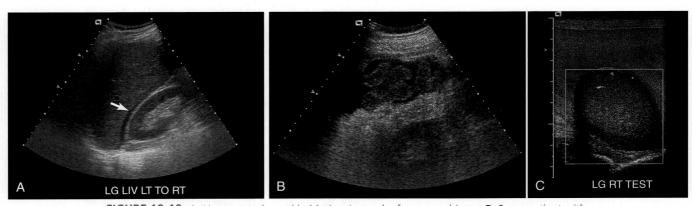

FIGURE 18-19 **A,** Hematoma *(arrow)* in Morison's pouch after a core biopsy. **B,** Same patient with free fluid along the left flank. **C,** The hematoma extended into the scrotal sac. Color Doppler verified that flow was present in the testicle.

imaging (MRI) scan directly into the ultrasound unit. This allows the sonographer to compare the MRI or CT scan directly with the ultrasound image in side-by-side images. As the ultrasound scan is being performed, the MRI or CT images move to the corresponding area, following the sonographer as they scan. Thus the same anatomy is seen in real-time on both the ultrasound image and the corresponding imported images (Figure 18-20). Another option allows fusing or superimposing of the two image sets on top of one another. Controls allow the ultrasound image or CT/MRI image to be given preference. For example, while locating the mass, the CT/MRI image may be emphasized, whereas the ultrasound image will be emphasized during the actual biopsy (Figure 18-21).

This technology uses an electromagnetic transmitter, which is placed near the area of scanning, and electromagnetic sensors that are connected to, or inside, the transducer. Both the electromagnetic transmitter and the transducer are connected to a position-sensing unit attached to the ultrasound machine. The position-sensing equipment allows the ultrasound unit to track the transducer's position as the sonographer scans, and with it the image position, within the electromagnetic field (Figure 18-22).

To begin, the MRI or CT data set must be imported into the ultrasound unit. This can either be done via the network or uploaded from a DVD (Figure 18-23). Next, the sonographer needs to register the ultrasound image with the CT or MRI data set. This is accomplished by choosing a common anatomic point that can be identified easily on both the ultrasound image and the MRI or CT data set. Some common reference points may be the bifurcation of a vessel, the border of an organ, or even an area inside the mass. Some units align the data sets after the sonographer obtains a three-dimensional (3D) sweep of the same area as the CT/MRI data set. After locking in these points, the machine builds a transformation matrix based on this information. This transformation matrix is then used to display the multiplanar reconstructed image from the 3D MRI or CT data set that corresponds to the current live ultrasound image. As the ultrasound transducer is moved, the CT/MRI images also move in the same direction. The images can then be displayed either side by side or in a blended, overlapping format. The ultrasound image can also be removed, allowing the sonographer to scan and see only the CT or MRI image. This can be helpful in allowing the sonographer to scan and locate the area using the other imaging

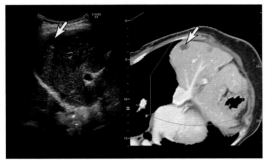

FIGURE 18-20 Fused studies of an ultrasound and CT demonstrating a simple liver cyst in the dome of the liver *(arrows)*.

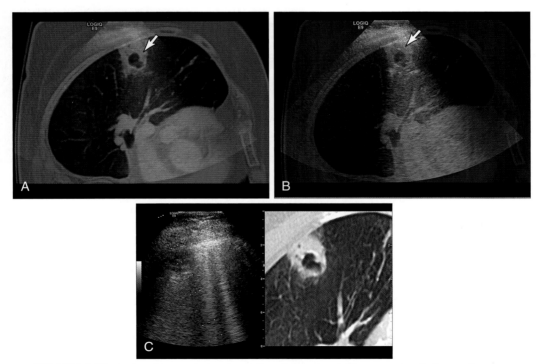

FIGURE 18-21 A, Fused imaged of a chest CT and ultrasound. The arrow is pointing to the mass. In this image, the CT has preference over the ultrasound image. **B,** Same two images, but this time the ultrasound has preference over the CT image. **C,** Side-by-side images used to guide the biopsy. This patient had adenocarcinoma of the lung.

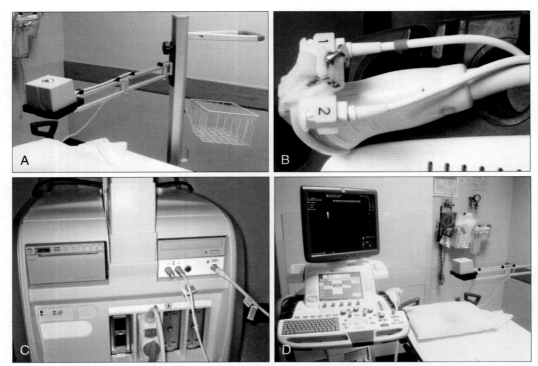

FIGURE 18-22 **A,** An electromagnetic transmitter unit. **B,** An example of sensors attached to the transducer. **C,** The cord from the transmitter unit and the paired cords from the transducer are plugged into the position sensing unit. **D,** The ultrasound unit and accessories needed to perform fusion imaging.

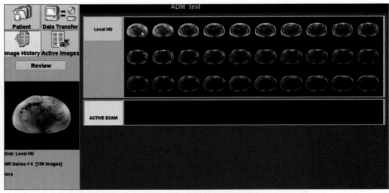

FIGURE 18-23 An MRI series that has been imported into the ultrasound unit.

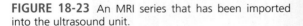

modality. Once the area of concern is located, the ultrasound image can be activated, and the sonographer can either remove the image from the other modality, scan in a fused method, or scan in a side-by-side format.

Once the two imaging modalities have been registered, the sonographer can use the CT or MRI scan to locate the area in question with ultrasound. If the area is not well seen by ultrasound, a marker can be placed on the MRI or CT image so that the radiologist knows where to obtain the specimen. Once this marker is placed on the MRI or CT image, a corresponding marker will appear on the ultrasound image (Figure 18-24). Another use for marking or targeting the mass is to quickly locate it when the transducer needs to be removed from the patient's skin. When the area that has been marked is on the screen, the marker will appear as a small square. As the

sonographer scans away from the area, the marker grows larger. For difficult lesions, marking the area on the scans allows the sonographer to rest his or her arm between passes or before the procedure begins, thus helping to prevent musculoskeletal injuries from prolonged holding of the transducer in one place. The sonographer can place the transducer back on the patient when the biopsy is ready to proceed, look for the marker, and adjust the scanning plane until the marker is small and the area of interest is displayed (Figure 18-25). This can be a time-saver when the transducer is removed from the patient's skin, especially for difficult-to-see lesions, as the tracking boxes will help the sonographer quickly return to the lesion with confidence. Fusion techniques are also helpful if multiple lesions are visible on the MRI or CT and there is a specific lesion that the clinician wants biopsied.

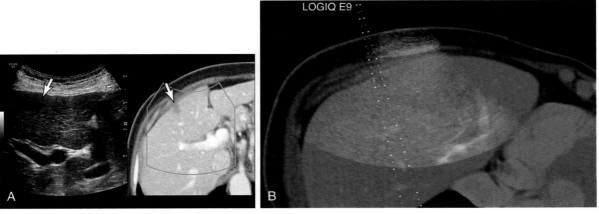

FIGURE 18-24 A, Very subtle liver mass *(arrow)* found on ultrasound with the aid of fusing the ultrasound with the imported CT scan. **B,** The biopsy was performed in a fused mode. The green box marks the liver mass. The biopsy specimen came back positive for metastatic colon cancer.

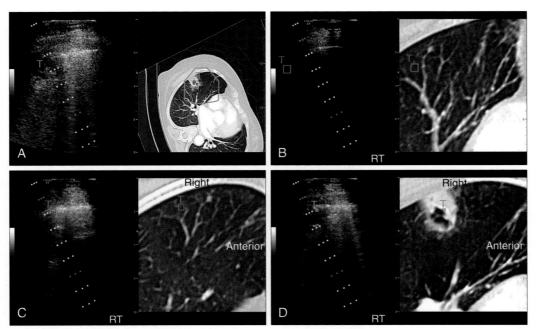

FIGURE 18-25 A, This lung lesion is found, the biopsy path determined, and a target marker placed on the CT image. The marker is duplicated on the ultrasound image *(small green T and +).* **B,** The sonographer removed the transducer while waiting for the procedure to begin to rest the arm. Upon placing the transducer back on the patient, the blue box and T appeared on both the CT and ultrasound image. This denotes that the lesion is close. **C,** As the sonographer scans closer to the lesion, the blue box gets smaller. **D,** The box is small and has turned green as the site marked on image A is now in view.

Fusion technology also allows special needles that have electromagnetic sensors embedded in them. By using a system consisting of a reusable sensor and a disposable needle, the radiologist will know exactly where the needle tip is at all times. This will help the radiologist to find the needle tip quickly if the needle is deflected or bends, as well as ensure that the needle is in the proper place for small or difficult-to-access masses. This technology will help the radiologist always know where the needle tip is during the insertion stage. Once the needle tip is in the proper location, the sensor is removed and the biopsy performed.

ULTRASOUND BIOPSY TECHNIQUES

1. Before beginning the procedure, the patient's medical history, laboratory values, and imaging studies should be reviewed and blood work checked. If the patient's PT, PTT, and INR are normal, the procedure can safely begin.
2. The next step is to explain the procedure to the patient, as a well-informed patient is usually more relaxed and cooperative. The patient must be informed of any potential risks, alternate methods of obtaining the same information, and what would be the course of the disease if the biopsy were not performed and the correct treatment cannot be planned. The

benefits of the procedure and what to expect during the procedure, especially the need for multiple passes, should be discussed, as well as any potential complications, including the possibility of a nondiagnostic procedure. The patient's role in the procedure should be explained: how the patient needs to keep still and to follow breathing instructions. A summary of all personnel in the room and their roles is given; the room can become crowded with the following people: sonographer, attending, fellow or resident, nurse, and possibly a cytopathology team. At this time the needs of the patient should be determined and sedatives ordered as needed. Patients need to be awake for the procedure so that they can stay in the needed position and control their breathing. Time should also be allowed for the patient to ask questions. The consent form is then signed and witnessed. The sonographer may serve as the witness. If the sonographer did not see the patient sign the form, he or she should show the signature to the patient and verify that it is the patient's signature.

3. After obtaining the patient's consent for the procedure, the next step in the process is to review any diagnostic imaging studies, such as an ultrasound, CT, MRI, or positron emission tomography (PET) scan. If possible, the image demonstrating the mass should be brought into the room. This is one of the advantages of fusion technology, as the images can be imported directly into the machine for

review without fusing the studies together. While the sonographer is reviewing or importing the images, the patient can be brought into the scanning/procedure room, changed into a gown, and have his or her vital signs taken. The nurse can also complete the preprocedural checklist at this time. Any additional equipment, such as a pulse oximeter, can be attached to the patient at this time.

4. Next, a limited ultrasound is performed to localize the mass and choose the optimal approach as well as the best transducer type and frequency (Figure 18-26). It is important to realize for a biopsy that the diagnostic process is complete and that the transducer type and frequency needed for the biopsy might not be the same as those used for a clinical examination. For example, it may be necessary to use a high-frequency linear array for a superficial liver or abdominal mass, and a mid- to low-frequency phased array transducer or even an endocavitary transducer for a subclavicular mass (Figure 18-27). Again, it is important to consider "approach to the mass or lesion" and not penetration and resolution. When appropriate, older units may be used for biopsies, freeing up newer machines for diagnostic studies. This is especially true for lower-resolution procedures such as paracentesis, thoracentesis, renal cores, and liver cores. The sonographer should determine multiple approaches, if needed, and review them with the radiologist. An X or a dot is marked on the skin with a marker, at the site where the

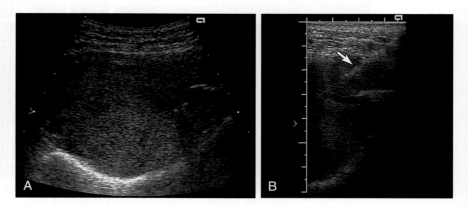

FIGURE 18-26 A, A large mediastinal mass is seen with a 5-MHz curved array transducer. **B,** This same patient is biopsied *(arrow)* using a 7-MHz linear array, as a hypoechoic area in the mass was better appreciated. This is the area from which positive cells were found. A primary mediastinal tumor was diagnosed.

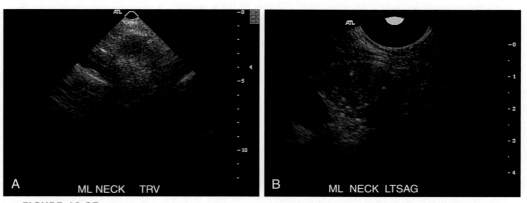

FIGURE 18-27 A, It proved difficult to image around the clavicle using a linear array transducer. To angle under the clavicle, a phased array transducer was first used. **B,** The same patient is now being evaluated with an endocavity transducer. This proved to be the best transducer, allowing an easy and safe path to the lymph node as well as the resolution to see the small calcifications. Metastatic thyroid cancer was diagnosed.

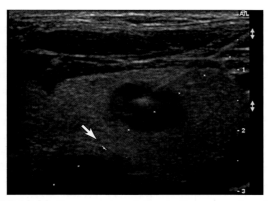

FIGURE 18-28 The arrow is pointing to the cursor along the biopsy line that determined the length of the needle needed to reach this point. As each mark represents 5 mm, the distance to the back wall of this thyroid lesion is 6.5 mm. A 9-cm needle length was used to perform the biopsy on this patient, who was determined to have a benign thyroid nodule compatible with an adenoma. Notice the slight needle deviation.

needle will pierce the skin. To determine the needle length required to reach the mass, measure the distance to the mass by placing a caliper at the bottom of the mass. This should be performed with the needle guidelines on the screen, as the machine will now take into account the length of the needle that is inside the needle guide, which is typically 2 to 4 cm (Figure 18-28). Common needle lengths are 6, 9, 15, and 20 cm. Usually it is best to have the sonographer on one side of the patient, preferably next to the ultrasound machine,

and the physician on the other side of the patient. Sometimes the best path requires the sonographer and physician to be on the same side of the patient. If this is the situation, the two of them will need to determine the best position so that they both can see the ultrasound monitor. One solution is for the sonographer to sit on a stool so that he or she is shorter than the radiologist. This allows the sonographer to still have access to the controls and see the monitor. Good ergonomics should be maintained. If the sonographer must scan from the opposite side of the stretcher, someone else will need to document the needle tip and adjust controls as needed, such as another sonographer or even a sonography student. The sonographer can also consider rearranging the relationship of the stretcher and machine to accommodate both the sonographer and the physician on the same side of the patient.

5. The national patient safety standards (found at www.jcaho.org) mandate that a "time-out" be performed before beginning any procedure. A member of the biopsy team should ask the patient to recite his or her full name and the reason that the patient is there. The patient's ID or history number is confirmed, as are the type and location of the procedure. The time-out needs to be documented, which may be part of the consent form. The words "time-out" can also be typed on the screen and an image documented as part of the ultrasound examination. This is helpful, as there will be preprocedural image, the "time-out" image documenting date and time, and then the needle-tip documentation images (Figure 18-29).

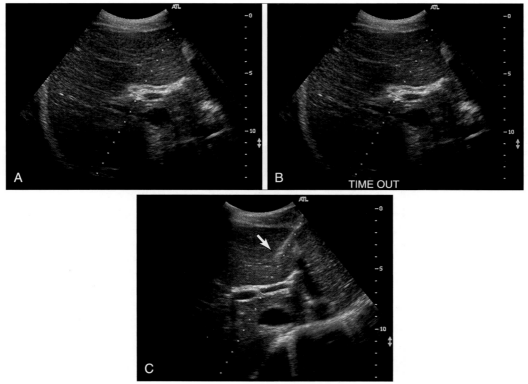

FIGURE 18-29 **A,** Preprocedural image for a liver core in a patient with hepatitis C demonstrating the needle path. **B,** Time-out verifying patient's name, ID number, and type of procedure. **C,** The procedure has begun. The arrow is pointing to the needle tip.

6. The radiologist/sonologist may start prepping the skin, usually after the time-out, while the sonographer preps and bags the transducer. Prepping the transducer often requires the assistance of another person, such as a nurse, a sonography student, a radiologist, or even another sonographer, to help maintain sterility of the transducer. Transducer preparation consists of attaching the needle guide to the transducer and covering the transducer with a sterile cover (Figure 18-30). Depending on the transducer, the needle guide may be covered by the sterile bag or it may also be sterile and placed over the sterile bag. Please note that the use of sterile bags and sterile guides varies among institutions. For example, one institution may bag the transducer and guide, keeping it sterile for a thyroid biopsy, whereas another may use the transducer and guide in a clean but not sterile fashion. After the transducer guide is attached, the correct size needle gauge insert is attached to the transducer guide. These guides are based on the gauge of the needle or catheter being used. These may need to be changed during the procedure. For example, a 22-gauge guide may be used during the FNA, but it may be changed to an 18-gauge guide for the core. Also, on a deep lesion, the radiologist may start with a 22-gauge needle but, because it keeps deviating, switch to a sturdier 20-gauge needle.

7. After the patient and transducer are prepped, sterile gel is used to rescan and check the mark. Once the area of the biopsy has been rechecked, local skin anesthesia is given, usually with a 25-gauge needle.

8. Next, deeper numbing is given along the needle path using the needle guide. This is important for patient comfort, especially on deep masses and liver masses, as the liver capsule is very sensitive. The transducer should stay on the anesthetized area to ensure that the needle is always passing through the numbed tissue (see Figure 18-17). Typically, a 9-cm, 22-gauge spinal needle is used for the deeper numbing. It is important that the physician squirt the lidocaine or numbing agent through the needle to push out any air inside the needle before inserting the needle into the patient. Otherwise, air will be introduced into the patient's tissue, obscuring the mass and the needle path. Patients should be reminded that they should not feel any sharp pain but that they may feel pressure. Some patients will complain of "pain" during the procedure when what they are really feeling is the pressure of the needle passing through their tissue. A good analogy is having a tooth filled. The patient feels the sensation of the drilling but not the sharp pain. Also, it is a good idea to let patients know that they may feel some pressure from the transducer as it is held steadily in place.

9. The sonographer holds the transducer as the radiologist performs the biopsy. In some institutions, the radiologist may be the person who holds the transducer while performing the biopsy. When a free-hand technique is used, the radiologist will usually hold the transducer. When a sonographer assists with the procedure, he or she will have one sterile hand, which is holding the transducer, while the other hand will be dirty, as it will be optimizing the controls, taking images to document the needle tip and procedure, and maybe even holding the patient's hand or patting the patient on the shoulder. The needle should be advanced in a swift motion while it is being tracked. Echogenic tip needles should be used, as the tip of the needle has been scored to produce an increase of scattered echoes, causing it to be echogenic. The shaft of the needle is echogenic, as it is a specular reflector, whereas the tip of the needle is more echogenic because it has been scored. Some needles have the stylet scored to enhance visualization of the needle (Figure 18-31).

10. For neck, chest, abdominal, and retroperitoneal biopsies, the patient is asked to stop breathing while the needle is inserted. A typical FNA pass lasts from 20 to 40 seconds. Patients who cannot hold their breath for this long should be instructed to breathe shallowly until the needle

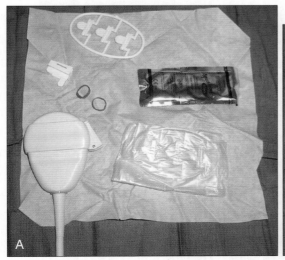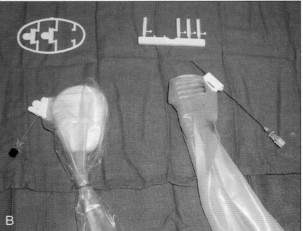

FIGURE 18-30 **A,** Transducer and sterile kit, which includes the bag, guide attachment, needle gauge inserts, rubber bands, and sterile gel. **B,** Prepped transducers.

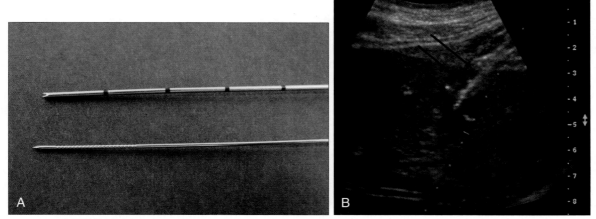

FIGURE 18-31 A, A biopsy needle with a scored stylet. **B,** Needle with an echogenic stylet *(arrows)* allowing easy visualization of the needle. This hypoechoic mass was a metastatic lesion from a colon primary.

is removed, as deep breaths may cause the needle to bend. The sonographer can be helpful by coaching and encouraging patients with their breathing and breath holding. When locating the mass, try to let patients breathe normally as much as possible, having them hold their breath to verify the selected path. This will allow the patient to be "fresh" for the biopsy and not out of breath already from the prescans. For masses that move a lot with breathing, it can be helpful to show patients the mass and biopsy line and how their breathing affects the location of the mass.

11. After the procedure is finished, the patient's skin is cleaned and a bandage placed over the biopsy site. A cold compress should also be placed over the biopsy site to reduce swelling and pain. The bag should be placed over the patient's gown or it can be wrapped in a towel or a few paper towels, as direct skin contact may be uncomfortable for the patient. The sterile bag and guide is removed from the transducer. Care should be taken not to accidentally throw the reusable guide in the garbage, as these guides are expensive. The sonographer should scan the area to look for any postprocedural complications such as a hematoma. Color or power Doppler can be used to ensure that there is no active bleeding. This is especially useful in renal biopsies. If an active bleed is discovered, the sonographer can use the transducer to apply pressure over the area to stop the bleeding. Usually the bleeding can be stopped within 5 to 10 minutes. If the bleeding cannot be stopped, interventional radiology should be contacted immediately (Figure 18-32).

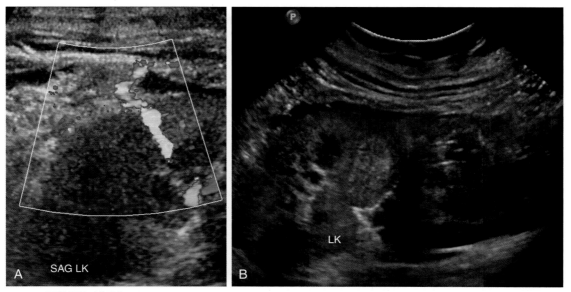

FIGURE 18-32 A, Color Doppler immediately after biopsy demonstrates active bleed into the perinephric space. **B,** After applying pressure for 15 minutes the bleeding stopped and the resulting hematoma is seen at the lower pole.

12. Before the patient leaves the room, the nurse will assess the patient's pain level and take vital signs. The sonographer should take the transducer and guide, remove the gel and blood, and perform high-level disinfection, according to the hospital's infection control policies and the recommendations of the transducer manufacturer.

13. The patient is then taken to a holding or observation area. Depending on the type of procedure, the patient may remain in this area between 15 and 120 minutes. If the patient's pain or discomfort increases, the sonographer should rescan to look for a hematoma (Figure 18-33). Stable patients can be discharged with appropriate instructions. Patients who have had chest procedures or procedures near the lungs will be sent to radiology for a chest x-ray to evaluate for a pneumothorax (Figure 18-34).

14. Typically, the nurse makes a follow-up phone call within the next 24 to 72 hours to ensure that the patient did not experience any complications.

THE SONOGRAPHER'S ROLE IN INTERVENTIONAL PROCEDURES

Interventional procedures can be challenging for everyone involved. A sonographer who has an interest in interventional ultrasound can be a valuable asset to the biopsy team. Sonographers may work closely with a radiologist, sonologist, or other physicians such as a nephrologist in native kidney biopsies, surgeons in kidney transplant or liver biopsies, or other clinicians for ascites taps or during **thoracentesis.**

Sonographer involvement has many benefits. Sonographers can locate the pathology and determine various approaches, offering recommendation for the best and safest needle path to the mass. Using their scanning skills, sonographers can optimize the image to locate subtle masses and use Doppler to ensure that there are no vessels in the needle path. The sonographer can place the patient in a variety of positions to determine the best approach. For example, by placing the patient in a left posterior oblique or left lateral decubitus position, the liver may drop into a more

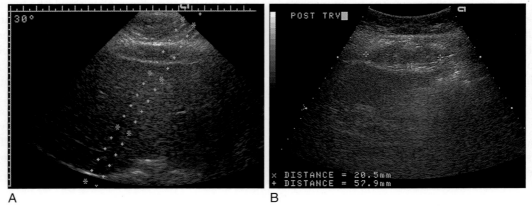

FIGURE 18-33 A, Prelive scan to determine the needle path in this patient with hepatitis C. Notice the prominent rectus abdominis muscle anterior to the liver. **B,** The patient developed a hematoma postbiopsy. Notice the similar appearance to the rectus abdominis muscle, which can be mistaken for a hematoma. It is recommended that a prebiopsy image be taken for a comparison.

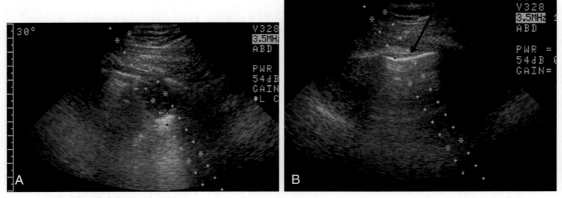

FIGURE 18-34 A, Pleural based lung lesion. **B,** The needle nicked the lung, causing a small pneumothorax *(arrow)*. Fortunately, an adequate specimen was obtained, which proved to be adenocarcinoma of the lung.

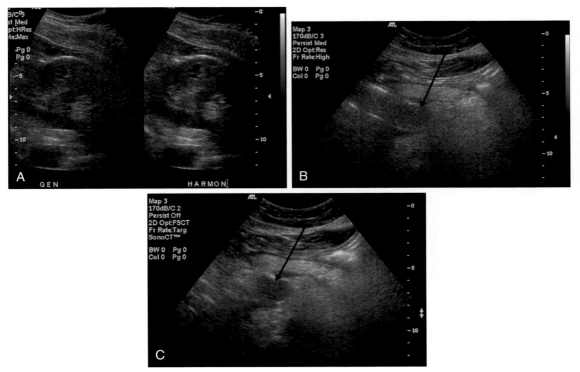

FIGURE 18-35 **A,** Cystic renal cell carcinoma *(arrow),* which was better visualized using harmonic imaging (Gen = normal image, Harmon = harmonic image). **B,** Image of a pancreas head mass *(arrow)* using normal imaging parameters. **C,** With compound imaging activated, the borders of the mass were better defined, leading to a successful biopsy and a diagnosis of adenocarcinoma of the pancreas.

subcostal position or a mass may roll away from a vessel. Placing the patient in a prone position may give better access to a renal mass. Knowledge of new technologies such as harmonic and compound imaging may facilitate finding or better defining the borders of the mass (Figure 18-35).

It is also important to use the proper transducer. This means choosing not only the right frequency but also the correct transducer type. Sometimes it may be better to use a transducer not normally associated in a routine examination for that area—for example, using an endocavitary transducer for a mediastinal or subclavicular mass or a phased array transducer to get to masses that require an intercostal approach in the chest (Figure 18-36). Because of

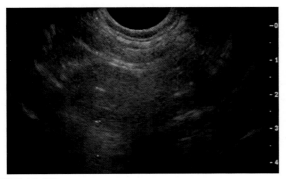

FIGURE 18-36 Using an endocavitary transducer gave better access and resolution on this metastatic supraclavicular node in a patient with a history of thyroid cancer.

the angle provided, a linear array may provide a safer choice in a pelvic node than a curved array. In the abdomen and pelvis, both a curved array and a phased array transducer should be evaluated. Different transducer types offer different angles and approaches to the mass.

Another aspect of preparing for the procedure is determining the effects of the patient's breathing on the mass. It is important to determine how much the mass moves with respiration and also how well and how long the patient can hold his or her breath. Determining this gives both sonographer and patient a chance to practice breathing so that the patient knows what is expected of him or her during the actual biopsy. The sonographer can also point out the mass on the screen and show the patient how breathing affects the location of the mass. They can then work together so that the patient can watch the screen and know how much of a breath to take so that the mass lines up on or between the dotted lines on the screen. Besides abdominal and chest masses, neck and thyroid masses can also move with respiration.

The sonographer should not be afraid to speak to the physician performing the procedure. For example, if the sonographer realizes that the needle is approaching a major vessel, he or she should calmly and professionally tell the physician to stop (Figure 18-37). Sonographers may also need to discuss and determine solutions to problems such as needle deviation. If a hematoma is forming, the sonographer may want to alert the physician so that he or she can decide whether to proceed or stop the procedure. Patients tend to talk to the

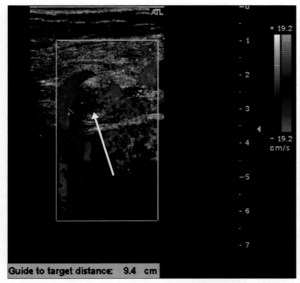

FIGURE 18-37 The sonographer must communicate to the physician if the needle deviates to any of the iliac vessels around this 1-cm node (*arrow*) in the pelvis. This node was positive in this HIV patient.

to be seen. This increased transducer pressure needs to be maintained during the procedure and requires another set of hands. This technique can also be used to minimize the distance between the skin and the mass on deep lesions (Figure 18-38).

The sonographer can assist and encourage the patient during the procedure. This can be valuable in helping the patient control breathing and giving the patient someone to talk to as needed. The sonographer can coach and support the patient emotionally, allowing the physician to concentrate on the procedure or discuss the specimen with the cytopathologist, if present. While the radiologist and nurse are busy with the specimen, the sonographer can talk to the patient to make sure that the patient is doing okay, look for signs of a complication, assure the patient that he or she is doing a great job, and, importantly, communicate to the patient what the next step will be.

Using their Doppler skills, the sonographer can locate vessels that may potentially traverse the needle path or be in close proximity to the mass. The sonographer can help guide the needle safely to deep retroperitoneal masses that may be near major vessels. Also, by using color or power Doppler, the sonographer can locate vessels in a mass, as this may represent areas of viable tumor tissue. This can be beneficial in masses that have necrotic areas (Figure 18-39).

Finally, the sonographer can be a time-saver for the busy physician. The sonographer can assist with probe preparation and with cleaning up. Sonographers can be scanning the next patient while the physician signs up the following patient or checks and dictates other studies. With a sonographer involved, a second physician may not be required for some procedures, thus allowing patient flow to continue in the department.

sonographer more, and their questions or fears can then be relayed to the physician. The sonographer can also gently remind the physician that the patient is holding his or her breath if the physician is taking a longer time than usual to obtain the specimen. Similarly, the sonographer can catch the signal that the patient needs to breathe and can let the physician know.

Importantly, a sonographer can be a second set of hands as needed to adjust imaging controls, freeze and unfreeze the image, and document the needle tip. When using biopsy guides, the sonographer can hold the transducer, freeing the physician's hands. This can be especially helpful when aspiration techniques are used. The sonographer can use the transducer to press bowel out of the way, allowing the mass

Experienced sonographers may find being involved with procedures a welcome change from routine scanning. It allows them to interact with the patient in a different way, be part of an important team, and bring into play all their scanning skills and knowledge.

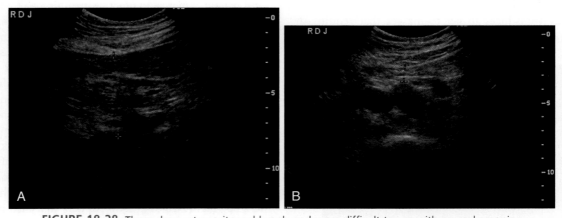

FIGURE 18-38 These deep retroperitoneal lymph nodes are difficult to see with normal scanning techniques. There is 5.4 cm of tissue between the abdominal wall and the anterior surface of the nodes. **B,** By applying pressure with the transducer, the distance from the abdominal wall and the nodes has decreased to 1.2 cm, allowing visualization of the nodes. This amount of pressure was applied during the biopsy, allowing a successful biopsy and a diagnosis of lymphoma.

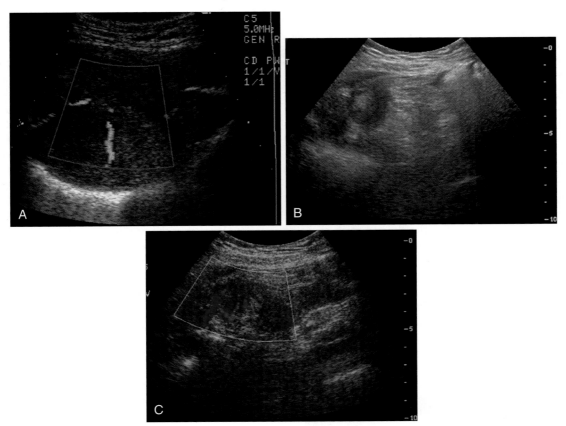

FIGURE 18-39 **A,** After several specimens showed only necrotic tissue, color Doppler was used to located flow within the mass. Viable tissue was found in this location, and a diagnosis of a mediastinal adenocarcinoma was made. **B,** Transverse image of the upper abdomen in a patient with a suspected hepatic flexure tumor. **C,** Using color Doppler, the colon mass was defined and an ultrasound-guided biopsy was performed confirming the suspicion of colon cancer.

FINDING THE NEEDLE TIP

The needle tip should appear as an echogenic dot on the ultrasound image. Visualizing the needle tip depends on several factors, including the type of needle (specially designed echogenic needles are better seen than normal needles), the gauge of the needle (larger-gauge needles cause brighter reflections), the transducer frequency (using the highest frequency possible), placement of the focal zone (which should be at or just below the level of the needle tip), using only one focal zone (multiple focal zones may decrease the frame rate), and the echogenicity of the mass (hypoechoic masses allow easier visualization of the needle than more echogenic masses) (Figure 18-40). The needle should be inserted quickly and steadily and the tip followed as

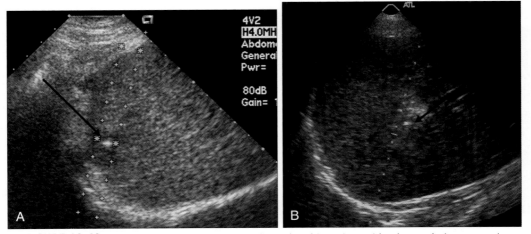

FIGURE 18-40 **A,** The needle tip is easily seen *(arrow)* in this patient with a hypoechoic metastatic lesion. **B,** The needle tip is hard to see *(arrow)* in this patient with a hyperechoic metastatic lesion.

it advances toward the mass. The needle may deviate out of the projected path and away from the ultrasound beam, causing loss of visualization of the needle tip. This deviation of the needle can be caused by the physician bending or tilting the needle as it is being advanced or by the tissue and muscle planes it is traversing (Figure 18-41). Echogenic needle tips or scored stylets improve needle and needle-tip visualization.

Tricks to try to see the needle tip include the following:
1. Moving the needle up and down in a bobbing motion.
2. Bobbing or jiggling the stylet inside the needle.
3. Scanning and angling the transducer in a superior and inferior motion. This is helpful when the needle is bent out of the plane of the sound beam.
4. Using harmonics or compound imaging.
5. A last resort is to remove the needle and start again, closely watching the displacement of the tissue as the needle advances.

At times the patient may move or breathe at the time that the biopsy core is fired, preventing the needle path from being visible for documentation. In these instances, the sonographer can scan the area and look for the needle track. This will be seen as an echogenic line caused by the air that is introduced into the tissue during the firing/cutting process (Figure 18-42).

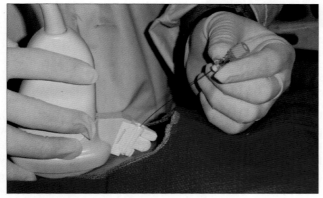

FIGURE 18-41 Notice that the needle is being inserted with bending, which causes the needle to bend out of plane and lose visualization of the needle tip.

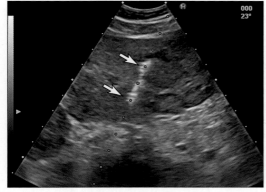

FIGURE 18-42 The patient breathed just as the biopsy gun was fired. The needle was not seen to document the location of the biopsy. By scanning the echogenic line from the needle track was located (*arrows*), allowing documentation of the biopsy area.

WHAT TO DO WHEN THE NEEDLE DEVIATES

Deviation of the needle from the projected path can be an issue and a challenge for the sonographer. The tissue and organs between the skin and the mass are usually the cause of this problem. For example, in pancreatic biopsies, the needle is often deflected as it passes through the posterior wall of the stomach. If it is a constant problem, the sonographer can overcorrect—that is, move the transducer more lateral or medial so that the path that the needle is following will intersect the mass. It is important that the sonographer verify that the correct size needle guide insert was used, because if the guide is too large, there will be some play within the needle guide that can cause this problem. As previously discussed, the sonographer should ensure that the guide on the transducer is set to the correct angle. Also, the sonographer should make sure that the transducer is perpendicular and that the needle guide touches the patient's skin. It is vital that the sonographer become familiar with the various transducers and guides, how they should be placed on the body, and how to correct or adjust their scanning as needed. If the problem persists, sometimes using a 20-gauge as opposed to a 22-gauge needle may correct the situation, as the larger-gauge needle is sturdier and does not bend as easily. In extreme cases, another pathway may need to be determined. The sonographer can also watch how the physician is inserting the needle to make sure that the needle is not bending as it is being inserted into the skin. Finally, the position of the tip of the needle can influence deviation on certain types of needles (see Figure 18-8, *B*). When the needle is inserted with the tip of the needle at the bottom (sometimes called bevel-up), the needle will encounter less resistance as it passes through the tissues; when bevel down, the needle may deviate as it passes through the same tissues.

Another problem is when a mass is pushed out of the way by the needle. This can be a problem with small nodes and masses. Again, the sonographer needs to understand how to counter these situations. Applying firm pressure with the transducer against the mass or trying to get the needle to approach the center of the mass so that it does not push the mass to the left or to the right can stabilize the mass and allow the needle to enter it. Sometimes another approach may be needed, which would require breaking down the sterile field and starting again. When any of these situations arise, the sonographer should be thinking of possible solutions to suggest. The physician can also try to quickly insert the needle or try to rotate the bevel of the needle into a different position.

BIOPSIES AND PROCEDURES BY ORGAN

Liver

The liver is one of the most common organs of which a biopsy is requested, either of a specific area or mass in the liver or for diffuse parenchyma abnormalities, such as hepatitis. Liver masses are amenable to ultrasound-guided biopsy in the majority of cases and can include metastatic masses, suspected hepatocellular carcinoma or other primary cancer, atypical benign lesions, and small abscesses (Figure 18-43). A biopsy of

a hypoechoic area in a cirrhotic liver may be requested, especially in a patient with elevated AFP, to differentiate it from a regenerating liver nodule. The inability to biopsy a liver mass can be caused by either the failure to visualize the mass or a lack of a safe approach to the mass. Whenever possible, a subcostal approach should be used to avoid the possibility of a pneumothorax or damage to the intercostal arteries. Intercostal biopsies also tend to be painful to the patient (Figure 18-44). Masses at the dome of the liver are easier to biopsy under ultrasound than CT, although a steep angle approach is often required. In some cases, scanning and biopsying in a sagittal plane is helpful. Core biopsies may be obtained on patients with hepatitis, cirrhosis, or increased liver function tests. Usually the left lobe of the liver is biopsied using a subcostal approach, as there are fewer major structures in the way, such as the gallbladder and porta hepatis. A biopsy of the left lobe in this group of patients is easier to perform and more comfortable for the patient than the traditional blind approach through the ribs of the right lobe. Specific complications of liver biopsies include pneumothorax for masses near the dome of the liver, bile leak, and hematomas (Figure 18-45). Use zoom

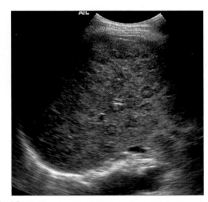

FIGURE 18-43 Patient with AIDS and multiple liver lesions. Biopsy was requested to determine the nature of the lesions. They were found to be amebic liver abscesses.

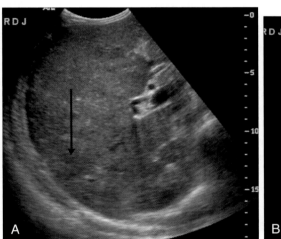
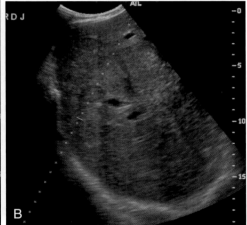

FIGURE 18-44 This liver lesion *(arrow)* could only be seen along the intercostal margin with the patient supine. **B,** With the patient in a right posterior oblique, the liver rolled out from under the ribs, allowing better visualization of the mass, and a subcostal approach could be used on this metastatic mass.

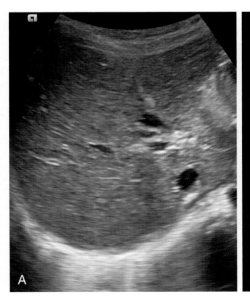
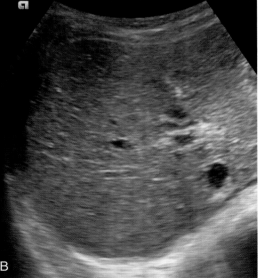

FIGURE 18-45 **A,** Prebiopsy image on a pediatric patient to evaluate for liver fibrosis in a patient with short gut syndrome. **B,** Immediately after this intercostal biopsy fluid was seen collecting in the subcapsule region with active bleeding seen. The sonographer applied pressure with the transducer in a subcostal approach while the physician applied pressure from an intercostal approach. Ten minutes later the bleeding had stopped and the patient did fine.

techniques for easier visualization of a small mass. Consider multiple patient positions to try to decrease the distance to the mass and to avoid intercostal approaches.

Pancreas

Most pancreatic mass biopsies are performed to confirm the diagnosis of adenocarcinoma, unresectable adenocarcinoma, or pancreatitis in patients with unusual imaging findings. Although the needle has to traverse the stomach or colon, complications are rare. Color Doppler is useful to map out vessels, especially if they are encased by the mass. Good specimens can usually be obtained near the biliary drainage tube, if the patient has one. A curved linear array transducer is preferred, as it can help display bowel gas with its large footprint. Pancreatic biopsies can be challenging because gas can move into the field and interfere with visualization of the mass, even after the biopsy has started. Other challenges include finding a safe path around the various vessels, deflection or bending of the needle as it goes through the stomach, and patient breathing, which can cause the pancreas to move with respirations (Figure 18-46). Pancreatitis is a potential complication of pancreatic biopsy.

Kidney

With current surgical techniques renal mass biopsies are increasing. Also, a biopsy of a renal mass may be requested to differentiate an incidental renal cell carcinoma from a renal metastasis in a patient with a known primary cancer or if the patient has a prior history of renal cell carcinoma. Atypical cysts, especially those with thick septations, need to be biopsied to differentiate between a cystic renal cell carcinoma and a benign complex cyst. Renal parenchymal biopsies are requested on patients with proteinuria, with nephrotic syndrome, or in renal failure. Because the disease process affects both kidneys, either kidney can be biopsied. The left kidney is preferred, as it offers a safer approach than the right, as the spleen is well above the left

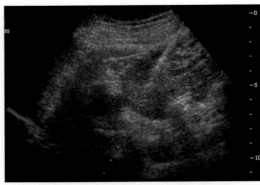

FIGURE 18-47 Renal core biopsy through the lower pole of the left kidney in this patient with proteinuria.

kidney, while the liver may be potentially in the way. These biopsies are performed with the patient prone, biopsying the lower pole of the left kidney, usually with an 18-gauge core needle. The sonographer should guide the needle through the parenchymal tissue, as the cortical tissue is needed to make the diagnosis (Figure 18-47). Specific complications of renal biopsies include perinephric hematoma and hematuria. The sonographer should evaluate the needle track area with color Doppler immediately after the biopsy to ensure that there is no active bleeding. If the patient develops hematuria, the bladder should be scanned for the presence of a clot. If a clot is discovered, the patient should be rolled into a steep oblique position to determine if the clot is mobile or attached to the bladder wall. This is important, as the clot may be positioned over the urethral opening, causing an outlet obstruction. For biopsies of renal masses, various patient positions should be evaluated including supine, decubitus, oblique, and prone (Figure 18-48).

Renal Transplants

Ultrasound is used to guide biopsies when there is elevation of the creatinine or when the cause of rejection needs to be

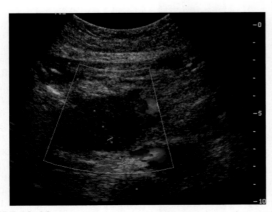

FIGURE 18-46 On this pancreatic head mass, the path was chosen to avoid the mesenteric vessels.

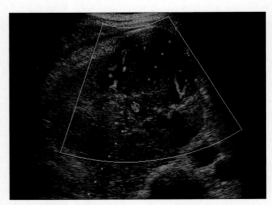

FIGURE 18-48 Biopsy of a right renal mass with the patient in a left lateral decubitus position. The diagnosis was metastatic disease from melanoma.

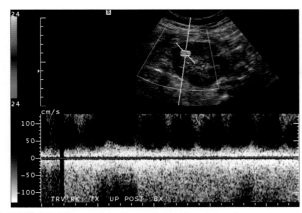

FIGURE 18-49 A postbiopsy image of this renal transplant demonstrates an arteriovenous fistula. Notice the mosaic color and turbulent Doppler flow.

determined for treatment. Locate the main renal vessels using color Doppler. Typically, the upper pole of the kidney is biopsied to avoid possible lacerations of the main renal vessels and ureter. It is also recommended that a color Doppler image of the entire kidney be obtained to use as a baseline in case there are complications such as an arteriovenous fistula (AVF) or pseudoaneurysm formation of intrarenal vessels. Ultrasound can also be used to direct drainage of perinephric fluid collections such as lymphoceles. Specific complications include hematomas, hematuria, and AVF (Figure 18-49).

Retroperitoneal Lymph Nodes

Most retroperitoneal masses, including para-aortic and pericaval lymph nodes, are amenable to ultrasound guidance. These can be technically challenging, especially with small masses and in larger patients, so the use of a needle guide is essential. Usually an anterior approach is preferred, and by applying a firm and steady pressure with the curved linear array transducer, overlying bowel loops and intraabdominal fat can be displaced (see Figure 18-38). This technique also reduces the depth at which the needle needs to be placed. To avoid major vessels and other structures, multiple biopsy transducers and guides may need to be evaluated to determine the safest path. Real-time monitoring of the needle tip ensures that the needle excursions during the biopsy stay within the node. In patients with suspected lymphoma, tissue needs to be obtained not only to diagnose lymphoma but also to determine the subtype, as this is critical for treatment. Usually part of the sample is sent for flow cytometric studies and a core may also be required. Specific complications include retroperitoneal hematomas. Because the sonographer may have to apply transducer pressure, the patient may feel more discomfort than usual from the increased pressure. The sonographer should explain this to the patient. Also, this increased pressure can add fatigue to the sonographer's wrist, hand joints, and shoulder. Therefore sonographers should relax the pressure and their grip on the transducer to reduce musculoskeletal injuries between passes.

Lung

Ultrasound guidance has been shown to be a safe alternative to CT for biopsy of pleural, parenchymal, or mediastinal masses abutting the chest wall. This technique is associated with a high success rate and lower complications than CT and is particularly valuable for small peripheral masses in close proximity to a rib and diaphragmatic masses where slight respiratory excursion can affect the position of the mass. The transducer is placed parallel to the intercostal space, and the needle is advanced in a single breath hold to minimize trauma to the pleura. The tip is monitored to ensure it does not slip out of the mass into normal aerated lung. Intraparenchymal tumors are generally not amenable to ultrasound guidance, unless they are within an area of consolidation or if the patient has a large pleural effusion that can be used as an acoustic window. Lung lesions can be challenging by ultrasound, and it is always helpful to have the CT films present for guidance. Fusion technology can assist in finding these masses quickly and accurately. These lesions are usually small and mobile with respiration. Creative positioning may be needed to get between ribs and around the scapula. The patient may need to be placed in an oblique, decubitus, or prone position. A pillow or sponges may be placed under the patient to spread the ribs apart. The patient's arm may also need to be adjusted to get the scapula out of the way in apical lesions. Transducer type also needs to be evaluated, as sometimes a phased array transducer provides better access than a linear array transducer (Figure 18-50). Remember that resolution is not as much an issue as is accessibility. Start with a small footprint phased array transducer, as it helps to image between the ribs and allows the sonographer to angle through the rib space. Once the lesion is located, the linear array transducer can be evaluated for path access. In lung biopsies, patient breathing is crucial because the lesion will move with respirations. The sonographer will need to evaluate the patient in various degrees of inspiration and expiration. These lesions can be challenging for the sonographer to find, as there are few landmarks to use. Specific complications include pneumothorax. If the patient starts to cough up blood (hemoptysis), the biopsy needs to stop immediately for patient safety.

Thyroid Gland

Thyroid biopsies can be helpful in distinguishing malignant masses from goiters or adenomas. Biopsies should be taken in various portions of the mass to confirm colloid or abnormal cells. The sonographer should look for small calcifications, as there is a higher percentage of positive cells in these areas (Figure 18-51). The sonographer should remember to evaluate if the thyroid gland moves with respiration. If it does, the patient should be told to hold his or her breath as the needle

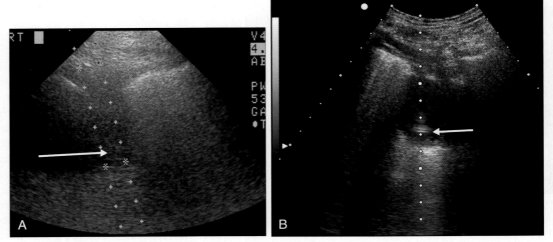

FIGURE 18-50 A, Pleura-based lung lesion *(arrow)*, which was difficult to access with this sector array transducer. **B,** Using this transducer with the biopsy guide, this lung mass was better defined and offered a safe approach. The arrow is pointing to the needle tip.

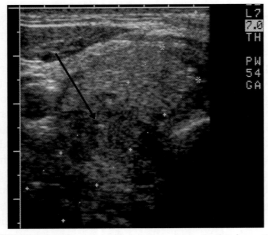

FIGURE 18-51 After several negative passes in this large thyroid nodule, positive cells were obtained in the area of the small calcifications *(arrow)*.

is inserted. Usually the patient can breathe shallowly during the biopsy process. Specific complications include neck pain and hematomas. Elastography may prove beneficial in finding areas of suspicion to improve biopsy results.

Neck Nodes and Masses

Biopsies of neck masses can easily be performed with ultrasound guidance. In a patient with a history of thyroid cancer, it is important to differentiate between malignant and benign lymph nodes. Round, homogeneous lymph nodes are usually suspicious for cancer as opposed to oval nodes with echogenic centers from a fatty hilum. Other causes of neck masses include lymphoma and submandibular gland tumors. Masses of the parotid gland can also be biopsied under ultrasound guidance. Large masses seen in a supraclavicular location may be difficult to access using a linear

array transducer. High-frequency curved arrays, phased arrays, or even an endocavitary transducer may give more access to these masses.

Musculoskeletal Biopsies

Ultrasound has also proven successful in biopsying masses in the extremities. These may be muscular in origin, such as a leiomyosarcoma or rhabdomyosarcoma, or from nerves, such as a schwannoma or neurofibroma. If a bony lesion has broken through the cortex, ultrasound can be used to guide the biopsy. Ewing's sarcoma, osteosarcoma, and metastatic disease from prostate cancer are some examples of bone cancers. Ultrasound is being widely used for nerve blocks and corticosteroid injections of various joints.

Pelvis

A variety of pelvic masses can be biopsied using ultrasound guidance. Pelvic lymph nodes can be seen and color Doppler used to identify the location of the iliac vessels (Figure 18-52). Perisacral masses may be seen with the patient supine, using a curved linear array transducer. If unable to see the mass with the patient supine, the radiologist should evaluate the CT or MRI to determine if a prone approach is possible. In females, pelvic masses or fluid collections should be evaluated with both a transabdominal approach and a transvaginal approach. Transvaginal biopsies are usually performed with the patient in stirrups.

Prostate Gland

Men with elevated PSA levels or palpable nodules found on a rectal digital examination may be referred for a prostate biopsy. If a full scan is needed before the biopsy, the biopsy guide should be placed on the transducer so that the probe does not need to be removed and reinserted. The patient is

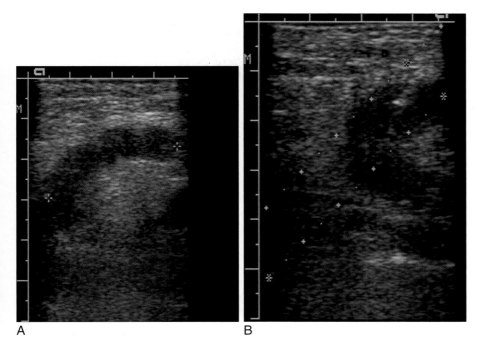

FIGURE 18-52 A, This lymph node exhibits the characteristic of a benign lymph node: oval in shape with a fatty hilum. **B,** The specimen came back positive for metastatic disease.

biopsied in the left lateral decubitus position. Because the biopsy is through the rectal wall, the patient should be placed on a broad-spectrum antibiotic the day before and usually 2 days after the biopsy to reduce the chance of infection. Some institutions may require a urine sample before the biopsy to evaluate for a urinary tract infection (UTI) because a UTI can become a urosepsis after biopsy, which may be life threatening. Because of the recent rises in postbiopsy infections, some institutions have started having their patients have a rectal swab to look for drug-resistant organisms. These are usually performed 5 to 14 days before the procedure. Transrectal prostate biopsies are considered clean procedures, not sterile procedures. Random samples are taken from the prostate gland as follows: one each from the apex, mid, and base of the peripheral zone and one through the central gland on both the right and left sides of the gland. Extra passes should also be obtained through any suspicious

hypoechoic area seen in the peripheral zone. For the peripheral zone area, the needle tip is placed on the edge of the prostate gland and fired. For central gland passes, the needle tip is placed inside the prostate gland, just inside the central gland. The number of passes obtained will vary among departments, with 8 to 10 total passes being a common number. MRI fused biopsies are performed on men with persistent elevating PSA levels and a normal traditional prostate biopsy. The MRI will demonstrate suspicious nodules that can be biopsied (Figure 18-53). On the patient where a rectal approach is not feasible because of rectal surgery, a transperineal biopsy can be performed. The best transducer is typically a phased array transducer, as a small footprint is required. The patient is placed in stirrups with the perineum exposed. The penis and scrotum need to be positioned out of the biopsy field and held in place with towels and tape. The patient is usually given IV sedation in

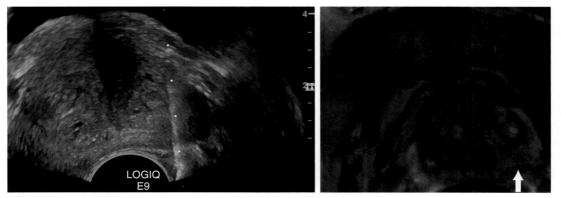

FIGURE 18-53 Prostate guided biopsy using MRI fusion technique. Patient's previous biopsies were normal yet PSA kept rising. MRI demonstrated a suspicious lesion *(blue arrow)*. Biopsy through this area found the prostate cancer with a Gleason grade of 5.

addition to plenty of local numbing. Because of the lack of resolution, two to three random specimens are obtained from both the right and left sides of the prostate gland. In a patient with a prostatic abscess, ultrasound is used to obtain a specimen from the abscess if the patient is not responding to antibiotic therapy. These patients are very tender, and care and gentleness need to be used when inserting the transducer.

FLUID COLLECTIONS AND ABSCESSES

Pleural Fluid

Patients who have pleural effusions may be marked for a thoracentesis and returned to the unit for the actual procedure, or they may have it performed under sonographic guidance. The patient should be scanned in the same position that the procedure will be performed, which is usually an upright position, through the back. In cases of loculated fluid, the procedure may be performed with the use of a needle guide (Figure 18-54). Care should be taken to identify the diaphragm and examine above the diaphragm so that the spleen or liver is not accidentally mistaken for a collection because of poor technical settings. Misidentification may happen because of air artifact and using reduced overall gain. A guide may not be necessary if the fluid is not complicated and the pocket is large enough. When just marking the patient who is having the tap performed blindly, it is important not to press too hard on the skin, as this will change the depth to the fluid and may cause the clinician not to advance the needle far enough to reach the fluid. The distance to the fluid and the distance to midpocket are usually measured. To scan between the ribs, a phased array or curved linear transducer is used (Figure 18-55). If unable to see any fluid in an upright position, the patient may be scanned supine to see if there is any fluid above the diaphragm. While the fluid is being drained, the patient may start to cough as

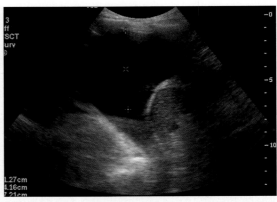

FIGURE 18-55 A marking for a thoracentesis to be performed without ultrasound guidance. The distance to the fluid is 1.27 cm and to midpocket it is between 4.16 and 7.21 cm.

the lung reexpands with air. After the procedure the patient may be sent for a chest x-ray to make sure that there is no pneumothorax.

Ascites

Ascites drainage is a common sonography request. Patients with intraabdominal fluid may be marked for an ascites tap (paracentesis) to have the procedure performed in their room or have the procedure performed under sonographic guidance. The entire abdomen and pelvis should be evaluated for the extent of fluid and to locate the largest area or "pocket" of fluid. To pool the fluid in the pelvis, the patient may be scanned in a reverse Trendelenburg position of 30 to 45 degrees. If the fluid is septated, the pocket is small, or if there are organs or bowel loops in the way, a guide may be used. During the procedure, the patient may be rolled into an oblique position so that the fluid drains to the dependent portion where the needle or centesis catheter is located. When marking the fluid, care should be taken to apply just enough pressure with the transducer to make contact with the skin, as pressure will influence the measurements to the fluid (Figure 18-56). If the procedure is to be performed on the floor blindly, the distance to the fluid and the distance to midpocket should be measured and reported (Figure 18-57). A postprocedural image should be taken to document the remaining amount of fluid (Figure 18-58).

Abscess Drainage

As mentioned, ultrasound can be used to drain abscesses and fluid collections from different locations in the body, including abdominal, pelvic, hepatic, perirenal, prostate, and peripancreatic. In some instances, only a small amount of fluid is removed to determine the organism that is causing the infection or to determine the proper type of antibiotics for treatment. Infected fluid is typically complex and may contain low-level echoes. Larger-bore needles from 16 to 18 gauge

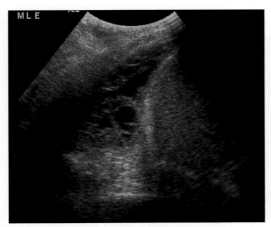

FIGURE 18-54 Because of the loculations in this pleural fluid, an ultrasound-guided thoracentesis was performed to remove fluid for cytology.

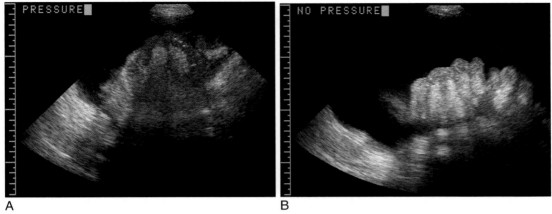

FIGURE 18-56 **A,** There is too much pressure from the transducer, giving the appearance that there is only a minimal amount of fluid in this area. **B,** The same patient with minimal transducer pressure demonstrates the true amount of fluid.

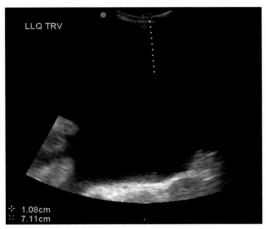

FIGURE 18-57 An example of marking for a paracentesis. The distance to the fluid is 1.08 cm, and it is 7.11 cm to about the middle of the fluid.

may be needed to remove the viscous fluid. Drains may be left in place and ultrasound or radiology used for follow-up as needed.

POINT-OF-CARE AND ABLATION TECHNIQUES

With the introduction of small, portable ultrasound units, sonography is being used outside the traditional areas of radiology, obstetrics, vascular medicine, and cardiology. These low-cost units are designed for ease of use and can be designed for specific applications including guidance for placing lines into various arteries and veins in the body. Physicians and nonphysicians such as internists, surgeons, emergency department personnel, residents, IV therapists, nurses, and interventional physicians are using these units for brachial IV guidance, performing the ascites tap in the patient's room, guiding superficial biopsies, and other applications. These procedures are performed by a nonsonologist without the assistance of either a sonologist or sonographer.

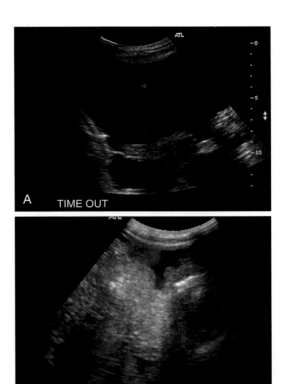

FIGURE 18-58 **A,** The predrainage image in this patient with a pelvic ascites. **B,** The postdrainage image demonstrating the residual fluid after the paracentesis.

Ultrasound guidance is also used in the operating room (OR) to verify the number and location of tumors, locate vessels, and determine resection approaches, as well as in guidance of biopsies on sedated patients, especially pediatric patients. The sonographer may be involved in setting up the equipment with the OR personnel, documenting

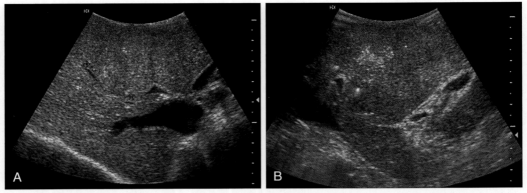

FIGURE 18-59 **A,** Liver lesion being measured before RF ablation. **B,** Same patient undergoing RF ablation. Notice the 60-cycle noise that is seen during the ablation. The bright echoes seen represent the microbubbles produced.

images, and assisting the surgeon with the identification of structures, because if more lesions are found on intraoperative ultrasound than are documented by MRI or CT, the surgery may be canceled. Some dedicated OR ultrasound units have ultrasound laparoscopic capabilities. The sonographer is a valuable member of the operating team and can assist the surgeon by offering ultrasound knowledge and skills. The problem is that OR cases can involve the sonographer for many hours or involve multiple trips to the OR as needed.

Ultrasound can be used for guidance for the various types of ablation procedures, which include radiofrequency (RF), cryoablation, laser, microwave, and high-intensity focused ultrasound (HIFU). The goal of ablation is to destroy the cancerous tissue while limiting the damage done to the normal tissue. Ablation procedures can be performed either in the OR or percutaneously through small incisions. These ablation therapies typically have fewer complications, as well as a shorter recovery time, than surgical resections. Ablation is used when the patient is not a candidate for surgery or on masses that are not resectable, and it can be used on various organs in the body including but not limited to the liver, kidney, breast, and prostate. Unfortunately, not all patients will be able to be treated with ablation and not all diseases or masses are amenable to this technique. On some patients, the procedure may be difficult to perform in a minimally invasive or safe manner.

Ablation utilizes cold or hot temperatures to kill cells. The extreme heating or cooling of the tissue results in death of the tissue. Most ablation techniques use heat to kill the cells. As the tissue is heated, dissolved gases, primarily nitrogen, are released from the cells forming microbubbles within the tissue. These microbubbles are visible by ultrasound and are seen as hyperechoic echoes. Seeing this streaming effect of the microbubbles assists in confirming the area that is being treated (Figure 18-59). The ablation area is roughly the diameter of the prongs, with different configurations available to create the proper size of ablation zone. Although ultrasound can be used for guidance,

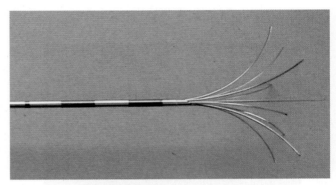

FIGURE 18-60 Deployed RF needle.

CT or MRI will be the imaging modality of choice for documenting the postablation area for residual tumor and for follow-up.

In RF ablation, the patient is grounded for the procedure by placing grounding pads on the appropriate place on the body, for example, the upper legs. When introduced, the expandable electrodes are collapsed within a 14- to 15-gauge needle. Once correctly positioned, the prongs or tines are deployed, resulting in a final configuration that resembles an umbrella (Figure 18-60). The needle is connected to an RF generator to create an electrical circuit. The tip of the probe releases a high-frequency current that heats and destroys the cancer cells. Tissue that is farther away from the prongs is heated by thermal conduction, with the temperature decreasing as the distance from the prongs increases. The temperature of the tissue will be the highest directly adjacent to the prongs and can reach about 100° C (212° F). Irreversible damage and cell death occur at temperatures over 60° C (140° F). The amount of tissue reaching these lethal temperatures depends on the type of tumor and the surrounding tissue. The body reabsorbs the destroyed cells. The procedure is performed under conscious sedation, although general anesthesia may be used. Each treatment session lasts between 10 and 30 minutes, depending on the size of the lesion. Tumors smaller than 7 cm have a greater

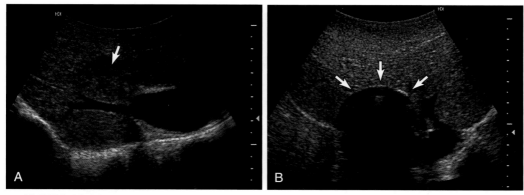

FIGURE 18-61 A, Precryoablation image. The arrow is pointing to the liver mass. **B,** The arrows are pointing to the ice ball that formed during the cryoablation.

success rate of being totally ablated than larger tumors. At the end of the procedure, the needle is withdrawn at a lower power output to prevent bleeding and seeding of the needle track. RF ablation is used in conjunction with other types of therapy such as chemotherapy. The advantages of RF ablation include low complication rate, reduced cost, and increased patient compliance. The hospital stay is short and most patients can resume normal activities within a few days. Complications are rare and are related to thermal injury to either the skin or nearby organs.

Unlike the other forms of ablation, which use heat to destroy the tissue, cryoablation uses extremely cold temperatures. Cryoablation uses repetitive freezing and thawing of tissue to produce cellular death and necrosis. Irreversible tissue destruction will occur at temperatures below $-20°$ to $-30°$ C ($-4°$ to $-22°$ F). Temperatures as low as $-160°$ C ($-256°$ F) can be achieved with cryoablation using liquid nitrogen and argon for the gases to freeze the tissue. As the tissues are frozen, crystals will form within, which causes the cells to expand. Both the formation of crystals and expansion of the cell wall cause cellular damage. Thawing the cell also results in cellular disruption and death. Just as in RF ablation, the body absorbs the destroyed cells. Different size and shape cryoprobes are available to map out the area to be treated.

Cryoablation is performed either in the OR with the patient open, or percutaneously using smaller diameter cryoprobes. Ultrasound is often used to guide the cryoprobe into position and to monitor the size of the ice ball. Once the cryoprobe is in place, the gases are released to freeze the tissue, followed by periods of tissue thawing. The development of the ice ball can be monitored using ultrasound with an accuracy of 1 to 5 mm (Figure 18-61). It is important that the ultrasound transducer does not touch the cryoprobe, as it will freeze the ultrasound transducer, causing it temporarily not to work.

There are several potential advantages of cryoablation over the various thermal ablation techniques. One main advantage is that the ice ball formed during the ablation process is highly visible with ultrasound, which allows precise control of the ablation area and limits injury to adjacent structures. A second advantage is that larger masses of up to 12 cm in size can be ablated with cryoablation. Some of the risks of cryoablation include freezing of nontarget tissues and internal bleeding.

NEW APPLICATIONS

As elastography and ultrasound contrast continue to evolve and get approval, they will have an impact on biopsies. Liver elastography may replace or greatly reduce the need for liver core biopsies in patients with parenchymal liver disease. Elastography may also help to identify abnormal tissue to aid in determining where to biopsy in such organs as the prostate and thyroid. Contrast may also help in reducing the need to biopsy masses with clear benign flow patterns, especially in the liver and kidney. These new technologies may help solve current issues so that more patients may have their procedure under ultrasound guidance, thus improving patient care and reducing costs to the health system.

 Key Pearls

- The main advantage of using ultrasound for guidance is to have continuous real-time visualization of the biopsy needle, which allows adjustment of the needle as needed during the procedure.
- The sonographer should look for indirect signs of the presence of a mass, such as displaced vessels, capsule bulges, or the presence of tumor vessels.
- Biopsies are used to confirm if a mass is benign, malignant, or infectious.
- Other indications include the need to differentiate between a metastatic and a second primary mass, to determine the cause of metastases in a patient with multiple primaries, to differentiate recurrent tumor from postoperative or therapy scarring, to differentiate malignancy from inflammatory or infectious disease, to determine metastatic

Continued

lymph adenopathy from lymphoma, and to characterize a benign mass.
- Other common reasons for a biopsy are to obtain a sample of the parenchyma in an organ to determine the severity or progression of a disease process such as hepatitis or renal failure or to determine the cause of rejection in a transplanted organ.
- Complications from an ultrasound-guided biopsy are usually minor and may include postprocedural pain or discomfort, vasovagal reactions, and hematomas.
- Serious complications, although rare, include bleeding, hemorrhage, pneumothorax, pancreatitis, biliary leakage, peritonitis, infection, and possibly death.

BIBLIOGRAPHY

Bernadino ME: Automated biopsy devices: significance and safety, *Radiology* 176:615-616, 1990.

Blavais M: Ultrasound-guided peripheral IV insertion in the ED: a two-hour training session improves placement success rates in one ED, *Am J Nurs* 105(10):54-57, 2005.

Charboneau JW, Reading CC, Welch TJ: CT and sonographically guided needle biopsy: current techniques and new innovations, *Am J Roentgenol* 154:1-10, 1990.

Cronan JJ: Percutaneous biopsy, *Radiol Clin North Am* 34(6):1207-1223, 1996.

Higgins H, Berger DL: RFA for liver tumors: does it really work? Available at www.theoncologist.alphamedpress.org/cgi/content/full/11/7/801. Accessed Feb 1, 2010.

Hinshaw JL, Laeseke PF, Lee FT, Durick NA: Image-guided tumor ablation: a technical overview of a less invasive cancer treatment. Available at www.cancernews.com/data/Article/454.asp. Accessed Feb 1, 2010.

Hopper KD: Percutaneous, radiographically guided biopsy: a history, *Radiology* 196:329-333, 1995.

Kliewer M, Sheafor D, Hertzberg B, et al: Percutaneous liver biopsy: a cost-benefit analysis comparing sonographic and CT guidance, *Am J Roentgenol* 173(5):1199-1202, 1999.

Ljung B-ME, Geller DA: Fine-needle aspiration techniques for biopsy of deep-seated impalpable targets: a primer for radiologists, *Am J Roentgenol* 171:325-328, 1998.

Manolakopoulos S, Triantos C, Bethanis S: Ultrasound-guided liver biopsy in real life: comparison of same-day prebiopsy versus real-time ultrasound approach, *J Gastroenterol Hepatol* 22(9):1490-1493, 2007.

Mauturen KE, Nghiem HV, Marrero J: Lack of tumor seeding of hepatocellular carcinoma after percutaneous needle biopsy using coaxial cutting needle technique, *Am J Roentgenol* 187:1184-1187, 2006.

Middleton WD, Hiskes SK, Teefey SA, Boucher LD: Small (1.5 cm or less) liver metastases: US-guided biopsy, *Radiology* 205:729-732, 1997.

Moore EH: Technical aspects of needle aspiration lung biopsy: a personal perspective, *Radiology* 208:303-318, 1998.

Nazarian L, Feld R, Johnson P, et al: Safety and efficacy of sonographically guided random core biopsy for diffuse liver disease, *J Ultrasound Med* 19:537-541, 2000.

Rockey D, Caldwell SH, Goodman Z: Liver biopsy, *Hepatology* 49(3):1017-1077, 2009.

Romics I: The technique of ultrasound guided prostate biopsy, *World J Urol* 22:353-356, 2004.

Sheafor DH, Paulson EK, Simmons CM, DeLong DM: Abdominal percutaneous interventional procedures: comparison of CT and US guidance, *Radiology* 207:705-710, 1998.

Takamori R, Wong LL, Dang C, Wong L: Needle tract implantation from hepatocellular cancer: is needle biopsy of the liver always necessary? *Liver Transpl Surg* 6:67-72, 2000.

Ward SC, Carey BM, Chalmers AG, Sutton J: The role of immediate cytological evaluation in CT-guided biopsy, *Clinical Radiology* 49:531-534, 1994.

Wood BJ, Khan MA, McGovern F, Harisinghani M, et al: Imaging guided biopsy of renal masses: indications, accuracy and impact on clinical management, *J Urol* 161(5):1470-1474, 1999.

Emergent Ultrasound Procedures

Sandra L. Hagen-Ansert

OBJECTIVES

On completion of this chapter, you should be able to:

- Discuss the advantages and disadvantages of sonography for the trauma patient
- Define the goal of sonography in the assessment of blunt trauma
- Describe the protocol for focused assessment with sonography for trauma (FAST)

- Describe the sonographic findings for aortic dissection, right upper quadrant pain, free fluid in the abdominopelvic region, acute pelvic pain, and scrotal trauma and torsion
- Identify the modalities commonly used to evaluate flank pain

OUTLINE

KEY TERMS

Diagnostic peritoneal lavage (DPL)
Focused assessment with sonography for trauma (FAST)

Hemoperitoneum
Incarcerated hernia
Intravenous urography (IVU)

Pseudodissection
Reducible hernia
Strangulated hernia

Sonography is well recognized as a powerful and efficient tool for the diagnosis and evaluation of the patient in the emergency department (ED). The development of smaller ultrasound equipment with improvement in transducer technology has enabled the sonographic examination to extend beyond the imaging departments and is especially prevalent in the ED. The implementation of educational curriculum changes in specialized residency programs and specialty practices has facilitated the integration of focused ultrasound into specific emergent settings. In emergent and critical situations the ED team must be able to efficiently and accurately assess the patient problem, and sonography is a tool that allows the team to quickly evaluate the patient.

The most common reasons people go to the ED include trauma, acute chest pain, shortness of breath, hypotensive, acute abdominal or pelvic pain, syncope, extreme nausea and vomiting, lacerations, and broken bones.

The primary focus of this chapter is to cover the more common emergent abdominal procedures that the sonographer is likely to encounter in a "call back" situation from the ED. The ED resident or emergency physician may have already performed a rapid survey of the area of interest and may call for a "formal, complete" ultrasound evaluation if further information is needed. Potential life-threatening emergencies such as abdominal emergencies, internal hemorrhage following blunt trauma, ectopic pregnancy, pericardial tamponade, and ruptured aortic aneurysm may be rapidly assessed with sonography.

ASSESSMENT OF ABDOMINAL TRAUMA

The assessment of the abdomen for possible sustained abdominal injury caused by blunt abdominal trauma is a common clinical challenge for physicians and emergency medicine physicians. The physical findings may be unreliable because of the state of patient consciousness, neurologic deficit, medication, or other associated injuries.

Diagnostic Peritoneal Lavage

Diagnostic peritoneal lavage (DPL) is used to sample the intraperitoneal space for evidence of damage to the viscera and blood vessels in patients with blunt abdominal trauma to decide which patients need exploratory laparotomy. For this procedure the patient is placed in the supine position and the urinary bladder is emptied by catheterization. The patient's stomach is emptied by a nasogastric tube because a distended stomach may extend to the anterior abdominal wall. The skin is anesthetized, and a small vertical incision is made. The incision is made either in the midline or at the paraumbilical site with multiple layers of tissue penetrated before the parietal peritoneum is located (Figure 19-1). Although peritoneal lavage has been used successfully to assess abdominal injuries, it is an invasive procedure that

takes at least 10 to 15 minutes and that carries a risk of bowel perforation, bladder penetration, vascular laceration, and wound complications. This procedure is inappropriate for alert patients in stable condition, who represent the majority of patients with blunt abdominal trauma. Peritoneal lavage decreases the specificity of subsequent ultrasonography or computed tomography (CT) because of the introduction of intraperitoneal fluid and air.

Computed Tomography

CT remains the radiology standard for investigating the injured abdomen but requires patient transfer and inevitable delay (bowel preparation). CT is usually performed in patients in whom intraabdominal injury is strongly suspected. Other indications for CT include equivocal findings of abdominal examination in stable patients, persistent abdominal pain, and decreasing hematocrit. CT is unsuitable for patients who are clinically unstable. The time required to complete a CT scan is variable; however, the sensitivity and specificity are high to detect fluid collections.

Ultrasound

The clinical utilization of sonography in the evaluation of blunt trauma has existed in Europe and Asia since the 1970s. North America and the United Kingdom did not incorporate its use until the 1990s. The development of smaller ultrasound systems and improved transducer technology has made this application grow. Using sonography as a screening procedure involves many factors that will be fast, accurate, portable, and noninvasive. A rapid survey with sonography may be made in less than 4 minutes. Disadvantages include the presence of subcutaneous or intraabdominal air, and obesity. Sonography is now well established as a noninvasive and easily repeatable tool to image many areas of the body (Box 19-1).

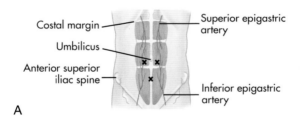

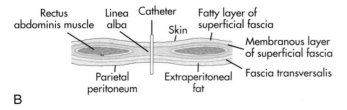

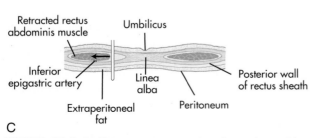

FIGURE 19-1 A, The two common sites for peritoneal lavage. **B,** Cross section of the anterior abdominal wall in the middle. Note the structures pierced by the catheter. **C,** Cross section of the anterior abdominal wall just lateral to the umbilicus.

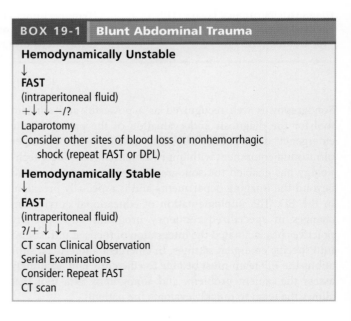

BOX 19-1	Blunt Abdominal Trauma

Hemodynamically Unstable
↓
FAST
(intraperitoneal fluid)
+↓ ↓ −/?
Laparotomy
Consider other sites of blood loss or nonhemorrhagic
  shock (repeat FAST or DPL)

Hemodynamically Stable
↓
FAST
(intraperitoneal fluid)
?/+ ↓ ↓ −
CT scan Clinical Observation
Serial Examinations
Consider: Repeat FAST
CT scan

FOCUSED ASSESSMENT WITH SONOGRAPHY FOR TRAUMA

Focused assessment with sonography for trauma (FAST) has become an extension of the physical examination of the trauma patient. This is a focused survey examination of the abdomen, pelvis, and pericardium to evaluate free fluid or pericardial fluid. The FAST examination is performed in the ED by properly trained and credentialed staff. In the context of traumatic injury, the timely diagnosis of potentially life-threatening hemorrhage found during the FAST examination is a decision-making tool to help determine the transfer to the operating room, CT scanner, or angiography suite.

> **Focused Assessment with Sonography for Trauma (FAST) Survey:**
> - Perihepatic and hepatorenal space
> - Perisplenic
> - Pelvis—cul-de-sac
> - Pericardium

The FAST evaluation survey is widespread, extending from the pericardial sac to the urinary bladder, and includes the perihepatic area (including Morison's pouch), perisplenic region (including splenorenal recess), paracolic gutters, and cul-de-sac (Figure 19-2). The visceral organs are assessed for heterogeneity and evaluated with color Doppler if necessary.

Accessibility and speed of performance are critical in the trauma setting. Onsite personnel who are educated in performing the ultrasound examination provide the highest success rate. Limitations of ultrasound include its dependence on operator skill and patient body habitus, which becomes particularly important if surgeons or emergency physicians with limited training perform the studies. Although CT remains the standard of reference for intraperitoneal and retroperitoneal assessment, this application is not available at the bedside.

Assessment of Blunt Trauma with Ultrasound

Ultrasound of the abdomen and pelvis is performed simultaneously with the physical assessment, resuscitation, and stabilization of the trauma patient. The examination usually takes less than 4 minutes. The goal is to scan the four quadrants, pericardial sac, and cul-de-sac for the presence of free fluid or hemoperitoneum. Ultrasound has been found to be highly sensitive for the detection of free intraperitoneal fluid, but it is not sensitive for the identification of organ injuries. If the patient is hemodynamically stable, the value of ultrasound is limited by the large percentage of organ injuries that are not associated with free fluid.

Protocol for Focused Assessment with Sonography for Trauma. The ultrasound examination is performed with the proper transducer according to the patient size.

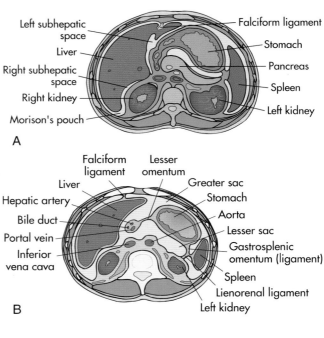

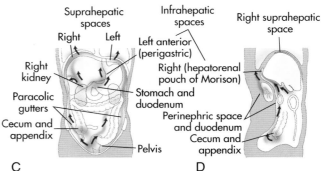

FIGURE 19-2 A, Transverse view of the perihepatic space and Morison's pouch. **B,** Transverse view of the perisplenic area and the splenorenal ligament. **C,** Anterior view of the collection of fluid in the abdomen and pelvic cavities. **D,** Sagittal view of the right abdomen shows how the fluid collects in the most dependent areas of the abdomen and pelvis.

The patient is usually in the supine position. The right and left upper quadrants of the abdomen, epigastrium, paracolic gutters, retroperitoneal space, and pelvis are evaluated with ultrasound (Box 19-2). If there is no contraindication to catheterization, the empty bladder is filled with 200 to 300 ml of sterile saline through a Foley catheter to ensure bladder distention to allow adequate visualization of the pelvic cavity. The examination is focused to look for the presence of free fluid, the texture of the visceral organs, and the pericardial sac around the heart.

The initial survey is directed in the subcostal plane with the transducer angled in a cephalic direction toward the four-chamber view of the heart to image the pericardial sac (Figure 19-3). The right upper quadrant is then evaluated, including the diaphragm, dome of the liver, subhepatic space (Morison's pouch), right kidney, and right flank (Figure 19-4). The liver is quickly scanned to look for texture abnormalities (Figure 19-5). The epigastrium is briefly examined (Figure 19-6). The transducer is then moved to the left upper quadrant to observe the diaphragm, spleen, left kidney, and left flank and to search for the presence of fluid (Figure 19-7). The pelvic cavity (with the bladder distended) is evaluated for the presence of free fluid in the cul-de-sac (Figure 19-8).

Sonographic Findings. In the trauma setting, free fluid usually represents **hemoperitoneum,** although it may also represent bowel, urine, bile, or ascitic fluid. Hemorrhage in the peritoneal cavity collects in the most dependent area of the abdomen (Figure 19-9). The fluid is usually hypoechoic or hyperechoic, with scattered internal echoes representing the

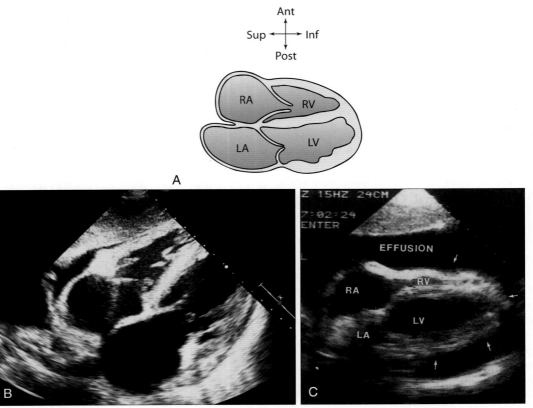

FIGURE 19-3 **A,** Subcostal view of the four chambers of the heart. The transducer is angled sharply in a cephalic direction in the subcostal area. Cardiac pulsations are noted and the four chambers of the heart should be seen. **B,** Normally, there is no significant fluid that separates the outer layer of the heart (epicardium) within the pericardial sac. **C,** Subcostal four-chamber view shows a tip of the left lobe of the liver anterior to the large pericardial effusion that fills the pericardial cavity.

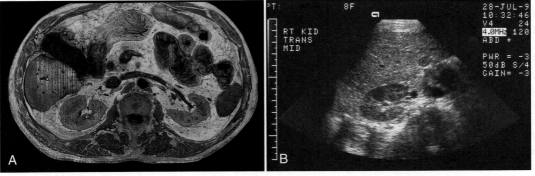

FIGURE 19-4 Gross anatomy **(A)** and transverse **(B)** images of the right upper quadrant and normal liver.

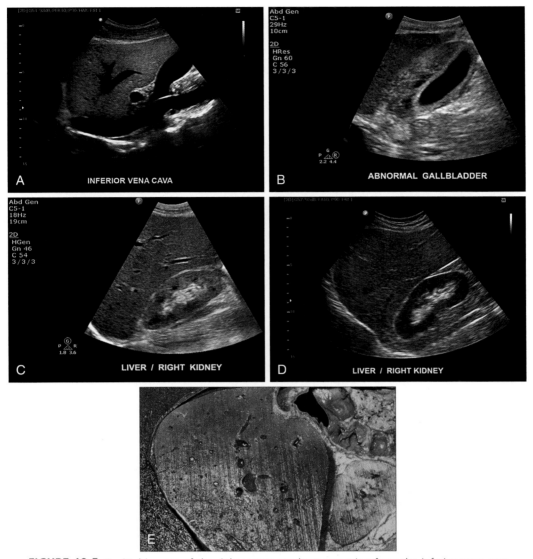

FIGURE 19-5 Sagittal images of the right upper quadrant sweeping from the inferior vena cava **(A)** to the inflamed gallbladder **(B)** to the lateral abdominal wall **(C** and **D)** demonstrate a good border between the liver and right kidney with no fluid in Morison's pouch. Gross anatomy **(E)** of the liver and right kidney.

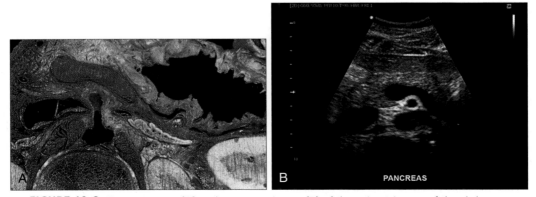

FIGURE 19-6 Gross anatomy **(A)** and transverse image **(B)** of the epigastric area of the abdomen. The horseshoe shape of the spine is the most posterior reflection with the aorta and inferior vena cava directly anterior. The celiac axis arises from the anterior wall of the aorta. The left lobe of the liver is identified anterior to the pancreas, which lies directly anterior to the prevertebral vessels (aorta, inferior vena cava, celiac axis, and splenic vein).

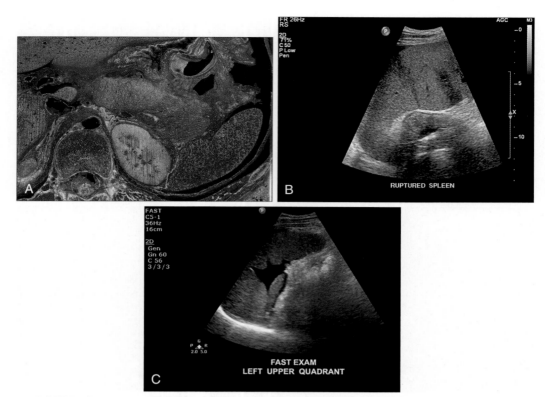

FIGURE 19-7 **A,** Gross anatomy of the left upper quadrant. **B,** Sagittal image of the diaphragm, enlarged ruptured spleen, and upper pole of the left kidney. **C,** Sagittal image of the left upper quadrant with fluid in the splenic hilum.

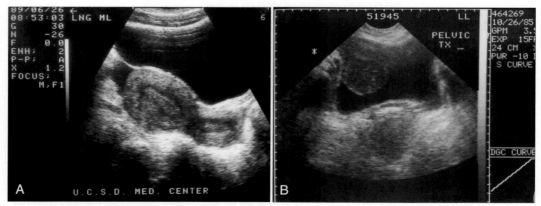

FIGURE 19-8 **A,** Normal sagittal pelvic image with a distended urinary bladder and uterus posterior. It is not uncommon to see a small amount of fluid in a female of menstrual age. **B,** Transverse image of the distended urinary bladder as it provides a window for the uterus and adnexal area.

blood, and conforms to the anatomic site it occupies. The most common site of fluid accumulation is the subhepatic space (Morison's pouch), regardless of the site of the injury (Figure 19-10). The next most common space is the pelvis. The blood in the pelvis may collect centrally in the pouch of Douglas or laterally in the paravesical space (Figure 19-11). When fluid is present, the poorly visualized loops of bowel are separated by triangular collections of fluid. If there is a massive hemoperitoneum, the intraperitoneal organs will float in the surrounding fluid.

If the collection of fluid is small, the surgeon may not want to do an immediate laparotomy. Close monitoring of the patient with either ultrasound or CT imaging may help to define the further extent of the injury after the patient stabilizes.

Parenchymal Injury

The ultrasound appearance of hepatic and splenic injury will vary with both the type and time of injury. Liver lacerations or

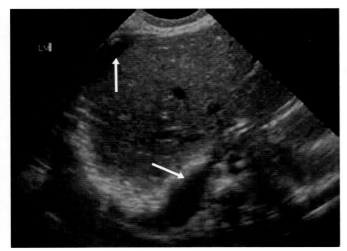

FIGURE 19-9 Transverse image of a patient with a fluid collection as seen posterior and anterolateral to the right lobe of the liver. Fluid will collect in the most dependent area of the abdomen and should not be confused with ascitic fluid.

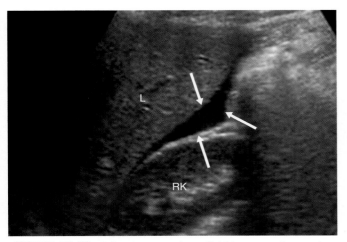

FIGURE 19-10 Right upper quadrant fluid is present in a patient after trauma. A small amount of fluid is seen in Morison's pouch anterior to the kidney. Fluid *(arrows)*; *L,* liver; *RK,* right kidney.

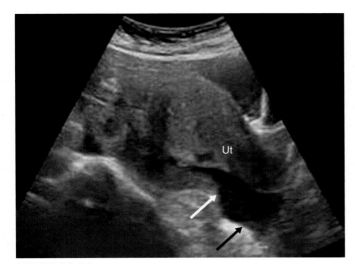

FIGURE 19-11 Sagittal images of a patient with fluid in the pouch of Douglas. Fluid *(arrows)*; *Ut,* uterus.

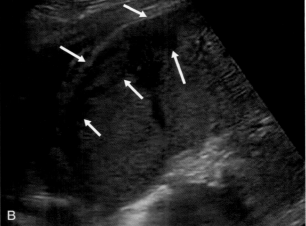

FIGURE 19-12 Images of a patient with a splenic hematoma *(arrows)* secondary to splenic trauma.

contusions are more easily detected with ultrasound than any other visceral abdominal injury. Such injuries appear as heterogeneous or hyperechoic. Hematomas and localized lacerations will appear initially hypoechoic with low-level echoes generated from the red blood cells, or echogenic, as the blood begins to coagulate, which over time will become more anechoic with the onset of hemolysis (Figure 19-12). Pitfalls of abdominal ultrasound include failure to show contained solid-organ injuries; injuries to the diaphragm, pancreas, and adrenal gland; and some bowel injuries. Therefore a negative ultrasound does not exclude an intraperitoneal injury, and close clinical observation or CT is warranted.

A brisk intraparenchymal hemorrhage may be identified as an anechoic region within the abnormal parenchyma, whereas a global parenchymal injury may project in the liver as a widespread architectural disruption with absence of the normal vascular pattern. An extensive splenic injury presents as a diffusely heterogeneous parenchymal pattern with both hyperechoic and hypoechoic regions.

The early diagnosis of parenchymal injury can affect patient treatment. The clinically stable patient with a hemoperitoneum and an obvious splenic injury seen on ultrasound can be taken directly to surgery. However, if extensive hepatic disruption is demonstrated, the surgeon may want further investigation with CT or even angiography before the surgery is performed.

Free Pelvic Fluid in Women. In female patients of reproductive age with trauma, free fluid isolated to the cul-de-sac is likely physiologic and clinical follow-up should suffice. Female patients with fluid elsewhere usually have a clinically important injury and require further evaluation.

Pitfalls and Limitations. As in other ultrasound procedures, obesity may prevent adequate visualization of the anatomic structures. In some cases the presence of subcutaneous emphysema precludes adequate ultrasound views. The presence of subcutaneous air from a pneumothorax that dissects into the abdominal cavity may collect over the liver or spleen.

An intraperitoneal clot is usually hyperechoic relative to the neighboring structures; occasionally, though, it is isoechoic, and intraperitoneal bleeding or parenchymal injury may go unrecognized.

Contained parenchymal injuries of the liver and spleen, as well as bowel injuries, may not be accompanied by hemoperitoneum and may therefore be missed if screening ultrasound alone is used to evaluate for blunt trauma. Ultrasound may not depict injuries to the diaphragm, the pancreas, the adrenal gland, and bone.

RIGHT UPPER QUADRANT PAIN

Acute Cholecystitis versus Cholelithiasis

One of the most frequent complaints in the ED is the onset of severe right upper quadrant pain. The patient may have other medical conditions, such as diabetes or peptic ulcer disease, which may contribute to the pain. A myocardial infarction may also present with radiating right upper quadrant pain. Thus a clinically focused physical examination in conjunction with historical and laboratory information should provide the information necessary for decision making. If the patient is female with symptoms of right upper quadrant pain with point tenderness, fever, and leukocytosis, acute cholecystitis should be ruled out. The most common cause of acute cholecystitis is cholelithiasis with a cystic duct obstruction.

Sonographic Findings. Sonographic findings of acute cholecystitis include an irregular, thickened gallbladder wall, a positive sonographic Murphy's sign, sludge, pericholecystic fluid, and a dilated gallbladder greater than 5 cm in transverse diameter (Figure 19-13). The presence of biliary stones within the inflamed gallbladder is recognized as tiny echogenic foci collected along the posterior wall with a well-demarcated acoustic shadowing in at least two planes. The sonographer

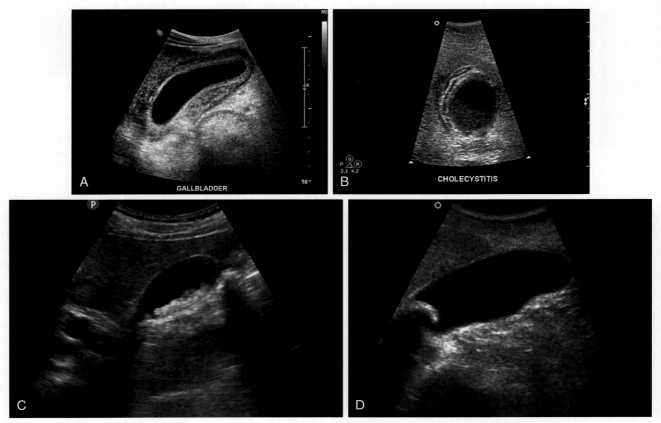

FIGURE 19-13 Sagittal **(A)** and transverse **(B)** images of the distended gallbladder with edema and wall thickening secondary to acute cholecystitis and sludge. **C,** Patient with chronic cholelithiasis shows an edematous thick-walled gallbladder with multiple small stones. **D,** Single large gallstone within the fundus of the gallbladder. This stone may obstruct the bile in the area of Hartmann's pouch, causing extreme right upper quadrant pain.

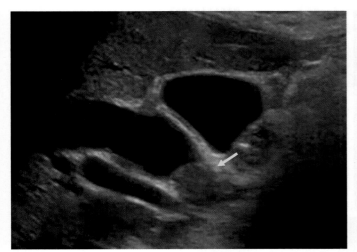

FIGURE 19-14 Prominent common bile duct is seen anterior to the portal vein in this sagittal image. Careful sweep of the transducer should demonstrate echo density *(arrow)* with shadowing if stones are present and large enough to be detected with sonography.

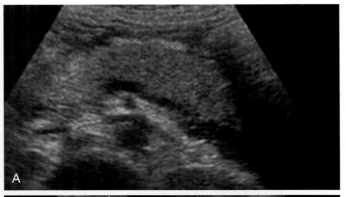

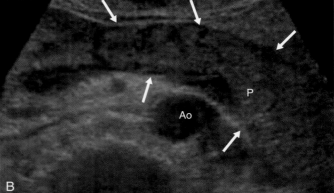

FIGURE 19-15 A, Acute epigastric pain may be secondary to pancreatitis with an enlarged pancreatic duct. **B,** Patient with diffuse pancreatitis shows the gland to be enlarged and edematous. *Ao,* aorta; *P,* pancreas.

must be careful to make sure the shadowing is secondary to gallstones and not to surrounding bowel gas. By holding the transducer carefully over the area of interest, the presence of peristalsis in the bowel may cause shifting of the dirty shadow. Alterations in the patient position will cause movement of the gallstones, with resultant movement of the acoustical shadow. If the stones are very small, they have a chance of becoming lodged within the neck of the gallbladder and may be too small to render an acoustical shadow. The gallbladder will show signs of inflammation. Cholesterol stones are usually smaller than the biliary stones and on sonography are less echogenic. They may be seen to "float" within the thick bile and demonstrate a "comet tail" artifact on sonography.

Biliary Dilation

The common bile duct (CBD) is demonstrated on sonography by identifying the portal vein. The duct is seen anterior and to the right of the portal vein on a transverse image and does not fill in with color Doppler (Figure 19-14). Recall that the hepatic artery is anterior and medial of the portal vein. The normal upper limit of the CBD is 6 mm, although with age this diameter may extend up to 10 mm in size. The presence of stones within the duct should be carefully assessed. The sonographer should look for echogenic foci with acoustical shadowing beyond the foci. Adjustment of gains should be made to delineate the CBD, and alterations in patient position may allow the visualization of the duct to be separated from bowel gas interference.

EPIGASTRIC PAIN

Pancreatitis

Midepigastric pain that radiates to the back is characteristic of acute pancreatitis. Pancreatitis occurs when the toxic enzymes

escape into the parenchymal tissue of the gland, causing obstruction of the acini, ducts, small blood vessels, and fat with extension into the peripancreatic tissue. Clinical findings of fever and leukocytosis are found along with elevated enzymes. The serum amylase levels increase within the first 24 hours of onset but fall rather quickly, whereas the lipase levels take longer to elevate (as much as 72 hours) and remain elevated for a longer period of time. Sonographic findings in acute pancreatitis show a normal to edematous gland that is somewhat hypoechoic to normal texture (Figure 19-15). The borders are irregular secondary to the inflammation. Increased vascular flow may be apparent because of the inflammatory nature of the disease.

Abdominal Aortic Aneurysm

The patient who presents with classic abdominal pain radiating to the back, with hypotension and a pulsatile abdominal mass, is not a diagnostic dilemma in the ED (Figure 19-16). Sonography can rapidly separate the emergent patient with a possible aortic dissection from the elderly patient with vague abdominal complaints or the middle-aged patient with symptoms that mimic nephrolithiasis. If a dissection is suspected, CT with contrast is generally more specific than sonography, as the full length of the aorta may be clearly imaged in a

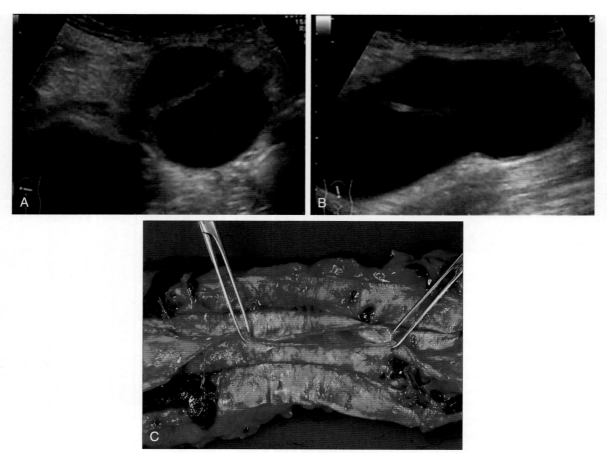

FIGURE 19-16 Dissection of the abdominal aortic aneurysm. **A,** This transverse image of the abdominal aorta demonstrates an enlarged aortic aneurysm just superior to the bifurcation of the vessel with a fine line within that represents the dissection. **B,** Sagittal image of the dilated aorta with the linear line representing the dissection. **C,** Gross pathology of a dissecting aortic aneurysm demonstrates the layers of the aortic wall separated by the blood.

matter of minutes without bowel gas interference. Sonography may identify the abdominal aortic aneurysm in relation to the renal vessels, which is important because in the event a dissection occurs, extension may extend into the renal arteries. Recall that the aorta and iliac arteries are measured from the outside margin of the wall on one wall to the outside margin on the other wall. This measurement should be performed in two planes, transverse and longitudinal. Most aneurysms occur at the level of the umbilicus, at the junction of the bifurcation into the iliac vessels. Aneurysms may expand in the transverse diameter and in the anteroposterior diameter. The sonographic examination may be inhibited by obesity, bowel gas interference, or extreme abdominal tenderness.

The sonographer should be aware of several pitfalls when scanning the abdominal aorta. If bowel gas precludes adequate visualization of the aorta from the anterior wall, the transducer may be directed from the lateral abdominal wall, using the liver or spleen as an acoustic window to image both the aorta and inferior vena cava. Alternately, the patient could be rolled into a decubitus position and imaged from the lateral wall. The true diameter of the aorta should

be measured with the transducer perpendicular to the vessel; an oblique or angled image would exaggerate the true aortic diameter. A small aneurysm does not preclude rupture. The sonographer should also assess for free intraperitoneal fluid when a patient with an acute abdominal aortic aneurysm is examined. Para-aortic nodes may be confused with the aorta, mimicking an aneurysm. These nodes often are anterior to the aorta, but they can be found posterior as well, encasing the aorta and displacing it from the vertebral body. The nodes are irregular in shape without luminal flow.

EXTREME SHORTNESS OF BREATH

Pericardial Effusion

The primary application of cardiac ultrasound in an emergent situation is to rule out the presence of pericardial effusion or to evaluate cardiac function in patients with sudden cardiac arrest. Body habitus and underlying pathologic conditions will affect the accessibility of the heart to sonographic evaluation. Patients with pulmonary hyperinflation have poor parasternal

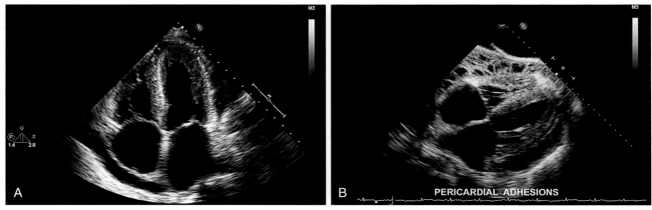

FIGURE 19-17 A, Apical four-chamber view shows a small separation between the right atrium and the diaphragm. This pericardial effusion is not large enough to cause compromise of the right side of the heart. **B,** Subcostal window shows a complex moderate size pericardial effusion representing adhesions from previous interventions.

windows but generally have adequate apical and subcostal windows.

Other emergent situations such as cardiac tamponade involve a more complex evaluation of the cardiac structures that requires high-end ultrasound equipment not commonly found in the ED. The diastolic collapse of right heart chambers in the presence of a moderate to large effusion may be indicative of tamponade. This is usually seen in the right atrial collapse or right ventricular collapse. Further Doppler evaluation of both the tricuspid and mitral valve inflow patterns with a respirator monitor is made to look for alterations of flow secondary to cardiac tamponade. The inferior vena cava should be assessed for dilation without respiratory collapse in patients with tamponade. Clinically, the presence of the pulsus tardus should be present in the setting of tamponade.

The evaluation of acute right ventricular dysfunction or acute pulmonary hypertension in the clinical setting of acute and unexplained chest pain, dyspnea, or hemodynamic instability is best evaluated with the use of high-end ultrasound equipment. In this case patients with suspected pulmonary embolism are usually referred for a rapid CT scan to demonstrate the presence of clot or thrombus lodged within the pulmonary arteries.

The sonographer should be aware that when a pericardial effusion is demonstrated, several observations should be made. The pericardial effusion usually appears as an anechoic or hypoechoic fluid collection within the pericardial space (Figure 19-17). With inflammatory, malignant, or hemorrhagic etiologies, this fluid may have a more complex echogenic texture. Fluid usually initially collects dependently. The size of the effusion is important to document. In the parasternal long axis view, the fluid is demonstrated within the pericardial sac beyond the epicardial border of the left ventricle. If the fluid collection is small (less than 1 cm between the epicardium and posterior border of the fluid in diastole), it may only be seen in the posterior of the heart. As the fluid increases, it becomes circumferential,

reflecting off the great vessels and not extending beyond the atrial appendage. A moderate size effusion measures between 1 and 2 cm in diastole, usually circumferential. Beyond 2 cm in diastole the fluid is considered large. The fluid should be assessed in multiple planes, short axis, apical four chamber, and subcostal views.

In the acute hemopericardium trauma patient with clotted blood, the fluid may have a soft echogenic to isoechoic texture compared with the myocardial texture, which would represent blood within the pericardial space. Hypoechoic fatty tissue found in the epicardial layer surrounding the heart may sometimes mimic pericardial effusion. It is important to note that a small, rapidly forming effusion may lead to tamponade, whereas extremely large, slowly forming effusions may be tolerated with minimal symptoms.

Care should also be taken not to confuse pleural effusions with a pericardial effusion (Figure 19-18). Patients with congestive heart failure who present with acute failure may have both pericardial and pleural effusion. Again in a long-axis

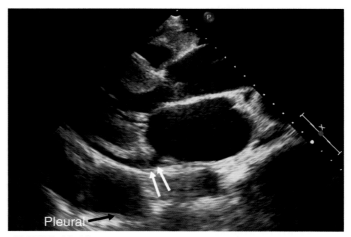

FIGURE 19-18 Pleural effusion is seen posterior to the descending aorta while pericardial effusion is anterior to the descending aorta.

view of the heart, the pericardial effusion will be seen posterior to the epicardial border of the left ventricular and anterior to the descending aorta. The pleural effusion will also be found in that similar area, but will be seen posterior to the descending aorta.

CHEST PAIN

Thoracic Aortic Dissection

A dissecting aortic aneurysm is a condition in which a propagating intramural hematoma actually dissects along the length of the vessel, stripping away the intima and, in some cases, part of the media. The resultant aortic dissection is a defect or tear in the aortic intima with concomitant weakness of the aortic media. At this point, blood surges into the media, separating the intima from the adventitia. This channel is called the "false lumen." This blood in the false lumen can reenter the true lumen anywhere along the course of the dissection. Most aortic dissections will occur at one of three sites: (1) at the root of the aorta with possible extension into the arch, descending aorta, and abdominal aorta; (2) at the level of the left subclavian artery, with extension into the descending aorta or abdominal aorta; and (3) only at the level of the ascending aorta (see Figure 8-43, *A* for an illustration of the aortic dissection).

Approximately 70% of dissections are located in the ascending aorta, 10% to 20% in the aortic arch, and 20% in the abdominal aorta. Most often, the dissection will propagate distally in the aorta into the iliac vessels, although proximal extension can occur.

Clinical Findings for Aortic Dissection. The typical presentation for an aortic dissection is that of a sudden onset of severe, tearing chest pain radiating to the arms, neck, or back (Box 19-3). Syncope occurs in a small percentage of patients. The complexity of the symptoms will depend on the extension of the dissection, the specific branches of the aorta involved, and the location of external rupture if present (Table 19-1). If the carotid artery is affected, hemiplegia may result. Involvement of the subclavian or iliac vessels will appear with decreased or absent pulses in the arms or legs.

The location of the pain may be a clue to the site of the dissection. If the pain centers in the anterior thorax, a proximal dissection may be present; severe pain in the interscapular area is more common with distal involvement.

BOX 19-3	Causes of Aortic Dissection

- Hypertension (70%–90%)
- Marfan syndrome (16%)
- Pregnancy
- Acquired or congenital aortic stenosis
- Coarctation of the aorta
- Trauma
- Iatrogenic (cardiac catheterization, aortic valve replacement)

TABLE 19-1	Common Emergency Conditions
Clinical Findings	**Sonographic Findings**
RUQ Pain: Cholecystitis	
RUQ pain	Thickened gallbladder wall
Fever	Positive Murphy's sign
Nausea, vomiting	Pericholecystic fluid
Leukocytosis	Dilated gallbladder
Epigastric Pain: Pancreatitis	
Midepigastric pain radiating to back	Normal to edematous gland
	Hypoechoic texture
Fever	Irregular borders
Leukocytosis	Increased vascular flow
↑ Amylase	
↑ Lipase	
Flank Pain: Urolithiasis	
Spasmodic flank pain	Echogenic foci with shadowing
Pain may radiate into pelvis	Hydronephrosis may be present
Hematuria	Look for ureteral jets in bladder
Fever	
Leukocytosis	
Thoracic or Abdominal Pain: Aortic Dissection	
Sudden onset of severe chest pain with radiation to arms, neck, or back	Aneurysm
	Look for flap at site of dissection
Syncope may be present	Look for false lumen
RLQ Pain: Appendicitis	
Intense RLQ pain	Distended, noncompressible appendix
Nausea, vomiting	
Fever	↑ Color flow
Leukocytosis	McBurney sign
Lower Abdominal Pain: Paraumbilical Hernia	
Asymptomatic to mild discomfort	Lower abdominal mass; look for peristalsis of bowel in hernia
Palpable mass	
Valsalva: shows exaggeration of mass	
Reduce sac with gentle pressure	

RLQ, Right lower quadrant; *RUQ,* right upper quadrant.

However, the majority of patients with distal dissection of the aorta have back pain. Occlusion of the visceral arteries may appear with abdominal pain.

Sonographic Findings. In the acute aortic dissection, time is of the essence and therefore magnetic resonance imaging (MRI) or contrast-enhanced CT is the imaging modality of choice for evaluating aortic dissections. In the stabilized patient with a suspected dissection, sonography may be performed. Because most dissections are seen in the ascending aorta, a transesophageal echocardiogram (TEE) will be performed by the cardiology department. If the dissection is suspected in the abdomen, an abdominal ultrasound may be requested.

On sonography, the classic finding is the visualization of the flap at the site of the dissection. An echogenic intimal membrane within the aorta or the iliac arteries may be seen to move freely with arterial pulsations on sonography if

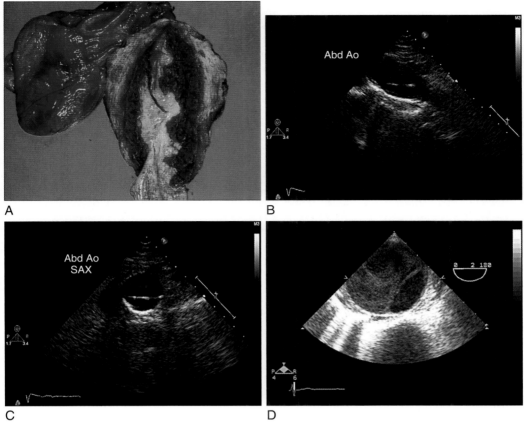

FIGURE 19-19 **A–D,** Type 1 aortic dissection. **B,** Sagittal view of aortic dissection. Note the linear line demarcating the site of dissection. **C,** Short axis *(SAX)* or transverse image. **D,** Transesophageal image of the dissection is shown as clear with homogeneous blood swirling in the thoracic aorta.

both the true and false lumens are patent (Figure 19-19). However, if the membrane is thick and the lumen is thrombosed, the membrane may not move. Color Doppler may demonstrate slow flow in both the true and false lumen. The flow is decreased or reversed in the false lumen. The sonographer should look for the presence of the intimal membrane with concomitant clotting in the iliac, celiac, and superior mesenteric arteries.

A **pseudodissection** on color flow demonstrates a turbulent blood flow pattern, indicating a hypoechoic thrombus near the outer margin of the aorta with an echogenic laminated clot. No intimal flap is seen with a pseudodissection.

FLANK PAIN

Urolithiasis

Flank pain caused by urolithiasis is a common problem in patients coming to the ED. Radiology plays a vital role in the evaluation of these patients through the use of **intravenous urography (IVU)**, ultrasonography, and limited noncontrast helical CT studies. The most sensitive and specific for the presence of stones are the IVU and helical CT. Traditional evaluation of the patient with flank pain consisted of conventional radiography followed by IVU with noniodinated contrast. In those patients unable to undergo IVU safely (i.e., patients with dye allergies, renal insufficiency, congestive heart failure, or suspected pregnancy), ultrasound is used to evaluate for secondary signs of obstruction, namely hydronephrosis. CT has largely replaced these other modalities with its ability to identify calculi and their location, determine the size, and guide the management.

Clinical Findings for Urolithiasis. Acute ureteral obstruction usually manifests as renal colic, a severe pain that is often spasmodic, increases to a peak level of intensity, and then decreases before increasing again. The pain can also manifest as steady and continuous. The pain usually begins abruptly in the flank and increases rapidly to a level of discomfort that often requires narcotics for adequate pain control. Over time, the pain may radiate to the lower abdomen and into the scrotum or labia as the stone moves into the more distal portion of the ureter.

Urinalysis is the initial laboratory examination. Hematuria is the common finding in 85% of the patients. However, if the stone completely obstructs the ureter, no hematuria will be present. Clinical symptoms such as fever, leukocytosis, and urine gram staining can help identify a superimposed urinary tract infection.

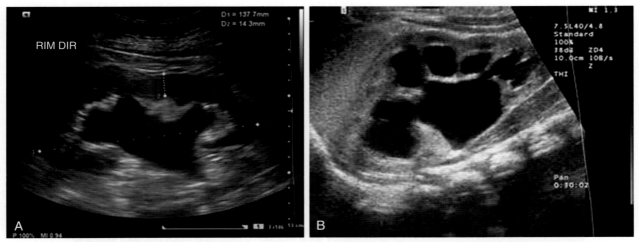

FIGURE 19-20 A, Patient with right flank pain presents with hydronephrosis secondary to a stone in the urinary system. **B,** Dilated collecting system and hydronephrosis of the right kidney.

▄ *Sonographic Findings.* The calculi imaged with sonography are highly echogenic foci with distinct acoustic shadowing. Stones as small as 0.5 mm may be seen. When obstruction occurs, ultrasound is effective in demonstrating the secondary sign of hydronephrosis (Figure 19-20). Overlying bowel gas in the pelvis may obscure the evaluation of the distal ureters. With the bladder distended, color Doppler is an excellent tool to image the presence of ureteral jets in the bladder. The transducer should be angled in a cephalic presentation through the distended urinary bladder. Color Doppler is turned on and the probe is held stationary to watch for the appearance of ureteral jets. The pulse repetition frequency should be decreased to assess the low velocity of the ureteral jet flow. The color gain should be turned up just enough to barely see color in the background. Usually within 2 to 3 minutes the jet will light up with color as the urine drains into the bladder (Figure 19-21). Be sure to look for the presence of both the right and left ureteral jet with this technique. Power Doppler may also be used to image the ureteral jets and is very effective.

The presence of hydronephrosis in a pregnant patient may be more problematic because it is not uncommon for the kidneys to become slightly hydronephrotic during the latter stage of pregnancy because the uterus enlarges and causes pressure on the ureter. This is seen especially in the right kidney because it lies lower than the left and is more likely to show minimal hydronephrosis. Therefore the appearance of ureteral jets may help to rule out the presence of obstruction secondary to calculi.

RIGHT LOWER QUADRANT PAIN

Appendicitis

Acute appendicitis is one of the most common diseases that necessitates emergency surgery and is the most common atraumatic surgical abdominal disorder in children 2 years of age and older. Appendicitis is the result of luminal obstruction and inflammation, leading to ischemia of the vermiform appendix. The early diagnosis of acute appendicitis is essential in the prevention of perforation, abscess formation, and postoperative complications. The classic clinical symptoms include exquisite lower abdominal pain, nausea, vomiting, fever, and leukocytosis. The quick-release maneuver is performed by applying pressure with the fingertips directly over the area of the appendix and then quickly letting go. With appendicitis, the patient will usually have rebound tenderness, termed *McBurney sign,* associated with peritoneal irritation.

The sonographer should use a high-frequency linear transducer to image the right lower quadrant. Careful explanation of the technique to the patient with care over the tender abdomen is essential in performing an adequate examination. The inflamed appendix will demonstrate a thickened edematous wall less than 2 mm thick (Figure 19-22).

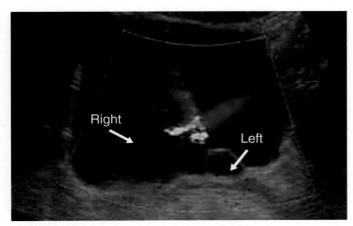

FIGURE 19-21 Normal ureteral jets in bladder as imaged with color flow Doppler.

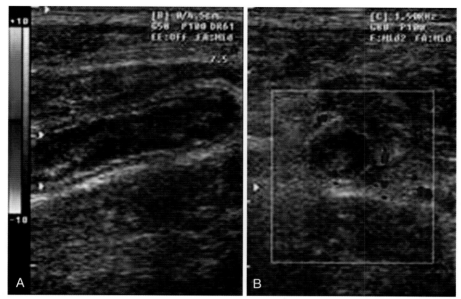

FIGURE 19-22 **Appendicitis.** Sagittal **(A)** and transverse **(B)** images of the inflamed appendix that was not compressed with the linear array transducer.

If the wall is asymmetric, perforation may have occurred and the search for fluid collections around the appendiceal area should be made. The inflamed appendix may also demonstrate a "target" lesion on transverse images demonstrating a hypoechoic, fluid-distended lumen, with a hyperechoic inner ring, and an outer hypoechoic ring representing the muscularis externa. There is a lack of peristalsis and compressibility of the inflamed appendix. Gradual pressure with the transducer is placed over the point of tenderness in an effort to displace the bowel to image the area of inflammation (see Table 19-1).

PARAUMBILICAL HERNIA

Another cause of abdominal pain and intestinal obstruction is the presence of an abdominal wall hernia. The hernia may be classified into one of three types: (1) **reducible hernia** is one in which the visceral contents can be returned to the normal intraabdominal location; (2) **incarcerated hernia** means the visceral contents cannot be reduced; and (3) **strangulated hernia** is an incarcerated hernia with vascular compromise.

A hernia forms when the abdominal wall muscles are weakened, which allows the viscera to protrude into the weakened abdominal wall. The weakest area of the abdomen is the site of the umbilicus, and this paraumbilical hernia occurs more often in females, whereas the inguinal hernia is more common in males (Figure 19-23, *A*).

Common causes of herniation include congenital defect or weakening of the abdominal wall, increased abdominal pressure secondary to ascites, abdominal mass, bowel obstruction, obesity, and repeated pregnancy. Strangulation of the colon and omentum is a complication of the hernia. Another complication of a hernia is rupture of the abdominal wall in severe chronic ascites.

Sonographic Findings. The real-time visualization of the bowel within the hernia provides critical information for the clinician. Sonography allows visualization of the peristaltic movement of the bowel during Valsalva maneuvers and determines the presence or absence of vascular flow within the defect. The sonographic criteria for a paraumbilical hernia include (1) demonstration of an anterior wall defect, (2) presence of bowel loops within the sac, (3) exaggeration of the sac during the Valsalva maneuver, and (4) reducibility of the sac with gentle pressure (Figure 19-23, *B*). Most paraumbilical hernias contain colon, omentum, and fat. The large intestine will display a complex pattern of fluid, gas, and peristalsis. Of course, the mesenteric fat is very echogenic. The high-frequency linear array transducer allows the sonographer to demonstrate a wide area of the abdominal wall. Reduced gain is necessary to demonstrate the layers of the abdominal wall and will be useful to see the distinction between the hernia, bowel, and muscular layers of tissue. Color flow will be required to determine the vascular flow within the hernia sac. The patient should be instructed to perform a Valsalva maneuver to determine the site of the wall defect and confirm the presence of the protruding hernia. It is important to visualize the peristalsis of the bowel loops within the hernia to confirm the diagnosis (see Table 19-1).

ACUTE PELVIC PAIN

The evaluation of the patient in acute pelvic pain can be challenging for the sonographer in the middle of the night. These patients usually appear in the ED when the pain is so intense that they cannot bear it any longer. The sonographer must

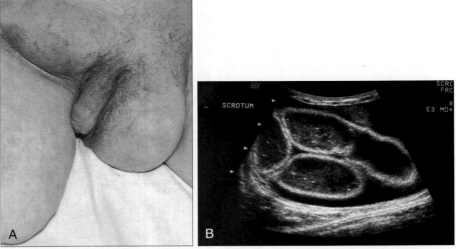

FIGURE 19-23 A, Right inguinal hernia that causes a bulging enlargement of the inguinal canal. **B,** Ultrasound evaluation in real-time shows the peristalsis of the multiple bowel loops in the swollen scrotal sac.

rule out acute pathology such as tubo-ovarian abscess, ruptured ovarian cyst, or ectopic pregnancy. Ovarian torsion is likewise an emergent situation for the patient with severe pelvic pain.

Sonography of Pelvic Structures

Sonography of the pelvic structures should include evaluation in at least two planes of the uterus, cul-de-sac, ovaries, fallopian tubes, and adnexal area. Transabdominal imaging with a full bladder will provide an overview of the entire pelvic area, whereas transvaginal imaging requires the bladder to be empty and allows exquisite detail of the uterus, ovaries, and fallopian tubes.

Uterus. On sonography the uterus should appear as a homogeneous structure with an echogenic line in the center representing the endometrial canal (Figure 19-24). The long axis plane should demonstrate the uterus from fundus to cervix with the endometrial cavity well demonstrated. The

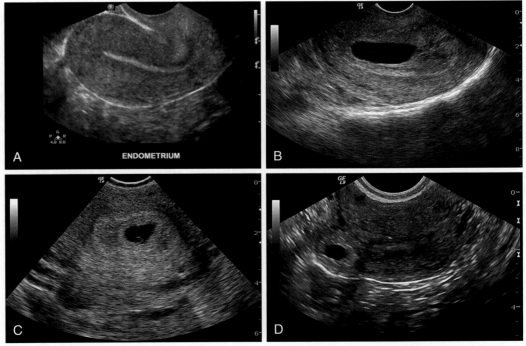

FIGURE 19-24 A, Transvaginal image of the normal uterus with the endometrial stripe. **B,** Blighted ovum shows dilation of the endometrium without products of conception. **C,** Tiny yolk sac is seen within the endometrial cavity in this very early pregnancy. **D,** The uterine cavity is normal; however, the gestational sac is lying outside the uterine cavity in the adnexal cavity.

entire uterus should be evaluated to look for inhomogeneity in texture that may represent degenerating fibroids or an interstitial pregnancy. Fibroids may cause significant pain and bleeding. A pregnancy that is within 5 to 7 mm from the edge of the myometrium is at risk for becoming an interstitial ectopic pregnancy. The presence of a normal gestational sac implanted high in the uterine cavity is the sign of an intrauterine pregnancy. Viability may be assessed with transvaginal ultrasound with demonstration of the fetal heart rate.

Cul-de-Sac. This area may normally contain a small amount of fluid in the healthy female that is dependent on her point in the menstrual cycle. However, large amounts of fluid are abnormal. An ectopic pregnancy that has ruptured may lead to increased amounts of fluid in the cul-de-sac. A pelvic inflammatory disease may also expand with pus into the cul-de-sac. Ascites or other free fluid secondary to trauma will accumulate in this dependent area of the pelvis.

Ovaries. The ovaries are best imaged with transvaginal sonography. Careful evaluation of the texture of the ovary should separate an enlarged ovarian cyst, ectopic pregnancy, or other ovarian masses that may lead to pelvic pain. Torsion of the ovary shows an enlarged edematous area with severe reduction of flow on color Doppler.

Fallopian Tubes. Again, the fallopian tubes are best imaged with transvaginal ultrasound, as they originate from the cornua of the uterus. The presence of enlarged anechoic to slightly heterogeneous tubes may signify hydrosalpinx or the presence of a tubo-ovarian abscess.

SCROTAL TRAUMA AND TORSION

Scrotal trauma presents a challenge to the sonographer because the scrotum is often painful and swollen. The trauma may be the result of a motor vehicle accident, athletic injury, direct blow to the scrotum, or a straddle injury. The most important goal of the sonographic examination is to determine whether a rupture has occurred. Rupture of the testis is a surgical emergency requiring a prompt diagnosis. If surgery is performed within 72 hours following injury, at least 90% of testes can be saved; this number decreases to 45% after 72 hours. Hydrocele and hematocele are both complications of trauma. Hematoceles contain blood and are also found in advanced cases of epididymitis or orchitis (Figure 19-25).

On sonography, findings associated with scrotal rupture include a focal alteration of the testicular parenchymal pattern, interruption of the tunica albuginea, irregular testicular contour, scrotal wall thickening, and hematocele. These findings may also be associated with abscess, tumor, or other clinical conditions, but when combined with a history of trauma, they suggest rupture.

Torsion of the spermatic cord occurs as a result of abnormal mobility of the testis within the scrotum. Torsion is a surgical emergency, and it is important to obtain diagnostic images as soon as possible. The abnormality is seen more frequently in the adolescent and young adult. The patient presents with a sudden onset of pain and swelling on the

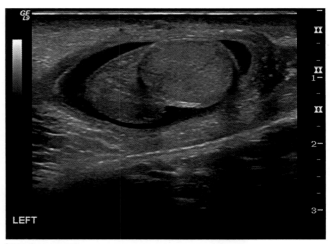

FIGURE 19-25 Acute scrotal pain with hydrocele and epididymitis.

affected side. On sonography, the early stages of torsion may show the testis to have a normal homogeneous pattern. After 4 to 6 hours, the testis becomes swollen and hypoechoic. The lobes within the testis are well identified during this time secondary to interstitial and septal edema. After 24 hours, the testis becomes heterogeneous as a result of hemorrhage, infarction, necrosis, and vascular congestion. The epididymal head appears enlarged and may have decreased echogenicity or become heterogeneous. Color Doppler is useful to differentiate torsion from epididymo-orchitis. An absence of perfusion in the symptomatic testis with normal perfusion demonstrated in the asymptomatic side is considered to be diagnostic of torsion.

EXTREMITY SWELLING AND PAIN

The evaluation of deep venous thrombosis in the patient with swelling of the proximal lower extremities may be made in the ED. There are essentially two types of evaluation: one is a superficial "compression" of the venous structures to see if there is an obstruction in the venous system, and the other is the thorough examination of the entire lower venous structures with gray scale, color, and spectral Doppler evaluation. The thrombosis may be acute, chronic, distal, or superficial in the venous system. Other causes of extremity pain and swelling include Baker's cyst (posterior swelling of the knee with extension into the lower calf), cellulitis, abscess, muscle hematoma, and fasciitis (Figure 19-26). Often the patient with extremity swelling presents with a swollen, tender extremity that is painful to the touch. Care must be taken to adequately evaluate the leg with gentle compression. The use of color and spectral Doppler allows the sonographer to determine the arterial from venous flow patterns to avoid the false-negative or false-positive result (Figure 19-27). In the obese patient, the large superficial veins may be mistaken for the deep veins and may prevent adequate compression of the venous structures. The unclotted thrombus may be isoechoic to slightly hypoechoic and thus not well seen in the lower-level equipment.

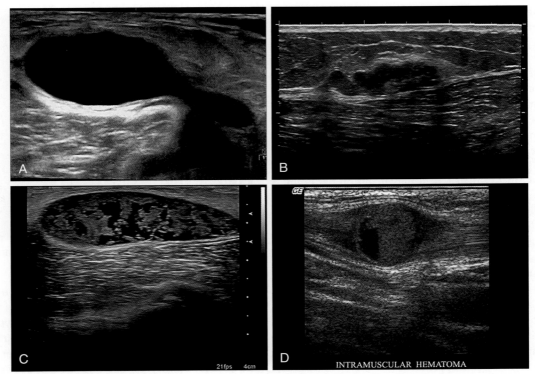

FIGURE 19-26 A, Baker's cyst. **B,** Musculo-fasciitis. **C,** Large Baker's cyst with complex fluid. **D,** Intramuscular hematoma.

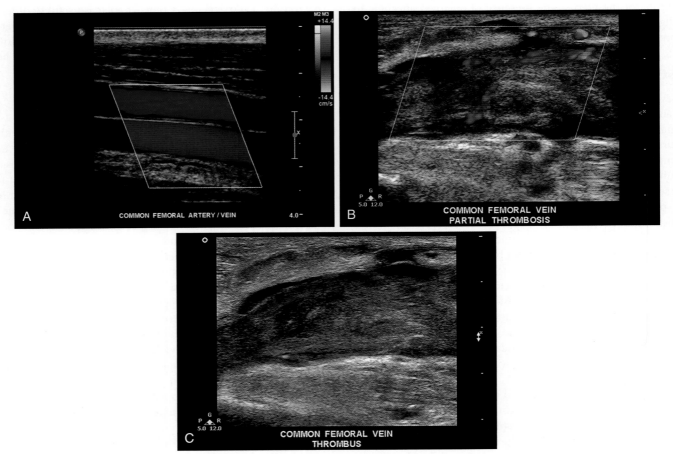

FIGURE 19-27 A, Sagittal color image of the normal femoral artery and vein. **B** and **C,** Large thrombosis of the common femoral vein.

The proximal deep veins of the lower extremity are those in which thrombus poses a significant risk of pulmonary embolization. These veins include the common femoral, superficial femoral, and popliteal veins. (Note that the superficial femoral vein is part of the deep system, not the superficial system.) The deep femoral vein is not considered to be a source of embolizing thrombi and is not included in the evaluation for deep venous thrombosis.

The sonographic evaluation is performed with a high-frequency linear array transducer using both real-time imaging and compression of the venous structures. The compression should be made with the vein directly under the transducer while watching for complete apposition of the anterior and posterior walls. If thrombus is present, complete compression will not be possible.

Other structures may be inflamed next to the venous structures as in cases of lymphadenopathy. The enlarged lymph nodes are hypoechoic with a small echogenic center and will not compress; these may be mistaken for thrombus within the venous structures.

The inferior vena cava and iliac veins should also be assessed for a possible source of emboli or thrombi, causing lower extremity pain and swelling.

 Key Pearls

- Diagnostic peritoneal lavage is used to sample the intraperitoneal space for evidence of damage to the viscera and blood vessels in patients with blunt abdominal trauma to decide which patients need exploratory laparotomy.
- Focused assessment with sonography for trauma (FAST) has become an extension of the physical examination of the trauma patient.
- The FAST examination is a focused survey examination of the abdomen, pelvis, and pericardium to evaluate free fluid or pericardial fluid.
- The FAST evaluation survey is widespread, extending from the pericardial sac to the urinary bladder, and includes the perihepatic area (including Morison's pouch), perisplenic region (including splenorenal recess), paracolic gutters, and cul-de-sac.
- Liver lacerations or contusions are more easily detected with ultrasound than any other visceral abdominal injury.
- Pitfalls of abdominal ultrasound include failure to show contained solid-organ injuries; injuries to the diaphragm, pancreas, and adrenal gland; and some bowel injuries.
- One of the most frequent complaints in the ED is the onset of severe right upper quadrant pain.
- Midepigastric pain that radiates to the back is characteristic of acute pancreatitis.
- The patient who presents with classic abdominal pain radiating to the back, with hypotension and a pulsatile abdominal mass, is not a diagnostic dilemma in the ED.

- Most aneurysms occur at the level of the umbilicus, at the junction of the bifurcation into the iliac vessels. Aneurysms may expand in the transverse diameter and in the anteroposterior diameter.
- The primary application of cardiac ultrasound in an emergent situation is to rule out the presence of pericardial effusion or to evaluate cardiac function in patients with sudden cardiac arrest.
- A dissecting aortic aneurysm is a condition in which a propagating intramural hematoma actually dissects along the length of the vessel, stripping away the intima and, in some cases, part of the media.
- Most aortic dissections will occur at one of three sites: (1) at the root of the aorta with possible extension into the arch, descending aorta, and abdominal aorta; (2) at the level of the left subclavian artery, with extension into the descending aorta or abdominal aorta; and (3) only at the level of the ascending aorta.
- The typical presentation for an aortic dissection is that of a sudden onset of severe, tearing chest pain radiating to the arms, neck, or back.
- Flank pain caused by urolithiasis is a common problem in patients coming to the ED.
- Acute appendicitis is one of the most common diseases that necessitates emergency surgery and is the most common atraumatic surgical abdominal disorder in children 2 years of age and older.
- Appendicitis is the result of luminal obstruction and inflammation, leading to ischemia of the vermiform appendix.
- Another cause of abdominal pain and intestinal obstruction is the presence of an abdominal wall hernia.
- Acute pelvic pain may indicate acute pathology such as tubo-ovarian abscess, ruptured ovarian cyst, ectopic pregnancy, or ovarian torsion.
- Scrotal trauma may lead to formation of a hydrocele or hematocele.
- Torsion of the spermatic cord occurs as a result of abnormal mobility of the testis within the scrotum. Torsion is a surgical emergency, and it is important to obtain diagnostic images as soon as possible.
- Thrombosis may be acute, chronic, distal, or superficial in the venous system. Other causes of extremity pain and swelling include Baker's cyst (posterior swelling of the knee with extension into the lower calf), cellulitis, abscess, muscle hematoma, and fasciitis.

BIBLIOGRAPHY

American College of Emergency Physicians: *Policy statement: emergency ultrasound imaging criteria compendium*, October 2014, pp. 1-55.
American Society of Echocardiography: *Focused cardiac ultrasound in the emergent setting: consensus statement of the American Society of Echocardiography* (website): http://www.asecho.org/wordpress/wp-content/uploads/2013/05/Focused-Cardiac-US-in-the-Emergent-Setting.pdf.

Bahner D, Blaivas M, Cohen HL, et al: AIUM practice guideline for the performance of the focused assessment with sonography for trauma (FAST) examination, *J Ultrasound Med* 27(2):313-318, 2008.

Branney SW, Moore EE, Cantrill SV, et al: Ultrasound based key clinical pathway reduces the use of hospital resources for the evaluation of blunt abdominal trauma, *J Trauma* 42(6):1086-1090, 1997.

Center for Devices and Radiological Health: *Initiative to reduce unnecessary radiation exposure from medical imaging,* Rockville, Md, 2010, Center for Devices and Radiological Health.

Cha JY, Kashuk JL, Sarin EL, et al: Diagnostic peritoneal lavage remains a valuable adjunct to modern imaging techniques, *J Trauma* 67(2):330-334, discussion 334-336, 2009.

Durston W, Carl ML, Guerra W, et al: Comparison of quality and cost-effectiveness in the evaluation of symptomatic cholelithiasis with different approaches to ultrasound availability in the ED, *Am J Emerg Med* 19(4):260-269, 2001.

Gonzalez RP, Ickler J, Gaschassin P: Complementary roles of diagnostic peritoneal lavage and computed tomography in the evaluation of blunt abdominal trauma, *J Trauma* 51:1128-1136, 2001.

Griffin XL, Pullinger R: Are diagnostic peritoneal lavage or focused abdominal sonography for trauma safe screening investigations for hemodynamically stable patients after blunt abdominal trauma? A review of the literature, *J Trauma* 62(3):779-784, 2007.

Heller M, Melanson S, Patterson J, Raftis J: Impact of emergency medicine resident training in ultrasonography on ultrasound utilization, *Am J Emerg Med* 17(1):21-22, 1999.

Hussain ZJ, Figueroa R, Budorick NE: How much free fluid can a pregnant patient have? Assessment of pelvic free fluid in pregnancy patients without antecedent trauma, *J Trauma* 70(6):1420-1423, 2011.

Jehle D, Davis E, Evans T, et al: Emergency department sonography by emergency physicians, *Am J Emerg Med* 8(5):469-470, 1990.

Korner M, Krotz MM, Degenhart C, et al: Current role of emergency US in patients with major trauma, *Radiographics* 28(1):225-242, 2008.

Labovitz AJ, Noble VE, Bierig M, et al: *Focused cardiac ultrasound in the emergent setting. A consensus statement of the American Society of Echocardiography and the American College of Emergency Physicians* (website): http://www.asecho.org/wordpress/wp-content/uploads/2013/05/Focused-Cardiac-US-in-the-Emergent-Setting.pdf.

Ma OJ, Gaddis G, Steele MT, et al: Prospective analysis of the effect of physician experience with the FAST examination in reducing the use of CT scans, *Emerg Med Australasia* 17(1):24-30, 2005.

Marx J, Isenhour J: Abdominal trauma. In Marx JA, Hockberger RS, Walls RM, et al, editors: *Rosen's emergency medicine: concepts and clinical practice,* ed 5, St. Louis, 2006, Mosby.

Moore CL, Molina AA, Lin H: Ultrasonography in community emergency departments in the United States: access to ultrasonography performed by consultants and status of emergency physician-performed ultrasonography, *Ann Emerg Med* 47(2):147-153, 2006.

Sheng AY, Dalziel P, Liteplo AS, et al: Focused assessment with sonography in trauma and abdominal computed tomography utilization in adult trauma patients: trends over the last decade, *Emerg Med Int* 2013:678380, 2013.

Sonographic Techniques in the Transplant Patient

Talisha Hunt

OBJECTIVES

On completion of this chapter, you should be able to:
- Understand the complexity of and criteria for receiving a transplant
- Gain knowledge of surgical techniques of liver, renal, and pancreatic transplants
- Identify the necessary imaging protocol needed for imaging the transplanted organ
- Recognize and define normal sonographic features of the transplant patient
- Recognize and define common and complex pathologies
- Know the importance of imaging in the immediate postoperative patient
- Identify and describe immediate complications after transplantation, and those that occur within the months and years to follow
- Understand how you can help donate life

OUTLINE

KEY TERMS

Model for End-Stage Liver Disease (MELD)
Organ Procurement and Transplantation Network (OPTN)

Pediatric End-Stage Liver Disease (PELD)
Posttransplant lymphoproliferative disorder (PTLD)
Renal autotransplantation

Simultaneous pancreas-kidney transplant (SPK)
United Network for Organ Sharing (UNOS)

WHO NEEDS A TRANSPLANT?

According to the **Organ Procurement and Transplantation Network (OPTN)**, there are 123,366 people who are in need of a transplant. Of these, 79,199 are actively waiting, and every 10 minutes, a new candidate is added to the national transplant waiting list. The average wait time is 5 to 7 years. With this severe shortage of donor organs, 21 people die each day on average while waiting for their transplant. In 2013, 28,954 patients received a transplant, which was an annual record, with 80% of these transplants coming from deceased donors. The majority of transplant recipients were age 50 and older during the past 10 years, with the most common age range between 50 and 64.

To ensure a successful transplant, each patient needs to receive the best of care from the entire transplant team. The team consists of clinical transplant coordinators, transplant physicians and surgeons, financial coordinators, and social workers. The **United Network for Organ Sharing (UNOS)** celebrated 30 years in 2014. UNOS maintains a centralized computer networking system for all organ procurement organizations and transplant centers while seeking to be fair and effective in selecting transplant candidates. The UNOS database can be accessed 24 hours a day. Once a patient is referred to a transplant center, the patient will have a series of tests, and his or her mental and physical health will be evaluated by a physician. The social support available to the patient is also a consideration. If the center accepts the candidate, the medical information will be entered into the national organ transplantation waiting list. Once a deceased donor is located, a transplant coordinator from an organ procurement organization will access the UNOS database. Each patient on the waiting list is matched with the donor characteristics using the computer. The computer will then display the ranked list of the candidates according to the OPTN organ allocation process. Factors in receiving a transplant include tissue match, blood type, immune status, length of time on the waiting list, and the distance between the donor and recipient. The organ is offered to the transplant team and candidate that are on top of the list. The person at the top does not always receive the organ because he or she may be too unhealthy or laboratory results indicate an incompatible match and rejection would likely occur. Once the patient is selected, he or she would be contacted for the transplant surgery to be scheduled and performed.

History and Criteria for Liver Transplantation

Patients who have severe liver disease require a liver transplant for survival. Acute liver failure is sudden and most commonly caused from a drug-induced injury such as an acetaminophen overdose. Chronic liver failure or end-stage liver disease is progressive over a period of months and years. Scar tissue is formed within the liver and normal functioning liver tissue is reduced, creating cirrhosis. The most common reason for transplantation in the United States is cirrhosis due to chronic hepatitis C, followed by alcohol abuse (Figure 20-1). Many other liver diseases can also cause the liver to fail resulting in the need for transplantation, including the following:

- Chronic hepatitis B and autoimmune hepatitis
- Nonalcoholic steatohepatitis, caused by fat and inflammation of the liver
- Hemochromatosis, due to iron overload within the liver
- Wilson disease, due to copper overload within the liver
- Budd-Chiari syndrome, caused by occlusion of the hepatic veins draining the liver
- Biliary diseases, including the following:
  - Biliary atresia, absent or blocked bile ducts and occurs only in infants
  - Alagille syndrome, blocked or malformed bile ducts and ductal paucity
  - Primary biliary cirrhosis, destruction of intrahepatic ducts
  - Primary sclerosing cholangitis (PSC), destruction of intrahepatic and extrahepatic ducts
- Cancer originating in the liver such as hepatocellular carcinoma (HCC), hepatoblastoma, and cholangiocarcinoma

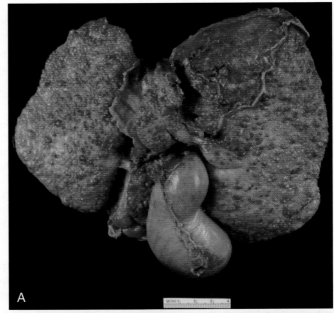

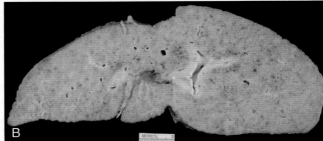

FIGURE 20-1 Pathology liver specimen of cirrhosis due to alcoholic liver disease. **A,** Surface nodularity is present. **B,** Cross-sectional slice.

Symptoms of liver disease include jaundice, fatigue, weight loss, itching, abdominal ascites, bleeding in the stomach from varices, confusion, black stools, nausea, and loss of appetite. A patient may not be a liver transplant candidate if he or she presents with severe irreversible illness, widespread cancer, human immunodeficiency virus/acquired immunodeficiency syndrome (HIV/AIDS), severe pulmonary hypertension, active infection, alcohol or drug abuse, or history of noncompliance.

Patients who are placed on the transplant waiting list receive a score that determines how urgently they need a new liver. Dr. Patrick Kamath originally developed the Mayo End-Stage Liver Disease Score at Mayo Clinic in 2001. With modification from UNOS, the **Model for End-stage Liver Disease (MELD)** scale for adults and **Pediatric End-stage Liver Disease (PELD)** for children under 12 years of age are still actively used today. MELD was initially used to predict death within 3 months in patients who had a transjugular intrahepatic portosystemic shunt (TIPS) performed. This scale was also found to be beneficial in predicting prognosis and prioritizing liver transplant recipients. MELD scores range from 6 to 40 and PELD scores range from negative values to 99. The scores identify the likelihood of death within 3 months without receiving a transplant. The higher the score denotes an increased need for a transplant. For example, a patient with a MELD score of 22 would have a 10% mortality risk at 3 months, whereas a patient with a score of 38 would have an 80% mortality risk. The MELD score is a mathematical calculation based on laboratory values of bilirubin (measurement of bile pigment), creatinine (kidney function), and international nationalized ratio (INR) (blood clotting ability).

$$MELD = [0.957 \times \log(creatinine) + 0.378 \times \log(bilirubin) + 1.12 \times \log(INR) + 0.643] \times 10$$

In 2002 there was an immediate decrease by 12% of the time spent on the waiting list, which also led to a reduction of almost 15% mortality. The mean waiting time in the MELD era went from 656 to 416 days. The reduction in mortality went from 2046 deaths in 2001 to 1364 by 2005.[1] The average wait time in the United States based on the MELD scores is 21 months for a MELD of 11 to 18, 4 months for a MELD of 19 to 24, and 20 days for a MELD greater than 25.[2]

The Milan criteria also play a role in liver transplantation. If a cirrhotic patient has HCC, the patient may be considered for a transplant if he or she has one HCC smaller than 5 cm, or up to three lesions smaller than 3 cm without vascular invasion or extrahepatic involvement. HCC is the most common primary malignant tumor in the liver and is the fifth most common cancer. There is a 10% to 50% chance of recurrence at 2 years and 70% at 5 years with liver resection. Transplantation and radiofrequency ablation (RFA) are potentially curative options.[3]

Dr. Thomas Starzl performed the first liver transplant on March 1, 1963. The 3-year-old patient with biliary atresia died due to uncontrolled bleeding. The first five transplant recipients died within 23 days. In 1967 the first successful liver transplant performed by Dr. Starzl in Denver, Colorado, survived 1 year. The patient died of recurrent HCC.[2] With the help of Sir Roy Caine, cyclosporine was introduced in 1979, improving survival rates significantly. In 1989 Starzl and colleagues reported that 1179 patients survived between 1 and 5 years after transplantation. Since the first transplant, more than 10,000,000 liver transplants have been performed worldwide with an 80% to 90% survival rate within the first year.[4] There are currently more than 125 transplant programs performing approximately 5000 to 6000 transplants each year.[2] As of June 15, 2012, 16,773 patients were awaiting a deceased liver transplant.[5]

In 2014 the average cost of receiving a liver transplant was $739,100. If a patient received a combined liver and kidney transplant, the cost was $1,190,300. These costs include 30 days pretransplant, procurement, hospital transplant admission, transplant physician, 180 days posttransplant discharge, and immunosuppressants.

History and Criteria for Renal Transplantation

The most common cause for needing a renal transplant is chronic end-stage renal disease or renal failure. Acute renal failure may also occur, requiring transplantation, but this is significantly uncommon. Symptoms of renal failure begin when the kidney only has 10% functioning tissue. Some signs and symptoms are decreased urine output, edema in the legs or feet, shortness of breath, fatigue, confusion, nausea, chest pain, heart arrhythmias, difficulty sleeping, itching, hypertension, loss of appetite, muscle cramps, and seizures or coma in severe cases. Depending on the cause of renal impairment, it may be treatable, yet some may show irreversible damage. Renal function is evaluated using blood laboratory values of blood urea nitrogen, creatinine, and glomerular filtration rate. With progressive loss of kidney function, patients will ultimately require dialysis to filter waste and remove excess fluid from the blood. Dialysis is the only means of survival until a renal transplant becomes available. Patients may not receive a transplant if they have widespread cancer, active infection, HIV/AIDS, liver or heart disease, history of noncompliance, or alcohol or drug abuse. The following are causes that can lead to renal failure and a need for transplantation:

- Hypertension and renal artery stenosis or renal vein thrombosis
- Diabetes mellitus: high blood glucose can damage the filtering system (diabetic nephropathy)
- Urinary tract obstruction such as renal stones or certain cancers
- Inherited kidney disease such as polycystic kidney disease
- Glomerulonephritis: inflammation of small filters, glomeruli
- Interstitial nephritis: inflammation of kidney tubules
- Hemolytic uremic syndrome: premature destruction of red blood cells
- Systemic lupus erythematosus: immune system attacks kidney as foreign object
- Scleroderma: hardening and tightening of the skin and connective tissue

- Vasculitis: inflammation of blood vessels
- Toxins such as alcohol, cocaine, or heavy metals
- Recurrent kidney infection
- Medication therapy used for other diseases
- Severe dehydration

On December 23, 1954, Dr. Joseph Murray performed the first successful kidney transplant at Peter Bent Brigham Hospital in Boston, Massachusetts. The surgery involved identical twins, Richard and Ronald Herrick, eliminating possible rejection.[6] In 1990 Dr. Murray won the Nobel Prize in Physiology of Medicine. Between 1954 and 1973, about 10,000 renal transplants were performed. More than 99,000 people were on the deceased kidney donor list as of June 15, 2012. Due to shortage of kidneys, the system of expanded criteria donors (ECD) was introduced in 2002. This includes the kidneys that once were considered not suitable. ECD kidneys are any donors older than 60 years or ages 50 to 59 years with two of the following conditions: hypertension, serum creatinine greater than 1.5 mg/dl, or cause of death from a cerebrovascular accident.[5]

In 2014 the average cost of receiving a renal transplant was $334,300. If a patient received a combined kidney and liver transplant, the cost was $1,190,300. The cost of a combined kidney and pancreas transplant was $558,600. These costs include 30 days pretransplant, procurement, hospital transplant admission, transplant physician, 180 days posttransplant discharge, and immunosuppressants.

History and Criteria for Pancreatic Transplantation

There are more than 15 million people in the United States who have diabetes mellitus, with 798,000 new patients diagnosed each year.[7] Patients receive a pancreas transplant in hopes to cure type 1 diabetes. In these patients, the pancreatic islet cells cannot produce enough insulin, resulting in dangerously elevated blood glucose. Insulin provides movement of the glucose in the blood into the muscles and fat to provide energy for the body. Initially, patients routinely receive insulin injections or take medications to help control blood glucose. Transplantation may be a consideration if glucose levels are poorly managed, if glucose levels show frequent insulin reactions, or if severe kidney damage occurs. It is common for a patient to receive a combined pancreas and renal transplant to ensure healthy organs are unlikely to be affected by the damage that comes from diabetes. High blood glucose can lead to many complications such as amputations, heart disease, stroke, vascular disease, blindness, nerve damage, or kidney damage.

Type 2 diabetes patients are not a consideration for pancreas transplant. In these patients, insulin is produced from the pancreas but the body develops insulin resistance, and a new pancreas will not be a cure in this case. Transplantation usually is not performed on a patient with cancer, active infection, HIV/AIDS, lung disease, obesity, severe heart disease, or an ongoing history of alcohol or drug abuse.

Dr. William Kelly and Dr. Richard Lillehei performed the first successful pancreas transplant combined with a kidney transplant on December 17, 1966, at the University of Minnesota.[7] The surgery was considered experimental until about 1990. There are about 1200 pancreas transplants performed each year in the United States, with 75% of cases being a **simultaneous pancreas-kidney transplant (SPK).** There have been more than 23,000 pancreas transplants reported to the International Transplant Registry.[8]

In the United States there were 3202 patients that were listed for a pancreas transplant as of February 2014. During the years of 2012 and 2013, there were 16,410 deceased donors with only 2826 pancreas allografts procured. This shortage of organs is due to lack of procurement or the pancreas is deemed unsuitable. The ideal donor is between 10 and 40 years of age with a body mass index (BMI) less than 27.5 kg/m^2, and with a cause of death not from cerebrovascular disease.[9] Recent studies have suggested organs from extended criteria donors can receive similar graft survival as the "ideal" donor. The accumulation of risk factors and extended cold ischemic time should be avoided when possible to ensure a healthy allograft.[10]

In 2014 the average cost of receiving a pancreas transplant was $317,500. The cost of a combined pancreas and kidney transplant was $558,600. These costs include 30 days pretransplant, procurement, hospital transplant admission, transplant physician, 180 days posttransplant discharge, and immunosuppressants.

LIVER TRANSPLANT

Surgical Technique of the Liver Transplant

The liver can be preserved between 12 and 16 hours on ice and using a special preservation solution. The shorter the ischemic time, the better the allograft function once transplanted. For every liver transplant, the donor and recipient are rechecked to verify a match. The blood type and compatibility need to be confirmed and the UNOS database per protocol as well. Before coming into the operating room, the team will discuss the risks, benefits, and alternatives with the patient and obtain consent. All institutions have certain protocols and techniques that they follow. The following will discuss the basic current practices at my institution.

Cadaveric Liver Donation. The patient is brought into the operating room confirming patient identification and procedure to be performed. Following general anesthesia and line placement, a Foley catheter is placed into the bladder. The abdomen is prepped and draped sterilely. Bilateral subcostal skin incisions are made and extended to the midline up to the xiphoid process. The scar resembles a "Mercedes sign." The diseased liver is mobilized, vessels clamped and ligated, and dissected free from the body cavity becoming "anhepatic." This diseased liver is sent for pathologic examination.

The procured liver is prepared on the "back table" for any reconstruction to occur, and submerged into a saline slush solution. Patients present with variant anatomy and that needs to be taken into consideration. Some may have normal anatomic variants such as additional veins or arteries to anastomose or vessels need to be trimmed down to size. Some may have short veins or arteries that are not long enough and require an interposition graft in which a deceased donor iliac artery or vein may be used. The iliac vein can act as a conduit between the recipient superior mesenteric vein and the donor portal vein. The iliac artery can be used as a conduit between the recipient infrarenal aorta and the donor hepatic artery.

Once the donor liver has been prepared, it is placed within the recipient's abdominal cavity and covered with laparotomy pads containing saline slush. Vent tubing is placed in the infrahepatic cava to prepare the suprahepatic cava for anastomosis. The upper caval anastomosis is sewn end-to-side with running sutures. The recipient portal vein is occluded with a clamp and flushed with glycine irrigant, and then an end-to-end portal vein anastomosis is sewn with sutures. The recipient common hepatic artery is flushed with heparinized saline, and occluded with a clamp. The donor and recipient common hepatic arteries are then sewn end-to-end using running sutures to create the arterial anastomosis. The arterial and portal venous clamps are removed and the liver flushed with blood to begin reperfusion. The surgeon examines all the anastomoses to ensure they are dry and do not have a leak and makes sure the patient is hemodynamically stable. At this point, a cholecystectomy is performed on the donor liver. A choledochodochostomy is sewn between donor and recipient common bile ducts using running sutures. The anastomosis is sewn over a polyurethane biliary stent or tube, which is brought out through the cystic duct stump. The catheter is then secured to the stump with a suture. Another option would be an end-to-side choledochojejunostomy using a suture over the jejunal biliary tube. In patients with PSC or retransplantation, a Roux-en-Y limb is created for reconstruction (Figure 20-2). The patient is rechecked for any significant bleeding. Drains are placed within the right and left subhepatic spaces and secured to the skin with stitches. Sponge, needle, and instrument counts are conducted before closure. If indicated, the patient will receive units of blood, platelets, or fresh frozen plasma. The incision is closed in two layers with a running layer suture on the midline and posterior fascia and then anterior fascia is closed. The skin is closed with staples. The wound is dressed with a dry sterile dressing and the patient is transported to the intensive care unit (ICU) when stable.

Living Donor Liver Donation. There is a shortage of organs available for donation. Living donor organ donation offers the alternative for ones waiting for a transplant and also increases the existing organ supply. A friend or family member may consider being a donor for their loved one. If the donor is not a match, there is a paired exchange program. The donor's organ would go to someone else for a better match rather than directly going to their friend or family member. The one needing the transplant will receive their organ in the exchange that meets their match.

The first adult living liver donor donation was performed in 1989, with currently more than 4000 performed in the United States. The 1-, 3-, and 5-year survival rates are 90%, 83%, and 78%, respectively.[2] Ultimately, a donor liver will regenerate to more than 85% of its original volume. Living donor transplantation has many ethical issues and has been a source of some controversy. Donors may experience a psychological syndrome due to the stress of surgery. Gokce

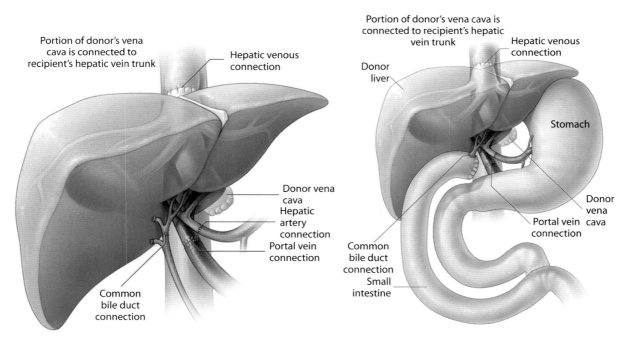

Duct-to-duct procedure (donor anatomy represented in gray)

Roux-en-Y procedure (donor anatomy represented in gray)

A

B

FIGURE 20-2 Illustration demonstrating anastomoses sites of cadaveric liver transplant **A,** Duct-duct procedure. **B,** Roux-en-Y procedure.*(Used with permission of Mayo Foundation for Medical Education and Research. All Rights reserved.)*

and colleagues showed that 21% of donors feel anxious about the complications and quality of life after surgery. The donor complication rate is 40% with incision infection, biliary leak, or stricture being the most common. Some donors develop complications that lead them to suicide or drug overdose.[11] Living donor liver transplants are optimal in urgent situations; however, 27.1% of living donors demonstrated one or more complications in the postoperative period.[12]

The surgical technique is very similar compared with a cadaveric liver. The allograft may demonstrate better function more quickly due to the decreased preservation time in a living donor. The recipient will receive part of a liver rather than a full organ, usually the right hepatic lobe. The patient is brought into the operating room confirming patient identification and procedure to be performed. Following general anesthesia and line placement, a Foley catheter is placed into the bladder. The abdomen is prepped and draped sterilely. Bilateral subcostal skin incisions are made and extended to the midline up to the xiphoid process. The scar resembles a "Mercedes sign." The diseased liver is mobilized, vessels clamped and ligated, and dissected free from the body cavity becoming "anhepatic." This liver is sent off for pathologic examination.

The procured liver is prepared on the back table for any reconstruction to occur, and submerged into a saline slush solution. Patients present with variant anatomy and that needs to be taken into consideration. Some may have additional veins or arteries to anastomose or vessels need to be trimmed down to size, or some may have short vessels and require an interposition graft. Once the donor liver is prepared, it is placed within the recipient's abdominal cavity and covered with laparotomy pads containing saline slush. The recipient's left middle hepatic vein trunk is stapled and the right hepatic vein is occluded using a clamp. The donor right hepatic vein opening is extended inferiorly on the vena cava, and two sutures are placed on the superior and inferior venotomy. The sutures are then placed through the donor right hepatic vein. An end-to-end

anastomosis is performed between the donor and recipient right hepatic vein and vena cava using running sutures. The recipient portal vein is flushed free of clot, and an end-to-end portal vein anastomosis is created using running sutures. Reperfusion of the liver is accomplished by releasing the venous and portal vein clamps. Following reperfusion, the perihepatic area is carefully inspected for hemostasis. If bleeding is noticed, the surgeon will control using additional sutures. The donor right hepatic artery is flushed with heparinized saline and occluded with a clamp. The recipient gastroduodenal artery is ligated and divided. The common hepatic artery is occluded with a clamp and divided in its distal portion. An end-to-end anastomosis is performed between the donor right hepatic artery and the recipient common hepatic artery using running sutures. Once arterial reperfusion is achieved, the perihepatic area is again carefully inspected for hemostasis. An end-to-end duct anastomosis is created. In patients with PSC or retransplantation, a Roux-en-Y limb is created for reconstruction. An end-to-side hepaticojejunostomy is performed using a running suture on the posterior layer and an interrupted suture on the anterior layer (Figure 20-3). Hemostasis is again ensured. Two drains are placed posterior to the liver and inferior to the incision. Sponge, needle, and instrument counts are conducted before closure. If indicated, the patient will receive units of blood, platelets, or fresh frozen plasma. The incision is closed with a running suture in the anterior and posterior layers and in the midline. Staples are used for skin closure. The wound is dressed with a dry sterile dressing and the patient is transported to the ICU when stable.

Evaluation of the Liver Allograft

As a sonographer, evaluate the liver transplant as a native liver. Assess the size, echotexture, contour, biliary tree, and vasculature, and look for any masses, fluid collections, or ascites. Institutions instill their own routine protocols on timing of examinations and specific images that are required.

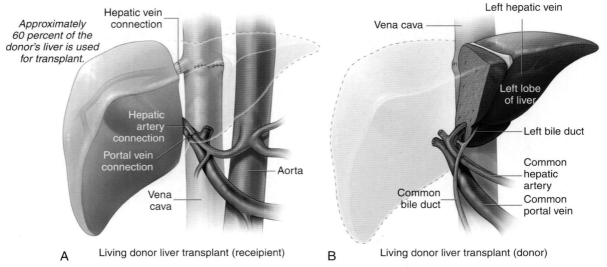

FIGURE 20-3 Illustration demonstrating anastomoses sites of living donor liver transplant. **A,** Liver transplant (recipient). **B,** Native liver (donor). *(Used with permission of Mayo Foundation for Medical Education and Research. All Rights reserved.)*

The following is the basis of what my institution practices. Once the patient has arrived to the ICU from the surgical suite, the sonographer will go portably to perform the "day 0" examination. Typically the patient will receive an ultrasound examination on postoperative day 1 and day 7 as well. The patient's liver function is closely monitored and if any issues arise, the transplant physicians will tailor their imaging requests. The patient usually has a follow-up ultrasound every 6 months to 1 year if there are no complications.

It is best to image using a 2.5- to 5.0-MHz curvilinear transducer and have the patient fasting 4 to 6 hours. Obese patients and livers with fatty infiltration will likely require lower frequencies. It is helpful to ask the patient to take a breath in and hold it if they are able to do so. This will give better visualization of the liver and reduce respiratory motion. Rolling the patient left lateral decubitus will also help aid visualizing the right lobe more clearly.

The sonographer should scan completely through the liver before taking any images using subcostal and intercostal approaches while adjusting the frequency, depth, gain, time-gain compensation (TGC), and focal zones as they go. Once the liver is fully accessed, the examination needs to include grayscale longitudinal and transverse images of the left and right hepatic lobes including the caudate lobe and vascular landmarks of the inferior vena cava (IVC), hepatic veins (HVs), and portal veins (PVs). The right lobe of the liver should be compared with the right kidney to evaluate the echogenicity. Document any pathology in two planes with and without measurements and include color Doppler flow. Knowing the type of transplant the patient received (i.e., living or cadaveric) is helpful before scanning because in living donor transplanted patients only the right lobe will be present. The donor liver receives a cholecystectomy during the surgical process and, as a result, no gallbladder images will be acquired. The biliary tree needs to be evaluated for intrahepatic and extrahepatic ductal dilation, wall thickening, biliary leaks, and stones or sludge. It is common for biliary stents to be present. Quadrant images need to be obtained checking for free fluid or signs of bleeding.

The Doppler portion is crucial for the transplanted liver. Venous and arterial color and spectral Doppler needs to be obtained looking for any signs of thrombus or stenosis. Ultrasound is commonly the first method of imaging in these patients, and the sonographer can help the physicians diagnose the patient and treatment will be administered quickly. The hepatic arteries (HAs) are not routinely included in the native liver examination, but they are very important to image in your transplanted patient. It is critical to angle correct in the left, right, and main HAs with pulsed-wave Doppler to accurately assess for stenosis. The sonographer will need to measure the peak systolic and end diastolic velocities to obtain the resistive index (RI) measurement. This is a common indirect Doppler technique to evaluate the HA. A low RI can be a strong indicator of a proximal stenosis the sonographer may not be able to otherwise identify or a presence of an arteriovenous fistula (AVF). A high RI may indicate rejection or hepatic venous congestion. These vessels are small in size, and the sonographer may choose to use the zoom feature on the ultrasound machine for better visualization. Although

sometimes it may be difficult to identify the anastomosis, attempt to evaluate the HA as proximally as possible. If a stenosis is present, the anastomotic site is the most common location. Color flow aliasing in the PVs, HVs, or IVC, should be further evaluated with spectral Doppler to help identify a narrowing. For all spectral Doppler, the angle should be parallel with the vessel that is being sampled and less than 60 degrees to avoid falsely elevated velocities. To increase diagnostic accuracy, all of the spectral waveforms should fill the spectral window while eliminating spectral aliasing.

When very slow flow is present in a vessel, a Doppler signal can be difficult to obtain and either the Doppler scale will need to be decreased or the color gain will need to be increased. Some ultrasound machines may have special settings to detect slow flow. These can often be found in other settings besides the abdominal settings such as those for detecting low flow in a lower extremity vein or the iliac vein. If these are not available, the renal artery setting can be helpful filling in the vessels as well. Sometimes the wall filter needs to be decreased if the very slow frequencies are rejected as "cluttered noise" (Figure 20-4).

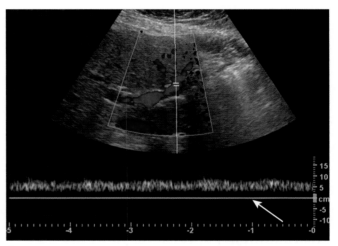

A

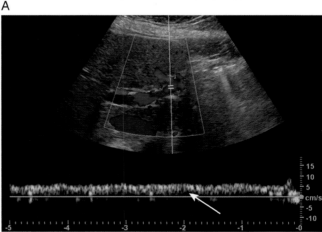

B

FIGURE 20-4 Wall filter settings. A, High wall filter is used and more noise is filtered on the spectral Doppler ultrasound. **B,** Low wall filter is used and can pick up more noise on the spectral Doppler ultrasound.

For obese patients, decreasing the gray-scale, color, and spectral Doppler frequencies will enable deeper penetration.

Normal Sonographic Findings of the Liver Transplant

On gray-scale imaging, the liver parenchyma should appear smooth and homogeneous being isoechoic relative to the right renal cortex. All vessels and biliary ducts should be anechoic. The HVs and IVC lack a distinct wall whereas the PVs, HAs, and ducts demonstrate echogenic walls running parallel from the liver hilum and branching within the liver. A normal common hepatic duct (CHD) ranges in diameter from 3 to 7 mm, and the common bile duct (CBD) can range from 5 to 9 mm. See Chapter 9 for a more detailed explanation of normal liver anatomy.

The Doppler portion of the transplanted liver examination is crucial to perform. Some vascular complications can only be diagnosed using color and spectral Doppler. The HA will be red on color imaging and the spectral waveform demonstrates a rapid systolic upstroke with continuous diastolic flow above baseline demonstrating a low-resistance waveform. The velocities should be below 200 cm/sec. A normal RI in the HA is in the range of 0.50 to 0.70. The PV flow should be toward the liver showing flow above the baseline with a red color. The spectral waveform of the PV has continuous flow with minimal respiratory changes. The IVC and HVs should be primarily blue in color with a phasic bidirectional spectral Doppler waveform representing changes in the cardiac cycle. The LHV can appear more pulsatile because you are in closer proximity to the heart (Figure 20-5). When measuring velocities using spectral Doppler imaging, turbulence or any velocity doubling or tripling in the vessel from one location to the next should not be seen.

Liver Allograft Imaging in the Immediate Postoperative Period

It is imperative to image the newly transplanted liver in the immediate postoperative period. Ultrasound is the initial modality of choice. There is no ionizing radiation and the cost is relatively inexpensive compared with computed tomography (CT) or magnetic resonance imaging (MRI). A skilled sonographer provides early detection of transplant complications and prevents misdiagnosis.

On the "day 0" ultrasound examination, the patient will be in the ICU and intubated. As a result, these patients will not be able to roll onto their side or help assist with their breathing. It is very helpful to image the patient without bandages on, if possible. This helps attain the best imaging windows possible and prevents missing pathology. Although this is not a sterile scanning environment, using sterile gel while the patient's incisions are healing can potentially reduce the risk of infection. It is common and helpful to have a member of the transplant team or surgeon present for this examination. They want to ensure that the allograft has adequate arterial and venous flow and look for signs of hemorrhage. If there is

an urgent complication noted, the surgeon can transfer the patient back to the operating room to correct the issue immediately. Not all complications are considered urgent, and a follow-up ultrasound will often be recommended within 24 hours to ensure stability or determine whether the issue has resolved or is getting worse. Urgent findings include, but are not limited to, HA thrombosis, PV, HV or IVC thrombus or occlusion, or active bleeding. It is very common to see postoperative fluid collections and these usually resolve on their own. Fluid collections will be monitored on serial ultrasound examinations making sure they are not enlarging and causing liver function problems. Another common finding involves the vasculature. Postoperative edema can create elevated blood flow velocities within the HAs or venous system. In this situation, the HAs can have an elevated RI and may demonstrate little or no diastolic flow. It may be common to see reversal of flow within the LPV due to the high flow volume state. Once the edema decreases, the vessels should return to their normal state (Figure 20-6). Once the ultrasound examination has been completed, the incision should be redressed to help prevent infection. If no complications arise during recovery in the transplant unit, the liver transplant patient is typically discharged from the hospital around postoperative day 5.

Liver Transplantation Complications in Routine Surveillance

Once patients receive their liver transplant, they are closely monitored with routine follow-up examinations and procedures. Blood levels to monitor hepatic function and coagulation studies are checked frequently: daily for 1 week, then 3 times a week, then 2 times a week, then once weekly for 4 months, then monthly. Ultrasound examinations are routinely performed on days 0, 1, and 7. If the transplant team is concerned with complications, the patient will often have more frequent follow-up ultrasounds. Long term, the liver transplant patient typically is followed with a yearly ultrasound.

It is common to perform a routine parenchymal biopsy around day 7 after transplantation, and some patients may require a biopsy yearly to ensure no disease recurrence and rule out rejection. If the patient is symptomatic with pain, fever, or elevated liver function tests (LFTs), a biopsy may be ordered if the ultrasound does not help provide a diagnosis (Figure 20-7).

Complications may arise while performing these biopsies. The most common complication is bleeding. The patient's INR and platelet counts are checked before the procedure. To reduce the risk of bleeding, patients are asked to stop taking anticoagulants 3 to 5 days before the procedure. Another risk of bleeding is elevated blood pressure or hypertension. Some patients may have known hypertension and be placed on an antihypertensive medication, and this should be taken as usual. Anxiety can significantly worsen hypertension as well in the acute setting. Blood pressures should not exceed 160/90 mm Hg. The radiologist or physician performing the biopsy may administer mild to moderate sedation to help calm the patient, reducing these pressures. Even after preventive measures, bleeding may still occur. Following the biopsy,

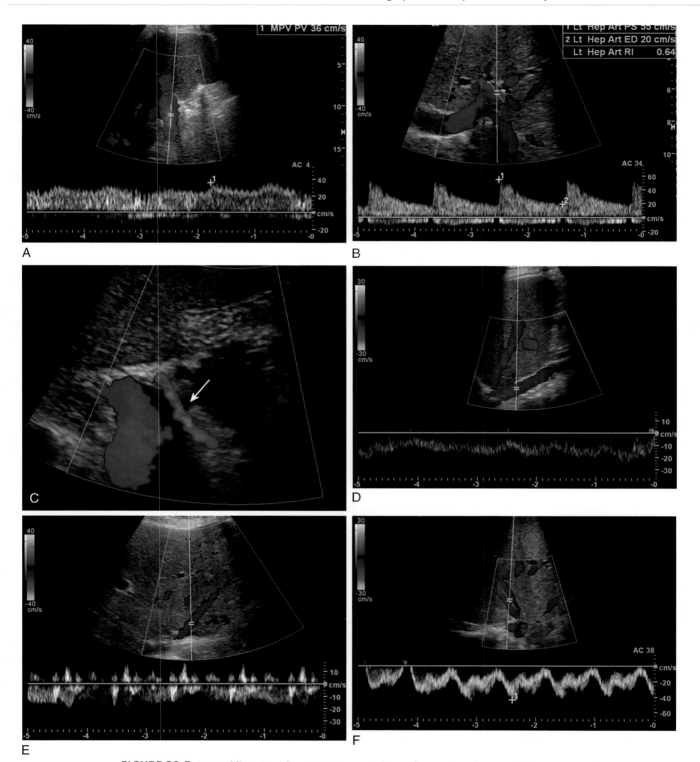

FIGURE 20-5 **Normal liver Doppler.** **A,** MPV spectral waveform using ultrasound shows a normal velocity with continuous hepatopetal flow. **B,** LHA spectral waveform using ultrasound shows a normal velocity and RI with a sharp systolic upstroke and continuous diastolic flow. **C,** MHA color Doppler ultrasound shows no signs of aliasing or narrowing and is widely patent. **D,** IVC spectral waveform using ultrasound shows phasic flow. **E,** LHV spectral waveform using ultrasound appears more pulsatile in relation to the heart. **F,** RHV spectral waveform using ultrasound shows phasic flow.

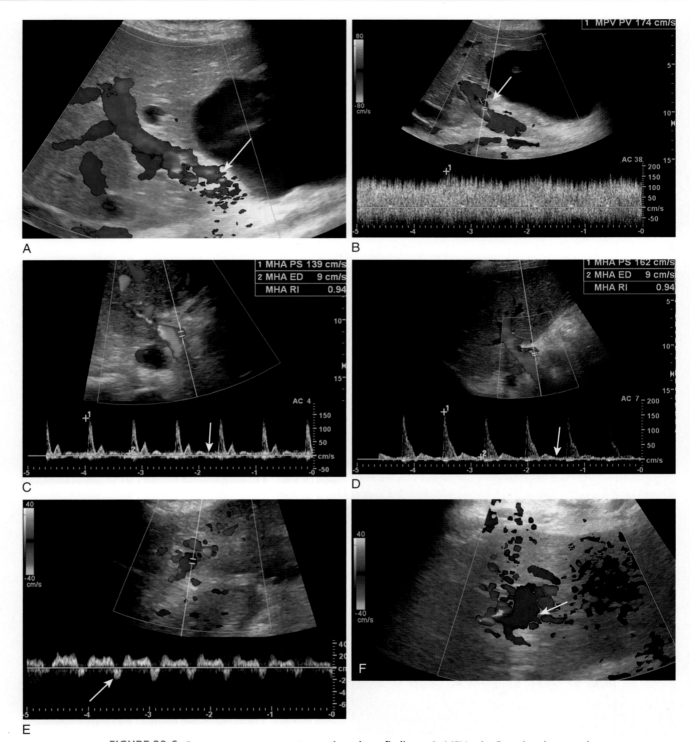

FIGURE 20-6 **Common temporary postoperative edema findings. A,** MPV color Doppler ultrasound shows aliasing. **B,** MPV spectral Doppler ultrasound shows turbulence and elevated velocities. **C** and **D,** MHA spectral Doppler ultrasound shows high resistance with little diastolic flow. **E,** LPV spectral waveform using ultrasound shows to-and-fro flow. **F,** LPV color Doppler ultrasound shows hepatofugal flow.

the physician should image the site assessing for a bleed. Arterial flow along the biopsy tract outside of the liver parenchyma may be visualized on ultrasound. Color and spectral Doppler should be used to document the bleed. At times, a large collection of lidocaine may collect mimicking a subcapsular

bleed. This area should be noted before the procedure so it is not confused with a postprocedural hematoma. The bleeding may be painful if it is associated with the liver capsule or painless. Most bleeds will stop on their own after applying moderate pressure over the biopsy tract. If the bleeding is severe, the

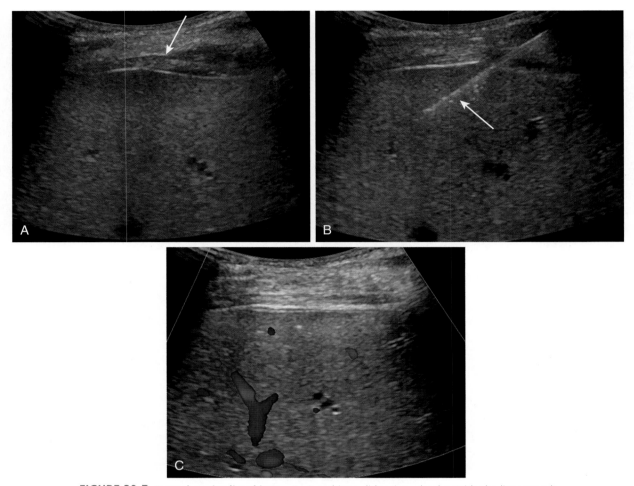

FIGURE 20-7   Normal routine liver biopsy. A, A prebiopsy lidocaine wheel outside the liver capsule visualized on ultrasound. **B,** Ultrasound-guided needle biopsy pass remaining away from large vessels. **C,** Ultrasound after biopsy shows no sign of bleeding on color imaging.

patient may become vasovagal and blood pressure may drop. Fluids should be given and the head should be lowered. If there is active bleeding that cannot be controlled, the patient may be transferred to the interventional radiology department for further imaging and possible embolization.

The biopsy needle is ultrasound guided to avoid major blood vessels and biliary ducts. At times, the needle path may cross small vessels for a potential risk creating an AVF or small intrahepatic ducts causing a bile leak forming a biloma (Figure 20-8). Another rare complication after biopsy is creating a hepatic artery pseudoaneurysm. You can visualize the to-and-fro waveform on spectral Doppler imaging. These findings are usually clinically insignificant, and will likely just be followed on serial ultrasound examinations. The radiologist can reduce these risks by avoiding the liver hilum.

Pathology of the Liver Transplant

Rejection. The most common cause for liver transplant failure is rejection. Acute rejection occurs within the first 10 days of transplantation. Some signs and symptoms include right upper quadrant pain, fever, tachycardia, hepatomegaly, and ascites. Liver function tests may be elevated and the patient may develop encephalopathy. Chronic rejection evolves over an extended part of time slowly deteriorating the liver graft, causing fibrosis. The ultrasound findings of rejection are often nonspecific and can include an elevated RI or periportal edema, most often requiring a liver biopsy for diagnosis.[13]

Infection and Abscesses. Intrahepatic abscesses are localized fluid collections of necrotic inflammatory tissue that contains purulent material and an infectious organism. Common signs and symptoms are fever, right upper quadrant pain, and jaundice. These abscesses are often seen secondary to a liver infarction. Patients who are on immunosuppressive medications who present with biliary stricture or arterial insufficiency are at increased risk for developing an infection. Infection is likely to spread to the chest and lungs in the immunocompromised patient.[14] On ultrasound imaging, an abscess will typically have thick walls and be hypoechoic and complex in appearance with an air-fluid level with poorly defined borders. Gas bubbles may be present within the abscess and will appear as a "dirty" shadow. Abscesses can have varied appearances

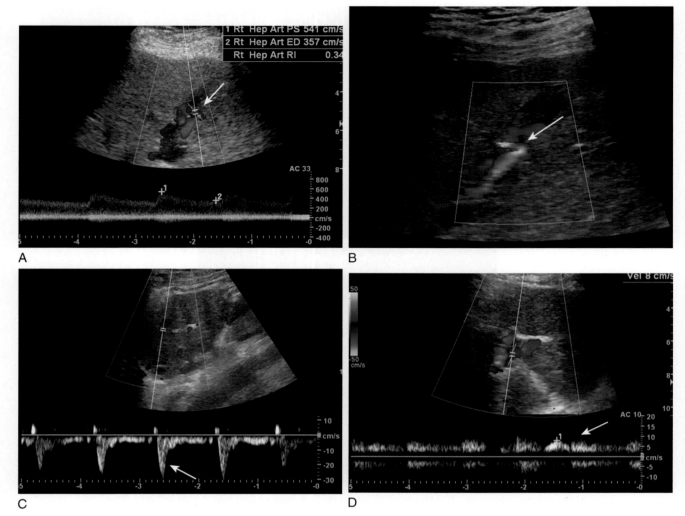

FIGURE 20-8 **Liver biopsy complications.** **A,** Spectral Doppler ultrasound shows an AVF between the RHA and RPV with an elevated velocity and low resistive waveform. **B,** Color Doppler ultrasound shows the connection of the RHA and RPV. **C,** LHV spectral Doppler ultrasound shows very pulsatile flow typically seen in an AVF. **D,** Very slow flow of the LPV on spectral Doppler ultrasound is also highly suggestive of an AVF.

though and may have internal septations or some may even appear solid mimicking a mass. The treatment of choice is usually a percutaneous drainage catheter using CT or ultrasound guidance and antibiotics (Figure 20-9).

Vascular Compromise

Hepatic Vein and IVC Thrombosis and Stenosis.
There is less than a 1% complication rate involving the IVC and HVs after transplantation. Thrombosis and stenosis is most common to occur at the anastomosis sites due to size discrepancy between the native and transplant vessels or suprahepatic caval kinking. Chronic IVC stenosis is more common in retransplanted or pediatric patients.[13] The IVC can be narrowed from extrinsic compression from postoperative edema or a large hematoma creating a stenosis. Color Doppler aliasing and tripling of the spectral Doppler waveform velocities demonstrating turbulence may be visualized. Hepatic vein dilation with a dampened monophasic waveform may also be visualized. Angioplasty with stent placement is

the treatment of choice (Figure 20-10). Stenosis of the HV mostly occurs in living donor transplants. A focal narrowing along with aliasing on color Doppler and a monophasic, turbulent waveform demonstrating elevated velocities on spectral Doppler imaging will be seen. IVC and HV thrombosis is caused from a hypercoagulable state and surgical factors. Intraluminal thrombus is identified filling the vessel with no color Doppler flow. There may be imaging features of Budd-Chiari syndrome (Figure 20-11). If the ultrasound examination is inconclusive, CT or MRI may be considered to confirm diagnosis.[13,14] These patients are typically treated with anticoagulants.

Portal Vein Thrombus and Stenosis.
Portal vein stenosis occurs in about 1% of patients after transplantation. Stenosis is usually found at the anastomosis site and may occur when there is a size discrepancy of the vessels.[13] On ultrasound imaging, the PV will demonstrate color and spectral Doppler aliasing, typically with a 3:1 ratio. Patients may

undergo balloon angioplasty, stent placement, or resection. Thrombosis of the PV occurs in about 3% of liver transplants.[14] This commonly results from mismatched caliber differences in the vessels, stretching of the PV near the anastomotic site, slow portal inflow, or hypercoagulable states.

Fresh thrombus appears echogenic and can be either occlusive or nonocclusive. Occlusive thrombus will demonstrate no flow with color or spectral Doppler (Figure 20-12). With nonocclusive thrombus, some flow will be visualized around the thrombus. As a thrombus ages, it typically becomes more

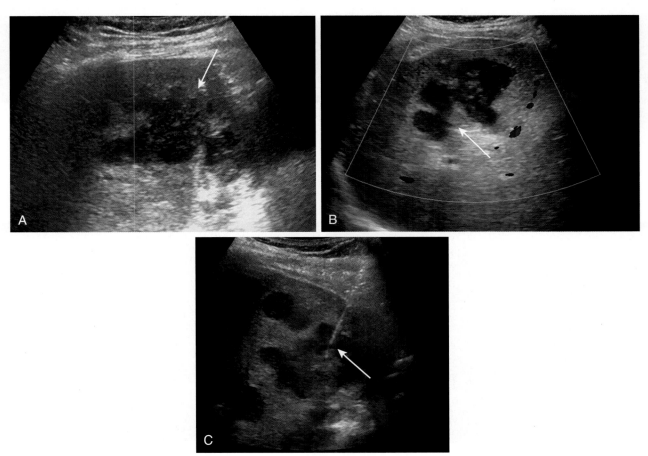

FIGURE 20-9 **Intrahepatic liver abscess. A,** Gray-scale ultrasound of the collection shows irregular, poorly defined borders with debris. **B,** Color Doppler ultrasound shows no flow within the complex collection. **C,** Ultrasound-guided percutaneous drain placement within the abscess.

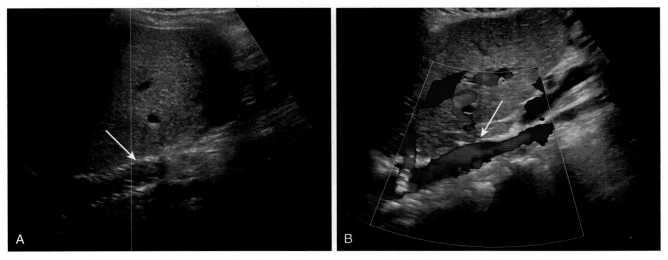

FIGURE 20-10 **IVC stenosis and stent placement. A,** Longitudinal gray-scale ultrasound shows a stent within the IVC. **B,** Color Doppler ultrasound within the stent shows no signs of aliasing or narrowing. *Continued*

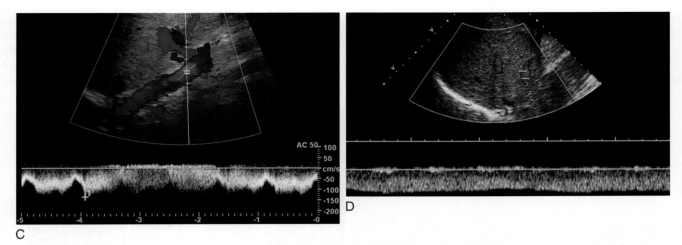

FIGURE 20-10, cont'd C, IVC spectral Doppler ultrasound shows normal velocities within the stent. **D,** Spectral Doppler ultrasound of an HV shows a flat monophasic waveform suggestive of IVC stenosis.

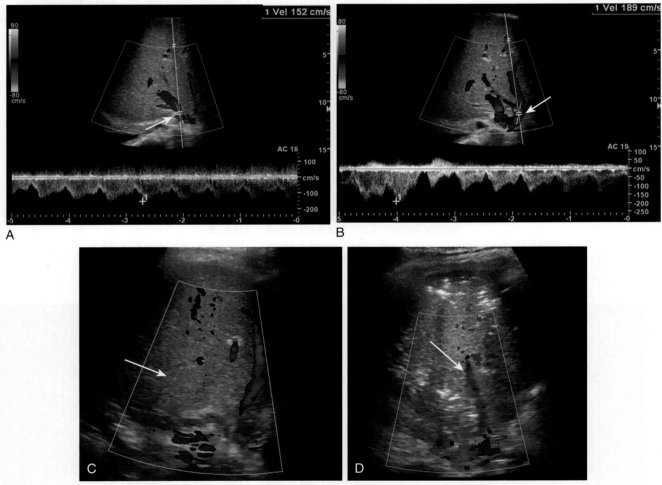

FIGURE 20-11 HV stenosis and thrombosis **A** and **B,** Spectral Doppler ultrasound of the RHV and MHV shows turbulence with elevated velocities near the anastomoses sites. **C** and **D,** Color Doppler ultrasound shows no flow within the RHV and MHV suggestive of complete thrombosis.

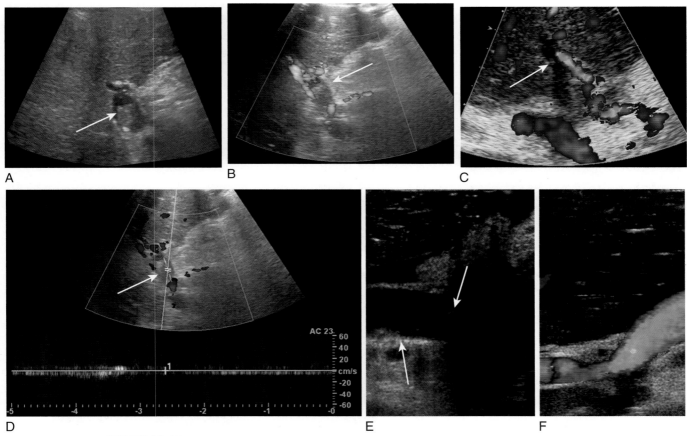

FIGURE 20-12 Acute PV occlusive thrombus immediately postoperative. A, Gray-scale ultrasound of MPV shows acute thrombus within the vessel. **B,** Power Doppler ultrasound shows no flow within the MPV. **C,** MPV shows no flow on color Doppler ultrasound. **D,** Spectral Doppler ultrasound shows no flow within the MPV. **E,** Intraoperative MPV gray-scale ultrasound shows a small amount of residual thrombus following a thrombectomy. **F,** Intraoperative color Doppler ultrasound shows the MPV widely patent following a thrombectomy.

anechoic. In the symptomatic patient, thrombectomy, thrombolysis, stent placement, or a venous graft may be necessary[13] (Figure 20-13). With chronic PV thrombosis, cavernous transformation can occur with the hepatic artery.

Hepatic Artery Stenosis. Hepatic artery stenosis occurs in 2% to 11% of liver transplant patients with a median time to diagnosis of 100 days. Risk factors include rejection, poor surgical technique, or clamp injury. The sonographer will notice color and spectral Doppler aliasing with turbulent flow. Pulsed-wave Doppler will demonstrate a low RI (less than 0.50) with a velocity greater than 200 cm/sec and a tardus parvus waveform. In the early postoperative period, less than 72 hours of transplantation, the RI can be elevated greater than 0.80, but usually will return to normal within a few days. The most common cause for this is postoperative edema. The increased hepatic artery resistance can be associated with an older donor age and an extended period of ischemic time. It is common to get an elevated false velocity measurement when the hepatic artery is tortuous. If the ultrasound examination is inconclusive, a CT angiography (CTA) or MR angiography (MRA) should be

considered. Treatment may include balloon angioplasty with stent placement or surgical revision[14] (Figure 20-14). If the stenosis is left untreated, it may lead to HA thrombosis, liver ischemia, biliary stricture, sepsis, and allograft loss. Early detection is critical to avoid the need for retransplantation.[13]

Hepatic Artery Thrombosis. The most common vascular complication of liver transplantation is HA thrombosis.[14] Thrombosis occurs in 4% to 12% of adults and 42% of children between postoperative days 15 and 132.[13,14] Risk factors include rejection, short warm ischemic time, end-to-end anastomosis, and pediatric transplantation. HA thrombosis and stenosis can lead to biliary ischemia because the HA is the only vascular supply to the biliary ducts. There will be absence of color and no flow on spectral Doppler imaging. On gray-scale, echogenic thrombus filing the HA lumen may be visualized. When there is slow flow present due to low cardiac output or arterial spasm, ultrasound may not detect flow leading to a false-positive diagnosis when the hepatic artery is patent. If the ultrasound is inconclusive, a CTA may ultimately be required. CT may demonstrate

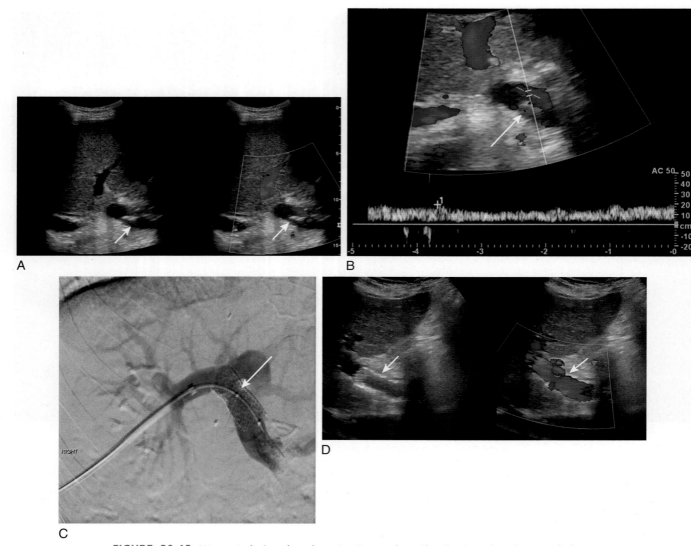

A

B

C

D

FIGURE 20-13 **PV nonocclusive thrombus. A,** Gray-scale and color Doppler ultrasound show thrombus along the wall with some flow within MPV. **B,** Spectral Doppler ultrasound of the MPV shows a patent segment flowing around the thrombus. **C,** Interventional radiology stent placement within the MPV. **D,** Gray-scale and color Doppler ultrasound show no signs of a filling defect within the stent.

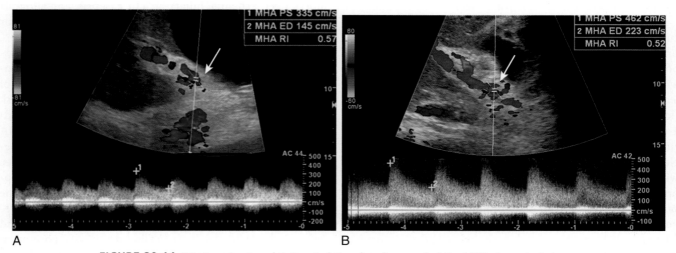

A

B

FIGURE 20-14 **HA stenosis. A** and **B,** Spectral Doppler ultrasound of the MHA shows turbulence and elevated velocities.

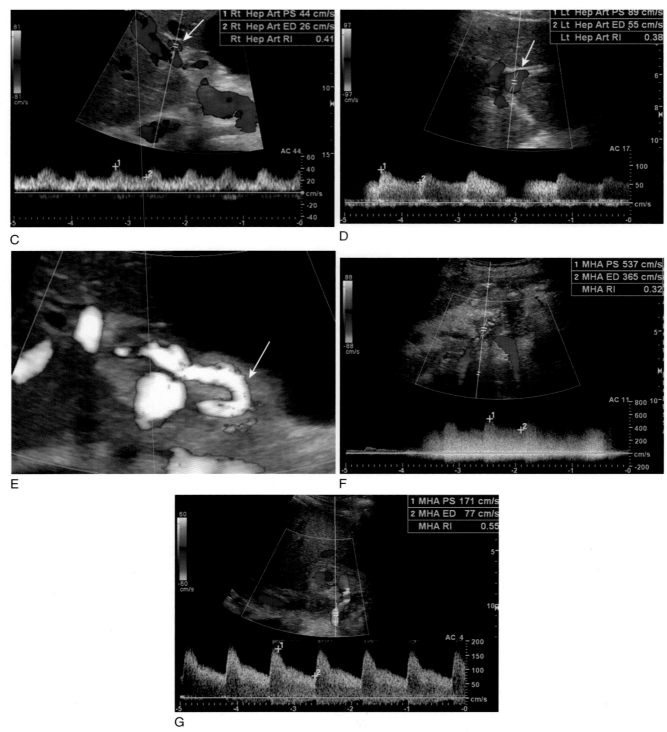

FIGURE 20-14, cont'd   C and **D,** Spectral Doppler ultrasound of the RHA and LHA shows a low RI concerning for a proximal stenosis. **E,** Power Doppler ultrasound of the MHA shows tortuosity in which elevated velocities may be present. **F,** Spectral Doppler ultrasound of a severe MHA stenosis at 537 cm/sec. **G,** Spectral Doppler ultrasound following an HA anastomosis reconstruction shows improvement.

areas of infarction as well. Treatment includes an emergent thrombectomy, but many cases ultimately require retransplantation[14] (Figure 20-15).

Infarction and Necrosis. In a native liver, it is rare for an infarction to take place. If the HA were to occlude,

collateral vessels would take over to give collateral flow to the liver. Within a transplant, development of collateral vessels is not usually possible as most of the collateral vessels are ligated during the surgical process. In 85% of cases, hepatic infarction is associated with HA complications with portal

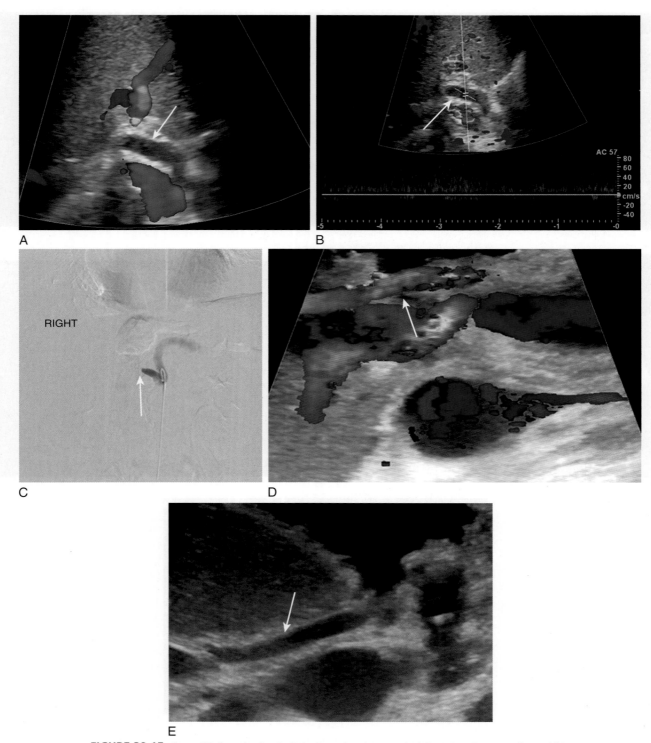

FIGURE 20-15 **Acute HA thrombosis. A,** Color Doppler ultrasound of the MHA shows no flow within the vessel. **B,** Spectral Doppler ultrasound of the MHA shows no flow within the vessel. **C,** Interventional angiogram shows no flow within the MHA. **D** and **E,** Intraoperative color Doppler and longitudinal gray-scale ultrasound shows no sign of thrombus and is widely patent following a thrombectomy.

vein occlusion being less likely. Ischemic areas within the liver can liquefy over time and may become infected and calcifications may be present.[13] Infarction usually appears hypoechoic and wedge shaped located along the periphery. Infarcts can be difficult to distinguish from focal abscesses

and an aspiration or biopsy may be needed for confirmation (Figure 20-16).

Hepatic Artery Pseudoaneurysms. Hepatic artery pseudoaneurysms are relatively uncommon and usually located at the anastomosis site or occur due to angioplasty

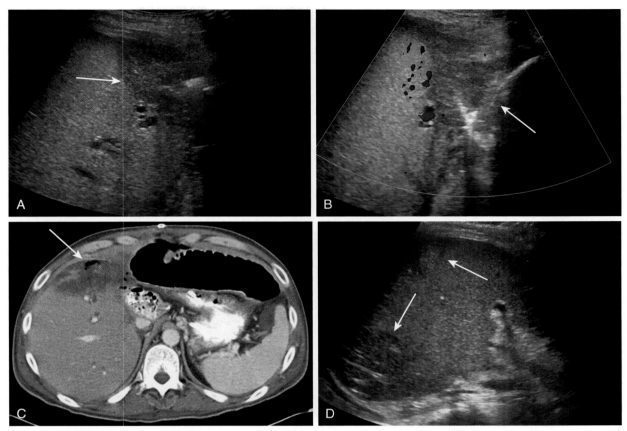

FIGURE 20-16 Hepatic infarction caused from previous HA thrombosis. A, Gray-scale ultrasound shows a hypoechoic wedge-shaped area along the periphery. **B,** Color Doppler ultrasound shows no flow within the infarcted segment. **C,** CT shows the peripheral infarction with a small amount of gas. **D,** Transverse gray-scale ultrasound of other infarcted areas within the liver.

complications. These may also be intrahepatic secondary to a liver biopsy, biliary procedures, or infection. Patients are most often asymptomatic. If the pseudoaneurysm ruptures, however, the patient may go into acute shock and a portal or biliary fistula can develop. Treatments for extrahepatic pseudoaneurysms include resection, coil embolization, or stent placement. The treatment option of choice for an intrahepatic pseudoaneurysm is coil embolization. On ultrasound imaging, a pseudoaneurysm appears as an anechoic structure often containing nonocclusive thrombus along the walls, and located along the course of the HA. On Doppler imaging, it fills with color and there is a disorganized, bidirectional flow pattern. A characteristic "yin-yang" pattern of flow on Doppler imaging has been described.[13,14] Pseudoaneurysms can be visualized using CTA or MRA. These appear as round masses at the anastomotic site and enhance avidly during the arterial phase. If slow flow is present, enhancement may only be noted during the portal or delayed venous phases[15] (Figure 20-17).

Biliary Complications. In about 5% to 15% of liver transplant patients, biliary complications occur. These typically occur within the first 3 months after transplantation.[14] Complications include biliary ductal obstruction, stenosis or stricture at the anastomosis, stone formation, biliary necrosis, sphincter of Oddi dysfunction, and recurrent biliary disease. Bile leaks and bilomas are also complications that are discussed later in this chapter. Biliary complications taken as a whole are the second most common cause of allograft dysfunction following rejection.[13]

Obstruction is the most common biliary complication usually caused from a stricture at the anastomosis but may also be secondary to choledocholithiasis.[13,14] The donor CBD will demonstrate postobstructive dilation in patients with choledocholithiasis. It is important to note that some patients may present with nonobstructive ductal dilation secondary to papillary dyskinesia and may be clinically insignificant. Imaging findings should be correlated with clinical findings and symptoms. Ultrasound is less reliable when mild ductal obstruction is present. As a result, MRI cholangiopancreatography is useful in detecting biliary obstruction. Most strictures are extrahepatic and near the anastomosis caused from fibrotic tissue scarring. These are usually treated with angioplasty with or without stent placement. As opposed to extrahepatic strictures, intrahepatic strictures are due to ischemia or cholangitis and treatment includes percutaneous biliary drain placement (Figure 20-18). Stones, sludge, and debris can be found in 5.7% of liver transplants.

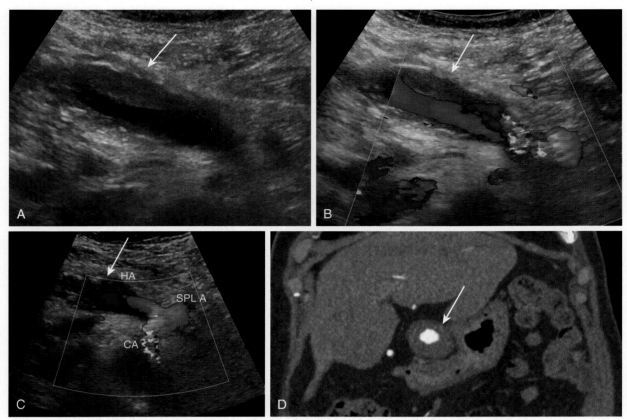

FIGURE 20-17 **HA pseudoaneurysm. A,** Longitudinal gray-scale ultrasound of a pseudoaneurysm measured at 3 cm. **B,** Color Doppler ultrasound shows thrombus along the arterial wall. **C,** Color Doppler ultrasound shows the relation between the splenic artery and celiac artery. **D,** CT shows a cross-sectional image of the MHA pseudoaneurysm with thrombus lining the arterial wall.

Altering the bile composition could be a predisposing factor for stone and sludge formation. Choledocholithiasis is usually treated with an endoscopic sphincterotomy and stone retrieval[14] (Figures 20-19 and 20-20). Biliary ductal ischemia is secondary to HA thrombosis or stenosis as the ducts are dependent on the HA for their only blood supply. Biliary necrosis occurs and biliary stenosis, bile leaks, and bilomas may follow. If angioplasty of the stenotic duct is not successful, retransplantation is often necessary.[13]

Fluid Collections

Bleeding and Hematomas. Hematomas are collections of blood and usually occur within the first 2 weeks

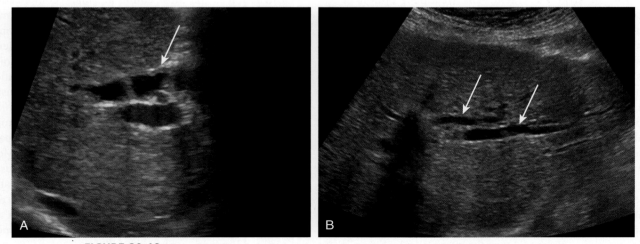

FIGURE 20-18 **Chronic cholangiopathy. A** and **B,** Gray-scale ultrasound of dilated ducts shows thickened walls and debris.

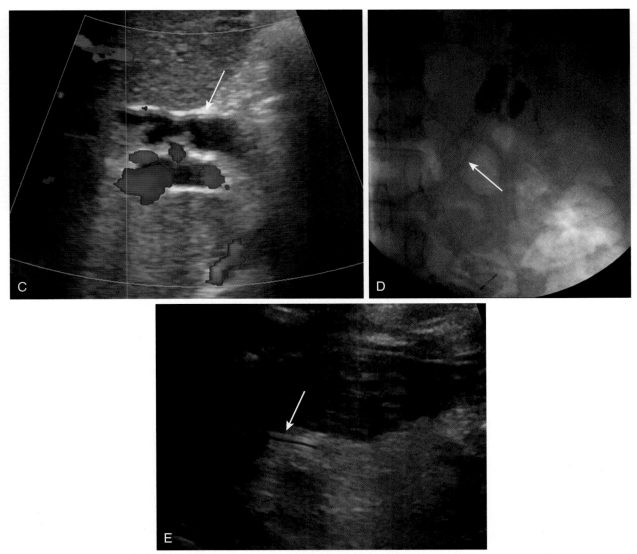

FIGURE 20-18, cont'd C, Color Doppler ultrasound shows no flow. **D,** ERCP shows changes of cholangitis and the stricture was balloon dilated and stent placement followed. **E,** Longitudinal gray-scale ultrasound of a biliary stent.

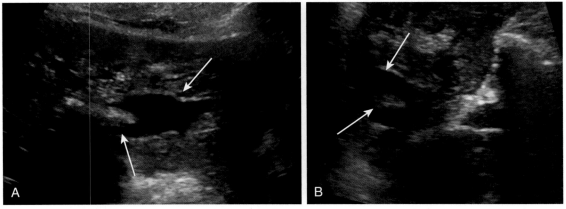

FIGURE 20-19 Intrahepatic ductal dilation with stones. A, Transverse gray-scale ultrasound shows shadowing from the stones. **B,** Longitudinal gray-scale ultrasound.

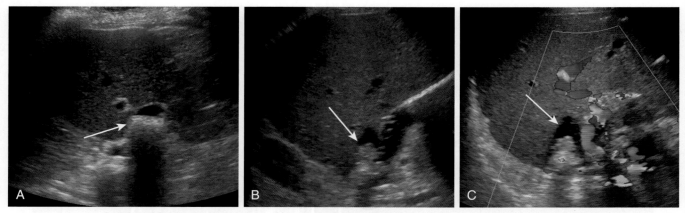

FIGURE 20-20 Cystic duct remnant with stones and debris. A, Transverse gray-scale ultrasound shows shadowing from the stones. **B,** Longitudinal gray-scale ultrasound. **C,** Color Doppler ultrasound shows "twinkle" artifact from stones.

postoperatively, and most are present and can be visualized on the "day 0" ultrasound examination. Hematomas are most common along the perihepatic spaces and near the vascular and biliary anastomoses sites. Most hematomas will resolve spontaneously with no intervention needed. At rare times, there may be an underlying infection within a hematoma and a percutaneous drainage catheter may need to be placed[13,14] Hematomas can have variable appearances as they age. They typically have irregular walls, are ovoid in shape, and decrease in size over time. Fresh hematomas have more internal echoes and can appear echogenic. As they age, they liquefy and become more anechoic and may contain septations[15] (Figure 20-21).

Seromas. Seromas are clear, serous fluid collections that are usually found within the first few days after transplantation.

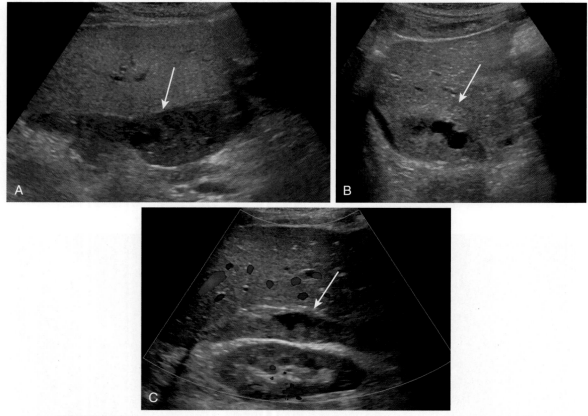

FIGURE 20-21 Postoperative hematoma. A, Longitudinal gray-scale ultrasound shows hypoechoic internal echoes consistent with a resolving hematoma. **B,** Transverse gray-scale ultrasound shows some liquefying components. **C,** Recurrent fresh echogenic hematoma following evacuation, color Doppler ultrasound shows no active bleed.

They are most common along the perihepatic spaces and near the vascular and biliary anastomoses sites. Most seromas will resolve spontaneously within a few weeks. On ultrasound, a seroma is a round, localized, anechoic, thin-walled fluid collection, which may contain debris or septations. Ultrasound is very sensitive to diagnose a fluid collection but not specific of contents. Unfortunately, blood, pus, lymph, bile, and serosanguineous fluid can have similar appearances on ultrasound, and ultimately CT or MRI is helpful in differentiating the collections. If there is concern the fluid collection is infected or creating mass effect on the vasculature, an aspiration may be performed[13] (Figure 20-22).

Lymphoceles. A surgical disruption of lymphatic channels causes lymph fluid leakage into the soft tissue space creating a lymphocele. These are typically found in the groin or retroperitoneal space. On ultrasound imaging, debris or septations within the fluid collection may be seen. Ultrasound is very sensitive to diagnose a fluid collection, although the contents are difficult to distinguish. CT or MRI is very helpful in differentiating among lymph, blood, bile, pus, or serosanguineous fluid.[13] The most common complication of venovenous bypass during liver transplantation is a lymphocele, which can be seen between 10% and 30%. Spontaneous resolution is rare. Treatment includes percutaneous drain placement used in conjunction with sclerotherapy. Surgical repair is the optimal choice of treatment. Methylene blue dye injected through the lymphatic system makes it possible to identify the leak source during an open repair. This complication fortunately is now only rarely seen, as the venovenous bypass is no longer routinely used for liver transplantation surgery.[16]

Bile Leak and Bilomas. Bile leaks occur in about 5% of liver transplant patients. These typically present in the early postoperative period with more than 70% within the first month of transplantation. Leaks are most often located at the biliary tube site with rare occurrences at the anastomotic site. Bile seeps into the peritoneal cavity and may form a contained perihepatic collection, or biloma. Treatment includes stent placement over the biliary leak and possibly placement of a percutaneous drainage catheter.[13] On ultrasound imaging, a biloma is a discrete, round, hypoechoic or anechoic fluid collection demonstrating no vascular flow. Ultrasound may have a difficult time differentiating biliary leaks from other fluid collections such as hematomas, abscesses, seromas, or ascites. Cholangiography and cholescintigraphy are sensitive and specific modalities that are helpful in biliary leakage evaluation[14] (Figure 20-23).

Free Fluid. Ascites is usually present in small amounts in the early postoperative period. It may contain debris or blood products. The ascites commonly resolves in 7 to 10 days following transplantation. If the patient is having pain and remains uncomfortable with a large amount of free fluid, a therapeutic paracentesis can be performed[15] (Figure 20-24).

Hepatocellular Carcinoma and Metastatic Disease. Patients who initially present with small HCC lesions with no extrahepatic involvement typically have a reasonable long-term survival following liver transplantation. Recurrence of HCC is seen in about 40% of patients after their transplant, however. This may occur when chronic cirrhosis is present or microscopic extrahepatic lesions are not identified at the time of transplantation. This may create distant metastasis in other organs.[17] The most common site of HCC recurrence is the lung followed by the liver.[13]

Ultrasound can be quite sensitive for detecting HCC, but the experience and skill of the sonographer are critical for localizing these smaller tumors. Their appearance is typically hypoechoic with variability in size. Some tumors may appear hyperechoic and can be misdiagnosed as a benign hemangioma. Ultrasound imaging is useful in evaluating presence of flow and detecting vascular invasion. A dedicated contrast CT or MRI is helpful identifying a benign verses a malignant process (Figure 20-25).

The most common malignancies after liver transplantation are skin cancer (excluding melanoma), Kaposi sarcoma, and non-Hodgkin's lymphoma. Long-term immunosuppression, a previous viral infection, chronic use of alcohol before transplantation, and acute rejection are risk factors contributing to malignant disease. Lymphoma may be seen intrahepatic or extrahepatic demonstrating a hypoechoic soft tissue mass or multiple liver lesions. The mass may encase the hilum affecting the vasculature or biliary tree.[13] Other metastasis from a different primary source may also be visualized (Figure 20-26).

Hepatitis Recurrence. Hepatitis C virus (HCV) reinfection occurs in nearly all patients who receive a liver transplant for HCV cirrhosis.[15] An infected liver will have a heterogeneous and coarsened echotexture on ultrasound imaging (Figure 20-27). Risk factors for recurrence include donor age, immunosuppression, cytomegalovirus infection, metabolic syndrome, and IL28B genotype. Donor age over 40 years old has a significant impact on HCV infection and graft loss. Ideally, patients awaiting a liver transplant with HCV are placed on antiviral medication to eradicate the viral process before transplantation. Recurrence following transplant is immediate and universal in patients who are viremic at the time of surgery. Viral levels 1 year after surgery are 10 to 20 times greater than pretransplant. Recurrence is often associated with rapid fibrosis leading to higher mortality and allograft loss rates. About 20% of these patients will develop cirrhosis within 5 years of transplantation.

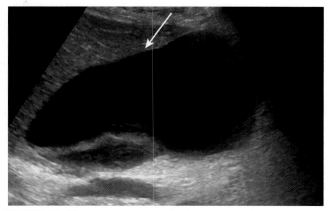

FIGURE 20-22 **Seroma.** Longitudinal gray-scale ultrasound shows a simple fluid collection.

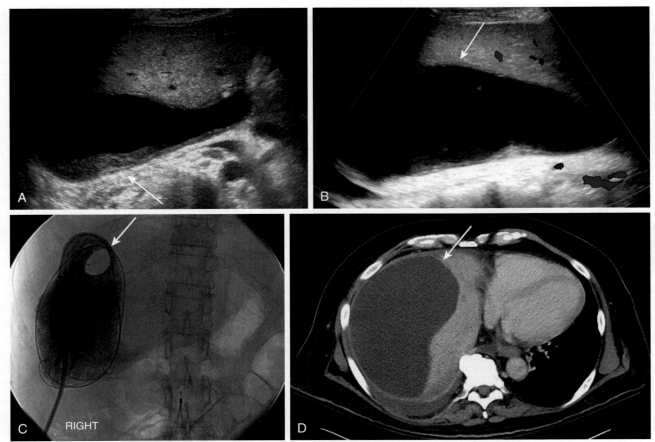

FIGURE 20-23 Biloma. A, Longitudinal gray-scale ultrasound shows a fluid collection with debris and posterior acoustic enhancement. **B,** Color Doppler ultrasound shows no flow within the collection. **C,** Interventional radiology sinogram shows a drain within the infected biloma. **D,** CT shows a large biloma caused from a biopsy complication.

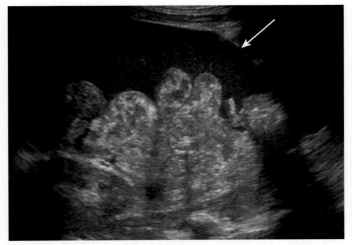

FIGURE 20-24 Debris-filled ascites due to hemorrhage on gray-scale ultrasound.

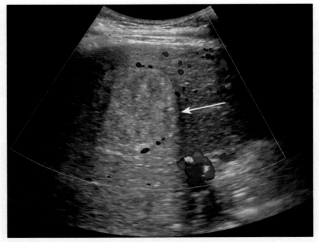

FIGURE 20-25 Primary HCC in recurrent hepatitis C. Color Doppler ultrasound shows no flow within but along the periphery of the mass.

Retransplantation remains controversial in these patients compared with other reasons for transplant loss such as primary nonfunction or hepatic arterial thrombosis.[18] Patients with coinfection of HIV and HCV are also debated in regards to receiving a liver transplant. The argument for transplantation in these patients is that HCV is more aggressive after liver transplantation in a patient with HIV and HCV, and is the major source of graft loss and death. In patients in whom HCV infection resolves, there is an 80% survival rate.[19]

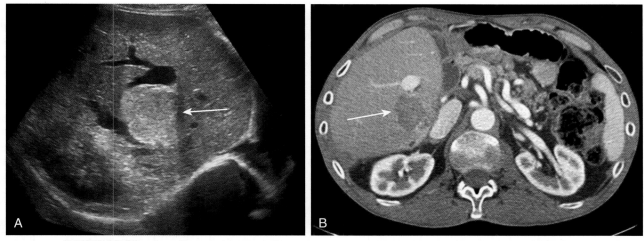

FIGURE 20-26 Islet cell metastasis. A, Transverse gray-scale ultrasound shows a hyperechoic mass within the right lobe of the liver. **B,** CT shows a mass with irregular borders within the right lobe of the liver.

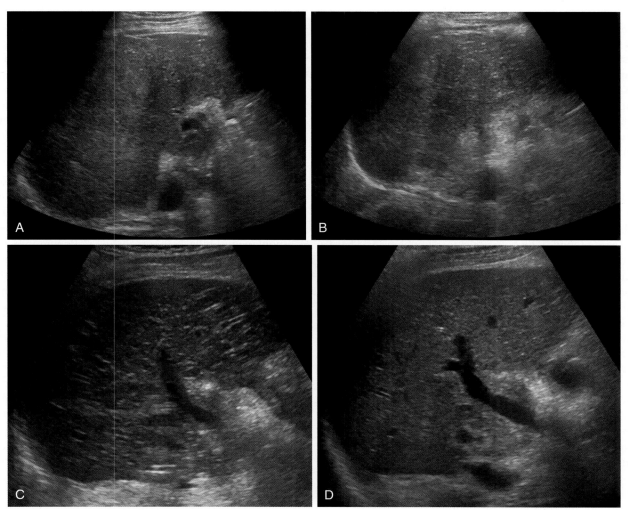

FIGURE 20-27 Hepatitis C recurrence. A, Longitudinal gray-scale ultrasound shows a coarsened liver parenchyma. **B,** Transverse gray-scale ultrasound of a heterogeneous liver. **C,** Immediate postoperative edema can have the appearance of chronic liver disease on gray-scale ultrasound. **D,** Longitudinal gray-scale ultrasound of the liver parenchyma returns to a normal appearance 1 day later.

Portal Venous Gas and Bowel Ischemia. Portal venous gas is a common finding on ultrasound during the early postoperative period following transplantation.[15,20] Beyond the early postoperative state, air visualized within the portal and mesenteric veins is associated with a poor prognosis. Some underlying causes of the portal venous gas are intestinal ischemia and necrosis (75% of patients), followed by ulcerative colitis (8%) and intraabdominal abscess (6%).[21] Bowel ischemia is an unfortunately common and dangerous condition, especially in the elderly. There is a high mortality rate of 75% to 90% of cases. Damage to the mucosal intestinal layer leads to overdistention of bowel loops and gas moves from the intestinal lumen to the mesenteric veins, through the portal veins, and into the liver parenchyma. Portal venous gas can be diagnosed on x-ray, CT, or ultrasound. Prompt treatment results in reducing the mortality rates. The prognosis is ultimately dependent on the underlying condition.[20] Using ultrasound, portal venous gas should be easily detectable on real-time imaging and should appear as echogenic foci flowing through the vein on gray scale. Clip stores can help aid in this diagnosis. On spectral Doppler, the turbulent flow can often be heard and sharp spikes can be seen on the venous waveform. In severe cases, echogenic foci can fill the entire liver parenchyma (Figure 20-28).

Posttransplant Lymphoproliferative Disorder. Posttransplant lymphoproliferative disorder (PTLD) is one of the most severe complications found in solid organ as well as stem cell transplantation. PTLD occurs in 1% to 20% of patients who receive a transplant. In one study, PTLD was found to occur in 0.8% of liver transplant patients.[22] Chronic use of immunosuppressant medication increases the risk of malignancies 2 to 5 times more than the general population. PTLD can range from benign reactive hyperplasia of tissue to malignant lymphoma. Most polymorphic masses are caused from the Epstein-Barr virus (EBV) occurring 60% to 80% and within 1 year of transplantation. Most of the monomorphic masses are found to be non-Hodgkin's lymphoma and have a B-cell origin. Treatment for EBV-induced PTLD includes reducing the dosages of immunosuppressant drugs to allow the natural immune system to help fight the disorder. Dose reduction has been found to be effective in 23% to 50% of cases. In patients who do not respond to reduction of immunosuppression, immunotherapy with monoclonal antibodies such as rituximab may be given. Success using this treatment is seen in 40% to 68% of cases.[22] If left untreated, mortality with PTLD can be as high as 71%. The location of PTLD can be focal or diffuse and more commonly is extrahepatic. On ultrasound imaging, PTLD usually appears as a hypoechoic soft tissue mass and may encase the hepatic hilum.[15]

Common Benign Findings. As a sonographer, the liver transplant is evaluated initially just as the native organ would be. Document any pathology visualized. The following are common findings that may be encountered within the liver and are not specific to transplantation.

Cysts. Simple hepatic cysts are benign liver lesions. They are common, occurring in 2% to 7% of the general population,[23,24] and can be diagnosed using CT, MRI, or ultrasound. Cysts can be focal or multiple, vary in size, and usually are found incidentally with most patients remaining asymptomatic. True cysts contain serous fluid with a thin wall.[23] On ultrasound evaluation, cysts appear round and anechoic with no color flow. The wall is thin with a well-defined border, and posterior acoustic enhancement can be visualized. Septations or debris may also be present.

Hemangiomas. Hepatic hemangioma (HH) is the most common benign liver tumor. It is hypervascular and supplied from the HA. Most are found incidentally and asymptomatic. HH can range from a few millimeters up to 40 centimeters, do not increase in size, and are found 0.4% to 20% within the general population. Symptoms are most common with large HH. Less than half of patients presenting with HH have significant symptoms, which include right upper quadrant pain, nausea, vomiting, loss of appetite, or fullness. HH can be diagnosed using ultrasound, CT, MRI, angiography, or nuclear medicine scans. On ultrasound, HH is a well-defined hyperechoic lesion demonstrating posterior acoustic enhancement with little or no Doppler flow. In patients with a hyperechoic fatty liver, HH may appear hypoechoic and can mimic a metastasis. Not all hyperechoic lesions are benign HH. Some of these lesions may represent hepatic metastasis or HCC and correlation with clinical history and other imaging modalities may be necessary. Typically there is no treatment necessary. Surgical resection of HH, RFA, or arterial embolization can be performed in rare circumstances when the clinical situation dictates.[25]

Pneumobilia. Pneumobilia is air within the biliary tree and suggests an abnormal connection of the intestinal tract with the biliary system or, less likely, infection from gas-forming bacteria. It is important to distinguish this relatively benign finding from the more ominous finding of portal venous gas. The most common causes of pneumobilia are recent biliary procedures such as an endoscopic retrograde cholangiopancreatography (ERCP), incompetent sphincter of Oddi, biliary-enteric surgical anastomosis, or a spontaneous biliary-enteric fistula.[26] Pneumobilia can be diagnosed on x-ray, CT, or ultrasound. Ultrasound is sensitive in detection, and echogenic foci movement within the biliary tree on real-time imaging on gray scale can be seen. These foci can produce a shadowing or reverberation artifact (Figure 20-29).

Fatty Liver and Focal Sparing. Fatty liver is a common condition affecting 20% to 30% of adults and 70% in diabetic patients. If left untreated, a fatty liver can lead to long-term illness and cirrhosis. Liver steatosis can be diffuse, focal, geographic, subcapsular, multifocal, or perivascular. Diagnosis can be made on CT, MRI, or ultrasound. Ultrasound is the first choice of imaging in chronic liver disease. Diffuse fatty liver is the most prevalent form involving the entire liver accumulated with fat. On ultrasound, the liver is hyperechoic or echogenic compared with the right kidney. It can be difficult to penetrate and a lower-frequency transducer is recommended. Focal fatty sparing is the geographic absence of fat within an otherwise diffusely fatty liver. This has a hypoechoic appearance and can mimic a mass. It tends to have a wedge-shaped margin with no mass effect on the vasculature or biliary tree[27].

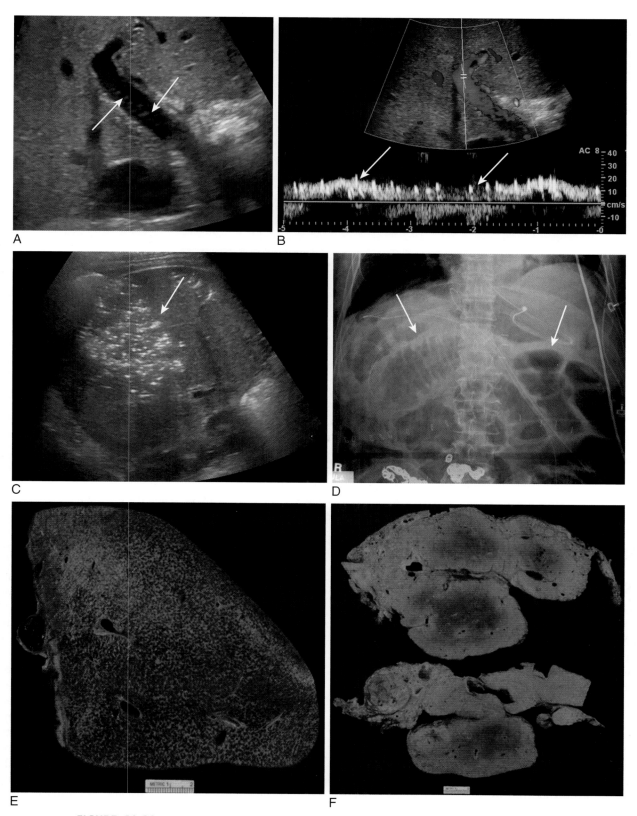

FIGURE 20-28 Portal vein gas. A, Longitudinal gray-scale ultrasound of an MPV shows gas bubbles flowing within the vessel. **B,** Spectral Doppler ultrasound of the MPV shows sharp spikes within the venous waveform. **C,** Severe PV gas on gray-scale ultrasound shows echogenic foci throughout the liver parenchyma. **D,** X-ray of thickened and dilated loops of bowel is suggestive of bowel ischemia. **E** and **F,** Pathology specimen of a necrotic liver.

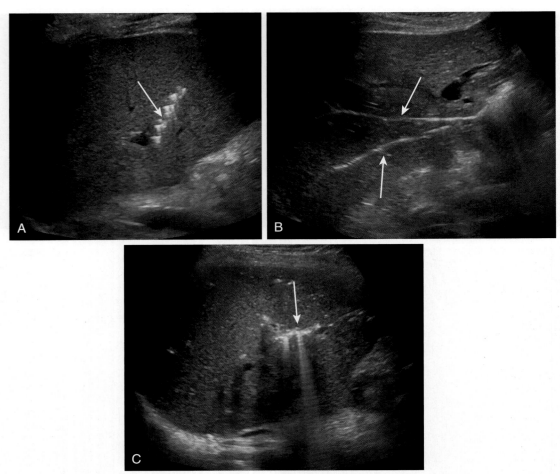

FIGURE 20-29 Pneumobilia. A, Longitudinal gray-scale ultrasound shows echogenic foci within the biliary tree. **B,** Transverse gray-scale ultrasound shows the echogenic air within the biliary tree of the right hepatic lobe. **C,** Transverse gray-scale ultrasound shows the reverberation artifact.

RENAL TRANSPLANT

Surgical Technique of the Renal Transplant

The kidney can be preserved between 24 and 48 hours on ice and using a special preservation solution. The shorter the ischemic time, the better the allograft function. For every transplant, the donor and recipient are rechecked to verify a match. The blood type and compatibility need to be confirmed as well as the UNOS database per protocol. Before coming into the operating room, the team will discuss the risks, benefits, and alternatives with the patient and obtain consent. All institutions have defined and specific protocols and techniques they follow. Every patient is unique, however, and individual surgeons will have different techniques they prefer.

Cadaveric Renal Donation. The 5-year survival rate for cadaveric transplantation from 1991 to 1995 was found to be 60%.[28] The patient is brought into the operating room confirming patient identification and procedure to be performed. Following general anesthesia and line placement, a Foley catheter is placed into the bladder. The abdomen is prepped and draped sterilely. The kidney back bench preparation includes removal of excess perinephric fat, the renal artery and vein are

freed from surrounding structures, the ureter is dissected, and the tributary vessels are ligated. The kidney is flushed with HTK solution, packed, and placed on ice until transplantation is ready to occur. A nephrectomy is not routinely performed and native kidneys remain in the retroperitoneum. Commonly, the renal transplant will be placed into the right iliac fossa. If combined renal and pancreas transplants are to be performed, the incision will be midline from about 5 cm above the umbilicus down to the pubis. The kidney typically will be placed in the left iliac fossa and the pancreas will be placed in the right iliac fossa. If the patient has a previous renal transplant, the surgeon will typically choose the opposite side for placement if there are no vascular contraindications.

A lower quadrant incision is made, and a retractor is placed. Colon is mobilized exposing the external iliac artery and vein. The vein and artery are clamped, and the renal vein is anastomosed end-to-side to the external iliac vein with a suture. Similarly, an end-to-side anastomosis is performed between the renal artery and external iliac artery using running sutures. Clamps are removed and the kidney is reperfused. The surgeon carefully looks for any bleeding points. After obtaining hemostasis, the ureter is spatulated and anastomosed to the anterior bladder wall using a running suture. This is done over a double-J stent, which is secured to the tip of the Foley catheter (Figure 20-30). A drain

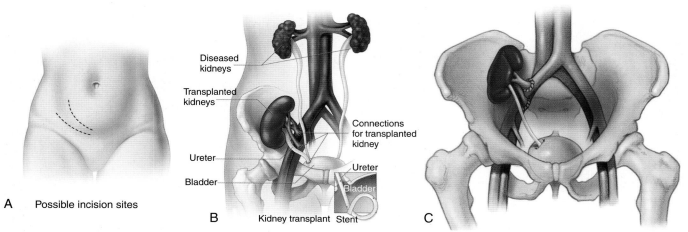

FIGURE 20-30 Illustrations demonstrating surgical technique of renal transplantation. A, Possible incision sites. **B,** Renal transplant in relation to the diseased native kidneys showing anastomotic sites. **C,** Right lower quadrant renal transplant shows the anastomoses.*(Used with permission of Mayo Foundation for Medical Education and Research. All Rights reserved.)*

may be placed before closure and secured to the skin with sutures. The abdomen is closed in two layers. Sponge, needle, and instrument counts are conducted before closure. If indicated, the patient will receive units of blood, platelets, or fresh frozen plasma. The wound is dressed with a dry sterile dressing and the patient is extubated and transferred to the recovery room and later moved into the ICU when stable.

Living Donor Renal Donation. The 5-year survival rate of living donor transplantation from 1991 to 1995 was found to be 75%.[28] Living donation provides better allograft survival compared with the deceased donation, especially in patients who have not begun dialysis yet. In 2004 living kidney donation celebrated 50 years using a kidney from an identical twin. Living donation has become the predominant form of renal transplantation with the annual number of living donors surpassing the number of deceased donors in 2001.[29]

The surgical technique and back bench table preparation are nearly exact compared with a cadaveric kidney. The allograft may demonstrate better function more quickly due to the decreased preservation time in a living donor. With the shortage of organs available for donation, living donor organ donation offers the alternative for those waiting for a transplant and also increases the existing organ supply. A friend or family member may consider being a donor for their loved one. If the donor is not a match, there is a paired exchange program. The donor's organ would go to someone else for a better match rather than directly going to their friend or family member. The one needing the transplant will receive their organ in the exchange for one that meets their need.

Autotransplantion. Renal autotransplantation was first performed in 1963 by James Hardy to repair a high ureteral injury during an aortic surgery. The patient's own kidney is removed from the retroperitoneum and reimplanted into the iliac fossa. The autotransplant is performed to help treat or manage ureteral injuries or stenosis due to retroperitoneal fibrosis, renovascular disease such as renal artery stenosis or aneurysms, renal cell carcinoma (RCC), ureteral cancer, severe cases of nephrolithiasis, and severe loin pain–hematuria syndrome when all other conventional methods have failed.[30] The surgical technique and back bench table preparation are similar compared with a cadaveric or living donor kidney.

Evaluation of the Renal Allograft

As a sonographer, the renal transplant is evaluated as a native kidney and renal artery examination would be, assessing the size, echotexture, and vasculature and looking for hydronephrosis, masses, fluid collections, or ascites. Institutions instill their own routine protocols on timing of examinations and certain images that are required. The following is the basis of what my institution practices. Once the patient has arrived at the recovery room from the surgical suite, the sonographer will go portably to perform the immediate postoperative examination. The patient's creatinine and urine output are closely monitored and if any issues arise, the transplant physicians will tailor their imaging requests. The blood values are evaluated weekly for the first 2 months, then every other week for 4 months, then monthly for 1 year, then every 3 months. The patient usually has a follow-up ultrasound every 4 to 6 months and then annually if there are no complications.

It is best to image using a 2.5- to 5.0-MHz curvilinear transducer and have the patient fasting 4 to 6 hours. Obese patients will require lower frequencies. The renal transplant is typically located in either the right or left lower quadrant and usually superficial. As a result, higher-frequency transducers are most commonly used. Breath holding is usually not necessary as respiratory motion of the pelvic structures is minimal. Depending on location, rolling the patient left lateral decubitus or right lateral decubitus may help move overlying bowel or bring the kidney to a more superficial position in the obese patient (Figure 20-31).

The sonographer should scan completely through the kidney before taking any images while adjusting the frequency, depth, gain, TGCs, and focal zones as they go. Once the renal transplant has been fully evaluated, the examination needs to include a length measurement along with medial and lateral gray-scale longitudinal images. Gray-scale transverse images of

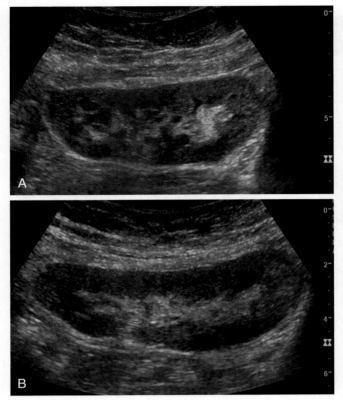

FIGURE 20-31 Renal transplant imaging using different patient positions. **A,** Longitudinal gray-scale ultrasound while the patient is supine. **B,** Longitudinal gray-scale ultrasound with the patient rolled onto the side brings the kidney more superficial.

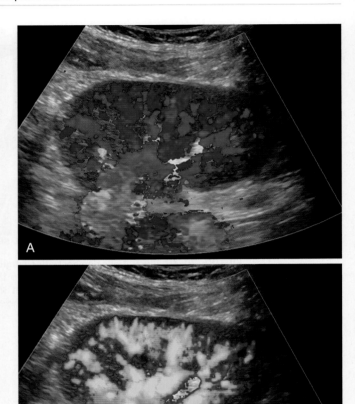

FIGURE 20-32 **Renal transplant perfusion. A,** Color Doppler ultrasound shows normal perfusion throughout the renal parenchyma. **B,** Power Doppler ultrasound shows normal perfusion throughout the renal parenchyma without direction of flow identification.

the upper, mid, and lower poles also need to be obtained. Document any pathology in two planes with and without measurements and include color Doppler flow. Longitudinal and transverse gray-scale images should be taken of the bladder assessing for masses, bladder distention, or signs of infection. Most patients will typically have a urinary catheter in place immediately after surgery and this should not be confused with a bladder mass. Quadrant images need to be obtained checking for free fluid or signs of bleeding.

The Doppler portion is crucial for the transplanted kidney. Venous and arterial color and spectral Doppler need to be obtained looking for any signs of thrombus or stenosis. Ultrasound is commonly the first method of imaging in these patients, critical in helping the physicians diagnose the patient and ensure treatment will be administered quickly. Color Doppler and power Doppler should be used to judge adequate perfusion throughout the kidney (Figure 20-32). The arcuate arteries within the parenchyma are evaluated in the upper, mid, and lower poles to obtain an RI measurement using the peak systolic and end-diastolic velocities. This is a common indirect Doppler technique to evaluate the arterial and venous flow. Angle correction is not necessary when obtaining an RI. The sweep speed can be increased, which will help spread the waveform over a period of 2 to 3 seconds. This helps magnify a particular part of the waveform for better interrogation and a more accurate measurement. A low RI can be a strong indicator

of a proximal stenosis that may not be able to be otherwise identified. A high RI may indicate rejection, renal venous congestion, or chronic small vessel disease. These vessels are small in size and magnifying the image may help with visualization. Color images of the renal artery (RA) and renal vein (RV) should be included. Adjusting the color scale appropriately is important so areas of aliasing can be identified in the areas of the highest velocities. When evaluating the RA, it is critical to angle correct with pulsed-wave Doppler to accurately assess for stenosis or else a falsely elevated velocity may be obtained. The sonographer should document the transplanted renal artery similar to a native renal artery, including spectral Doppler with velocity measurements in the distal, mid, and proximal RA and at the anastomosis between the iliac artery and RA. The iliac artery and vein at the anastomosis and proximal to it should be evaluated and documented with spectral Doppler as well. If a stenosis is present, the anastomotic sites are the most common location. Some patients may have peripheral vascular disease, and an inflow stenosis may be identified affecting flow into the kidney allograft. A stenosis may undergo a balloon angioplasty with possible stent placement (Figure 20-33). For all spectral

A normal RI in the arcuate artery is in the range of 0.60 to 0.70 with borderline values between 0.70 and 0.80. The RV drains the kidney showing flow below the baseline with a blue color. The spectral waveform of the RV and iliac vein has continuous monophasic flow with minimal respiratory changes. The iliac artery and CFA should demonstrate a triphasic waveform with spectral Doppler imaging (Figure 20-37). When measuring velocities using spectral Doppler imaging, turbulence or any doubling or tripling of velocities in the vessel from one location to the next should not be seen.

Renal Allograft Imaging in the Immediate Postoperative Period

It is imperative to image the newly transplanted kidney in the immediate postoperative period. Ultrasound is routinely used for this initial examination. The cost of sonography imaging is relatively low compared with CT or MRI and without the use of ionizing radiation. A skilled sonographer can provide pertinent images to the physician to help aid in diagnosis and transplant complications. Emergent findings can be treated quickly when the patient is routinely monitored with imaging.

During the postoperative ultrasound examination, the patient will be in the recovery unit while the general anesthesia is wearing off. As a result, these patients will not be able to roll onto their side or help assist with their breathing. Sometimes the patient may become combative or confused. Reassure the patient that surgery is over and he or she is recovering. One of the common statements from patients is that they need to urinate. Again, reassure these patients that they are okay and that they have a catheter in place to help them. The nurses can give a medication to relieve this sensation as well. It is very helpful to have the patient's bandages taken off. This helps obtain the best imaging windows possible and prevents missing pathology.

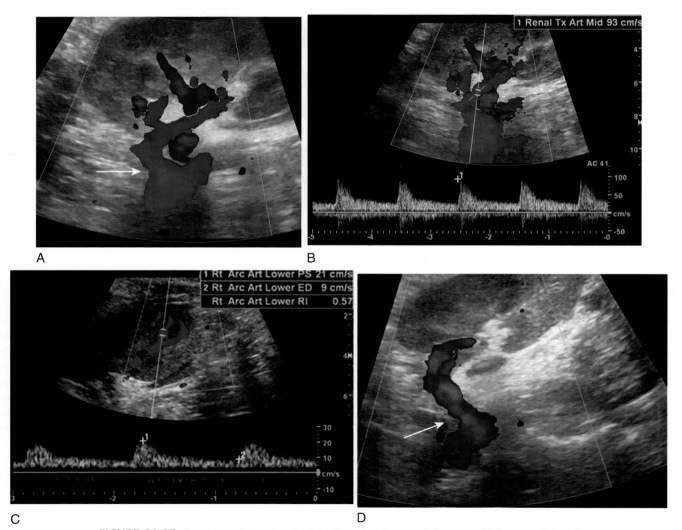

FIGURE 20-37 **Normal renal Doppler. A,** Color Doppler ultrasound shows a widely patent RA and anastomosis site without evidence of narrowing or focal stenosis. **B,** Spectral Doppler ultrasound shows a normal RA waveform with a sharp systolic upstroke and continuous diastolic flow without elevated velocities. **C,** Spectral Doppler ultrasound of the renal lower pole arcuate artery shows a normal RI with a sharp systolic upstroke and continuous diastolic flow. **D,** Color Doppler ultrasound shows a widely patent RV and anastomosis site draining the kidney without evidence of narrowing or focal stenosis.

Continued

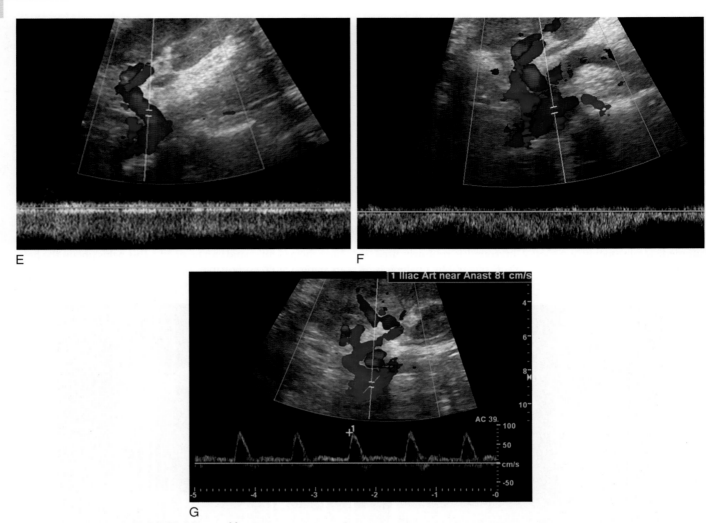

FIGURE 20-37, cont'd E, Spectral Doppler ultrasound of the RV near the anastomosis shows continuous monophasic flow. **F,** Spectral Doppler ultrasound of the iliac vein shows continuous monophasic flow. **G,** CFA on spectral Doppler ultrasound shows a triphasic waveform without elevated velocities.

Although this is not a sterile scanning environment, using sterile gel while the patient's incisions are healing can potentially reduce the risk of infection. It is common to have a member of the transplant team or surgeon present for this examination. The physician wants to ensure the allograft has adequate arterial and venous flow and look for signs of hemorrhage. If there is an urgent complication noted, the surgeon could transfer the patient back to the operating room to correct the concerning issue immediately. Not all complications are considered urgent, and the radiologist likely will recommend a follow-up ultrasound within 24 hours to ensure stability or determine whether the issue has resolved or is getting worse. Urgent findings include the following: (1) RA severe stenosis or kinking of vessel affecting the flow within the renal parenchyma; (2) RA, RV, CFA, iliac artery or vein thrombus, or occlusion; or (3) an identified source of active bleeding. It is very common to see postoperative fluid collections and these usually are self-limited and resolve on their own. Fluid collections will be monitored in serial ultrasound examinations making sure they are not enlarging or causing renal function problems. Another common finding

involves the vasculature. Postoperative edema can create elevated blood flow velocities within the RA or RV and the arcuate arteries can have an elevated RI as well, demonstrating little or no diastolic flow. Once the edema decreases, the vessels usually return to a normal appearance. Once the ultrasound examination has been completed, remember to redress the incision with clean bandages or ask the patient's nurse to help assist. If the patient is stable and no complications arise during the recovery in the transplant unit, the patient is typically discharged from the hospital on postoperative day 3.

Renal Transplantation Complications in Routine Surveillance

It is common to perform routine protocol parenchymal biopsies around 4 months after transplantation followed by 1 year, 5 years, and 10 years. If the patient is symptomatic with pain, fever, or elevated creatinine, a biopsy may be ordered sooner. If a virus or rejection is discovered from the pathology results, the patient will be treated with medication for 1 month

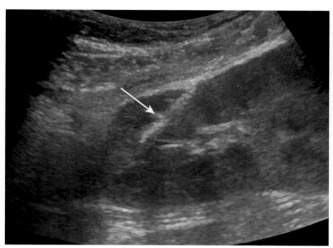

FIGURE 20-38 Normal routine renal biopsy. Ultrasound-guided needle biopsy is aimed in the lateral renal cortex of the upper pole.

and then another biopsy will take place to evaluate the treatment plan (Figure 20-38).

Biopsy complications may occur, with bleeding being the most common. The patient's INR and platelet counts are checked immediately before the biopsy. Patients are asked to stop taking anticoagulants 3 to 5 days before the procedure. Elevated blood pressure or hypertension is also a risk factor for bleeding. Some patients with known hypertension should take their antihypertensive medication as usual. Patients may come to the department showing anxiety. This may elevate the blood pressure as well. Pressures should not exceed 160/90 mm Hg. The radiologist or physician performing the biopsy may administer mild to moderate sedation to help relax the patient reducing the blood pressure. Even after preventive measures, bleeding may still occur. A hematoma can form outside of the kidney capsule, and the patient may or may not develop pain (Figure 20-39). Most bleeds will stop on their own after applying moderate pressure over the biopsy tract. If the bleeding is severe, the patient may become vasovagal and the blood pressure may drop. The patient's head should be lowered and saline fluids given. If there is active bleeding that cannot be controlled, the patient may be transferred to the interventional radiology department for further imaging and possible coil embolization (Figure 20-40).

The biopsy needle is ultrasound guided to avoid major blood vessels and the collecting system. At times, the needle path may cross small vessels for a potential risk of creating an AVF. Inadvertent damage to the collecting system or ureter can also create a urine leak forming a urinoma. The radiologist will typically aim as lateral as possible within the cortex to retrieve enough glomeruli for the pathologist to evaluate while staying away from the renal hilum. Creating an AVF occurs in about 10% of patients. Depending on size and renal function, the AVF may be routinely followed or may be treated with embolization. Spectral Doppler will demonstrate a high velocity with a low resistive waveform. The renal vein will typically show arterialization near the fistula site[32] (Figure 20-41).

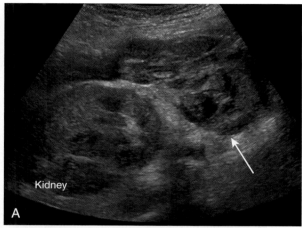

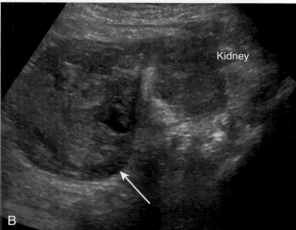

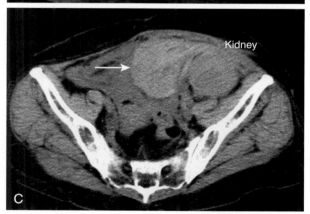

FIGURE 20-39 Renal biopsy hematoma complication. A, Longitudinal gray-scale ultrasound shows a large hematoma that followed a renal biopsy. **B,** Transverse gray-scale ultrasound shows a large hematoma that occurred after a renal biopsy. **C,** CT imaging shows a large hematoma following a renal biopsy.

Pathology of the Renal Transplant

Rejection and Acute Tubular Necrosis. Causes of graft dysfunction include rejection, acute tubular necrosis (ATN), and drug nephrotoxicity. Chronic parenchymal disease and chronic rejection will eventually lead to renal failure. The most common complications immediately postoperative and within

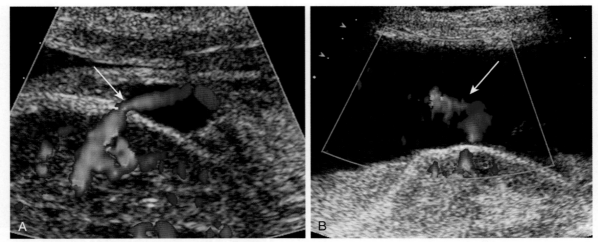

FIGURE 20-40 Renal biopsy active bleeding complication. A, Color Doppler ultrasound shows an active bleeding site along the biopsy tract into the abdomen. **B,** Color Doppler ultrasound shows an active site of bleeding in a patient with ascites that could not be controlled by applying pressure to the biopsy site.

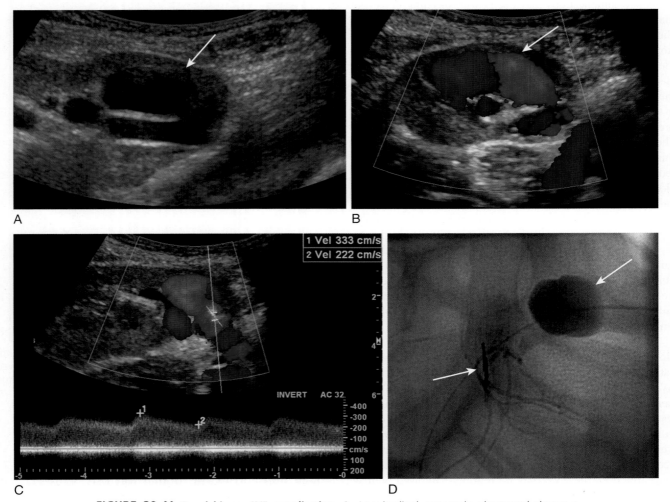

FIGURE 20-41 Renal biopsy AVF complication. A, Longitudinal gray-scale ultrasound shows a large AVF of the lower renal pole caused from a biopsy site. **B,** Transverse color Doppler ultrasound shows the flow within the AVF. **C,** Spectral Doppler ultrasound shows a low resistive waveform and the elevated velocity within the AVF. **D,** Interventional radiology shows a large AVF using coil embolization as treatment.

the first year of transplantation are acute rejection and ATN. The kidney will usually be enlarged and edematous. A nonspecific finding of elevated RIs between 0.80 and 0.90 can be an indicator of dysfunction. A biopsy is required for diagnosis and differentiation of other pathologies. In the early stages following transplantation, acute rejection is the most common cause of hypertension. About 50% of patients will develop hypertension after receiving their kidney transplant[32] (Figure 20-42).

Infection and Abscesses. More than 80% of renal transplant recipients develop at least one infection within the first

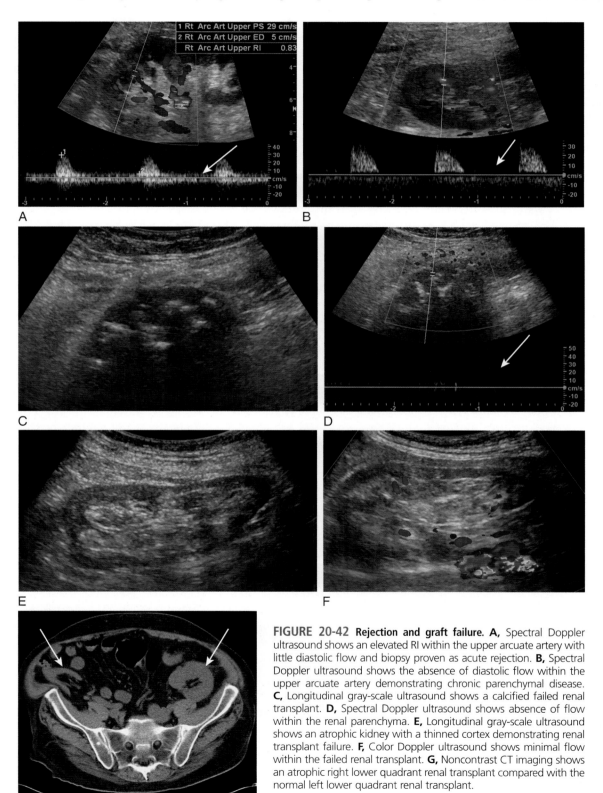

FIGURE 20-42 Rejection and graft failure. A, Spectral Doppler ultrasound shows an elevated RI within the upper arcuate artery with little diastolic flow and biopsy proven as acute rejection. **B,** Spectral Doppler ultrasound shows the absence of diastolic flow within the upper arcuate artery demonstrating chronic parenchymal disease. **C,** Longitudinal gray-scale ultrasound shows a calcified failed renal transplant. **D,** Spectral Doppler ultrasound shows absence of flow within the renal parenchyma. **E,** Longitudinal gray-scale ultrasound shows an atrophic kidney with a thinned cortex demonstrating renal transplant failure. **F,** Color Doppler ultrasound shows minimal flow within the failed renal transplant. **G,** Noncontrast CT imaging shows an atrophic right lower quadrant renal transplant compared with the normal left lower quadrant renal transplant.

year. These can include pneumonia, wound infections, or urinary tract infections. Patients may present with fever or pain over the allograft. Peritransplant abscesses are uncommon and usually occur within the first few weeks after transplantation. These may be treated with percutaneous drain placement along with antibiotics. Any peritransplant fluid collection should be considered infected in the symptomatic patient. Acute pyelonephritis can also mimic acute rejection. Focal pyelonephritis can be an isolated area of increased or decreased echogenicity with nonspecific findings. Emphysematous pyelonephritis contains gas within the collecting system. The gas produces shadowing or reverberation artifacts. Fungus balls may also been seen within the collecting system. These masses appear echogenic with weak shadowing. Debris or low-level echoes within a dilated

collecting system suggests pyonephrosis in a patient who presents with fever[33] (Figure 20-43).

Urinary Obstruction and Stones. Urinary obstruction is seen in about 2% of renal transplant recipients and almost always within the first 6 months after transplantation. The most common site of obstruction is at the site of ureteral implantation into the bladder. Ureteral stenoses are found in the distal third in more than 90% of these patients. Narrowing distally may be due to scarring caused from ischemia or rejection, surgical technique, or kinking. Other causes of obstruction include pelvic fibrosis, stones, papillary necrosis, fungus balls, clots, or extrinsic compression from a mass or fluid collection. Clinically the patient will have elevated creatinine levels making it difficult to distinguish from chronic rejection. Ultrasound is very sensitive for detecting hydronephrosis, the

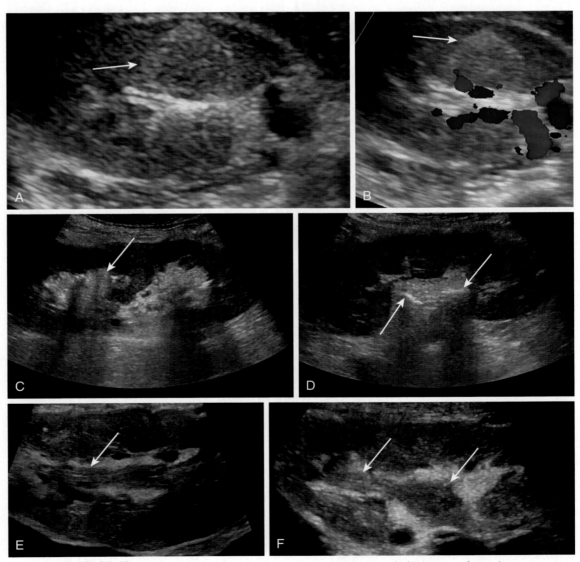

FIGURE 20-43 Renal infection. A, Transverse gray-scale ultrasound shows an echogenic area demonstrating focal pyelonephritis that can mimic a mass. **B,** Color Doppler ultrasound shows no flow within the focally infected area. **C** and **D,** Longitudinal gray-scale ultrasound shows gas within the collecting system creating shadowing and demonstrating emphysematous pyelonephritis. **E** and **F,** Longitudinal gray-scale ultrasound shows thick debris and pus within the collecting system demonstrating pyonephrosis in the febrile patient.

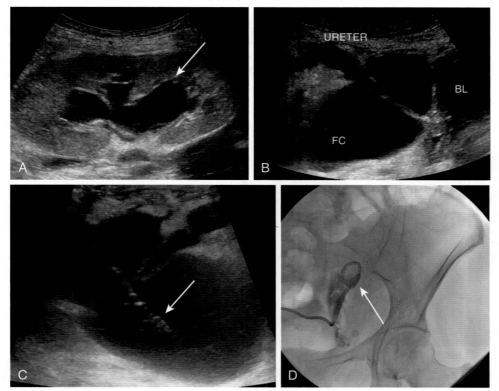

FIGURE 20-44   Urinary obstruction. A, Longitudinal gray-scale ultrasound shows moderate hydro-nephrosis. **B,** Gray-scale ultrasound shows a pelvic fluid collection compressing the ureter. **C,** Ultra-sound guided drain placement into the fluid collection. **D,** Sinogram performed to check drain placement.

dilation of the urinary collecting system (Figure 20-44). A percutaneous nephrostomy tube helps relieve the obstruction allowing for balloon dilation and stent placement. Dilation is successful in 90% of cases and may prevent the need for long-term stent placement, which can increase the risk of infection in the immunocompromised patient. Stents are usually removed after 10 days.[32,33]

Renal transplant recipients are at a higher risk for developing urinary calculi. If the patient's renal function is quickly declining, renal stones are considered. About 1% to 2% of patients develop a significant stone and require treatment. Percutaneous neph-rostolithotomy or electrohydraulic lithotripsy may be used.[33] Stones and calculi can usually be visualized on ultrasound if large enough. You will visualize echogenic foci within the collecting system, ureter, or bladder, which may demonstrate shadowing or "twinkle" artifact on color Doppler imaging (Figure 20-45).

Vascular Compromise

Renal Vein Stenosis and Thrombosis. Renal vein thrombosis is a rare complication that usually occurs within the first week of transplantation and is seen in less than 5% of pa-tients. Clinical concerns include low urinary output and pain or swelling over the renal allograft. Slow flow, extrinsic compres-sion, or a narrowing at the anastomosis may be a precursor to develop thrombus. On gray-scale imaging, the kidney may be edematous from venous congestion, and thrombus may be visualized within the vein lumen. On color and spectral Doppler,

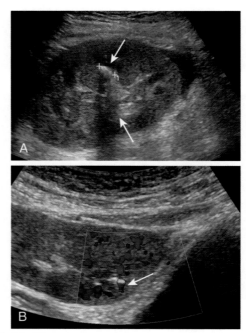

FIGURE 20-45   Renal stones. A, Longitudinal gray-scale ultra-sound shows a stone with posterior shadowing. **B,** Color Doppler ultrasound shows "twinkle" artifact associated with the renal stone.

there will be absence of flow within the vein. There will often be increased resistance within the arterial system and demonstrate reversal of diastolic flow on spectral Doppler. Nonocclusive thrombus may also be observed with little venous flow along with a monophasic waveform (Figure 20-46). CT or MRI may be helpful in diagnosis if thrombus is not directly visualized. Acute renal vein thrombosis is an urgent finding and the patient should undergo thrombectomy to avoid allograft loss. Infarction

may occur due to late diagnosis and a nephrectomy may ultimately be required to prevent subsequent infection.[32,33] Renal vein stenosis usually occurs near the anastomosis site. The sonographer should look for color aliasing and doubling velocities within the vein on spectral Doppler. This should be routinely monitored to ensure stability or resolution. Commonly this is visualized in the immediate postoperative state due to surrounding soft tissue edema (Figure 20-47).

Renal Artery Stenosis and Thrombosis. Renal artery stenosis is one of the most common vascular complications and usually occurs within the first year following transplantation. The stenosis may be related to the surgical technique and occur at the anastomosis or may be caused from atherosclerosis in the donor artery. The artery may also have a kink due to positioning. About 80% of end-stage renal disease patients develop hypertension. After transplantation, nearly two thirds have improvement in their hypertension.[33] Patients who have multiple renal arteries have a slight increased risk of stenosis.[32] On ultrasound imaging, color flow will demonstrate aliasing in the area of stenosis. Blood flow velocities exceeding 250 cm/sec and an RA to iliac artery ratio above 3.0 strongly suggest stenosis.

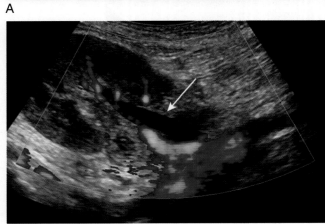

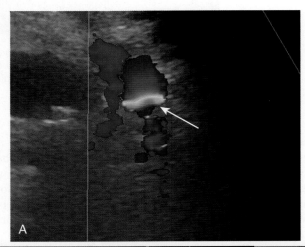

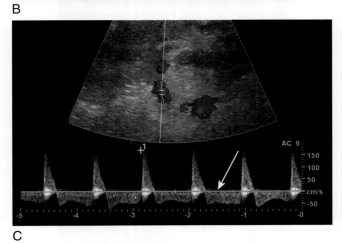

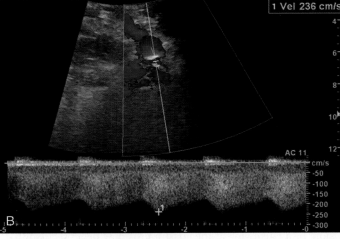

FIGURE 20-46 Renal vein thrombosis. A, Longitudinal gray-scale ultrasound shows an echogenic edematous kidney demonstrating venous congestion. **B,** Power Doppler ultrasound shows absence of flow within the RV. **C,** Spectral Doppler ultrasound within the RA shows reversal of diastolic flow consistent with RV thrombosis.

FIGURE 20-47 Renal vein stenosis. A, Color Doppler ultrasound shows aliasing within the RV near the anastomosis. **B,** Elevated velocities are visualized indicating a narrowing within the RV on spectral Doppler ultrasound.

Tardus parvus arcuate artery waveforms are indicative of a proximal stenosis as well. Within the immediate postoperative period, it is common to visualize elevated blood flow velocities due to soft tissue edema, but this usually resolves within a few days and does not usually affect renal function. This should be routinely monitored to ensure stability or resolution. Treatment of choice when needed is percutaneous transluminal angioplasty with or without stent placement. Success rates have been seen in 73% of patients. This typically reduces blood pressure and creatinine levels in 1 day[33] (Figure 20-48). Arterial thrombus and thrombosis is a rare but very severe complication that usually leads to renal allograft loss. Early detection within 24 hours can salvage the transplant using fibrinolysis treatment.[34]

Infarction and Necrosis. Segmental infarction within the transplant is a result of vascular thrombosis, hyperacute rejection, kinking of the artery, dissection, or anastomotic occlusion (Figure 20-49). Patients present with no urinary output and may have swelling or pain over the allograft. Infarcts may be diffuse or focal and have a hypoechoic wedge-shaped appearance on ultrasound. No color flow is visualized within the infarcted area. Power Doppler is useful in detecting slow flow. With complete vascular obstruction, there will be no arterial or venous flow identified within the renal transplant. Early detection is crucial to salvage the allograft by means of interventional or surgical techniques.[32,33]

Pseudoaneurysms. A pseudoaneurysm is a focal disruption of the artery with no direct communication with a vein and can occur in any vessel. On ultrasound, a pseudoaneurysm appears as a round cystic structure and demonstrates disorganized "yin-yang" color flow within. On spectral Doppler imaging, a to-and-fro waveform may be noted. A pseudoaneurysm can be due to surgical technique, trauma, or infection. Depending on size and location, these can be observed over time or treated surgically.[32]

Fluid Collections

Bleeding and Hematomas. It is common for patients to develop a hematoma, a collection of blood, in the immediate postoperative period with an overall incidence of 4% to 8%. Hematomas may also be caused from trauma or at a biopsy site and these usually resolve on their own.[35] Subcapsular hematomas may compress the parenchyma and affect renal function[32] (Figure 20-50). Large hematomas may displace the kidney or cause compression of the ureter, and hydronephrosis may develop. On ultrasound,

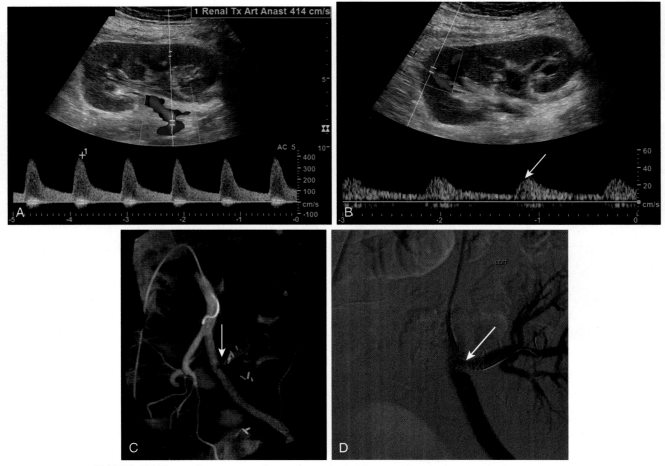

FIGURE 20-48 Renal artery stenosis. A, Elevated velocities near the RA anastomotic site are seen on spectral Doppler ultrasound. **B,** The upper arcuate artery shows a tardus parvus waveform with a dampened systolic upstroke on spectral Doppler ultrasound. **C,** Three-dimensional angiography shows a severe RA stenosis near the anastomosis. **D,** Interventional radiology successfully placed an RA stent for treatment.

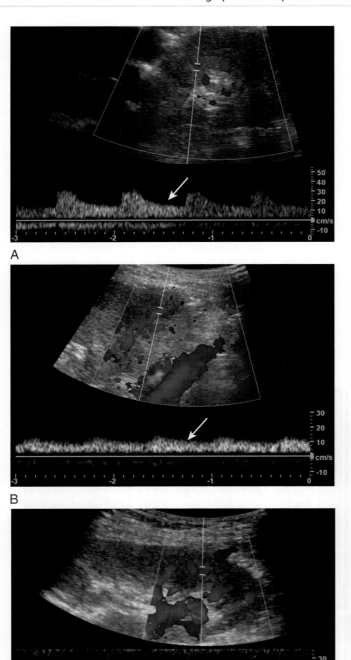

A

B

C

FIGURE 20-49 Surgical ligation of an accessory RA. A, Spectral Doppler ultrasound of a normal upper arcuate artery. **B,** Spectral Doppler ultrasound of the lower pole arcuate artery shows a low RI with high diastolic flow. **C,** Spectral Doppler ultrasound of the lower pole arcuate artery on a follow-up examination appears to return to normal as collateral flow helped establish more flow.

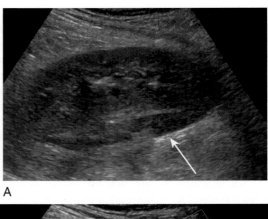

A

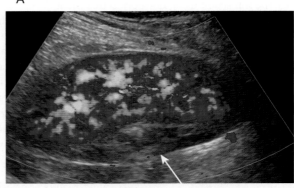

B

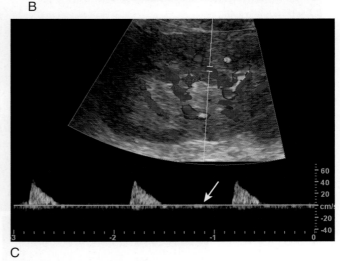

C

FIGURE 20-50 Hematoma. A, Longitudinal gray-scale ultrasound shows a subcapsular hematoma posteriorly. **B,** Longitudinal power Doppler ultrasound shows mass effect on the renal parenchyma. **C,** Spectral Doppler ultrasound of the mid arcuate artery shows no diastolic flow consistent with impaired renal function.

hematomas appear as a complex fluid collection and may have debris or septations. Fresh blood has an echogenic appearance whereas old hematomas become anechoic. If an infectious source is suspected, an aspiration can be obtained. If there is no infection present, drain placement is typically not recommended, as there is an increased risk of infection.[33]

Seromas. Seromas are clear, serous fluid collections that are typically found within the early postoperative period and are most common along the vascular anastomoses sites. A seroma will usually resolve on its own with no treatment. If there is concern that the fluid collection is infected or if it is creating a mass effect on the vasculature or the ureter, an aspiration may be performed. A seroma is a round, localized, anechoic, thin-walled fluid collection, which may contain debris or septations on ultrasound imaging. Ultrasound is very sensitive to diagnose a fluid collection but it remains difficult to determine the contents. CT or MRI may be helpful in differentiating the collections[13] (Figure 20-51).

Lymphoceles. The most common peritransplant fluid collection is a lymphocele occurring in 0.5% to 20% of cases. These are usually an early complication seen within the first 2 months following transplantation but can also develop years later. A surgical disruption of lymphatic channels causes lymph fluid leakage into the soft tissue space, creating a lymphocele. These are typically found medial to the transplant and are the most common fluid collection that causes hydronephrosis. Lymphoceles may also compress the iliac or femoral vein, causing leg edema.[33] On ultrasound imaging, you may see debris or septations within the fluid collection. Ultrasound is very sensitive to diagnose a fluid collection but as with other fluid collections is not specific for the contents.[13] Spontaneous resolution is rare. Treatment includes percutaneous drain placement in conjunction with sclerotherapy with a 97% success rate. Frequent aspirations increase the risk of infection and may require a drain placement along with antibiotic medications. Lymphoceles commonly recur after simple aspiration and ultimately may need surgical repair[33] (Figure 20-52).

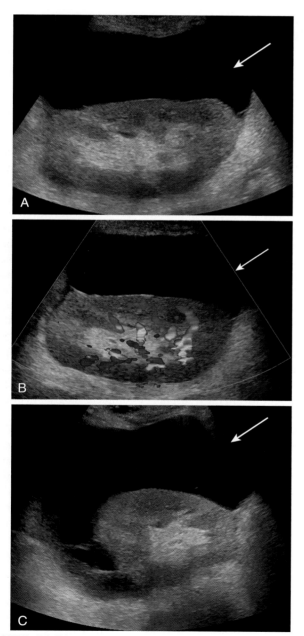

FIGURE 20-51 **Seroma. A,** Longitudinal gray-scale ultrasound shows a simple fluid collection anterior to a echogenic kidney. **B,** Color Doppler ultrasound shows absence of flow within the collection. **C,** Transverse gray-scale ultrasound demonstrates a mostly simple seroma with some debris.

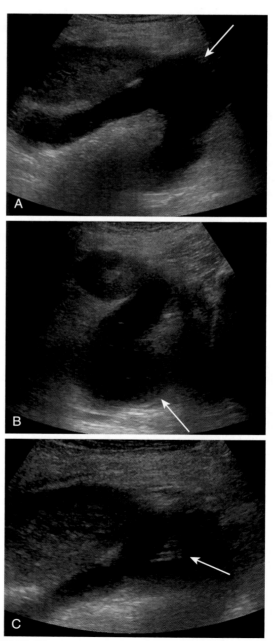

FIGURE 20-52 **Lymphocele. A,** Longitudinal gray-scale ultrasound shows a fluid collection with minimal debris. **B,** Transverse gray-scale ultrasound shows a fluid collection with minimal debris. **C,** Ultrasound-guided drain placement within the recurrent lymphocele.

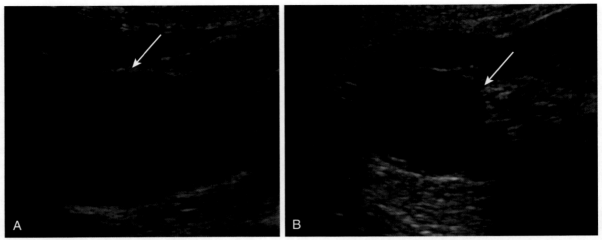

FIGURE 20-53 **Urinoma. A,** Longitudinal gray-scale ultrasound shows a simple fluid collection with no debris or septations. **B,** Transverse gray-scale ultrasound shows a simple fluid collection medial to the transplant.

Urine Leak and Urinomas. Urine leaks and urinomas are rare complications and usually found within the first 2 weeks after transplantation. Urine may leak from the renal pelvis, ureter, or ureteroneocystostomy site due to ureteral necrosis. Urine seeps into the peritoneal cavity forming a contained fluid collection, a urinoma. Urinomas can vary in size and are typically visualized between the kidney and bladder. On ultrasound, a urinoma appears as an anechoic, well-defined fluid collection with no septations, and rapidly increases in size (Figure 20-53). The patent may present with little or no urine output and have fullness or pain over the allograft. Large urinomas may rupture, creating urinary abdominal ascites and increasing the risk for infection and abscess formation. Early detection and treatment reduces the patient mortality rate. Treatment includes ultrasound-guided aspiration and percutaneous nephrostomy tube and stent placement. Stents should remain in place for 6 to 8 weeks to allow complete healing of the ureter. If the ureter fails to heal, ureteral reimplantation may be necessary.[33]

Renal Cell Carcinoma. Renal cell carcinoma (RCC) is rare within a renal transplant. Renal transplant tumors may be transmitted from donors, metastasis from the native kidneys, or new carcinomas arising after transplantation. A study reported 4.6% of posttransplant cancers were found to be renal carcinomas with 10% within the allograft itself.[36] Long-term immunosuppression increases the risk 100 times the normal risk for developing a malignancy and occurs in about 6% of patients. The most common malignances are skin cancers and lymphoma. Patients with glomerulopathy and recurrent glomerulonephritis cause microhematuria and increase the risk of developing neoplasms. Ultrasound imaging of renal cell carcinomas typically demonstrates a solid heterogeneous mass with a well-defined border that may contain cystic components in some cases. CT or MRI may be helpful in diagnosis. It is recommended that the native kidney be evaluated when an RCC is suspected. A final diagnosis can be made performing a mass biopsy.

Treatment includes removal of the renal allograft or percutaneous ablation[33] (Figure 20-54).

Transitional Cell Carcinoma. Transitional cell carcinoma (TCC) of the urinary tract occurs more often in the transplanted patient compared with the general population and is seen in about 0.07% to 1.9% of patients. TCC is rare within the transplanted patient and only a few cases have been published. The BK virus and human papillomavirus (HPV) have been shown to carry an increased risk of TCC. Most of these tumors are found within the bladder, but can occur anywhere along the urinary tract. TCC within the transplanted patient tend to be more aggressive, rapidly progressive, poorly differentiated, and more fatal in comparison with the general population. Ultrasound may note an irregular mass within the bladder demonstrating vascular flow (Figure 20-55). Final diagnosis is typically made with cystoscopy and biopsy. Treatments may include a radical cystectomy or nephroureterectomy in cases that involve the native upper tract. If TCC is present within the transplant, a complete allograft nephrectomy needs to be performed.[37]

Posttransplant Lymphoproliferative Disorder. PTLD occurs in 1% to 20% of patients who receive a transplant. In one study, PTLD was found to occur in 0.8% of renal transplant patients.[22] PTLD is the most severe complication found in solid organ and stem cell transplantation. Patients who are taking immunosuppressant medication increase the risk of malignancies 2 to 5 times more than the general population. PTLD can present as benign reactive hyperplasia of tissue to fulminant lymphoma. Most polymorphic masses are caused by the Epstein-Barr virus (EBV) occurring 60% to 80% and within 1 year of transplantation. Most of the monomorphic masses are found to be non-Hodgkin's lymphoma and have B-cell origin. Reducing immunosuppressant drugs is a recommended treatment in those patients with EBV-induced PTLD, effective in 23% to 50% of cases. Some patients may not positively respond to the reduction of immunosuppression, therefore immunotherapy with monoclonal antibodies

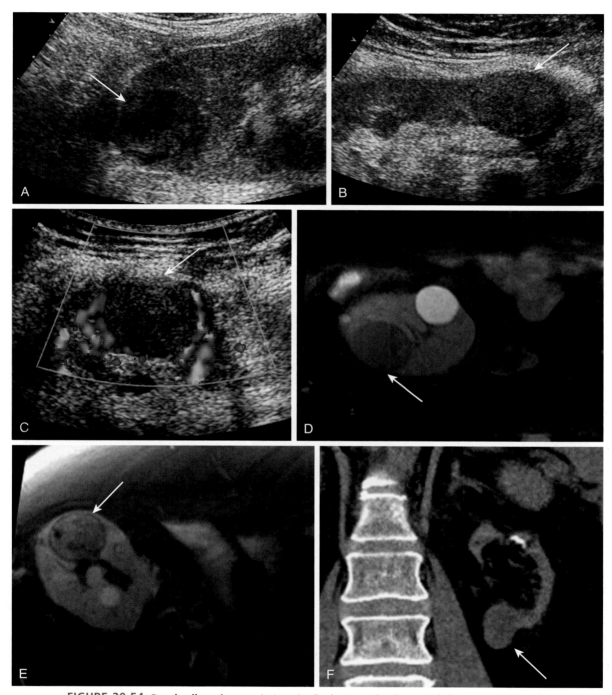

FIGURE 20-54 Renal cell carcinoma. A, Longitudinal gray-scale ultrasound shows an upper pole solid hypoechoic mass. **B,** A lower pole solid mass is also seen on longitudinal gray-scale ultrasound. **C,** Color Doppler ultrasound shows splaying of vascularity around one of the masses. **D,** MRI shows the upper pole mass. **E,** The lower pole mass is visualized on MRI. **F,** After metastatic RCC was found in the renal transplant, CT shows a suspicious solid mass within the left native kidney on the lower pole.

such as rituximab is given. From 40% to 68% of cases have shown success using this treatment.[22] PTLD can occur in any solid organ or viscera.[32] The most common sites of involvement are the lymph nodes followed by the liver, brain, and lung. If the small intestine is involved, the patient presents with a generalized disease.[33] On ultrasound imaging, PTLD usually appears as a hypoechoic soft tissue mass and may be found near the renal hilum[32] (Figure 20-56).

Common Benign Findings. As a sonographer, the renal transplant is evaluated in a similar fashion as the native organ. The following are common findings that may be encountered within the kidney and are not specific to transplantation.

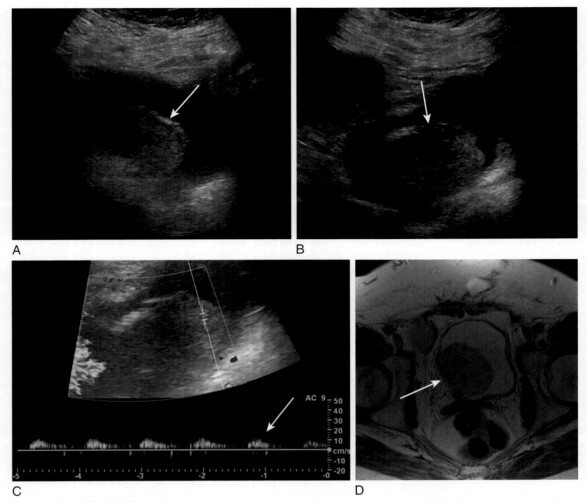

FIGURE 20-55 Transitional cell carcinoma. A, Transverse gray-scale ultrasound shows a solid hypoechoic mass with irregular borders within the bladder. **B,** Longitudinal gray-scale ultrasound of the solid bladder mass. **C,** Spectral Doppler ultrasound shows arterial vascular flow within the mass. **D,** MRI shows a large mass adhering to the bladder wall.

Cysts. Renal cysts are a common benign finding. They have well-defined margins, thin walls, and are anechoic with posterior acoustic enhancement on ultrasound examination. Some may have thin septations or demonstrate debris representing a hemorrhagic cyst. If a thick irregular wall or internal vascularity is noted, the possibility of an RCC should be raised and further evaluated with other imaging modalities or biopsy. Cysts typically remain asymptomatic and are incidental findings. Renal cysts increase with age and occur in 40% of the population who have a CT scan.[38] One study reported that cystic lesions found within the transplant did not cause dysfunction or related complications. An ultrasound or CT scan is commonly recommended for routine follow-up.[39]

Angiomyolipomas. Angiomyolipoma (AML) is the most common benign kidney lesion. It is composed of adipose tissue, smooth muscle, and vessels occurring in 0.1% to 0.22% of patients. AMLs are usually sporadic but can be associated with tuberous sclerosis, an autosomal dominant genetic disorder with other systemic findings. AMLs tend to be asymptomatic and incidental findings. AML is the second

most common cause of retroperitoneal hemorrhage due to the potential risk of rupture, especially when larger than 4 cm. On ultrasound examination, AML is highly echogenic and may produce posterior shadowing. Treatment is usually not necessary unless the lesion is large enough for potential rupture or to cause renal failure. Embolization is the treatment of choice. An AML should not be a contraindication as a renal transplant donor.[40]

PANCREATIC TRANSPLANT

Surgical Technique of the Pancreatic Transplant

The pancreas can be preserved up to 12 hours on ice and using a special preservation solution (e.g., UW, HTK, or Celsior). Shorter ischemic time leads to better allograft function. For every transplant, the donor and recipient are rechecked to verify a match. The blood type and compatibility need to be confirmed, as well as the UNOS database per protocol. Before

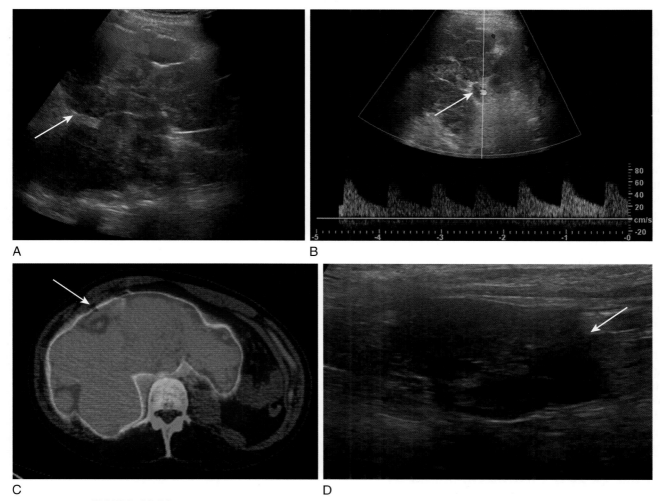

A

B

C

D

FIGURE 20-56 Posttransplant lymphoproliferative disease. **A,** Transverse gray-scale ultrasound shows a large solid mass with irregular margins in the right lower quadrant. **B,** Spectral Doppler ultrasound shows arterial blood flow within the mass. **C,** PET/CT shows a large mass with FDG avid uptake in the right lower quadrant. **D,** Longitudinal gray-scale ultrasound shows an overall decreased size of the mass after chemotherapy treatment.

coming into the operating room, the team will discuss the risks, benefits, and alternatives with the patient and obtain consent. All institutions have certain protocols and techniques they follow. Every patient has a unique situation, and the surgeons have different techniques they prefer.

Cadaveric Pancreatic Donation. The patient is brought into the operating room confirming patient identification and procedure to be performed. Following general anesthesia and line placement, a Foley catheter is placed into the bladder. The abdomen is prepped and draped sterilely. A primary midline incision is made. The subcutaneous tissues and rectus fascia are divided to enter the peritoneum, and the colon is mobilized to the hepatic flexure. The surgeon may choose a right lower quadrant or a left lower quadrant location. The right lower quadrant is typically the preferred choice. The distal vena cava (IVC) and common iliac artery and vein are dissected free from surrounding tissues.

The back bench table preparation includes performing a splenectomy, oversewing the stapled ends of the duodenum

and the root of the mesentery using running sutures. The portal vein, superior mesenteric artery (SMA), and splenic artery (SA) are dissected free from surrounding tissues. A donor iliac artery bifurcation (Y graft) is anastomosed to the SMA and SA using continuous sutures. Once prepared, the pancreas is repacked and placed on ice containing UW solution while awaiting transplantation.

Before vascular clamps are placed, the patient receives intravenous heparin. An end-to-side anastomosis is created between the donor portal vein and the recipient common iliac vein and IVC confluence. An end-to-side anastomosis is created between the common channel of the iliac Y graft and the common iliac artery of the recipient using continuous sutures. The clamps are released and the pancreas is reperfused. The surgeon will carefully look at the anastomosis sites and check for bleeding. If bleeding points are identified, they are controlled using sutures. The pancreas is then laid underneath the colon. A side-to-side anastomosis is fashioned between the terminal ileum and the allograft duodenum using sutures for the outer and inner layers. If needed, a drain may be placed near the pancreas bed. Once hemostasis has been achieved, the muscular fascia is closed with running sutures, and the skin is closed using staples (Figure 20-57). Sponge, needle, and instrument counts are conducted before closure. If indicated, the patient will receive units of blood, platelets, or fresh frozen plasma. The wound is dressed with a dry sterile dressing and the patient is extubated and transferred to the recovery room and later moved into the ICU when stable.

Pancreatic Islet Cell Transplantation. Islet cells can be transplanted using minimally invasive techniques versus a full pancreatic organ transplant allowing lower morbidity rates. Clinical trials have demonstrated restoration of the beta islet cell function and subsequent insulin production to regulate the blood glucose. For an autotransplant, islet cells are retrieved from the patient and a pancreatectomy is performed due to chronic pain such as pancreatitis or, rarely, trauma. For an allotransplant, the islet cells come from a donor. These cells are isolated and purified and then the islet cell clusters are infused into the hepatic sinusoids using a catheter in the portal vein. There is risk of portal vein thrombosis during this procedure. Posttransplant limitations include not being able to image these patients to determine function. These patients are monitored checking blood glucose level, renal function, lipid levels, and liver function.[41] There have been 471 patients that have received islet cell transplants from 1999 to 2004.[42]

Evaluation of the Pancreatic Allograft

As a sonographer, the pancreas transplant is evaluated as a native pancreas would be, but with some additional Doppler imaging. Assessing the echotexture and vasculature and looking for any masses, fluid collections, or ascites are important. Institutions have their own routine protocols on timing of examinations and specific images that are required.

Once the patient has arrived to the recovery room from the surgical suite, the sonographer will go portably to perform the immediate postoperative examination. The patient's amylase, lipase, and glucose are closely monitored and if any issues arise, the transplant physicians will tailor their imaging requests. These blood values are evaluated weekly for the first 2 months, then every other week for 4 months, then monthly for 1 year, then every 3 months. The patient usually only has a follow-up ultrasound if the patient is symptomatic or develops surgical complications.

It is best to image using a 2.5- to 5.0-MHz curvilinear transducer and have the patient fasting 4 to 6 hours. Obese patients will require lower frequencies. The pancreatic transplant is placed in either the right or left lower quadrant and typically superficial. As a result, higher-frequency transducers are most commonly used. Breath holding is usually not necessary as respiratory motion is limited. Depending on location, rolling the patient left lateral decubitus or right lateral decubitus will help move overlying bowel or bring the

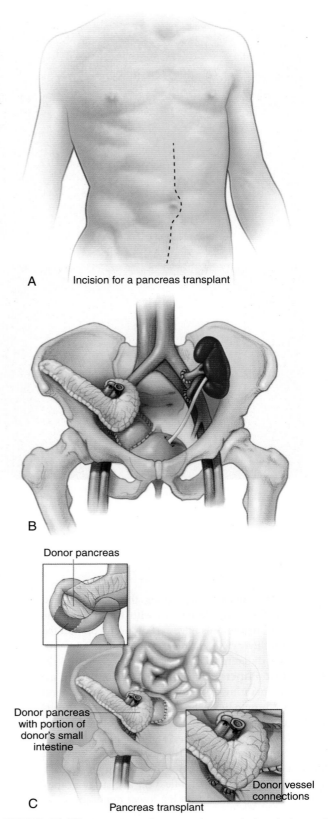

A Incision for a pancreas transplant

B

Donor pancreas

Donor pancreas with portion of donor's small intestine

Donor vessel connections

C Pancreas transplant

FIGURE 20-57 Illustrations demonstrating surgical technique of pancreatic transplantation. **A,** Incision site. **B,** The pancreas transplant is shown in relation to a possible combined renal transplant demonstrating the anastomoses sites. **C,** The pancreas transplant anastomoses are demonstrated. *(Used with permission of Mayo Foundation for Medical Education and Research. All Rights reserved.)*

pancreas to a more superficial position in the obese patient. Most of these patients are very thin due to type 1 diabetes and obesity is less likely to be a problem.

The sonographer should scan completely through the pancreas before taking any images while adjusting the frequency, depth, gain, TGCs, and focal zones. Once the pancreatic transplant has been fully accessed, the examination needs to include a few representative gray-scale longitudinal images. Gray-scale transverse images of the upper, middle, and lower thirds also need to be obtained. Document any pathology in two planes with and without measurements and include color Doppler flow. Quadrant images need to be obtained checking for free fluid or signs of bleeding.

The Doppler portion is crucial for the transplanted pancreas. Venous and arterial color and spectral Doppler needs to be obtained looking for any signs of thrombus or stenosis. Ultrasound is commonly the first method of imaging in these patients, and the skilled sonographer can help the physicians diagnose the patient and treatment will be administered quickly. Color Doppler and power Doppler should be used to ensure adequate perfusion throughout the pancreatic tissue (Figure 20-58). The intraparenchymal arteries and veins within the pancreas are evaluated in the upper, middle, and lower thirds. The sonographer should obtain an RI measurement using the peak systolic and end-diastolic velocities on these arterial waveforms. This is a common indirect Doppler

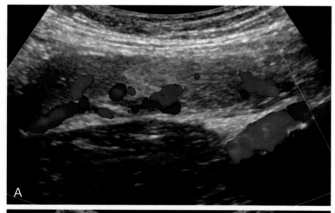

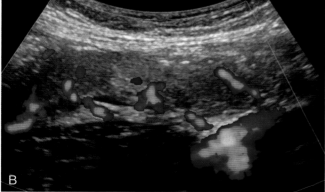

FIGURE 20-58 Pancreatic parenchymal perfusion. A, Normal perfusion using color Doppler ultrasound. **B,** Power Doppler ultrasound shows adequate perfusion.

technique to evaluate the arterial and venous flow. Angle correction is not necessary while obtaining the RI. Adjusting the sweep speed will spread the waveform over a period of 2 to 3 seconds, which will help magnify a particular part of your waveform for better interrogation and a more accurate measurement. A low RI is a strong indicator of a proximal stenosis that might not otherwise be able to be identified. A high RI may indicate rejection or venous congestion. Color images of the pancreatic artery and pancreatic vein should be included. Adjusting the color scale appropriately will help identify the highest velocities. When evaluating the pancreatic artery, it is critical to angle correct with pulsed-wave Doppler to accurately assess for stenosis. Spectral Doppler with velocity measurements in the distal, mid, proximal pancreatic artery and at the anastomosis between the iliac artery and pancreatic artery should also be included. The iliac artery and vein at the anastomosis and proximal to it should be evaluated and documented with spectral Doppler as well. If color flow aliasing in the pancreatic vein or iliac vein is visualized, angle correcting during your spectral Doppler images is important and will be helpful in identifying a focal narrowing. For all spectral Doppler, the angle should be parallel to the vessel that is being sampled and less than 60 degrees to ensure an accurate velocity measurement. The common femoral artery (CFA) should be documented to ensure adequate flow to the leg. All of the waveforms should fill the spectral window while eliminating aliasing.

Slow flow may be present within the vessels, and this can make it difficult to obtain a Doppler signal at times. The sonographer should try decreasing the color Doppler scale, and increase the color gain. Using a slow flow setting such as a lower extremity vein or iliac vein model can be very useful if available on the ultrasound machine. The renal artery setting can also be helpful filling in the vessels as well. If the very slow frequencies are rejected as "cluttered noise," the wall filter needs to be decreased. If the patient is obese, decreasing the gray-scale, color, and spectral Doppler frequencies will enable deeper penetration.

Normal Sonographic Findings of the Pancreatic Transplant

On gray-scale imaging, the pancreas parenchyma should appear homogeneous and hypoechoic relative to the mesenteric fat. The pancreas will appear different than the native organ and typically it has a "blob" appearance, and the borders can be difficult to visualize at times. The bowel can be confused with the transplant at times and looking for peristalsis can help differentiate (Figure 20-59). The pancreatic duct is usually not visualized unless it is abnormally dilated. The duct should measure less than 3 mm. See Chapter 12 for a more detailed explanation of the normal pancreatic anatomy.

The Doppler portion of the transplanted pancreas examination is crucial to perform. Some vascular complications can only be diagnosed using color and spectral Doppler. The pancreatic artery (Y graft of SMA and splenic artery) will be red

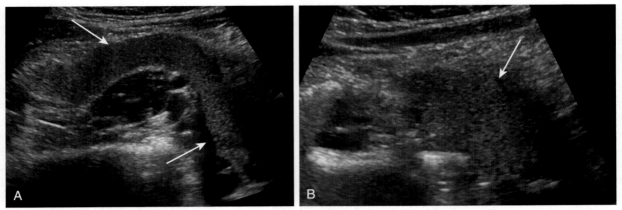

FIGURE 20-59 Normal pancreas. A, Longitudinal gray-scale ultrasound shows a normal-appearing pancreatic transplant. **B,** Transverse gray-scale ultrasound shows normal pancreatic tissue separate from the neighboring bowel loops.

on color imaging bringing flow into the pancreas, and the spectral waveform demonstrates a rapid systolic upstroke with continuous diastolic flow above baseline demonstrating a low-resistance waveform. The velocities should be below 200 cm/sec. A normal RI in the intraparenchymal artery should be below 0.80. The pancreatic vein drains the pancreas showing flow below the baseline with a blue color. The spectral waveforms of the intraparenchymal, pancreatic, and iliac vein have continuous monophasic flow with minimal respiratory changes. The iliac artery and CFA should demonstrate a classic triphasic waveform with spectral Doppler imaging. When measuring velocities using spectral Doppler imaging, turbulent flow or doubling or tripling of velocities in a vessel should not be seen as it indicates potential focal stenosis (Figure 20-60).

Pancreatic Allograft Imaging in the Immediate Postoperative Period

It is imperative to image the newly transplanted pancreas in the immediate postoperative period. Ultrasound is the initial modality of choice. There is no ionizing radiation and the cost is relatively inexpensive compared with CT or MRI. These patients will be closely monitored and scanned routinely so there will be no delay in treatment if needed. A skilled sonographer provides early detection of transplant complications and prevents misdiagnosis.

The patient will be in the recovery unit while the general anesthesia is wearing off during the initial ultrasound examination. These patients will not be able to roll onto their side or help assist with breathing techniques if needed. Sometimes the patient may be confused or combative. Reassure your patient that surgery is over and the patient is recovering. The patient's dressings should be removed to help attain the best imaging windows possible and prevent missing pathology. Even though this is not necessarily a sterile scanning environment, using sterile gel while the patient's incisions are healing can potentially reduce the risk of infection. It is common to have a member of the transplant team or a surgeon present for this examination. This is very helpful to the sonographer to understand the surgical technique performed and variant anatomy of the patient. The physician would like to ensure the allograft has adequate arterial and venous flow and look for signs of hemorrhage. If there is an urgent complication noted, the surgeon could transfer the patient back to the operating room to correct the concerning issue immediately. Not all complications are considered urgent, and the radiologist may recommend a follow-up ultrasound within 24 hours to ensure stability or determine whether the issue has resolved or is getting worse. Urgent findings include, but are not limited to, the following: severe stenosis of the pancreatic artery or kinking of the vessel affecting the flow within the pancreatic parenchyma; thrombus or occlusion of the CFA, iliac artery, or pancreatic artery or vein; or an identified source of active bleeding. It is very common to see postoperative fluid collections and these usually spontaneously resolve. Fluid collections will be monitored in serial ultrasound examinations, making sure they are not enlarging or causing pancreatic function problems. Commonly, postoperative edema can create elevated blood flow velocities within the pancreatic artery and vein, and the intraparenchymal arteries can have an elevated RI as well, demonstrating little or no diastolic flow. Once the edema decreases, the vessels return to their normal state. If the patient is stable and no complications arise during the recovery in the transplant unit, the patient is typically discharged from the hospital between postoperative days 5 and 7.

Pancreatic Transplantation Complications in Routine Surveillance

It is common to perform routine protocol parenchymal biopsies around 4 months after transplantation followed by 1 year, 5 years, and 10 years. If the patient is symptomatic with pain and fever or has elevated amylase, lipase, or glucose, a biopsy may be ordered. If rejection is discovered from the pathology results, the patient will be treated with medication for 1 month and then another biopsy will take place to evaluate the treatment plan. If the patient clinically has pancreatitis, the biopsy will not be performed, as this could potentially aggravate the pancreatic tissue more (Figure 20-61).

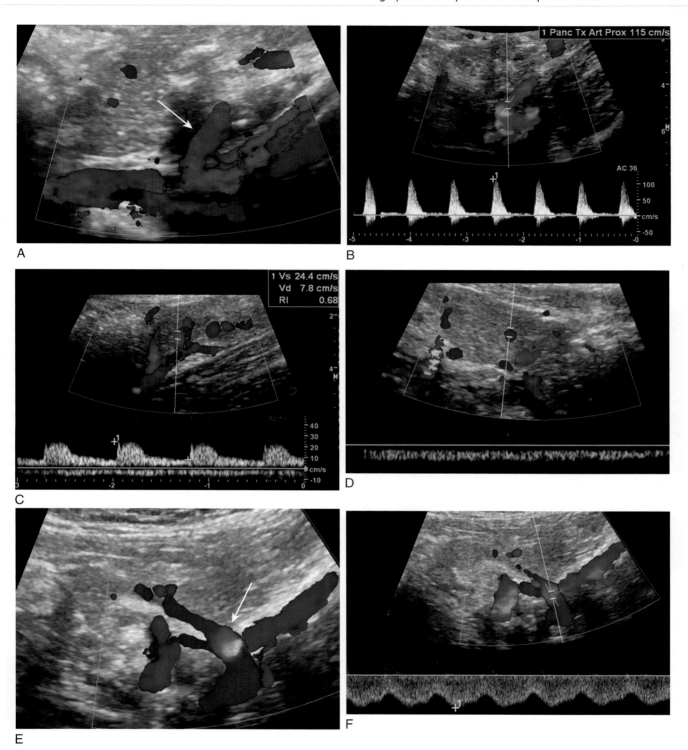

FIGURE 20-60 **Normal pancreas Doppler.** **A,** A widely patent pancreatic artery is identified without areas of aliasing or narrowing using color Doppler ultrasound. **B,** Spectral Doppler ultrasound shows a normal high resistive waveform within the pancreatic artery without presence of an elevated velocity. **C,** Spectral Doppler ultrasound of a normal waveform and RI within an intraparenchymal artery. **D,** Spectral Doppler ultrasound of a normal monophasic waveform within an intraparenchymal vein. **E,** Color Doppler ultrasound shows a normal pancreatic vein and anastomosis without evidence of aliasing or narrowing. **F,** Spectral Doppler ultrasound shows a normal monophasic venous waveform within the pancreatic vein near the anastomosis.

Continued

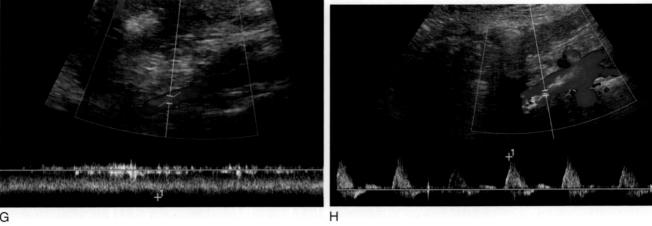

G

H

FIGURE 20-60, cont'd G, The iliac vein seen on spectral Doppler ultrasound has a normal mono-phasic venous waveform. H, The CFA visualized on spectral Doppler ultrasound has a classic triphasic waveform.

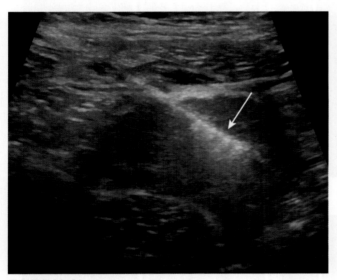

FIGURE 20-61 **Routine pancreatic biopsy.** Ultrasound-guided nee-dle biopsy staying clear of nearby bowel and pancreatic hilum.

While performing these biopsies, there are potential risks of complications. Bleeding is the most common complication observed. The patient's INR and platelet counts are checked before the procedure and patients are asked to stop taking anticoagulants 3 to 5 days before the procedure. Elevated blood pressure or hypertension is an associated risk factor for bleeding. If the patient currently takes antihypertensive medication routinely, this should be taken as usual. Patients may become anxious about the procedure, thereby elevating the blood pressure. Pressures should not exceed 160/90 mm Hg. The radiologist or physician performing the biopsy may choose to administer mild to moderate sedation to help relax the patient, reducing these pressures. Bleeding may still occur after preventive measures are taken. You may see a hematoma form outside of the pancreatic tissue, and the patient may or may not develop pain. Usually bleeding will cease on its own after applying moderate pressure over the biopsy tract. If the bleeding is severe, the patient may become vasovagal and the blood pressure may drop.

It is helpful to lower the head of the patient and give IV fluids as necessary. If there is an active bleed that cannot be controlled, the patient could be transferred to the interventional radiology department for further imaging and possible coil placement.

The biopsy needle is ultrasound guided to avoid major blood vessels and the pancreatic duct, although this can be difficult to visualize. At times the needle path may cross small vessels for a potential risk of creating an AVF, or damage to the duct can create a pancreatic leak forming a pseudocyst. The radiologist will aim away from the hilum of the pancreas and stay clear of the nearby bowel. If overlying bowel seems to be a problem, obtaining a biopsy using ultrasound guidance or CT may be beneficial to use for guidance by accurately visualizing the bowel (Figure 20-62).

Pathology of the Pancreatic Transplant

Rejection. Rejection is the primary cause of allograft loss, occurring between 5% and 25%. Hyperacute rejection is rare and occurs immediately postoperative, and causes

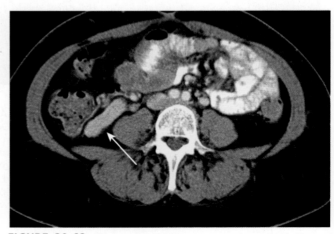

FIGURE 20-62 CT imaging of the pancreas transplant. Normal pancreatic transplant on CT covered by overlying bowel.

thrombosis and graft loss. Acute rejection usually occurs 1 to 3 weeks following transplantation. If left untreated, infarction may occur resulting from an autoimmune vasculitis. Chronic rejection is the major long-term cause of graft failure after the first 6 months, occurring in 4% to 10% of patients. It may be due to multiple episodes or partially treated acute rejection, resulting in fibrosis and atrophy of the pancreas. An elevation of serum glucose, amylase, and lipase poorly correlates with the severity of rejection. Ultrasound findings are nonspecific and may demonstrate pancreatic enlargement and a heterogeneous echotexture in the acute stages (Figure 20-63). With chronic rejection, the pancreas is markedly atrophied and may not be visualized on ultrasound (Figure 20-64). Percutaneous biopsy is required for diagnosis and grading either with ultrasound or CT guidance.[43]

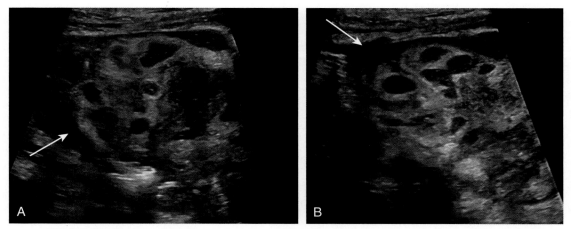

FIGURE 20-63 Acute rejection. A, Transverse gray-scale ultrasound shows an enlarged heterogeneous pancreas. **B,** An enlarged pancreas with heterogeneous echotexture is visualized on longitudinal gray-scale ultrasound.

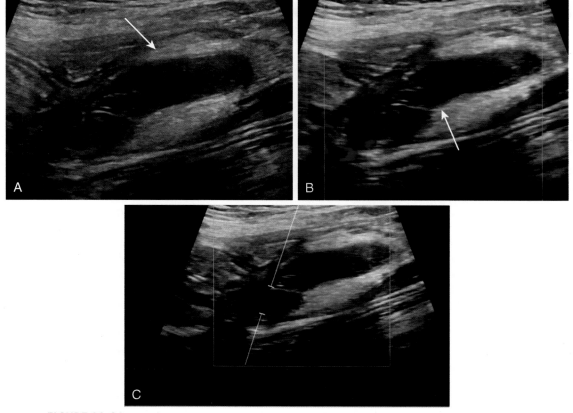

FIGURE 20-64 Chronic rejection and failure. A, Longitudinal gray-scale ultrasound shows an atrophic echogenic pancreas. **B,** Color Doppler ultrasound shows no flow within the dilated pancreatic vein. **C,** Absence of pancreatic venous flow is seen on spectral Doppler ultrasound.

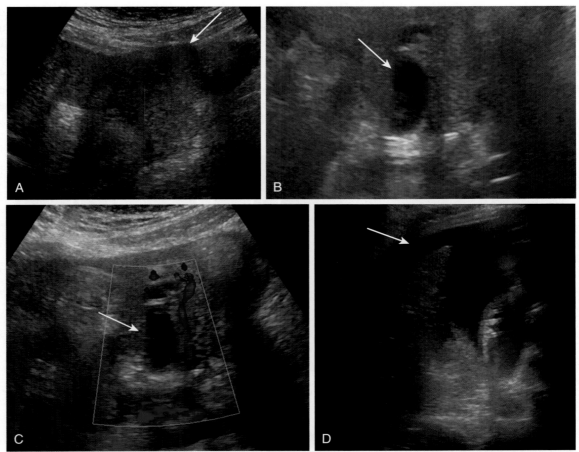

FIGURE 20-65 Pancreatitis with elevated amylase and lipase levels. A, Longitudinal gray-scale ultrasound shows mild enlargement of the inhomogeneous pancreas. **B,** Longitudinal gray-scale ultrasound shows a small fluid collection representing a pseudocyst. **C,** Color Doppler ultrasound shows no vascular flow within the collection. **D,** Gray-scale ultrasound shows new abdominal ascites.

Pancreatitis. Pancreatitis is the second most common complication following transplantation.[44] Within the first 4 weeks of transplantation, mild pancreatitis is present in about 35% of patients. This is usually caused from reperfusion injury. The patient may develop pain over the allograft, and elevated serum amylase and lipase are usually noted. Nonspecific ultrasound findings include pancreatic enlargement and heterogeneous echotexture. Ultrasound may visualize a pseudocyst, free fluid, infarction, or necrosis[43] (Figure 20-65).

Infection and Abscesses. Infection at the surgical site occurs in 50% of patients. Superficial infections are more common and can be treated with antibiotics. Deep infections are associated with greater morbidity, mortality, and allograft loss. Percutaneous drain placement is the treatment of choice for localized abscesses. An infected collection may be filled with debris or presence of gas on ultrasound creating a "dirty" shadow.[43] Abscesses typically demonstrate thicker, irregular walls, and are associated with adjacent inflammatory tissue. At times, abscess formation may be associated with enteric leakage. Hyperemia may be present within the abscess wall or surrounding soft tissue using color Doppler.[45] It is sometimes difficult to determine the contents, and aspiration is beneficial for diagnosis and treatment. CT or MRI may also be helpful aiding in diagnosis[43] (Figure 20-66).

Vascular Compromise

Pancreatic Venous and Arterial Thrombosis. Acute pancreatic transplant thrombosis occurs in 2% to 10% of patients and is more common on the venous side but can be visualized within the arterial system as well. Venous thrombosis is the second most common cause of allograft failure and is typically seen within the first 6 weeks following transplantation. Patients may present with elevated glucose and amylase, and note pain and swelling over the allograft. If detected early, the patient may be sent to the operating room to attempt to salvage the pancreas. Thrombectomy and thrombolysis are limited treatment options to short segments of thrombosis without developing necrosis. Some risk factors of thrombosis include severe pancreatitis, arterial wall injury, or superior mesenteric and splenic arterial and venous stump thrombus. Stump thrombus may be incidental and usually

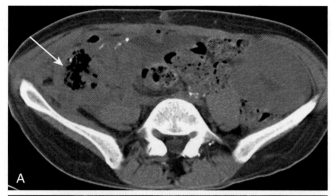
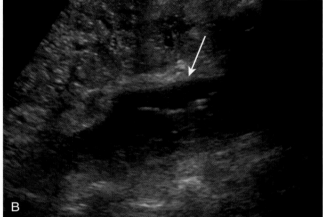

FIGURE 20-66 Abscess. A, CT imaging shows an infected collection near the pancreas transplant. **B,** Gray-scale ultrasound shows the drainage catheter within the abscess.

does not interfere with pancreatic function. If treatment is not successful or the thrombosis is found too late in the disease process, extensive thrombosis can lead to necrosis requiring an emergent pancreatectomy to reduce the risk of infection and mortality. With an arterial occlusion, collateral vessels may develop preserving the tissue and function. Echogenic thrombus filling the vessel lumen with no flow identified on color or spectral imaging is demonstrated using ultrasound. With the presence of venous thrombosis, the arterial waveforms usually demonstrate high resistance with reversal in diastole (Figures 20-67 and 20-68). If necrosis and infarction develop, the pancreas will be enlarged and hypoechoic with lack of blood flow. The pancreas may become atrophic and echogenic with chronic thrombosis and may be difficult to visualize on ultrasound. CTA or MRA may be beneficial aiding in diagnosis when the ultrasound remains inconclusive.[43]

Pancreatic Arterial and Venous Stenosis. Stenosis may uncommonly develop at the pancreatic arterial or venous anastomoses sites. Many patients are found to have peripheral vascular disease. As a result, inflow may be compromised due to a proximal stenosis. If a stenosis is identified, balloon angioplasty and stenting may be performed. The artery or vein may kink or twist on itself. As with other transplants, it is common to see elevated velocities in the

immediate postoperative examination due to edema. On ultrasound, assess for color flow aliasing and turbulence with velocity measurement doubling on spectral Doppler[43] (Figure 20-69).

Pseudoaneurysms. A pseudoaneurysm is a focal disruption of the artery with no direct communication with a vein and can occur in any vessel. On ultrasound, it appears as a round cystic structure and demonstrates disorganized "yin-yang" color flow within. On spectral Doppler imaging, a to-and-fro waveform is typically seen. These complications are rare and can be due to surgical technique, infection, pancreatitis, or biopsy. A pseudoaneurysm is typically asymptomatic but may be associated with a high risk of bleeding and allograft loss. Treatment depends on size and location and most can usually be followed conservatively. Some cases may require surgical or interventional treatments.[32,43]

Fluid Collections

Bleeding and Hematomas. Fluid collections are the most common complication following pancreatic transplantation, with the most common being a hematoma. Fresh hematomas usually appear echogenic with well-defined borders and absent of blood flow. Over a period of time, the hematoma may develop debris and septations and then liquefy, becoming anechoic. Hematomas typically spontaneously resolve without treatment. Percutaneous drain placement may only be needed when the collection is proven infectious by obtaining a diagnostic aspiration. CT or MRI may also be helpful aiding in diagnosis.[45]

Seromas. Seromas are clear, serous fluid collections that are usually found within the first few days of transplantation, being most common along the vascular anastomoses sites. Usually seromas will resolve spontaneously within a few weeks. If there is concern that it is part of an infectious process or creating a mass effect and compressing vasculature, an aspiration may be performed. A seroma is described as a round, localized, anechoic, thin-walled fluid collection, which may contain debris or septations found on ultrasound imaging. Fluid collections are easily identified on ultrasound, but not specific determining the contents. CT or MRI can be very helpful in differentiating the collections.[13,45]

Lymphoceles. A surgical disruption of lymphatic channels causes lymph fluid leakage into the soft tissue space, creating a lymphocele. These are typically found medial to the transplant. Lymphoceles may also compress the iliac or femoral vein causing leg edema.[33] Debris or septations within the fluid collection may be visualized on ultrasound. Ultrasound is very sensitive to diagnose a fluid collection but not specific of the contents because blood, pus, lymph, and serosanguineous fluid appear very similar. CT or MRI is helpful in differentiating the collections.[13,45] Spontaneous resolution is rare, and treatment is required. Percutaneous drain placement along with sclerotherapy has been shown to have a 97% success rate. The risk of infection increases with each aspiration and may require a drain placement along with antibiotic medications. Lymphoceles commonly

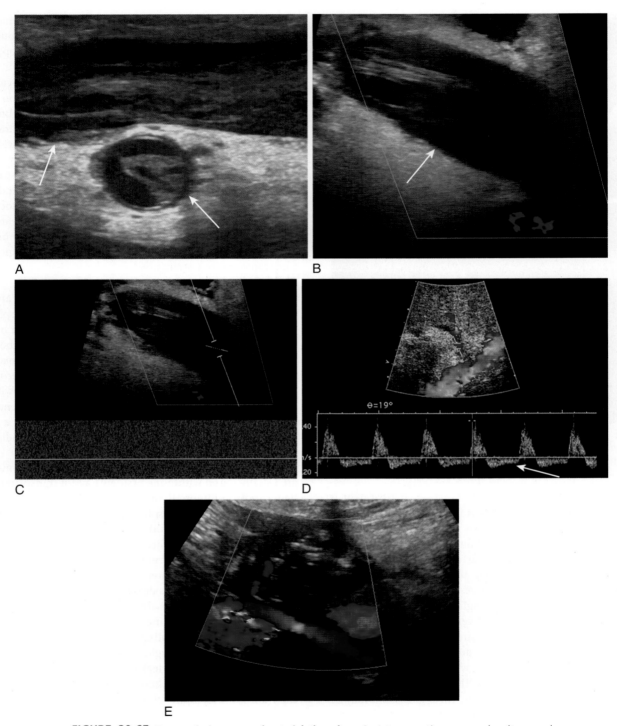

FIGURE 20-67 Pancreatic venous and arterial thrombus. A, Intraoperative gray-scale ultrasound shows thrombus within the longitudinal vein and transverse of the artery. **B,** Intraoperative color Doppler shows absence of flow within the pancreatic vein. **C,** Intraoperative spectral Doppler shows no venous flow present. **D,** Spectral Doppler ultrasound of the pancreatic artery shows reversal of diastolic flow consistent with pancreatic vein thrombus or occlusion. **E,** Color Doppler ultrasound could not identify a pancreatic vein.

recur after a simple aspiration and ultimately may need surgical repair.[33]

Pancreatic Fistulas and Pseudocysts. Following pancreatic transplantation, fistulas or leakage has been reported in as many as 30.8% of cases. This may be related to

ischemia-reperfusion injury, and usually does not significantly impair allograft function or survival.[46] A pseudocyst may ultimately develop. Pseudocysts may be caused from multiple episodes of pancreatitis and are usually found within the pancreatic parenchyma or surrounding tissues. Abscess

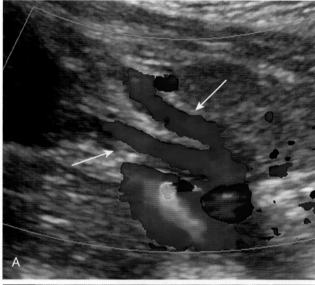

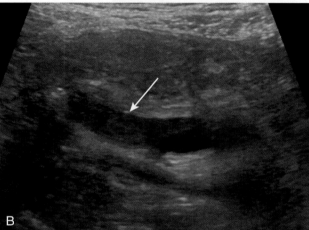

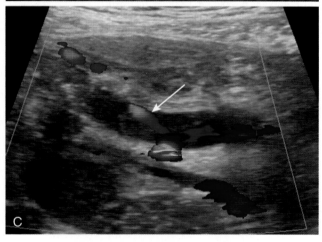

FIGURE 20-68 Pancreatic artery stump thrombus. A, Color Doppler ultrasound shows the normal branches, SMA, and splenic artery of the Y graft. **B,** Gray-scale ultrasound shows arterial thrombus in the blind end of the SMA or splenic artery. **C,** Color Doppler ultrasound shows the incomplete filling of blood flow within the stump of the branch.

formation may be a complication related to the pseudocyst, but usually has a simple appearance. On ultrasound, pseudocysts appear anechoic, with well-defined borders and thin walls with occasionally layering debris[13,45] (Figure 20-70).

Cysts. As technology advancements continue to improve, pancreatic cystic neoplasms are now found more frequently. A subset of pancreatic cystic neoplasms has been shown to have malignant potential. Studies that have used CT and MRI to identify these cysts have reported that 2.5% of the population have them and are asymptomatic and incidentally noted. Ten percent of people 70 years or older have a pancreatic cyst. Some cysts may be observed over time to ensure stability or some patients may continue on for a fine-needle aspiration and/or surgical resection. Most cysts are anechoic and thin walled, with well-defined borders and posterior acoustic enhancement with some containing debris and no vascular flow within on ultrasound imaging. A concerning cystic lesion would contain mural nodules or solid components with vascularity noted.[47]

Pancreatic Adenocarcinoma. Pancreatic adenocarcinoma is the fourth most common cause of cancer-related deaths with only 5% of patients surviving 5 years. The only treatment is complete resection of the tumor with less than 20% having a possible cure on new diagnosis. Unfortunately, many patients do not develop symptoms until the later stages of disease when metastases are already present. Early detection is essential with various imaging modalities, including ultrasound, MRI, or CT. On ultrasound, a hypoechoic mass with pancreatic ductal dilation is very suspicious for pancreatic adenocarcinoma. Unfortunately, ultrasound has a low sensitivity (50% to 90%) for detecting these lesions in the native pancreas.[48]

Posttransplant Lymphoproliferative Disorder. PTLD occurs in 1% to 20% of patients who receive a transplant.[22] In one study, PTLD was found to occur in 6.1% of pancreas transplant patients diagnosed between 1.3 months and 6.1 years.[49] PTLD is the most severe complication found in solid organ and stem cell transplantation. Patients who are on long-term use of immunosuppressant medication have an increased risk of malignancies 2 to 5 times more than the general population. PTLD can be in the form of benign tissue hyperplasia or present as malignant lymphoma. Most polymorphic masses are caused from the EBV, occurring 60% to 80% and within 1 year of transplantation. Most of the monomorphic masses are found to be non-Hodgkin's lymphoma and have B-cell origin. In 23% to 50% of cases, treatment has been shown to be successful in the EBV patients by reducing the immunosuppressants. Patients have better outcomes when diagnosed in the early stages of PTLD. Immunotherapy with monoclonal antibodies such as rituximab may be given to patients as another treatment option with a 40% to 68% success rate.[22] PTLD can occur in any solid organ or viscera.[32] In 39% to 40% of cases, PTLD involves the lymph nodes and liver, followed by the gastrointestinal tract in 33%, and it is considered rare to involve the pancreas itself (10%). On ultrasound imaging, PTLD usually appears as a hypoechoic soft tissue mass and demonstrates lymphadenopathy (Figure 20-71).[43]

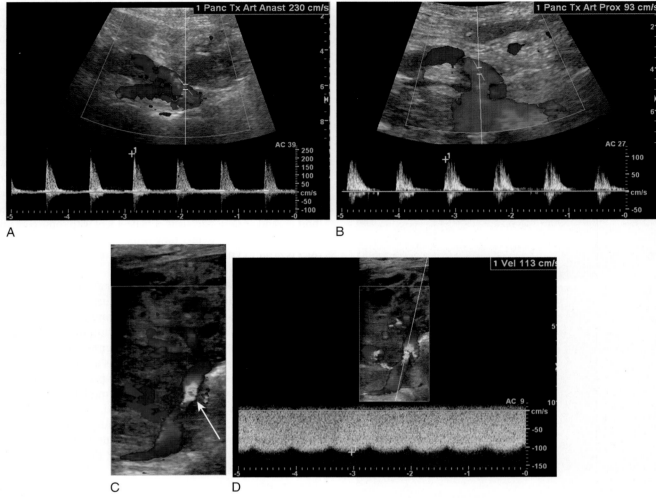

A

B

C   D

FIGURE 20-69 Pancreatic artery and vein stenosis. A, Spectral Doppler ultrasound shows elevated velocities near the anastomosis likely due to postoperative edema. **B,** Spectral Doppler follow-up ultrasound shows the velocities decreased over a period of time. **C,** Color Doppler ultrasound shows aliasing identifying a narrowing within the pancreatic vein. **D,** Elevated velocities are documented near the anastomosis site of the pancreatic vein on spectral Doppler ultrasound.

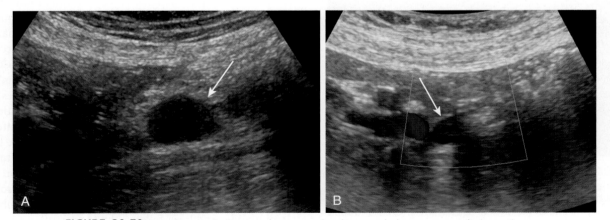

FIGURE 20-70 Pseudocyst. A, Transverse gray-scale ultrasound shows an anechoic cystic area with some debris within and posterior acoustic enhancement. **B,** Color Doppler ultrasound shows absence of flow within the pseudocyst.

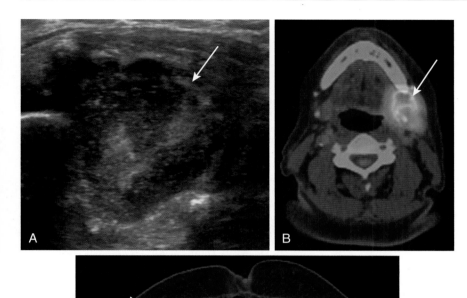

FIGURE 20-71 Posttransplant lymphoproliferative disease. A, Transverse gray-scale ultrasound shows a solid left submandibular mass. **B,** PET/CT demonstrates a left submandibular FDG avid mass. **C,** PET/CT also shows colon involvement.

LEARN HOW YOU CAN HELP DONATE LIFE

At the completion of this chapter, you may have a new insight into what receiving a transplant is like. It is a very long and challenging struggle with a failing organ in the hope you can live to see the next day. If you are interested in more information about becoming an organ donor or would like to share with others, visit donatelife.net. Please consider the gift of life and how you can affect someone's loved one.

 Key Pearls

- Transplant ultrasound requires specialized knowledge of transplant anatomy in order to detect pathology and monitor transplant viability.
- A standardized protocol for how and when to image transplants is important for each institution to develop in collaboration with the transplant surgeons.
- With the shortage of transplants, specialized imaging, of which ultrasound is the prime modality, is critical to maintaining healthy and viable transplants.

REFERENCES

1. Kamath PS, Kim WR: The model for end-stage liver disease (MELD), *Hepatology* 45(3):797-805, 2007.
2. Bachir NM, Larson AM: Adult liver transplantation in the United States, *Am J Med Sci* 343(6):462-469, 2012.
3. Kornberg A: Liver transplantation for hepatocellular carcinoma beyond Milan criteria: multidisciplinary approach to improve outcome, *ISRN Hepatol* 2014:25, 2014.
4. Meirelles RF Jr, Salvalaggio P, Rezende MB, et al: Liver transplantation: history, outcomes and perspectives, *Einstein (Sao Paulo)* 13(1): 149-152, 2015.
5. Smith JM, Biggins SW, Haselby DG, et al: Kidney, pancreas and liver allocation and distribution in the United States, *Am J Transplant* 12(12):3191-3212, 2012.
6. Leeson S, Desai SP: Medical and ethical challenges during the first successful human kidney transplantation in 1954 at Peter Bent Brigham Hospital, Boston, *Anesth Analg* 120(1):239-245, 2015.
7. Han DJ, Sutherland DE: Pancreas transplantation, *Gut Liver* 4(4):450-465, 2010.
8. Hampson FA, Freeman SJ, Ertner J, et al: Pancreatic transplantation: surgical technique, normal radiological appearances and complications, *Insights Imaging* 1(5-6):339-347, 2010.
9. Fridell JA, Powelson JA, Kubal CA, et al: Retrieval of the pancreas allograft for whole-organ transplantation, *Clin Transplant* 28(12): 1313-1330, 2014.
10. Maglione M, Ploeg RJ, Friend PJ: Donor risk factors, retrieval technique, preservation and ischemia/reperfusion injury in pancreas transplantation, *Curr Opin Organ Transplant* 18(1):83-88, 2013.
11. Yang X, Gong J: The value of living donor liver transplantation, *Ann Transplant* 17(4):120-124, 2012.

12. Cheng YF, Ou HY, Yu CY, et al: Interventional radiology in living donor liver transplant, *World J Gastroenterol* 20(20):6221-6225, 2014.

13. Caiado AH, Blasbalg R, Marcelino AS, et al: Complications of liver transplantation: multimodality imaging approach, *Radiographics* 27(5):1401-1417, 2007.

14. Singh AK, Nachiappan AC, Verma HA, et al: Postoperative imaging in liver transplantation: what radiologists should know, *Radiographics* 30(2):339-351, 2010.

15. Zamboni GA, Pedrosa I, Kruskal JB, Raptopoulos V: Multimodality postoperative imaging of liver transplantation, *Eur Radiol* 18(5):882-891, 2008.

16. Rao AR, Chui AK, Shi LW, et al: Technique for repair of lymphocele after liver transplantation using patent blue dye, *Transplant Proc* 32(7):2221-2222, 2000.

17. Zimmerman MA, Ghobrial RM, Tong MJ, et al: Recurrence of hepatocellular carcinoma following liver transplantation: a review of preoperative and postoperative prognostic indicators, *Arch Surg* 143(2):182-188, discussion 188, 2008.

18. deLemos AS, Schmeltzer PA, Russo MW: Recurrent hepatitis C after liver transplant, *World J Gastroenterol* 20(31):10668-10681, 2014.

19. Miro JM, Stock P, Teicher E, et al: Outcome and management of HCV/HIV coinfection pre- and post-liver transplantation. A 2015 update, *J Hepatol* 62(3):701-711, 2015.

20. Abboud B, El Hachem J, Yazbeck T, Doumit C: Hepatic portal venous gas: physiopathology, etiology, prognosis and treatment, *World J Gastroenterol* 15(29):3585-3590, 2009.

21. Sivrioglu AK, Incedayi M, Saglam M, Sonmez G: Portomesenteric venous gas and pneumatosis intestinalis due to intestinal ischaemia, *BMJ Case Rep* 2013. doi:10.1136/bcr-2013-009214.

22. Petrara MR, Giunco S, Serraino D, et al: Post-transplant lymphoproliferative disorders: from epidemiology to pathogenesis-driven treatment, *Cancer Lett* 369(1):37-44, 2015.

23. Mortele KJ, Ros PR: Cystic focal liver lesions in the adult: differential CT and MR imaging features, *Radiographics* 21(4):895-910, 2001.

24. Horton KM, Bluemke DA, Hruban RH, et al: CT and MR imaging of benign hepatic and biliary tumors, *Radiographics* 19(2):431-451, 1999.

25. Bajenaru N, Balaban V, Savulescu F, et al: Hepatic hemangioma—review, *J Med Life* 8(Spec Issue):4-11, 2015.

26. Sherman SC, Tran H: Pneumobilia: benign or life-threatening, *J Emerg Med* 30(2):147-153, 2006.

27. Decarie PO, Lepanto L, Billiard JS, et al: Fatty liver deposition and sparing: a pictorial review, *Insights Imaging* 2(5):533-538, 2011.

28. Cecka JM: The UNOS Scientific Renal Transplant Registry, *Clin Transpl* 1-14, 1996.

29. Davis CL, Delmonico FL: Living-donor kidney transplantation: a review of the current practices for the live donor, *J Am Soc Nephrol* 16(7):2098-2110, 2005.

30. Azhar B, Patel S, Chadha P, Hakim N: Indications for renal autotransplant: an overview, *Exp Clin Transplant* 13(2):109-114, 2015.

31. Chen CH, Hsieh SR, Shu KH, Ho HC: Salvage of external iliac artery dissection immediately after renal transplant, *Exp Clin Transplant* 11(3):274-277, 2013.

32. Weber TM, Lockhart ME: Renal transplant complications, *Abdom Imaging* 38(5):1144-1154, 2013.

33. Akbar SA, Jafri SZ, Amendola MA, et al: Complications of renal transplantation, *Radiographics* 25(5):1335-1356, 2005.

34. Rouviere O, Berger P, Beziat C, et al: Acute thrombosis of renal transplant artery: graft salvage by means of intra-arterial fibrinolysis, *Transplantation* 73(3):403-409, 2002.

35. Sharfuddin A: Renal relevant radiology: imaging in kidney transplantation, *Clin J Am Soc Nephrol* 9(2):416-429, 2014.

36. Banshodani M, Kawanishi H, Marubayashi S, et al: De novo renal cell carcinoma in a kidney allograft 20 years after transplant, *Case Rep Transplant* 2015:679262, 2015.

37. Hevia V, Gomez V, Alvarez S, et al: Transitional cell carcinoma of the kidney graft: an extremely uncommon presentation of tumor in renal transplant recipients, *Case Rep Transplant* 2013:196528, 2013.

38. Carrim ZI, Murchison JT: The prevalence of simple renal and hepatic cysts detected by spiral computed tomography, *Clin Radiol* 58(8):626-629, 2003.

39. Grotemeyer D, Voiculescu A, Iskandar F, et al: Renal cysts in living donor kidney transplantation: long-term follow-up in 25 patients, *Transplant Proc* 41(10):4047-4051, 2009.

40. Abboudi H, Chandak P, Kessaris N, Fronek J: A successful live donor kidney transplantation after large angiomyolipoma excision, *Int J Surg Case Rep* 3(12):594-596, 2012.

41. Pileggi A: Islet transplantation. In De Groot LJ, Beck-Peccoz P, Chrousos G, et al, editors: *Endotext,* South Dartmouth, MA, 2000, MDText.com, Inc.

42. Shapiro AM, Lakey JR, Paty BW, et al: Strategic opportunities in clinical islet transplantation, *Transplantation* 79(10):1304-1307, 2005.

43. Vandermeer FQ, Manning MA, Frazier AA, et al: Imaging of whole-organ pancreas transplants, *Radiographics* 32(2):411-435, 2012.

44. Nadalin S, Girotti P, Konigsrainer A: Risk factors for and management of graft pancreatitis, *Curr Opin Organ Transplant* 18(1):89-96, 2013.

45. Heller MT, Bhargava P: Imaging in pancreatic transplants, *Indian J Radiol Imaging* 24(4):339-349, 2014.

46. Woeste G, Moench C, Hauser IA, et al: Incidence and treatment of pancreatic fistula after simultaneous pancreas kidney transplantation, *Transplant Proc* 42(10):4206-4208, 2010.

47. Farrell JJ: Prevalence, diagnosis and management of pancreatic cystic neoplasms: current status and future directions, *Gut Liver* 9(5):571-589, 2015.

48. Lee ES, Lee JM: Imaging diagnosis of pancreatic cancer: a state-of-the-art review, *World J Gastroenterol* 20(24):7864-7877, 2014.

49. Issa N, Amer H, Dean PG, et al: Posttransplant lymphoproliferative disorder following pancreas transplantation, *Am J Transplant* 9(8):1894-1902, 2009.

PART III

Superficial Structures

Breast

Deziree Rada

OBJECTIVES

On completion of this chapter, you should be able to:
- Describe breast anatomy and sonographic layers
- Discuss breast physiology
- Explain the difference between breast screening and breast imaging
- Summarize the indications for the use of ultrasound in breast imaging
- Describe the correct sonographic technique for imaging the breast
- Know how to use methods of identifying and labeling breast anatomy and masses
- Identify the sonographic characteristics associated with benign and malignant breast masses
- Identify the mammographic characteristics associated with malignant breast masses
- Discuss ultrasound-guided interventional procedures

OUTLINE

Historical Overview
Emerging Sonographic Technologies
  Elastography
  Automated Whole-Breast Sonography
  Three-Dimensional Imaging
Anatomy of the Breast
  Normal Anatomy
  Sonographic Appearance
  Parenchymal Pattern

Vascular Supply
Lymphatic System
The Male Breast
Physiology of the Breast
Breast Evaluation Overview
  Breast Screening
  Breast Evaluation
Sonographic Evaluation of the Breast
  Indications for Sonographic Evaluation

Technique
Sonographic Characteristics of Breast Masses
Pathology
  Differential Diagnosis of Breast Masses
  Benign Conditions
  Malignant Conditions
  Ultrasound-Guided Interventional Procedures

KEY TERMS

Acini
Adenosis
Antiradial
Apocrine metaplasia
Areola
Atypical hyperplasia
Axilla
Breast
Breast cancer
Breast cancer screening

Breast Imaging Reporting and Data System (BI-RADS)
Breast self-examination (BSE)
Clinical breast examination (CBE)
Cooper's ligaments
Fibroadenoma
Gynecomastia
Infiltrating (invasive) ductal carcinoma
Mammary layer

Paget's disease
Peau d'orange
Radial
Retromammary layer
Sentinel node
Spiculation
Subcutaneous layer
Tail of Spence
Terminal ductal lobar units (TDLUs)

One out of eight American women will develop **breast cancer.** It is the most common type of cancer among women in the United States and is the second leading cause of cancer death among women between the ages of 40 and 59. It is estimated that the lifetime risk of breast cancer development is approximately 12%. Early detection of breast cancer is vital, because cancer can be difficult to eradicate once it has spread.

Ultrasound evaluation of the breast plays a significant role in the early detection and characterization of breast masses and provides real-time guidance during interventional breast procedures. This chapter presents an overview of breast anatomy, physiology, sonographic evaluation techniques, and breast pathology with emphasis on breast cancer diagnosis and staging.

HISTORICAL OVERVIEW

John Wild published the first paper on breast ultrasound in 1951. This early paper described the A-mode technique of ultrasound imaging. Advancements in ultrasound equipment design allowed increased tissue characterization, and by 1970, gray-scale ultrasound technique had significantly improved diagnostic accuracy. Dedicated whole-breast ultrasound units were tested as a potential screening method for the detection of breast cancer. This effort, unfortunately, failed. Whole-breast ultrasound imaging units gave way to smaller units with handheld transducers for breast evaluation. Although ultrasound was not an effective primary tool in breast cancer screening, its usefulness as an adjunctive tool to mammography for breast lesion characterization has become increasingly evident. Screening mammograms have long been considered the gold standard for breast cancer screening, although accumulating evidence suggests that ultrasound screening in conjunction with mammography may be beneficial in patients with very dense tissue, complicated mammograms, or very high risk factors for breast cancer.

Most clinical laboratories today use high-resolution, real-time sonography as an adjunct to mammographic screening. Although screening the entire breast with ultrasound is not routinely done, most ultrasound laboratories currently perform the breast examination within a localized area to characterize palpable lesions or suspicious areas seen on a mammogram. High-frequency 10- to 15-MHz transducers have the optimum resolution and the short-to-medium focus necessary for obtaining high-quality images of the breast parenchyma. The high frame rates available with real-time ultrasound systems in use today facilitate ultrasound guidance during interventional procedures of the breast, including cyst aspirations, core biopsies, preoperative localization techniques, and vacuum-assisted biopsies for small lesion diagnosis and removal.

EMERGING SONOGRAPHIC TECHNOLOGIES

Technical improvements over the past 30 years have led to advances in breast imaging. Aside from advances in gray-scale imaging, there have been significant software and hardware developments that have enhanced breast imaging. These new technologies not only provide additional information about the breast, but have the potential to change the way breast sonograms are performed.

Elastography

Introduced in 1991, elastography, also known as elasticity imaging, has recently shown its usefulness in improving the diagnosis of diseases in many parts of the body. This technology produces images based on the relative stiffness of tissues and maps their elastic properties. By applying compression to the breast, elastography is able to produce images, which show the differences in firmness in breast tissue. Breast cancers, generally firmer than benign lesions, appear darker when compared with surrounding

tissue or as red in commonly seen green/red color scale. Although elastography appears as a promising adjunct to gray-scale imaging, it is still being studied for its value in improving diagnostic performance. With researchers actively redesigning elastography hardware and software, elastography may soon show its benefits in diagnostic sonographic breast imaging.

Automated Whole-Breast Sonography

When used on a localized area of the breast, sonography is an important tool in a patient's diagnosis. As previously mentioned, whole-breast sonography is not routinely done for screening purposes due to it being completely operator dependent. It is difficult to have exact documentation of the entire breast with a handheld device projecting a small field of view. In response to this issue, there has been commercial interest in developing an automated ultrasound system for the breast.

Automated whole-breast sonography may be performed with the patient supine or upright, depending on the design of the equipment. This water path system allows the breast to be compressed, which provides excellent visualization of the mammary tissue. The automated transducer has the ability to obtain images over the entire breast. The machine then correlates the B-mode data and appropriately places the lesion oriented to the nipple and quadrant of the breast. Finally, the data are then put together in a series of sonographic gray-scale cine images, which form a whole-breast image.

Three-Dimensional Imaging

Three-dimensional (3D) imaging has been successfully used in other areas of sonography such as obstetrics and gynecology. Currently its diagnostic capabilities are comparable to two-dimensional (2D) imaging producing sensitivities and specificities that are close statistically. Unlike 2D imaging, 3D offers images of the coronal plane. In this plane, masses can be described in two new sonographic patterns: compression and converging, also known as *retraction*. Clinical findings show that the compression patterned masses have an oval shape and are associated with benign lesions, whereas the converging pattern masses appear with spiculations and are associated with malignant tumors.

ANATOMY OF THE BREAST

Normal Anatomy

The **breast** is a modified sweat gland located in the superficial fascia of the anterior chest wall. The major portion of the breast tissue is situated between the second and third rib superiorly, the sixth and seventh costal cartilage inferiorly, the anterior axillary line laterally, and the sternal border medially. In many women, the breast extends deep toward the lateral upper margin of the chest and into the **axilla**. This extension is referred to as the axillary tail of the breast, or the **tail of Spence** (Figure 21-1).

The surface of the breast is dominated by the nipple and the surrounding **areola**. A few women may have ectopic

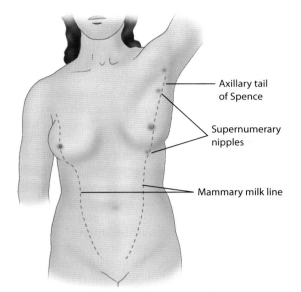

FIGURE 21-1 The mammary milk line is the anatomic line along which breast tissue can be found in some women. The axillary tail of Spence is an extension of breast tissue into the axilla that is present in some women.

breast tissue or accessory (supernumerary) nipples. Ectopic breast tissue and accessory nipples are usually located along the mammary milk line, which extends superiorly from the axilla downward and medially in an oblique line to the symphysis pubis of the pelvis.

Sonographically, the breast is divided into three layers located between the skin and the pectoralis major muscle on the anterior of the chest wall. These layers are the **subcutaneous layer,** the **mammary** (glandular) **layer,** and the **retromammary layer** (Figure 21-2 and Box 21-1). The subcutaneous and

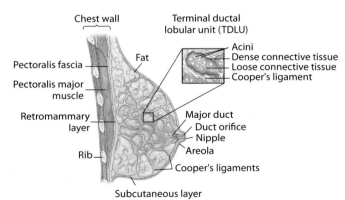

FIGURE 21-2 Breast anatomy. Fifteen major ductal systems are present within the breast. Each gives rise to many separate terminal ductal lobular units (TDLUs) containing the terminal ducts, at least one lobule, and the separate acinar units (milk-producing glands) within each lobule. Each TDLU is surrounded by varying amounts of loose and dense connective tissue. The TDLU represents the site of origin of nearly all pathologic processes of the breast. Cooper's ligaments surround and suspend each of the TDLUs within the surrounding fatty tissue. The ligaments extend to the subcutaneous layer of the skin and the deep retromammary layer next to the pectoralis fascia overlying the chest wall.

BOX 21-1   Breast Anatomy

Subcutaneous layer: thin layer
- Fatty tissue
- Cooper's ligaments

Mammary layer: functional portion of the breast
- 15 to 20 lobes radiate from the nipple.
- Lactiferous ducts carry milk from acini to the nipple.
- Terminal ductal lobular unit is made up of acini and terminal ducts.
- Fatty tissue is interspersed between lobes.
- Cooper's ligaments extend from the retromammary fascia to the skin and provide support.

Retromammary layer: thin layer
- Fatty tissue
- Cooper's ligaments

Pectoralis major muscle
Pectoralis minor muscle
Ribs
Chest wall

retromammary layers are usually quite thin and consist of fat surrounded by connective tissue septa. Although fat is often highly echogenic in other parts of the body, it is the least echogenic tissue within the breast. The fatty tissue appears hypoechoic, and the ducts, glands, and supporting ligaments appear echogenic (Figure 21-3).

The mammary/glandular layer includes the functional portion of the breast and the surrounding supportive (stromal) tissue. The functional portion of the breast is made up of 15 to 20 lobes, which contain the milk-producing glands, and the ductal system, which carries the milk to the nipple. The lobes emanate from the nipple in a pattern resembling the spokes of a wheel. The upper outer quadrant of the breast contains the highest concentration of lobes. This concentration of lobes in the upper outer quadrant of the breast is the reason why most

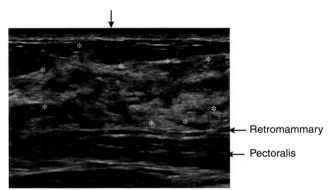

FIGURE 21-3 Sonographic layers of breast tissue. The three layers of breast tissue are bordered by the skin and chest wall muscles *(arrows)*. The subcutaneous fat layer and the retromammary fat layer are usually very thin *(arrowheads)*. The mammary layer *(asterisks)* varies remarkably in thickness and in echogenicity, depending on location within the breast (most glandular tissue is located in the upper outer quadrant) and the patient's age, hormonal status (e.g., pubertal, mature, gravid, lactating, postmenopausal), and inherited breast parenchymal pattern.

tumors are found here, as most tumors originate from within the ducts. The lobes of the breast resemble a grapevine branch; the major duct branches into smaller branches called lobules. Each lobule contains **acini** (milk-producing glands; singular *acinus*), which are clustered on the terminal ends of the ducts like grapes on a vine. Literally hundreds of acini are present within each breast (Figures 21-4 and 21-5). The terminal ends of the duct and the acini form small lobular units referred to as **terminal ductal lobular units (TDLUs),** each of which is surrounded by both loose and dense connective tissue. The TDLUs are invested within the connective tissue skeleton of

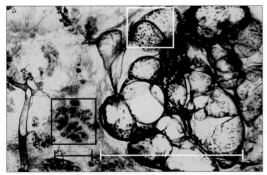

FIGURE 21-4 Galactogram (contrast injected retrograde into a single ductal system) showing opacification of individual glands (terminal ductal lobular units [TDLUs]). Normally, TDLUs are 2 mm or less in diameter. The TDLU is the site of origin of most pathologic processes within the breast.

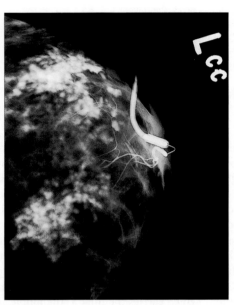

FIGURE 21-5 Three-dimensional histology showing normal terminal ductal lobular units (TDLUs) and dilated TDLUs. Normal TDLUs are usually no larger than 2 mm. Fibrocystic condition and other pathologic processes can cause marked enlargement of the TDLU. Note the difference between the normal TDLU within the black box and the dilated TDLU filling the right half of the image. The white box shows a single dilated acinus within the enlarged TDLU, showing cellular changes of apocrine metaplasia (one of the tissue changes of fibrocystic condition recognized by pathologists), and causing the lining cells to enlarge and overproduce fluid.

the breast (see Figures 21-2, 21-4, and 21-5). Normal TDLUs measure 1 to 2 mm and usually are not differentiated sonographically. The TDLU is significant in that nearly all pathologic processes that occur within the breast originate here. The space between the lobes is filled with connective and fatty tissue known as *stroma*. These stromal elements are located both between and within the lobes and consist of dense connective tissue, loose connective tissue, and fat. The connective tissue septa within the breasts form a fibrous "skeleton," which is responsible for maintaining the shape and structure of the breast. These connective tissue septa are collectively termed **Cooper's ligaments;** they connect to the fascia around the ducts and glands and extend out to the skin.

The pectoralis major muscle lies posterior to the retromammary layer. It originates at the anterior surface of the medial half of the clavicle and anterolateral surface of the sternum and inserts into the intertubercular groove on the anteromedial surface of the humerus (Figure 21-6). The lower border of the pectoralis major muscle forms the anterior margin of the axilla. The pectoralis minor muscle lies superolateral and posterior to the pectoralis major. The pectoralis minor courses from its origin near the costal cartilages of the third, fourth, and fifth ribs to where it inserts into the medial and superior surface of the coracoid process of the scapula. These muscles sonographically appear as a hypoechoic interface between the retromammary layer of the breast and the ribs (see Figure 21-6). Although most lesions are found within the glandular tissue of the breast, it is important to evaluate tissue all the way to the chest wall.

Sonographic Appearance

The boundaries of the breast are the skin line, nipple, and retromammary layer. These generally give strong, bright echo reflections. The areolar area may be recognized by its slightly lower echo reflection compared with the nipple and the skin. The internal nipple may show low to bright reflections

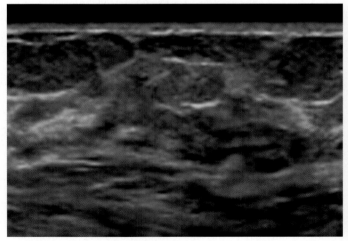

FIGURE 21-6 The hypoechoic pectoralis muscle *(arrows)* is seen between the retromammary layer and the ribs.

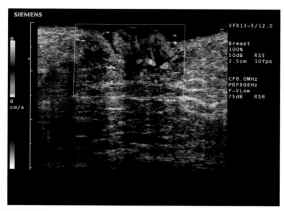

FIGURE 21-7 Shadow from the areolar area prevents imaging directly posterior to the nipple. The transducer should be moved away from the nipple area to image the mammary and retromammary layers.

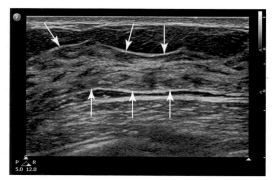

FIGURE 21-9 Mammary-glandular layer lies between the subcutaneous fatty layer anteriorly and the retromammary layer posteriorly (arrows).

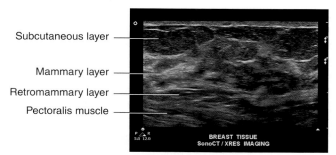

Subcutaneous layer ——
Mammary layer ——
Retromammary layer ——
Pectoralis muscle ——

FIGURE 21-10 The retromammary layer is similar in echogenicity and echo texture to the subcutaneous layer.

with posterior shadowing, and it has a variable appearance (Figure 21-7).

Subcutaneous fat generally appears hypoechoic, whereas Cooper's ligaments and other connective tissue appear echogenic and are dispersed in a linear pattern (Figure 21-8). Cooper's ligaments are best identified when the beam strikes them at a perpendicular angle; compression of the breast often enhances the ability to visualize them.

The mammary/glandular layer lies between the subcutaneous fatty layer anteriorly and the retromammary layer posteriorly (Figure 21-9). The fatty tissue interspersed throughout the mammary/glandular layer dictates the amount of intensity reflected from the breast parenchyma. If little fat is present, a uniform architecture with a strong echogenic pattern (because of collagen and fibrotic tissue) is seen throughout the mammary/glandular layer. When fatty tissue is present, areas of low-level echoes become intertwined with areas of strong echoes from the active breast tissue. Analysis of this pattern becomes critical to the final diagnosis, and one must be able to separate lobules of fat from a marginated lesion.

The retromammary layer is similar in echogenicity and echotexture to the subcutaneous layer, although the boundary echoes resemble skin reflections (Figure 21-10). The pectoral

muscles appear as low-level echo areas posterior to the retromammary layer. The ribs appear sonographically as hyperechoic rounded structures with dense posterior shadowing. They are easily identified by their occurrence at regular intervals along the chest wall.

Several normal structures within the breast can appear abnormal, unless care is taken to prevent this during the sonographic examination. The ducts immediately behind the nipple frequently cause acoustic shadowing and can be mistaken for a suspicious breast mass. Angling of the transducer in the retroareolar tissue will usually improve visualization and eliminate doubt. The distinction of a subtle isoechoic or hypoechoic sonographic mass from normal fibroglandular tissue in the breast can sometimes be troublesome. The adipose or fatty tissue can situate itself in and among the areas of glandular tissue and, in some scanning planes, can mimic isoechoic or hypoechoic masses. It is helpful to turn on the structures to see if they are consistent or lengthen out within the scanning plane. To see whether a structure will lengthen out geometrically, one should rotate the transducer 90 degrees during real-time. In the case of a true sonographic mass, the mass will maintain its shape in both dimensions, confirming its 3D character, whereas glandular tissue elements will elongate and appear less like a mass.

Parenchymal Pattern

The size and shape of the breasts vary remarkably from woman to woman. Some women have more glandular tissue,

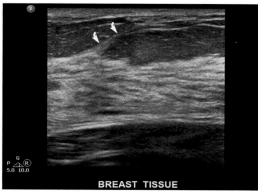

FIGURE 21-8 Subcutaneous fat is hypoechoic, whereas Cooper's ligaments appear echogenic within the subcutaneous layer (arrows).

some have less. Some have more fatty tissue than others, and some have more connective tissue, thus resulting in firmer breasts. Some women have very little breast tissue. The size and shape of the breasts also vary over time because of changes that occur during the menstrual cycle, with pregnancy and breast-feeding, and during menopause. Most differences in breast size between women are due to the amount of fatty tissue within the breasts.

The involutional changes that occur in the breast throughout life affect the appearance and pattern of the breast parenchyma. Involution is hallmarked in breast imaging by the remodeling process that causes glandular tissue to be slowly replaced by fatty tissue. This accounts for differences in the size, shape, and architecture of breast tissue.

Generally, in a young woman, fibrous tissue elements predominate, and the resulting appearance on mammography and ultrasound is a dense echogenic pattern of tissue (Figure 21-11). In a pregnant or lactating woman, the glandular portions of the breast proliferate remarkably in both density and volume, creating interfaces that are less echogenic. As a woman ages, the glandular breast tissue undergoes cell death and is remodeled by the infiltration of fatty

tissue. The tissue is progressively replaced by fat and, with the onset of menopause, the ducts atrophy, resulting in a mammographic and sonographic pattern with less fibrous tissue elements (Figure 21-12). This fatty breast is most difficult to image by sonography, as all three layers of the breast appear hypoechoic, with less distinction between the layers. Sonographically, cancers can be difficult to differentiate in the fatty breast because most cancers appear hypoechoic and can be difficult to differentiate from normal breast tissue. Although sonography of the fatty breast is difficult, mammography images this type of breast very well.

Vascular Supply

The main arterial supply to the breast comes from the internal mammary and the lateral thoracic arteries. More than half of the breast—mainly the central and medial portions—is supplied by the anterior perforating branches of the internal mammary artery. The remaining portion—the upper outer quadrant—is supplied by the lateral thoracic artery; intercostals and subcapsular and thoracodorsal arteries contribute in lesser ways to the blood supply.

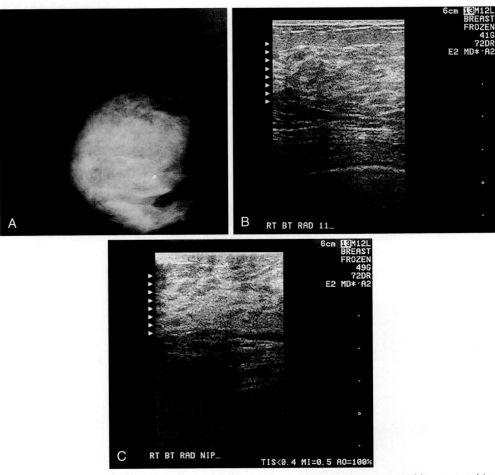

FIGURE 21-11 **Dense breast.** **A,** Example of dense breast tissue on mammogram. Mammographic technique emphasizes tissue contrast. As a result, the skin often is not visible on routine images. The skin is separated in this case by nearly 2 cm from the outer margins of the dense mammary layer. **B,** Example of ultrasound appearance of dense breast tissue. **C,** Example of variation in breast tissue pattern at different locations even within the same breast.

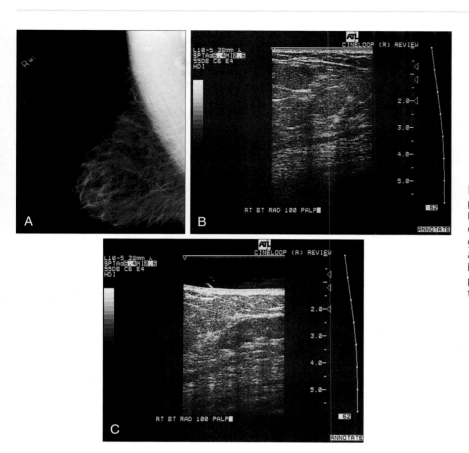

FIGURE 21-12 **Fatty breast. A,** Example of predominantly fatty tissue on mammogram. **B,** Example of ultrasound appearance of predominantly fatty tissue. Note the loss of sonographic detail in the deeper layers of the breast and chest wall. Fat deflects the ultrasound beam and degrades detail. **C,** Example of improved visualization of skin and subcutaneous tissues with a stand-off pad.

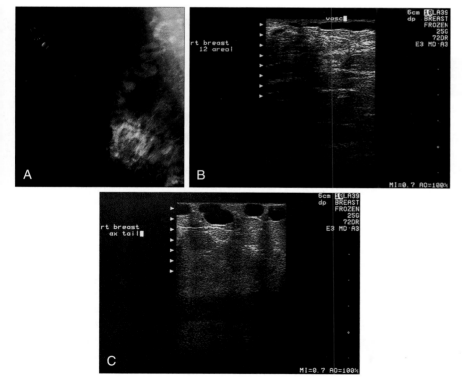

FIGURE 21-13 **Dilated veins in the breast. A,** Mammographic image of a breast showing markedly dilated surface veins in an elderly woman. **B** and **C,** Ultrasound images of veins just under the skin of the breast in the same patient. In cases in which there is doubt, color flow mapping or Doppler techniques will easily confirm the vascular nature of these dilated tubular structures and will distinguish them from dilated ducts.

Venous anatomy largely parallels the arterial anatomy in the deep breast. However, venous drainage is mainly provided by unpaired superficial veins that can be seen sonographically just under the skin. These surface veins are often enlarged with superior vena cava syndrome or chronic venous thrombosis of the subclavian vein, as well as when arteriovenous shunts are placed in patients with chronic renal insufficiency. Figure 21-13 shows an example of a grossly dilated surface vein in the breast. When there is doubt concerning the vascular nature of a long, tubular, anechoic structure on breast ultrasound, such as the distinction between a dilated duct and a vessel, color flow vascular imaging or Doppler ultrasound techniques can easily resolve this situation.

Lymphatic System

Lymphatic drainage from all parts of the breast generally flows to the axillary lymph nodes. The flow of lymph is promoted by valveless lymphatic vessels that allow the fluid to mingle and proceed unidirectionally from superficial to deep nodes of the breast. The flow of lymph moves from the intramammary nodes and deep nodes centrifugally toward the axillary and internal lymph node chains. It has been estimated that only about 3% of lymph is eliminated by the internal chain, whereas 97% of lymph is removed by the axillary chain.

Part of the standard surgical therapy of invasive breast cancer involves axillary lymph node dissection. This is vital in the staging and management of breast cancer because nodal status affects the patient's prognosis and is important in guiding adjunctive therapy. Although most tumors can infiltrate and spread via the axillary lymph nodes, they may begin their infiltration by using alternative lymph channels, such as the internal mammary chain within the chest, across the midline to the contralateral breast, deep into the interpectoral (Rotter's) nodes, or into the supraclavicular nodes (Figures 21-14, 21-15, and 21-16).

The Male Breast

In males, the nipple and the areola remain relatively small. The male breast normally retains some ductal elements beneath the nipple, but it does not develop the milk-producing lobular and acinar tissue. The ductal elements usually remain small but can hypertrophy during puberty and later in life under the influence of hormonal fluctuations, disease processes, or medications. This condition, in which the ductal elements hypertrophy, is called benign **gynecomastia** (Figure 21-17). Imaging with mammography and ultrasound is often requested to exclude breast cancer as a cause.

Although breast cancer is uncommon in males, it does occur. Approximately 1300 new cases are diagnosed each year within the United Sates. The occurrence approximates 1% of the incidence in women. Box 21-2 lists male patients who have an increased risk for breast cancer.

PHYSIOLOGY OF THE BREAST

The primary function of the breast is fluid transport. The breast includes fat, ligaments, glandular tissue, and a ductal system that work together to provide fluid transport. The ductal system is critical in the transport of fluids within the breast. The ductal system is also where many pathologic conditions originate.

An important function of the breast during the reproductive years is to make milk from nutrients and water taken

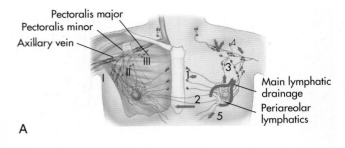

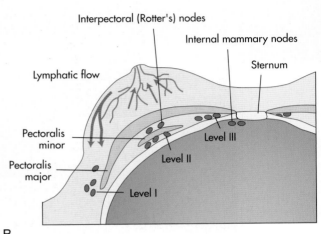

FIGURE 21-14 Lymphatic drainage of the breast. A, General position of the major axillary lymphatic groups I, II, and III in relation to the pectoralis major and minor muscles of the chest wall. On the right side of the figure, the major lymphatic flow from the periareolar plexus toward the axilla is shown. Alternative routes of lymphatic flow include *(1)* retromammary nodes, *(2)* contralateral flow to the opposite breast, *(3)* interpectoral (Rotter's) nodes located between the pectoralis major and minor muscles, *(4)* supraclavicular nodes, and *(5)* diaphragmatic nodes. **B,** Same information in cross section.

from the bloodstream. Milk is produced within the acini and is carried to the nipple by the ducts. During lactation, the transport of milk depends on the action of the two epithelial cells that make up the ductal network: luminal cells, which secrete the milk components into the ductal lumen, and myoepithelial cells, which contract to aid in the ejection of milk.

The female breast is remarkably affected by changing hormonal levels during each menstrual cycle and is further affected by both pregnancy and lactation (breast-feeding). Breast development begins before menarche and continues until the female is approximately 16 years old. During this time, the ductal system proliferates under the influence of estrogen. During pregnancy, acinar development is accelerated to enable milk production by estrogen, progesterone, and prolactin. Prolactin is a hormone produced by the pituitary gland that stimulates the acini to produce and excrete milk. Prolactin levels usually rise during the latter part of pregnancy, but milk production is suppressed by high levels of progesterone. Expulsion of the placenta after the birth of a baby causes a drop in circulating progesterone, initiating milk production within the breasts. The physical stimulation of suckling by the baby initiates the release of

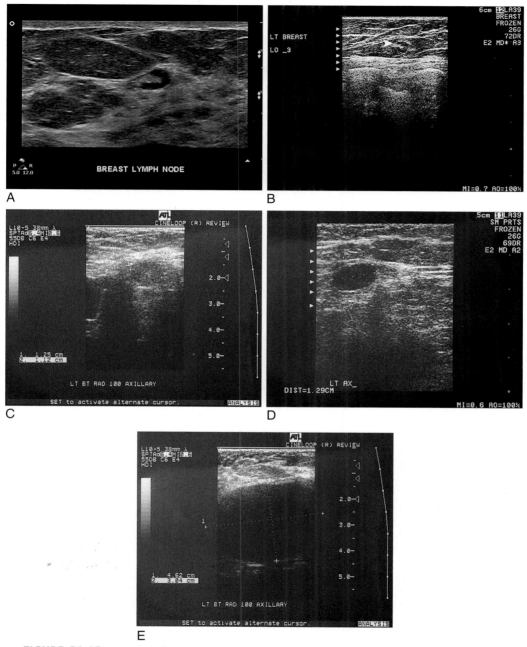

FIGURE 21-15 Normal and abnormal lymph nodes. A and **B,** Sonographic images of a normal lymph node showing a smooth homogeneously hypoechoic cortex and an echogenic fatty internal hilum. **C–E,** Images of abnormal lymph nodes. Signs of suspicion for metastatic involvement of lymph nodes include an irregular, inhomogeneous cortex and loss of the fatty hilum. **C,** Lymph node that has nearly lost the fatty hilum and has a poorly defined but relatively homogeneous cortex. This may be a reactive lymph node or one with early metastatic involvement. **D,** Similar lymph node that has completely lost its fatty hilum but has a smooth homogeneous cortex. **E,** Large hypoechoic mass that has no sonographic characteristics of a normal lymph node. This mass was sampled by ultrasound-guided core biopsy, confirming a low axillary lymph node nearly completely replaced with metastatic cancer.

oxytocin (produced by the hypothalamus and released by the pituitary gland), which further incites prolactin secretion, stimulating additional milk production. Full maturation of the acini occurs during lactation and is thought to be mildly protective against the development of breast cancer.

At the end of lactation, the breast tissue parenchyma involutes. Breast evaluation by mammography can be difficult in a dense, lactating breast; therefore mammographic screening of the breast usually is not performed until at least 6 months after cessation of lactation.

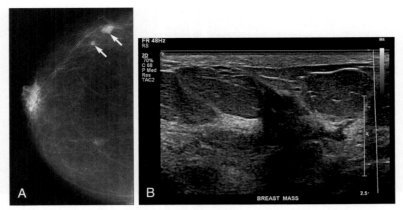

FIGURE 21-16 Metastatic spread of breast cancer to the opposite breast. A, Mammogram showing several moderate- to low-density, relatively benign-appearing masses *(arrows)* in a patient with a history of mastectomy for cancer in the opposite breast. **B,** Image of one of the masses shows a solid mass with an irregular, poorly defined margin and heterogeneous echogenicity. These lesions were all metastatic lesions from the opposite breast, likely from an alternative route of lymphatic spread across the midline.

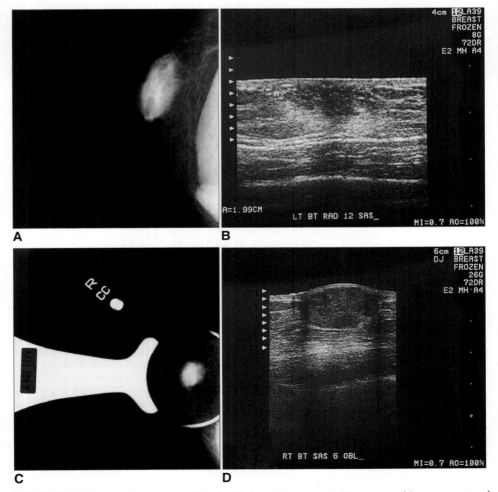

FIGURE 21-17 Two male patients with palpable breast masses. A, Mammographic appearance of benign gynecomastia. This condition is nearly as often unilateral as bilateral. **B,** Ultrasound example of the frequently masslike appearance of gynecomastia. **C,** Mammography example of male breast cancer. **D,** Sonographic image with stand-off pad of palpable suspicious breast mass in elderly male. Note the heterogeneous echogenicity and the elevation of skin over the mass.

BOX 21-2 | Male Patients at Increased Risk for Breast Cancer

Klinefelter's syndrome
Male-to-female transsexual
History of prior chest wall irradiation (especially for Hodgkin's lymphoma)
History of orchitis or testicular tumor
Liver disease
Genetic predisposition (*BRCA2* gene mutation, breast cancer in female relatives, p53 mutation)

BREAST EVALUATION OVERVIEW

Breast Screening

The primary purpose of breast screening is the detection and diagnosis of breast cancer in its earliest and most curable stage. Accurate identification of benign breast lesions during cancer screening is also important for good care because it can save the patient from unnecessary surgical procedures and resultant tissue scarring.

Three general categories of diagnostic breast imaging are available, two of which involve breast ultrasound. These three categories include breast cancer screening (generally performed by physical breast evaluation with mammography), diagnostic interrogation (consultation, problem solving, workup), and interventional breast procedures (histologic diagnosis and/or localization).

Breast cancer screening is recommended in women without clinical signs of breast cancer (Box 21-3). According to the American Cancer Society, breast cancer screening involves monthly **breast self-examination (BSE)**, regular **clinical breast examination (CBE)** by a physician or other health care provider, and annual screening mammography. Monthly BSE is best performed at the end of menses and should begin at age 20. CBE should be performed once every 3 years from ages 20 to 39 and at least yearly from age 40 on. Screening mammography should be performed yearly starting at age 40. BSE and CBE are important steps in breast cancer screening because 70% of cancers are found as lumps felt during BSE and CBE. BSE and CBE may also identify other signs or symptoms of possible breast cancer that require further evaluation by diagnostic breast imaging (Box 21-4).

Mammography, sonography, and magnetic resonance imaging (MRI) are the primary imaging tools used for diagnostic breast evaluation. Mammography provides a sensitive method of screening for breast cancer, whereas ultrasound and MRI are used to provide additional characterization and further interrogation of breast lesions that are not well visualized by mammography. The mammographic signs of breast cancer are listed in Box 21-5. Because ultrasound examination is performed by scanning in cross-sectional planes, it is difficult to adequately screen the entire breast in most patients. Ultrasound may be used for screening purposes in young, dense breasts, which are difficult to penetrate by mammography; to evaluate palpable masses that are not visible on a mammogram; and to image the deep juxtathoracic tissue not normally visible by mammography. Ultrasound is also useful in differentiating structures within uniformly

BOX 21-4 | Clinical Signs and Symptoms of Possible Breast Cancer

New or growing dominant, discrete breast lump
- Hard, gritty, or irregular surface
- Usually (but not always) painless
- Does not fluctuate with hormonal cycle
- Different from "lumpy" breast texture
Unilateral single-duct nipple discharge
- Spontaneous, persistent; serous or bloody
Surface nipple lesions
- Nonhealing ulcer
- Focal irritation
New nipple retraction
New focal skin dimpling or retraction
Unilateral new or growing axillary lump
Hot, red breast
Note: Although these clinical signs and symptoms may indicate the presence of breast cancer, it is important to understand that in most cases the cause is not cancer, but rather a benign condition.

BOX 21-3 | Breast Cancer Screening

Breast self-examination (BSE)
- Monthly beginning at age 20
Clinical breast examination (CBE) by a health care provider
- Ages 20 to 39: every 3 years
- Ages 40 on: yearly
Screening mammography
- Yearly starting at age 40
Exceptions: Personal history of breast cancer, first-degree relative (mother or sister) with premenopausal breast cancer, atypical hyperplasia or lobular carcinoma in situ on prior breast biopsy, and known breast cancer gene mutation (*BRCA1* or *BRCA2*)

BOX 21-5 | Signs of Breast Cancer on Mammography

Primary Signs

Common	Irregular (spiculated), high-density mass
	Clustered pleomorphic microcalcifications
	Focal distortion (with no history of prior biopsy, infection, or trauma)
Less common	Focal asymmetric density (with associated palpable lump or solid sonographic mass)
	Developing density

Secondary Signs

Common	Nipple or skin retraction
	Skin thickening
	Lymphedema pattern
	Increased vascularity

dense breast tissue in which mammography is limited (e.g., in differentiating solid, round masses from fluid-filled cysts and in visualizing tissue adjacent to implants or other structures that limit visualization by mammography). MRI is also a useful tool in breast imaging but is prohibitively expensive for screening purposes. Because a strong magnetic field is used to create images, not all patients are good candidates for MRI (e.g., patients with pacemakers or artificial joints). Patients who suffer from uncontrolled claustrophobia are also not good candidates for MRI.

Breast Evaluation

The overall goal of breast evaluation is the proper classification of a breast lesion according to the level of suspicion for breast cancer. Thorough evaluation takes into account the results of both the breast imaging assessment and the clinical assessment. The appropriate next step in patient management is dictated by the level of suspicion for cancer in any breast lesion and takes into account the age and individual risk factors for each particular patient. Risk factors for breast cancer are listed in Box 21-6.

Clinical Assessment. It is important to recognize clinical signs or symptoms of possible breast cancer (see Box 21-4). Patients with clinical indications of breast cancer generally undergo diagnostic breast interrogation. Diagnostic imaging of the breast is tailored to the patient's age and specific clinical problem. Clinical history and examination of the patient with a breast problem (Box 21-7) help determine the next diagnostic step. In the patient with no signs or symptoms of possible breast cancer, screening mammography is typically the first diagnostic test performed.

Screening Mammography. In women age 40 and over who are asymptomatic (without clinical signs of possible breast cancer), annual screening by mammography is recommended. Usually less than 10% of these women will have abnormalities detected on the screening examination that require further workup. When a breast lesion is identified by

BOX 21-6	Risk Factors for Breast Cancer

Female gender
Increasing age
Family history of breast cancer
Personal history of breast cancer
- First-degree relative (mother, sister, daughter)
- Premenopausal breast cancer
- Multiple affected first- and second-degree relatives
- Associated cancers (ovarian, colon, prostate)
Biopsy-proven atypical proliferative lesions
- Lobular neoplasia (lobular carcinoma in situ)
- Atypical epithelial hyperplasia
Prolonged estrogen effect
- Early menarche
Late menopause
Nulliparity
Late first pregnancy

BOX 21-7	Clinical Evaluation of the Patient with a Breast Problem

History
- Patient age
- Risk factors for breast cancer
- Onset and duration of mass
- Relation to menstrual cycle
Breast examination (for palpable mass)
Location of mass
- Clock face or quadrant
Characteristics of mass:
- Size
- Shape (round, oval, lobular, irregular)
- Surface contour (smooth, irregular)
- Consistency (soft, rubbery, firm, hard, gritty)
- Mobility (movable, fixed)

mammography, it is normally described using guidelines contained within the **Breast Imaging Reporting and Data System (BI-RADS).** BI-RADS was developed by the American College of Radiology (ACR). A key component of this system is an overall outcome assessment category that indicates the suspicion of malignancy (Table 21-1). Figures 21-18, 21-19, 21-20, and 21-21 present mammographic and sonographic examples of various BI-RADS category masses.

Diagnostic Breast Interrogation. Diagnostic breast interrogation (consultation, workup, problem solving) is performed on all patients who present with any clinical signs of possible breast cancer found on CBE or BSE, and on patients who are recalled for additional evaluation because of an abnormal screening mammogram. Diagnostic mammography

TABLE 21-1	American College of Radiology BI-RADS Assessment Categories for Mammographic Masses	
BI-RADS Category/ Recommended Action	**Description**	
1. Negative	Nothing to comment on. Breasts are symmetric; no masses, architectural distortion, or suspicious calcifications.	
2. Benign finding(s)	Involuting, calcified fibroadenomas, multiple secretory calcifications, fat-containing lesions.	
3. Probable benign finding(s)/initial short-term follow-up	Noncalcified circumscribed solid mass; focal asymmetry; cluster of round (punctate) calcifications. Less than 2% chance of malignancy.	
4. Suspicious abnormality/consider biopsy	Findings do not have classic appearance of malignancy but have wide range of probability of malignancy greater than those in Category 3.	
5. Highly suggestive of malignancy/appropriate action needed	Classic breast cancers with a 95% or greater likelihood for malignancy.	

Used with permission of the American College of Radiology.

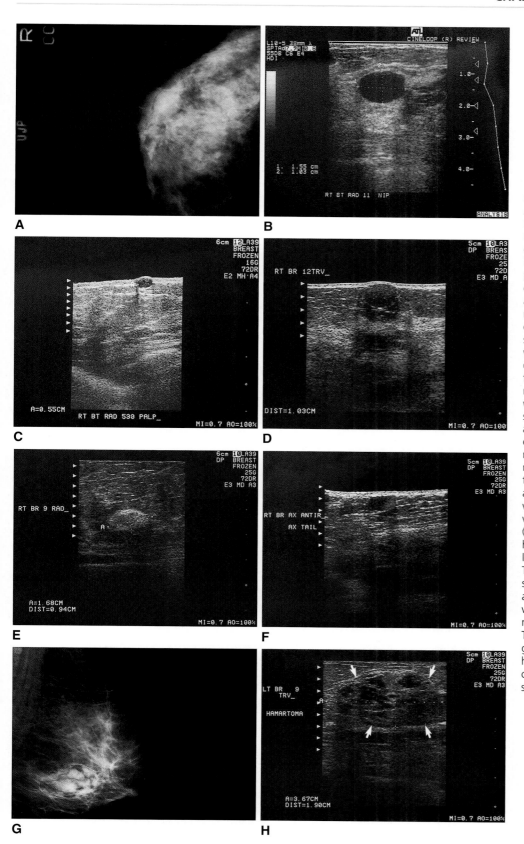

FIGURE 21-18 Examples of benign (BI-RADS category 2) masses. A, Smooth, benign-appearing mammographic mass. **B,** Same mass on ultrasound showing classic features of a simple cyst. **C,** Example of a sebaceous cyst. Note the smooth, hypoechoic appearance and classic location within the skin. **D,** Example of an isoechoic mass abutting the dermis. This is an epidermal inclusion cyst, often indistinguishable from a sebaceous cyst. These lesions appear within the skin or at the junction of the dermis and the subcutaneous fatty layer. **E,** Vague, low-density mammographic mass correlated with this echogenic mass on ultrasound. Echogenic masses are nearly always benign, but the level of suspicion should be determined by the mammographic appearance. **F,** Small mass on mammogram in this hospitalized patient on warfarin appears as a small, superficial complex cyst with a "fluid-fluid" level consistent with a small, resolving hematoma (a galactocele in a lactating patient has a similar appearance, but is located within the mammary layer). This superficial hematoma may resolve completely or may evolve into an oil cyst. **G,** Mammographic mass with mixed fatty and soft tissue elements, surrounded by a thin capsule. This is a breast hamartoma. **H,** Sonographic appearance of the same hamartoma. Note that its high fat content makes differentiation from surrounding fatty tissue difficult.

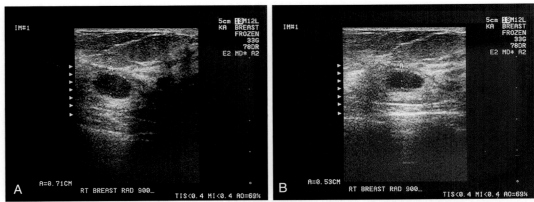

FIGURE 21-19 **Example of probably benign (BI-RADS category 3) mass. A,** Sonographic appearance of a smooth, benign-appearing mass with homogeneous echogenicity, wider than tall, showing low-level posterior acoustic enhancement. This image is taken without applied compression. **B,** Same mass with applied compression, showing the decreased anteroposterior dimension. Most benign masses are soft and compressible.

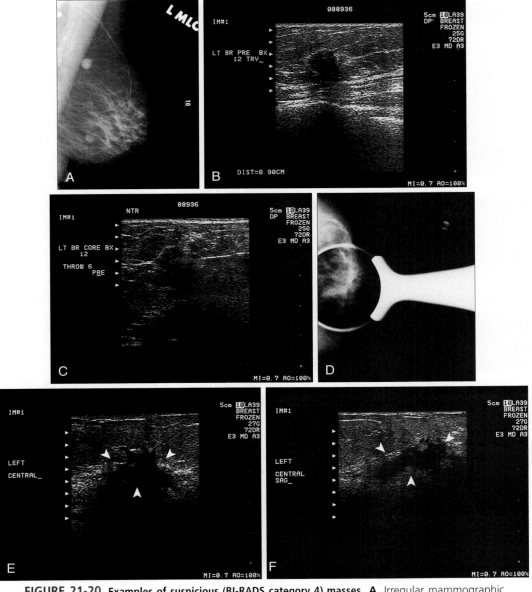

FIGURE 21-20 **Examples of suspicious (BI-RADS category 4) masses. A,** Irregular mammographic mass that had shown interval growth. **B,** Sonographic appearance of the same mass, with a heterogeneous echogenicity but only a slightly irregular margin. Weak posterior acoustic shadowing can be seen. **C,** Fourteen-gauge core-biopsy needle traversing the mass. Pathologic condition confirmed an infiltrating ductal carcinoma. **D,** Mammographic area of focal distortion that persisted with detail imaging. Transverse **(E)** and sagittal **(F)** ultrasound images confirm a 3D area of focal distortion. The patient had no history of previous surgery, injury, or infection in this breast to explain the distortion.

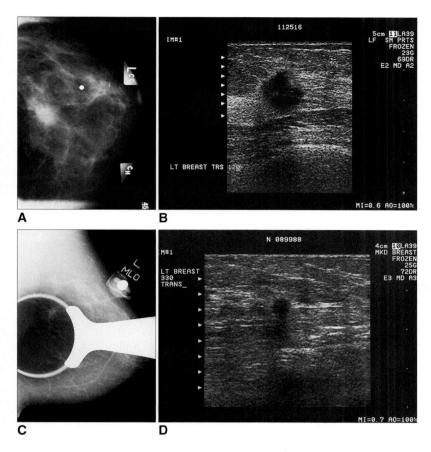

FIGURE 21-21 Example of highly suspicious (BI-RADS category 5) mass. A, Magnification view of a palpable lump showing a spiculated, highly suspicious mammographic mass. **B,** Sonographic image of the same mass. Note the heterogeneous echogenicity, poorly defined and irregular margin, and "higher than wide" appearance, which does not change with most cancers even with applied compression. **C,** Spot compression mammogram of a small spiculated mass. **D,** Ultrasound image showing a small mass with features similar to those in **B.**

involves specialized detailed views to analyze specific areas of the breast in question. In at least one third of cases, adjunctive ultrasound of the breast is used to further evaluate questionable mammographic or clinical findings (see later discussion). **Interventional Breast Procedures.** In some breast lesions, interventional procedures are necessary for definitive diagnosis. A common example is a smooth, benign-appearing mass identified by mammography that correlates with a hypoechoic sonographic lesion but does not meet the criteria for interpretation as a simple cyst. Cyst aspiration can be performed to determine whether the lesion is a complex cyst or truly a solid mass. Under real-time sonographic guidance, a needle is guided into the lesion in an attempt to aspirate fluid. Successful fluid aspiration is diagnostic of a complex cyst. The same approach can be used to guide fine-needle aspiration for cytology, core-needle biopsies for histology, and preoperative needle wire localization of masses for surgery, and for the injection of radioactive tracers for **sentinel node** identification and mapping.

In some cases, a patient has a clinical sign or symptom of possible breast cancer, and yet diagnostic breast imaging shows no abnormality. The most common clinical scenario is the patient with a breast lump and negative breast imaging. If no imaging correlation can be identified to explain the patient's breast lump, the patient must be managed clinically, which means that she is examined sequentially through at least one menstrual cycle. In the overwhelming majority of cases, the breast lump will improve or resolve completely, confirming the diagnosis of clinical fibrocystic condition. If

the breast lump does not improve or continues to grow, surgical biopsy is performed.

SONOGRAPHIC EVALUATION OF THE BREAST

Indications for Sonographic Evaluation

The sonographer must have basic clinical information regarding any patient who is referred for breast ultrasound. Pertinent clinical information includes the patient's age, risk factors for breast cancer (see Box 21-6), and symptoms, and the location and clinical impression of any breast lumps. Any history of trauma to the breast or previous breast surgery is also helpful. Inspection of the breast during the ultrasound examination often reveals pertinent findings. For example, the examiner should make note of any surface nipple erosion (possible **Paget's disease**), nipple or skin retraction, skin thickening (edema, scarring, or **peau d'orange**), scars, signs of inflammation (induration and erythema), or contusion. Sonography is normally used as an adjunct to mammography but may be the initial method of imaging when a breast lump is palpable; it may also be used in a young patient with dense breasts, in a pregnant or lactating patient, in a patient with breast augmentation, or in a patient with a difficult or compromised mammogram.

Palpable Breast Lump. Patients are often referred for breast ultrasound because of a palpable breast lump. Pertinent clinical information that should be provided by the referring physician includes size and location of the lump, when it was noticed, and its relation to the menstrual cycle. The physician's clinical impression (e.g., suspicion of cancer, probable fibrocystic condition, possible abscess) can help focus the sonographer's examination. The sonographer can often feel the mass of concern while scanning the breast. This can help guide the examination and over time will lead to improved expertise on the part of the sonographer in differentiating lesions. For example, a dominant cyst is frequently round or oval (long axis toward nipple), smooth, soft (some cysts under tension can be firm and are usually very tender), and easily movable. Fibroadenomas are usually similar in shape, but are often firm and rubbery in consistency and homogeneously solid on ultrasound. Breast cancer, by contrast, will generally be painless (although some cancers are associated with focal pain), lobular or irregular in shape, uneven in surface contour (sometimes gritty in texture), and fixed or poorly movable (Box 21-8).

Young Patient with Dense Breasts. Ultrasound is the primary tool in breast imaging for all women younger than age 30, according to most authors. Mammography is added as necessary on a limited basis between ages 20 and 30, mainly to rule out microcalcifications (a sign of possible breast cancer that may not be visible by ultrasound). Mammography is rarely indicated for patients younger than age 20 and, in some centers, younger than age 25. The three main reasons for this are that breast cancer is rare in women younger than 25 years, that breast tissue at this age is generally denser and more difficult to analyze by mammography, and that young breast tissue is more sensitive to damage from radiation.

Most breast masses that arise during the teen years are fibroadenomas (Figure 21-22). Other common causes of

BOX 21-8	Differential Diagnoses
Smooth Mass	
Common	Simple cyst
	Complex cyst
	Fibroadenoma
	Lymph node
	Oil cyst
Less common	Galactocele
	Seroma
	Hematoma
	Phyllodes tumor
	Cancer
Focal Distortion	
Common	Postsurgical scar
	Fibrocystic condition
	Cancer
Less common	Prior infection
	Old hematoma
	Degenerating fibroadenoma
Uncommon	Fibrocystic condition
Palpable Breast Lump with Negative Breast Imaging	
Common	Fibrocystic condition
Less common	Resolving trauma
Uncommon	Cancer

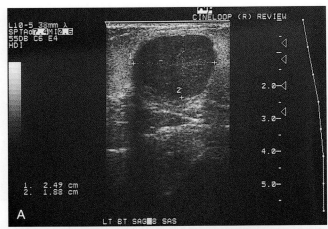

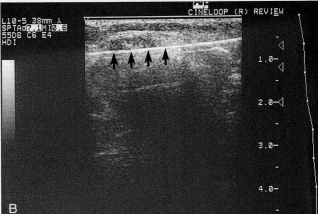

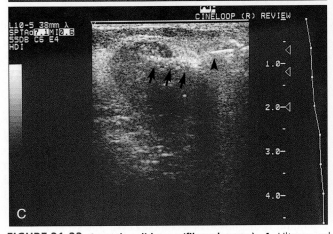

FIGURE 21-22 Smooth, solid mass (fibroadenoma). A, Ultrasound image of a growing palpable mass in a teenage female. This was one of several similar masses. Fibroadenomas are frequently multiple and often run in families. Note the hypoechoic, homogeneous echogenicity of the mass, and the low-level posterior acoustic enhancement and edge refraction. **B,** The patient was referred for large core-needle biopsy for diagnosis. This ultrasound image shows the 14-gauge core-biopsy needle in postfire position traversing the superficial portion of the mass. The approximate area of the sample notch from which tissue is obtained is indicated by the *arrows.* Multiple passes are made to ensure adequate sampling and a reliable tissue diagnosis. **C,** Note the echogenic core biopsy tract within the mass *(arrows).* Fresh hemorrhage along the needle tract caused the echogenic appearance. The prefire position of the needle adjacent to the mass, in preparation for the next tissue sampling, is also visible *(arrowhead).*

breast lumps include the developing breast bud immediately behind the nipple (which must never be mistaken for an abnormal mass and surgically removed) or a dominant cyst. Less commonly, a hyperplastic lymph node, abscess, hematoma, or giant fibroadenoma can present before age 20. Malignant breast lesions in patients younger than 20 years are extremely rare. When they do occur, they generally are not of breast origin, but rather are metastatic or of soft tissue origin (such as soft tissue sarcomas). If a young patient has a rapidly enlarging or painful mass, surgical excision should be considered.

Pregnant or Lactating Patient. Sonography is the primary tool for breast imaging in a pregnant patient. Mammography is added (with abdominal shielding) to allow accurate characterization of a breast mass as necessary. Diagnostic evaluation of a breast mass (including biopsy if indicated) should not be delayed because of the pregnancy.

Most masses that present in a pregnant or lactating patient are benign fibroadenomas. These can often enlarge rapidly because of the marked increase in circulating hormone levels during pregnancy and lactation. The increase in circulating hormones, however, can have a similar effect on breast cancers. In patients who develop breast cancer during pregnancy, cancers are often diagnosed at a later stage than in the nonpregnant patient.

Other breast problems that may arise during pregnancy or lactation include mastitis, abscesses, cysts, or galactoceles (cysts containing milk). In the case of a galactocele, a fat-fluid level may be visible both by mammography and by ultrasound, but more commonly, this lesion appears as a complex cyst. Galactoceles or cysts can be aspirated easily under ultrasound guidance.

Patient with Breast Augmentation. Sonographic evaluation of the breast in a patient who has had breast augmentation or reconstruction with silicone implants has been shown to be of benefit. Mammography is often limited in its ability to image beyond the implant, whereas ultrasound has the ability to evaluate the tissue surrounding the implant, search for the presence of defects in the membrane, and look for leakage into the breast parenchyma. An intracapsular implant rupture occurs when there is a breach of the membrane surrounding an implant, but the silicone that leaks out is still confined within the fibrous scar tissue, which forms a "capsule" around the implant. As the implant collapses and the membrane folds inward, a series of discontinuous echogenic lines parallel to the face of the transducer may be seen and are referred to as the "stepladder sign" or "linguine sign" (Figure 21-23). Caution must be used when evaluating internal echoes within an implant because the internal architecture of an implant may appear heterogeneous as a result of reverberation artifacts and/or a mixture of the gel with other fluids that may have been injected into the implant during surgery, giving a false-positive stepladder sign. An implant rupture allowing extracapsular leakage of silicone into the tissue sonographically appears as an indistinctly marginated area of increased echogenicity along the margin of the implant, with dirty posterior acoustic shadowing and the presence of noise. The depiction of an extracapsular rupture has

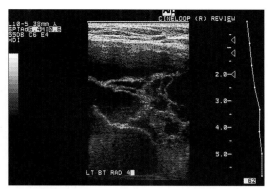

FIGURE 21-23 Seroma. This chronic seroma (noninfected fluid collection) has been repeatedly aspirated in this patient with previous silicone implants that ruptured. Note the thick septations (synechiae) within the seroma.

been described as having a "snowstorm" appearance. Ultrasound is often the first choice among imaging procedures to examine the implant. If the image is unclear, MRI may be used to further define the area in question.

Patient with a Difficult or Compromised Mammogram. For some patients, breast imaging by mammography is limited in its sensitivity (as in the case of very dense breast tissue) or in its ability to visualize the breast tissue (as in the case of retroglandular breast implants) (Figure 21-24). Distinguishing between scar tissue and breast cancer is difficult with mammography. With more women having breast reduction surgeries, these reduction scars, along with previous open biopsy scars, form tissue that is distorted and is difficult to distinguish from breast cancer distortion of normal tissue.

For other patients, examination of breast tissue is compromised because of postsurgical or postradiation changes (Figures 21-25 and 21-26). This is a common situation in the patient who has had breast-conserving therapy for early-stage breast cancer located close to the chest wall or in the axillary tail near the armpit. As technologic advances in ultrasound continue to improve its sensitivity and specificity, the routine use of adjunctive breast ultrasound and mammography in certain high-risk or complicated patients is being advocated (Box 21-9). Although sonography is an invaluable aid to breast imaging, it should not be used as a substitute for mammography because microcalcifications and focal distortion, two of the three principal signs of breast cancer seen by mammography, are often difficult to visualize with ultrasound.

Technique

Scanning is performed using the real-time technique. In most laboratories and clinics, hard copy images are produced to document the examination. The image first must be optimized using electronic focusing, overall gain, and time gain compensation adjustment. The goal is to balance the image from the low-level echoes of the subcutaneous fat to the low-level echoes of the retromammary fat. This should result in an image that clearly shows all levels of the breast from the skin

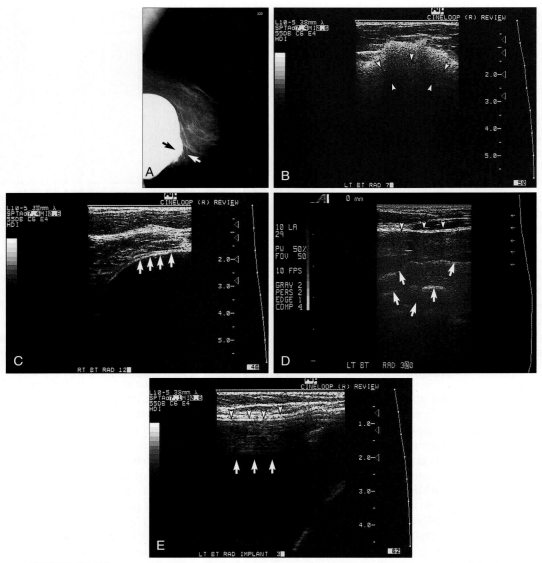

FIGURE 21-24 Ruptured silicone breast implants. A, Mammogram showing retroglandular implant with extracapsular silicone *(arrows)*. **B,** Ultrasound image of the same case showing typical "snowstorm" appearance of free extracapsular silicone *(arrowheads)*. **C,** Ultrasound image of normal intact silicone implant. Note the anechoic appearance of the silicone and the double echogenic margin of the implant perpendicular to the incident sound waves *(arrows)*. **D** and **E,** Two ultrasound images of the same silicone breast implant taken at separate times showing intracapsular rupture. **D,** Note the echogenic fibrous capsule *(arrowheads)* that is no longer a double line, but only a single line. Note the nonparallel echogenic interfaces *(arrows)* within the silicone. These interfaces represent portions of the collapsed and ruptured envelope surrounded by silicone still contained within the fibrous capsule. Compare this appearance with **(E),** the same patient at an earlier time, showing the double echogenic interface *(arrowheads)*. Note the faint parallel lines under the echogenic capsule *(arrows)* representing reverberation artifact.

level through the echogenic breast core and the deeper echogenic chest wall layers. Moderate compression applied with the transducer during scanning will improve detail and decrease the depth of tissue that the ultrasound beam must traverse. In the case of a negative breast ultrasound examination, the usual practice is to record representative images of each quadrant, the subareolar ducts, or specific radial images of the breast, depending on the protocol of the imaging center.

Positioning. Patients are usually scanned in the supine position with the use of a handheld, high-resolution transducer. The patient is positioned with her arm behind her head on the side of the breast to be examined. This spreads the breast tissue more evenly over the surface of the chest and provides a more stable scanning surface and easier access to the axilla. When the medial portion of the breast is scanned, a supine position works well. For the lateral margin of the

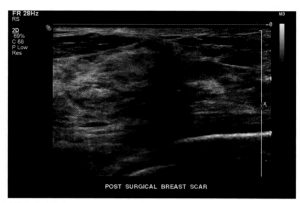

FIGURE 21-25 Postsurgical breast scar causes interruption in the ultrasound beam at the site of the scar (area of shadowing).

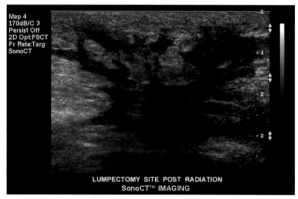

FIGURE 21-26 Lumpectomy site after radiation demonstrates an irregular area that appears to be "masslike" without defined borders in the breast.

BOX 21-9	Breast Ultrasound Applications

Further characterization of mammographic masses
Evaluation of a palpable breast lump
Young patient with dense breasts
Pregnant or lactating patient
Patient with breast augmentation
Difficult or compromised mammogram
Image-guided procedures

breast, the patient can be rolled slightly toward the opposite side (approximately 30 to 45 degrees) and stabilized with a cushion under her shoulder and hips.

If a lesion identified on a mammogram cannot be located sonographically, it may be helpful to sit the patient upright and position the breast in the same positions used to obtain the mammogram. This allows easier localization and a similar frame of reference.

Scanning Technique. When examining for a palpable mass or for correlation with an abnormal mammogram, some centers scan only the area of interest. For example, if a mass in the upper inner quadrant of the right breast is seen on the mammogram, then only the upper inner quadrant of the right breast will be scanned by ultrasound. This is a more specific approach to lesion evaluation, results in fewer cases of false-positive sonographic findings, and is more cost effective than scanning the entire breast. Other centers, however, routinely scan the entire breast. Breast scanning points to remember are listed in Box 21-10.

When a patient is evaluated for a palpable breast mass or for a specific abnormality seen on a mammogram, the abnormality is first located with a preliminary scan. It is helpful to mark the external skin over the mass. The transducer orientation should remain the same as with conventional ultrasound examination (i.e., the patient's right side is oriented to the left of the screen on transverse images, and the notch of the transducer is directed cephalad on longitudinal images). The mass is then thoroughly scanned in orthogonal planes (90 degrees apart) for evaluation of the lesion in three dimensions. This can be recorded using sagittal and transverse images or using radial/antiradial transducer positions (Figure 21-27). Use of radial/antiradial positions is unique to the breast and can often pick up subtle abnormalities extending toward the nipple along the ductal system from the mass. All dominant solid masses are generally recorded with 3D measurements (length, width, and height) to facilitate management decisions and future follow-up.

Annotation. Labeling sonographic images of the breast is extremely important in the identification and correlation of breast images with images from other modalities. Most imaging centers have traditionally used the quasi-grid pattern. This views the breast as a clock face. Directly above the nipple on either breast is 12 o'clock. Right medial breast and left lateral breast are 3 o'clock. Directly below the nipple bilaterally is 6 o'clock, and right lateral breast and left medial breast are 9 o'clock, respectively (Figure 21-28). Other imaging centers might divide the breast into 4 quadrants indicating if they are in the upper or lower, and outer or inner portion of the breast.

Annotation of locating a breast mass varies depending on the imaging center. After determining an o'clock position,

BOX 21-10	Breast Scanning Points to Remember

Image optimization (image tissue from skin through chest wall equally)
Lesion location and annotation methods
- Clock face
- Quadrant
- Distance from nipple
- "1, 2, 3 . . . A, B, C" method
Three-dimensional measurement methods
- Sagittal/transverse
- Radial/antiradial
Ultrasound pitfalls
- Pseudomass
- Infiltrative pattern
- Large, fatty breast

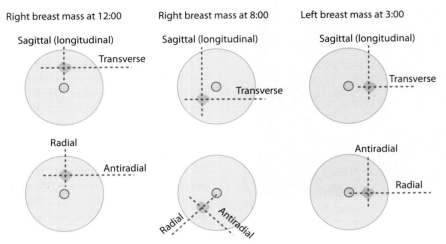

Right breast mass at 12:00   Right breast mass at 8:00   Left breast mass at 3:00

FIGURE 21-27 Examples of sagittal and transverse, plus radial and antiradial, transducer positions.

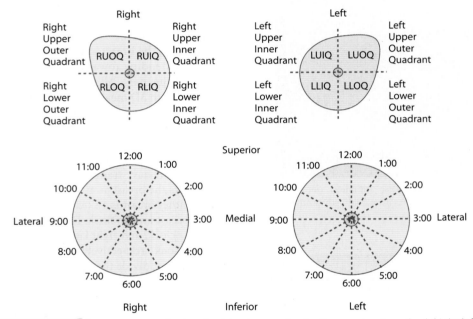

FIGURE 21-28 Breast anatomy is described by two methods: the quadrant method (right/left, upper/lower, and inner/outer quadrants) and the clock face method.

many imaging centers will further subdivide the breast with three concentric circles, with the center being the nipple (Figure 21-29, *A*). This will help identify the location of the breast mass by identifying how far the lesion is from the nipple. The first ring circles one third of the breast tissue, encompassing the area just outside the nipple, or zone 1. The second ring is about two thirds of the breast surface from the nipple, or zone 2. The final ring is to the breast periphery, or zone 3. Lesions located close to the nipple are labeled "A," lesions in the middle of the breast are labeled "B," and lesions located at the outer margin of the breast are labeled "C" (Figure 21-29, *B* and *E*).

Another approach to annotating a pathologic condition is by noting the distance the mass is from the nipple in centimeters. Images may be annotated as "N + 5 cm" indicating a lesion is 5 centimeters from the nipple. Should the nipple be

in the same image, calipers may be used to measure the distance from the nipple.

Finally, the depth of any pathologic condition is documented. The breast again is divided into thirds from the skin to the pectoralis major. Depth A is the most superficial third of the breast, depth B is the middle layer, and depth C is the deepest third of the breast. Superficial lesions located close to the skin surface are labeled "1," lesions in the middle of the breast are labeled "2," and deeper lesions located toward the chest wall are labeled "3."

With solid lesions, it is important to document the orientation of the mass, in addition to its location. The orientation of a lesion is determined by aligning the transducer with the longest axis of a lesion and identifying whether the long axis is oriented in a **radial** or **antiradial** plane. This is important because malignancies tend to grow within the

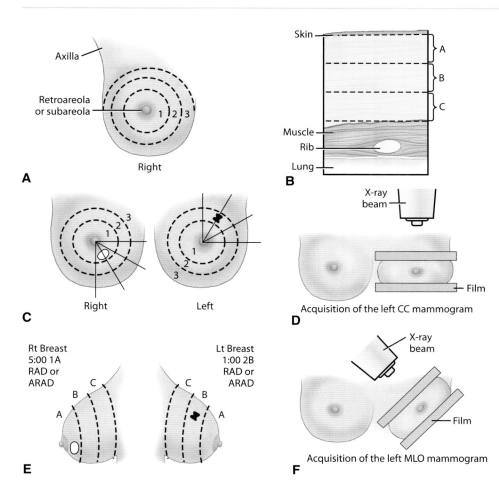

FIGURE 21-29 A, Zones of the breast are shown. **B,** Documentation of depth of tissue. **C,** Localization of mass in the right breast. **D,** Anterior and posterior mammogram of the breast. **E,** Longitudinal view of the breast mass. **F,** Medial to lateral mammogram acquisition.

ducts and often follow the ductal system in a radial plane toward the convergence at the nipple. The various methods of annotation described earlier can be combined to relay a specific location and orientation of a lesion. For example, a lesion labeled "RT BREAST 2:00 B3 RAD" can be relocated easily for follow-up; this lesion in the right breast is deeply situated toward the chest wall in the 2 o'clock position approximately midway between the nipple and the outer margin of the breast, and its long axis is oriented radially toward the nipple.

Sonographic Characteristics of Breast Masses

Sonographic evaluation of a breast lesion normally begins with determination of whether a lesion is cystic or solid (Box 21-11). The distinction between a cyst and a solid mass is extremely important for management purposes; a cyst that meets the criteria of a simple cyst on ultrasound is universally considered benign. Solid masses, however, have a malignant potential. Although a vast majority of solid masses are benign, further characterization of a solid lesion is necessary.

To be considered a simple cyst, a lesion must meet several criteria on ultrasound: It must be devoid of internal echoes (anechoic), show smooth inner margins with an imperceptible capsule, and demonstrate posterior acoustic enhancement (Table 21-2). Cysts within the breast can be multilocular with thin internal septations. In the case of simple cysts, no further workup is usually necessary. In some cases, however, these cysts will be painful or disturbing to the patient (Figure 21-30). Aspiration can be performed quickly and easily under ultrasound guidance.

If the cyst has internal echoes, wall irregularity, mural nodularity or septation, shadowing, nonuniform internal echoes, or any other feature not associated with a simple cyst, it is by definition a complex cyst, and aspiration and/or biopsy should be considered. Complex cysts are often indistinguishable from homogeneous solid sonographic masses because of their thick proteinaceous fluid content. Other complex cysts have thick or irregular capsules, a possible intracystic mass, or dependent debris. Cysts with layering calcifications or floating crystals (these can be seen moving on real-time scanning) are benign, although careful ultrasound technique is required to distinguish these cysts from those requiring further evaluation.

The usual approach to a small, smooth, round or oval, benign-appearing solid mass in low-risk patients favors close-interval follow-up breast imaging. Color Doppler has been successfully used to interrogate solid masses to check for increased vascular flow. The demonstration of increased

BOX 21-11	Sonographic Characteristics of Breast Lesions

Simple cyst
- Smooth walls
- Anechoic
- Posterior enhancement

Complicated cyst
- Wall thickening or irregularities
- Septations
- Internal echoes

Solid mass
- Margins
  Benign: smooth, rounded
  Malignant: indistinct, fuzzy, spiculated
- Disruption of breast architecture
  Benign: grow within tissue, causing compression of the tissue adjacent to the mass
  Malignant: grow through tissue without compressing adjacent tissue and may cause retraction of the nipple or dimpling of the skin
- Shape
  Benign: rounded or oval, large lobulations (fewer than three)
  Malignant: sharp, angular microlobulations (three or more)
- Orientation
  Malignant: taller than wide highly suspicious; radial growth suspicious for intraductal lesions
- Internal echo pattern
  Benign: isoechoic, hyperechoic
  Malignant: hypoechoic, weak internal echoes, clustered microcalcifications
- Attenuation effects
  Benign: posterior enhancement
  Malignant: strongly attenuating
- Mobility
  Benign: some mobility
  Malignant: firmly fixed
- Compressibility
  Benign: fatty tumors are usually compressible
  Malignant: rigid, noncompressible
- Vascularity
  Malignant: hypervascular; feeder vessel may be identified

TABLE 21-2	Sonographic Characteristics of Common Lesions

Mass	Characteristics
Simple cyst	Oval or round, anechoic, imperceptible capsule, posterior acoustic enhancement, edge refraction shadowing, often compressible
Fibrocystic changes	Multiple cysts, well circumscribed, thin walls, increased fibrous stroma
Complex cyst	Irregular or thickened wall, mural nodule, fluid levels, debris, particulate echoes, variable degrees of shadowing
Benign fibroadenoma	Oval or gently lobular, hypoechoic, uniform echogenicity, smooth, distinct margins, wider than tall, posterior acoustic enhancement, edge refraction shadow
Lipoma	May be large, smooth walls, hypoechoic (isoechoic with fat), posterior acoustic enhancement, easily compressible
Fat necrosis	Irregular, complex mass with low-level echoes; may have posterior acoustic shadow, separate from breast parenchyma
Abscess	Hypoechoic, complex lesion, posterior enhancement, thick walls, fluid levels
Cystosarcoma phyllodes	Large, hypoechoic tumor, well-defined margins, decreased through-transmission, fine or coarse internal echoes, variable amounts of shadowing
Intraductal papilloma	Intracystic lesion with fibrovascular stalk
Malignant	Irregular, spiculated, indistinct, or angular margins, hypoechoic, heterogeneous echogenicity, taller than wide, posterior acoustic shadowing, noncompressible, hypervascular with feeder vessel
Ductal carcinoma	Calcifications and ductal enlargement with extension within the ducts in situ (DCIS)
Invasive ductal	Begins in the ducts, invades the fatty tissue of the breast carcinoma (IDC)
Lobular carcinoma in situ	Confined to the gland, difficult to distinguish sonographically
Invasive lobular carcinoma	Begins in the lobule, extends into the fatty tissue; often bilateral, multicentric, or multifocal

vascular flow could accelerate the need for biopsy of these masses.

Tissue diagnosis is suggested in high-risk patients or patients with larger masses. The size cutoff for tissue diagnosis versus follow-up varies. In a low-risk patient with a single, dominant, smooth, solid mass, follow-up is offered for masses with a diameter of up to 1 cm. Some physicians recommend following lesions up to 1.2 or even 1.5 cm in size, especially in the case of multiple bilateral masses. In a high-risk patient or in a patient who is not comfortable waiting on follow-up for an answer, tissue diagnosis can be pursued more aggressively. Options include fine-needle aspiration cytology, large-core needle biopsy, vacuum-assisted biopsy, and surgical excisional biopsy (Figure 21-31). High-quality sonographic imaging of a solid breast mass is accurate in characterizing a lesion as probably benign or probably malignant in a majority of cases

(see Table 21-2). It is important, however, to realize that there is significant overlap in the appearance of benign and malignant lesions; ultrasound cannot be used as a substitute for tissue diagnosis when sonographic findings are indeterminate or when a biopsy is indicated by clinical examination or patient history.

Margins. The margins of a mass should be investigated carefully. A technique called *fremitus* can be used to identify and confirm the margins of a mass. Fremitus is a palpable tremor or vibration of the chest wall. Using power Doppler, have the patient hum. The vibrations of the chest wall will carry through to the breast tissue, creating a power Doppler signal. The lesion is normally void of signal, making it easier to identify its margins. This technique can be useful in

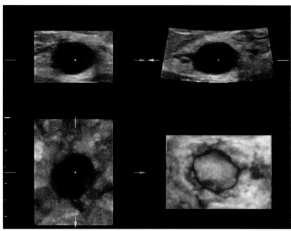

FIGURE 21-30 Symptomatic cyst. Simple cyst on ultrasound (notice the lack of internal echoes and the smooth internal margin, imperceptible capsule, strong posterior acoustic enhancement, and edge refraction) is large enough to create a painful lump in the patient's breast.

confirming the presence of a mass when in doubt, identifying multifocal masses, differentiating diffuse masses, and locating palpable masses that are isoechoic with the breast parenchyma.

Benign lesions usually have smooth, rounded margins (Figure 21-32, *A–C*). Malignant tumors are aggressive and tend to grow through tissue via finger-like extensions termed **spiculation** (Figure 21-32, *D*). Spiculated margins are the ultrasound finding with the highest positive predictive value of malignancy and correlate with mammographic spiculation. Sonographic spiculations appear as small lines that radiate outward from the surface of a mass. They are typically alternating hypoechoic and hyperechoic lines. Ductal extensions project radially from the tumor and are oriented toward the nipple. Small extensions may not be visible sonographically, but may make the margins of a lesion appear indistinct or fuzzy.

Disruption of Breast Architecture. Benign tumors are usually slow growing and do not invade surrounding tissue.

They tend to grow horizontally within the tissue planes, parallel to the chest wall. Larger benign lesions often cause compression of tissue adjacent to the mass, implying that the mass is pushing against adjacent breast tissue, as opposed to infiltrating it.

Malignant lesions, on the other hand, tend to grow right through the normal breast tissue. As malignant masses enlarge, they may cause retraction of the nipple or dimpling of the skin as the spiculations pull on Cooper's ligaments (Figure 21-33).

Shape. A rounded or oval shape is usually associated with benign lesions; sharp, angular margins are associated with malignancy. Mild undulations in contour can be seen in benign masses such as fibroadenomas; however, microlobulations (very small 1- to 2-mm lobulations) are more often associated with malignancy. Lobulations associated with benign fibroadenomas are usually large, rounded lobulations and do not exceed three in number. Microlobulations associated with malignancy are usually smaller, sharper, and more numerous.

Orientation. The normal tissue planes of the breast are horizontally oriented. Benign lesions tend to grow within the normal tissue planes, and their long axis lies parallel to the chest wall. These lesions are noted to be "wider than tall." Malignant lesions are able to grow through the connective tissue and may have a vertical orientation when the breast is imaged from anterior to posterior. If a mass measures longer in the anteroposterior dimension (height) than in the transverse or sagittal plane (width), it has a vertical orientation, is usually described as "taller-than-wide," and is suspicious for malignancy.

Internal Echo Pattern. Lesions that appear isoechoic with the breast parenchyma or have echoes equivalent to or brighter than that of fat are most often benign. A solid lesion that is hypoechoic relative to the normal breast parenchyma is more suspicious for malignancy. Malignant lesions tend to be highly hypoechoic relative to fat and usually have weak internal echoes. They are often associated with dense posterior shadowing, making the lesion difficult to penetrate.

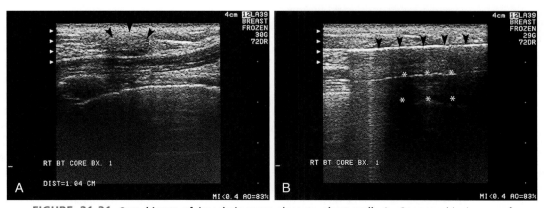

FIGURE 21-31 Core biopsy of isoechoic mass close to chest wall. A, Sonographic image of an isoechoic mass *(arrowheads)* located immediately adjacent to the pectoralis muscle *(arrows)*. **B,** Core-biopsy needle *(arrowheads)* is directed parallel to the chest wall. Note the loss of information posterior to the needle caused by acoustic shadowing and reverberation echoes *(asterisks)*.

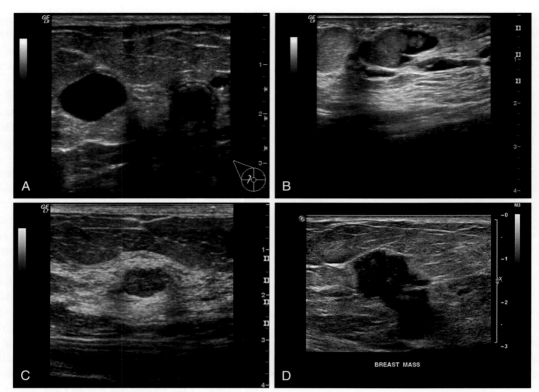

FIGURE 21-32 **Benign lesions of the breast. A,** Cyst. **B,** Complex. **C,** Fibroadenoma. **D,** Malignant solid mass with spiculation.

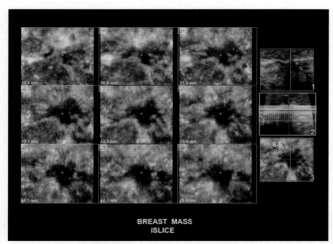

FIGURE 21-33 Malignant lesions interrupt the normal breast architecture as they spread throughout the tissue, as shown on this tomographic presentation.

Microcalcifications within a solid mass are associated with a breast malignancy. Ultrasound is less sensitive than mammography in the detection of microcalcifications due to the heterogeneous appearance of normal breast tissue. Microcalcifications seen with ultrasound are typically very small echogenic foci that do not create shadows because of their small size. Although calcifications are not visualized frequently by sonography, their detection in a hypoechoic mass is suspicious for malignancy.

Attenuation Effects. Enhancement behind a lesion is normally caused by a weakly attenuating structure; it usually indicates that the lesion is made up of fluid and is a characteristic associated with benign lesions. Most solid lesions, with the exception of a fibroadenoma, will not enhance.

Shadowing behind a solid breast mass is another suspicious sonographic sign for malignancy because malignant tumors tend to be highly attenuating. Posterior shadowing should not be confused with edge or refraction shadowing, in which shadowing occurs at the curved edge of a smooth, benign mass.

Mobility. Benign lesions normally demonstrate a limited degree of mobility or may roll away as they are palpated. Because of the spiculations associated with malignancy, malignant lesions are normally very fixed or rigid in their position.

Compressibility. If pressure applied by the transducer causes the lesion to compress or change shape, the lesion is probably benign and most likely represents a fat lobule. Malignant lesions normally are very hard and noncompressible.

Vascularity. Doppler interrogation of a breast lesion is an essential element of the study. Although breast lesions are not associated with consistent resistance patterns on Doppler ultrasound, malignant masses often demonstrate increased vascularity within the lesion and often have a feeder vessel, which can be identified on careful evaluation. Vessels that penetrate a mass are highly suspect for malignancy and should be checked using color or power Doppler to ascertain the number and to look for intratumoral vessels.

PATHOLOGY

The most common pathologic lesions of the female breast are, in order of decreasing frequency, fibrocystic disease, carcinoma, fibroadenoma, intraductal papilloma, and duct ectasia. Benign lesions are the most common breast lesions, representing 70% of proved lesions in biopsies after they are removed. Several parameters, including the patient's age, physical characteristics of the mass, and previous medical history, must be considered when a dominant mass has been palpated. Lesions common to younger women are fibrocystic disease and fibroadenomas. Older or postmenopausal women are more likely to have intraductal papilloma, duct ectasia, and cancer.

Differential Diagnosis of Breast Masses

Symptoms of breast masses include pain, a palpable mass, spontaneous or induced nipple discharge, skin dimpling, ulceration, and nipple retraction. Benign processes are usually associated with pain, tumor, and nipple discharge. Skin dimpling or ulceration and nipple retraction nearly always result from cancer. Benign tumors are rubbery, mobile, and well defined (as seen in a fibroadenoma), whereas malignant tumors are often stone hard and irregular with a gritty feel. Soft tumors usually represent a lipoma (fat tissue). Cystic masses are like a balloon of water, well delineated but not as mobile as fibroadenomas because they form part of the breast parenchyma, whereas a fibroadenoma has a capsule.

Benign Conditions

Cysts. Cysts are commonly seen in women 35 to 55 years of age. Symptoms include history of changing with the menstrual cycle, pain (especially when the cyst is growing rapidly), recent lump, and tenderness. Small cysts may not regress completely and may persist from one cycle to the next.

Fibrocystic Condition. Fibrocystic changes produce histologic alterations in the terminal ducts and lobules of the breast in both epithelial and connective tissue. Fibrocystic changes are usually accompanied by pain or tenderness in the breast and represent normal physiologic processes of breast tissue that fluctuate under the influence of normal female hormonal cycles. These processes become magnified in some patients to the point of causing symptoms that are upsetting to the patient (mainly pain and tenderness or recurrent cysts). In some cases, *fibrocystic condition (FCC)* causes changes that are frankly worrisome for breast cancer. In all age-groups, the most common diagnosis at breast biopsy is FCC. These biopsies are prompted by a growing or dominant clinically suspicious breast lump.

The terms *fibrocystic condition* and *fibrocystic change* (use of the term *fibrocystic disease* is discouraged) actually encompass many different processes under a single term. An abundance of inaccuracy and confusion results from using the term *fibrocystic condition*. In some cases, FCC may refer to the normal hormonal fluctuations in breast texture. At the other end of the spectrum, a surgical biopsy may be undertaken because of a growing suspicious breast lump. In a few cases, a biopsy reveals tissue changes that mean the patient is at increased risk for subsequent development of breast cancer.

Clinical signs and symptoms of FCC include the lumps and mastalgia, which the patient might particularly feel in the outer portion of the breasts. This feeling may fluctuate with every monthly cycle. In most cases, both breasts are equally involved. In some cases, FCC may affect just one area of one breast. This can be frightening for the patient and is a frequent cause of referral for diagnostic breast imaging.

Imaging signs of FCC may be visible on the mammogram or breast ultrasound. On mammogram, FCC may cause diffuse benign microcalcifications, **adenosis,** and multiple round masses. Sonographically, FCC may include scattered calcifications and cystic changes, which include simple cysts, complicated cysts, clustered cysts, and clustered microcysts (Figure 21-34).

Many separate tissue processes of FCC are recognized by the pathologist in reviewing breast tissue under a microscope, including **apocrine metaplasia,** fibrosis, epithelial ductal hyperplasia, and sclerosing adenosis. In correlating the pathologic results of a breast biopsy with the indication for biopsy (i.e., palpable breast lump, suspicious mammographic or sonographic mass, or clustered microcalcifications), it is very important for the physician to document that the pathologic results are concordant with the targeted lesion. If a breast biopsy was performed because of suspicious microcalcifications, for example, the pathology report should state that microcalcifications were seen. If no microcalcifications were seen on pathology slides, then this is a discordant result, and further investigation will be required.

In an attempt to create a more clinically relevant classification of tissue processes under the enormous and confusing heading of fibrocystic condition, these processes have been separated into three categories: (1) nonproliferative lesions (no increased risk of subsequent development of breast cancer); (2) proliferative lesions without atypical cells (mildly elevated risk of subsequent breast cancer); and (3) proliferative lesions with atypical cellular changes (moderately increased risk of subsequent breast cancer). Any woman with an atypical proliferative breast lesion (especially lobular neoplasia) who also has

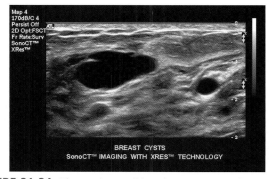

FIGURE 21-34 Fibrocystic condition shows two sonolucent structures within the breast.

TABLE 21-3	Fibrocystic Condition: Common Breast Lesions—Risk of Subsequent Breast Cancer
Classification	**Description**
Nonproliferative lesions: no increased risk	Cyst Apocrine metaplasia Fibroadenoma Ductal ectasia Mild epithelial ductal hyperplasia Benign microcalcifications
Proliferative lesions without atypical features: mildly increased risk (1.5–2×)	Moderate or florid epithelial ductal hyperplasia Sclerosing adenosis Radial scar (complex sclerosing lesion) Intraductal papilloma
Proliferative lesions with atypical features: moderately increased risk (4–6×)	Atypical ductal hyperplasia Atypical lobular hyperplasia Lobular neoplasia (alternative term for lobular carcinoma in situ)

Note: Patients with an atypical proliferative lesion and a first-degree relative with breast cancer are at even greater risk for subsequent breast cancer.

a family history of a first-degree relative with breast cancer will have double the risk of subsequent breast cancer compared with the patient with an atypical proliferative lesion alone (Table 21-3).

Fibroadenoma. The most common benign breast tumor is **fibroadenoma,** and it occurs primarily in young women. Fibroadenomas may be found in one breast or in both breasts. The growth of a fibroadenoma is stimulated by estrogen. Under normal circumstances, hormonal influences on the breast (estrogen) result in the proliferation of epithelial cells in lactiferous ducts and in stromal tissue during the first half of the menstrual cycle. During the second half of the cycle, this condition regresses, allowing breast tissue to return to its normal resting state. In certain disturbances of this hormonal mechanism, regression fails to occur, resulting in the development of fibrous and epithelial nodules that become fibroadenomas, fibromas, or adenomas, depending on the predominant cell type. They may also be related to pregnancy and lactation.

Clinically, a fibroadenoma is firm, rubbery, freely mobile, and clearly delineated from the surrounding breast tissue (Figure 21-35). It is round or ovoid and smooth or lobulated, and usually does not cause loss of contour of the breast unless it develops to a large size. It rarely causes mastodynia, and it does not change size during the menstrual cycle. Fibroadenomas tend to grow very slowly. A sudden increase in size with acute pain may be the result of hemorrhage within the tumor. However, a growth greater than 20% within 6 months may suggest a phylloides tumor, which warrants further investigation. Calcification may follow hemorrhage or infarction; thus the tumor may have calcifications and may mimic the

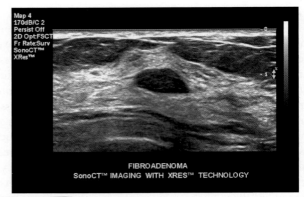

FIGURE 21-35 Fibroadenoma. Smooth, ovoid, solid mass with a low-level internal echo pattern.

appearance of a carcinoma on mammography. Sonographically, fibroadenomas have benign characteristics with smooth, rounded margins and low-level homogeneous internal echoes and may demonstrate intermediate posterior enhancement. Fibroadenomas are normally hypoechoic, but occasionally are hyperechoic to the fat within the breast.

Lipoma. A pure lipoma consists entirely of fatty tissue. Other forms of lipoma consist of fat with fibrous and glandular elements interspersed (fibroadenolipoma). A lipoma may grow to a large size before it is clinically detected. It is usually found in middle-aged or menopausal women. Clinically, on palpation, a large, soft, poorly demarcated mass is felt that cannot be clearly separated from the surrounding parenchyma. No thinning or fixation of the overlying skin is noted. Sonographically, it may be difficult or impossible to detect a lipoma in a fatty breast. Lipomas typically have smooth walls, are hypoechoic, and appear similar to fat. They often demonstrate posterior enhancement and are easily compressible.

Fat Necrosis. Injury to breast fat may cause a common benign inflammatory process known as fat necrosis. Injuries include trauma to the breast, surgery, radiation treatments, or plasma cell mastitis or may be related to an involutional process or other disease present in the breast, such as cancer. It is more frequently found in older women. Clinical palpation reveals a spherical nodule that is generally superficial under a layer of calcified necrosis. A deep-lying focus of necrosis may cause scarring with skin retraction and thus may mimic carcinoma. Sonographically, fat necrosis may appear a number of ways. It may appear as a solid lesion, as a complex mass with mural nodules or echogenic bands, as an anechoic mass with either posterior acoustic enhancement or with shadowing, or without a visible mass. This variability may mimic a malignant lesion; however, it is separate and distinct from the rest of the breast parenchyma.

Acute Mastitis. Acute mastitis may result from infection, trauma, mechanical obstruction in the breast ducts, or other conditions. It often occurs during lactation, beginning in the lactiferous ducts and spreading via the lymphatics or blood. Acute mastitis causes an enlarged, reddened, tender breast, and is often confined to one area of the breast. Diffuse mastitis results when infection is carried via the blood or breast lymphatics and thus affects the entire breast. Patients are treated initially with antibiotics and are referred for breast imaging when acute inflammatory symptoms are sufficiently reduced to allow good quality mammography and breast ultrasound to rule out inflammatory breast cancer as a cause.

Chronic Mastitis. An inflammation of the glandular tissue is considered to be chronic mastitis. This is very difficult to differentiate by ultrasound; the echo pattern is mixed and diffuse with sound absorption. The condition is usually found in elderly women. Thickening of the connective tissue results in narrowing of the lumina of the milk ducts. The cause is inspissated intraductal secretions, which are forced into the periductal connective tissue. Clinically, the patient usually has a nipple discharge; frequently, the nipple has retracted over a period of years. Palpation reveals some subareolar thickening, but no dominant mass.

Abscess. Abscesses may be single or multiple. Acute abscesses have a poorly defined border, whereas mature abscesses are well encapsulated with sharp borders. A definite diagnosis cannot be made from a mammogram alone, and either an aspiration or core needle biopsy is necessary to determine a diagnosis. An aspiration or biopsy is necessary to determine a diagnosis, but clinical findings help diagnose breast abscesses. Patients may present with pain, swelling, and reddening of the overlying skin. The patient may be febrile, and swollen painful axillary nodes may be present. Sonographic findings may show a diffuse, mottled appearance of the breast, irregular margins, posterior enhancement, and low-level internal echoes (Figure 21-36). If associated with mastitis, skin thickening is almost always present, and edema leads to diffusely increased echogenicity of the breast tissue. Color or power Doppler of the breast may be helpful to document hyperemia associated with increased vascularity, which may tip the scales toward abscess rather than hematoma.

Cystosarcoma Phyllodes. Cystosarcoma phyllodes is a rare, predominantly benign breast neoplasm. It accounts for less than 1% of all breast neoplasms, yet it is the most frequent sarcoma of the breast. It is more commonly found in women in their 50s and usually is unilateral. It may arise from a fibroadenoma.

Many patients may notice that a small breast mass that has been present for a long time suddenly begins to grow rapidly. Although it is considered a benign lesion, 27% of these tumors are malignant, and 12% metastasize.

When the tumor is small, it is well delineated, firm, and mobile, much like a fibroadenoma. As it enlarges, the surface may become irregular and lobulated. Skin changes can develop from increasing pressure. Edema may produce a skin change. Increasing pressure causes trophic changes and eventual skin ulcerations. Infection and abscess formation may be a secondary complication. The tumor never adheres to adjacent soft tissue or underlying pectoral muscle; therefore dimpling of the skin or fixation of the tumor is not observed. Sonographic findings include a large, hypoechoic tumor with well-defined margins and decreased through-transmission. Internal echoes may be fine or coarse with variable amounts of shadowing.

Intraductal Papilloma. An intraductal papilloma is a small, benign tumor that grows within the acini of the breast. It occurs most frequently in women 35 to 55 years of age. The predominant symptom is spontaneous nipple discharge arising from a single duct. When the discharge is copious, it is usually preceded by a sensation of fullness or pain in the areola or nipple area that is relieved as the fluid is expelled. It has a "raspberry-like" configuration on the mammogram and in this way helps to promote correlation between the mammogram and the sonogram.

Papillomas are usually small, multiple, and multicentric. They consist of simple proliferations of duct epithelium projecting outward into a dilated lumen from one or more focal points (Figure 21-37), each supported by a vascular stalk from which it receives the blood supply. Trauma may rupture the stalk, filling the duct with blood or serum. Papillomas may grow to a large size and thus become palpable lesions. They are somewhat linear, resembling the terminal duct, and are usually benign.

Malignant Conditions

Malignancies generally develop over a long time. It is not unusual for several years to pass from the first appearance of

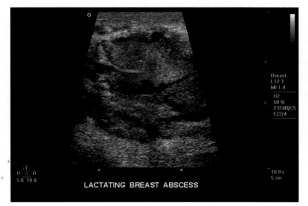

FIGURE 21-36 Lactating breast abscess shows a diffuse mottled appearance of the breast with irregular margins and posterior enhancement.

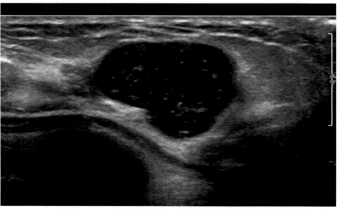

FIGURE 21-37 Complex cyst with debris

atypical hyperplasia to the final diagnosis of in situ cancer. Malignant cells grow along a line of least resistance, such as in fatty tissue. In fibrotic tissue, most cancer growth occurs along the borders. Lymphatics and blood vessels are frequently used as pathways for new tumor development. If the tumor is encapsulated, it continues to grow in one area, compressing and distorting the surrounding architecture. When the carcinoma is contained and has not invaded the basal membrane structure, it is considered in situ. Most cancer originates in the terminal ductal lobular units, whereas a smaller percentage originates in the glandular tissue. The breast lobules are concentrated in the upper outer quadrant of the breast, and so it is not surprising that a majority of breast cancers (50%) are found there, followed by lesser incidence in the retroareolar area (17%), upper inner quadrant (15%), lower outer quadrant (10%), and lower inner quadrant (5%). Multifocal masses are least common and occur in approximately 3% of cases.

Cancer of the breast is of two types: sarcoma and carcinoma. Sarcoma refers to breast tumors that arise from supportive or connective tissues. Sarcomas tend to grow rapidly and invade fibrous tissue. Carcinoma refers to breast tumors that arise from the epithelium, in the ductal and glandular tissue, and usually has tentacles. Other malignant diseases affecting the breast result from systemic neoplasms, such as leukemia or lymphoma.

Breast carcinomas are generally categorized by two factors: where the cancer cells originate (ductal or lobular) and whether the cancer is prone to spreading (noninvasive or invasive). Most breast carcinomas begin within the ducts of the breast and are called ductal or intraductal carcinomas. Breast cancers that form in the lobules are called lobular carcinomas. Carcinomas that do not normally spread outside of the duct or lobule are called noninvasive, noninfiltrating, or in situ cancer, whereas cancers that spread into nearby tissue are said to be invasive or infiltrating.

Ductal Carcinoma In Situ. Ductal carcinoma in situ (DCIS) is also known as intraductal carcinoma. DCIS is characterized by excessive growth of abnormal epithelial cells within the duct. These abnormal cells have not yet spread through the walls of the ducts into the fatty tissue of the breast, hence the term *in situ* (Figure 21-38). Because these are confined to the duct and have not spread, they usually have a 100% cure rate with treatment. However, if left untreated an estimated 14% to 53% of DCIS will process to invasive cancer, which penetrates the basement membranes. Calcifications and ductal enlargement with extension within the ducts are common (Figure 21-39).

Invasive Ductal Carcinoma. Invasive ductal carcinoma (IDC) accounts for nearly 80% of breast cancers. Similar to DCIS, these cancers begin in the ducts, but in contrast to DCIS, they invade the fatty tissue of the breast and have the potential to metastasize via the bloodstream or the lymphatic system. It is important to get a definitive diagnosis and begin treatment before cancer spreads to other organs.

Lobular Carcinoma In Situ. Lobular carcinoma in situ (LCIS) is not considered a "cancer" because it has a low malignant potential. LCIS is often referred to as *lobular neoplasia* and is classified as a precancerous growth that begins in the lobule. LCIS is confined to the gland and does not penetrate through the wall of the lobule. LCIS does not usually form a distinct mass and therefore can be difficult to pick up with the use of only mammography and ultrasound screening. Women with LCIS are at higher risk of developing invasive breast cancer later on.

Invasive Lobular Carcinoma. Invasive lobular carcinoma (ILC) begins in the lobule, where it extends into the fatty tissue of the breast. Similar to IDC, ILC has the potential to metastasize and spread to other parts of the body. ILC is the second most common type of invasive tumor, accounting for 10% to 15% of all breast cancers. ILC is often bilateral, multicentric, or multifocal (Figure 21-40). Compared with IDC, ILC carries a poorer prognosis.

Breast cancers are considered multifocal when more than one tumor is identified and when they are located within the same quadrant or ductal system and are within 5 cm of each

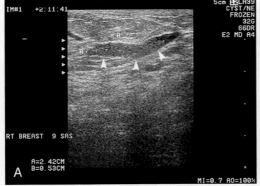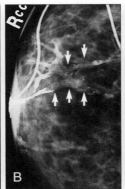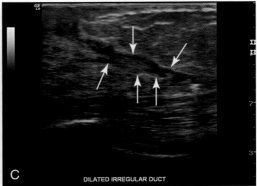

FIGURE 21-38 Intraductal masses. A, Sonographic image shows a large intraductal mass in a patient with a unilateral single-duct discharge (*arrowheads*). **B,** Magnification view from a galactogram, in which contrast was injected retrograde into the duct orifice from which the discharge was expressed. Note the large filling defect (*arrows*). **C,** Sonographic image from another patient showing a small intraductal mass (*arrows*). Most intraductal masses are benign papillomas. It is generally difficult, however, to distinguish an intraductal papilloma from an early intraductal cancer.

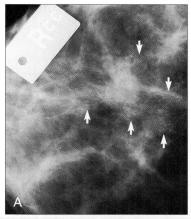

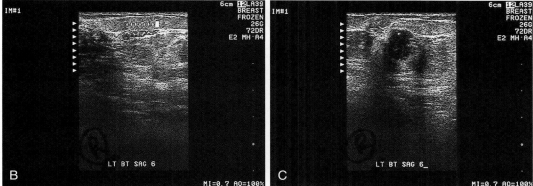

FIGURE 21-39 Suspicious microcalcifications (DCIS) and occult infiltrating ductal carcinoma. **A,** Magnification mammogram image of pleomorphic (irregular shapes) suspicious microcalcifications identified on screening mammogram in this asymptomatic young woman. No mass was visible on the mammogram. **B,** Sonographic demonstration of echogenic microcalcification within a dilated duct *(arrows).* **C,** Image of the same breast showing an unsuspected sonographic mass with suspicious features (note that the mass is taller than wide, shows an irregular indistinct margin, and shows asymmetric posterior shadowing and heterogeneous echogenicity). Ultrasound-guided large-needle core biopsy proved infiltrating malignancy. This altered the patient's management, requiring a mastectomy and axillary node dissection for staging.

other. Breast cancers are considered multicentric when they are located in different quadrants and are located at least 5 cm apart. Multifocal lesions tend to be of the same cell type histologically, whereas multicentric lesions are more likely to be of two different cell types.

The more favorable cancers remain localized to the breast longer, and treated patients have a 75% survival rate after 10 years. They represent only 10% to 12% of all breast cancers. This group includes medullary, intracystic papillary, papillary, colloid, adenoid cystic, and tubular carcinomas. Other malignant tumors that have a better than average prognosis after treatment include malignant cystosarcoma phyllodes and stromal sarcomas, because they rarely metastasize to regional nodes.

Definitive identification of a tumor type can be made only by histologic (tissue) examination. Although many solid lesions have definite malignant characteristics, crossover of benign and malignant characteristics is often seen on ultrasound, and the nature of the lesion is indeterminate by sonographic evaluation alone. It is not uncommon for

malignant lesions to have a benign appearance on ultrasound, thus making it extremely important to consider the patient's risk factors and clinical history when considering the differential diagnosis. The following is a brief description of the more common malignancies affecting the breast.

Comedocarcinoma. Intraductal solid carcinoma in which the lactiferous ducts are filled with a yellow pastelike material that looks like small plugs (comedones) when sectioned is called comedocarcinoma. Histologically, the ducts are filled with plugs of an epithelial tumor that have a central necrosis, giving rise to the pastelike material. Both invasive and noninvasive forms exist.

Noninvasive forms may lack any clinical or palpatory findings. If a nipple discharge occurs, it is more frequently clear than bloody (unlike papillary carcinoma, in which bloody discharge is typical). The patient may complain of pain or the sensation of insects crawling on the breast. With early invasion, minimal thickening of the surrounding breast tissue may be palpated. In the advanced

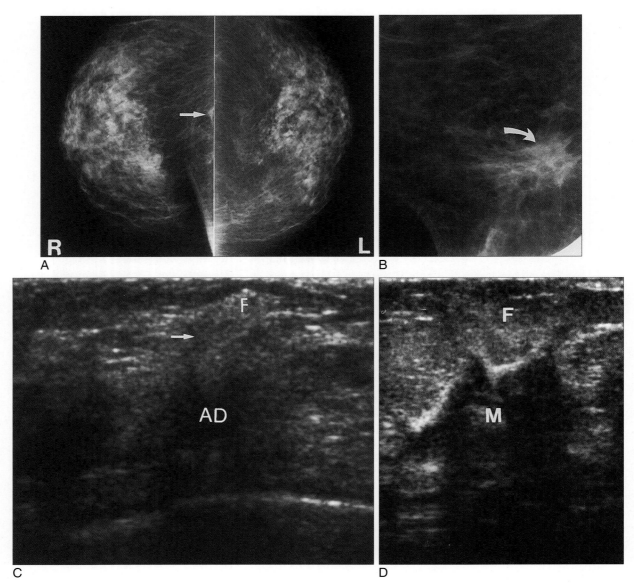

FIGURE 21-40 Infiltrating lobular carcinoma. A, Craniocaudal view of both breasts shows portion of nodular density *(arrow)* in posterior central right breast. **B,** Spot compression magnification view shows wispy area *(arrow)* of parenchymal density in the inframammary fold corresponding to the nodule on the craniocaudal view. **C,** Sonogram of area of mammographic abnormality shows hypoechoic, ill-defined area of architectural distortion *(AD)* with infiltration *(arrow)* into the adjacent fibroglandular parenchyma *(F);* ultrasound-guided biopsy confirmed the diagnosis of infiltrating lobular carcinoma. **D,** In another patient with vague thickening on self-examination, a mammogram showed dense glandular tissue but no focal mass. Ultrasound demonstrates an extensive hypoechoic angular mass *(M)* occupying nearly two thirds of the breast. *F,* Fibroglandular tissue.

stage, clinical signs include nipple retraction, dominant mass, and fixation.

Microcalcifications are commonly seen on mammography and may be picked up sonographically. Intraductal carcinomas have malignant characteristics, including irregular margins, a diffuse internal echo pattern, and attenuation with shadowing.

Juvenile Breast Cancer. Juvenile breast cancer is similar to ductal carcinoma in situ and invasive ductal carcinoma as found in adults. Generally, it occurs in young females,

between 8 and 15 years of age, and has a good prognosis when treated early.

Papillary Carcinoma. Papillary carcinoma is a tumor that initially arises as an intraductal mass. It may also take the form of an intracystic tumor, which is rare. The early stage of papillary carcinoma is noninvasive. The tumor occasionally arises from a benign ductal papilloma. It is associated with little fibrotic reaction.

Both intraductal and intracystic forms exist, and these represent 1% to 2% of all breast carcinomas. The earliest

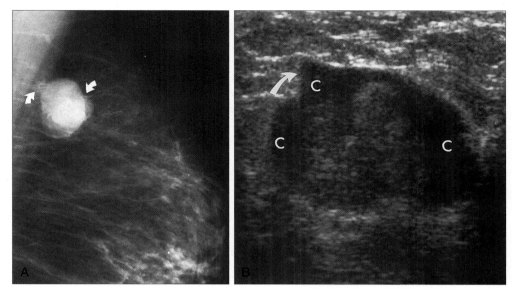

FIGURE 21-41 Papillary carcinoma. A, Mediolateral oblique view of the left breast shows well-circumscribed mass containing area of increased density. Slight marginal irregularity is seen *(arrows).* **B,** Circumscribed complex mass with anterior protuberance *(curved arrow).* Central area of echogenicity is surrounded circumferentially by what most likely represents the cystic component *(C)* of this in situ papillary carcinoma with stromal invasion.

clinical sign of intraductal papillary carcinoma is bloody nipple discharge. Occasionally, a mass can be palpated as a small, firm, well-circumscribed area and may be mistaken for a fibroadenoma (Figure 21-41). Nodules of blue or red discoloration may be found under the skin with central ulceration. A diffusely nodular appearance overlying the skin is a special variant of multiple intraductal papillary carcinoma. Intracystic papillary carcinoma is clinically indistinguishable in its early stages from a cyst or fibroadenoma. When the tumor has invaded through the cyst wall, it is palpable as a poorly circumscribed mass. Papillary carcinoma typically has a more favorable prognosis than other types of carcinoma.

Paget's Disease. Paget's disease arises in the retroareolar ducts and grows in the direction of the nipple, spreading into the intraepidermal region of the nipple and areola, and has a rashlike appearance that may be confused with a melanoma. Any ulceration, enlargement, or deformity of the nipple and areola should suggest Paget's disease. This is a relatively rare tumor, accounting for 2.5% of all breast cancers. It typically occurs in women over 50 years of age. Differential diagnosis includes benign inflammatory eczematous condition of the nipple, because palpatory findings frequently are not present. The primary ductal cancer may be quite deep or embedded in fibrotic tissue. Sonographically, Paget's disease will present as a retroareolar mass with irregular margins, heterogeneous internal echoes, and attenuation with posterior shadowing.

Scirrhous Carcinoma. Scirrhous carcinoma is a type of intraductal tumor with extensive fibrous tissue proliferation (very dense fibrosis). Focal calcification may also be present. Histologically, the cells are found in narrow files or strands, clusters, or columns and may form lumina with varying frequency.

Scirrhous carcinoma is the most common form of breast cancer and often has no specific histologic findings or patterns; therefore it is often classified as ductal carcinoma that is not otherwise specified. The classic clinical signs include a very firm nodular, frequently nonmovable mass, often with fixation and flattening of overlying skin and nipple retraction. The retraction is a result of an infiltrative shortening of Cooper's ligaments caused by productive fibrosis (see Figure 21-22). Fixation and retraction of the nipple may be the result of a subareolar carcinoma, but may also be caused by benign fibrosis of the breast. It is important to note that some patients normally have inverted nipples. The size of the cancer may vary from a few millimeters to involvement of nearly the entire breast. The deep-lying scirrhous carcinoma may grow into and become fixed to the thoracic wall. A bloody discharge is rare with this tumor.

Medullary Carcinoma. Medullary carcinoma is a densely cellular tumor that contains large, round, or oval tumor cells. It usually is a well-circumscribed mass, with the center frequently necrotic, hemorrhagic, and cystic (Figure 21-42). Medullary carcinomas are relatively rare, accounting for less than 5% of breast cancers. The age of occurrence is slightly lower than for the average breast cancer, with a majority of cases occurring in women younger than 50 years old. Medullary carcinomas are usually well circumscribed, are often large, and resemble fibroadenoma with a fairly benign appearance. Discoloration of the overlying skin is often seen as a clinical finding, and bilateral occurrence is more frequent with medullary carcinoma than with other cancers.

Colloid Carcinoma. Colloid carcinoma (mucinous) is a relatively rare type of ductal carcinoma that accounts for approximately 3% of breast carcinomas. The cells of the tumor produce secretions that fill lactiferous ducts or stromal tissues in which the tumor cells are invading. Clinically, the tumor presents in older women as a slow-growing, smooth, and not particularly firm mass on palpation. The sonographic appearance is often similar to a fibroadenoma with smooth margins and posterior enhancement. The echotexture

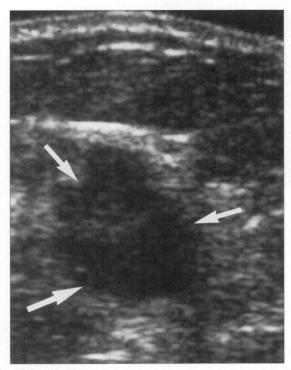

FIGURE 21-42 Medullary carcinoma. Sonogram depicts lobulated mass *(arrows)* with ill-defined margins, low-level internal echoes, and a small amount of posterior acoustic enlargement.

has been described as having a "salt and pepper" appearance (Figure 21-43).

Tubular Carcinoma. Tubular carcinoma represents an extremely well-differentiated form of **infiltrating (invasive) ductal carcinoma** usually less than 2 cm in dimension. Tubular carcinoma occurs in women with an average age of 50 and has a favorable prognosis with a low rate of recurrence or metastasis. Death is rare. Tubular carcinoma typically has poorly circumscribed margins and a hard consistency (Figure 21-44).

Ultrasound-Guided Interventional Procedures

Ultrasound is an important guide for many diagnostic and interventional procedures in the breast. These include cyst aspiration, fine-needle aspiration cytology, abscess or seroma drainage, large-core needle biopsy, vacuum-assisted needle biopsy, ultrasound-guided preoperative needle wire localization for surgical excision, and injection of a radiopharmaceutical agent for sentinel node identification and biopsy (Box 21-12). Sterile coupling gel is available commercially, as are sterile plastic transducer sleeves. It is possible and more cost effective to use isopropyl alcohol as a coupling agent during procedures.

When ultrasound is used to guide any diagnostic or interventional procedure in the breast, the high-frequency, narrow-beam linear array transducer is a valuable tool. Even narrow-gauge needles (22 or 25 gauge) can be seen and accurately guided into cysts or masses. The key to visualizing the needle is to keep it oriented as nearly parallel to the transducer face as possible. Accuracy in placing the needle tip within the target lesion is also aided when the lesion is kept in the field of vision along with the needle (Figure 21-45).

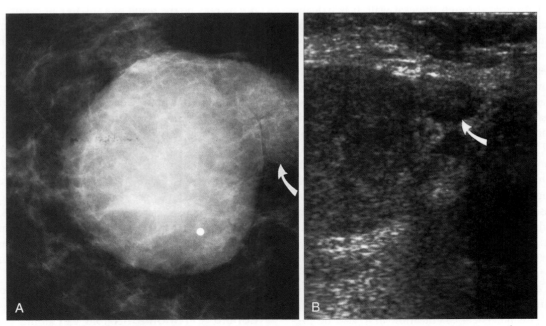

FIGURE 21-43 Mucinous (colloid) carcinoma. A, Spot compression mammographic view of palpable (denoted by radiopaque marker) circumscribed mass. A satellite nodule suggestive of diverticulum is seen laterally *(curved arrow).* **B,** Sonography of a portion of the mass shows that the sonographic margins are well defined and the diverticulum-like satellite *(curved arrow)* is easily seen. This homogeneous mass shows posterior acoustic enhancement.

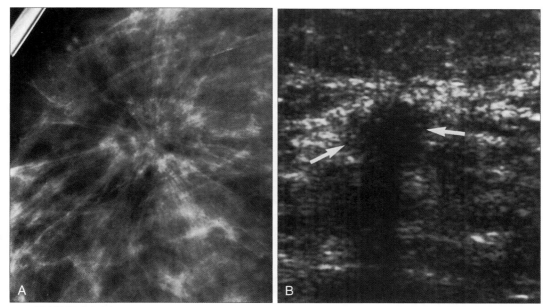

FIGURE 21-44 Tubular carcinoma. A, Magnified mammographic view shows mass with central radiolucent areas and very long radiating spiculation, suggesting radial scar. **B,** Sonogram depicts 0.7-cm, solid, hypoechoic mass with irregular, poorly defined margins *(arrows)* and posterior acoustic attenuation—common features of carcinoma.

BOX 21-12	Ultrasound-Guided Interventional Procedures

Cyst aspiration
Fine-needle aspiration cytology
Drainage procedures
Preoperative needle (wire) localization
Large-core needle biopsy
Vacuum-assisted needle biopsy
Sentinel node biopsy

This protects the patient, because the main hazard for the patient is inadvertent piercing of the chest wall. Puncture of the lung resulting in a pneumothorax can occur in some cases with asthenic patients (especially those with emphysema, in which case the lung may protrude between ribs). If care is taken to maintain the needle parallel to the transducer face, the needle tip will remain parallel to the chest wall, and this will help prevent potential complications.

Another important consideration in planning needle procedures in the breast is the approach. When dealing with any breast lesion that has the potential for malignancy, selection of the needle approach can have consequences in future therapeutic and reconstructive surgical procedures. Although the shortest approach from skin to target lesion has been advocated in the past for preoperative needle wire localizations and is often the favored route for ultrasound-guided core biopsy, a more horizontal approach will often facilitate a better cosmetic outcome for the patient if a mastectomy is necessary. Preprocedure consultation with the referring surgeon concerning the approach for needle wire localizations and core biopsies will ensure the best final outcome for the patient.

Cyst Aspiration. Cyst aspiration is a common interventional technique used in the breast. The cystic fluid is usually

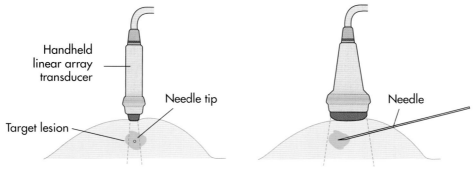

FIGURE 21-45 Placement of the needle tip is facilitated by keeping it in the field of vision and as parallel as possible to the transducer surface.

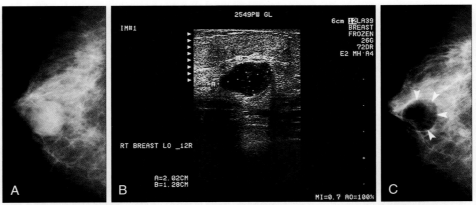

FIGURE 21-46 Complex cyst. A, Mammogram shows a smooth, benign-appearing dominant mass. **B,** Ultrasound shows a lobular, smooth, hypoechoic lesion with weak posterior acoustic enhancement. Cyst aspiration attempt under ultrasound guidance was done to assess this lesion as cystic or solid. Benign cyst fluid was obtained, and a pneumocystogram (air injected through the aspiration needle into the cyst cavity with a postaspiration mammogram) was performed. **C,** Postaspiration view of a normal pneumocystogram *(arrowheads)* after successful aspiration of a complex cyst. Pneumocystography can be used to exclude the possibility of an intracystic mass and may prevent or retard cyst recurrence.

"straw colored" when it is withdrawn, unless it is tinged with blood. The two main indications are a symptomatic cyst (one large enough to create a palpable lump or to cause a patient pain) and a hypoechoic lesion on ultrasound that does not meet criteria for a simple cyst (Figure 21-46). In the latter situation, aspiration determines whether the lesion is simply a complex cyst or a solid mass. This distinction is important for patient management. Occasionally, cyst aspiration will be undertaken because cysts are so large or so numerous that visualization of breast tissue by mammogram is significantly compromised.

Fine-Needle Aspiration Cytology. Fine-needle aspiration cytology (FNAC) uses a fine needle (usually 25 gauge) and an aspiration technique intended to harvest individual cells for diagnosis. The technique is used in the United States and many other countries. It is fast, easy for the patient, and generally very cost effective. The single greatest problem in FNAC is obtaining an adequate specimen. Another limitation in FNAC is the requirement for a specially trained and experienced pathologist (cytopathologist)—not available in many centers. This technique has not been as popular in the United States in part because of the somewhat greater inaccuracy of FNAC diagnosis (especially in fibrous malignant lesions and in proliferative benign lesions) and because of the greater availability of the more accurate (although more invasive) large-core needle biopsy.

Drainage Procedures. When clinically indicated, most cases of breast abscess, seroma, or hematoma will be easily palpated and drained in a simple office procedure by a breast surgeon or other physician. In some cases, the physician or surgeon may request ultrasound guidance. These lesions differ from simple cysts in that they typically require a larger needle (at least 18 gauge); have thicker, more fibrous capsules; have thicker fluid, often with abundant cellular debris; and frequently have numerous fibrous synechiae within the

lesion that can interfere with complete evacuation of contents. The goal in therapy of a breast abscess is complete eradication of the abscess, usually accomplished through a combination of drainage and antibiotic therapy. Seromas and hematomas are fluid accumulations within the breast that are not infected. These lesions have similar imaging characteristics (smooth mammographic mass, complex cyst on ultrasound). They differ in the quantity of blood and blood by-products within the fluid. They usually are encountered during healing from surgical procedures and are not infrequently seen after lumpectomy or following a large-core needle biopsy. In some cases blunt trauma may lead to a hematoma, and occasionally a foreign body reaction or an implant rupture may cause a seroma.

Preoperative Needle Wire Localization. Ultrasound offers a quick method for placement of a percutaneous needle wire assembly for preoperative localization of a nonpalpable breast lesion for surgical excision (Figure 21-47). Ultrasound guidance offers a significant advantage in complicated cases, such as localization of a lesion adjacent to a breast implant (Figure 21-48), a lesion close to the chest wall, or a lesion in other areas not easily approached under mammographic guidance.

Large-Core Needle Biopsy. Ultrasound offers a fast and easy method for guiding large-core needle biopsy of solid masses. Patient comfort is enhanced, procedure time is often shorter, and ultrasound guidance is more cost effective in general than prone stereotactic procedures. It should be noted, however, that stereotactic guidance is still the preferred method for evaluation of clustered pleomorphic microcalcifications, which are difficult to see by ultrasound. An exception to this rule is illustrated in Figure 21-49, in which ultrasound scanning of a patient with multiple suspicious microcalcifications noted on a screening mammogram revealed an unsuspected solid mass. Ultrasound-guided core

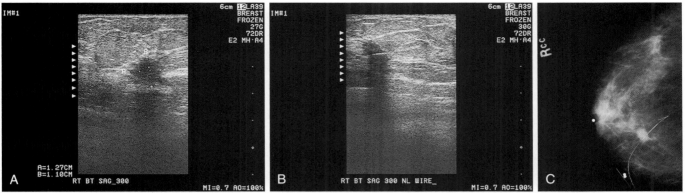

FIGURE 21-47 Preoperative needle wire localization of spiculated cancerous mass. A, Ultrasound image shows a sonographic mass with suspicious features. **B,** Ultrasound image shows the echogenic wire through the center of the mass. **C,** Mammogram taken after wire placement shows the hook wire through the center of the cancerous mass. This wire placement aids the surgeon in identifying and removing tissue around the target mass.

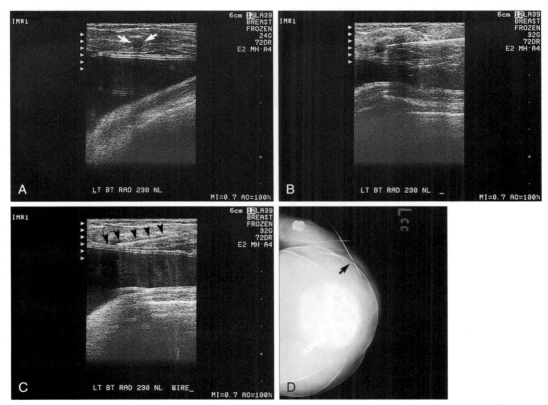

FIGURE 21-48 Preoperative needle wire localization of sonographic mass adjacent to saline breast implant. A, Ultrasound image shows a small, solid mass *(arrows)* near the anterior margin of the patient's intramammary saline implant. **B,** Under ultrasound guidance, the needle wire assembly can be guided carefully through the mass, avoiding inadvertent piercing of the implant. **C** and **D,** Mammogram and ultrasound performed after wire placement show the position of the wire adjacent to the implant. The wire *(arrowheads)* did not pierce the implant. The arrow identifies the approximate position of the target mass (not visible on mammogram).

biopsy of the solid mass revealed infiltrating malignancy, which altered the patient's management.

Vacuum-Assisted Needle Biopsy. A relatively new breast biopsy technique is vacuum-assisted breast biopsy. This type of biopsy is a percutaneous procedure that relies on stereotactic mammography or ultrasound imaging for

guidance. Stereotactic mammography is performed using computers to pinpoint the exact location of a breast mass taken from two different angles. The computer coordinates help the physician guide the needle to a position posterior to the mass. Ultrasound may also be used to guide the needle and allows the physician to observe the biopsy

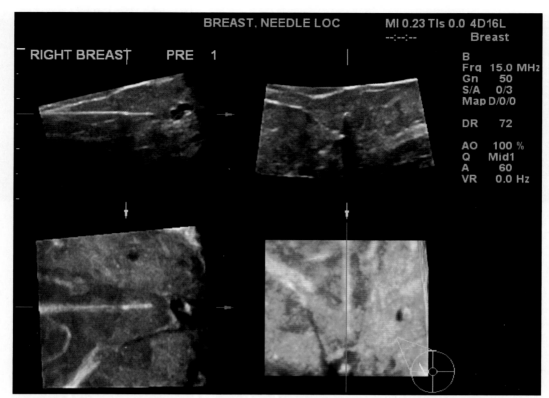

FIGURE 21-49 Ultrasonic guidance for a needle biopsy may aid the clinician in accurate needle placement when the suspected mass is large enough to be imaged with sonography. The needle is shown as the linear bright straight line as it approaches the solid mass. Three-dimensional imaging assures the clinician that the needle is correctly placed within the lesion for biopsy.

procedure in real-time. Vacuum-assisted biopsy is a minimally invasive procedure that allows the removal of multiple larger tissue samples with a single insertion of the needle. A special biopsy probe and needle are used. The needle used in a vacuum-assisted biopsy is generally of a larger gauge than needles used for core biopsies and has a special cutting blade at its tip to make the needle easier to insert. The opening of the needle (aperture) is located along the side of the needle on the distal end. Under ultrasound guidance, the needle is inserted immediately posterior to the tumor. Once sampling is initiated, a vacuum pulls the tumor into the opening on the needle, and a rotating cutting blade slices the tissue. The tissue sample is sent to a special chamber in the biopsy probe, where it can be retrieved without removal of the needle. This technique allows multiple tissue samples to be taken with minor rotations of the needle. It is also possible to completely remove smaller masses by taking multiple samples.

Sentinel Node Biopsy. Standard surgical therapy for breast cancer has, for many years, involved a full level I and at least a partial level II axillary lymph node dissection. This results in a small but significant rate of morbidity from lymphedema or nerve damage, or, in severe cases, loss of arm and shoulder function. An important step forward in surgical therapy for breast cancer involves sentinel node biopsy. In this procedure, the superficial subcutaneous tissues around

the tumor bed and/or the areola are injected with methylene blue dye and/or radioactive-labeled solution (usually technetium-labeled filtered sulfur colloid). Both of these substances are taken up by the lymphatics and transported to the first, or *sentinel*, lymph node along the axillary node chain. This lymph node is then identified in surgery and is carefully analyzed for evidence of metastasis. This is generally followed by a limited axillary node dissection. Early experience with this procedure shows an excellent accuracy rate for detecting lymph node metastases, which results in a reduced rate of morbidity and a faster recovery for the patient.

 Key Pearls

- Sonographically, the breast is divided into three layers located between the skin and the pectoralis major muscle on the anterior of the chest wall. These layers are the subcutaneous layer, the mammary (glandular) layer, and the retromammary layer.
- The fatty tissue appears hypoechoic, and the ducts, glands, and supporting ligaments appear echogenic.
- The terminal ends of the duct and the acini form small lobular units referred to as terminal ductal lobular units, each of which is surrounded by both loose and dense connective tissue.

- These connective tissue septa are collectively called Cooper's ligaments; they connect to the fascia around the ducts and glands and extend out to the skin.
- Lymphatic drainage from all parts of the breast generally flows to the axillary lymph nodes.
- The primary function of the breast is fluid transport.
- Three general categories of diagnostic breast imaging are available, two of which involve breast ultrasound. These three categories are breast cancer screening (generally performed by physical breast evaluation with mammography), diagnostic interrogation (consultation, problem solving, workup), and interventional breast procedures (histologic diagnosis and/or localization).
- The overall goal of breast evaluation is the proper classification of a breast lesion according to the level of suspicion for breast cancer.
- Most breast masses that arise during the teen years are fibroadenomas.
- Breast problems that may arise during pregnancy or lactation include mastitis, abscesses, cysts, or galactoceles (cysts containing milk).
- Sonographic evaluation of a breast lesion normally begins with determination of whether a lesion is cystic or solid.
- Cysts within the breast can be multilocular with thin internal septations.
- If the cyst has internal echoes, wall irregularity, mural nodularity or septation, shadowing, nonuniform internal echoes, or any other feature not associated with a simple cyst, it is by definition a complex cyst, and aspiration and/or biopsy should be considered.
- Benign lesions usually have smooth, rounded margins.
- Malignant tumors are aggressive and tend to grow through tissue via finger-like extensions called speculation. As malignant masses enlarge, they may cause retraction of the nipple or dimpling of the skin as the spiculations pull on Cooper's ligaments.
- A rounded or oval shape is usually associated with benign lesions; sharp, angular margins are associated with malignancy.
- The normal tissue planes of the breast are horizontally oriented. Benign lesions tend to grow within the normal tissue planes, and their long axis lies parallel to the chest wall. These lesions are noted to be "wider than tall."
- Malignant lesions are able to grow through the connective tissue and may have a vertical orientation when the breast is imaged from anterior to posterior.
- Lesions that appear isoechoic with the breast parenchyma or have echoes equivalent to or brighter than that of fat are most often benign.
- A solid lesion that is hypoechoic relative to the normal breast parenchyma is more suspicious for malignancy.
- Microcalcifications within a solid mass are associated with a breast malignancy.
- Most solid lesions, with the exception of a fibroadenoma, will not enhance.

- Benign lesions normally demonstrate a limited degree of mobility or may roll away as they are palpated.
- If pressure applied by the transducer causes the lesion to compress or change shape, the lesion is probably benign and most likely represents a fat lobule. Malignant lesions normally are very hard and noncompressible.
- Vessels that penetrate a mass are highly suspect for malignancy and should be checked using color or power Doppler to ascertain the number and to look for intratumoral vessels.
- Symptoms of breast masses include pain, a palpable mass, spontaneous or induced nipple discharge, skin dimpling, ulceration, and nipple retraction.
- Skin dimpling or ulceration and nipple retraction nearly always result from cancer.
- Benign tumors are rubbery, mobile, and well defined (as seen in a fibroadenoma), whereas malignant tumors are often stone hard and irregular with a gritty feel.

BIBLIOGRAPHY

American College of Radiology (ACR): *Breast imaging reporting and data system (BI-RADS®) atlas,* ed 4, Reston, 2003, American College of Radiology.

Booi RC, Carson PL, O'Donnell M, et al: Diagnosing cysts with correlation coefficient images from 2-dimensional freehand elastography, *J Ultrasound Med* 26:1201-1207, 2007.

Cho SH, Park SH: Mimickers of breast malignancy on breast sonography, *J Ultrasound Med* 32:2029-2036, 2013.

Handel ER, Jackson VP: Other sonographically guided interventional procedures. In Bassett LW, Jackson VP, Fu KL, Fu YS, editors: *Diagnosis of diseases of the breast,* ed 2, Philadelphia, 2005, Saunders.

Hashimoto BE: New sonographic breast technologies, *Semin Roentgenol* 46(4):292-301, 2011. doi:10.1053/j.ro.2011.08.001

Ikeda D: *Breast imaging: the requisites,* St Louis, 2005, Mosby.

Iorfida M, Maiorano E, Orvieto E, et al: Invasive lobular breast cancer: subtypes and outcome, *Breast Cancer Res Treat* 133:713-723, 2012.

Jesinger RA: Breast anatomy for the interventionalist, *Tech Vasc Interv Radiol* 17(1):3-9, 2014.

Kim SJ, Park YM, Jung SJ, et al: Sonographic appearances of juvenile fibroadenoma of the breast, *J Ultrasound Med* 33:1879-1884, 2014.

Norton K, Wininger M, Bhanot G, et al: A 2D mechanistic model of breast ductal carcinoma in situ (DCIS) morphology and progression, *J Theor Biol* 263:393-406, 2010.

Nwariaku FE: Sentinel lymph node biopsy, an alternative to elective axillary dissection for breast cancer, *Am J Surg* 176:529, 1998.

Romrell LJ, Bland KI: Anatomy of the breast, axilla, chest wall, and related metastatic sites. In Bland KI, Copeland EM, editors: *The breast: comprehensive management of benign and malignant diseases,* ed 4, Philadelphia, 2010, Saunders.

Schwartz T, Cyr A, Margenthaler J: Screening breast magnetic resonance imaging in women with atypia or lobular carcinoma in situ, *J Surg Res* 193:519-522, 2015.

Seymour MT, Moskovic EC, Walsh G, et al: Ultrasound assessment of residual abnormalities following primary chemotherapy for breast cancer, *Br J Cancer* 76:371, 1997.

Veronesi U, Paganelli G, Viale G, et al: Sentinel lymph node biopsy and axillary dissection in breast cancer: results in a large series, *J Natl Cancer Inst* 91:368, 1999.

Wilhelm MC, Langenburg SE, Wanebo HJ: Cancer of the male breast. In Bland KI, Copeland EM, editors: *The breast: comprehensive management of benign and malignant diseases,* ed 4, Philadelphia, 2010, Saunders.

Wilson M, Remlinger R, Wilson A: Critical thinking for sonographic breast imaging, *J Diagn Med Sonogr* 26(5):226-237, 2010.

Thyroid and Parathyroid Glands

Janette Wybo and Sandra L. Hagen-Ansert

OBJECTIVES

On completion of this chapter, you should be able to:
- Discuss the embryology of the thyroid and parathyroid glands
- Describe the normal anatomy and physiology of the thyroid and parathyroid glands
- Define the relational anatomy of the thyroid and parathyroid glands
- Discuss the laboratory values and clinical findings of the thyroid and parathyroid glands
- Describe the sonographic examination of the thyroid and parathyroid glands
- Differentiate the sonographic features of pathologic conditions found in the thyroid and parathyroid glands

OUTLINE

KEY TERMS

Abscess
Adenoma
Branchial cleft cyst
Calcitonin
Endemic goiter
Euthyroid
Follicular adenoma
Follicular carcinoma
Graves' disease
Goiter
Hashimoto's thyroiditis
Hyperthyroidism

Hypothyroidism
Isthmus
Longus colli muscle
Medullary carcinoma
Multinodular goiter (MNG)
Nontoxic (simple) goiter
Papillary carcinoma
Parathyroid hormone (PTH)
Parathyroid hyperplasia
Primary hyperparathyroidism
Pyramidal lobe
Secondary hyperparathyroidism

Sternocleidomastoid muscles
Strap muscles
Subacute (de Quervain's) thyroiditis
Thyroglossal duct cyst
Thyroid-stimulating hormone (TSH)
Thyrotoxicosis
Thyrotropin-releasing hormone (TRH)
Thyroxine (T_4)
Toxic goiter
Triiodothyronine (T_3)

The thyroid gland is an organ of the endocrine system that maintains body metabolism, growth, and development through the synthesis, storage, and secretion of thyroid hormones. A hormone triggers a reaction in a specific, targeted cell. Thyroid hormones include triiodothyronine (T_3), thyroxine (T_4), and calcitonin. The primary hormones, **triiodothyronine (T3)** and **thyroxine (T4)**, stimulate cell metabolism, which is the body's ability to break down food and convert it to energy. The third hormone, **calcitonin,** plays a minor role to regulate blood calcium levels. Disorders of the thyroid may result from thyroid gland dysfunction, which is regulated by the pituitary and hypothalamus glands (located in the brain).

The thyroid is located on the anterior lower neck on either side of the midline and is not easily palpated by physical examination. General enlargement of the thyroid gland is called a **goiter.** A localized enlargement is a *nodular goiter,* and multiple thyroid nodules are described as a **multinodular goiter (MNG).** Both insufficient and excessive secretion of thyroid hormones may cause thyroid gland enlargement.

Since the thyroid gland is superficial, high-resolution sonography is used to evaluate the gland. The examination is easy to perform and is well tolerated by patients. Sonography of the thyroid is used to evaluate gland size, shape, and echogenicity and determine the sonographic appearance of a palpable lesion (i.e., solid or cystic, complex or calcified) and whether the lesion is single or multiple. The nodule size and location and the evaluation of the adjacent anatomy (i.e., lymph node adenopathy) may be imaged. Color Doppler, power Doppler, and pulsed wave Doppler are used to determine vascularity. Thyroid sonography will not determine the physiology of the thyroid gland. The functional state is better determined by nuclear medicine scintigraphy and laboratory measurements of the thyroid hormones present in the blood. Interventional procedures under sonographic guidance, including fine-needle aspiration (FNA) biopsy, are important applications of sonography. Sonographic evaluation of the parathyroid gland and other lesions of the neck will also be presented in this chapter.

EMBRYOLOGY OF THE THYROID GLAND

The thyroid gland is the first endocrine gland to develop in the human embryo. It develops at the floor of the primitive pharynx at the same location of the base of the tongue. The developing thyroid gland will migrate inferiorly along the anterior neck region to the lower neck anteriorly to the trachea. The migration may leave behind embryonic remnants or ectopic thyroid tissue that should atrophy, but may form developmental cysts.

ANATOMY OF THE THYROID GLAND

The thyroid gland is located inferior to the thyroid cartilage (Adam's apple) in the anteroinferior neck. The gland has an "H" or "U" configuration and consists of right and left lobes that consist of upper, middle, and lower poles that are connected across the midline by a thin bridge of thyroid tissue called the **isthmus.** The isthmus straddles the trachea anteriorly, whereas the paired lobes extend on either side of the trachea, bounded laterally by the common carotid arteries and internal jugular veins. When present, the **pyramidal lobe** arises from the isthmus and tapers superiorly just anterior to the thyroid cartilage and may be seen in 15% to 30% of patients (Figure 22-1). The pyramidal lobe is most commonly visualized in pediatric patients and usually atrophies with age. A fascia surrounds the thyroid, trachea, esophagus, and parathyroid glands (Figure 22-2).

The thyroid gland is made up of two types of cells: follicular and parafollicular cells. Follicular cells make up the majority of thyroid tissue and secrete the main thyroid hormones triiodothyronine (T_3) and thyroxine (T_4). The follicular cells require an adequate supply of iodine in order to produce the correct amount of thyroid hormones. The parafollicular cells (also called C cells) secrete calcitonin.

Size

The size and shape of the thyroid gland vary with gender, age, and body surface area with females having a slightly larger gland than males (Table 22-1). In tall individuals, the lateral lobes of the thyroid have a longitudinally elongated shape on sagittal scans, whereas in shorter individuals, the gland is more oval shaped. As a result, the normal dimensions of the gland have a wide range of variability. The lobes are normally equal in size. At age 1 year, the mean length is 25 mm, anteroposterior (AP) diameter is 12 to 15 mm, and width is 10 to 15 mm. In the normal adult, the thyroid gland measures 40 to 60 mm in length, 20 to 30 mm in AP diameter, and 15 to 20 mm in width. The isthmus is the smallest portion of the gland with an AP diameter of 4 to 6 mm. The gland is considered enlarged when the thyroid lobe AP diameter measures greater than 20 mm and when the isthmus measures 10 mm or greater.

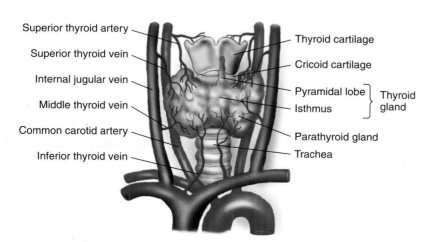

FIGURE 22-1 Anterior view of the thyroid and parathyroid glands.

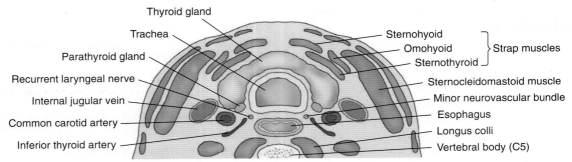

FIGURE 22-2 Cross section of the thyroid region showing the thyroid gland and the vascular and muscular relationships to one another.

TABLE 22-1	Size of the Thyroid	
Dimension	Adults	Children
Length	40–60 mm	20–30 mm
Anteroposterior	20–30 mm	12–15 mm
Width	15–20 mm	10–15 mm
Volume	10–12 ± 3 ml	

Due to shape variations, the thyroid volume is more useful to determine gland enlargement. The method commonly used to calculate thyroid volume is based on the ellipsoid formula with a correction factor (length × width × thickness × 0.523 for each lobe). The normal mean thyroid volume is 10 to 12 ± 3 ml. The volume in males is slightly more than in females. Volume measurement can be used to assess the need for surgery, calculate iodine-131 dosage for treatment of **thyrotoxicosis** (a toxic condition resulting from excessive amounts of thyroid hormones occurring in extreme hyperthyroidism), or evaluate the response to suppression treatments.

Relational Anatomy

Anterior. Along the anterior surface of the thyroid gland lie three **strap muscles,** including the sternohyoid, sternothyroid, and omohyoid, with the anterolateral **sternocleidomastoid muscles** (see Figure 22-2).

Lateral. Directly lateral to each thyroid lobe are the common carotid artery, internal jugular vein, and vagus nerve within the carotid sheath.

Posterior. Along the posterior border adjacent to thyroid tissue lie the superior and inferior parathyroid glands along with the anastomosis between the superior and inferior thyroid arteries. The **longus colli muscle** is posterior and lateral to each thyroid lobe along the anterior surface of the cervical vertebrae (see Figure 22-2).

Medial. Medial anatomy consists of the larynx, the trachea, and the inferior constrictor muscle of the pharynx. The esophagus is considered an anatomically midline structure but is usually found sonographically to the left of midline lateral to the trachea (see Figure 22-3). It is identified by the target appearance in the transverse plane and confirmed during real-time evaluation by its peristaltic movements when the patient swallows.

Blood Supply

The thyroid gland is supplied by four arteries and considered highly vascular. Two superior thyroid arteries branch from the external carotid arteries and descend to the upper poles

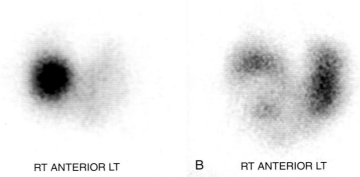

A   RT ANTERIOR LT   B   RT ANTERIOR LT

FIGURE 22-3 A, Scintigraphy of the thyroid gland demonstrating a "hot" nodule. **B,** Scintigraphy of the thyroid demonstrating a "cold" nodule.

of the thyroid. Two inferior thyroid arteries arise from the thyrocervical trunk of the subclavian arteries and ascend to the lower poles of the thyroid. Corresponding superior thyroid veins drain into the internal jugular veins, and the inferior thyroid veins drain into the brachiocephalic veins (see Figure 22-1).

THYROID PHYSIOLOGY AND LABORATORY DATA

The role of the thyroid is to maintain normal body metabolism, physical and mental growth, and development by the synthesis, storage, and secretion of thyroid hormones. Every cell in the body depends on thyroid hormones for regulation of their metabolism. The mechanism for producing thyroid hormones is through iodine metabolism. The thyroid follicular cells are the only cells in the body that can absorb iodine. Through a series of chemical reactions, the thyroid produces triiodothyronine (T_3) and thyroxine (T_4). Most endocrine glands do not store their hormones, but thyroid hormones are stored in the colloid material of the gland to be secreted when needed into the blood. In terms of amount of hormone secretion, T_4 is more abundant at 80%, whereas T_3 is 20% of secretion, but T_3 is more potent.

When thyroid hormones are needed in the body, they are released into the bloodstream by the action of thyrotropin, or **thyroid-stimulating hormone (TSH),** which is produced by the pituitary gland. The secretion of TSH is regulated by **thyrotropin-releasing hormone (TRH),** which is produced by the hypothalamus. The level of TRH is controlled by the basal metabolic rate in a negative feedback system. Low concentration of thyroid hormones causes a decrease in the basal metabolic rate, which results in an increase in TRH. This causes an increased secretion of TSH and a subsequent increase in the release of thyroid hormones. When the blood level of thyroid hormones is returned to normal, the basal metabolic rate returns to normal and TSH secretion stops. In summary, the hypothalamus signals the pituitary gland to tell the thyroid gland to produce more or less thyroid hormones.

Calcitonin decreases the concentration of calcium in the blood by first acting on bone to inhibit its breakdown of calcium. When less calcium is being resorbed into the blood, less calcium moves out of the bone into the blood with a decrease in blood calcium levels. Calcitonin secretion will increase after any concentration of blood calcium increases.

Euthyroid, Hypothyroidism, and Hyperthyroidism

Euthyroid. When the thyroid is producing the correct amount of thyroid hormones, it is considered to be normal or **euthyroid.**

Abnormal thyroid hormone secretion is classified as either primary, if caused by inherent dysfunction of the thyroid gland, or secondary, if there is failure of the pituitary or hypothalamus glands to correctly stimulate the thyroid gland to release hormones or possibly a pituitary mass.

Hypothyroidism. Undersecretion of thyroid hormones is called **hypothyroidism** and is the most common thyroid disorder. In the adult, it can be referred to as *myxedema.* Hypothyroidism can occur spontaneously from inability of the thyroid to produce the proper amount of thyroid hormones or a problem with the pituitary gland. Most commonly (75%), hypothyroidism is caused by a chronic thyroid inflammatory process called Hashimoto's thyroiditis. The inflammatory process can also be the result of an autoimmune response that damages a large percentage of thyroid cells where it is inadequate to produce sufficient hormones. Other causes include medications or radiation exposure to the head or neck. Radiation treatments to the neck and upper chest are associated with certain types of lymphoma. Box 22-1 lists the common disorders associated with hypothyroidism.

Clinical signs and symptoms of hypothyroidism include weight gain, hair loss, increased subcutaneous tissue around the eyes, lethargy, intellectual and motor slowing, cold intolerance, constipation, and a deep husky voice. Medical treatment with synthetic thyroid hormone can successfully treat, manage, and reverse the condition. A rare, more severe complication of hypothyroidism could lead to a life-threatening coma.

Hyperthyroidism. The oversecretion of thyroid hormones is called **hyperthyroidism.** This occurs when the entire gland is not functioning properly, usually from diffuse enlargement or localized nodule or **adenoma** causing overproduction of thyroid hormones called **Graves' disease.** Box 22-2 lists the common disorders associated with hyperthyroidism.

Clinical signs and symptoms of hyperthyroidism include weight loss, increased appetite, high degree of nervous energy, irritable, tremor, excessive sweating, heat intolerance, palpitations, impaired fertility, and exophthalmos (protruding eyes). An extreme form of hyperthyroidism is thyrotoxicosis.

BOX 22-1	Disorders Associated with Hypothyroidism

Common
Chronic inflammatory process (most common Hashimoto's thyroiditis)
Endemic iodine deficiency

Uncommon
Hyperfunctioning thyroid cancer
Thyroid-stimulating hormone–secreting pituitary adenoma
Neonatal thyrotoxicosis associated with maternal Graves' disease

Tests of Thyroid Function

Laboratory Tests. The most common laboratory test to evaluate thyroid function is serum thyroxine (T_4). This test reflects the amount of T_4 or thyroxine in the blood and is considered a good screening test of thyroid function. Serum triiodothyronine (T_3) reflects the amount of triiodothyronine in the blood. Measurements of both thyroid hormones may be used to give a more accurate picture of thyroid function. The TSH (serum thyrotropin) laboratory test will also indicate thyroid function and may be the first to elevate as an indication of hypothyroidism. Often the TSH level is opposite the T_4 and T_3 levels with thyroid dysfunction (i.e., low TSH with elevated T_4 and T_3 indicates hyperthyroidism). If the TSH, T_3, and T_4 levels are all low, this could indicate pituitary dysfunction or pituitary mass from secondary hypothyroidism. The laboratory findings associated with common thyroid disorders are listed in Box 22-3.

Calcitonin helps to maintain homeostasis of blood calcium levels and helps prevent increased amounts of calcium in the blood (hypercalcemia). Additionally, calcitonin is not a common indicator of thyroid function, but can be a laboratory test for medullary carcinoma with elevated calcitonin used as a tumor marker.

Nuclear Medicine or Scintigraphy. Scintigraphy can be used to determine the thyroid function with two tests that can be performed together: iodine uptake scan and thyroid scan. For an iodine uptake scan, a capsule containing a small amount of radioactive iodine (called a radiotracer) is ingested by mouth. The amount of radioactivity accumulated in the thyroid gland is measured at multiple time points for up to 24 hours by a gamma camera. In comparison with normal thyroid uptake, patients with hyperthyroidism have a higher percentage of radioactivity in the thyroid gland; a lower percentage of radioactivity is present with hypothyroidism.

The thyroid scan will detect the amount of radioactive tracer to image the thyroid gland and demonstrate the thyroid size, shape, and position. In addition, if the thyroid has a concentrated amount of radioactivity, this will be imaged as a "hot" (hyperfunctioning) nodule (Figure 22-3, *A*). An area of the thyroid with lower concentration of the radioactive tracer will demonstrate absence of uptake as a "cold" (nonfunctioning) nodule (Figure 22-3, *B*). The majority (80% to 85%) of nodules in a thyroid scan are demonstrated as a cold nodule with the remaining (15% to 20%) seen as a hot nodule. Hot nodules are considered to be benign. Cold nodules have the potential to be malignant, but only 10% to 15% of cold nodules are shown to be malignant with FNA biopsy.

Other imaging modalities for thyroid include computed tomography (CT) and magnetic resonance imaging (MRI) to determine thyroid size, shape, position, and imaging characteristics of masses within the gland and neck area.

SONOGRAPHIC EVALUATION OF THE THYROID GLAND

No patient preparation is required for thyroid sonography. The sonographer should review the examination indication and the available imaging results (i.e., previous thyroid sonography, scintigraphy, CT, or MRI). A thorough patient clinical history should be obtained before the sonographic examination. Pertinent information includes results of the physician's physical examination (e.g., palpable nodule or goiter), pain/duration, history of hyperthyroidism, hypothyroidism, thyroiditis and symptoms related to thyroid disorders, thyroid medications, or surgery. If the patient has a previous history of cancer, along with prior history of radiation or surgery to the neck and upper chest, this should be noted in the examination record. If the patient has a palpable mass, ask the patient to indicate the location or obtain a description of the palpable area from the ordering physician.

The examination procedure should always be explained to the patient before scanning. The patient is placed in the supine position with a pillow or pad under both shoulders to provide moderate hyperextension of the neck with chin elevated to place the thyroid more horizontal and bring the inferior portion of the gland more superior for visualization. If the lower pole of the thyroid is still difficult to view, having the patient swallow will move the entire gland superiorly.

BOX 22-3 | **Laboratory Findings with Common Thyroid Disorders**

Laboratory Test	Normal Thyroid (Euthyroid)	Hyperthyroidism	Primary Hypothyroidism	Secondary Hypothyroidism (Possible Pituitary Dysfunction or Mass)
T_4, T_3	Normal	High	Low	Low
TSH	Normal	Low	High	Low

Having the patient elevate the chin superiorly and turn to the opposite side will enable better visualizing of each lobe. It is important to be conscious of elderly patients or those who may experience dizziness or neck strain and make positioning adjustments as needed.

A high-frequency (7 to 15 MHz) linear-array transducer should be used, selecting the highest frequency to penetrate the entire thyroid and surrounding musculature. Each lobe and isthmus should be carefully surveyed in transverse and longitudinal planes. The survey should also extend superior, inferior, and lateral of the thyroid gland to identify and document any enlarged cervical lymph nodes (Figure 22-4). The transverse survey is completed scanning from above to below the thyroid to note gland symmetry. Multiple transverse images of the superior, mid, and inferior levels of each lobe are imaged and labeled accordingly (Figure 22-5). Virtual convex, split screen, or panoramic features may provide imaging of larger glands (Figure 22-6).

Transverse and longitudinal survey of the isthmus is completed with images recorded and labeled. Transverse imaging landmarks include the trachea, common carotid artery, and internal jugular vein. The trachea is noted in the midline posterior to the isthmus with posterior shadowing. The common carotid artery is a circular, pulsatile structure directly lateral and adjacent to the gland. The oval-shaped internal jugular vein lies lateral to the common carotid artery (see Figure 22-6).

To locate the longitudinal scan plane of the thyroid gland, it is helpful to align the longitudinal axis of the common carotid artery and slide medially. Longitudinal survey is completed by scanning from the lateral to internal jugular vein to the midline isthmus. Multiple longitudinal images of the lateral, mid, and medial portions of each lobe are imaged individually and labeled accordingly (see Figure 22-4). On longitudinal scans, landmarks include the recurrent laryngeal nerve and inferior thyroid artery, which may be seen between the thyroid lobe and esophagus on the left and between the thyroid lobe and longus colli muscle on the right.

During the examination, obtain three measurements of each lobe for volume calculations at maximum length, AP, and width of gland. The AP measurement of isthmus should be imaged in the transverse plane (Figure 22-7). Examination protocol should also include color Doppler images of both transverse and longitudinal planes of the middle portion of the thyroid demonstrating gland vascularity (see Figure 22-6, *B*). A low pulse repetition frequency is chosen for the color Doppler scale to distinguish all vascular structures. Power Doppler or pulsed wave Doppler may also contribute information on vascular hemodynamics and should be obtained as needed.

Normal sonographic appearance of the thyroid gland is fine homogeneous echotexture that is slightly more echogenic than the surrounding musculature. The thyroid capsule

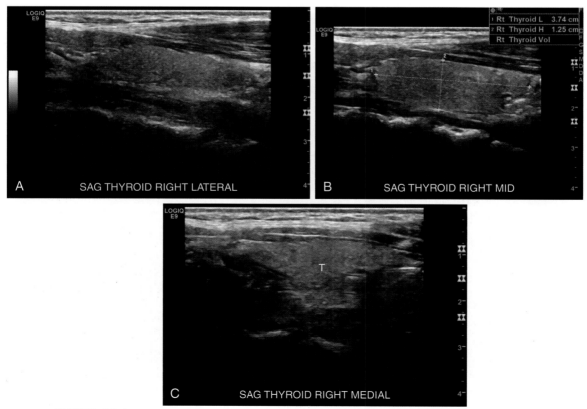

FIGURE 22-4 **Longitudinal images of the normal thyroid gland. A,** Long, lateral. *T,* Thyroid. **B,** Long, mid. Measurement of the length and anteroposterior dimension of the gland. **C,** Long, medial. *T,* Thyroid.

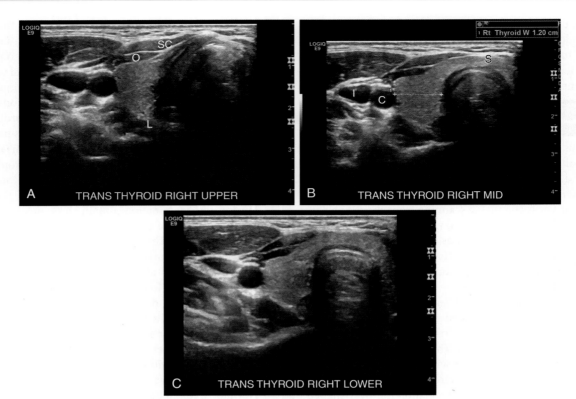

FIGURE 22-5 Transverse images of the normal thyroid gland. A, Trans, superior. **B,** Trans, mid. *O,* Omohyoid muscle; *S,* sternohyoid muscle; *SC,* sternocleidomastoid; *L,* longus colli muscle; *I,* internal jugular vein; *C,* carotid artery. Measurement of the width of the gland. **C,** Trans, inferior.

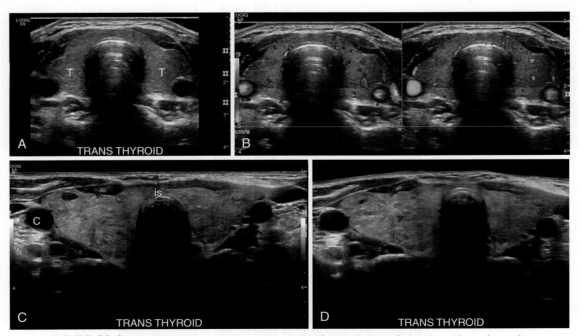

FIGURE 22-6 Normal image. A, transverse image of both lobes of the thyroid to show the comparable homogeneity of each lobe. *C,* Carotid; *T,* thyroid; *is,* isthmus. **B,** Color and power Doppler of both lobes. **C,** Split-screen transverse image of both lobes. **D,** Panoramic image of both lobes.

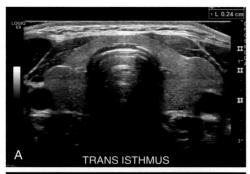

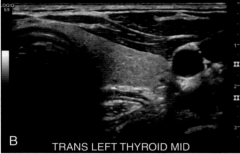

FIGURE 22-7 **A,** The isthmus *(arrows)* is shown in the transverse view at the inferior border of the thyroid gland. **B,** Transverse image of the esophagus located posterior to the thyroid and the left side of trachea.

is imaged as a thin, hyperechoic line that outlines the gland from surrounding relational anatomy. The air-filled trachea is demonstrated as a curvilinear structure with acoustic shadowing. Multiple, tiny vascular structures may be seen as tubular anechoic structures more apparent at the periphery and upper and lower poles within the gland representing the superior and inferior thyroid arteries and veins. Normal pulsed Doppler spectrum will demonstrate peak systole velocities of 20 to 40 cm/sec in the major thyroid arteries and 15 to 30 cm/sec in intraparenchymal arteries.

The surrounding musculature of the thyroid gland is hypoechoic compared with the normal thyroid parenchyma. The strap muscles are anterior to the gland with the larger sternocleidomastoid muscle imaged more anterolateral to the gland. The hypoechoic longus colli muscle is found posterior to each lobe of the thyroid (see Figure 22-5). The recurrent laryngeal nerve and the inferior thyroid artery pass in the angle between the trachea, esophagus, and thyroid lobe. The esophagus is adjacent to the trachea with a hypoechoic rim surrounding an echogenic center more commonly visualized slightly to the left of the midline, next to the trachea with peristalsis noted in real-time with patient swallowing (see Figure 22-7).

CONGENITAL ABNORMALITIES OF THE THYROID GLAND

Congenital abnormalities of the thyroid gland include aplasia, hypoplasia, and ectopic locations of the thyroid gland. Aplasia is congenital absence of gland and may affect one lobe, the isthmus, or the entire gland. Complete

absence of the thyroid gland has a severe impact on physical and mental development. Hypoplasia refers to underdevelopment of any part of the gland and may be associated with congenital hypothyroidism.

Ectopic locations may be present along the path of embryonic descent if the thyroid migrates too little or too far. Most commonly, ectopic tissue may be present posterior to the tongue (sublingual or lingual thyroid). Other ectopic locations include larynx (prelaryngeal thyroid) or mediastinum (substernal thyroid). Scintigraphy is best for visualization of ectopic thyroid tissue.

PATHOLOGY OF THE THYROID GLAND

Pathology identified in the thyroid and adjacent neck structures should always be documented in both longitudinal and transverse scan planes. The gland measurements and volume should be obtained and parenchyma defined as homogeneous or heterogeneous. If a nodule is visualized, the location should be noted in relationship to gland (e.g., right thyroid transverse upper; left thyroid long lateral) and also measured in three dimensions. The sonographic appearance should be demonstrated and echogenicity described (e.g., hypoechoic, hyperechoic, and whether cystic, complex cystic, solid, and/or presence and type of calcifications). In addition, the nodule borders should be described as ill defined or well defined and whether a hypoechoic halo is surrounding the nodule. It is not uncommon for sonography to demonstrate multiple nodules in a gland. Vascularity should also be demonstrated with color or power Doppler and possibly pulsed wave Doppler.

Nodular Thyroid Disease

Nodular Hyperplasia, Multinodular Goiter, and Adenomatous Hyperplasia. Approximately 80% of nodular thyroid disease is due to hyperplasia or compensatory hypertrophy forming micronodules and macronodules of the gland. This can lead to overall enlargement (goiter) or multiple nodules (MNG) (Figure 22-8) that may be unilateral or bilateral,

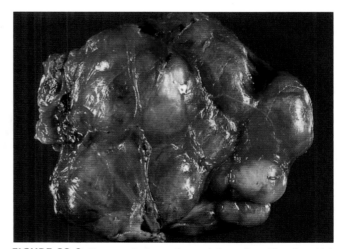

FIGURE 22-8 **Gross pathology of a nodular goiter.** The thyroid is enlarged with nodules that vary in size and shape.

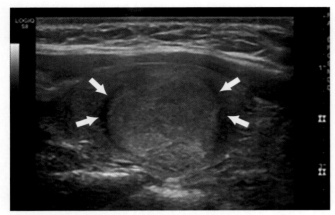

FIGURE 22-9 The heterogeneous appearance is well seen within the adenoma with well-defined, discrete borders. The hypoechoic halo is shown surrounding the lesion (arrows).

TABLE 22-2	Thyroid Findings: Nodular Thyroid Disease	
Clinical Findings	**Sonographic Appearances**	**Differential Considerations**
Nontoxic Simple Goiter		
Thyroid enlargement	Sometimes smooth, sometimes nodular; possible compression of surrounding structures	Thyroiditis Hypothyroidism Neoplasm
Toxic Multinodular Goiter		
Thyroid enlargement	Enlarged inhomogeneous gland; can have focal scarring, focal ischemia, necrosis, and cyst formation	Neoplasm Cyst
Graves' Disease		
Diffuse toxic goiter	Diffusely homogeneous and enlarged	Neoplasm Ophthalmopathy Cutaneous manifestations Hyperthyroidism
Thyroiditis		
Swelling and tenderness of the thyroid; later, hypothyroidism	Homogeneous enlargement with nodularity; later, inhomogeneous	Neoplasm
Benign Lesions Cysts		
Solitary nodules or multiple nodules	Anechoic areas, echogenic fluid, or moving fluid levels	Toxic multinodular goiter
Adenoma		
Usually euthyroid or hyperthyroidism	Compression of adjacent structures; fibrous encapsulation; ranges from anechoic to hyperechoic; may have halo	Graves' disease

seen more commonly in women with increasing age. When evaluated microscopically, most benign nodules are classified as hyperplastic, adenomatous, and colloid type nodules (Figure 22-9).

The most common cause of thyroid disorders worldwide is iodine deficiency, which leads to nodule and goiter formation. Often the gland is able to keep up with the demand and provide normal release of thyroid hormones. However, in some cases, the gland lags behind the demand and the patient develops hypothyroidism. In the first stage, hyperplasia occurs; in the second stage, colloid involution occurs. Progression of this process leads to an asymmetric and multinodular gland with areas of hemorrhage and calcification.

An **endemic goiter** may affect large groups of people in a specific geographic area where iodine levels in the soil, food, and water are low (e.g., mountainous areas or the Great Lakes region). Certain types of food (cabbage, turnips, and other related vegetables) when ingested in large quantities may increase blood synthesis of T_3 and T_4, but increase TSH secretion from the pituitary gland. This dietary deficiency can cause hyperplasia and hypertrophy and can promote goiter formation in the thyroid gland. Iodized salt as a dietary supplement usually corrects the iodine deficiency. In areas not deficient in iodine, autoimmune processes (Graves' disease or Hashimoto's thyroiditis) are believed to be the basis for most cases of thyroid disease.

A **toxic goiter** is condition where nodular enlargement causes hyperactivity of the thyroid gland and hyperthyroidism. **Nontoxic (simple) goiter** occurs when nodular enlargement is not associated with thyroid dysfunction (hypothyroidism or hyperthyroidism).

Clinical Findings. A goiter may first present visibly as an anterior protrusion on the neck on thin patients. The clinician may palpate an enlarged thyroid during a physical examination. A goiter may become very large, compressing the esophagus with difficulty swallowing (dysphagia), pressure on the trachea (inspiratory stridor) or neck veins (venous distention), or laryngeal nerve (hoarseness). Patients may also present with clinical symptoms of hypothyroidism or

hyperthyroidism. Table 22-2 lists the common findings, sonographic appearances, and differential considerations for nodule thyroid disease.

Sonographic Findings. Sonographic appearance of nodular thyroid disease will vary. There can be diffuse symmetric gland enlargement (Figure 22-10) or localized discrete nodule(s). Enlargement can involve both lobes and isthmus with several nodules, described as an MNG (Figure 22-11), or one lobe (Figure 22-12). Nodules can also vary in echogenicity (i.e., isoechoic, hyperechoic, and complex cystic) due to fibrosis, colloid, focal scarring, ischemia, cystic degeneration, or calcification formation. Nodules may present as poorly circumscribed or well defined and encapsulated by a thin, peripheral hypoechoic halo due to surrounding compressed tissue and should be documented. Hyperfunctioning nodules usually demonstrate increased perinodular and intranodular vascularity on color or power Doppler as seen in Figure 22-11, B.

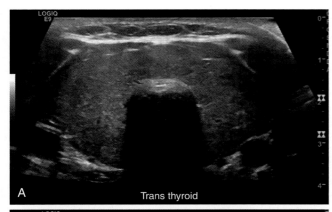

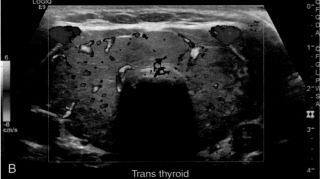

FIGURE 22-10   A, A patient with a goiter demonstrating diffusely enlarged thyroid gland. **B,** Vascularity of the diffusely enlarged thyroid gland.

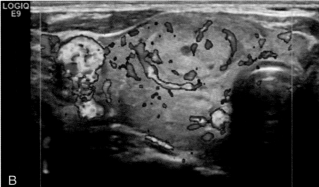

FIGURE 22-11   A, Multinodular goiter is seen as an inhomogeneous enlarged tissue mass within the thyroid gland. **B,** Increased vascularity is shown in a patient with a multinodular goiter.

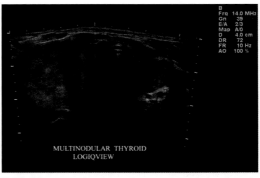

FIGURE 22-12 Transverse panoramic image of multinodular goiter shows an inhomogeneous pattern. The right lobe is more than twice the size of the left lobe.

Benign Lesions

A discrete, palpable nodule of the thyroid gland is the most common indication for a thyroid sonography. Nodular thyroid disease is frequently encountered in the adult population, with up to 7% found to have benign nodule, with women affected more frequently than men. Sonography is useful to locate the palpable nodule and describe sonographic appearance.

Cyst. A true epithelial-lined cyst within the thyroid is uncommon and considered benign. Most represent cystic degeneration of a follicular adenoma. Cystic component may represent serous fluid, colloid fluid, or hemorrhage and may contain blood or debris within the nodule.

Sonographic Findings. A true thyroid cyst demonstrates the sonographic appearance of a simple cyst as round, anechoic, and well defined, with thin echogenic walls and distal acoustic enhancement (Figure 22-13, *A*). Colloid cyst will demonstrate a cyst with a tiny echogenic focus (Figure 22-13, *B*) and often demonstrates a comet tail artifact. Hemorrhage cyst may demonstrate low-level echoes with possible fluid and debris level with possible wall irregularities and internal septation(s) (Figure 22-13, *C*). Vascularity should always be obtained on all thyroid masses with color Doppler images. Thyroid carcinoma could present as complex cystic nodule, so FNA biopsy would be necessary to evaluate any suspicious cystic masses.

Adenoma. A **follicular adenoma** is a benign thyroid neoplasm that represents 5% to 10% of all nodular diseases of the thyroid. It is 7 times more common in females than in males (Figure 22-14). Other rarer subtypes of follicular adenomas that are distinguished histologically include fetal adenoma, embryonal adenoma, and Hurthle cell adenoma. A Hurthle cell adenoma should be further evaluated when found after FNA because 15% to 25% will have malignant cells found within the adenoma after excision.

The adenoma is often solitary and slow growing unless hemorrhage occurs that could cause sudden and painful enlargement. Most patients with a thyroid adenoma do not have thyroid dysfunction (euthyroid), and less than 10% develop hyperthyroidism (toxic nodule). Rarely, a toxic nodule may cause extreme hyperthyroidism or thyrotoxicosis and would require immediate treatment. Sonography cannot distinguish between a toxic and nontoxic adenoma.

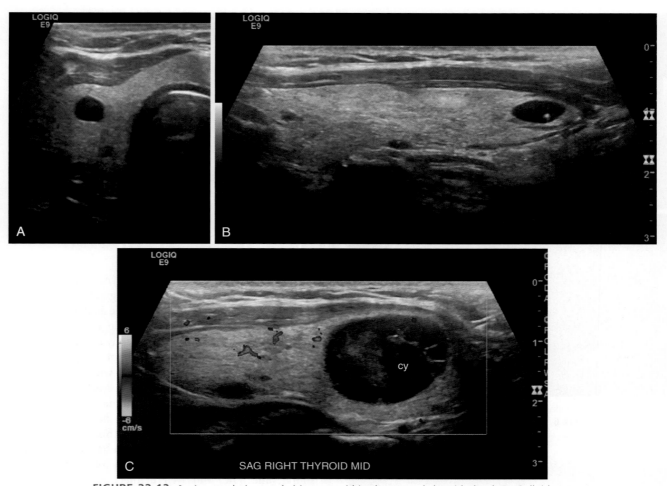

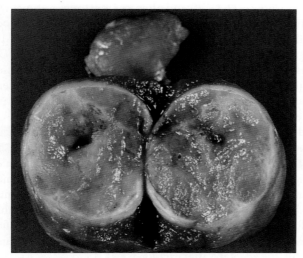

FIGURE 22-13 **A,** An anechoic cyst *(cy)* is seen within the normal thyroid gland. **B,** Colloid cyst with echogenic focus. **C,** Hemorrhagic cyst with color Doppler.

FIGURE 22-14 **Gross pathology of follicular adenoma.** The nodule is well circumscribed with a fibrous capsule separating it from the normal parenchyma.

Sonographic Findings. Adenomas have a broad spectrum of sonographic appearances. They are most often solitary, homogeneous, and variable in size and range in echogenicity from anechoic, hypoechoic, isoechoic, to hyperechoic. The presence of a thin hypoechoic rim or halo due to compressed tissue surrounding the adenoma is a relatively consistent finding with a benign adenoma (Figure 22-15, *A*). However, it is not always present or may be seen less commonly (10% to 24%) with malignancy. Adenomas may contain anechoic areas from hemorrhage or cystic degeneration and may be irregular in outline. Calcification along the rim with an "eggshell" appearance with shadowing can also be demonstrated with an adenoma (Figure 22-15, *B–D*). Rim calcification with shadowing may obscure visualization. Color or power Doppler will demonstrate enhanced blood flow patterns along the peripheral borders or within the lesion but not specific to separate a benign from malignant process.

Malignant Lesions

Carcinoma of the thyroid is rare. A solitary nodule may be malignant in a small percentage of cases, but the risk of malignancy decreases with the presence of multiple nodules. A solitary markedly hypoechoic thyroid nodule with the presence of cervical lymphadenopathy on the same side suggests malignancy. A prior history of neck or upper chest radiation is associated with the most common type of thyroid malignancy.

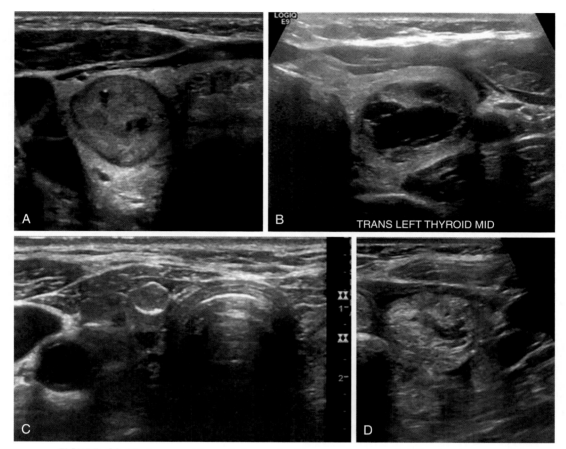

FIGURE 22-15 Sonographic variations of adenomas. A, A well-defined adenoma with a cystic component with a hypoechoic halo is seen on the right lobe. **B,** Complex cystic adenoma. **C,** Large eggshell calcification within a thyroid adenoma. **D,** Well-defined echogenic adenoma.

Clinical Findings. Thyroid malignancy is associated with the presence of a painless, palpable, hard, firm solitary nodule. If more advanced, the patient may present with compression of adjacent structures with hoarseness, cough, dysphagia, or dyspnea.

Sonographic Findings. Sonographic appearance of thyroid cancer is highly variable, making the distinction between benign and malignant nodules by sonography alone difficult. As stated previously, a malignant lesion is most often single, but could be multiple; it may be variable in size, solid, partially cystic, or a largely cystic mass. Generally, the sonographic characteristic that suggests malignancy is a solitary, solid mass that is markedly hypoechoic compared with strap muscles, with irregular or microlobulated margins that may be taller than wide. Additionally, there are often small, punctate internal microcalcifications (less than 2 mm). Microcalcifications are present in 50% to 80% of thyroid carcinoma. Increased vascularity may be noted with color Doppler with a more disorganized internal flow pattern (Figure 22-16). Definitive diagnosis would need to be determined by FNA biopsy.

Papillary Carcinoma. The most common of the thyroid malignancies is **papillary carcinoma,** which comprises approximately 70% of all thyroid cancers. It is considered the least aggressive type of tumor with excellent prognosis if found early and a 20-year survival rate above 90% (Figure 22-17). Females are affected 3 times more often than males and usually seen between the ages of 20 and 40. There is a higher incidence with clinical history of neck or upper chest radiation. The major route of spread of papillary carcinoma is through the lymphatic system to the nearby cervical lymph nodes with metastatic cervical adenopathy seen in approximately 20% to 50% of patients when diagnosed.

Sonographic Findings. Sonographic characteristics of papillary carcinoma include solid texture with marked hypoechogenicity when compared with strap muscles (reported in 90% of cases). Incomplete halo or ill-defined borders surrounding the nodule, "taller than wide," internal microcalcifications that appear as tiny, punctate hyperechoic foci (less than 2 mm with or without acoustic shadowing), and increased vascularity with color or power Doppler are seen in 90% of cases. Papillary carcinoma may also present as complex cystic in appearance. Ipsilateral cervical lymph node metastasis seen in about 20% to 50% of cases (see Figure 22-16).

Follicular Carcinoma. Follicular carcinoma is the second most common type (10% to 20%) of well-differentiated

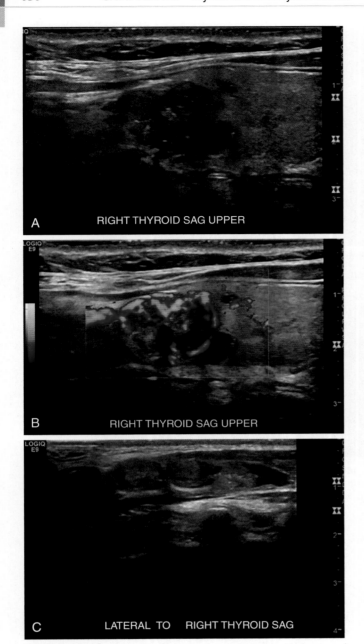

FIGURE 22-16 **A,** Papillary carcinoma on biopsy. **B,** Increased vascularity demonstrated with power Doppler. **C,** Enlarged cervical lymph nodes seen with papillary carcinoma.

thyroid cancer. It affects females 3 times more often than males, is seen between the ages of 40 and 60, and is not associated with prior neck and upper chest radiation. There are two types of follicular carcinoma: minimally invasive and widely invasive. The minimally invasive type is well encapsulated, which is best differentiated histologically from benign follicular adenoma by the demonstration of focal invasion of capsular blood vessels of the fibrous capsule. The widely invasive type is not encapsulated and will demonstrate invasion of the tumor blood vessels into adjacent thyroid tissue. Follicular carcinoma

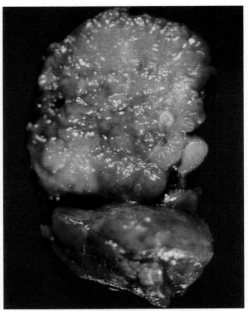

FIGURE 22-17 **Gross pathology of papillary carcinoma.** Large solid tumor mass nearly replaced one lobe of the thyroid gland.

spreads through the bloodstream rather than by the lymphatic system with metastases to bone, lung, brain, and liver. Lymph node involvement is less common (10%). Follicular carcinoma usually presents as a solitary thyroid mass and may not be differentiated pathologically with FNA biopsy and may require surgical removal of the entire nodule to confirm diagnosis. It is more aggressive than papillary cancer with a 20-year mortality rate of approximately 20% (Figure 22-18).

Sonographic Findings. Sonographic features are similar to benign follicular adenoma, but malignancy should be suspected with presence of thick irregular halo and tortuous internal blood vessels with increased vascularity with color or power Doppler. These findings along with cervical lymphadenopathy are characteristics, but not specific, for follicular carcinoma (Figure 22-19).

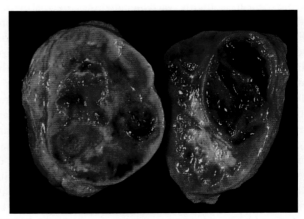

FIGURE 22-18 Gross pathology of follicular carcinoma shows a well-circumscribed tumor.

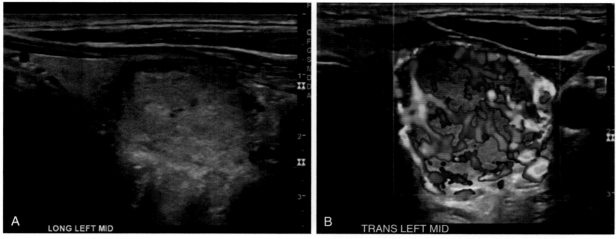

FIGURE 22-19 **A,** Solitary lesion representing a follicular carcinoma on biopsy. **B,** Increased vascularity is seen within the mass.

Medullary Carcinoma. Medullary carcinoma accounts for 5% of thyroid cancers. This cancer derives from the parafollicular or C cells of the thyroid that secrete calcitonin. Calcitonin will be elevated and used as a laboratory tumor marker. This has only a slightly higher female-to-male ratio of 3:2 and is not associated with prior neck or upper chest radiation exposure.

It may also be familial (20%) and associated with other disorders such as multiple endocrine neoplasia type 2 (MEN 2) syndrome and subtypes. MEN 2 syndrome is a hereditary condition associated with three primary types of endocrine tumors: medullary thyroid cancer, parathyroid tumors, and adrenal medullary tumors. A higher incidence of metastatic involvement of the cervical lymph nodes (80%) and liver metastasis have been reported, yielding a worse prognosis (Figure 22-20).

Sonographic Findings. Medullary carcinoma will appear sonographically similar to papillary carcinoma as a solid mass that is marked by hypoechogenicity and calcifications (Figure 22-21). Hypervascularity may also be noted. Careful

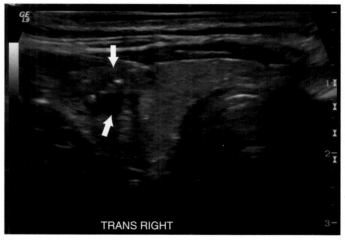

FIGURE 22-21 Solitary lesion representing a medullary carcinoma on biopsy *(arrows).*

evaluation of the liver and entire neck area for cervical lymph node metastasis should be completed.

Anaplastic Carcinoma. Anaplastic carcinoma (*anaplastic* means undifferentiated) is rare, accounts for less than 2% of thyroid cancers, and is considered most deadly. It is considered undifferentiated because it may be associated with papillary or follicular carcinomas. It is 2 times more common in men and usually occurs after age 60. It may be seen many years after radiation exposure to the neck or upper chest with lung metastasis seen in 50% of patients along with 90% cervical lymph node involvement. It is usually diagnosed at stage IV when found, and the 5-year mortality rate is 90% to 95%.

Clinically, the patient presents with a rapidly enlarging, hard, fixed mass and commonly dyspnea, dysphagia, hoarseness, and cough. It grows quickly with local invasion of the surrounding neck structures and widespread

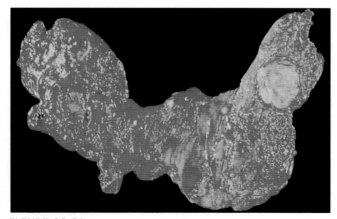

FIGURE 22-20 Gross pathology of medullary carcinoma shows a well-defined mass in the thyroid gland.

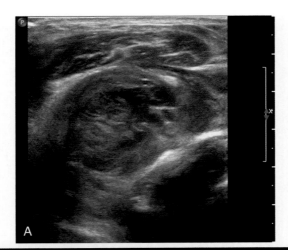

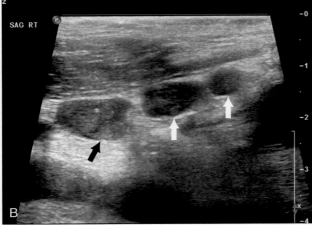

FIGURE 22-22 A, Large solitary lesion representing an anaplastic carcinoma causing enlargement of the thyroid gland. **B,** Several enlarged cervical lymph nodes noted with anaplastic carcinoma *(arrows).*

metastasis. It usually causes death by compression and asphyxiation due to invasion into the trachea.

Sonographic Findings. Anaplastic thyroid carcinoma presents as a large, hypoechoic mass with encasement and invasion of surrounding structures and vasculature of the neck. Careful evaluation of the liver and entire neck area for cervical lymph node metastasis should be completed (Figure 22-22). CT and MRI may be more accurate to demonstrate the entire extent of the mass.

Lymphoma. Lymphoma within the thyroid is primarily non-Hodgkin's type and accounts for 4% of all thyroid malignancies. It affects older females 4 times more often than men. In many cases, the patient has a preexisting chronic lymphocytic thyroiditis (Hashimoto's disease) with subclinical or overt hypothyroidism. Clinically the patient has a rapidly growing neck mass, possibly with partial airway obstruction (dyspnea). Prognosis is good if found in early stages, but poor if found in a more advanced stage.

Sonographic Findings. Lymphoma is characterized by a large, nonvascular, hypoechoic, and lobulated solid mass. There may be large areas of cystic necrosis within the tumor

along with encasement of adjacent neck vessels. The adjacent thyroid parenchyma may be heterogeneous secondary to associated chronic thyroiditis.

Thyroid Metastasis. The thyroid gland is not a common site for metastasis and usually occurs later in spread of the neoplasm. When found, it is usually from melanoma, breast, or renal cell carcinoma.

Sonographic Findings. Metastasis can present as a solitary, well-defined hypoechoic nodule or diffuse gland involvement. There are no distinctive sonographic features, but it should be questioned if there is a known primary carcinoma and a new thyroid mass is sonographically demonstrated.

Elastography. A new sonographic application, elastography is used to evaluate the tissue stiffness. There are several methods to evaluate the stiffness of normal tissue and solid thyroid lesions, such as strain elastography, acoustic radiation force impulse, and shear wave elastography. Medical studies are being used to investigate and validate whether elastography methods can be used to manage thyroid nodules and limit the number of FNAs. Figure 22-23 shows elastography images demonstrating soft areas as blue and hard areas as red within the thyroid gland.

Diffuse Thyroid Disease

Several diseases of the thyroid are characterized by diffuse involvement of the gland causing enlargement (goiter) without palpable nodules. Conditions that produce diffuse enlargement of the gland include Graves' disease, thyroiditis,

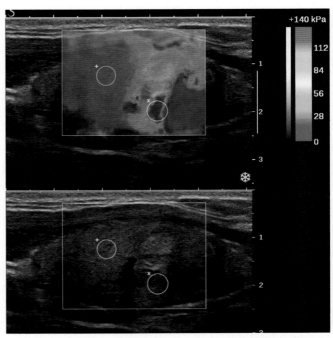

FIGURE 22-23 Elastography images that demonstrate soft areas of blue and hard areas of red of nodules within the thyroid gland.

and colloid or adenomatous goiter. Specific diagnosis is made on the basis of clinical and laboratory findings and possibly FNA biopsy. Sonography is usually not indicated with a diffusely enlarged gland; however, it may be indicated if a suspected thyroid mass is present.

Graves' Disease. Graves' disease is an autoimmune disorder and the most common (85%) cause of hyperthyroidism. With Graves' disease, the immune system attacks the thyroid gland and causes it to produce thyroid hormones. It occurs 5 to 8 times more frequently in women than men and usually is seen after 30 years of age. Graves' disease is characterized by a triad of clinical findings: hypermetabolism, diffuse toxic goiter, and exophthalmos (bulging eyes due to inflammatory infiltration of the tissue surrounding the orbit). Exophthalmos is also clinically characterized by the presence of protruding, staring eyes with decreased movement. The patient also presents with an enlarged thyroid associated with diffuse hyperplastic goiter (Figure 22-24). There may also be thickening of the dermis of the legs (pretibial areas) and dorsum of the feet. Laboratory tests will demonstrate elevated serum T_3 and T_4, but very low TSH.

Uncontrolled acute hyperthyroidism may cause a severe complication of Graves' disease called thyrotoxicosis, thyrotoxic crisis, or thyroid storm. It usually occurs after recent infection or surgery and may be life threatening due to resulting hyperthermia, tachycardia, heart failure, and delirium.

◥ Sonographic Findings. Graves' disease can demonstrate a normal thyroid gland appearance or present as an enlarged and inhomogeneous gland because of large intraparenchymal vessels. In young patients, the gland may be hypoechoic secondary to extensive lymphocytic infiltration or predominant cellular parenchyma that is devoid of colloid substance. The overactivity of Graves' disease often demonstrates increased vascularity on color Doppler imaging, leading to the term *thyroid inferno* (Figure 22-25).

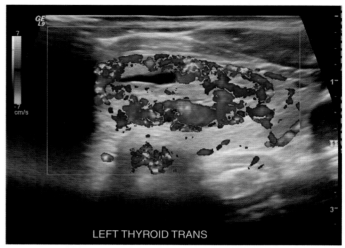

FIGURE 2-25 Diffusely enlarged heterogeneous gland with increased color Doppler in a patient with Graves' disease.

Spectral Doppler may show low resistive flow with peak systolic velocities greater than 70 cm/sec.

Thyroiditis. Thyroiditis is a group of disorders that include inflammation of the thyroid gland with several causes, such as bacteria or viral infections, postpartum, post–radiation ablation technique, drug induced, or related to autoimmune abnormalities. All usually result in hypothyroidism. Types of thyroiditis include acute suppurative thyroiditis, subacute granulomatous thyroiditis (de Quervain's disease), and chronic lymphocytic thyroiditis (Hashimoto's disease). Clinical findings may vary from mild to severe swelling and tenderness of the thyroid followed later by symptoms of hypothyroidism.

◥ Sonographic Findings. The appearance can change with acute to chronic disease progression. With acute disease the thyroid is hypoechoic, is enlarged, and may have increased color flow visualized. Sonography can be used to determine whether an abscess is present and location. An abscess usually appears as an irregular, ill-defined, hypoechoic, heterogeneous mass with internal debris, possible septation(s), and could have gas present with shadowing. Chronically, the thyroid will become more inhomogeneous and fibrotic with nodular borders.

Subacute (de Quervain's) Thyroiditis. Subacute (de Quervain's) thyroiditis is probably caused by a viral infection of the thyroid, which results in diffuse inflammation of the thyroid with dysphagia, fever, pain, tenderness, enlargement, and malaise. The disease has a gradual or fairly abrupt onset and the pain may be severe. De Quervain's thyroiditis may cause transient hyperthyroidism, but in a period of weeks or a few months, the swelling and pain subside with the gland returning to normal function.

◥ Sonographic Findings. May demonstrate an enlarged and hypoechoic thyroid with normal or decreased vascularity secondary to diffuse edema of the gland. The process could also present as focal hypoechoic regions within the thyroid gland.

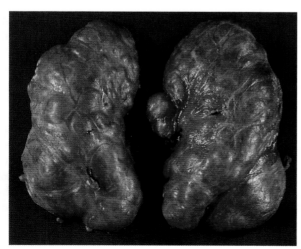

FIGURE 22-24 Gross pathology of a patient with Graves' disease shows symmetric enlargement of the thyroid gland.

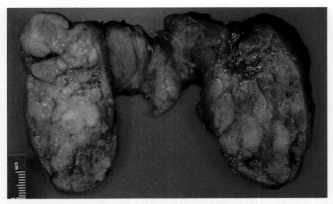

FIGURE 22-26 **Gross pathology of a patient with Hashimoto's thyroiditis.** The enlarged gland is multinodular with multiple lymphoid infiltrates.

Hashimoto's Thyroiditis. **Hashimoto's thyroiditis** is the most common form of thyroiditis. It is associated with a destructive autoimmune disorder, which leads to chronic inflammation of the thyroid. The outstanding clinical feature is a painless, diffusely enlarged gland seen most often in young or middle-aged women. The entire gland may be involved, with an inflammatory reaction with enlargement that is not necessarily symmetric (Figure 22-26). Eventually, the gland becomes severely compromised with resultant hypothyroidism. Laboratory tests will demonstrate low serum T_3 and T_4, but elevated TSH levels.

Sonographic Findings. Sonographic findings demonstrate heterogeneous gland enlargement with micronodulation with ill-defined hypoechoic areas (pseudolobules) (Figure 22-27). Color Doppler shows normal to decreased flow velocity, although occasionally the "thyroid inferno" with a high peak systolic velocity (PSV) is seen when hypothyroidism develops. Adjacent cervical lymphadenopathy may also be demonstrated.

EMBRYOLOGY OF THE PARATHYROID GLAND

The parathyroid glands are derived from endoderm germ cell tissue in the embryo. The parathyroid glands begin as separate paired glands. The superior parathyroid glands develop in the primitive pharyngeal region and migrate inferiorly to the dorsal aspect of the upper to middle portion of the thyroid gland. The paired inferior parathyroid glands develop in the area of the thymus gland and also migrate, but during migration the parathyroid glands should normally lose their connection with the thymus gland and rest at the inferior dorsal aspect of thyroid gland. Normal migration occurs in 60% of patients, with the remaining having ectopic location of parathyroid glands that can extend from the submandibular to the mediastinal region. Other ectopic locations are retrotracheal, intrathyroid, and along the carotid sheath (Figure 22-28).

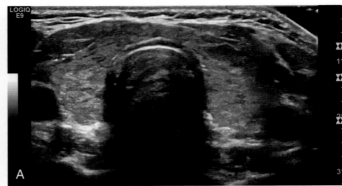
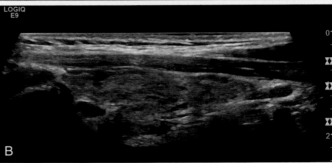

FIGURE 22-27 **A,** Image of heterogeneous, irregular thyroid gland seen in a patient with Hashimoto's thyroiditis. **B,** Sagittal image of prominent lymph nodes noted posterior and inferior to the thyroid gland seen with Hashimoto's thyroiditis.

ANATOMY OF THE PARATHYROID GLAND

The parathyroid glands are endocrine organs normally located on the posterior surface of the thyroid gland. Most people have four parathyroid glands, but some individuals could have three or five parathyroid glands. The four parathyroid glands are paired and embedded within the fascia surrounding the thyroid gland. Two lie posterior to each superior pole of the thyroid, and the other two lie posterior to the inferior pole (see Figure 22-1).

Normal parathyroid glands are small, flat, and disc shaped with normal size up to $5 \times 3 \times 1$ mm. Due to their small size and position, normal parathyroid glands are commonly not demonstrated sonographically.

PARATHYROID PHYSIOLOGY AND LABORATORY DATA

The parathyroid glands are considered the calcium-sensing organs of the body. Total body calcium is stored in bone in the form of phosphate with only a smaller portion of calcium in the blood. The parathyroid glands produce **parathyroid hormone (PTH)** to control the serum calcium concentration using a feedback mechanism. When the serum calcium level decreases, the parathyroid glands are stimulated to release PTH. When the serum calcium level increases the parathyroid hormone level decreases. Abnormalities are initially suspected clinically when routine laboratory screening

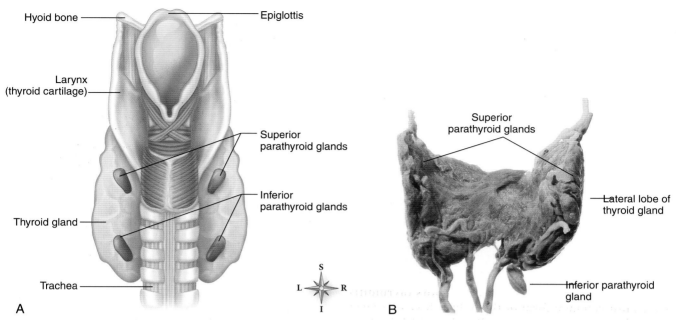

FIGURE 22-28 Variations of parathyroid gland locations.

demonstrates an elevated serum calcium level (hypercalcemia), elevated urine calcium level (hypercaluria), and low serum phosphorous levels (hypophosphatemia). It is important to note that elevated serum calcium levels may be associated clinically with other conditions including chronic renal failure and vitamin D deficiency that would also elevate serum calcium (secondary hyperparathyroidism). PTH acts on several target organs (skeletal system, kidneys, and intestines) to increase calcium absorption into the blood. The elevated serum calcium levels could be asymptomatic or lead to abdominal and/or musculoskeletal pain. It could also lead to the formation of renal stones (nephrolithiasis), ulcers, pancreatitis, or bone pain related to loss of bone calcium (osteopenia or osteoporosis). There can also be a clinical manifestation that is neurologic with increased depression, nervousness, confusion, and headaches. The primary physician may order a PTH laboratory test to look for abnormal PTH elevation that, along with elevated serum calcium levels, could indicate primary hyperparathyroidism.

Nuclear Medicine Scintigraphy

A nuclear medicine test called a *sestamibi parathyroid scan* is often completed to try to locate abnormally functioning parathyroid gland(s). The patient is given a radiopharmaceutical (Tc-99m sestamibi) and then imaged along with delay scan to note any increased uptake to the parathyroid gland(s). If available, sestamibi parathyroid scan results should be evaluated and correlated with sonography examination findings (Figure 22-29). One of the advantages of a nuclear medicine examination is to locate increased activity from an ectopic parathyroid gland that

cannot be imaged by sonography, especially if it is within the mediastinum.

SONOGRAPHIC EVALUATION OF THE PARATHYROID GLAND

Correct sonographic imaging of parathyroid abnormalities requires use of a high-resolution (7- to 15-MHz) linear-array transducer. A thorough clinical history is obtained that includes previous diagnosis of parathyroid disease, kidney stones, ulcer, pancreatitis, and/or osteoporosis. It is also important to determine whether the patient has chronic renal failure or is receiving renal dialysis that could explain abnormal laboratory data (secondary hyperparathyroidism). The referring physician should also provide recent laboratory values on serum calcium and PTH levels. On clinical examination, enlarged parathyroid glands are usually soft and not palpable and have no association with dysphagia.

The examination should always be explained to the patient. The patient is then placed supine with a pillow or pad placed under the shoulders to hyperextend the neck. To investigate all locations for enlarged parathyroid glands and possible ectopic glands, the entire anterior and lateral neck should be surveyed. This should extend superiorly from the submandibular region to inferiorly to the sternal notch in transverse and longitudinal planes and laterally to the internal jugular veins with representative images recorded. Attention should be focused on the areas adjacent to the superior and inferior poles of both thyroid glands. To detect the inferior parathyroid glands, the patient should be asked to swallow to elevate the thyroid gland superiorly during real-time scanning. It is important to note that the parathyroid glands will

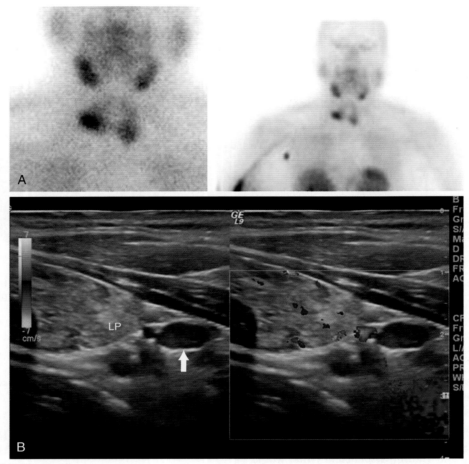

FIGURE 22-29 A, Scintigraphy demonstrating increased uptake associated with parathyroid adenoma. **B,** Longitudinal image of a typical parathyroid adenoma with two-dimensional and color Doppler. Parathyroid adenoma *(arrow)*. *LP,* Lower pole of thyroid gland.

move with the thyroid gland when swallowing because they are located within the same fascia. Due to their small and flat shape and their close proximity to the thyroid, visualization of the normal parathyroid gland(s) is a challenge.

In transverse images, a prominent longus colli muscle located posteriorly to the thyroid may be confused with an enlarged parathyroid gland and should be evaluated with the opposite side for muscle symmetry. In addition, longitudinal images will be differentiated when the muscle elongates into the linear muscle appearance. If present, cervical lymph nodes that are located near the thyroid borders can be confused for an enlarged parathyroid gland. This can be differentiated by the demonstration of the echogenic hilum and central flow that is present in the sonographic appearance of normal lymph nodes. In addition, the minor neurovascular bundle, consisting of the inferior thyroid artery and recurrent laryngeal nerve, may be confused for the parathyroid glands. Longitudinal images can often eliminate this confusion by identifying the bundle's tubular appearance along with color or power Doppler demonstration of vascular flow.

PATHOLOGY OF THE PARATHYROID GLAND

Primary Hyperparathyroidism

Primary hyperparathyroidism is an endocrine disorder caused by the increased function of the parathyroid gland. It is more commonly seen after age 40, affecting women 2 to 3 times more than men. Primary hyperparathyroidism is characterized by abnormal secretion of PTH, which then signals more calcium to be released into the blood. Laboratory findings include hypercalcemia, hypercaluria, and elevated PTH levels with hypophosphatemia. Most patients are asymptomatic without manifestation of primary hyperparathyroidism, such as nephrolithiasis, abdominal or musculoskeletal pain, or osteopenia. The role of sonography is to determine whether primary hyperparathyroidism is caused by a parathyroid adenoma, parathyroid hyperplasia, or, rarely, carcinoma of the parathyroid gland.

Adenoma. A parathyroid adenoma (PTA) is a benign, solid mass and the most common (80% to 85%) cause of primary hyperparathyroidism. The exact cause is unknown. PTAs are usually oval and solitary (Figure 22-30), but could involve one or more of four parathyroid glands causing enlargement. Because surgical removal is the only definitive treatment, location of an enlarged parathyroid gland within the complex anatomy of the neck will significantly aid the surgeon by indicating the

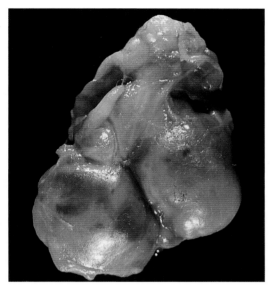

FIGURE 22-30 Gross pathology of parathyroid adenoma. The gland is enlarged and nodular.

affected side and whether the PTA is demonstrated superior or inferior to thyroid gland.

Sonographic Findings.   Parathyroid adenomas are oval, hypoechoic, homogeneous, and usually solid (Figure 22-31). They can often become more oblong, tubelike, or bilobar in shape. Smaller adenomas are usually less than 3 cm in size with larger adenomas measuring 5 cm or greater in length. Superior PTAs are usually located adjacent to the posterior aspect of the superior to mid portion of the thyroid, but inferior parathyroid adenomas are more variable and could extend inferiorly from the lower pole of the thyroid to the sternal notch. Color and power Doppler may show vascularity to the gland that is usually more peripheral or a peripheral vascular arc pattern. This will help to differentiate from central hilum flow seen in hyperplastic regional lymph nodes. Less commonly, a PTA may have cystic components or calcifications. Pitfalls to be aware of in diagnosing parathyroid enlargement include recognition of normal cervical structures, longus colli muscle, esophagus, and vasculature, which could result in false-positive findings. An inferior PTA may be visualized by having the patient swallow and will demonstrate movement with the thyroid gland to help confirm identification. The parathyroid gland may also be ectopic, making it difficult to locate by sonography. Common locations are mediastinal, retrotracheal, intrathyroidal, and carotid sheath/undescended.

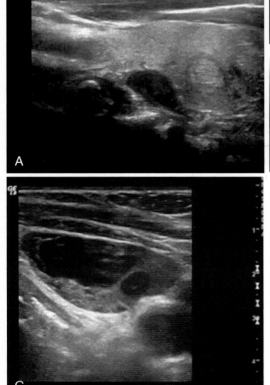

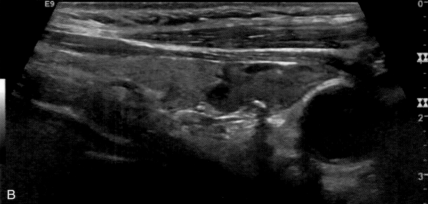

FIGURE 22-31 Sonographic variations of parathyroid adenomas. A, Parathyroid adenoma located along the posterior border of the upper pole of the thyroid. **B,** Irregular parathyroid adenoma with calcification and shadowing. **C,** Complex cystic parathyroid adenoma inferior to the thyroid gland.

Parathyroid Hyperplasia. Approximately 10% to 15% of patients with primary hyperparathyroidism have parathyroid hyperplasia. **Parathyroid hyperplasia** is defined as enlargement and hyperfunction of the parathyroid gland with no apparent cause. Only one gland may be significantly enlarged, with the remaining glands only mildly affected, or all glands may be enlarged (Figure 22-32).

◾ *Sonographic Findings.* Noting enlargement of several glands will help differentiate hyperplasia from multiple parathyroid adenomas (Figure 22-33). If adjacent glands become enlarged, it becomes more difficult to separate the enlarged glands with sonography.

Parathyroid Carcinoma. Only 1% of patients with primary hyperparathyroidism have a parathyroid carcinoma. The histologic differentiation of adenoma and carcinoma is very difficult. Metastasis to regional lymph nodes or distant organs or local occurrence must be present for cancer to be diagnosed. Clinically, most parathyroid cancers are small and irregular, but as they enlarge will become firm or hard masses and adhere to or invade surrounding structures. It is seen equally in males and females. Laboratory findings of parathyroid cancer will usually demonstrate very high serum calcium levels.

◾ *Sonographic Findings.* The sonographic appearance of parathyroid cancer is usually larger, more irregular in shape, or with a lobulated contour. Gland orientation may be taller than wide, more heterogeneous, with increased vascularity or internal cystic components. Because a large adenoma may have some of these same sonographic findings, the diagnosis of malignancy may not be made until surgical removal. Metastases to regional nodes or distant organs, capsular invasion, and local recurrence are more reliable to diagnose parathyroid cancer by sonography.

Secondary Hyperparathyroidism Secondary hyperparathyroidism occurs when the serum PTH level is increased due to chronic hypocalcemia. Increased PTH level is not caused by a dysfunction of the parathyroid gland, but stimulated by a compensatory reaction by the hypocalcemia usually from chronic renal failure, vitamin D deficiency or rickets, or intestinal malabsorption syndromes. Laboratory findings will demonstrate elevated PTH levels with low calcium levels. Secondary hyperparathyroidism may demonstrate enlargement of all four parathyroid glands.

MISCELLANEOUS NECK MASSES

When a palpable neck mass is present, the role of sonography is to determine the origin of the mass by demonstration of the location, sonographic characteristics, and vascularity of the mass.

Developmental Cysts

Thyroglossal Duct Cyst. The most common congenital cystic anomaly is **thyroglossal duct cyst,** which is usually located (70%) in the midline of the neck anterior to the trachea or within 2 cm of the midline. During embryology, a narrow, hollow tract connects the thyroid lobes to the flow of the pharynx between the base of the tongue, at or below the level of the hyoid bone. This tract should atrophy with age. If the tract persists, it creates a potential space for fluid to collect into a cystic mass anywhere along the tract from above to below the level of the hyoid bone. It is usually seen in the pediatric population with 90% found before age 10.

◾ *Sonographic Findings.* The thyroglossal duct cyst may have the same sonographic characteristics of a cyst, often oval or spherical in shape and located in the midline. The cyst may often be more complex cystic in appearance and rarely larger than 2 or 3 cm (Figure 22-34).

Branchial Cleft Cyst. **Branchial cleft cyst** is a congenital cystic mass that is located in the lateral portion of the neck.

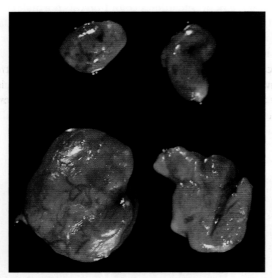

FIGURE 22-32 Gross pathology of parathyroid hyperplasia with enlargement of all four parathyroid glands.

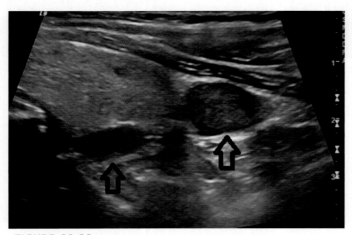

FIGURE 22-33 Sonographic images that demonstrates enlargement of two parathyroid glands *(arrows)* in the lower pole of the thyroid.

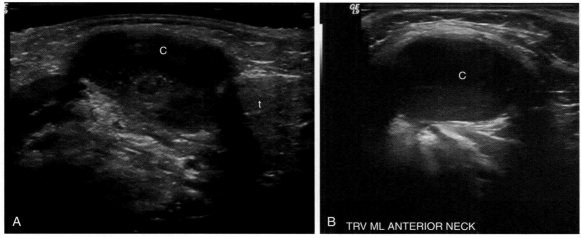

FIGURE 22-34 A, Sagittal image of a thyroglossal duct cyst *(C)* located in the midline superior to the thyroid gland *(t)*. **B,** Transverse image superior to the thyroid gland demonstrating a thyroglossal duct cyst *(C)* in the midline.

It may vary in location, but usually is found laterally in the submandibular region. During embryonic development, the branchial cleft is a slender tract extending from the pharyngeal cavity to an opening near the auricle or into the neck. A diverticulum may extend laterally from the pharynx or medially from the neck and fill with fluid causing a cyst formation. It is usually single, but 2% to 3% are bilateral, and it is found more often in older children or young adults.

Sonographic Findings. The branchial cleft cyst appearance can vary; although primarily cystic, it may present as complex or solid components with low-level echoes, particularly if it has become infected (Figure 22-35).

Abscess. An abscess can arise in any location of the neck and can have acute onset and progress quickly. Common clinical presentation of neck abscess is pain, erythema, edema, and fever, with a palpable mass. Sonography is also used to discern the nature of the palpable mass and involvement of adjacent anatomy. Sonography may also be used to guide for percutaneous needle aspiration and imaging after surgical or medical treatment.

Sonographic Findings. An abscess can range in its sonographic appearance from primarily fluid filled to completely echogenic. Most commonly, an abscess will appear as a complex cystic mass with low-level echogenicity and irregular walls (Figure 22-36). Presence of air within and ring-down artifact or shadowing will confirm the suspected etiology of the mass as an abscess. Chronic abscesses may be particularly difficult to demonstrate because there are usually indistinct margins

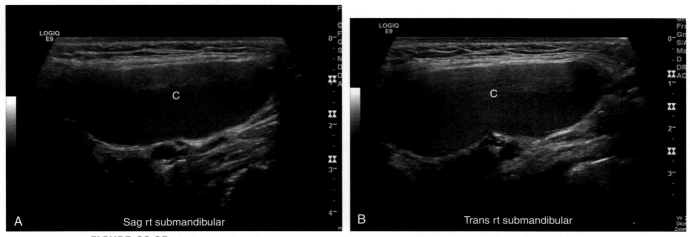

FIGURE 22-35 A, Longitudinal image at the angle of the mandible demonstrating a branchial cleft cyst *(C)* located inferior to the angle of the mandible. **B,** Transverse image of the branchial cleft cyst *(C)*.

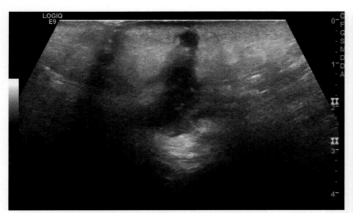

FIGURE 22-36 Sonographic image that demonstrates an irregular, complex cystic neck abscess.

and they are more isoechoic with the surrounding neck anatomy.

Cervical Lymphadenopathy. *Lymphadenopathy* is a localized or generalized enlargement of the lymph nodes. A lymph node can become prominent due to reactive hyperplasia, but could be enlarged due to neoplasm, metastasis, or an inflammatory process. Sonography can be an important imaging modality to assist tumor staging and careful evaluation of the neck regions for cervical lymphadenopathy with postthyroidectomy patients.

◣ *Sonographic Findings (Normal Lymph Node).* Sonographic appearance of a normal lymph node is oval in shape with a symmetric, homogeneous, thin outer cortex and an echogenic central hilum. Size typically does not exceed 1 cm (Figure 22-37, *A*). Color or power Doppler settings should be lowered to demonstrate flow entering the hilum.

◣ *Sonographic Findings (Lymphadenopathy).* Appearance may vary, but cervical lymphadenopathy will usually demonstrate a more rounded shape or more lobulated shape and loss of the echogenic hilum. The cortex may be thickened and symmetric or show localized asymmetry with lobulated or irregular boarders. Color may also demonstrate increased vascularity or avascularity to lymph node (Figure 22-37, *B* and *C*). Less commonly, lymphadenopathy may present with calcification(s) and a more complex cystic appearance from necrosis. Presence of multiple enlarged nodes is abnormal. Differentiation between inflammation, neoplasm, or metastatic processes is confirmed with FNA biopsy.

Postthyroidectomy Neck Sonography. Sonography plays an important role in the evaluation and management of patients after total thyroidectomy for thyroid cancer. A detailed scanning technique is being requested more often by endocrinologists and surgeons to detect potential regional recurrences or metastases. The sonographer will carefully evaluate and image the neck region to map the level and compartment of any enlarged lymph nodes. Sonography can also be invaluable as guidance for FNA of suspicious lymph nodes.

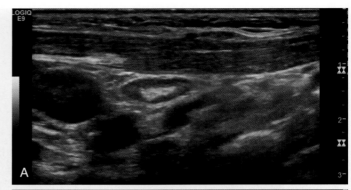

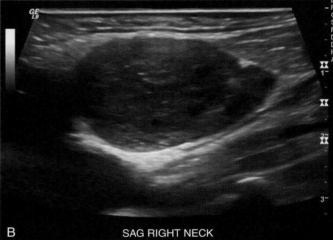

SAG RIGHT NECK

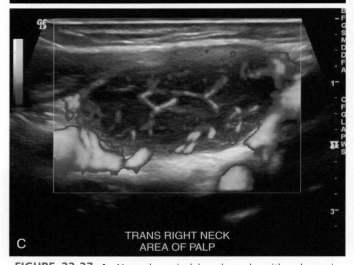

TRANS RIGHT NECK
AREA OF PALP

FIGURE 22-37 A, Normal cervical lymph node with echogenic hilum. **B,** Enlarged, hypoechoic, lobulated abnormal lymph node. **C,** Increased vascularity noted within an enlarged lymph node with power Doppler.

> **Key Pearls**
>
> - Sonography is excellent modality when clinically indicated for high-resolution evaluation of the thyroid gland for gland size, shape, location, and parenchyma echogenicity.

- Sonography can visualize the nature of palpable nodules as simple cyst, complex cystic, or solid and document associated calcifications.
- Thyroid pathology that includes inflammatory processes and benign and malignant conditions can be demonstrated by sonography but cannot be reliably differentiated.
- Sonographic characteristics that are suspicious for malignant thyroid nodule are a solid mass that is markedly hypoechoic with irregular margins that may be taller than wide. Visualization of microcalcifications and increased vascularity may be noted with color Doppler with a more disorganized internal flow pattern.
- Interventional procedures often use sonographic guidance for fine-needle aspiration of thyroid nodules.
- The parathyroid gland is often not visualized by high-resolution sonography unless enlarged, most often due to the presence of parathyroid adenoma, hyperplasia, or carcinoma of gland.
- Sonography can play an important role for the surgeon to locate enlarged parathyroid gland(s) before surgical removal of the abnormal gland(s).

BIBLIOGRAPHY

Barreda R, Kaude JV, Fagein M, et al: Hypervascularity of nontoxic goiter as shown by color-coded Doppler sonography, *Am J Roentgenol* 156:199, 1991.

Brander A, Viikinloski P, Nichels J, et al: Thyroid gland: US screening in a random adult population, *Radiology* 181:683-687, 1991.

Brant W, Helms C: *Fundamentals of diagnostic radiology,* ed 4, Philadelphia, 2012, Lippincott Williams & Wilkins.

Brkljacic B, Cuk V, Tomic-Brzak H, et al: Ultrasonic evaluation of benign and malignant nodules in echographically multinodular thyroids, *J Clin Ultrasound* 22:71, 1994.

Chang DG, Yang PC, Yu CJ, et al: Differentiation of benign and malignant cervical lymph nodes with color Doppler sonography, *Am J Roentgenol* 162:956-960, 1994.

Chheda H: *Sestamibi scan—technical details.* Available at http://www.parathyroid.com/sestamibi-technical.htm. Accessed Nov 29, 2011.

Clark KJ, Cronan JJ, Scola FH: Color Doppler sonography: anatomic and physiologic assessment of the thyroid, *J Clin Ultrasound* 23: 215-223, 1995.

Esseig G, Meyers A: *Parathyroid physiology.* Available at http://emedicine.medscape.com/article/874690. Accessed Nov 7, 2014.

Gladziwa U, Ittel TH, Dakshinamurty KV, et al: Secondary hyperparathyroidism and sonographic evaluation of parathyroid gland hyperplasia in dialysis patients, *Clin Nephrol* 38:162, 1992.

Goldberg B, McGahan J: *Atlas of ultrasound measurements,* ed 2, Philadelphia, 2006, Elsevier.

Hennemann G: Non-Toxic Goiter, *Clin Endocrinol Metab* 8:167, 1999.

Holmes EC, Morton DL, Ketcham AS: Parathyroid carcinoma: a collective review, *Ann Surg* 169:631, 1999.

Hopkins CR, Reading CC: Thyroid and parathyroid imaging, *Semin Ultrasound CT MR* 16:279-295, 1995.

Kawamura D, Lunsford B: *Diagnostic medical sonography: abdomen and superficial structures,* ed 3, Philadelphia, 2012, Lippincott Williams & Wilkins.

Kerr L: High-resolution thyroid ultrasound: the value of color Doppler, *Ultrasound Q* 12:21, 1994.

Kohri K, Ishikawa Y, Kodama M, et al: Comparison of imaging methods for localization of parathyroid tumors, *Am J Surg* 164:140-145, 1992.

Kuntz KM: Neck mass. In Henningsen C, editor: *Clinical guide to ultrasonography,* St. Louis, 2004, Mosby.

Meola M, Barsotti M, Lenti C, et al: Color-Doppler in the imaging work-up of primary hyperparathyroidism, *J Nephrol* 12:270, 1999.

Montazemi M: There is a mass in the neck (presentation). Sonography for SDMS-Society of Diagnostic Medical Sonography, 2012.

Rosai J: *Rosai and Ackerman's surgical pathology,* ed 9, St. Louis, 2004, Mosby.

Rumack C, Wilson S, Charboneua JW, et al: *Diagnostic ultrasound,* ed 4, Philadelphia, 2005, Elsevier.

Sargis R: *Thyroid gland overview: a major player in regulating your metabolism.* Available at www.endocrineweb.com. Accessed Mar 23, 2015.

Solbiati L, Cioffi V, Ballarati E: Ultrasonography of the neck, *Radiol Clin North Am* 30:941, 1992.

Takashima S, Morimoto S, Ikezoe J, et al: Primary thyroid lymphoma: comparison of CT and US assessment, *Radiology* 171:439, 1995.

Thibodeau G, Patton K: *Structure and function of the body,* ed 14, St. Louis, 2012, Elsevier.

Van Herle AJ, Rich P, Ljung BME, et al: The thyroid nodule, *Ann Intern Med* 196:221, 1992.

23

Scrotum

Cindy A. Owen

OBJECTIVES

On completion of this chapter, you should be able to:
- Identify the normal anatomy of the scrotum
- Explain the vascular supply to the scrotal contents
- Describe patient positioning, scanning protocol, and technical considerations for an ultrasound examination of the scrotum
- Discuss the role of color and spectral Doppler in scrotal imaging
- Describe the ultrasound characteristics of scrotal pathology

OUTLINE

Anatomy of the Scrotum
    Vascular Supply
    Patient Positioning and Scanning
       Protocol
Technical Considerations
Scrotal Pathology
    Acute Scrotum

Extratesticular Masses
Varicocele
Scrotal Hernia
Hydrocele, Pyocele, and
    Hematocele
Sperm Granuloma

Benign Testicular Masses
Malignant Testicular Masses
Lymphoma and Leukemia
Congenital Anomalies

KEY TERMS

Centripetal arteries
Cremasteric artery
Cremasteric muscle
Cryptorchidism
Deferential artery
Ejaculatory ducts
Epididymal cysts
Epididymis
Epididymitis
Hematocele
Hydrocele

Mediastinum testis
Pampiniform plexus
Pudendal artery
Pyocele
Recurrent rami
Rete testis
Scrotum
Seminal vesicles
Septa testis
Spermatic cord
Spermatoceles

Testicle
Testicular arteries
Testicular vein
Tunica albuginea
Tunica vaginalis
Urethra
Varicocele
Vas deferens
Verumontanum

Ultrasound is the imaging modality of choice for evaluating the scrotum. High-frequency ultrasound imaging, combined with color and spectral Doppler, quickly and reliably provides valuable information in the assessment of scrotal pain or mass. In particular, color Doppler has a central role in the evaluation of suspected testicular torsion because it can demonstrate absence of flow in the affected testis. Color Doppler also plays a key role in the evaluation of testicular infection by demonstrating hyperemic flow on the affected side. Ultrasound imaging accurately differentiates intratesticular from extratesticular masses and cystic from solid masses. Advances in the development of ultrasound equipment have provided improved spatial and contrast resolution, reduced speckle artifact, and increased sensitivity to the display of scrotal perfusion. The steady progress in ultrasound image quality has enhanced our ability to clearly define the scrotal anatomy and to more accurately depict and differentiate abnormalities. This chapter covers the pertinent anatomy of the scrotum and its contents, including the vascular supply. The ultrasound scanning protocol is discussed along with tips on scanning techniques and potential pitfalls. A review of the disease processes affecting the scrotum is provided, including a description of sonographic findings.

ANATOMY OF THE SCROTUM

The testes are symmetric, oval-shaped glands residing in the **scrotum.** In adults, the testis measures approximately 3 to 5 cm in length, 2 to 4 cm in width, and approximately 3 cm in height. Each testis is divided into more than 250 to 400 conical lobules containing the seminiferous tubules. These tubules converge at the apex of each lobule and anastomose to form the rete testis in the mediastinum. The rete testis drains into the head of the epididymis through the efferent ductules (Figure 23-1). Sonographically, the testes appear as smooth, medium-gray structures with a fine echo texture.

The epididymis is a 6- to 7-cm tubular structure beginning superiorly and then coursing posterolateral to the testis. It is divided into head, body, and tail. The head is the largest part of the epididymis, measuring 6 to 15 mm in width. It is located superior to the upper pole of the testis (Figure 23-2). It contains 10 to 15 efferent ductules from the rete testis, which converge to form a single duct in the body and tail. This duct is known as the ductus epididymis. It becomes the vas deferens and continues in the spermatic cord. The body of the epididymis is much smaller than the head. It is difficult to see with ultrasound on normal individuals. It follows the posterolateral aspect of the testis from the upper to the lower pole. The tail of the epididymis is slightly larger and is positioned posterior to the lower pole of the testis. The appendix of the epididymis is a small protuberance from the head of the epididymis. Postmortem studies have shown the appendix epididymis in 34% of testes unilaterally and 12% of testes bilaterally. The normal epididymis usually appears as isoechoic or hypoechoic compared with the testis, although the echo texture is coarser.

At the upper pole of the testis, the appendix testis is attached. It is located between the testis and the epididymis. Postmortem studies have shown the appendix testis to be present in 92% of testes unilaterally and 69% bilaterally (Figure 23-3).

The testis is completely covered by a dense, fibrous tissue termed the **tunica albuginea.** The posterior aspect of the tunica albuginea reflects into the testis to form a vertical

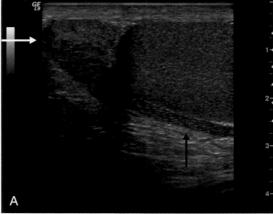

A

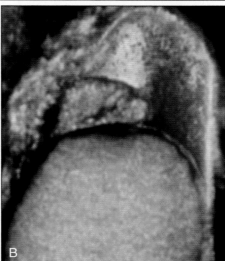

B

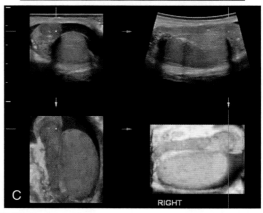

C   RIGHT

FIGURE 23-2 A, Sagittal ultrasound scan of a normal epididymis and testis. The head of the epididymis is seen superior to the upper pole of the testis *(white arrow).* The body of the epididymis is seen posterior to the testis *(black arrow).* Note the coarse echo texture of the epididymis compared with the fine texture of the testis. **B,** Three-dimensional (3D) view rendered in the coronal plane demonstrates the relationship of the normal epididymal head to the superior pole of the testis. **C,** 3D view shows orthogonal planes of enlarged epididymis in patient with epididymitis. An axis point *(small white dot)* is placed on the epididymal head to demonstrate the same point in three orthogonal views. The 3D data set allows manipulation of the volume in an infinite number of imaging planes. This allows the sonographer to adjust the display, so that the entire length of the epididymis can be demonstrated.

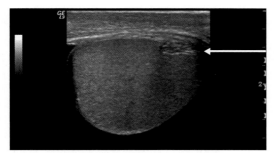

FIGURE 23-1 Transverse ultrasound scan of the normal rete testis. With the use of high-resolution imaging and transducer frequencies of 10 MHz or greater, the normal rete testis can sometimes be depicted with ultrasound. It appears as tiny tubules adjacent to the epididymal head and the testis mediastinum *(arrow).*

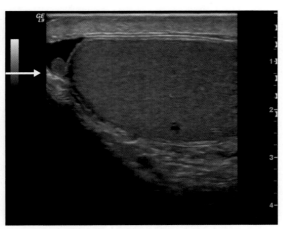

FIGURE 23-3 Sagittal ultrasound scan of the normal testis demonstrates the appendix testis as a small structure superior to the testis *(arrow)*. The appendix testis is isoechoic to the testis. A small hydrocele improves the visibility of the appendix testis.

septum known as the **mediastinum testis.** Multiple septa **(septa testis)** are formed from the tunica albuginea at the mediastinum. They course through the testis and separate it into lobules. The mediastinum supports the vessels and ducts coursing within the testis. The mediastinum is often seen on ultrasound as a bright hyperechoic line coursing craniocaudad within the testis (Figure 23-4). The **tunica vaginalis** lines the inner walls of the scrotum, covering each testis and epididymis. It consists of two layers: parietal and visceral. The parietal layer is the inner lining of the scrotal wall. The visceral layer surrounds the testis and epididymis. A small bare area is posterior. At this site, the testicle is against the scrotal wall, preventing torsion. Blood vessels, lymphatics, nerves, and spermatic ducts travel through the area (see Figure 23-1). The space between the layers of the tunica vaginalis is where hydroceles form. It is normal to see a small amount of fluid in this space.

The **vas deferens** is a continuation of the ductus epididymis. It is thicker and less convoluted. The vas deferens dilates at the terminal portion near the **seminal vesicles.** This portion is termed the *ampulla* of the deferens. The vas deferens joins the duct of the seminal vesicles to form the **ejaculatory duct,** which, in turn, empties into the **urethra.** The junction of the ejaculatory ducts with the urethra is termed the **verumontanum.** The urethra courses from the bladder to the end of the penis. In men, the urethra transports both urine and semen outside the body.

The vas deferens, testicular arteries, venous pampiniform plexus, lymphatics, autonomic nerves, and fiber of the cremaster form the **spermatic cord.** The cord extends from the scrotum through the inguinal canal and internal inguinal rings to the pelvis. The spermatic cord suspends the testis in the scrotum.

Vascular Supply

Right and left **testicular arteries** arise from the abdominal aorta just below the level of the renal arteries. They are the primary source of blood flow to the testis. The testicular arteries descend in the retroperitoneum and enter the spermatic cord in the deep inguinal ring. Then they course along the posterior surface of each testis and pierce the tunica albuginea, forming the capsular arteries, which branch over the surface of the testis. With high-frequency ultrasound imaging, the capsular artery is sometimes seen as a hypoechoic linear structure on the surface of the testis. Color Doppler can be used to confirm its identity (Figure 23-5). The capsular arteries give rise to **centripetal arteries,** which course from the testicular surface toward the mediastinum along the septa. Before reaching the mediastinum, they curve backward, forming the **recurrent rami** (centrifugal arteries) (Figure 23-6). These centrifugal arteries branch farther into arterioles and capillaries. With sensitive color Doppler settings, the recurrent rami may be seen giving a candy cane appearance (Figure 23-7).

FIGURE 23-4 A, Three-dimensional (3D) view showing the mediastinum testis in orthogonal planes with the septa. This image was obtained with a 3D transducer sweeping in the sagittal plane *(upper left)*. The transverse image is derived from the 3D volume and is displayed upper right. 3D view allows visualization of the coronal plane *(lower left)*. The coronal plane is rarely imaged with traditional two-dimensional imaging. A rendered view of the testis is seen in the lower right. **B,** 3D coronal view demonstrating the layers of the tunica vaginalis *(arrows)*. This is well demonstrated because of the presence of a hydrocele. Hydroceles form between the parietal and visceral layers of the tunica vaginalis.

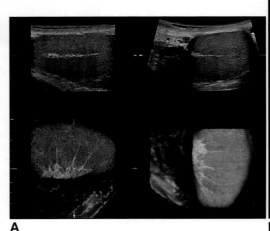

A

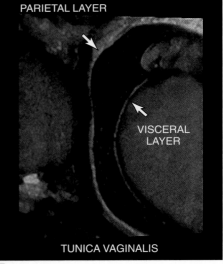

B

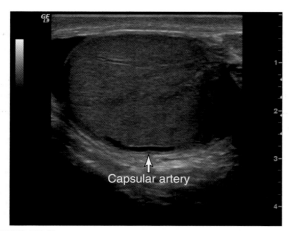

FIGURE 23-5 Transverse ultrasound view of the testis depicting the capsular artery in a patient with orchitis. The capsular artery is seen as an anechoic structure coursing along the surface of the testis *(arrow)*.

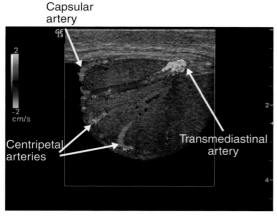

FIGURE 23-6 Color Doppler image of the testis depicting the capsular artery giving rise to centripetal arteries. A transmediastinal artery is seen coursing from the mediastinum to the testicular surface. It then branches across the top of the testis as capsular arteries. The flow direction in the transmediastinal artery *(blue)* is opposite that in the centripetal arteries *(red)*. The centripetal arteries rise from the capsular arteries with a flow direction through the testis toward the mediastinum, whereas the blood flow in the transmediastinal artery courses from the mediastinum to the testicular capsule.

In approximately one half of normal testes, a transmediastinal (or transtesticular) artery is visualized coursing through the mediastinum toward the testicular capsule. A large vein is often identified adjacent to the artery (Figure 23-8). On color Doppler, the transmediastinal artery will have a different color than the centripetal arteries because its flow is directed away from the mediastinum and toward the capsule. On reaching the testicular surface opposite the mediastinum, the transmediastinal artery courses along the capsule as capsular arteries. Spectral Doppler waveforms obtained from the capsular, centripetal, or transmediastinal arteries show a low-resistance waveform pattern in normal individuals (Figure 23-9). Box 23-1 diagrams arterial branching in the testicles.

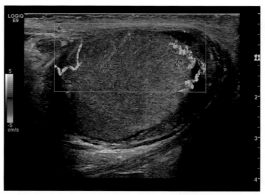

FIGURE 23-7 Color Doppler image of the testis depicting the recurrent rami. A centripetal artery is seen coursing from the testicular capsule. Before reaching the mediastinum, it turns backward in a candy cane pattern, forming the recurrent rami.

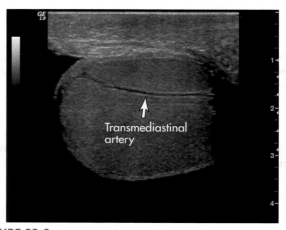

FIGURE 23-8 Transverse ultrasound image shows a normal transmediastinal artery coursing from the mediastinum to the testicular capsule. It appears as an anechoic or hypoechoic tube. Transmediastinal arteries are seen in approximately 50% of testes.

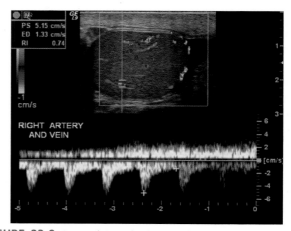

FIGURE 23-9 Spectral Doppler image showing the normal low-resistance waveform pattern of the intratesticular arteries. A low-resistance waveform demonstrates forward flow during both systole and diastole. In this image, the Doppler sample volume includes both a transmediastinal artery and its accompanying vein. The venous and arterial flow signals are on opposite sides of the Doppler baseline, as their flow is in opposite directions.

BOX 23-1   **Testicular Arterial Branching**

Testicular artery
↓
Capsular artery
↓
Centripetal artery
↓
Recurrent rami

The **cremasteric artery** and **deferential artery** accompany the testicular artery within the spermatic cord to supply the extratesticular structures. They also have anastomoses with the testicular artery and may provide some flow to the testis. The cremasteric artery branches from the inferior epigastric artery (a branch of the external iliac artery). It provides flow to the **cremasteric muscle** and peritesticular tissue. The deferential artery arises from the vesicle artery (a branch of the internal iliac artery). It mainly supplies the epididymis and vas deferens. The scrotal wall is also supplied by branches of the **pudendal artery.**

Venous drainage of the scrotum occurs through the veins of the **pampiniform plexus.** The pampiniform plexus exits from the mediastinum testis and courses in the spermatic cord. It converges into three sets of anastomotic veins: testicular, deferential, and cremasteric. The right **testicular vein** drains into the inferior vena cava, and the left testicular vein joins the left renal vein. The deferential vein drains into the pelvic veins, and the cremasteric vein drains into tributaries of the epigastric and deep pudendal veins.

Patient Positioning and Scanning Protocol

Scrotal Protocol. High-resolution ultrasound imaging is the primary screening modality for most testicular pathology. Applications include inflammatory processes of the testes and epididymis, tumors, trauma, torsion, hydrocele, varicocele, hernias, spermatoceles, and undescended testes.

1. Patient preparation: none.
2. Transducer selection: 8- to 12-MHz linear array.
3. Patient position: supine (Valsalva maneuver or upright position to check for varicocele).
4. Images and observations should include the following:
   - Gray scale.
   - Long testicle (include medial, mid, and lateral).
   - Long epididymis.
   - Anteroposterior (AP) and long measurements of above anatomy.
   - Transverse scan of each testis (upper, mid, lower).
   - Transverse scan of head of epididymis.
   - Include AP and transverse measurements of the middle pole of the testicles.
   - If possible, a split-screen image should be obtained to compare the echogenicity of each testis.
   - Images of the extratesticular area should be obtained to determine the presence of hydrocele, hernia, or other conditions.

Doppler flow analysis of the scrotal area:
- When indicated, color and pulsed Doppler analysis of intratesticular flow with resistance measurements should be obtained.
- The scanning instrument should be optimized for slow flow detection (e.g., decrease pulse repetition frequency/scale, lower filters, increase gain or power).

Ultrasound examination of the scrotum is performed with the patient in the supine position. The penis is positioned on the abdomen and covered with a towel. The patient is asked to place his legs close together to provide support for the scrotum. Alternatively, a rolled towel placed between the thighs can support the scrotum. It is often unnecessary to place a towel for support if the legs are positioned close together. This may be more comfortable for the patient in pain.

A generous amount of warmed gel is applied to the scrotum to ensure adequate probe contact and eliminate air between the probe and the skin surface. Rarely, a stand-off pad may be necessary to improve imaging of very superficial structures such as a tunica albuginea cyst. However, with the use of high-frequency probes (10 to 14 MHz), this is usually not necessary. Instead of a stand-off pad, an extra-thick mound of gel may be adequate to improve near-field imaging.

Before beginning the scrotal ultrasound, it is necessary to determine clinical findings. Was this patient referred because of a palpable mass, scrotal pain, swollen scrotum, or other reason? It is important to ask the patient to describe his symptoms, including history, location, and duration of pain. Can he feel a mass? If so, ask the patient to find the lump. Then place the probe exactly over this location to examine the site. Did the patient experience trauma? When did the trauma occur? Ask him to describe what happened. Has he had a vasectomy? When? Not only is this information helpful in guiding the examination, but it is important to the interpreting physician and gives confidence to the patient regarding the quality of the ultrasound study. Box 23-2 lists important tips when performing an ultrasound examination of the scrotum.

Scrotal ultrasound is always a bilateral examination, with the asymptomatic side used as a comparison for the symptomatic side. To begin, it is best to perform a brief survey scan to determine what abnormalities, if any, are present. Each testis is scanned from superior to inferior and is carefully examined to determine whether abnormal findings are present. The size, echogenicity, and structure of each testis are evaluated. The testicular parenchyma should be uniform with

BOX 23-2   **Sonographer Tips**

- Explain procedure and preparation to patient, and then allow the patient to get ready in private.
- Be sure to take an image of right and left testicles together for comparison in both gray-scale and color Doppler.
- Perform Valsalva maneuver when a varicocele is suspected.
- Sensitize color Doppler for slow flow when evaluating torsion.
- Torsion is a surgical emergency; perform the examination in a timely manner.

equal echogenicity between sides. Think of these questions as you scan: Is the parenchyma homogeneous or heterogeneous? Is there a mass? If so, is it cystic or solid? Is it intratesticular or extratesticular? Is one testis much larger than the other? Which side is swollen, or is one side shrunken? All testes should appear similar in size and shape. Is the epididymis normal? Is the skin thickened? Turn on color Doppler to assess the flow. Is there an absence of flow in the testis, or is it hyperemic? How does the color Doppler compare between sides? Testes should show about the same amount of flow when the same color Doppler setup is used. Check the flow in each epididymis. Again, compare between sides. They should be similar. After the survey scan, images are obtained that demonstrate the findings.

Representative images are obtained in at least two planes—transverse and sagittal—with additional imaging planes scanned as needed to demonstrate the findings. In transverse, images are taken that show the superior, mid, and inferior portions of each testis. The width of the testis is measured in the midtransverse view. A transverse view of the head of the epididymis is included. Superior to the epididymal head, an image is obtained to demonstrate the area of the spermatic cord. In the sagittal plane, images are taken to show the medial, mid, and lateral portions. A long axis measurement of testicular length is obtained in the midsagittal image. Again, additional images may be taken to demonstrate abnormal areas. An image is obtained of the epididymal head superior to the **testicle**. The body and tail of the epididymis can be demonstrated coursing posteriorly on each side. Scrotal skin thickness is evaluated and compared from side to side. At least one image is taken to show both testes at the same time, so the interpreting physician can compare size and echogenicity (Figure 23-10). Additional views may be taken in patients with suspected varicocele. These include upright positioning and the Valsalva maneuver. Color and spectral Doppler are used in all examinations, with representative images taken to demonstrate both arterial and venous flow in each testis. Table 23-1 lists the scanning protocols for scrotal ultrasound.

TABLE 23-1	Ultrasound Scrotal Scan Protocol
Transverse Image	**Sagittal Image**
Spermatic cord area	Spermatic cord area
Epididymal head	Epididymal head with superior testis
Superior testis	Long axis midtestis with measurement
Mid testis with measurement	Medial long axis
Inferior testis	Lateral long axis
Transverse view showing both testes	Color Doppler of epididymal head
	Color Doppler of mid testis
	Spectral Doppler of artery
	Spectral Doppler of vein

Note: In patients with suspected varicocele, additional views include upright view of spermatic cord with and without Valsalva maneuver.

TECHNICAL CONSIDERATIONS

High-frequency linear-array transducers are preferred for scrotal imaging because they provide the best spatial resolution. However, the field of view is limited with linear arrays. Occasionally, a larger field of view is required to measure anatomy or display anatomic relationships. Ultrasound systems provide numerous methods to meet this need, including virtual convex imaging, panoramic imaging, stitching images together, and using a curved-array transducer.

Real-time imaging of the scrotum is performed with a high-frequency linear-array probe of at least 7.5 MHz. Because high-frequency transducers have better spatial and contrast resolution compared with lower-frequency transducers, they are preferred for scrotal imaging. Probes with frequencies of 10 to 15 MHz are usually best. Because there is a tradeoff between frequency and penetration, the highest frequency providing adequate penetration should be used. In patients with considerable wall edema and thickening, frequencies as low as 5 to 7.5 MHz may be necessary to adequately penetrate the testis.

Many ultrasound systems have a trapezoid or virtual convex feature that can be selected with the linear-array probe. This is very helpful for measuring the long axis of the testis, or when an abnormal area cannot be entirely imaged with the standard linear format (Figure 23-11, *A*). It is best to use this feature selectively instead of routinely, because steering the beam to create the wider format has a negative impact on image quality; steering widens the distance between scan lines and degrades lateral resolution.

In cases of large hydroceles, hematomas, or swelling, an even larger field of view may be required. In these cases, a panoramic tool may be useful. This tool allows the image to build as the probe is moved over the skin surface. A very long image can be obtained that shows anatomic relationships (Figure 23-11, *B*). Images may also be stitched together in a combined mode. The first image is obtained in one window; then the probe is moved, and another image is obtained by attempting to match the boundaries of the

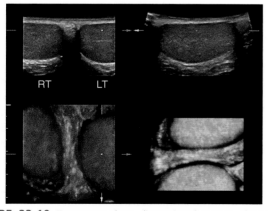

FIGURE 23-10 Transverse three-dimensional sweep obtained at the midline in a normal patient demonstrating both testes. The size, echogenicity, and texture are similar between sides. It is advisable to obtain an image like this in all cases to allow comparison between the testes.

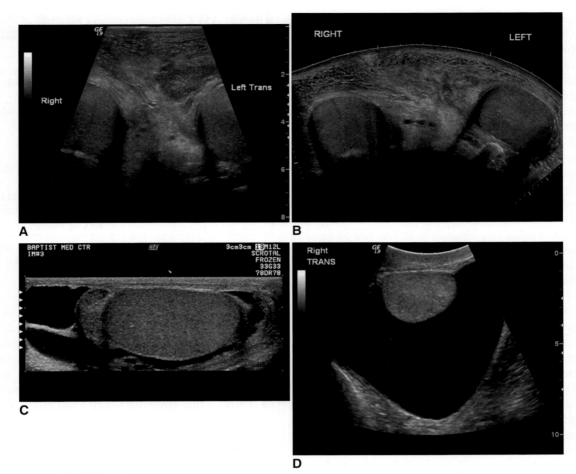

FIGURE 23-11 A, Transverse ultrasound scan of a scrotal hematoma using a virtual convex to create a sector or trapezoidal format using a linear-array probe. The field of view is enlarged to allow better depiction of the size and location of the hematoma compared with the testes. This feature is useful for measuring testicular length and showing abnormal areas that are too large to view with the standard linear format. However, because the scan lines are steered to create this image, lateral resolution is decreased compared with the standard format. **B,** Transverse ultrasound view of the same scrotal hematoma using a panoramic setting. This feature allows the image to build as the transducer is moved across the anatomy. It is very useful for showing large masses and anatomic relationships. **C,** Sagittal ultrasound image in a patient with epididymitis and hydrocele. The image was obtained by stitching together two images in a combined mode. This is another useful tool when a larger field of view is necessary to demonstrate anatomy. **D,** Sagittal ultrasound image of the testis surrounded posteriorly by a large hydrocele. The linear-array format could not display the entire hydrocele, so a 7-MHz curved-array transducer was used to better demonstrate a pathologic condition.

first image (Figure 23-11, *C*). Another way to obtain a larger field of view is to use a 5- to 7.5-MHz curved-array transducer for a portion of the examination to demonstrate the entire scrotal contents. Again, this should be done selectively to obtain the necessary images and should be followed by a return to the high-frequency linear-array probe for further evaluation of each testis (Figure 23-11, *D*).

Most modern ultrasound scanners offer additional features that enhance the quality of the ultrasound image. These features include, but are not limited to, compound imaging, harmonics, extended field-of-view imaging, virtual convex, speckle reduction algorithms, and use of multiple focal zones (Table 23-2). All of these controls may be adjusted to improve image quality.

Color and spectral Doppler play an important role in scrotal ultrasound. The typical color/spectral Doppler frequencies used for scrotal ultrasound are between 4 and 8 MHz. The upper frequency range is used to improve sensitivity to slow flow. This is important in evaluation of testicular torsion or tumor vascularity. Penetration is decreased with higher frequencies, so it is important to make sure that the color penetrates to the depth of interest. Color and spectral Doppler findings on the symptomatic side are always compared with the asymptomatic side.

Power Doppler is often used as a way to quickly get to a sensitive setting that will demonstrate slow flow. Power Doppler shows the amplitude or power of the moving signal, whereas color Doppler shows the frequency shift. Power Doppler does

TABLE 23-2	Scanning Features		
Feature	**What Is It?**	**Advantage**	**Disadvantage**
Harmonics	Selective reception of penetration (uses frequencies generated within tissue)	Improved contrast resolution Improved visibility of low-level echoes Reduction of artifacts	Less harmonic penetration (uses higher frequency)
Compound imaging	Uses multiple-angled firings to create one image	Improved border definition Reduced speckle Less angle dependence	Slowed frame rate Loss of some beneficial artifacts (i.e., shadowing, refraction, and enhancement)
Speckle reduction algorithms	Sophisticated algorithms applied to the image to reduce speckle (salt and pepper appearance of ultrasound image)	Improved contrast resolution Improved conspicuity of masses	None
Extended field of view imaging	Image builds up as probe is moved across anatomy	Improved ability to show anatomic relationships of structures too large to fit in linear-array format	May be difficult to perform on uncooperative patient or over sharply curving interface
Trapezoid or virtual convex imaging	Steering of linear-array probe to create sector format	Larger field of view with linear-array probes	Reduced lateral resolution
Multizone focus	Use of multiple focal zones to create an extended area of focus on one image	Improved lateral resolution	Slowed frame rate

not demonstrate flow direction or aliasing, and to some offers a more straightforward display of blood flow. Presets for power Doppler are often set at a lower pulse repetition frequency (PRF) than color Doppler because aliasing is not an issue, so pushing the power Doppler button may show more flow with fewer adjustments to the controls. This often provides a quick way to get to a more sensitive flow setting. Persistence is usually much greater with power Doppler, requiring a steady hand and slower movement of the probe. To further enhance power Doppler, the same parameters are adjusted as for color Doppler.

Familiarity with color Doppler controls is very important when performing scrotal ultrasound. The sonographer may need to adjust some of the following color Doppler parameters throughout the study to enhance the visibility of scrotal perfusion (Table 23-3):

- *Gain*—The color gain control is used to amplify the reflected color Doppler signal. Whenever the expected amount of color is not visible in the image, the color gain should be increased until noise is present. Once color noise is visible, the gain can be decreased until it just disappears. At this point, the color gain setting is optimized.
- *Scale/pulse repetition frequency (PRF)*—The PRF is the number of pulses transmitted in 1 second. This important color parameter affects the sensitivity of the system in

TABLE 23-3	Color/Power Doppler Parameters	
Parameter	**What Is It?**	**How to Adjust**
Gain	Amplification of selected frequency shift signal	Turn up until noise is present and then decrease until noise goes away
Pulse repetition frequency (PRF)	PRF is the number of pulses transmitted per second; sets the Nyquist limit; main control affecting sensitivity to flow	Adjust on the asymptomatic side so that flow is visible without too much flash or motion artifact; decrease to improve sensitivity to slow flow; increase to reduce aliasing
Wall filter	Color signals received below the wall filter setting do not appear on the image	Decrease to improve sensitivity and to reduce flash/motion artifact
Line density	Density of scan lines contained within the color box	Turn up to improve lateral resolution of vessels; turn down to increase frame rate
Threshold	Level of gray-scale brightness that is allowable to be overwritten by color when both gray-scale and color information are obtained for the same pixel location within the image	Turn up so that color information is prioritized compared with gray-scale information; if the threshold (also known as color/write priority) is set too low, small intratesticular vessels will not be filled with color
Packet size	Number of pulses on each color scan line sensitivity	Turn up to improve signal-to-noise ratio and turn down to improve frame rate
Color box size	Region of interest that is color encoded within the image	Set just over the area of interest; increasing color box size or depth will slow frame rate

displaying slow flow. It also sets the point at which color aliasing occurs (Nyquist limit). The control has different names depending on the ultrasound equipment being used. It is variably named scale, PRF, or flow rate. The PRF is reduced to improve sensitivity to slow flow. This is critical when ruling out testicular torsion. If the PRF is set too high, slow flow may not be visible. When the PRF is set too low, excessive color aliasing occurs, which makes it impossible to determine flow direction or to assess flow quality. Neither of these factors is significant in scrotal ultrasound, so it is common to use low PRF settings. However, flash artifact from patient motion is more apparent with very low PRFs and may make scanning difficult. It is recommended to adjust the PRF so that the asymptomatic testicular flow is well demonstrated without excessive flash artifact. Then compare the same settings on the contralateral side (Figure 23-12).

- *Wall filter*—The wall filter acts as an electronic eraser. Color echoes that fall below the filter cutoff do not appear on the image display. The wall filter is adjusted downward to enhance flow sensitivity. It is turned up to reduce flash artifact. On most ultrasound systems, the wall filter is automatically adjusted with the PRF. But in some instances, it may be beneficial to make further adjustments.
- *Line density*—The line density is the number or density of scan lines contained within the color box. It affects the lateral resolution of the color display. As line density is increased, lateral resolution is improved. The size of the intratesticular arteries is displayed more accurately when line density is high. Frame rate becomes slower as line density is increased, because more transmitted pulses are required to create each image frame. If the frame rate becomes too slow, the line density can be decreased. The user must choose the tradeoff between resolution and frame rate (Figure 23-13).

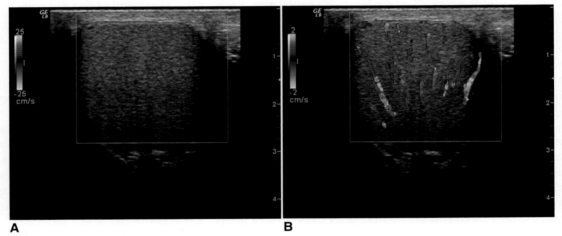

FIGURE 23-12 A, Transverse color Doppler image of a normal testis. Almost no color signal is apparent in the testis because of the high pulse repetition frequency (PRF) setting. The velocity scale values adjacent to the color bar show a velocity sensitivity of 25 cm/sec. **B,** Image of the same testis, using a much lower PRF setting. The velocity scale shows a flow sensitivity of 2 cm/sec. Many intratesticular vessels can now be seen with color Doppler.

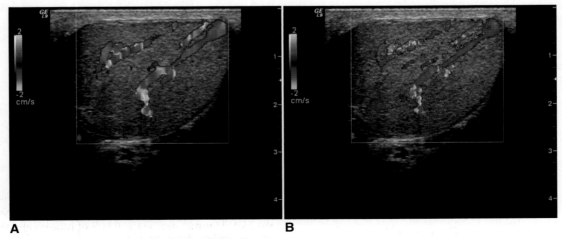

FIGURE 23-13 A, This image was obtained at a low line density setting. The vessels appear wider than expected (poor lateral resolution). **B,** When the line density is increased, the vessel size is more accurately displayed. Frame rate is slower because more scan lines are present within the same-sized color box.

- *Threshold or Color/Tissue Priority*—The B/color threshold is used to determine whether a gray scale or a color pixel is displayed in any given location on the image. Color and power Doppler images are color overlays on top of an existing gray-scale image. A problem arises when gray-scale and color information is received for the same pixel location. The threshold control allows the user to prioritize either gray scale or color. For ultrasound of most small parts, including scrotal imaging, it is best to set the threshold so that color is prioritized. Based on the setting, when color and gray-scale information is received for an identical pixel location, the one displayed is determined by the brightness (amplitude) of the gray-scale dot and the frequency shift and/or power level of the color signal. This feature is not as important when looking at large vessels, such as the common carotid artery, because the vessel lumen typically does not contain gray-scale information, and color can be freely displayed in those pixels. However, in small parts imaging, most vessels are so small that the lumen is not visible or may contain gray-scale echoes caused by volume averaging. In these instances, color will not be displayed unless the threshold control is set to a level that prioritizes color.
- *Packet size*—The packet size is the number of sound pulses transmitted on each scan line within the color box. The packet size is usually set between 8 and 20 pulses for each scan line. The packet size affects the signal-to-noise ratio, improving color sensitivity when more pulses are used. The frame rate gets slower as the number of packets (pulses) is increased on each scan line. The packet size can be reduced to raise the frame rate when necessary, or increased to improve color sensitivity. The key factor affecting color sensitivity, however, is the PRF.
- *Color box/region of interest*—The color box or region of interest is the area within the gray-scale image where flow is color encoded. The width of the color box affects the frame rate. If the color box is very wide, more scan lines are required to complete each image frame. This means that a greater number of pulses must be transmitted. This takes more time, so the frame rate is reduced. Color box depth also affects frame rate. When the color box is placed deep in the image, the round-trip time for the sound is increased. This slows down the frame rate.

An understanding of the factors affecting color frame rate, sensitivity, and resolution allows the sonographer to optimize the color parameters for each clinical situation. Most systems have specific presets for each ultrasound application. Selection of the scrotal preset will set the color parameters near an optimal setting for a typical normal examination. However, the user must further adjust the controls to enhance the visibility of scrotal perfusion in abnormal states.

SCROTAL PATHOLOGY

Table 23-4 lists the pathology and sonographic appearance associated with scrotal trauma, infection, and fluid collection. Although the sonographer is not responsible for the interpretation of ultrasound images, an understanding of the various

TABLE 23-4	Scrotal Infection, Trauma, and Fluid Collections
Pathology	**Sonographic Appearance**
Infection	
Epididymitis	Enlarged epididymis
	Heterogeneous texture
	Hypoechoic, may contain hyperechoic areas
	Blood flow in the epididymis
Focal orchitis	Hypoechoic area within testis
	Blood flow in the testis
Diffuse orchitis	Enlarged, hypoechoic testis
	Echogenicity of the whole testis
Trauma	
Rupture	Irregular contour
	Focal alteration in echogenicity
Hematoma	Heterogeneous area
	Becomes hyperechoic as the blood clot ages
	Avascular
Torsion	Gray-scale image of testis normal when duration <4 hours
	Testis enlarged and hypoechoic 4–12 hours
	Testis heterogeneous after 24 hours
	Absence of testicular flow
Fluid Collections	
Hydrocele	May be anechoic, but often contains low-level echoes
	Surrounds anterolateral aspect of testis
Spermatocele	Located in head of epididymis
	May contain internal echoes and/or septations
	Smooth walls
	Posterior acoustic enhancement
Epididymal cyst	May be located anywhere in epididymis
	Usually small, anechoic
	Ultrasound cannot differentiate between spermatocele and epididymal cyst
	Posterior acoustic enhancement
Varicocele	Tortuous, dilated veins
	Increased size with Valsalva maneuver or patient standing
	Dilated veins fill with color on Valsalva maneuver
	Spectral Doppler confirms venous flow
Hematocele	Contains low-level echoes
	May contain septations and loculations

differential considerations is useful to fully evaluate the lesion. Table 23-5 lists many of the common and uncommon masses or fluid collections found within or surrounding the testes.

Acute Scrotum

Scrotal Trauma. Scrotal trauma presents a challenge to the sonographer because the scrotum is often painful and swollen. Trauma may be the result of motor vehicle accident, athletic injury, direct blow to the scrotum, or straddle injury. The most important goal of the ultrasound examination in testicular trauma is to determine whether a rupture has

TABLE 23-5	Differential Considerations: Extratesticular Fluid Collections or Masses
Scrotal Masses	
Common:	Hydrocele
	Varicocele
	Ascites
	Hematocele
	Spermatocele
	Epididymitis
Uncommon:	Cysts
	Pyoceles
	Herniated bowel
	Metastasis
	Polyorchidism
	Extratesticular
	Seminoma
Extratesticular Cystic Mass	
Common:	Hematocele
	Spermatocele
Uncommon:	Pyocele
	Epididymal cyst
	Herniated bowel
Hypoechoic Lesion	
Common:	Seminoma
	Embryonal cell carcinoma
	Choriocarcinoma
	Mixed cell tumor
	Lymphoma
	Leukemia
Uncommon:	Teratoma
	Torsion
	Metastasis
	Epididymal tumor
	Abscess
Enlarged Testicle	
Common:	Tumor
	Edematous testis caused by trauma
	Torsion
Uncommon:	Myeloma of testicle
	Idiopathic macro-orchidism
Enlarged Epididymis	
Common:	Epididymitis
	Sperm granuloma
Uncommon:	Polyorchidism
	Lipoma
Hypoechoic Band in Testis	
Common:	Normal mediastinum testis
	Normal vessels

occurred. Rupture of the testis is a surgical emergency that requires prompt diagnosis. If surgery is performed within 72 hours following injury, up to 90% of testes can be saved, but only 45% can be saved after 72 hours. Hydrocele and hematocele are both complications of trauma. However, neither is specific to trauma. Hematoceles contain blood and are also found in advanced cases of epididymitis or orchitis.

Sonographic Findings. The sonographic findings associated with scrotal rupture include focal alteration of the testicular parenchymal pattern, interruption of the tunica albuginea, irregular testicular contour, scrotal wall thickening, and **hematocele.** These findings may also be associated with abscess, tumor, or other clinical conditions. When combined with a history of trauma, they suggest rupture.

The sonographic appearance of hematoceles varies with age. An acute hematocele is echogenic with numerous, highly visible echoes that can be seen to float or move in real-time. Over time, hematoceles show low-level echoes and develop fluid-fluid levels or septations. The presence of a hematocele does not confirm rupture. Hematoceles result from bleeding of the pampiniform plexus or other extratesticular structures.

Hematomas associated with trauma may be large and may cause displacement of the associated testis. Hematomas appear as heterogeneous areas within the scrotum. They tend to become more complex over time, developing cystic components. Hematomas may involve the testis or epididymis, or they can be contained within the scrotal wall. Because hematomas are avascular, color Doppler is helpful in identifying them as areas with no flow (Figure 23-14).

Other uses of color Doppler in testicular trauma include identification of blood flow disruption across the surface of the testis. This is an indication of rupture. Color Doppler can aid in separating a normally vascularized testis from one that is disrupted by hematoma. Epididymitis may result from trauma, and color Doppler imaging can be used to identify the associated increased vascularity in the **epididymis.** Torsion may also be associated with trauma. Color Doppler is used to confirm absence of flow in the testis with torsion.

Epididymo-orchitis. Epididymo-orchitis is infection of the epididymis and testis. It most commonly results from the spread of a lower urinary tract infection via the spermatic cord. Less common causes include mumps, syphilis, tuberculosis, viruses, trauma, and chemical causes. Epididymo-orchitis

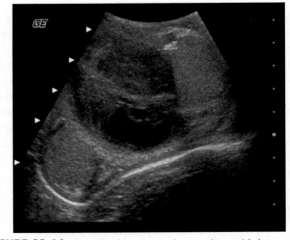

FIGURE 23-14 Complex hematoma in a patient with hemophilia following scrotal trauma. Transverse ultrasound scan of both testes shows a large heterogeneous mass adjacent to the left testis. Color Doppler (*not shown*) demonstrated the mass to be avascular.

represents the most common cause of acute scrotal pain in adults. The epididymis is the organ primarily involved with infection, which spreads to the testis in about 20% to 40% of cases. Orchitis almost always occurs secondary to epididymitis. Patients typically have increasing scrotal pain over 1 or 2 days. The pain may be mild or severe. Symptoms may also include fever and urethral discharge.

Sonographic Findings. **Epididymitis** appears as an enlarged, hypoechoic gland. If secondary hemorrhage has occurred, the epididymis may contain focal hyperechoic areas. Hyperemic flow is confirmed with color Doppler (Figure 23-15). The normal epididymis shows little flow with color Doppler. The amount of color flow signal should be compared between sides. The affected side shows significantly more flow than the asymptomatic epididymis. It is important to use the same color Doppler settings when comparing the amount of flow between sides.

With epididymitis, Doppler waveforms demonstrate increased velocities in both systole and diastole. A low-resistance waveform pattern is present (see Figure 23-15). If the infection is isolated to the epididymis, the testis will appear normal. When orchitis has developed, ultrasound imaging will show an enlarged testis. The infection may be focal or diffuse, and affected areas may appear hypoechoic compared with surrounding tissue. Focal areas of infection within the testis will result in a heterogeneous appearance on ultrasound. A diffusely infected testis will appear enlarged and homogeneous with a hypoechoic echogenicity (Figure 23-16). Up to 20% of cases will have a normal appearing epididymis and testis on ultrasound. Ultrasound gray-scale findings associated with epididymo-orchitis are not specific and may also be seen with torsion or tumor. Color and spectral Doppler are key tools in differentiating between epididymo-orchitis and torsion in the patient with acute scrotal pain.

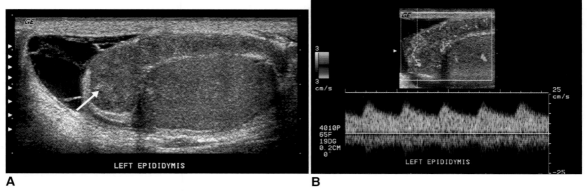

FIGURE 23-15   A, Sagittal ultrasound image in a patient with severe epididymitis shows an enlarged epididymis with a heterogeneous echo texture. Focal hyperechoic areas *(arrow)* within the epididymis may represent hemorrhage. A complex hydrocele with numerous septations is shown near the epididymal head. **B,** Color Doppler shows hyperemic flow within the epididymis. A Doppler waveform obtained from the epididymal head shows increased diastolic flow associated with inflammation.

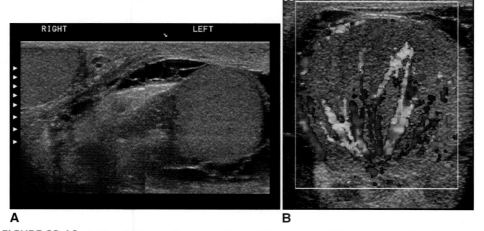

FIGURE 23-16   A, Orchitis in a patient presenting with severe scrotal pain and swelling. Transverse stitched ultrasound scan shows an enlarged left testis and a normal right testis. A complex hydrocele surrounds the left testis. Marked skin thickening is present on the left side compared with the normal right side. **B,** Color Doppler shows hyperemic flow.

Epididymo-orchitis causes hyperemic flow with a significantly greater number of visible vessels on color Doppler compared with the asymptomatic side. Hyperemic flow is seen in the epididymis and testis when both are involved but is isolated to the epididymis when the testis is normal. Documentation of findings on ultrasound must include an image showing both testes, so the size and echogenicity can be compared. It is also recommended to obtain an image with the color box opened wide enough to show portions of both testes, so that the amount of flow between sides can be easily compared.

Other findings associated with epididymitis and epididymo-orchitis include scrotal wall thickening and **hydrocele.** Hydroceles are found around the anterolateral aspect of the testis. They may appear anechoic or may contain low-level echoes. Complex hydroceles may be associated with severe epididymitis and orchitis. These have thick septations and contain low-level echoes. In severe cases, a pyocele may be present. A **pyocele** occurs when pus fills the space between the layers of the tunica vaginalis. It usually contains internal septations, loculations, and debris. This same appearance may be noted following trauma or surgery.

In severe cases of orchitis, testicular infarction may occur. The swollen testis is confined within a rigid tunica albuginea. Excessive swelling can cause obstruction to the testicular blood supply. Color Doppler will show decreased or absent flow compared with the contralateral testis. With decreased flow, spectral Doppler waveforms will have high resistance with little or no diastolic flow. A Doppler waveform demonstrating reversed diastolic flow is a serious finding, indicating threatened testicular infarction (Figure 23-17). Infarction can affect the entire testis or may be confined to a focal area. With focal infarction, color will show perfusion only in portions of the testis that have an absence of color signals in the affected areas. Gray-scale imaging will depict a heterogeneous pattern. Areas of infarction tend to appear hypoechoic compared with the surrounding testicular parenchyma. If the entire testis becomes infarcted, findings cannot be differentiated from testicular torsion.

Torsion. Torsion of the spermatic cord occurs as a result of abnormal mobility of the testis within the scrotum. An anomaly termed the *bell clapper deformity* is the most common cause of this condition. Normally, the testis and epididymis are surrounded by the tunica vaginalis, except at the bare area where they are attached to the posterior scrotal wall. The bell clapper anomaly occurs when the tunica vaginalis completely surrounds the testis, epididymis, and distal spermatic cord, allowing them to move and rotate freely within the scrotum. This movement is similar to that of a clapper inside a bell, hence the name. Torsion results when the testis and epididymis twist within the scrotum, cutting off the vascular supply within the spermatic cord. Up to 60% of patients with torsion will have an anatomic anomaly on both sides. Undescended testes are 10 times more likely to be affected by torsion than

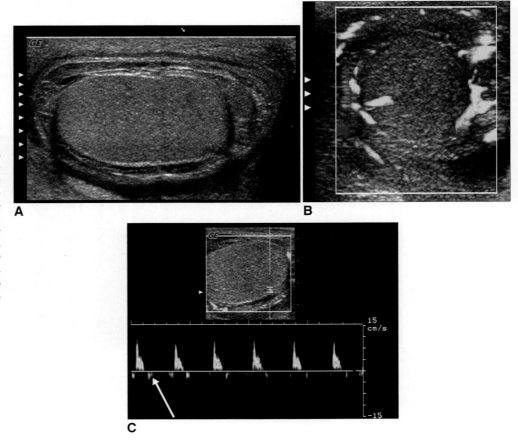

FIGURE 23-17 A, Severe epididymo-orchitis in patient with scrotal pain, swelling, and edema. The testis is swollen against a rigid tunica albuginea. Scrotal skin thickening is evident. **B,** Power Doppler shows hyperemic perfusion surrounding the testis but little intratesticular flow, despite the use of sensitive Doppler settings. **C,** Spectral Doppler waveform of an intratesticular artery demonstrates a high-resistance waveform. Reversed flow is seen in diastole *(arrow).* This is a serious finding, indicating threatened infarction.

normal testes. Torsion compromises blood flow to the testis, the epididymis, and the intrascrotal portion of the spermatic cord. Venous flow is affected first, with occluded veins causing swelling of the scrotal structures on the affected side. If torsion continues, the arterial flow is obstructed, and testicular ischemia follows.

Torsion of the spermatic cord is a surgical emergency. It is important to obtain diagnostic images as quickly as possible because the salvage rate of the testis depends on the elapsed time since torsion. If surgery is performed within 5 to 6 hours of the onset of pain, 80% to 100% of testes can be salvaged. Between 6 and 12 hours, the salvage rate is 70%, but after 12 hours, only 20% will be saved. The degree of torsion (or number of twists) also affects testicular salvage.

Torsion is the most common cause of acute scrotal pain in adolescents. Although it is more common in young adults and adolescents, torsion can occur at any age, with peak incidence at age 14. Patients with torsion most often present with sudden onset of scrotal pain accompanied by swelling on the affected side. The severe pain causes nausea and vomiting in many patients. Patients with torsion frequently report previous episodes of scrotal pain. The clinical differentiation between torsion and epididymo-orchitis is difficult in that patients have similar symptoms. Ultrasound plays a key role in helping to differentiate these entities.

Sonographic Findings. Gray-scale findings on ultrasound depend on how much time has passed since the torsion occurred. In early stages, scrotal contents may have a normal sonographic appearance. After 4 to 6 hours, the testis becomes swollen and hypoechoic (Figure 23-18). The lobes within the testis are usually well identified during this time as a result of interstitial and septal edema. After 24 hours, the testis becomes heterogeneous as a result of hemorrhage, infarction, necrosis, and vascular congestion (Figure 23-19).

The epididymal head appears enlarged and may have decreased echogenicity or may become heterogeneous. In some cases, the twisted spermatic cord knot may be seen as a round or oval extratesticular mass that can be traced back to normal spermatic cord. Other findings may include scrotal skin thickening and reactive hydrocele.

Because ultrasound gray-scale findings are similar to those noted with epididymo-orchitis, Doppler evaluation in testicular torsion is very important. Color Doppler imaging is used to make diagnostic images of torsion. Absence of perfusion in

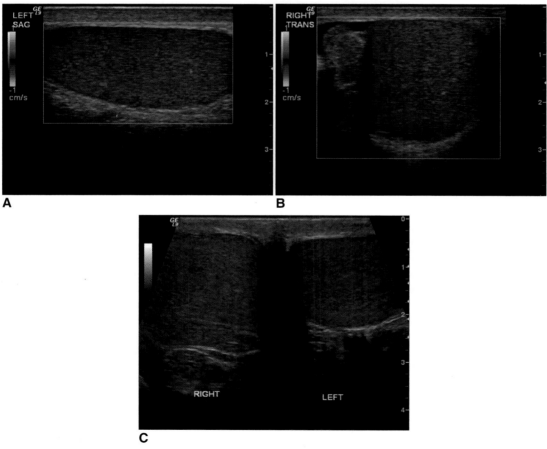

A

B

C

FIGURE 23-18 Testicular torsion in an adolescent patient with sudden onset of right testicular pain, accompanied by nausea and vomiting. **A,** Color Doppler shows normal flow within the parenchyma of the left testis. **B,** The right testis and epididymis are avascular with color Doppler imaging, with the same settings used to show flow on the asymptomatic side. **C,** Transverse ultrasound image showing both testes in right testicular torsion. The right testis is swollen and hyperechoic compared with the normal left testis.

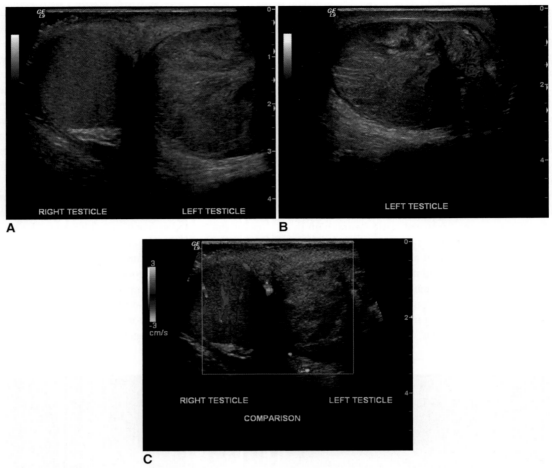

FIGURE 23-19 Left spermatic cord torsion in adolescent with a history of scrotal pain of duration greater than 24 hours. **A,** Transverse ultrasound image showing both testes. The left testis is enlarged and heterogeneous. **B,** Sagittal ultrasound image of the left testis. The infarcted testis has a mixed echo pattern caused by the hemorrhage, necrosis, and vascular congestion associated with spermatic cord torsion exceeding 24 hours. **C,** Transverse color Doppler image showing normal perfusion to the right testis with absence of detectable signal on the left side. Paratesticular blood flow is increased around the abnormal testis.

the symptomatic testis with normal perfusion on the asymptomatic side is considered to be diagnostic of torsion. Color or power Doppler parameters must be adjusted for optimal detection of slow flow. The PRF and wall filter should be set at a low level. Flow around the ischemic testis will appear normal or decreased.

Spontaneous detorsion can produce a very confusing picture both clinically and by ultrasound. Depending on how long the testis was torsed and how long it has been since relief was attained, the intratesticular flow may be minimal or hyperemic. Extratesticular flow is usually increased. This is very difficult to differentiate from epididymo-orchitis.

Torsion of the appendix epididymis and the appendix testis also occurs and further complicates the clinical picture. The clinical presentation is similar to that of testicular torsion and epididymo-orchitis. Ultrasound may show a small, hypoechoic mass located between the head of the epididymis and the superior testis. Color Doppler shows increased flow around the mass. Hemorrhage may cause the mass to appear hyperechoic.

Extratesticular Masses

Epididymal Cysts, Spermatoceles, and Tunica Albuginea Cysts.
Cysts are benign fluid collections that may be located within the testis or in the extratesticular structures. Most scrotal cysts are extratesticular. Extratesticular cysts are found in the tunica albuginea or epididymis. These include spermatoceles, epididymal cysts, and tunica albuginea cysts. **Spermatoceles are cystic dilations of the efferent ductules of the epididymis.** They are always located in the epididymal head. Spermatoceles contain proteinaceous fluid and spermatozoa. They may be seen more often following vasectomy.

Epididymal cysts are small, clear cysts that contain serous fluid (Figure 23-20). They can be found anywhere within the epididymis. Small cysts are sometimes found between the layers of the tunica vaginalis or between the tunica vaginalis and the tunica albuginea. All three entities are generally asymptomatic, although they may be palpable and may cause the patient to be concerned.

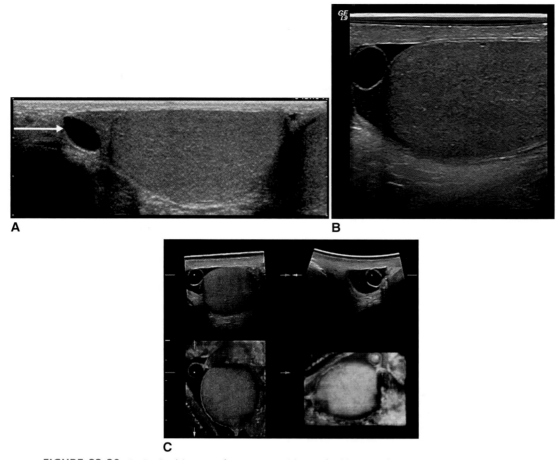

A **B** **C**

FIGURE 23-20 A, Sagittal image of a patient with a palpable scrotal mass. This image was obtained by scanning directly over the palpable area. It shows a fluid-filled mass with posterior acoustic enhancement located in the head of the epididymis *(arrow)*. This finding is consistent with both spermatocele and epididymal cyst. **B,** Conventional two-dimensional sagittal image demonstrated a cystic mass slightly superior and lateral to the right testis. **C,** Three-dimensional volume from the same patient showing orthogonal planes and surface rendering *(lower right)* demonstrated smooth walls and confirmed the extratesticular location of the cyst near the epididymal head. The coronal plane image *(lower left image)* demonstrated a stalk connecting the cyst to the epididymal head, confirming the diagnosis of a pedunculated cystic appendix epididymis.

▶ *Sonographic Findings.* Spermatoceles may be seen as simple cysts or multilocular cystic collections that contain internal echoes. Epididymal cysts appear as simple fluid-filled structures with thin walls and posterior acoustic enhancement. Ultrasound imaging cannot reliably differentiate epididymal cysts from spermatoceles. Tunica albuginea cysts are usually small and appear as anechoic, thin-walled structures on ultrasound. They can become large and cause displacement and distortion of the testis. This helps to differentiate them from hydroceles, which do not distort the testis.

Varicocele

A **varicocele** is an abnormal dilation of the veins of the pampiniform plexus (located within the spermatic cord). Varicoceles are usually caused by incompetent venous valves within the spermatic vein. These are called primary varicoceles. They are more common on the left. This is probably due to the mechanics pertaining to the left spermatic vein and the left renal vein. The spermatic vein empties into the left renal vein at a steep angle, which may inhibit blood flow return. The left renal vein can become compressed between the aorta and the superior mesenteric artery. Secondary varicoceles are caused by increased pressure on the spermatic vein. This may be the result of renal hydronephrosis, an abdominal mass, or liver cirrhosis. An abdominal malignancy invading the left renal vein may cause a varicocele with noncompressible veins. Any noncompressible varicocele in a man older than 40 years of age should prompt a search for a retroperitoneal mass.

Varicoceles have a relationship with impaired fertility. They are more common in infertile men. Treatment of the varicocele has been shown to improve sperm count in up to 53% of cases, but controversy surrounds the treatment of varicoceles for infertility. Uncommonly, varicoceles may extend within the testis. These will be located near the mediastinum. Intratesticular varicoceles have unknown clinical significance, but it is possible that they will affect male fertility by the same mechanism as extratesticular varicoceles.

🔹 *Sonographic Findings.* Ultrasound imaging of a varicocele shows numerous tortuous tubes of varying sizes within the spermatic cord near the epididymal head. The tubes may contain echoes that move with real-time imaging. This represents slow venous flow (Figure 23-21, *A* and *B*). Varicoceles measure more than 2 mm in diameter. They tend to increase diameter in response to the Valsalva maneuver. Scanning with the patient in an upright position will enhance the visibility of a varicocele because the veins will become more distended. Some authors advocate using a standing position routinely; others believe that supine scanning with the Valsalva maneuver and color Doppler imaging is adequate. With either protocol, color and spectral Doppler are used to confirm the presence of venous flow and to demonstrate retrograde filling with the Valsalva maneuver (Figure 23-21, *C*). Color Doppler settings must be sensitized for slow flow to detect the venous signal in varicoceles. Flash artifact may be a problem with color Doppler imaging during a Valsalva maneuver. It is helpful to instruct the patient to hold as still as possible during the maneuver and to carefully adjust the color settings so that the PRF and wall filter are sensitized, but not so low that flash artifact fills the screen with a small movement.

Intratesticular varicocele has the sonographic appearance of straight or serpiginous channels coursing from the mediastinum into the testicular tissue. Color and spectral Doppler are used to identify these channels as dilated veins. On grayscale imaging, the appearance can mimic that of tubular ectasia of the rete testis. Color Doppler will differentiate between intratesticular varicocele and tubular ectasia of the rete testis, as the latter shows no flow (Figure 23-22).

Scrotal Hernia

Hernias occur when bowel, omentum, or other structures herniate into the scrotum. Clinical diagnosis is usually sufficient, but ultrasound imaging is helpful when findings are equivocal. The bowel is the most commonly herniated structure, followed by the omentum.

🔹 *Sonographic Findings.* Peristalsis of the bowel, seen on real-time imaging, confirms the diagnosis of a scrotal hernia (Figure 23-23). This can be captured on videotape or as a cine clip for the interpreting physician to review. Unfortunately, peristalsis may not always be visible. Fluid-filled bowel loops

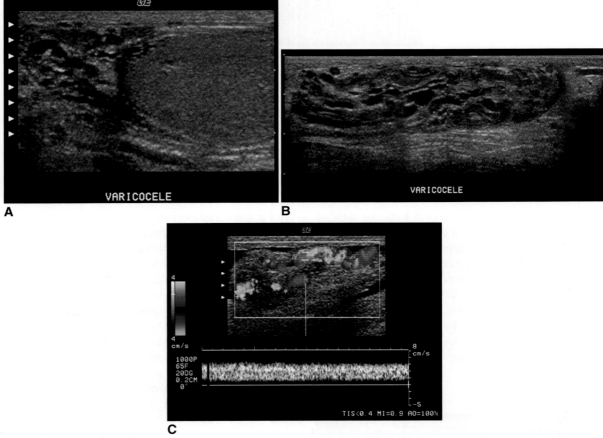

FIGURE 23-21 Varicocele in patient being evaluated for infertility. **A,** Sagittal view of the testis shows dilated tubular structures superiorly. **B,** Stitched ultrasound image shows prominent serpiginous venous channels forming a large varicocele on the left. **C,** Doppler ultrasound with Valsalva maneuver shows venous flow within the dilated vascular channels, confirming the diagnosis of varicocele.

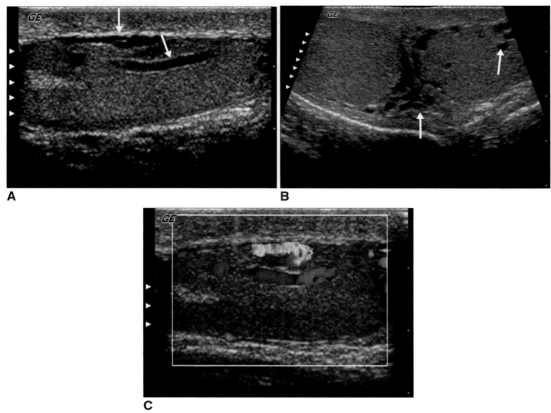

FIGURE 23-22 Intratesticular varicocele. **A,** Sagittal ultrasound image shows prominent connecting tubes with the testis *(arrows)*. **B,** Transverse ultrasound image of both testes shows an intratesticular and extratesticular varicocele on the left side *(arrows)*. **C,** Color Doppler is used to detect flow within the dilated intratesticular veins during Valsalva maneuver.

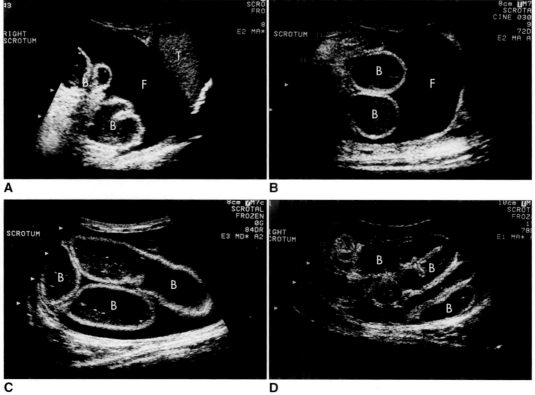

FIGURE 23-23 A–D, Small bowel herniated into the scrotum, representing scrotal hernia. Peristalsis was noted on real-time imaging. *B,* Bowel; *F,* fluid; *T,* testicle.

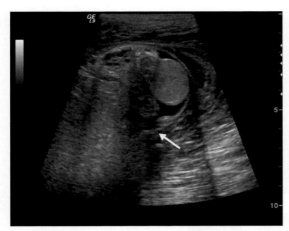

FIGURE 23-24 Scrotal hernia. Sagittal ultrasound image in a patient with chronic heart failure and scrotal edema. A large amount of edema is seen in the tissue surrounding the normal testis. A small hydrocele is present. A large hernia is seen protruding into the scrotum and displacing the testis inferiorly (arrow). The hyperechoic appearance of the hernia suggests omental fat content.

are easily recognizable by ultrasound. Air-filled loops and loops that contain solid stool are more difficult to recognize. On ultrasound, air appears as bright echoes with a dirty acoustic shadow or ring artifact. Omental hernias appear brightly echogenic because of the omental fat (Figure 23-24).

Hydrocele, Pyocele, and Hematocele

A potential space exists between the visceral and parietal layers of the tunica vaginalis. This space is the place where a hydrocele, pyocele, or hematocele will develop. Normally, a small amount of fluid is present in this cavity, and this should not be confused with the presence of a hydrocele. A hydrocele contains serous fluid and is the most common cause of painless scrotal swelling. Hydroceles may have an unknown cause (idiopathic) but are commonly associated with epididymo-orchitis and torsion. They may also be found in patients following trauma or development of a neoplasm. Hydroceles associated with neoplasms tend to be smaller than those associated with other causes. Pyoceles and hematoceles are much less common than hydroceles.

A pyocele is a collection of pus. Pyoceles occur with untreated infection or when an abscess ruptures into the space between the layers of the tunica vaginalis. Hematoceles are associated with trauma, surgery, neoplasms, or torsion. They are collections of blood.

Sonographic Findings. A hydrocele displays a fluid-filled collection located outside the anterolateral aspect of the testis. Hydroceles may be anechoic but most often contain some low-level echoes as a result of cellular debris (Figure 23-25). The display of low-level echoes is enhanced by high-frequency transducers and harmonic imaging. Hydroceles are more likely to appear anechoic with transducer frequencies below 7 MHz, or when low dynamic range settings are used. Hydroceles associated with infection show more internal echoes and septations. Sonographically, pyoceles and hematoceles are

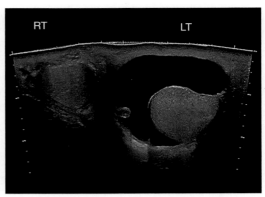

FIGURE 23-25 Idiopathic hydrocele formation in patient with scrotal swelling and tenderness. Panoramic view shows the normal right testis. The left testis is compressed because of the large hydrocele.

indistinguishable. They both contain internal echoes, thickened septations, and loculations (Figures 23-26 and 23-27). Ultrasound depiction of air within the space indicates an abscess, although an abscess may occur without the presence of air.

Sperm Granuloma

Sperm granulomas occur as a chronic inflammatory reaction to extravasation of spermatozoa. They are most frequently seen in patients with a history of vasectomy. A sperm granuloma may be located anywhere within the epididymis or the vas deferens.

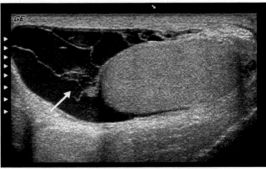

A

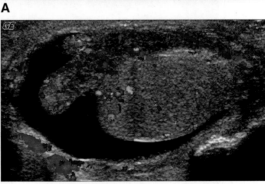

B

FIGURE 23-26 Pyocele formation in patient with severe, untreated epididymo-orchitis. A, Sagittal ultrasound image shows the multiseptated fluid collection containing internal debris (arrow). B, Color Doppler image shows increased perfusion in the epididymis, testis, and surrounding tissue.

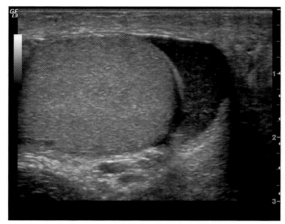

FIGURE 23-27 Hematocele in patient from the emergency department with scrotal trauma. Sagittal ultrasound image shows a small fluid collection with numerous bright echoes.

The main role of ultrasound imaging is to determine whether the mass is intratesticular or extratesticular. Extratesticular masses have a much lower rate of malignancy compared with intratesticular masses. Sperm granulomas cannot be reliably differentiated from epididymal tumors by ultrasound imaging. However, a clinical history of vasectomy will help to target the differential diagnosis. Additionally, sperm granulomas are often painful. This aids in their differentiation from epididymal tumors, which are usually painless.

Sonographic Findings. Sonographic imaging shows a well-defined solid mass that may appear hypoechoic or isoechoic to the epididymis. These masses are often heterogeneous (Figure 23-28). Calcifications are not commonly present. Increased flow may be seen with color Doppler when inflammation is present.

Benign Testicular Masses

Tubular Ectasia of the Rete Testis. The **rete testis** is located at the hilum of the testis where the mediastinum resides. Tubular ectasia of the rete testis is an uncommon, benign condition. It is

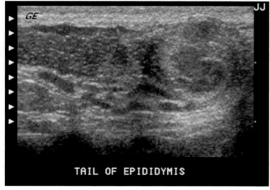

FIGURE 23-28 Painful epididymal mass in patient with history of vasectomy. Sagittal ultrasound image of epididymis shows a small, heterogeneous mass in the tail of the epididymis, possibly representing a sperm granuloma.

associated with the presence of a spermatocele, an epididymal or testicular cyst, or other epididymal obstruction on the same side as the dilated tubules. It is more commonly seen in patients 45 years of age or older.

Sonographic Findings. The normal rete testis may not be clearly depicted with ultrasound imaging. High-resolution imaging sometimes allows visualization of the normal rete testis as very tiny tubular structures near the mediastinum. Tubular ectasia appears as prominent hypoechoic channels near the echogenic mediastinum testis (Figure 23-29). Color Doppler can confirm the avascular nature of the tubules. Tubular ectasia has a similar sonographic appearance to intratesticular varicocele. These conditions can be differentiated using Doppler interrogation because the varicocele will demonstrate slow venous flow. To demonstrate slow flow, the color Doppler must be sensitized by using a low PRF and wall filter setting. The Valsalva maneuver should be used to enhance flow if a varicocele is present. If these and other adjustments are not made to the color controls, flow within a varicocele may not be detected, and results may be misinterpreted.

Cyst. Intratesticular cysts were once thought to be uncommon but are seen more often with more frequent use of ultrasound imaging. Cysts are common in men older than 40 years of age and have an association with extratesticular spermatoceles. They are located near the mediastinum. They may be single or multiple and of variable size. Cysts are incidental findings on sonography and do not require treatment.

Sonographic Findings. The sonographic appearance of cysts is the same throughout the body. Simple cysts are anechoic with posterior acoustic enhancement and a smooth border (Figure 23-30).

Microlithiasis. Microlithiasis is an uncommon condition characterized by tiny calcifications within the testis. These microcalcifications are smaller than 3 mm. Microlithiasis is usually a bilateral condition. It has been reported to have an association with testicular malignancy, but the exact nature of this is unknown. Annual follow-up of patients with testicular microlithiasis is recommended by some to exclude the development of neoplasm. Microlithiasis has also been associated with cryptorchidism, Klinefelter's syndrome, infertility, varicoceles, testicular atrophy, and male pseudohermaphroditism.

Sonographic Findings. The sonographic appearance of testicular microlithiasis is of multiple bright, nonshadowing foci scattered throughout the testis (Figure 23-31). The microliths may be numerous or few but are not considered to be abnormal unless more than five appear on any single image (Figure 23-32).

Malignant Testicular Masses

Table 23-6 lists the sonographic findings for solid malignant masses.

Germ Cell Tumors. Testicular cancer is not common, accounting for only 1% of cancers in men, but it is the most common malignancy in men between 15 and 35 years of age. Fortunately, testicular cancer is one of the most curable forms of cancer. It is more common in white men than black men.

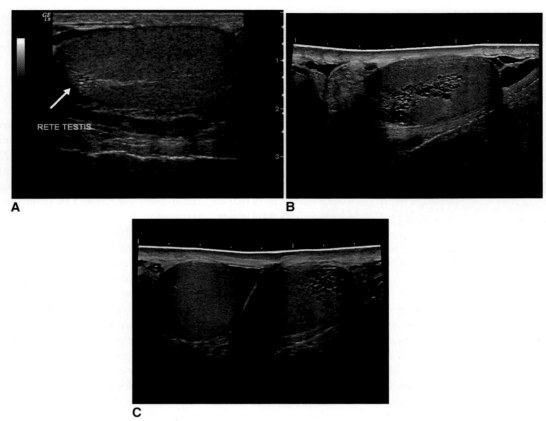

FIGURE 23-29 A, Mild dilation of the rete testis in patient with spermatocele. Sagittal ultrasound image shows enlarged tubular structures located near the mediastinum testis. **B,** Sagittal panoramic view on the same patient demonstrates the dilated tubules of the rete testis in the area of the testicular mediastinum. **C,** Panoramic transverse image through the right and left testis shows dilation of the rete testis on the left in a patient with a large spermatocele (not shown).

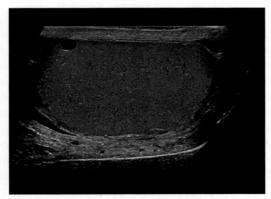

FIGURE 23-30 Simple testicular cyst. Sagittal ultrasound image was obtained using virtual convex to obtain a wide field of view. A small, simple cyst is shown in the superior pole of the testis. Note the smooth borders and the posterior acoustic enhancement.

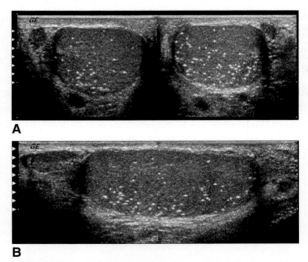

FIGURE 23-31 Testicular microlithiasis. A, Stitched transverse ultrasound image showing both testes with numerous brightly echogenic foci throughout. **B,** Sagittal ultrasound image showing testis with fewer microliths.

Testicular cancer occurs most frequently between ages 20 and 34 years. Undescended testes are 2.5 to 8 times more likely to develop cancer.

Most patients have no other symptoms except a painless lump, testicular enlargement, or vague discomfort in the scrotum. The primary goal of the ultrasound examination in testicular tumors is to determine mass location and differentiate between cystic and solid composition. Extratesticular masses are usually benign, whereas intratesticular masses are more likely to be malignant. Intratesticular cysts are benign masses, but care must be taken to ensure that a cyst is simple because some testicular cancers contain cystic components. Some benign conditions may mimic malignancy. These include hematoma, orchitis

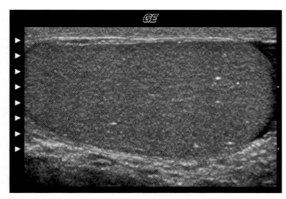

FIGURE 23-32 Sagittal ultrasound image showing testis with fewer microliths. More than five microcalcifications per image is considered abnormal. Note the absence of shadowing.

TABLE 23-6	Solid Malignant Masses
Tumor	**Sonographic Findings**
Seminoma	Hypoechoic lesion
	Smooth, well-defined borders
Embryonal cell carcinoma	Small hypoechoic mass
	Areas of increased echogenicity due to calcification
	Irregular borders
	May contain cystic areas
Teratoma	Complex mass, usually cystic and/or solid
	Well-defined borders
	Acoustic shadowing
Choriocarcinoma	Irregular borders
	Complex lesion
	Metastasis usually seen
Metastasis	Solid hypoechoic lesion (uncommonly may appear as hyperechoic or mixed echogenicity)
Lymphoma and leukemia	Enlarged testis
	Diffuse or focal areas of decreased echogenicity
Chronic lymphocytic leukemia	Well circumscribed
	Anechoic
	Through-transmission

(especially when focal), abscess, infarction, and sperm granuloma. Obtaining a thorough patient history is very important because it will help to differentiate between these conditions.

In general, testicular tumors are divided into germ cell and non–germ cell tumors. Germ cell tumors are associated with elevated levels of human chorionic gonadotropin and alpha-fetoprotein. Approximately 95% of all testicular tumors are of germ cell type and are highly malignant. Non–germ cell tumors are generally benign. The most common type of germ cell tumor is seminoma, followed by mixed embryonal cell tumors and teratocarcinomas. Other less common germ cell tumors include yolk sacs, choriocarcinomas, teratomas, and other combinations of these cell types. The sonographer must remember that although testicular masses can be clearly described and differentiated using ultrasound, the examination cannot confirm the histology of the neoplasm. However, the sonographic features of a mass may suggest a certain type of tumor.

Sonographic Findings. Ultrasound is nearly 100% sensitive for detecting tumors. Sonographically, most tumors appear as focal, hypoechoic masses (see Table 23-6). Seminomas tend to be homogeneous, hypoechoic masses with a smooth border (see Figures 23-27, 23-33, and 23-34). They often do not contain calcification or cystic components. In comparison, embryonal cell carcinoma is heterogeneous and is less well circumscribed. It may contain areas of increased echogenicity resulting from calcification, hemorrhage, or fibrosis (see Figure 23-28). Cystic components are found in up to one third of embryonal cell carcinomas (Figure 23-35). Embryonal cell tumors are more aggressive than seminomas, often invading the tunica albuginea and distorting the testicular contour. Teratomas may show dense foci that produce acoustic shadowing. They are normally heterogeneous but have well-defined borders. Teratomas are usually benign in children but malignant in adults. Choriocarcinoma has a varied sonographic appearance because of mixed cell types. Its appearance is determined by the dominant cell type, but it typically has irregular borders (see Figure 23-29). Ultrasound imaging cannot differentiate malignant from benign masses. Neither color Doppler nor Doppler waveforms can reliably distinguish between flow patterns of benign and malignant tumors.

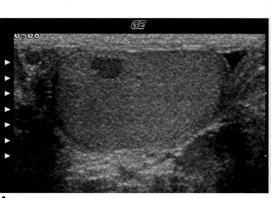

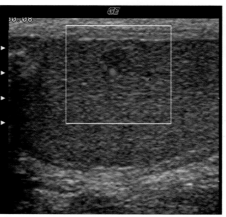

FIGURE 23-33 **Small seminoma. A,** Sagittal ultrasound image shows a small, hypoechoic mass within the testis. Note the presence of a small hydrocele. **B,** Color Doppler shows increased vascularity to the mass.

A   B

FIGURE 23-34 **Germ cell testicular tumor. A,** Transverse ultrasound image shows heterogeneous echo texture throughout the testis. The tumor is primarily hypoechoic. **B,** Color Doppler shows distortion of the normal vessel architecture within the testis. Increased flow is seen within the mass. **C,** Power Doppler clearly shows the distorted vasculature of the testis within the mass. **D,** Spectral Doppler waveforms obtained within the mass show low resistance with prominent end-diastolic velocities characteristic of tumor flow. Doppler waveforms have not been shown to reliably differentiate between benign and malignant flow patterns.

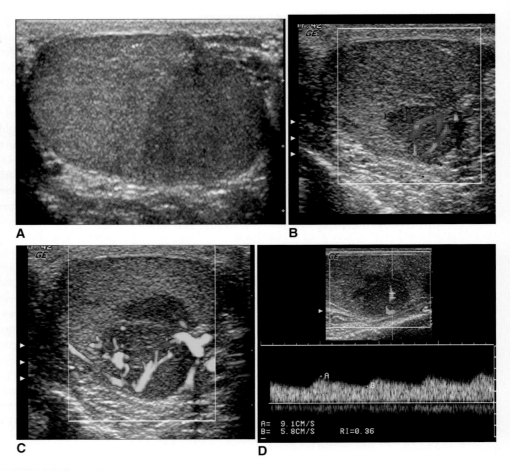

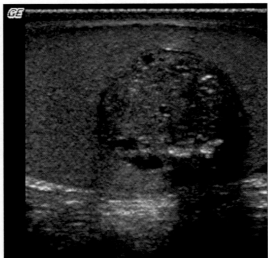

FIGURE 23-35 Heterogeneous testicular tumor. Sagittal ultrasound image of a testicular tumor containing calcium and cystic components. Although this pattern is not specific, it is typical of embryonal cell tumor.

Metastasis. Metastasis to the testicle is rare, normally occurring later in life. The primary tumor may originate from the prostate or kidneys; less common sites include lung, pancreas, bladder, colon, thyroid, and melanoma. Metastasis to the testicle is bilateral, with multiple lesions found.

▨ *Sonographic Findings.* Sonographically, metastasis appears as a solid hypoechoic mass, although it has been reported as hyperechoic or a mixture of both (see Table 23-6).

Lymphoma and Leukemia

Malignant lymphoma makes up 1% to 7% of all testicular tumors and is the most common bilateral secondary testicular neoplasm affecting men older than 60 years.

Leukemic involvement of the testicle is the next most common secondary testicular neoplasm, most often found in children. Of children with leukemia, 8% have been reported to have testicular involvement.

Clinically, patients may experience weight loss, anorexia, and weakness. The testicle may become enlarged, and the tumor may be bilateral or unilateral.

▨ *Sonographic Findings.* Sonographically, lymphoma and leukemia appear similar. The testes may appear homogeneously hypoechoic or may contain multiple focal areas of decreased echogenicity (see Table 23-6). Chronic lymphocytic leukemia may appear as a focal, well-circumscribed, anechoic mass with through-transmission. Increased vascularity is seen with color Doppler imaging.

Congenital Anomalies

Cryptorchidism (Undescended Testicle). During fetal growth, the testes first appear in the retroperitoneum near the

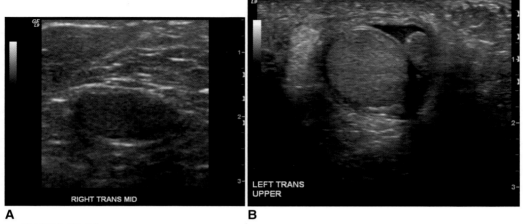

FIGURE 23-36 Undescended right testicle **(A)** with normal left testicle **(B)**. The undescended testis is smaller and hypoechoic compared with the normal left testis. The right testicle was located within the right inguinal canal.

kidneys. They descend into the scrotum from the inguinal canal shortly before birth or early in the neonatal period. The terms *undescended testis* and **cryptorchidism** describe a condition in which the testis has not descended into the scrotum and cannot be brought into the scrotum with external manipulation. The undescended testis may be located in the abdomen, inguinal canal, or other ectopic location. In most cases (up to 80%), the testis is found in the inguinal canal and is usually palpable. Because the testes do not descend until late in pregnancy, this condition is more common in premature babies. Cryptorchidism is bilateral in 10% to 25% of cases.

Surgical treatment of an undescended testicle by freeing it from the structures and implanting it into the scrotum is known as *orchiopexy*. If orchiopexy is not performed at an early age, multiple complications can occur. Exposure of the testis to higher temperatures than that found in the scrotum can prohibit spermatogenesis and result in infertility. Undescended testes are much more likely to develop testicular cancer. The risk of cancer is not reduced by orchiopexy, but it does allow the testis to be more easily palpated, so that a lump may be detected and treated earlier. Testicular torsion is also more common with undescended testes.

 Sonographic Findings. On ultrasound, the undescended testis is smaller and less echogenic than the normal testis. It is usually oval with a homogeneous texture (Figure 23-36). Rarely, the mediastinum is seen.

Testicular Ectopia. Testicular ectopia is a very rare condition. Unlike an undescended testicle, an ectopic testicle cannot be manipulated into the correct path of descent. The most common site for the ectopic testicle to rest is the superficial inguinal pouch. Other sites include the perineum, femoral canal, suprapubic area, penis, diaphragm, and the other scrotal compartment.

Anorchia. Anorchia is rare. Unilateral anorchia, or monorchidism, is found in 4% of patients with a nonpalpable testis. It is more common on the left side, and definitive diagnosis depends on surgical diagnosis. Causes include intrauterine testicular torsion and other forms of decreased vascular supply

to the testicle in utero. Bilateral anorchia is found in only 0.6% to 1.0% of patients with a nonpalpable testis. Patients have a male XY genotype. On physical examination, the scrotum is an empty, hypoplastic sac with a micropenis. These patients also have delayed onset of puberty, usually caused by an imbalance of hormones.

Polyorchidism (Testicular Duplication). Polyorchidism is a very rare disorder, with only 80 cases reported. It is more common on the left side (75%) and is bilateral in 5% of cases. Testicular duplication is usually found in the scrotum, but has also been found in the inguinal canal or retroperitoneum. The incidence of malignancy, cryptorchidism, inguinal hernia, and torsion is increased with polyorchidism. The duplicated testis is usually small, and its efferent spermatic system is completely absent.

Key Pearls

- The testes are symmetric, oval-shaped glands residing in the scrotum.
- Sonographically, the testes appear as smooth, medium-gray structures with a fine echo texture.
- The epididymis is a 6- to 7-cm tubular structure beginning superiorly and then coursing posterolateral to the testis.
- Right and left testicular arteries arise from the abdominal aorta just below the level of the renal arteries.
- Venous drainage of the scrotum occurs through the veins of the pampiniform plexus.
- The sonographic findings associated with scrotal rupture include focal alteration of the testicular parenchymal pattern, interruption of the tunica albuginea, irregular testicular contour, scrotal wall thickening, and hematocele.
- Epididymo-orchitis is infection of the epididymis and testis and most commonly results from the spread of a lower urinary tract infection via the spermatic cord.

Continued

- Torsion of the spermatic cord occurs as a result of abnormal mobility of the testis within the scrotum. An anomaly termed the *bell clapper deformity* is the most common cause of this condition.
- Cysts are benign fluid collections that may be located within the testis or in the extratesticular structures. Most scrotal cysts are extratesticular.
- A varicocele is an abnormal dilation of the veins of the pampiniform plexus (located within the spermatic cord). Varicoceles are usually caused by incompetent venous valves within the spermatic vein.
- Hernias occur when bowel, omentum, or other structures herniate into the scrotum.
- A potential space exists between the visceral and parietal layers of the tunica vaginalis. This space is the place where a hydrocele, pyocele, or hematocele will develop.
- A hydrocele contains serous fluid and is the most common cause of painless scrotal swelling. Hydroceles may have an unknown cause (idiopathic) but are commonly associated with epididymo-orchitis and torsion.
- A pyocele is a collection of pus. Pyoceles occur with untreated infection or when an abscess ruptures into the space between the layers of the tunica vaginalis.
- Sperm granulomas occur as a chronic inflammatory reaction to extravasation of spermatozoa. They are most frequently seen in patients with a history of vasectomy.
- The rete testis is located at the hilum of the testis where the mediastinum resides. Tubular ectasia of the rete testis is an uncommon, benign condition. It is associated with the presence of a spermatocele, an epididymal or testicular cyst, or other epididymal obstruction on the same side as the dilated tubules.
- The sonographic appearance of testicular microlithiasis is of multiple bright, nonshadowing foci scattered throughout the testis.
- Extratesticular masses are usually benign, whereas intratesticular masses are more likely to be malignant.
- In general, testicular tumors are divided into germ cell and non–germ cell tumors.
- Germ cell tumors are associated with elevated levels of human chorionic gonadotropin and alpha-fetoprotein.
- Seminomas tend to be homogeneous, hypoechoic masses with a smooth border.
- Embryonal cell carcinoma is heterogeneous and is less well circumscribed. It may contain areas of increased echogenicity resulting from calcification, hemorrhage, or fibrosis; it may also have cystic components.
- Teratomas may show dense foci that produce acoustic shadowing. They are normally heterogeneous but have well-defined borders.
- Malignant lymphoma makes up 1% to 7% of all testicular tumors and is the most common bilateral secondary testicular neoplasm affecting men older than 60 years.
- The terms *undescended testis* and *cryptorchidism* describe a condition in which the testis has not descended into the scrotum and cannot be brought into the scrotum with external manipulation.
- Surgical treatment of an undescended testicle by freeing it from the structures and implanting it into the scrotum is known as *orchiopexy*.

BIBLIOGRAPHY

American College of Radiology: *ACR standard for performance of scrotal ultrasound examination*, 2001. Available at www.acr.org.
Berman JM, Beidle TR, Kunberger LE, et al: Sonographic evaluation of acute intrascrotal pathology, *Am J Roentgenol* 166:857-861, 1996.
Black JAR, Patel A: Sonography of the abnormal extratesticular space, *Am J Roentgenol* 167:507-511, 1996.
Bree RL, Hoang DT: Scrotal ultrasound, *Radiol Clin North Am* 34:1183, 1996.
Dambro TJ, Stewart RR, Carroll BA: The scrotum. In Rumack CM, Wilson SR, Willi J, editors: *Diagnostic ultrasound*, vol 1, ed 2, St Louis, 1998, Mosby.
Dogra VS, Gottlieb RH, Oka M, et al: Sonography of the scrotum, *Radiology* 227:18-36, 2003.
Feole JB, Lee FT Jr: Doppler sonography in testicular and scrotal imaging, *Curr Opin Urol* 8:87, 1998.
Figler TJ, Olson MC, Kinzler GJ: Polyorchidism and rete testis adenoma: ultrasound and MR findings, *Abdom Imaging* 21:470, 1996.
Horstmann WG, Middleton WD, Melson GL: Scrotal inflammatory disease: color Doppler sonographic findings, *Radiology* 179:55, 1991.
Morse MJ, Whitmore WF: Neoplasm of the testis. In Walsh P, editor: *Campbell's urology*, ed 7, Philadelphia, 1998, Saunders.
Oh C, Nisenbaum HL, Langer J, et al: Sonographic demonstration, including color Doppler imaging of recurrent sperm granulomas, *J Ultrasound Med* 19:333-335, 2000.
Older RA, Watson LR: Tubular ectasia of the rete testis: a benign condition with a sonographic appearance that may be misinterpreted as malignant, *J Urol* 152:477-478, 1994.
Prando D: Torsion of the spermatic cord, *Ultrasound Q* 18:41-57, 2002.
Ragheb D, Higgins JL: Ultrasonography of the scrotum, technique, anatomy, and pathologic entities, *J Ultrasound Med* 21:171-185, 2002.
Weiss AJ, Kellman GM, Middleton WD, et al: Intratesticular varicocele: sonographic findings in two patients, *Am J Roentgenol* 158:1061-1063, 1992.

24

Musculoskeletal System

Susan Raatz Stephenson

OBJECTIVES

On completion of this chapter, you should be able to:

- Identify the normal anatomic location and function of the tendon, ligament, muscle, nerve, and bursa
- Know the advantages and disadvantages of sonographic artifacts in musculoskeletal imaging
- Summarize the basic sonographic examinations of the shoulder, wrist, knee, ankle, and foot
- Distinguish normal anatomy from common pathologic conditions

OUTLINE

KEY TERMS

Acromioclavicular (AC) joint
Anisotropy
Aponeuroses
Bursa
Cartilage interface sign
Clapper-in-the-bell sign
Comet-tail artifact
Dorsiflexion
Epineurium
Fasciculi

Guyon's canal
Ligament
Muscle
Myelin
Naked tuberosity sign
Nerves
Pennate
Perineurium
Phalen's sign
Plantar flexion

Refractile shadowing (edge artifact)
Seroma
Synovial sheath
Tendinitis
Tendon
Thompson's test
Tinel's sign
Volar

In the early 1990s, a radiologist asked me to try to image a torn suprapatellar tendon. It was difficult to image the torn tendon because of technologic limitations and our inexperience in musculoskeletal ultrasound imaging. Musculoskeletal imaging is now gaining in popularity in the United States, following in the wake of magnetic resonance imaging (MRI). However, ultrasound of the musculoskeletal system has been widely used outside of the United States.

Many things have changed since then, both in the delivery of medical care and in the production of sonographic images. The decrease in medical reimbursements has forced the development of less expensive modalities to complement or replace computed tomography (CT) or MRI. Ultrasound

equipment manufacturers have also continued to improve and refine technology, and this has resulted in improved soft tissue imaging. The 5- or 7-MHz transducer commonly used in the 1990s is hardly acceptable for scanning superficial structures today. Current transducers create images with frequencies as high as 17 MHz.

This chapter is intended to provide a solid foundation for basic musculoskeletal ultrasound. Imaging of the muscular system is not limited to the muscles themselves, but also includes the tendons, nerves, ligaments, and bursa. Other areas of musculoskeletal imaging include the joints, pediatric imaging, bone, skin, many disease processes, foreign bodies, and postoperative scanning. Add the joint-specific scanning of shoulder, knee, ankle, elbow, and wrist, and you begin to understand that musculoskeletal ultrasound imaging is a significant area that we have just begun to explore.

ANATOMY OF THE MUSCULOSKELETAL SYSTEM

Normal Anatomy

Skeletal muscle contains long organized units called *muscle fibers.* The characteristic long fibers are under voluntary control, allowing us to contract a **muscle** and move a joint. The blood vessels, lymphatics, and nerves follow the fibrous partitions between the bundles of muscle.

Several different types of muscles are present in the human body. Muscles have fibers that run parallel to the bone, have a fan shape, or form a **pennate** pattern. These feather-like muscle patterns run oblique to the long axis of the muscle and are unipennate, bipennate, multipennate, or circumpennate. Think of a feather and how the fibers grow from a central section. Half of this feather is unipennate, whereas the whole feather is bipennate. A multipennate muscle is a division of several feather-like sections in one muscle, and the circumpennate is the convergence of fibers to a central tendon (Figure 24-1, *A*). The deltoid muscle is an example of a unipennate muscle; it has feather-like fascicles with a unipennate, bipennate, or multipennate attachment (Figure 24-1, *B*). The gastrocnemius muscle in the calf is a bipennate muscle in which the fibers

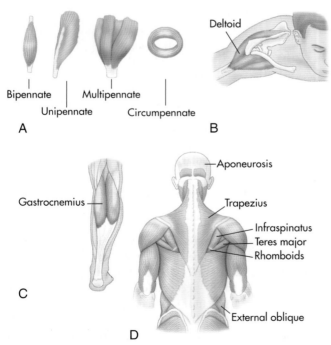

FIGURE 24-1 **Different types of muscle. A,** Unipennate, bipennate, multipennate, and circumpennate muscle patterns. **B,** The deltoid muscle is an example of a unipennate muscle and has feather-like fascicles with a unipennate, bipennate, or multipennate attachment. **C,** The gastrocnemius muscle in the calf is a bipennate muscle, whose fibers have a central origin. **D,** The large, flat muscles of the external oblique or the trapezius attach with a large, flat aponeurosis.

have a central origin (Figure 24-1, *C*). The large, flat muscles of the external oblique or the trapezius attach with a large, flat aponeurosis (Figure 24-1, *D*).

Attachment of the muscle occurs at the proximal and distal portions of the bundle. This attachment, a collection of tough collagenous fibers, is a **tendon.** These attachments may be cordlike or flat sheets called **aponeuroses.** This type of attachment occurs in flat muscles, such as the rectus abdominis in the abdomen. The elastic tendon consists of collagen fibers that enable it to stretch and flex around structures. This avascular structure heals slowly and has a whitish appearance. Because of the lack of vascularity, tendons heal slowly; this is why an injury can incapacitate a patient.

Tendons occur with or without a **synovial sheath.** This tubular sac surrounding a tendon has two layers. Fluid separates the two layers of the sheath and is found in the shoulder, hand, wrist, and ankle. This sheath plays an important role in imaging these structures with sonography. The biceps tendon of the shoulder is one example of a tendon with a synovial sheath. Other tendons, such as the Achilles and patellar, lack this sheath and have a surrounding fat layer or loose connective tissue, which makes this type of tendon more difficult to image with sonography.

The support and strength of a joint are due in part to the **ligaments.** These short bands of tough fibers connect bones to other bones. This type of connective tissue is especially important in the knees, ankles, and shoulders.

The saclike structure surrounding joints and tendons that contains a viscous fluid is the **bursa.** This potential space provides an area for synovial fluid to aid in the reduction of friction between two musculoskeletal structures, such as tendon and bone or ligament and bone. For example, two of the knee joints that have such a bursa are the patellofemoral and femorotibial joints. The suprapatellar pouch has a continuous connection with the joint cavity but is often referred to as a bursa. The knee joint itself has nine bursae—three located anterior and six on the popliteal side of the joint.

Nerves are the conduits for impulses to and from the muscles and the central nervous system. Muscle action is under the control of the muscle system with the nerves in contact with the muscle through motor end plates. Elements of the nerves include the nerve fibers, arranged into bundles (**fasciculi**) and surrounded by dense insulating sheaths of **myelin** (forms the sheath of Schwann cells) and connective tissue.

Normal Sonographic Appearance

Imaging of the musculoskeletal system can be overwhelming because so many different muscles, attachments, ligaments, and tendons can be seen. All joints contain similar anatomic structures, and tendons and ligaments have the same sonographic imaging characteristics whether they are part of an ankle or a shoulder. Muscle attachments also have a similar sonographic appearance. The first step in sonographic imaging of any musculoskeletal structure is knowledge of the normal appearance.
Tendons. MRI has been the modality of choice for physicians in the United States when diagnosing musculoskeletal problems. The advent of high-resolution ultrasound has challenged the superiority of MRI for imaging tendons, especially when the

examination is performed by a skilled sonographer using high-quality equipment. The evolution of real-time ultrasound allows demonstration of the full range of motion of the tendon. The high resolution of modern transducers also allows imaging of the fine tendon fibers and comparison of normal versus abnormal using dual imaging techniques.

The tendon occurs in two forms: with and without a synovial sheath (Figure 24-2). Wrapped around the tendon, the

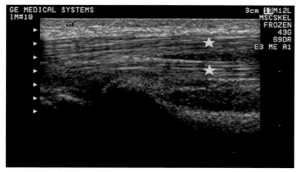

FIGURE 24-2 Superficial and deep flexor tendons *(stars)* have a surrounding synovial sheath that allows smooth motion of the pulley system of the hand. Tendon movement can be seen in real-time with movement of the fingers.

smooth inner layer of this tubular sac lies in close contact with the tendon. Between this inner layer and an outer layer, a small amount of thick mucinoid material helps facilitate movement. The biceps tendon is one example of a sheath-covered tendon that images well (Figure 24-3). The thickness of this sheath measures only a couple of millimeters and is sonographically imaged as a hypoechoic halo surrounding the tendon. Inflammation of this sheath and tendon often aids in imaging and diagnosing problems with this tendon. Acute disease may reveal a sheath that is thicker than the contained tendon. Areas of high stress in the hand, wrist, and ankle also contain tendons with sheaths.

Paratenon, a loose areolar connective tissue, fills the fascial compartment of the tendon lacking a synovial sheath. The dense epitendineum, another layer of connective tissue, closely adjoins the tendon. The epitendineum images as an echogenic layer adjacent to the tendon. The lack of density differences in these interfaces makes the tendon somewhat difficult to image. Fortunately, many of the tendons without a synovial sheath are large and image relatively well. The accompanying bursa may also be abnormal, thus enhancing the tendon. Examples of this type of tendon include the Achilles, patellar, proximal gastrocnemius, and semimembranosus tendons (Figure 24-4).

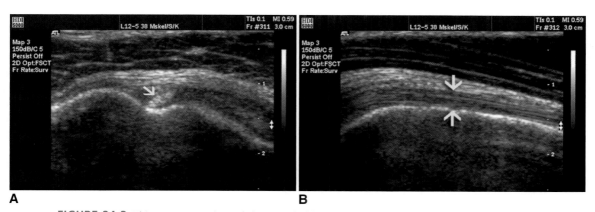

FIGURE 24-3 This transverse view of the rounded biceps tendon **(A)** images the tendon as a hyperechoic structure sitting within the bicipital groove of the humerus *(arrow)*. The longitudinal view **(B)** has the characteristic pattern seen with tendons encased within a synovial sheath *(arrows)*.

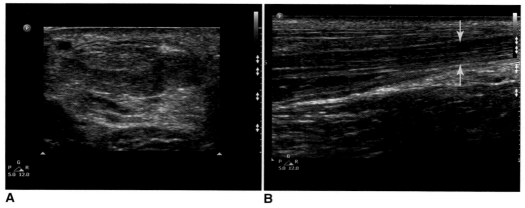

FIGURE 24-4 A cross section or transverse view of the distal Achilles tendon **(A)** demonstrates the characteristic oval appearance. The tendon changes shape with decreased use, becoming round in the sedentary individual. The lack of synovial sheath is evident on the longitudinal image of the tendon **(B)**. The slight increase in echogenicity *(arrows)* on each side of the tendon is the epitendineum.

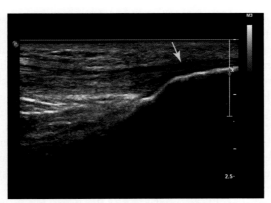

FIGURE 24-5 The normal Achilles tendon insertion *(arrow)* images at that insertion on the calcaneus and mimics cartilage found in other parts of the body.

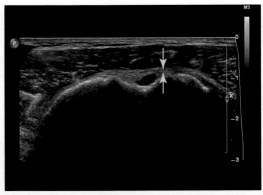

FIGURE 24-6 The coracohumeral ligament *(between arrows)* helps maintain the proper location of the long biceps tendon within the bicipital groove. This biceps tendon demonstrates tenosynovitis and inflammation of the tendon and sheath, which results in a hypoechoic appearance.

Interwoven and interconnected collagen fibers found in the tendon run in a parallel path. The numerous interfaces of the collagen fascicles provide a strong linear reflector that images well with ultrasound. The higher the frequency of the imaging transducer, the better these fibers image—a fact that underscores the need for a transducer of 7 MHz or greater. This normal fibrillar hypoechoic pattern and imaging detail become very important when diagnosing abnormalities.

Care must be taken when imaging the tendon because even a slight rotation off axis may produce an image that incorrectly suggests tendinitis. Both transverse and longitudinal planes help image the tendon, along with a side-by-side (dual) comparison of the contralateral side.

The tendon insertion site has its own sonographic characteristics. The joining of the tendon to the bone (enthesis) occurs with a narrow band of fibrocartilage. This avascular structure is approximately 1 cm long and images longitudinally as a triangular hypoechoic area in the distal tendon. Familiarity with the normal sonographic appearance is important because injury to this area of the tendon results in thickening of the insertion site (Figure 24-5).

Ligaments. Ligaments are thin, superficial structures, which makes them difficult to image. This superficial location requires the use of a higher-frequency transducer—10 MHz or greater—and possibly a stand-off pad to aid in imaging ligaments outside the joint. Critical to ligament identification is the equipment parameter adjustment. Adding too much gain to the image using overall gain or time gain compensation (TGC) results in loss of detail due to the strong bone reflections. Unlike imaging in other areas of the body, longitudinal imaging of the ligament is the only method used to image injuries. Transverse planes are of little help when imaging the ligament because they blend with the surrounding fat. The difficulty of imaging the ligament is helped by using a dual or side-by-side technique to compare normal and abnormal anatomy.

Many ligaments in the large joints of the body image well as hyperechoic straplike structures (Figure 24-6). One exception is the cruciate ligament within the knee joint, which appears hypoechoic. The large joints include the hip, shoulder, ankle, wrist, and knee. Part of the difficulty associated with imaging the ligament is the lack of a contiguous structure, such as muscle, to aid in location. The dense fibers have a slightly less regular appearance and may help hold a tendon in place. Usually the ligament measures 2 to 3 mm thick and images as a hypoechoic band with a homogeneous appearance. These ligament structures are found close to both ends attaching to the bony cortex.

One ligament—the medial collateral ligament (MCL) or tibial collateral ligament, which connects the medial femoral condyle to the medial proximal tibia—deviates from the usual ligament appearance. This wide, smooth ligament is about 9 cm long and has deep and superficial portions. The external superficial portion consists of connective tissue appearing as a dense band that connects the medial femoral condyle to the proximal tibia. The deep layer connects the medial meniscus to the femur and tibia.

Sonographic imaging of the MCL reveals a three-layer structure. The superficial and deep layers have a hypoechoic-separating layer. Loose connective tissue forms the middle layer, which provides a potential space for bursas in some individuals (Figure 24-7).

Muscle. Discussions of muscle often include references to the origin and insertion of the muscle. The proximal portion of the muscle is considered the origin, whereas the insertion is the distal end. A muscle with two or more heads has an origin in more than one place on the bone. Most of us do not think in terms of origins and insertions, so for the purpose of this discussion, we will talk in terms of the location or attachment of the muscle.

To begin to learn the normal appearance of a muscle, it is easy to use the large quadriceps muscle located in the anterior thigh or the posterior calf muscles. Skeletal muscle imaged on a longitudinal plane appears homogeneous with multiple, fine parallel echoes (Figure 24-8). Connective tissue surrounding the fiber bundles produces these echogenic bands. The main portions of the muscle fibers are hypoechoic and radiate toward a central tendon or aponeurosis (Figure 24-9). The transverse plane discloses a less organized pattern of fine punctate echoes scattered through the

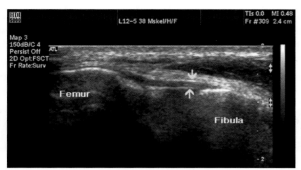

FIGURE 24-7 The fibular collateral ligament connects the fibula to the lateral side of the femur. This hypoechoic linear structure *(arrows)* passes over the lateral meniscus and has a slightly oblique course.

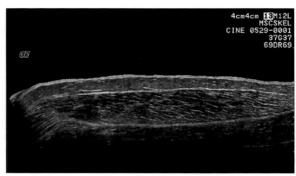

FIGURE 24-10 Panoramic imaging allows global study of this normal gastrocnemius muscle.

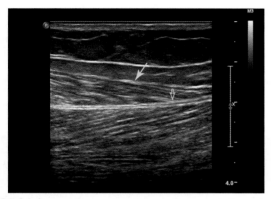

FIGURE 24-8 The bipennate gastrocnemius muscle has echogenic obliquely oriented connective tissue *(solid arrow)* between the muscle bundles. A small central tendon *(open arrow)* serves as the anchor for these bundles.

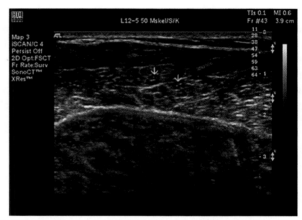

FIGURE 24-11 Small punctate echogenicities *(arrows)* image on the transverse muscle.

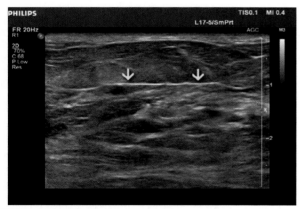

FIGURE 24-9 The dense aponeurosis tissue that connects the muscle to bone images is an echogenic linear structure *(arrows)*.

muscle bundle. Encasing the muscle is a connective tissue fascia that has a bright echogenic appearance (Figures 24-10 and 24-11). This fascia layer, although brighter than the sheathed muscle fibers, has less echogenicity than subcutaneous fat or tendons.

The muscle bundle contains nerves, fascia, tendons, fat, and fibrous connective tissue surrounding the muscle. The epimysium continues into the muscle, developing into the perimysium, which separates the bundles into muscle fibers. These hypoechoic structures, compared with the muscle fibers, help differentiate muscles. The sonographic appearance of muscle can be deceiving in some areas, such as the hand, because of the similarity of echo texture to a mass or tenosynovitis. Careful scanning and transducer rotation help image the pennate structure of the muscle, aiding in identification of a possible normal muscle variant.

Normal dynamics of the muscle images easily in real-time because contraction of the muscle increases muscle thickness and hypoechogenicity. In addition, echogenic connective tissue bands increase in obliquity. Sustained contraction of the muscle has the same sonographic appearance as muscle bundles found in the athletic patient. This decreased echogenic muscle, as a result of hypertrophy, is normal for this patient population. Compression of the muscle with the transducer condenses the tissue, resulting in an increase in muscle echogenicity.

Transducer orientation is another factor that influences muscle echogenicity. Ensuring a longitudinal and transverse plane with good contact helps negate the possibility of introducing artifactual information. It is helpful to scan the contralateral normal side to ensure technique or to ensure that normal variants do not result in a misdiagnosis.

Nerves. The normal nerve has a hyperechoic appearance compared with muscle but is hypoechoic compared with tendons. The echogenicity depends on the surrounding structures and is not constant within the body. The longitudinal plane reveals a fibrillar pattern with parallel inner linear echoes similar to the tendon. In transverse imaging, the nerve fibers appear hypoechoic, with a hyperechoic **perineurium** surrounding each fiber. The collagenous **epineurium**—the outer layer of the nerve—appears as a hyperechoic layer (Figures 24-12 and 24-13).

Differentiating nerves from tendons is a simple task when you contrast the two structures. Real-time imaging shows tendons that move when the corresponding joint or muscle contracts. The nerve will remain stable within the muscle tissue. Sonographic artifacts (anisotropy) are not as evident on the nerve as they are on the tendon, and nerves are imaged best with a transducer of 10 MHz or higher. Power Doppler is especially helpful because vessels accompany the nerves. Table 24-1 lists the nerves that are identifiable with sonography.

Bursa. The small sac between two moving surfaces, usually tendon and bone, is the bursa. These fluid-filled cavities facilitate the movement of tendons or muscles over bony projections. The minute amount of viscous fluid contained within the bursa helps reduce friction between moving parts of the joint (Figures 24-14 and 24-15). The major bursa of the body is the subacromial-subdeltoid bursa,

TABLE 24-1	Nerves Identifiable with Sonography
Lower Limb	**Location**
Sciatic	Posterior thigh lateral to the hamstring muscle
Popliteal	Popliteal fossa superficial to the popliteal artery and vein
Upper Limb	**Location**
Suprascapular	Deep to the trapezius to the infraspinatus fossa
Median	Medial to the biceps tendon and brachial artery, elbow, right side of the carpal tunnel
Radial	Between the brachioradialis and brachialis muscles
Ulnar	Median epicondyle of the elbow, medial to the ulnar artery in Guyon's canal

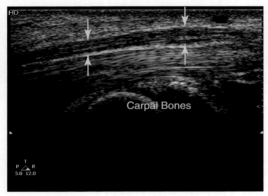

FIGURE 24-12 The median nerve runs on the ventral side of the forearm and wrist, supplying the muscles of the superficial layers of the forearm and hand. The hypoechoic nerve *(right arrows)* sits just anterior to the echogenic deep flexor tendon of the index finger *(left arrows).*

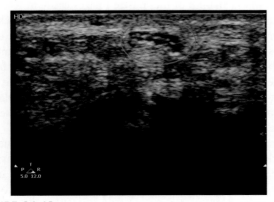

FIGURE 24-13 This transverse scan of the median nerve reveals the hyperechoic nerves with hypoechoic nerve fiber fascicles.

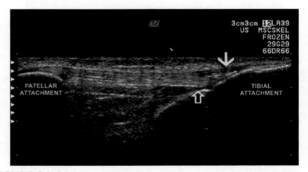

FIGURE 24-14 This normal infrapatellar tendon has multiple bursae, which usually blend in with surrounding tissue. One lies between the skin and fascia anterior to the tibial tuberosity *(arrow),* and a deep bursa lies between the patellar ligament and the tibial tuberosity *(open arrow).* The knee itself has a total of nine bursae located in and around the joint.

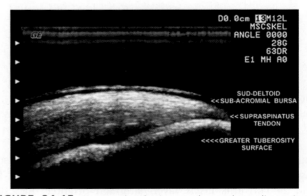

FIGURE 24-15 New technologies, such as three-dimensional imaging, have the ability to remove surrounding tissue signals from the data set. This capability makes this modality ideal for imaging of the bursa. This subdeltoid-subacromial bursa image clearly demonstrates the external synovial layer with hypoechoic lubricating fluid.

TABLE 24-2	Normal Sonographic Appearance		
Anatomy	**General Sonographic Appearance**	**Longitudinal Appearance**	**Transverse Appearance**
Tendon	Hyperechoic linear structure Dynamic with movement of corresponding joint/muscle	Cordlike	Oval, round, or cuboid
Ligament	Isoechoic, weakly hyperechoic	Striated structures connecting bone to bone	Difficult to image on the transverse plane
Nerve	Hypoechoic to tendons Hyperechoic to muscle Cannot be mobilized with movement Posterior enhancement lacking	Cordlike tubular structure	Hypoechoic with fascicles
Muscle	Muscular bundles—hypoechoic Perimysium, epimysium, fascia, fat plane—hyperechoic	Parallel echogenic linear appearance within hypoechoic muscle tissue; may appear featherlike depending on the type of muscle imaged	Punctate echogenic areas within the hypoechoic muscle
Bursa	Thin, hypoechoic structure that merges with the surrounding fat	Thin linear hypoechoic structure adjacent to a tendon	Normal bursae are difficult to image on the transverse plane

found in the shoulder, covering the deep surface of the deltoid muscle.

Two types of bursas are found in the body: communicating and noncommunicating. This categorization helps explain the relationship of the bursa to the joint space. One communicating bursa sonographers often see is Baker's cyst, which is located in the medial popliteal fossa. This bursa, located between the semimembranosus and medial gastrocnemius tendons, has a connecting neck to the bursa contained within the knee joint. Usually, sonographers image bursas that do not communicate with the joint space. An example of a superficial noncommunicating type of bursa is the prepatellar bursa.

In the normal patient, the bursae are difficult to image because they often blend in with surrounding tissue and fat. The thin film of viscous fluid found within the bursa contributes to the hypoechoic appearance of the structure because the walls are too thin to image. These potential spaces will appear on ultrasound in the presence of an inflammatory process caused by fluid accumulation. Any bursa larger than 2 mm is enlarged and needs to be compared with the normal contralateral side.

Table 24-2 summarizes the normal sonographic appearance of tendons, ligaments, nerves, muscle, and bursae.

ARTIFACTS

Sonographers and sonologists have the daily challenge of separating artifacts from useful image information. All equipment manufacturers program in some basic assumptions about the interaction between tissue and sound: that the speed of sound is 1540 m/sec, that the area imaged is within the central beam, and that sound travels out and back in a straight line. Artifacts occur when these basic assumptions are not met, and something is created that is not real, is erroneously positioned, has improper brightness, or is absent from the image. Many manufacturers have developed technology to reduce and often eliminate some types of artifacts caused by compound and harmonic imaging.

Musculoskeletal imaging displays the same gamut of artifacts seen in other areas of the body. The superficial nature of musculoskeletal structures, often anterior to the highly reflective bone, causes artifacts to become more of a problem. Some artifacts aid in identifying pathologic conditions and structures; however, others hinder and even mimic disease.

Several artifact types—anisotropy, reverberation, time-of-flight artifact, and refractile shadowing—are important in musculoskeletal ultrasound. Understanding how artifacts occur and how to correct images increases both diagnostic confidence and image accuracy.

Anisotropy

The anisotropic phenomenon is one that occurs not only in sonography but also in other professions, such as astronomy, geology, and chemistry. **Anisotropy** occurs when the sound beam misses the transducer on the return because of the curve of the structure (Figure 24-16). The angle and direction of the reflected beam depend on the angle of incidence.

The reflection coefficient is a function of the angle and becomes a problem when the reflected beam misses the receiver. The nonperpendicular tissue interfaces return echoes at an angle that does not return to the transmitting transducer, creating an imaging challenge. This results in differing image properties depending on the angle of incidence.

The loss of definition of the curved upper pole of the right kidney is one example of this artifact. The muscle, ligaments, and nerves also image as an anisotropic reflector because of the plane they occupy, with tendons having the most pronounced anisotropy in musculoskeletal imaging. This loss of image requires a heel-to-toe rocking of the transducer to create the optimal 90-degree angle (Figures 24-17 and 24-18).

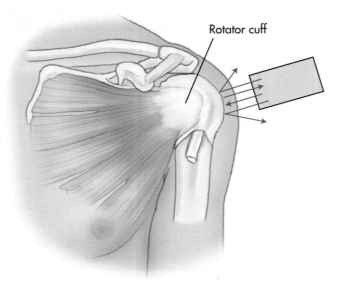

Rotator cuff

FIGURE 24-16 A perpendicular or 90-degree angle of the sound beam to the reflecting tissue surface results in the greatest amount of reflection and optimal images. At nonperpendicular incidence, part of the incident sound beam misses the transducer, resulting in the display of decreased brightness of returning echoes.

Reverberation

A reflective surface reverberates sound and may be beneficial or detrimental. We often experience this phenomenon without realizing its impact. Our senses use reverberation as a clue to the location of structures in a room through reflection of sound back to our ears. Any acoustic environment, such as an auditorium, relies on reverberation to transmit sound.

The same is true of sound transmitted into the body. The initial sound beam transmits and returns. Multiple delayed reflections from strong tissue boundaries, such as bone, result in a linear artifact that *decreases* in intensity with depth. This collection of reflected sound is superimposed over the primary signal, often adding distracting information to the image (Figure 24-19).

Reverberation is not always a detrimental process. One type of artifact, comet tail, results from reverberation from metal, such as clips, sutures, staples, or a foreign object such as a BB. This type varies slightly from the traditional reverberation, which bounces between the transducer face and the strong reflector. The **comet-tail artifact** is a function of the sound bouncing between two closely placed reflectors within the imaged structure. In the case of a pin surgically

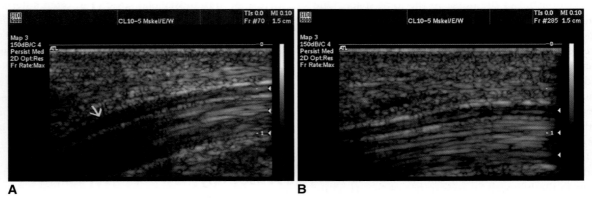

A   B

FIGURE 24-17 These images of the median nerve and the deep flexor tendon illustrate the effects of anisotropy. **A,** A large artifact occurred because the angle of incidence is not 90 degrees, resulting in a hypoechoic appearance of the tendon and nerve *(arrow)*. **B,** Rocking the transducer or repositioning the structure allows the angle of incidence to be closer to 90 degrees, thus reducing or eliminating the artifact.

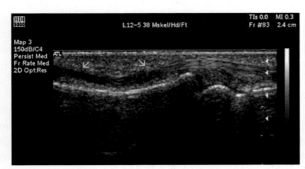

FIGURE 24-18 Change in direction of the imaged structure (digital flexor tendon) causes multiple areas of anisotropy *(arrows)* due to changes in the angle of incidence.

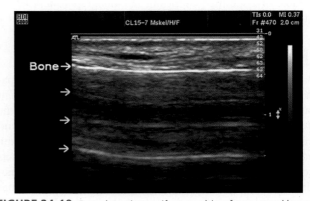

Bone→

FIGURE 24-19 Reverberation artifact resulting from sound bouncing between the strongly reflecting bone and the transducer face.

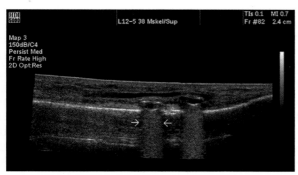

FIGURE 24-20 Comet-tail artifact *(arrows)* seen posterior to tibial pins placed to stabilize a tibial fracture. Note the widening of the posterior reverberation, which is due to reverberation within the metal pins. This widening is common with metal placed within musculoskeletal structures and is still a comet-tail artifact even though it does not narrow in the distal area.

placed within a bone, the reflecting surfaces are the anterior and posterior borders of the hardware. The ringing occurs within the metal object, and each time the sound returns to the anterior border, some of the sound escapes. The resultant artifact resembles a comet tail, hence its name (Figure 24-20).

Refractile Shadowing

The bending of the transmitted sound beam to an oblique path occurs often and is seen as **refractile shadowing (edge artifact)** on the sonographic image. This change in direction of the sound beam results in a hypoechoic band posterior to the structure. Another cause of refractile shadowing is a tissue impedance mismatch different than the average speed of sound within soft tissue (1540 m/sec). This is seen at the edge of a round or oval ligament or as the result of a traumatic tear of a musculoskeletal structure (Figures 24-21 and 24-22). Most commonly seen with a complete tendon tear, the angles formed from the retracted tendon cause refractile shadowing. This shadowing is often used to determine the distance

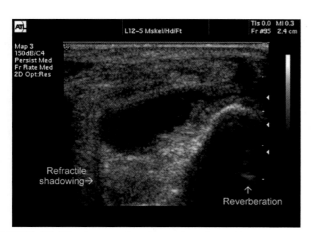

FIGURE 24-21 This ganglion located in the ankle demonstrates refractile shadowing.

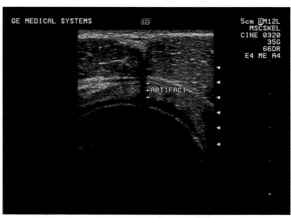

FIGURE 24-22 Refractile shadowing from a normal structure anterior to the area of interest (supraspinatus tendon) makes it difficult to diagnose abnormalities.

between ligaments by measuring from one artifact edge to the other.

Time-of-Flight Artifact

Time-of-flight, or speed-of-sound, artifacts occur when the returning sound wave has passed between two tissues with markedly different speeds. This misrepresentation of the return time results from the assumption that the speed of sound is a constant 1540 m/sec. If the speed of sound is less than the average in tissue, the artifact appears to be farther away from the transducer. Faster speed results in the artifact being closer to the transducer on the image. Creation of this type of false information occurs most commonly with musculoskeletal ultrasound when imaging obese patients at a muscle-fat interface (Figure 24-23).

The speed-of-sound artifact displaces the image in the anteroposterior (axial) plane. When this speed artifact is coupled with refraction, a structure displays with an incorrect shape. For example, think of a wall of bricks. If one section fails and drops down, the result is that one section is

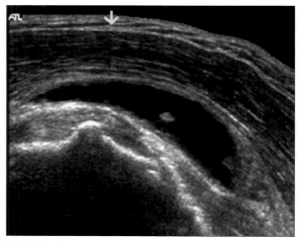

FIGURE 24-23 This panoramic image of a rotator cuff tear demonstrates the very subtle time-of-flight artifact.

TABLE 24-3	Correction Techniques for Artifacts
Artifact	**Correction Technique**
Anisotropy	Heel-to-toe rocking of the transducer creates a perpendicular angle of incidence, removing the anisotropy.
Reverberation	Anterior reverberation can be minimized with the use of a stand-off pad or by changing the angle of incidence.
Refractile	Use of newer technologies, such as compound shadowing imaging or tissue harmonics, helps reduce or eliminate this artifact. Changing the angle of incidence may move the artifact out of the region of interest.
Time of flight	May not be able to eliminate as a result of tissue artifact sound properties. Change the angle of incidence to demonstrate surrounding tissue.

asymmetric from the surrounding areas. Do not mistake this very subtle artifact with a transducer crystal malfunction. A mechanical failure produces a decrease in image information that begins at the transducer face, but the time-of-flight artifact affects only the image.

Table 24-3 lists the techniques for correcting the artifacts discussed previously.

SONOGRAPHIC EVALUATION OF THE MUSCULOSKELETAL SYSTEM

Sonographic imaging of the joints begins with the proper choice of transducers. Superficially located joints and structures image well with high-frequency transducers of 5 MHz or higher. The more superficial the imaged structure is, the higher the transducer frequency must be to ensure maximal detail; however, larger joints, such as the shoulder, may require a lower frequency to penetrate the musculoskeletal structures.

Positioning of the joint of interest is an important part of the examination. The patient should be placed in a comfortable position that allows the sonographer to maintain correct scanning ergonomics to prevent development of musculoskeletal problems. A final consideration is the dynamic portion of the examination. It is often helpful to be able to move the joint to confirm the imaged structure. Space must be allowed for a full range of motion for the imaged joint.

Rotator Cuff

The American Institute for Ultrasound Medicine (AIUM) recommends middle frequencies of 7 and 10 MHz for imaging shoulder structures; however, deeper rotator cuff structures may require a frequency of 5 MHz. Shoulder anatomy is complex, with numerous bursae, muscles, and tendons surrounding the joint. A basic sonographic examination of the structures found in the rotator cuff includes 11 images. Comparison with the contralateral normal shoulder

is always helpful in determining the absence or presence of a pathologic condition.

The biceps tendon is one of the easiest structures to image in the adult shoulder. Similar to any examination, documentation includes both longitudinal and transverse views. Begin by having the patient sit erect on a rotating chair with a back. The rotation of the chair allows quick and easy readjustments to the shoulder. To begin the examination of the biceps tendon, place the patient with a slight internal rotation of the shoulder. To obtain this position, have the patient place the arm on the lap with the fingers of the hand facing the opposite shoulder (Figure 24-24).

Begin the examination by facing the patient and checking the transducer orientation to prevent confusion during scanning. The structures will change with the particular shoulder being imaged. When facing the patient and imaging the right shoulder, the lateral anatomy displays on the left side of the image and the medial anatomy on the right side of the screen. When scanning posterior shoulder structures, the image corresponds to the patient position.

Begin the examination with the 3- to 5-mm-thick biceps tendon. This tendon is easily located in the transverse plane and images as an echogenic oval structure within the bicipital groove of the humerus. This groove, located between the greater and lesser tuberosities, coupled with the overlying transverse ligament, maintains the biceps tendon location. Once identified, images at several different levels help determine normalcy. A small amount of fluid—less than 1.5 mm—is a normal finding. Care must be taken to use minimal transducer pressure because small amounts of fluid may be compressed out of the imaging plane (Figure 24-25). A longitudinal image of the tendon requires some rocking of the transducer to obtain images with minimal anisotropic artifacts. When scanning the biceps tendon, take note of the fibrillar pattern of the

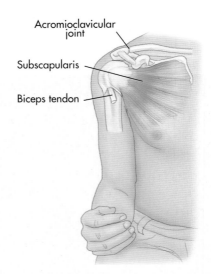

FIGURE 24-24 The subscapularis, the biceps tendon, and the acromioclavicular joint image easily from the anterior approach. This is considered a neutral position for the shoulder.

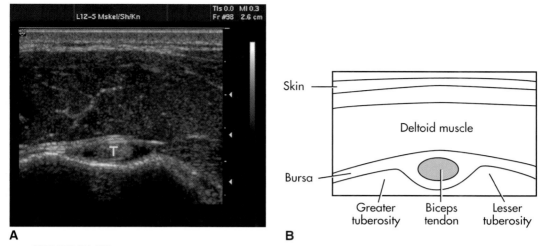

FIGURE 24-25 A, The transverse view of the normal biceps tendon has the echogenic tendon *(T)* within the bicipital groove. The anechoic effusion of tenosynovitis surrounding the tendon aids in visualization. **B,** Diagram of the anatomy.

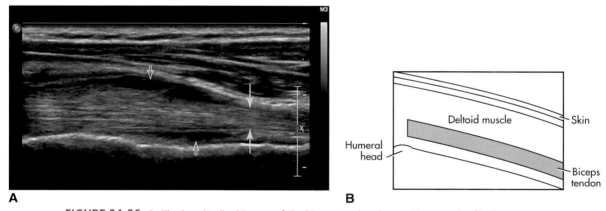

FIGURE 24-26 A, The longitudinal image of the biceps tendon *(arrows)* images the fibrillar pattern seen with tendons. The small amount of effusion *(open arrows)* seen posterior to the tendon indicates mild tenosynovitis. **B,** Diagram of the anatomy.

normal tendon because disruptions indicate a possible pathologic condition (Figure 24-26).

Finding the subscapularis tendon begins by imaging the biceps tendon on the transverse plane at the level of the humeral head. Using the biceps tendon as a landmark, angle the transducer anteromedially while locating the subscapularis. The transverse view images the tendon as an oval soft tissue structure. Note that the transverse view of the tendon requires a longitudinal transducer orientation (Figure 24-27). Externally rotating the arm while scanning aids in visualization of the tendon and determination of normal movement. This tendon inserts into the lesser tuberosity at an angle requiring slight rotation to obtain the longitudinal view (transverse transducer position).

The next structure to be located is the 3- to 7-mm supraspinatus tendon located laterally and posteriorly from the biceps tendon. This bandlike tendon has a medium-level echo texture and originates from the greater tuberosity of the

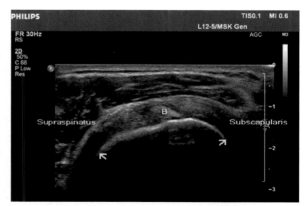

FIGURE 24-27 The biceps tendon *(B)* is a good landmark to locate the subscapularis and supraspinatus tendons. This image shows the transverse tendon between the anteromedially located subscapularis tendon and the posterolateral supraspinatus. Note the anisotropy artifact *(arrows)* seen as the tendons curve with the humeral head.

humerus. The acromion limits the field of view, necessitating careful transducer and patient positioning. A portion of the tendon, called the critical zone and located 1 cm posterolateral to the biceps tendon, is the most likely location for injury. Care must be taken here because improper scanning results in a false-positive or false-negative finding. The dual- or split-screen function allows for normal versus injured shoulder comparisons, which help to pinpoint tears.

Initial transverse and longitudinal views begin with the patient's arm in a neutral position; however, after localization of the tendon, the arm is repositioned into the Bouffard or Crass position (Figure 24-28). Whether the shoulder can be externally rotated into these positions depends on the patient's ability to place the arm behind the back or on the hip. This stresses the tendons of the rotator cuff, helping to emphasize any abnormalities. Another benefit is that the supraspinatus moves anterior and out from under the acromion, allowing better visualization of the tendon (Figures 24-29 through 24-32).

The infraspinatus tendon is the next structure to be imaged; two methods are available to localize the tendon. The first involves rotating the patient to gain access to the posterior shoulder and positioning the hand on the patient's opposite shoulder. The posterior glenoid labrum is a good landmark to help find the anteriorly located infraspinatus tendon (Figure 24-33). A second method has the patient's arm in the same position used in imaging the biceps tendon, locating the supraspinatus tendon, moving posterior and parallel to the scapular spine, and locating the infraspinatus tendon at its attachment to the posterior greater tuberosity of the humerus. Fluid imaged superficial to the infraspinatus tendon indicates bursal fluid, whereas posterior fluid indicates joint effusion. Take note of the humeral head contours because irregularities indicate a pathologic condition.

Although injury to the teres minor tendons is uncommon, imaging ensures complete visualization of the infraspinatus tendon because of their close proximity. This tendon lies parallel to the scapular spine and inferior to the infraspinatus tendon. To differentiate the infraspinatus tendon from the teres minor, pay close attention to the plane of the tendon fibers. Horizontal fibers indicate the infraspinatus, whereas the teres minor is on an oblique plane. The teres minor appears as a trapezoidal structure inferior to the infraspinatus tendon.

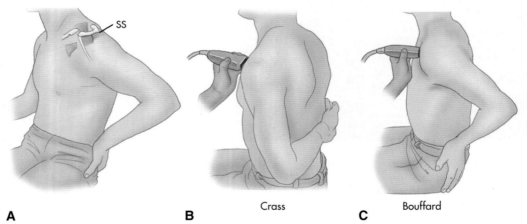

A   **B**   Crass   **C**   Bouffard

FIGURE 24-28 Once the supraspinatus (SS) has been located in the neutral position **(A),** move the hand to position the patient in the Crass **(B)** or Bouffard **(C)** position.

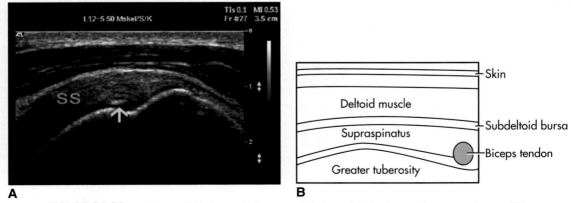

FIGURE 24-29 **A,** The medially located biceps tendon (arrow) helps locate the supraspinatus (SS). Scan this tendon from the acromion to the greater tuberosity to locate any echogenicity changes or the presence of fluid. **B,** Diagram of the anatomy.

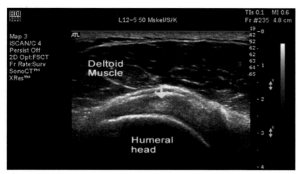

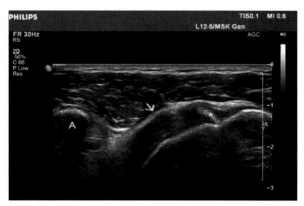

FIGURE 24-30 This transverse scan of the supraspinatus shows the tendon *(arrow)* to be mildly hyperechoic.

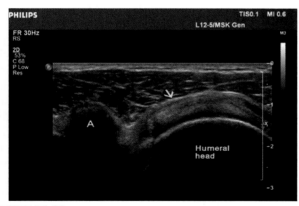

FIGURE 24-31 This image has the arm in a neutral position. To locate the supraspinatus, use the biceps tendon *(star)* as a landmark, and then rotate the transducer until the acromion *(A)* comes into view. The supraspinatus tendon *(arrow)* appears between these two structures. Note the anisotropy artifact that hinders visualization of part of the tendon.

FIGURE 24-32 This image shows the supraspinatus tendon *(arrow)* seen extending to the acromion *(A)* with the shoulder internally rotated into the Bouffard position. Most of the anisotropic artifact disappears because the tendon is closer to parallel to the transducer.

During examination of rotator cuff structures, it is important to note any bursal thickening, tendon calcifications, bony irregularities, loose bodies, or fluid collections. Many other non–rotator cuff structures can also be imaged, such as the **acromioclavicular (AC) joint.** Because of the superficial location of the AC, joint separations are easily imaged, especially

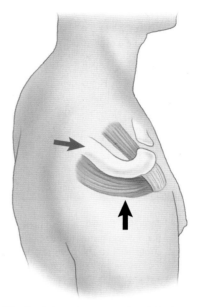

FIGURE 24-33 The infraspinatus tendon *(black arrow)* lies lateral and inferior to the scapular spine *(green arrow)*.

compared with a normal contralateral joint. As with any other portion of the body, soft tissue masses and injury, foreign body localization, and fluid collections are easily identified (Figures 24-34 and 24-35).

Box 24-1 lists the main indications for shoulder sonography. Box 24-2 lists the minimum shoulder views of the rotator cuff.

Carpal Tunnel

The wrist joint is easily examined because of its accessibility, size, and lack of overlying bony structures. This ease of imaging implies that the wrist is an uncomplicated joint to image; however, familiarity with wrist anatomy reveals a very complex set of structures. The complexity of the wrist is underscored by the fact that some orthopedic surgeons specialize in just this one joint.

Positioning of the wrist entails placing the arm at a 90-degree angle with the palm pronated or supinated on the lap of the patient (Figure 24-36). Placing a small rolled-up towel under the wrist when examining the palmar **(volar)** portion of the wrist places the joint in a neutral position. The towel also helps dorsal imaging of the wrist when the hand is palm down. These positions allow imaging of carpal tunnel structures, ganglion and synovial cysts, tears of the triangular fibrocartilage, tenosynovitis, and any other tumors. Another benefit of sonographic imaging of the wrist is the ability to demonstrate the dynamics of the wrist and associated masses with finger movement. The smaller wrist joint requires a higher-frequency transducer in the 10- to 20-MHz range. Manufacturers also offer transducers with smaller footprints, which allow easier scanning than some of the larger linear transducers.

The carpal tunnel is located between the carpal bones and the flexor retinaculum on the palmar side of the wrist.

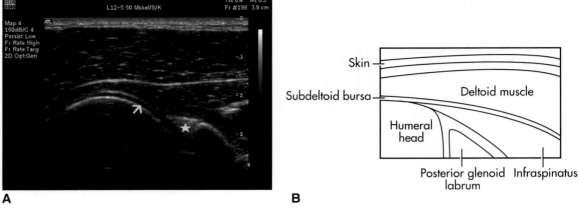

FIGURE 24-34 A, The posterior glenoid labrum *(star)* is a triangular hyperechoic structure deep to the infraspinatus tendon. The humeral head cartilage *(arrow)* images as a thin, hypoechoic layer superficial to the bony surface. **B,** Diagram of the anatomy.

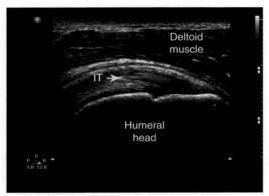

FIGURE 24-35 The infraspinatus tendon *(IT)* has a triangular appearance at the attachment to the posterior greater tuberosity. This image helps determine the echogenic consistency of the tendon when coupled with external and internal rotation maneuvers.

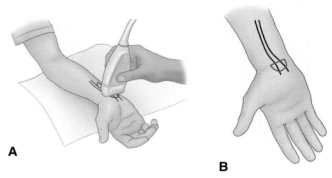

FIGURE 24-36 A, The wrist can be positioned on a pillow on the patient's lap to aid in imaging the volar structures. **B,** The retinaculum *(red),* a strong fibrous structure, attaches to the pisiform on the lateral side and the hook of the hamate.

BOX 24-1	Indications for Shoulder Sonography

- Shoulder pain or swelling
- Pain with joint rotation
- Weakness with arm elevation
- Trauma
- Decreased range of motion
- Evaluation of soft tissue masses

BOX 24-2	Minimum Shoulder Views of the Rotator Cuff

View: 1/2: Biceps longitudinal and transverse
View: 3/4: Subscapularis longitudinal and transverse
View: 5/6/7/8: Supraspinatus in neutral and internal rotation
View: 9/10: Infraspinatus/posterior glenoid labrum
View: 11: Teres minor

This fibro-osseous space contains the median nerve, the flexor pollicis longus, and the eight tendons that connect the digital muscles to the wrist (flexor digitorum tendons). The ulnar artery and veins indicate the medial border of the carpal tunnel, whereas the most lateral structures are the radial artery and veins. The flexor retinaculum forms the anterior border by attaching to the scaphoid tubercle, trapezium ridge, pisiform bone, and hook of the hamate. The median nerve, which is of particular interest when diagnosing carpal tunnel syndrome, lies superficial and toward the radial side of the tunnel. **Guyon's canal** is a tunnel on the ulnar side of the wrist formed by the hook of the hamate and pisiform bones. The ulnar nerve may be compressed at this site in long-distance cyclists, by falling on the wrist, or by repetitive wrist actions.

The transverse imaging plane is the easiest approach to use to begin an examination of the carpal tunnel. Locating the ulnar artery at the wrist crease helps orientation and subsequent identification of wrist structures. Care must be taken to maintain a perpendicular scan plane to reduce anisotropic effects. Use of large amounts of gel or a stand-off pad may help in imaging the anterior structures of the wrist. The flexor digitorum tendons are a hypoechoic structure just posterior to the median nerve. Fibrillary hyperechoic tendon patterns help differentiate the median nerve because the nerve is hypoechoic with a hyperechoic border. The rounded or oval median nerve flattens as it continues through the carpal tunnel (Figure 24-37).

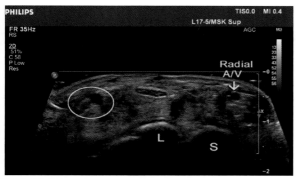

FIGURE 24-37 This image taken from the volar side of the wrist at the crease demonstrates the complicated anatomy from this view. Large amounts of gel allow for imaging with minimal artifact on the lateral curved edges. Guyon's canal *(circle)* contains the ulnar vein and vessels demarcating the medial carpal tunnel border. The lunate *(L)* and scaphoid bone *(S)* mark the posterior boundaries of the carpal tunnel. Laterally, the radial artery and vein mark this border. The median nerve is slightly flattened at this level, which is a normal finding.

The longitudinal nerve images as a parallel structure superficial to the flexor digitorum tendons. The nerve sheath appears as a continuous hyperechoic structure on the anterior and posterior borders of the nerve. Tendons located posterior to the median nerve have the characteristic hyperechoic fibrillar pattern seen with tendons in other areas of the body (Figure 24-38).

Box 24-3 lists the main indications for wrist sonography.

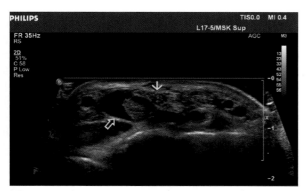

FIGURE 24-38 This image taken proximal to Figure 24-37 demonstrates a rounder median nerve *(solid arrow)*. The flexor pollicis longus tendon and the beginning of the muscle *(open arrow)* appear as a hypoechoic structure.

BOX 24-3	Indications for Wrist Sonography

- Masses
- Loss or decrease of digital mobility
- Pain and swelling
- Trauma
- Foreign body location
- Numbness of the middle and index fingers
- Weakness or clumsiness of the hand
- Tingling with nerve percussion (Tinel's sign)
- Pain with wrist flexion when sustained for a minute or longer (Phalen's sign)

Achilles Tendon

The Achilles tendon is named after a figure in Greek mythology. Achilles' mother wished to have her son invulnerable to all weapons, so she dipped him in the waters of the river Styx. The only portion that was not bathed in the water was his heel, resulting in a vulnerable spot. A poison arrow would later pierce the unprotected heel during the Trojan wars, resulting in Achilles' death.

This large, strong fibrous tendon connects the gastrocnemius and soleus muscles to the calcaneus. Although this tendon (as with any tendon) has many variations, approximately two thirds of the tendon originates from the gastrocnemius muscle and one third from the soleus muscle. This tendon helps move your foot downward, push off when walking, and rise up on your toes. Injury to this tendon can make it impossible to walk without pain.

A limited blood supply increases risk of injury to the Achilles tendon and slows the healing process. The longitudinal arteries that run the length of the gastrocnemius and soleus muscles provide the blood supply. The poorest blood supply is above the insertion of the tendon into the calcaneus, which is also the most frequent site of tendon tears. Chances of rupture and inflammation increase with age as the result of a diminishing blood supply.

A connective tissue sheath called the paratenon surrounds the Achilles tendon. This allows a gliding action of 2 to 3 cm with movement, and the tendon may thicken with increased activity. The lack of a true synovial sheath results in a less echogenic border between the tendon and the surrounding tissue.

The largest tendon of the body, the Achilles tendon may develop tendinitis in the athletic patient. Any activity that involves jumping and sudden stops and starts will stress the tendon. Female athletes who wear high-heeled shoes and then change into sneakers to exercise also increase their risk of tendinitis. Overstretching the tendon can result in a partial or complete tear, with the most common site being the distal tendon at the area of decreased blood flow (2 to 6 cm from the calcaneus).

Fortunately, the Achilles tendon is relatively easy to scan because of its echo characteristics and location. To begin the examination, position the patient prone with the foot hanging over the edge of the cart or bed. The foot may also be supported on a pillow or sponge for easier scanning and patient comfort. Patients who are unable to lie prone may be scanned while on their side if the injured Achilles tendon is on the upside.

The size of this tendon allows imaging with a 5-MHz linear transducer. Scan the tendon from the origin at the gastrocnemius and soleus muscles to the insertion on the calcaneus. A complete scan includes transverse and sagittal views and measurements of the transverse tendon. The anteroposterior (AP) diameter of the normal tendon is approximately 5 to 6 mm, varying with patient gender and body habitus. Measurement of the AP tendon diameter on the longitudinal plane tends to overestimate the distance because of the oblique course of the tendon. **Dorsiflexion** and **plantar**

flexion of the foot, best imaged on the sagittal plane, increase the chances of imaging an Achilles tendon tear. The **Thompson's test** (plantar flexion with squeezing of the calf) may be used to evaluate the integrity of the Achilles tendon. The patient kneels on the examination table with the feet hanging off; the examiner then squeezes the calf while observing for plantar flexion. The result is positive if no movement of the foot is noted; this indicates an Achilles tendon rupture.

When scanning the patient in the prone position, special attention must be given to the hypoechoic Kager's fat pad or pre-Achilles fat pad located deep in the Achilles tendon. Displacement of this triangular fat pad is one radiographic marker for the Achilles tendon and can serve as a landmark during the sonographic examination. Scanning the contralateral side also aids in determining normalcy of the tendon (Figures 24-39 and 24-40).

Box 24-4 lists the indications for Achilles tendon sonography.

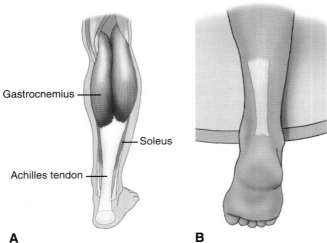

FIGURE 24-39 A, Achilles tendon imaging extends from the origin at the gastrocnemius and soleus muscles to the insertion on the calcaneus. **B,** Placing the patient prone with the foot over the cart edge allows easy access to the tendon and dorsal and plantar flexion of the foot.

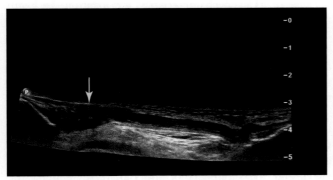

FIGURE 24-40 Panoramic or extended field of view imaging allows imaging of a greater length of the Achilles tendon. This ensures comparison of the echo texture in different areas of the tendon. Kager's fat pad *(arrow)* images as a hypoechoic structure.

BOX 24-4	Indications for Achilles Tendon Sonography

- Abnormal Thompson's test (toes point toward the plantar surface of the foot when the calf is squeezed.)
- Trauma
- Displacement of Kager's fat pad on a radiograph
- Knot or bulge over the proximal tendon
- Audible pop or snap followed by a sharp pain
- Inability to stand on toes
- Swelling
- Heel pain for longer than 4 weeks
- Decreased strength or mobility
- Postoperative monitoring

PATHOLOGY OF THE MUSCULOSKELETAL SYSTEM

Familiarity with the sonographic appearance of injury, inflammation, and chronic problems allows a confident diagnosis of musculoskeletal problems. Some pathology occurs with increased frequency in a specific joint, but the same problem images similarly in the tendons, ligaments, and muscles, regardless of location.

Shoulder Biceps Tendon Subluxation/Dislocation

The dislocation (also called *subluxation*) of the biceps tendon from the bicipital groove may be due to a problem with the transverse humeral ligament, abnormal development of the bicipital groove or supraspinatus, and/or subscapularis tears. The most common dislocation is deep to the subscapularis anterior to the glenohumeral joint capsule. This medial dislocation results in an empty groove that may fill with granulation and fibrous tissue. Rotating the arm from a neutral to external position allows real-time imaging of the tendon dislocation or subluxation (Figures 24-41 and 24-42).

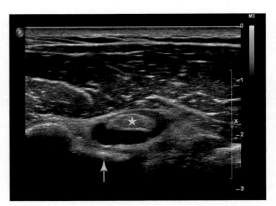

FIGURE 24-41 Subluxation and complete or incomplete dislocation of the biceps tendon *(star)* out of the bicipital groove *(arrow)* of the humerus.

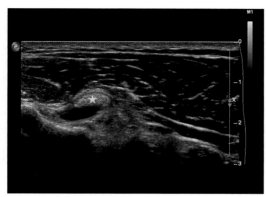

FIGURE 24-42 Complete dislocation of the biceps tendon *(star)* outside of the biceps groove of the humerus.

Rotator Cuff Tears

Tears of the rotator cuff may be classified as partial-thickness or full-thickness tears (Figure 24-43). The two types are differentiated through determination of abnormal communication between the glenohumeral joint and the subacromial bursa. The full-thickness tear has this communication, although the partial-thickness tear does not.

Rotator cuff problems may occur as an acute or chronic process. Biceps tendon ruptures, falls, and shoulder dislocations are a few causes of an acute rotator cuff tear. A chronic process occurs as a cumulative progression of injury from activities involving placing the arms over the head. This may be due to actions such as placing items on high shelves, playing tennis, swimming, or rock climbing. This microtrauma, due to impingement of the tendon between the humeral head and the acromion, results in cuff degeneration and an eventual tear. Rotator cuff tears are divided into three stages—stage I: swelling and mild pain; stage II: inflammation and scarring; and stage III: partial or complete tears of the rotator cuff.

The supraspinatus, similar to all tendons of the shoulder, is a straplike tendon with three dimensions. Tears in width,

length, and thickness occur in tendons, and a complete examination includes a description of the tear in all planes. A tear located on the sagittal plane of the tendon images as a disruption on the thickness or AP dimension of the tendon. This is only part of the picture, and an orthogonal image will identify the location and extent of the tear on the width of the tendon.

Another consideration is that the curved tendons will have an increased chance of producing an anisotropic artifact, which will appear similar to a tear. Moving the patient's arm to an internal rotation or an extended position changes the imaging plane and helps not only to reduce the artifact, but to accentuate the defect.

Partial-Thickness Tear. The partial-thickness tear may involve the bursal or articular cuff surface or the intrasubstance material. An intrasubstance tear is very rare. Tears begin in the critical zone of the anterolateral supraspinatus tendon and image as focal disruptions of the tendon fibers. This zone is located 1 cm from its insertion into the greater tuberosity. When injured, the acute tendon tear images as an anechoic defect in the rotator cuff. A chronic tear may image as an area of hyperechogenicity caused by mixing of blood and bursal granulation tissue in the frayed tendon area. Diffuse thinning of the tendon is another indication of a chronic partial-thickness tear.

The most common type of tear is the articular cuff surface defect. The following criteria help in establishing the presence of a partial-thickness tear:

1. A critical zone focus of mixed hyperechoic and hypoechoic echo texture (focal discontinuity).
2. Bursal or articular extension of any hypoechoic areas imaged in two orthogonal planes.
3. An irregularity of the anterior greater tuberosity is seen in up to three fourths of partial-thickness tears. These may appear as bone cortex defects, fragmentation, and/or spurring.
4. Decreased thickness of the tendon with chronic partial-thickness tears.

Fluid seen within the biceps tendon indicates the possibility of an articular surface tear. The presence of large amounts of fluid in the subacromial-subdeltoid bursa raises the chance of a nonvisualized full-thickness tear.

Hypoechoic concave bursal surface tears are the next most common type of partial rotator cuff tears (Figure 24-44). These defects, close to the joints and bursa, are tender to palpation.

Box 24-5 lists the sonographic criteria for partial-thickness tears.

Full-Thickness Tear. A tear of the rotator cuff that involves the full thickness and full width of the tendons is considered a full-thickness tear. Retraction of multiple tendons occurs with a separation of 2 to 4 cm between the torn tendon ends. The frequency of tendon tearing in descending order occurs in the supraspinatus, infraspinatus, and subscapularis, and, very rarely, the teres minor.

Images of the tear on sagittal and transverse planes not only confirm the full-thickness tear, but also provide for measurement between the torn tendon edges (Figures 24-45 through 24-47).

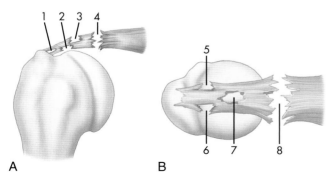

FIGURE 24-43 Coronal view **(A)** and view from above **(B)** showing tears of the supraspinatus tendon. These tears can occur anywhere along the tendon and range from an intrasubstance tear *(1)* to a complete full-thickness, full-width tear *(8)*. The range includes partial-thickness humeral surface tear *(2)*, partial-thickness bursal surface tear *(3)*, full-thickness tear *(4)*, full-thickness tear posteriorly (partial width) *(5)*, full-thickness tear posteriorly (partial width) *(6)*, and full-thickness tear centrally (partial width) *(7)*.

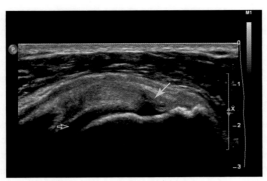

FIGURE 24-44 This bursal side partial-thickness tear *(solid arrow)* has a hypoechoic appearance compared with the surrounding rotator cuff. Fluid, blood, and debris collect in the bursa, producing an anechoic structure *(open arrow)*.

BOX 24-5	Sonographic Criteria for Partial-Thickness Tears

- Critical zone of the supraspinatus imaging with a hypoechoic or hyperechoic focus
- Articular or bursal extension of a hypoechoic lesion on two orthogonal planes
- Hypoechoic or echogenic line within the cuff substance
- Anterior greater tuberosity regional irregularities
- Effusions of the biceps tendon sheath
- Concave subdeltoid bursal surface

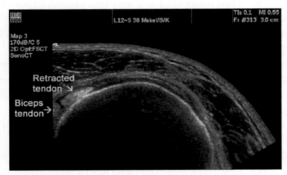

FIGURE 24-45 This complete full-thickness tear (complete rupture) panoramic image shows the biceps tendon retraction in the far left of the image. The deltoid muscle is located anterior to the greater tuberosity.

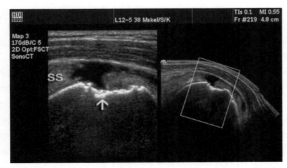

FIGURE 24-46 This magnification and panoramic image shows a complex subdeltoid bursa representing hemorrhage after a rotator cuff tear. The retracted supraspinatus *(SS)* leaves a space for fluid and blood to collect. Note the irregularity of the biceps groove *(arrow)*.

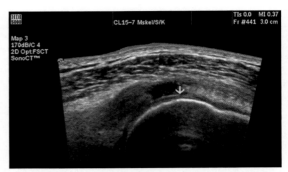

FIGURE 24-47 The cartilage interface sign *(arrow)* is the echogenic anterior linelike border of the cartilage surrounding the humeral head. This is seen through the anechoic or hypoechoic complete rotator cuff tear.

The largest distance measurement is used to classify the tear. The **cartilage interface sign** is the echogenic line on the anterior surface of the cartilage surrounding the humeral head. The four classifications of rotator cuff vary with the author; the criteria listed here are a composite of published categorizations:

1. Partial-thickness tear
2. Small full-thickness tear 1 to 2 cm in AP dimension over the greater tuberosity
3. Large full-thickness tear of 2 to 4 cm
4. Complete tears of greater than 4 cm

During the real-time examination, perform a simple compression test over the area of concern. The normal tendon cannot be compressed; however, the injured tendon flattens as the torn edges move apart. Long-standing cuff injury may also result in atrophy or nonvisualization of a muscle. Rupture of the subscapularis tendon results in retraction of muscle between the scapula and the chest wall. Fatty infiltration of the supraspinatus and infraspinatus fossae changes the echo appearance of this area, giving a false appearance of normalcy and underscoring the importance of scanning the normal contralateral side. The **naked tuberosity sign** is defined as the deltoid muscle on the humeral head; it is seen with a full-thickness tear of the rotator cuff.

Joint effusion around the biceps tendon combined with subacromial-subdeltoid (SASD) bursitis results in the double effusion sign. This is a specific sign of a rotator cuff tear and has been quoted as having a positive predictive value as high as 95%. Arm extension and internal rotation help image lateral greater tuberosity bursal fluid. Light transducer pressure is important because a heavy scan technique may compress the fluid into other nonimaged areas of the joint. This indirect sign is important enough to warrant complementary imaging of arthroscopy or MRI.

Box 24-6 lists the primary and secondary sonographic signs of a full-thickness tear.

Tendinitis

One of the most common tendon abnormalities is inflammation due to age-related elasticity loss, disease such as

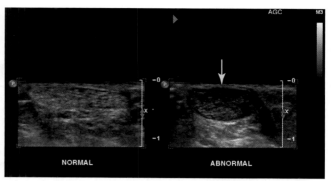

FIGURE 24-49 Comparison of the normal with the injured tendon reveals a focal area of inflammation *(arrow)*.

BOX 24-6 Primary and Secondary Sonographic Signs of a Full-Thickness Tear

Primary Signs
- Naked tuberosity sign
- Tendon edge atrophy in a chronic tear
- Retracted tendons
- Fiber discontinuity with interposed fluid
- A cleft in the cuff of hypoechoic or anechoic echo texture
- Distended SASD bursa in direct communication with the joint
- Compressed tendon
- Absence of the rotator cuff
- Deltoid muscle or SASD bursa herniation into the rotator cuff

Secondary Signs
- Long head biceps tendon effusion
- Double effusion sign
- Erosion of the greater tuberosity of the humerus
- Cartilage interface sign
- Glenohumeral joint effusion

SASD, Subacromial-subdeltoid.

rheumatoid arthritis, overuse, or acute trauma. **Tendinitis** occurs in any tendon, but is seen more often in the shoulder, wrist, heel, and elbow. This inflammatory condition has a characteristic clinical symptom of pain at the tendinous insertion into the bone, a palpable mass in the area of pain, and a decreased range of movement. Treatment is important because chronic tendinitis may lead to weakening of the tendon, resulting in rupture (Figure 24-48).

Sonography images tendinitis well because of changes in the inflamed area in surrounding tissue (Figure 24-49). Acute tendinitis (also called *tenosynovitis*) involves not only the tendon but also the surrounding synovial sheath. Imaging demonstrates an increase in fluid within the synovial sheath, appearing as a halo effect on the transverse image (Figure 24-50). The normal synovial sheath appears as a hypoechoic halo around the tendon. Fluid surrounding the tendon may be anechoic or complex because of debris. To differentiate complex fluid from edema, tap the area or increase the output power to encourage movement of the debris.

A focal or diffuse decrease in echogenicity within the tendon fibers is one sonographic sign of tendinitis. This hypoechoic area also demonstrates increased Doppler flow in the periphery, caused by hyperemia. These areas of injury may be very subtle; comparing the normal side versus the abnormal side helps confirm the diagnosis (see Figure 24-49). Any discrepancy in thickness measurements greater than 1.5 mm is highly suspicious of a focal lesion.

De Quervain's tendinitis is one form of tendinitis with which many sonographers and sonologists may be inherently familiar. This type of tendon inflammation results in symptoms of pain over the thumb side of the wrist and may even result in an audible creaking called *crepitus*. Continuous use of the hand and thumb in a twisting, pinching, or grasping fashion increases the chances of developing swelling on the thumb side of the wrist. During the acute phase of this disease, sonographic imaging of the large abductor pollicis longus and small extensor pollicis brevis tendon reveals hypoechoic tendons and synovium. As the process becomes chronic, fibrosis forms, increasing echogenicity. Fibrosis results in restriction of the tendons through the dorsal compartment of the hand, leading to an inability to move the thumb away from the rest of the hand or to straighten the thumb after grasping.

Box 24-7 lists the sonographic features of tendinitis.

Muscle Tears

Ultrasound demonstrates traumatic muscle injury through its ability to reveal subtle changes in the internal structure of the muscle. A tear is the most common pathologic condition of the muscles of the limbs, although other sites are also affected. A muscle strain related to exertion does not image with ultrasound because of the lack of a lesion; however, imaging of this type of pain-related problem helps differentiate a tear from a strain. Two types of tears occur in the muscle: distraction (indirect) and compression (direct) tears. Abrupt stretching of the muscle beyond the maximum length results in distraction tears. These are usually due to sudden interruption of a movement, such as kicking, or improper body alignment. External force resulting in a crush injury is considered a compression tear. This type of trauma, which results from

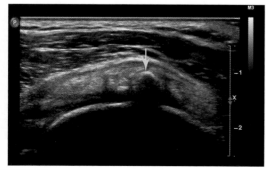

FIGURE 24-48 Intratendinous calcifications *(arrow)*, as seen in this rotator cuff, are a common finding with chronic tendinitis.

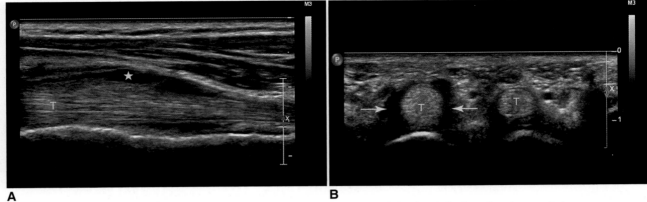

A   B

FIGURE 24-50 A, Tenosynovitis of the extensor tendons of the hand displays the characteristic anechoic fluid *(star)* surrounding the tendon *(T)*. **B,** The fluid within the tendon sheath creates a halo effect *(arrows)* around the tendon on the transverse image.

BOX 24-7	Sonographic Features of Tendinitis

- Focal or diffuse hypoechogenicity
- Enlargement of the tendon in a focal or diffuse pattern
- Echogenic tendon fibrils within the area of inflammation
- Calcifications with chronic tendinitis
- Increased color or power Doppler signal in the periphery
- Coexisting bursitis
- Synovial sheath fluid

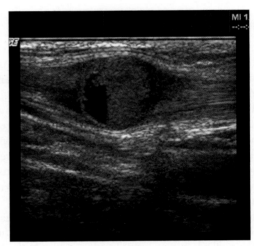

FIGURE 24-51 This intramuscular hematoma images an organized clot with a heterogeneous appearance.

muscle crushing against the underlying bone, ranges from a bruise to a large hematoma. Hematomas also occur with muscle injury and have a variable sonographic appearance. This characteristic of a muscle injury helps determine the extent of the underlying damage. The new hematoma is a hyperechoic mass structure that pushes the muscle fibers apart. Often diffuse and ill defined, the acute hematoma images as an area of enlargement with increased echogenicity within the muscle fibers. Within a few days, the hematoma becomes organized; this often increases detection (Figure 24-51). As the hematoma ages, it liquefies into a hypoechoic to anechoic mass, and a **seroma,** an accumulation of serous fluid within tissue, forms within the defect in a few weeks. Healing of this type of injury results in a hyperechoic fibrous scar or calcifications within the muscle after reabsorption of the serous material. The hematoma that conforms to the fibrous layers may also mimic deep vein thrombosis within the calf or arm muscles.

The sonographic appearance of a muscle tear varies with the type of injury. A tear of the full thickness of the muscle images with the torn muscle end outlined by fluid. The muscle belly will appear thicker with a whorled circular pattern compared with the contralateral side (Figure 24-52). As the hematoma resolves, it becomes smaller, and echogenicity is increased.

A complete tear of a muscle has a straightforward appearance of a retracted hyperechoic muscle surrounded by a hematoma **(clapper-in-the-bell sign).** The partial tear

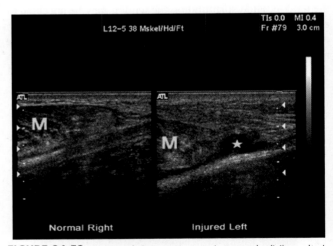

FIGURE 24-52 A tear of the gastrocnemius muscle *(M)* results in a hematoma *(star)* at the area of the injury. Comparison of the normal and injured sides confirms the muscle tear, which may be seen in athletes participating in jumping activities.

TABLE 24-4	Sonographic Appearance of Muscle Tear Grades
Muscle Tear Grade	**Sonographic Appearance**
I (elongation injury)	Normal, flame-shaped focal fiber discontinuity, small hematoma (<1 cm)
II (partial rupture)	<⅓ of muscle fibers disrupted, hematoma <3 cm, interfascial hematoma, hypoechoic gap within the muscle that changes position with transducer pressure
III (complete rupture)	>⅓ rupture of muscle resembling a soft tissue mass, hematoma >3 cm, large interfascial hematoma

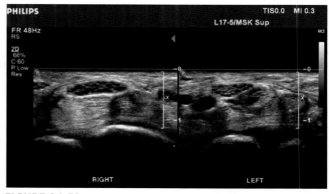

FIGURE 24-53 The right median nerve is notably flattened in this symptomatic patient. The left median nerve is also mildly flattened.

may be as subtle as a discontinuity of the muscle fibers and septa or as obvious as a hematoma with echoic debris. This type of tear may be difficult to separate from the earlier mentioned edge artifact because of the similar appearance. The true torn muscle with irregular margins will maintain the same sonographic appearance at different angles of incidence, whereas the edge artifact will appear only with the 90-degree angle. Examination of the injured muscle includes images with the muscle contracted and at rest in both longitudinal and transverse planes. An area of rupture may also image with a hyperechoic halo surrounding the jagged rupture margins. As the muscle heals, the edges of the tear increase in echogenicity and thickness. The normal muscle architecture becomes evident with healing. The hyperechoic linear, stellate, or nodular scar or an intramuscular cyst provides evidence of an abnormal healing process.

Table 24-4 lists the sonographic appearance of muscle tears by grade.

Carpal Tunnel Syndrome

Carpal tunnel syndrome (CTS) is primarily entrapment or compression neuropathy of the median nerve. Occupations that require repetitive motion produce repetitive stress on the nerve, resulting in the pain and paresthesias characteristic of this syndrome. Continued use of the same muscle group results in hypertrophied muscles, and repeated trauma to the tendon sheath may cause enlargement (traumatic synovitis). This increase in size of the muscle and tendon sheath results in tunnel narrowing (Figure 24-53). We are most familiar with the repetitive causes of CTS, but this group of problems can have other causes, including pregnancy, chronic renal failure, diabetes mellitus, rheumatoid arthritis, amyloidosis, and tenosynovitis. Extrinsic causes include accessory muscles, soft tissue masses, and ganglions.

The patient suffering from CTS typically presents with numbness of the middle and index fingers, weakness or clumsiness of the hand, and pain. The clinical examination is positive for **Tinel's sign** or **Phalen's sign,** and weakness is seen in the affected hand.

BOX 24-8	Sonographic Appearance of Median Nerve Compression

- Focal or diffuse proximal enlargement
- Increased cross-sectional area (>15 mm²)
- Three flattening ratios of the median nerve in distal carpal tunnel
- Tenosynovitis with >4 mm dorsal bowing of the flexor retinaculum

Normal median nerves are elliptical and flatten with distal progression. The transverse scan on a patient with CTS reveals a nerve that flattens in the distal tunnel and nerve swelling in the distal tunnels; at the level of the distal radius and palmar, bowing is seen in the flexor retinaculum. Because of the varied cross-sectional area, calculation of the area is helpful in determining the presence of an increase in the median nerve. This area estimate uses the formula for the ellipse (area = π(D1 × D2)/4). Any cross-sectional area greater than 15 mm² at the level of the proximal tunnel is considered diagnostic for an increased median nerve.

Box 24-8 describes the sonographic appearance of median nerve compression.

 Key Pearls

- Skeletal muscle contains long organized units called muscle fibers.
- Muscles have fibers that run parallel to the bone, have a fan shape, or form a pennate pattern.
- These feather-like muscle patterns run oblique to the long axis of the muscle and are unipennate, bipennate, multipennate, or circumpennate.
- Attachment of the muscle occurs at the proximal and distal portions of the bundle. This attachment, a collection of tough collagenous fibers, is a tendon.
- These attachments may be cordlike or flat sheets called aponeuroses. This type of attachment occurs in flat

Continued

muscles, such as the rectus abdominis in the abdomen. Tendons occur with or without a synovial sheath. This tubular sac surrounding a tendon has two layers.

- The support and strength of a joint are due in part to the ligaments. These short bands of tough fibers connect bones to other bones.
- The saclike structure surrounding joints and tendons that contains a viscous fluid is the bursa. This potential space provides an area for synovial fluid to aid in the reduction of friction between two musculoskeletal structures, such as tendon and bone or ligament and bone.
- Nerves are the conduits for impulses to and from the muscles and the central nervous system.
- Anisotropy occurs when the sound beam misses the transducer on the return because of the curve of the structure. The angle and direction of the reflected beam depend on the angle of incidence.
- The comet-tail artifact is a function of the sound bouncing between two closely placed reflectors within the imaged structure. In the case of a pin surgically placed within a bone, the reflecting surfaces are the anterior and posterior borders of the hardware.
- The bending of the transmitted sound beam to an oblique path occurs often and is seen as an edge artifact (refractile shadowing) on the sonographic image. This change in direction of the sound beam results in a hypoechoic band posterior to the structure.
- Time-of-flight, or speed-of-sound, artifacts occur when the returning sound wave has passed between two tissues with markedly different speeds.
- The Achilles tendon is a large, strong fibrous tendon that connects the gastrocnemius and soleus muscles to the calcaneus. This tendon helps move your foot downward, push off when walking, and rise up on your toes. Injury to this tendon can make it impossible to walk without pain.
- Thompson's test (plantar flexion with squeezing of the calf) may be used to evaluate the integrity of the Achilles tendon.
- The dislocation (also called *subluxation*) of the biceps tendon from the bicipital groove may be due to a problem with the transverse humeral ligament, abnormal development of the bicipital groove or supraspinatus, and/or subscapularis tears.
- Rotator cuff problems may occur as an acute or chronic process. Biceps tendon ruptures, falls, and shoulder dislocations are a few causes of an acute rotator cuff tear.
- One of the most common tendon abnormalities is inflammation due to age-related elasticity loss, disease such as rheumatoid arthritis, overuse, or acute trauma. Tendinitis occurs in any tendon, but is seen more often in the shoulder, wrist, heel, and elbow.

- A complete tear of a muscle has a straightforward appearance of a retracted hyperechoic muscle surrounded by a hematoma (clapper-in-the-bell sign).
- The carpal tunnel is located between the carpal bones and the flexor retinaculum on the palmar side of the wrist. Carpal tunnel syndrome is primarily entrapment or compression neuropathy of the median nerve.

BIBLIOGRAPHY

American Institute of Ultrasound in Medicine: *AIUM practice guidelines for the performance of a shoulder ultrasound examination,* Laurel, MD, 2007, AIUM.

Bianchi S: Ultrasound of the peripheral nerves, *Joint Bone Spine* 75: 643-649, 2008.

Bradley M, O'Donnell P: *Atlas of musculoskeletal ultrasound anatomy,* Cambridge, 2007, Greenwich Medical Media Limited.

Dondelinger R, editor: *Peripheral musculoskeletal ultrasound atlas: a CD-ROM atlas,* New York, 2001, Thieme.

Fessell D, Jacobson J: Ultrasound of the hindfoot and midfoot, *Radiol Clin North Am* 46:1027-1043, 2008.

Finlay K, Friedman L: Ultrasonography of the lower extremity, *Orthop Clin North Am* 37:245-275, 2006.

Grainger A: Internal impingement syndromes of the shoulder, *Semin Musculoskelet Radiol* 12:127-135, 2008.

Harvey C, Hart J, Lloyd C, Barbar S: Musculoskeletal ultrasound in adults, *Br J Hosp Med* 69:M100-M103, 2008.

Jacobson J: *Fundamentals of musculoskeletal ultrasound,* Philadelphia, 2007, Elsevier.

Jamadar D, Jacobson J, Caoili E, et al: Musculoskeletal sonography technique: focused versus comprehensive evaluation, *Am J Roentgenol* 190:5-9, 2008.

Kremkau F: *Diagnostic ultrasound: principles and instruments,* ed 7, Philadelphia, 2006, Saunders.

Lew H, Chen C, Wang T, Chew K: Introduction to musculoskeletal diagnostic ultrasound: examination of the upper limb, *Am J Phys Med Rehabil* 86:310-321, 2007.

Lin J, Fessell D, Jacobson J, et al: An illustrated tutorial of musculoskeletal sonography: part 3, lower extremity, *Am J Roentgenol* 175:1313-1321, 2000.

Ly J, Bui-Mansfield L: Anatomy of and abnormalities associated with Kager's fat pad, *Am J Roentgenol* 182:147-154, 2004.

Moore K, Dalley A, Agur A: *Clinically oriented anatomy,* ed 6, Philadelphia, 2010, Lippincott Williams & Wilkins.

O'Neill J, editor: *Musculoskeletal ultrasound: anatomy and technique,* New York, 2008, Springer.

Peetrons P: Ultrasound of muscles, *Eur Radiol* 12:35-43, 2002.

Schmidt W, Backhaus M: What the practicing rheumatologist needs to know about the technical fundamentals of ultrasonography, *Best Pract Res Clin Rheumatol* 22:981-999, 2008.

Tagliafico A, Rubino M, Autuori A, et al: Wrist and hand ultrasound, *Semin Musculoskelet Radiol* 11:95-104, 2007.

Torriani M, Kattapuram S: Dynamic sonography of the forefoot: the sonographic Mulder sign, *Am J Roentgenol* 180:1121, 2002.

van Holsbeeck M, Introcaso J: *Musculoskeletal ultrasound,* ed 2, St Louis, 2001, Mosby.

Walker F, Cartwright M, Wiesler E, et al: Ultrasound of nerve and muscle, *Clin Neurophysiol* 115:495-507, 2004.

Wiesler E, Chloros G, Cartwright M, et al: The use of diagnostic ultrasound in carpal tunnel syndrome, *J Hand Surg Am* 31:726-732, 2006.

Winter T, Teefey S, Middleton W: Musculoskeletal ultrasound: an update, *Radiol Clin North Am* 39:465-483, 2004.

Zagzebski J: *Essentials of ultrasound physics,* St Louis, 1997, Mosby.

PART IV

Pediatrics

689

Neonatal and Pediatric Abdomen

Kathryn E. Zale

OBJECTIVES

On completion of this chapter, you should be able to:

- Understand the different pediatric stages/ages and how to increase patient cooperation
- List the more common hepatobiliary, pancreatic, and splenic reasons for acute abdominal pain in the pediatric population
- List the more common acquired and hereditary diseases and how pediatric sonography can monitor the associated chronic or malignant processes

- List the causes of jaundice in the neonate and pediatric patient
- Distinguish obstructive from nonobstructive jaundice
- List the common primary hepatic tumors in children
- List the most common gastrointestinal surgical conditions in the pediatric population
- Describe the sonographic appearance of the pathologic conditions discussed in this chapter

OUTLINE

Examination Preparation
Normal Anatomy and Sonographic Findings
Hepatobiliary, Pancreatic, and Splenic Pathology
    Common Presenting Diseases

    Abdominal Tumors
Gastrointestinal Pathology
    Common Surgical Conditions
    Other Surgical Conditions

KEY TERMS

Acholic (stools)
Appendectomy
Appendicitis
Appendicolith
Atretic
Beckwith-Wiedemann syndrome
Biliary atresia
Choledochal cyst
Extracorporeal membrane
  oxygenation (ECMO)
Hemihypertrophy

Hypertrophic pyloric stenosis (HPS)
Hypomotility
Inspissated
Intussusception
Kasai portoenterostomy
McBurney's point
Midgut malrotation
Mucosa
Neonatal intensive care unit (NICU)
Neuroblastoma
Nonalcoholic steatohepatitis

Pancreatic lipomatosis
Projectile vomiting
Pyloric canal
Pyloromyotomy
Scintigraphy
Short bowel syndrome
Target (donut) sign
Ultrasound first
Umbilical vein catheter
Ventriculoperitoneal shunt
Wilms' tumor (nephroblastoma)

Sonography is often the first imaging procedure used to evaluate the neonatal and pediatric abdomen. Pediatric sonography is a powerful imaging specialty, providing excellent visualization of an infant's or child's anatomy while not subjecting them to ionizing radiation, iodized contrast material, or anesthesia. Furthermore, it is portable, inexpensive, relatively painless, and generally well tolerated. It is important to relay that children often have different diseases than adults with their own features; therefore this chapter focuses on the more common, as well as critical, abdominal

diagnoses specific to the pediatric population. Abdominal conditions discussed here are primarily focused on hepatobiliary and gastrointestinal disorders, but some pancreatic and splenic diseases are also discussed. Hepatobiliary, splenic, and pancreatic pathology is presented as nonneoplastic (a broad spectrum from abdominal pain, acquired and hereditary diseases, to neonatal jaundice) and neoplastic (liver masses). Common surgical conditions of the gastrointestinal system, such as appendicitis, intussusception, and hypertrophic pyloric stenosis, are also covered. Many of these diagnoses will require surgical treatment, and using the **ultrasound first** approach may, in some cases, obviate the need for more testing or imaging. Finally, although this section focuses on diseases specific to the neonate and child, pediatric sonographers must also have in-depth comprehension of adult pathology. Obesity is not just a challenge among the adult population, and the increase of childhood obesity may come along with the earlier onset of adult disease processes (e.g., nonalcoholic fatty liver disease). Additionally, pediatric hospitals may follow patients affected by childhood diseases for life (e.g., cystic fibrosis and myelomeningoceles).

EXAMINATION PREPARATION

Gaining the trust of the patient and the patient's family is critical to facilitating the examination. Patience and preparation cannot be stressed enough. It is imperative to remember that children are not just small adults, and one way to prepare is to be mindful of the patient's developmental stage (mentally, physically, and emotionally), along with a basic understanding of his or her normal age-group. With the aim of minimizing patient discomfort and optimizing image quality, the information listed in Table 25-1 should be kept in mind. Also, with increasing conditions such as attention-deficit/hyperactivity

TABLE 25-1	Pediatric Stages, Ages, and Tips	
Stage	**Age**	**Scanning Considerations**
Preterm infants	Less than 37 weeks of gestation	• Use 9–12 MHz curved array or linear transducer • Extra infection control measures are critical in this delicate population; use gel packets if possible to decrease contamination risks • Susceptible to hypothermia; always use warm gel, but be sure it is not too hot • Remove gel as soon as possible; it gets cold quickly • Keep preemie securely wrapped in a blanket when not scanning • Observe and note any and all monitors in the **neonatal intensive care unit (NICU)**; always ask nurse for permission before starting

Neonates
 	
Infants
	First 28 days of life
	First year of life after the first 28 days
		• Use 7.5–9 MHz curved array or linear transducer
		• Use warm gel and be sure it is not too hot
		• Wrap blankets around infant as needed
		• Use good infection control techniques
		• Let mother hold child until calm
		• Neonates and infants up to 6 months old
		  • Use pacifier, cuddling, or changing diaper when necessary to keep comfortable
		  • Feeding okay if not contraindicated or after biliary evaluation and pancreas completed in full abdominal study
		  • Glycogen and water bottles should be handy (dip binky into sugar solution; may repeat while scanning until able to give milk/formula)
		  • Palpate abdomen when muscles are relaxed
		  • Have plenty of distractions ready (e.g., noisy bright-colored toys, keys, singing)
		• Older infants over 6 months old (in addition to above infant information)
		  • Separation and stranger anxiety developing, keep parents near, examine on parent's lap if necessary
		  • Smile and talk to infant throughout examination

Toddlers/preschoolers	Between 1 and 5 years old	• Use 5–7.5 MHz linear, curved array, or sector • Tell the child what you are doing at each step • Provide positive feedback when cooperating • Give them choices when possible; may prefer the cold gel • Let the child touch the gel beforehand • Offer to scan favorite doll/teddy first to reduce anxiety • Have plenty of distractions ready (e.g., stickers, televisions, mobiles, or ultrasound itself—"watch the movies") • If toddler becomes too stressed, give the child a rest • Feasible to allow child to lie next to mother on stretcher to continue examination
School-age children	Between 6 and 12 years old	• Use 5–7.5 MHz curved array or sector • Usually understand and cooperative at this age; explain what you are doing and why • Distract with questions about favorite color, pets, classes, etc. • Provide positive feedback when cooperating • Develop modesty at this age, so be sure to explain procedure before child undresses
Teenagers/adolescents	Between 12 and 18 years old	• Use 2–5 MHz curved array or sector • Provide privacy for undressing if required • Provide chaperone when parent or accompanying adult is unavailable • Adolescents have a lot of concerns about their developing bodies; provide reassurance when appropriate

TABLE 25-2	Pediatric Considerations
Condition/Issue	**Considerations**
Attention-deficit/hyperactivity disorder (ADHD)	One of the most common childhood disorders, average onset is 7 years old, affects 9% of children ages 13–18, with boys at risk 4× > girls. Children with ADHD suffer from inattentiveness, hyperactivity, and impulsivity. Be clear and consistent, focus on the positive, providing praise/rewards when following the rules.
Autism spectrum disorder (ASD)	Occurs in 1/68 children in the United States, affecting boys 4–5× > girls. Inhibits a child's ability to interact socially, usually plays alone or shows little eye contact. Usually diagnosed by age 3, though sometimes later. No "mold" most with ASD fit into, so since different from child to child, it is important to carefully observe the parents' interaction and be very clear in directions and sensitive to touching issues often displayed.
Family dynamics/structure	It is well known the nuclear family is on the decline, and many different family dynamics/structures exist. Never just assume the person with the child is the parent/grandparent, etc., and be respectful of all family types.
Childhood abuse	May take on the form of sexual abuse, physical abuse, or neglect. Physical abuse and neglect by caregivers has not declined in recent years, among some trends showing overall child abuse is down. As a health care worker you are *obligated under law* to report ANY suspicion of abuse.
Food allergies	Allergies are on the rise along with roughly 30%–35% of all children affected. As health care workers with direct contact with children it is especially important to wash hands after handling potential allergens and keep our clothes clean of them as well; even a small amount of peanut dust may send a child who is very allergic to peanuts into anaphylactic shock.
Childhood obesity	Increasing prevalence—has doubled in children and quadrupled in adolescents in the past 30 years. In children ages 6–11 years old obesity rates rose from 7% in 1980 to 18% in 2012. At increased risk for cardiovascular disease. Greater risk for bone and joint problems, sleep apnea, and social and psychological issues stemming from stigmatization and poor self-esteem.
Critically ill and dying infant/child	Perhaps the most difficult part of scanning in pediatrics is dealing with the critically ill or dying patient. In these cases it becomes increasingly important to have a child-centered approach and respect for the family, keeping in mind they are under an immense amount of stress. It is also equally important to acknowledge one's own feelings in order to perform examinations without them interfering in providing quality patient care.

disorder (ADHD), autism, Down syndrome, cerebral palsy, and childhood obesity among our society, it is important to take these considerations, and others, to heart when dealing with children. Table 25-2 provides more information on some of these issues in pediatrics.

The sonographer should first allow sufficient time to calmly explain the examination to the parents and to the child who is old enough to comprehend the proceedings. Recruiting the parent(s) is an invaluable resource and can help reassure and quiet the patient. Therefore parents are highly encouraged to be present during the examination. Talking to the patient in age-appropriate terms will also facilitate the examination. Speaking with a soft voice, one should keep steady eye contact and concentrate on the child. Additionally, it is best to make eye contact on the child's level if possible, as towering over them (and wearing white coats) can be intimidating. It is also best to start the examination in a well-lit room, as not to scare the child. Sedation and immobilization techniques are generally not required or recommended. Toys, books, keys, televisions, mobiles, and a variety of other distracting devices can help to quiet the frightened young child. A good attitude and a dose of fun can go a long way too. A pacifier may likewise serve well when examining infants. Formula feeding is not recommended if the child is a surgical candidate. Some laboratories offer glucose "sugar" water or Pedialyte feedings when examining a neonate for pyloric stenosis.

Patient preparation will depend on the type of abdominal examination being performed and emergent status. In order to image the biliary system completely, it is recommended that feeding be withheld for a short time according to the age of the patient (Box 25-1). Adequate distention of the urinary bladder is also desirable in many situations (see Box 25-1). This not only allows assessment of the bladder itself but also facilitates identification of dilated distal ureters, free peritoneal fluid, the pelvic reproductive organs, and pelvic masses. A urine-filled bladder may also help localize gastrointestinal abnormalities, such as appendicitis and intussusception. In females, pelvic structures are examined with a well-filled, but not overly distended, bladder.

BOX 25-1	Pediatric Ultrasound Examination Prep

Abdominal Ultrasound
Nothing by mouth (NPO), age specific (see below)
0–2 years = NPO 4 hours
3–8 years = NPO 6–8 hours
>9 years = NPO 8–10 hours

Pelvic Ultrasound
Full urinary bladder
<3 years: Push fluids 1 hour before examination.
3–6 years: Drink 8 oz of fluid 1 hour before examination and encourage child not to void.
5–12 years: Drink 12–16 oz of fluid 1 hour before and refrain from voiding.
>13 years: Drink 32 oz of fluid 1 hour before examination and refrain from voiding.

Pediatric scanning will require some technical changes as well. Because imaging infants and children involves countless different body habitus, it is not unusual to utilize a wide array of probe frequencies and footprints. The provided information on transducer selection is merely a guideline, and the highest-frequency transducer and smallest footprint for the area being imaged is best. Avoid "shooting the table" or including nondiagnostic information posterior to the spine; that 5 MHz just used on an adolescent will provide poor diagnostic images on an infant. However, if the optimal frequency is unavailable use sequential focusing and zoom instead of decreasing depth for better resolution. And, as always, optimize. To improve child cooperation, it is usually best to put the gel on the probe instead of directly on the patient. It will also be necessary to learn how to acquire images quickly when imaging infants and young children, and cine clips can serve well in depicting difficult anatomy or pathology in the unruly child. Protocol scanning is not always advised, or possible, in the case of a critically ill preemie or uncooperative child. Careful consideration is necessary to determine a child's patience and/or ability to withstand an examination; therefore modifying protocols to tailor to these individuals is necessary. Finally, before beginning any pediatric examination, a review of the medical record and any previous imaging (paying close attention to ultrasound transducer selection and settings) will aid in providing a more thorough and time-efficient study.

NORMAL ANATOMY AND SONOGRAPHIC FINDINGS

In contrast to many adult abdominal ultrasound examinations, the neonatal/pediatric evaluation is rarely limited to the right upper quadrant, and a full abdominal examination is in order. A limited abdominal ultrasound examination is relegated for follow-up examinations or the emergent acute abdomen for gastrointestinal conditions. As an example to underscore the importance of a complete abdominal evaluation, palpation alone is not accurate enough to diagnose an enlarged liver or spleen; and hepatosplenomegaly is a common presentation for newly diagnosed leukemia, the most common childhood cancer, among many other conditions. Ultrasound is the modality of choice to document organ size and other abnormalities in the pediatric abdomen. Therefore it is important to be well acquainted with the normal pediatric abdomen, as well as document organ growth and properly utilize size charts.

In the upper abdomen the pancreas should be examined for normal size and echotexture, without evidence of peripancreatic fluid or adenopathy, dilation of the distal common bile duct, or dilation of the pancreatic duct (Figure 25-1). The pancreatic head should measure 1.0 to 2.2 cm; the body, 0.4 to 1.0 cm; and the tail, 0.8 to 1.8 cm. The pancreatic duct should not exceed 1 to 2 mm. The size of the pancreas should increase with the child's age (Table 25-3). The normal texture is homogenous and is hypoechoic compared with the normal

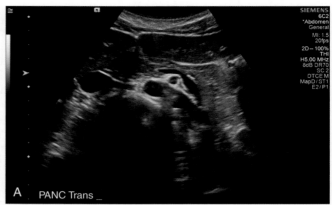

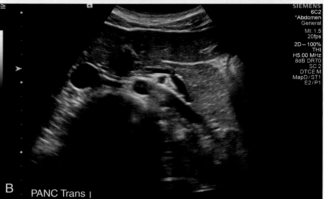

FIGURE 25-1 Normal pediatric pancreas seen in transverse plane. Evaluation of the pancreas is unremarkable without evidence of focal mass. **A,** Uncinate process, head, and body of pancreas are well visualized. **B,** Tail of the pancreas seen in its entirety. (*Images courtesy Nationwide Children's Hospital, Columbus, OH.*)

TABLE 25-3	Normal Dimensions of the Pancreas as a Function of Age		
Maximum Anteroposterior (AP) Dimensions of Pancreas in cm (standard deviation).			
Patient Age	**Head**	**Body**	**Tail**
Neonates	1.0 (0.4)	0.6 (0.2)	1.0 (0.4)
1 mo–1 yr	1.5 (0.5)	0.8 (0.3)	1.2 (0.4)
1–5 yr	1.7 (0.3)	1.0 (0.2)	1.8 (0.4)
5–10 yr	1.6 (0.4)	1.0 (0.3)	1.8 (0.4)
10–19 yr	2.0 (0.5)	1.1 (0.3)	2.0 (0.4)

Data from Siegel MJ, Martin KW, Worthington JL: Normal and abnormal pancreas in children: US studies, *Radiology* 165:15-18, 1987.

liver texture, as little fatty tissue has yet invaded the islets of Langerhans.

The size and texture of the liver should be evaluated (Figure 25-2). The right hepatic lobe should not extend more than 1 cm below the costal margin in a young infant without pulmonary hyperaeration and should not extend below the right costal margin in older infants and children. The echogenicity is normally low to medium homogeneity with clear definition of the portal venous vasculature. The

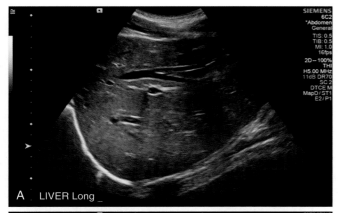

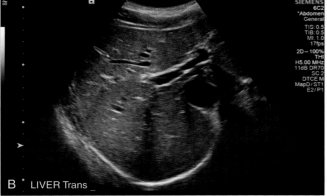

FIGURE 25-2 **Normal pediatric liver.** The liver is normal in size and contour without focal mass or marginal irregularity. **A,** Longitudinal right lobe of the liver showing normal hepatic veins. **B,** Transverse right lobe of the liver showing right and left portal vein split, and gallbladder in transverse. *(Images courtesy Nationwide Children's Hospital, Columbus, OH.)*

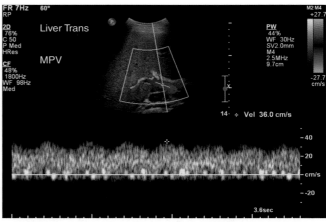

FIGURE 25-3 **Normal pediatric portal vein.** The portal vein is normal in size with hepatopedal phasic flow patterns shown with color Doppler and angle-corrected pulsed Doppler. *(Image courtesy Nationwide Children's Hospital, Columbus, OH.)*

BOX 25-2   Normal Sonographic Measurements

Pancreas (Size Increases with Age)
- Head: 1.0–2.2 cm
- Body: 0.4–1.0 cm
- Tail: 0.8–1.8 cm
- Duct: 1–3 mm (see text for specific age ranges)

Liver
- Infant: right lobe should not extend >1 cm below costal margin
- Older infants and children: right lobe should not extend below right costal margin

Portal Vein Diameter
- Neonates: 3–5 mm
- Children <10 yr: 8.5 mm
- Children >10 yr: 10 mm
- Adolescents up to age 20: 7–13 mm

Biliary Ducts
- Neonates: CBD <1 mm
- Infants (up to 1 yr): CBD <2 mm
- Older children (1–10 yr): CBD <4 mm
- Adolescents: CBD <6–7 mm

Gallbladder Length
- Infants (under 1 yr): 1.5–3 cm
- Older children: 3–7 cm

Spleen Length (Upper limits)
- Small-for-date neonates: 3.0 cm (mean)
- Infants
  - (0–3 mo): 6.0 cm
  - (3–6 mo): 6.5 cm
  - (3–12 mo): 7.0 cm
- Toddlers
  - (1–2 yr): 8.0 cm
  - (2–4 yr): 9.0 cm
- Children
  - (4–6 yr): 10.0 cm
  - (6–8 yr) 10.5 cm
  - (8–10 yr): 11.0 cm
  - (10–12 yr): 11.5 cm
- Older children (>12 yr): 12.0 cm

---

right hemidiaphragm and pleural space should be evaluated as well.

The diameter of the portal vein is helpful in determining the presence of portal hypertension (Figure 25-3) and increases in size with age and weight (Box 25-2). Color, as well as pulsed-wave, Doppler should be used to determine flow direction and patency. Pulsatility of the portal vein is reported as being 94% sensitive for identifying portal hypertension, and a to-and-fro or hepatofugal flow pattern may emerge. Portal hypertension may also be suspected when portal flow peak systolic velocities are low (drop below 20 cm/sec). Elevated peak systolic velocities in the hepatic artery with velocities greater than 3 times the portal vein flow may also indicate portal hypertension in the pediatric patient.

Careful evaluation of the biliary system should be made to exclude ductal dilation (Figure 25-4). The common bile duct should measure less than 1 mm in neonates, less than 2 mm in infants up to 1 year old, less than 4 mm in older children, and less than 7 mm in adolescents and adults (see Box 25-2). The gallbladder size and wall thickness should be assessed. In infants under 1 year of age the gallbladder length is 1.5 to 3 cm, and in older children it is 3 to 7 cm. The length of the gallbladder should not exceed the length of the kidney.

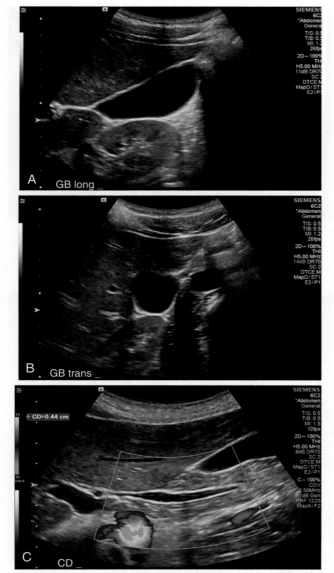

FIGURE 25-4 Normal pediatric gallbladder and common bile duct. Gallbladder is unremarkable without wall thickening, pericholecystic fluid, or cholelithiasis. No ductal dilation is seen. **A,** Longitudinal gallbladder. **B,** Transverse gallbladder. **C,** Common bile duct measurement is within normal limits for this adolescent patient. *(Images courtesy Nationwide Children's Hospital, Columbus, OH.)*

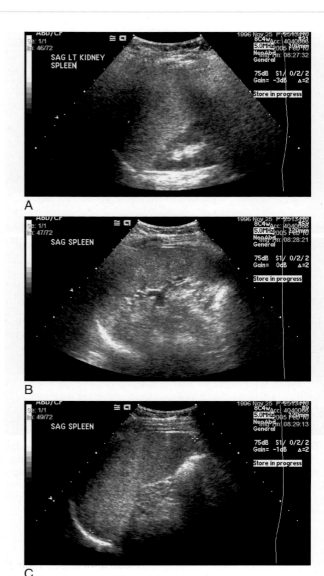

FIGURE 25-5 Normal pediatric spleen. The spleen is normal in size, contour with echogenicity measuring 10.9 cm in greatest pole-to-pole diameter, within this patient's normal age limits. No focal masses are seen. **A,** Sagittal spleen and left kidney. **B,** Sagittal spleen with hilum. **C,** Sagittal spleen with measurement of the long axis.

Careful evaluation of the normal gallbladder should show a smooth-walled anechoic structure without internal echoes. Pericholecystic fluid should not be present.

The splenic size and texture should be evaluated (Figure 25-5). The upper limits of normal splenic length range from 6.0 cm in infants less than 3 months old to 12 cm in children over 12 years of age. Polysplenia, as with any anatomic anomaly, should be ruled out. The left hemidiaphragm and pleural space should be evaluated when viewing the spleen as well.

Finally, the retroperitoneal area should be closely evaluated throughout the abdominal sonographic evaluation, as most malignant abdominal masses arise from the retroperitoneum in both infants and children. The inferior vena cava

(IVC) and aorta vessels are documented. Proper positioning and relationship should be established to rule out situs inversus and both vessels should be free of any thrombus. This is a critical finding. Lymph nodes are not normally visualized and abnormal when detected. They can be indicated in lymphomas, as well as malignant abdominal and pelvic masses.

In the lower abdomen normal bowel peristalsis should be observed, bowel should not appear thickened (2 to 3 mm in distended bowel and 4 to 6 mm in collapsed bowel), and it should be free of any pelvic mass or free fluid. Free fluid is often abnormal, with the exception of a little free fluid in the menstruating female or a patient with a **ventriculoperitoneal shunt.** If a shunt is present, the tip should be documented to rule out development of an abdominal cerebrospinal fluid pseudocyst.

HEPATOBILIARY, PANCREATIC, AND SPLENIC PATHOLOGY

A wide variety of pathologies may be seen within the pediatric abdomen and it is important to remember that the cause may arise from any of the body's systems, so what we rule out can be just as important as what we rule in. Given the wide range of ages and developmental stages within the pediatric population, it is vital to be cognizant of the general disease processes as well as the sonographic appearance of the presenting pathology.

Nonneoplastic disease entities of the neonatal/pediatric abdomen may be acute, chronic, congenital, or acquired. The presenting clinical issue and associated underlying causes will be presented in this section.

Common Presenting Diseases

Acute Abdominal Pain. Acute abdominal pain is one of the most common complaints among children, and a very usual reason for the pediatric abdominal ultrasound. There are many underlying surgical and nonsurgical conditions, which vary according to age, associated symptoms, and pain location. The most common nonsurgical condition is gastroenteritis, and the most common surgical condition is appendicitis. Gastrointestinal conditions (see Gastrointestinal Pathology later in this chapter) are often the underlying cause, but other reasons for acute abdominal pain in the child include trauma, pancreatitis, splenic sequestration, and choledocholithiasis.

Trauma. Accidents (unintentional injuries) are the leading cause of mortality for children in all age-groups (followed by congenital malformations, deformations, chromosomal abnormalities, and homicide in ages 1 to 4 years old and cancer and suicide in ages 5 to 14 years old). Blunt abdominal trauma (caused by motor vehicle accidents, falling down, and child abuse) is more common than penetrating trauma and may cause laceration of abdominal organs, bowel perforation, ischemia of organs due to vascular injury, and intramural hematoma. In neonates, traumatic delivery or resuscitation efforts may cause liver or splenic injury. Children have incomplete rib ossification, making the liver the most commonly injured abdominal organ (versus spleen in adults); and in 50% of cases involving the liver, other abdominal organs are affected too, especially the spleen. The pancreas (Figure 25-6) and duodenum may also be injured.

The focused assessment with sonography in trauma (FAST) ultrasound examination is often used in the immediate detection of fluid, and then nearly 97% of children are treated conservatively through careful follow-up imaging. Ultrasound can play an important role in this follow-up imaging in children. Hepatic subcapsular hematomas may be observed, as well as parenchymal hematomas, lacerations, and fractures. Liver lacerations will usually appear slightly echogenic in the acute stage and will become more hypoechoic or cystic in the following days. Pseudoaneurysms and bilomas may also develop as later complications. Complex appearance, gas due to tissue necrosis, and calcifications may also be depicted sonographically in an aging liver hematoma.

Pancreatitis. Acute and chronic pancreatitis in childhood can cause significant morbidity and mortality. Often, acute inflammation is due to trauma or structural abnormalities, multisystemic disease, or drugs and toxins, but in 23% of children the cause is idiopathic. According to American College of Radiology (ACR) guidelines, ultrasound should be the first imaging modality in acute pancreatitis. It allows for the exclusion of extrapancreatic disease, such as gallstones or choledocholithiasis. The most useful diagnostic finding is an enlarged pancreatic duct, which should measure less than 1.5 mm (1 to 6 years old), less than 1.9 mm (7 to 12 years old), and less than 2.2 mm (13 to 18 years old). Pancreatic enlargement or swelling is present in up to half of patients with acute pancreatitis. Peripancreatic fluid and fluid collections (pseudocyst), as well as peripancreatic fatty infiltration, may be present.

Chronic inflammation of the pancreas is more often caused by cystic fibrosis (see Acquired and Hereditary Diseases, following), fibrosing pancreatitis, hereditary chronic pancreatitis, or inborn errors of metabolism. In chronic pancreatitis, the pancreas may appear echogenic with calcifications (both shadowing and nonshadowing).

Splenic Sequestration Syndrome. Splenic sequestration syndrome presents with rapid splenic enlargement and an acute fall in hematocrit. It causes extreme pain and, if left untreated, can be fatal. Often it occurs in children under 2 years old with sickle cell disease, but it can occur in older children with blood disorders or neonates/infants on **extracorporeal membrane oxygenation (ECMO).** Ultrasound will reveal a grossly enlarged spleen with peripheral low echogenicity foci (corresponding hemorrhage on magnetic resonance imaging), but with internal blood flow preserved.

Choledocholithiasis. The incidence of gallstones in children, though still uncommon, has been increasing over the past few decades. The widespread use of ultrasound in detecting asymptomatic cholelithiasis and increasing childhood obesity are key reasons for this trend. In neonates and infants causes of cholelithiasis or choledocholithiasis include sepsis, total parenteral nutrition, and diuretics. Fetal gallstones, however, will often resolve spontaneously within the first year of life. In older children causes include hemolytic anemia (such as sickle cell disease), cystic fibrosis, and small bowel diseases. Echogenic foci may be detected within the lumen of the gallbladder or anywhere along the biliary tract. Distal ductal dilation may be present as well. Documenting gallstone mobility is encouraged. Also, color Doppler may aid in producing "twinkle" artifact in a nonmobile focus, as up to half of pediatric biliary stones are calcified, especially among those with hemolytic disease.

Acquired and Hereditary Diseases. Often, acquired and hereditary diseases need to be carefully monitored or screened in the pediatric population. Some hereditary diseases may predispose an infant or child to developing certain cancers (e.g., Beckwith-Wiedemann syndrome's increased risk of hepatoblastoma) or chronic conditions (cystic fibrosis's high association with chronic pancreatitis). Common abdominal

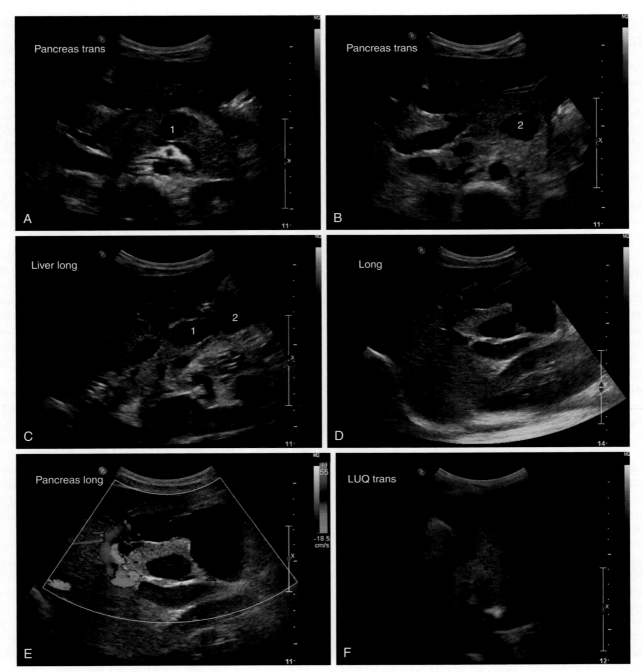

FIGURE 25-6 Transected pancreas. An 11-year-old having increasing abdominal pain, not easing with pain medication, several days after blunt trauma to the abdomen from handlebars on her bike. Fluid collections are seen within the pancreas, as well as peripancreatic and perisplenic fluid. Gallbladder with sludge was noted and no free fluid was seen in the lower quadrants. **A,** Transverse view of the pancreas showing first fluid collection in the body (labeled *1*). **B,** Transverse view, more inferior and lateral depicting a second fluid collection (labeled *2*). **C,** Longitudinal view of both fluid collections in pancreas (labels *1* and *2*). **D,** Large (7.5 cm by 4.7 cm) peripancreatic fluid collection seen in inferior longitudinal view. **E,** Peripancreatic fluid with Color Doppler. **F,** Perisplenic fluid in transverse view. *(Images courtesy Nationwide Children's Hospital, Columbus, OH.)*

disorders associated with acquired and hereditary disease in children are described here.

Hepatobiliary Disease

Fatty Liver. Once only seen in adults, nonalcoholic fatty liver disease (NAFLD) is now considered one of the most prevalent chronic liver diseases in children, with an estimated 3% to 10% of the pediatric population affected (mostly adolescents). This is directly linked to increased obesity among children and resulting fatty deposition within the liver. It may lead to **nonalcoholic steatohepatitis.** Sonographically, the same four general categories of fatty liver classification (absent, mild, moderate, and severe) are used in children, as with adults. Elastography is becoming increasingly used in conjunction with the standard liver sonogram in pediatrics to assess liver tissue stiffness. This can aid in selecting children who should undergo a liver biopsy, which is the gold standard to definitively diagnose and determine NAFLD extent.

Cirrhosis and Portal Hypertension. Although less common than their adult counterparts, cirrhosis and portal hypertension are found in the pediatric population. The cause of cirrhosis in children is often divided into four categories: (1) biliary (biliary atresia, Alagille syndrome, alpha-1 antitrypsin deficiency, and cystic fibrosis); (2) metabolic (Wilson's disease); (3) postnecrotic cirrhosis (neonatal, postviral, or autoimmune hepatitis); and (4) unknown causes. Sonographically this disease displays the same adult characteristics, such as abnormal liver surface, with increased echogenicity and nodular changes of the parenchyma being the most specific. If portal hypertension is suspected, it is imperative to Doppler not only the main portal vein, but also the right and left intrahepatic veins, as hepatofugal flow may only be involved with one of these.

Cholangitis. Infection of the biliary tract can occur in children and is often associated with congenital or immune-related biliary abnormalities and immunodeficiency states. It may also result from surgery, such as correction of biliary atresia (Kasai procedure) or liver transplantation. Often the cause is bacterial, but it may be parasitic, viral, or fungal in an immune-suppressed child. Ultrasound is the modality of choice and it is used to identify underlying structural bile duct abnormalities or identify causes of bile flow obstruction.

Primary sclerosing cholangitis, a distinct type, is increasingly being found in children. It is a chronic condition with unknown cause, although 70% to 80% of those afflicted also have inflammatory bowel disease. This progressive cholestatic disease may result in cirrhosis, portal hypertension, and ultimately liver failure. Intrahepatic or extrahepatic duct dilation may be present on ultrasound, along with cirrhotic liver changes and splenomegaly.

Pancreatic Disease. Pancreatic pathology in children may be associated with Beckwith-Wiedemann syndrome, von Hippel–Lindau disease, autosomal dominant polycystic kidney disease, cystic fibrosis, and Shwachman-Diamond syndrome. The last two often present with **pancreatic lipomatosis** and resulting pancreatic insufficiency. Beckwith-Wiedemann syndrome is associated with pancreaticoblastomas (solid malignant tumor), whereas von Hippel–Lindau and polycystic kidney disease present with associated cysts or lesions within the pancreas.

Cystic Fibrosis. Cystic fibrosis (CF) is an autosomal recessive disease involving abnormal chloride metabolism, which often affects exocrine glands (i.e., sweat glands, pancreatic exocrine glands) leading to increased viscosity. As with many inherited disorders, many different organs and systems can be involved. CF frequently affects the biliary epithelium resulting in end-stage liver cirrhosis and pancreatic

atrophy. Serious liver disease affects 13% to 25% of children with CF; however, pancreatic disease is more prevalent in children, affecting 85% to 90% of CF pediatric patients. As normal pancreatic tissue is replaced by fatty tissue, due to blocked ducts, ultrasound often reveals increased echogenicity. Cyst formation, calcifications, and atrophy of the pancreas may also be seen.

Splenic Disease. The spleen is implemented in many acquired and hereditary childhood diseases, as it is part of the body's immune response and blood formation. Splenomegaly may be seen in children affected by diseases such as mononucleosis, hemolytic anemias (sickle cell disease), leukemias (Figure 25-7), lymphomas, liver cirrhosis, and cat-scratch fever or disease.

Cat-Scratch Disease. Cat-scratch disease is a bacterial disease spread by cats when a child is scratched or bitten, and often appears within 1 to 2 weeks following the incident. Although self-limiting, fever and lymphadenopathy occur. Abdominal reactive lymph nodes may be seen with ultrasound. Both hepatic and splenic round, hypoechoic, well-defined nodules are often visualized (Figure 25-8). Histologically, the lesions may be vascular proliferative lesions (peliosis) or necrotizing granulomatous lesions. It may take a month or two for them to resolve radiographically. Contrast-enhanced ultrasound may help better define such lesions. A thorough history is important to rule out other more serious etiologies, such as malignancies (lymphoma or metastasis) or granulomatous disease (tuberculosis, sarcoidosis). Previous contact with a cat or kitten is vital to the diagnosis, so a thorough history is important.

Neonatal Jaundice. During the first few weeks of life many neonates, especially preemies, experience transient jaundice due to an excess of bilirubin at birth and a liver not quite ready for the task of conjugating it. Unconjugated hyperbilirubinemia occurs in approximately 60% of normal term infants and in 80% of preterm infants. However, persistent jaundice beyond the 2-week postdelivery date is abnormal. The cause may be difficult to

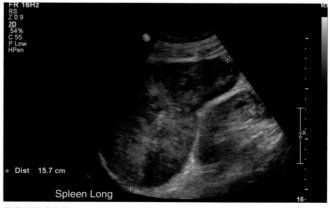

FIGURE 25-7 Splenomegaly in 17-year-old male with leukemia. Intensive care unit patient with acute lymphoblastic or lymphocytic leukemia (ALL), the most common childhood leukemia, presents with portal hypertension and splenomegaly; spleen measures 15.7 cm in longitudinal dimension. The diseased spleen is enlarged and grossly inhomogeneous. *(Image courtesy Nationwide Children's Hospital, Columbus, OH.)*

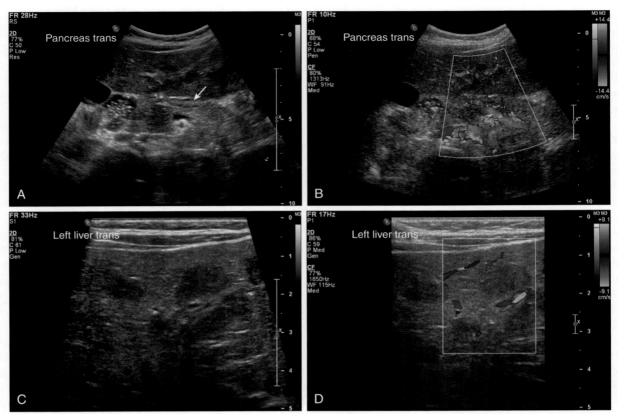

FIGURE 25-8 Cat-scratch disease. A, Reactive lymph node anterior to pancreas in transverse view *(arrow)* in a 2-year-old patient with cat-scratch disease. **B,** Color Doppler of peripancreatic node. **C,** Multiple round, hypoechoic nodules seen throughout liver, shown here with high-frequency transducer. **D,** Color Doppler of liver lesion. *(Images courtesy Nationwide Children's Hospital, Columbus, OH.)*

define because clinical and laboratory features may be similar in hepatocellular jaundice (often treated medically) and obstructive jaundice (usually necessitates surgery). Sonographic evaluation, however, may differentiate between obstructive versus nonobstructive jaundice. In the case of bile obstruction, biliary atresia, or metabolic diseases it is important that the neonate is treated early before cirrhosis occurs, and a diagnosis must be made soon after delivery. Furthermore, jaundice may be caused by either extrahepatic or intrahepatic obstruction to bile flow. The extrahepatic obstruction in the neonate includes conditions such as choledochal cyst, biliary atresia, or spontaneous perforation of the bile ducts. The intrahepatic causes of neonatal jaundice include hepatitis and metabolic disease. Systemic diseases that cause cholestasis include heart failure, shock, sepsis, neonatal lupus, histiocytosis, and severe hemolytic disease.

Sonography may be ordered to differentiate among the three most common causes for neonatal jaundice: hepatitis, biliary atresia, and choledochal cyst. With each of these conditions, the liver appears coarse and echogenic on ultrasound; various other conditions (e.g., hepatic inflammatory, obstructive, and metabolic processes) have a similar sonographic appearance. Other studies, such as hepatic **scintigraphy** or liver biopsy, may be necessary to further narrow down the differential considerations. Ultrasound is useful in demonstrating the gallbladder with **inspissated**

bile and biliary duct stones. Jaundice in infants and children may be due to cirrhosis, benign strictures, and neoplastic processes.

A number of differentials for persistent neonatal jaundice are possible, so clinical and laboratory workup is necessary to identify the underlying infectious, metabolic, or structural causes. Laboratory workup may include liver function tests, evaluation for hepatitis B antigen, TORCH infections, which include toxoplasmosis, other (syphilis, varicella-zoster, parvovirus B19), rubella, cytomegalovirus (CMV), and herpes to rule out maternal disease, workup for sepsis, metabolic screening, and sweat test. See Table 25-4 for clinical findings, sonographic findings, and differential considerations for the diseases and conditions discussed here.

Causes and Diagnosis of Neonatal Jaundice. The three most common causes of jaundice in the neonatal period are hepatitis, biliary atresia, and choledochal cyst.

Neonatal Hepatitis. Neonatal hepatitis is an infection of the liver that occurs within the first 3 months after birth. There are a number of causes of neonatal hepatitis, including infections, metabolic disorders, familial recurrent cholestasis, metabolism errors, or idiopathic causes. The infection reaches the liver through the placenta, via the vagina from infected maternal secretions, or through catheters or blood transfusions. Transplacental infection occurs most readily during the third

TABLE 25-4	Most Common Causes of Neonatal Jaundice	
Clinical Findings	Sonographic Findings	Differential Considerations
Neonatal Hepatitis		
Hepatomegaly	Liver normal or enlarged	Biliary atresia
Jaundice when obstruction is present	Liver parenchyma echogenic with decreased vascularization of peripheral portal venous structures When severe, gallbladder may be small in size	
Biliary Atresia		
Persistent jaundice Acholic stools Dark urine Distended abdomen	Liver may be enlarged Echogenicity of liver parenchyma may be normal or increased with slight decrease in visualization of portal structures Intrahepatic ducts not dilated Polysplenia may be present	Neonatal hepatitis
Choledochal Cyst		
Jaundice Pain Palpable mass may be present	Fusiform dilation of the common bile duct with associated intrahepatic ductal dilation	Duplicated gallbladder Liver cyst Fluid in duodenum

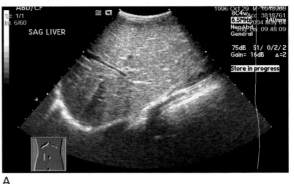

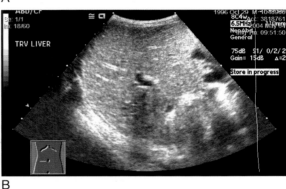

FIGURE 25-9 Liver size and texture should be evaluated in a patient with hepatitis. The liver may appear normal or enlarged, often with a more coarse and echogenic echotexture. **A,** Sagittal liver. **B,** Transverse liver.

trimester of pregnancy via TORCH infections. Bacterial hepatitis is most common secondary to an upward spread of organisms from the vagina, infecting endometrium, placenta, and amniotic fluid. During delivery, direct contact with the viruses of herpes, CMV, human immunodeficiency virus (HIV), and *Listeria* may lead to hepatitis. Blood transfusions may contain the hepatitis virus, Epstein-Barr virus, or HIV. In addition, bacterial hepatitis or abscess formation may be obtained from an **umbilical vein catheter** after delivery.

Sonographic Findings. Liver may be normal sized or enlarged (Figure 25-9). The parenchyma pattern is hyperechoic with decreased visualization of the peripheral portal venous structures. The biliary ducts and gallbladder are not enlarged. If the hepatocellular dysfunction is severe, the gallbladder may be small in size because of the decreased production of bile. The differential of neonatal hepatitis and biliary atresia may be difficult when the gallbladder is small; therefore nuclear scintigraphy will allow visualization of the biliary function.

Biliary Atresia. **Biliary atresia** is the narrowing or underdevelopment of the biliary ductal system. This serious disease is seen more commonly in males and may result from inflammation of the hepatobiliary system. Biliary atresia may affect the intrahepatic or extrahepatic ducts and may or

may not involve the gallbladder, although the latter is the most common form with absence of the gallbladder. However, sonographers should recognize the "pseudogallbladder," or abnormally shaped gallbladder, sometimes seen in neonates with biliary atresia.

The clinical features of biliary atresia in the neonate include persistent jaundice, **acholic** stools, dark urine, and distended abdomen from hepatomegaly. Early surgical intervention (**Kasai portoenterostomy**) is often necessary to prevent serious complications, which include cirrhosis, liver failure, and subsequent death. Biliary atresia remains the leading cause of liver transplants in children.

Sonographic Findings. Sonographic findings in a neonate with biliary atresia may vary depending on the type and the severity of the disease (Figure 25-10). The liver size may be normal or enlarged. The echogenicity of the liver parenchyma may be normal or increased with slight decrease in visualization of the peripheral portal venous vasculature (indicative of fibrosis). The intrahepatic ducts are not dilated, although a remnant duct may be identified with some types of atresia. A small hyperechoic focal triangular area often referred to as the "triangular cord" sign may be seen anterior to the portal vein bifurcation on an oblique transverse view, which is a hypoplastic fibrotic remnant of the biliary structure.

A normal-sized gallbladder may be seen when the **atretic** common bile duct is distal to the insertion of the cystic duct. However, if there is a gallbladder present with biliary atresia, it is often the small "pseudogallbladder," which appears as a

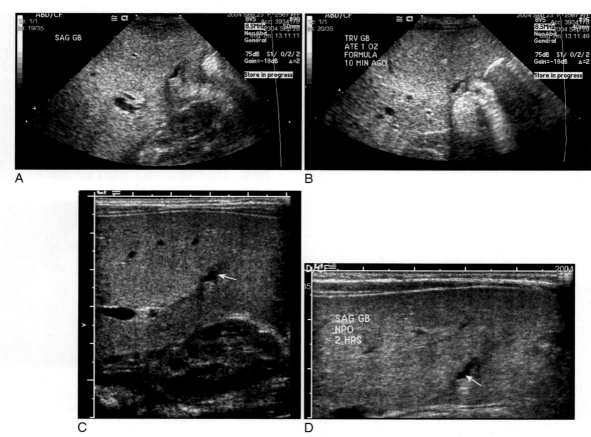

FIGURE 25-10 Biliary atresia. A 5-day-old infant with direct hyperbilirubinemia of unknown origin with liver congestion, inflammation, and ductal blockage. The liver is enlarged with a fairly homogeneous appearance. The neonate had eaten just before the study and the gallbladder was contracted and measured less than 1 cm. The patient was scanned after 2 hours and the gallbladder did not change in appearance. The common bile duct was not identified. **A,** Sagittal gallbladder. **B,** Transverse gallbladder after patient had 1 oz of formula. **C,** Sagittal gallbladder *(arrow)* utilizing higher-frequency linear transducer. **D,** Sagittal gallbladder *(arrow);* no change seen after patient NPO for 2 hours.

fluid-filled structure less than 15 mm in length within the interlobar fissure region, often without a normal gallbladder wall. However, a small gallbladder is nonspecific, as mentioned earlier, and may be seen with either hepatitis or biliary atresia. A decrease in the gallbladder size after a milk feeding, however, suggests normal patency of the common hepatic and common bile ducts and would suggest neonatal hepatitis in this case.

The abdomen should be closely evaluated for the presence of polysplenia if there is suspicion for biliary atresia because there is a high association of this abnormality. There are also known associations of situs inversus, interrupted IVC, or enlarged hepatic artery. Signs of end-stage liver disease (i.e., ascites, hepatofugal flow, and collateral venous channels) should also be documented. Ultrasound has a very high accuracy differentiating biliary atresia from other causes of increased conjugated hyperbilirubinemia if all of these sonographic features are carefully evaluated.

Choledochal Cyst. A **choledochal cyst** is an abnormal cystic dilation of the biliary tree, which most frequently affects the common bile duct. There are five types of choledochal

cysts, with type I being the most common. The basic choledochal cysts are presented here:

Type I—Fusiform dilation of the common bile duct (CBD)
Type II—One or more diverticula of the CBD
Type III—Dilation of the intraduodenal portion of the CBD (choledochocele)
Type IV—Dilation of the intrahepatic and extrahepatic ducts
Type V—Caroli's disease (see Chapter 10) with dilation of intrahepatic ducts

The neonate clinically presents with jaundice and pain. A palpable mass may be felt in the right upper quadrant. Sonography is used to differentiate the presence or absence of a gallbladder, dilation of the ductal system, and the presence or absence of a mass (Figure 25-11). When a choledochal cyst is present, there is usually fusiform dilation of the common bile duct with associated intrahepatic ductal dilation.

Causes and Diagnosis of Pediatric Jaundice. There are several causes of jaundice in the pediatric patient, including hepatocellular disease, hepatic neoplasms, cholelithiasis and choledocholithiasis, and cirrhosis. Only hepatic neoplasms will be presented. See Chapters 9 and 10 for further discussion of the other abnormalities.

Abdominal Tumors

Pediatric abdominal masses are often differentiated based on a patient's age (neonate/young infant versus older infant and child) and symptoms (symptomatic versus asymptomatic). Usually, but certainly not always (as in the case of ovarian torsion), abdominal masses of the gastrointestinal tract are symptomatic and others asymptomatic. In all age-groups the majority of neoplasms arise from the retroperitoneum, particularly the kidneys.

Less often masses may arise from the adrenals, reproductive organs (ovarian cysts, teratomas, hydrocolpos, hydrometrocolpos), gastrointestinal tract (lymphoma), liver, and biliary tract (choledochal cysts). Pancreatic masses are rare, but seen in infants and young children the pancreaticoblastoma may be suspected, which presents as a large, hypoechoic, solitary mass.

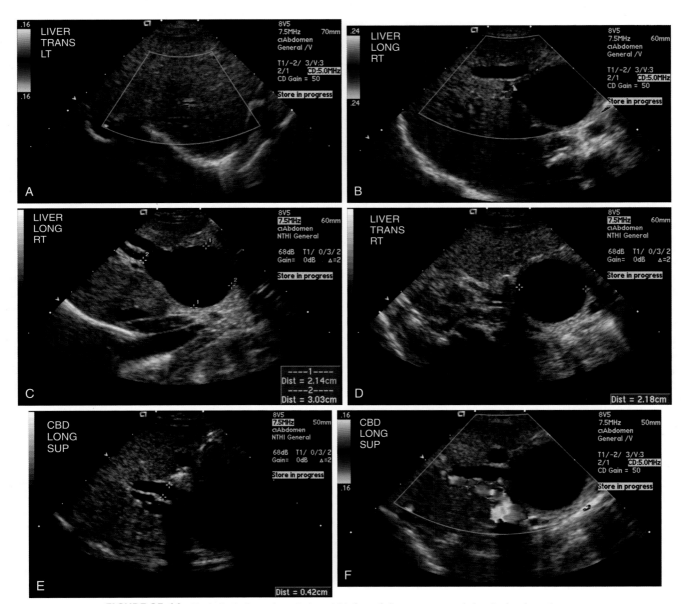

FIGURE 25-11 Choledochal cyst in a 5-day-old infant, follow-up to an abdominal polycystic mass on prenatal ultrasound. The gallbladder is seen without evidence of gallstones or wall thickening. A thin-walled fluid collection is seen in the right upper quadrant (RUQ) measuring 2 × 3 × 2.2 cm. The cystic mass is separate from the gallbladder and does not demonstrate flow. RUQ cyst is connected to the common bile duct (CBD), consistent with a choledochal cyst type II. **A,** Transverse left liver demonstrating slightly dilated central hepatic ducts with color Doppler. **B,** Sagittal right liver showing large cystic area posterior and inferior to the CBD. **C,** Sagittal measurement of cyst. **D,** Transverse measurement of cyst. **E,** Dilated CBD measuring 4 mm. **F,** Supine position showing CBD connection to cyst, while color Doppler shows CBD separate from vascular structures.
Continued

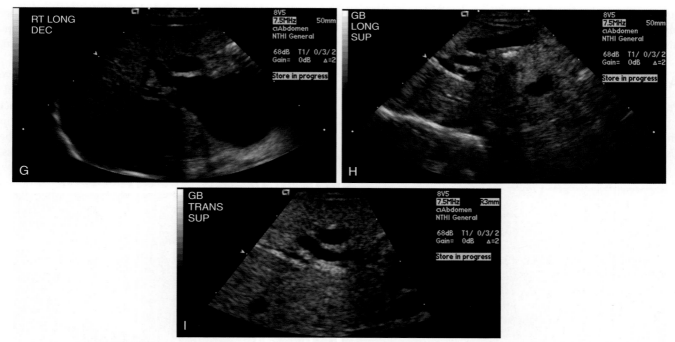

FIGURE 25-11, cont'd G, Decubitus position showing CBD connection to cyst. **H,** Sagittal gallbladder. **I,** Transverse gallbladder. *(Images courtesy Nationwide Children's Hospital, Columbus, OH.)*

In adolescent girls and young women, the often-large solid pseudopapillary tumor, also called the solid and pseudopapillary epithelial neoplasm (SPEN), may be indicated.

Liver Tumors. Primary liver tumors, although more common in children, only account for 5% to 6% of all intraabdominal masses and 1% to 4% of all solid tumors in the pediatric population. However, two thirds of all childhood hepatic tumors are malignant. Sonography plays an important role, not only in their detection, but also defining the origin, size, number, Doppler flow characteristics, IVC involvement, location for potential resection, and response to therapy. The two most common neoplasms (Table 25-5) in the pediatric population often present as an asymptomatic mass and are the hepatoblastoma and infantile hepatic vascular tumors (infantile hemangioendotheliomas).

Malignant Liver Tumors. The distinction of the benign from malignant mass with sonography is not possible; only histologic diagnosis is definitive. However, the clinical history, laboratory results, and sonographic findings may provide a differential for the clinician. The two most common malignant tumors in childhood are the hepatoblastoma and hepatocellular carcinoma. The undifferentiated sarcoma and biliary rhabdomyosarcoma are rare. Metastases to the liver may arise from **neuroblastoma**, Wilms' tumor, leukemia, or lymphoma.

Hepatoblastoma. Hepatoblastoma is the most common primary malignant disease of the liver and occurs most frequently in children under 4 years of age, with the majority occurring in children under 1 year of age. It is the third most common pediatric abdominal malignancy after **Wilms' tumor** (**nephroblastoma**) and **neuroblastoma** (see Chapter 26). It is

sometimes considered the infantile form of hepatocellular carcinoma. The tumor may be familial. Hepatoblastoma has been associated with **Beckwith-Wiedemann syndrome, hemihypertrophy,** familial adenomatous polyposis, precocious puberty, congenital anomalies, fetal alcohol syndrome, and very low birth weight (generally defined as less than 1500 g).

Pathologically the tumor is single, solid, large, or mixed echogenicity, and poorly marginated, with small cysts and rounded or irregularly shaped deposits of calcium. The tumor may show areas of necrosis, hemorrhage, and calcification (Figure 25-12). It usually does not show diffuse infiltration; the remaining liver may be normal. The intrahepatic vessels are displaced or amputated by the mass. Color Doppler is useful to detect high-velocity flow in the malignant neovasculature.

Clinical findings include a palpable abdominal mass and a highly elevated serum alpha-fetoprotein level. Patients may be symptomatic with fever, pain, anorexia, and subsequent weight loss. The prognosis of the tumor is dependent on the resectability of the mass.

Sonographic Findings. The sonographic appearance of the hepatoblastoma shows hepatomegaly with a large solitary mass (Figure 25-13). Calcifications are common. The heterogeneous mass is predominantly solid; however, there may be hypoechoic areas with necrosis or hemorrhage. The fleshy areas around the mass are often mildly hyperechoic. It becomes important to identify the hepatic vessels, as hepatic and portal venous thrombosis may be present. The Doppler flow pattern in the lesion shows a high-velocity, low-resistance flow pattern.

Hepatocellular Carcinoma. Hepatocellular carcinoma, also known as hepatoma, is the second most common malignant

TABLE 25-5	Most Common Hepatic Neoplasms	
Clinical Findings	Sonographic Findings	Differential Considerations
Hepatoblastoma		
Most common malignant tumor of the liver	Hepatomegaly	Hepatocellular carcinoma
	Calcification may occur	Adenoma
	Solitary heterogeneous mass	Focal nodular hyperplasia
Less than 4 years of age	Portal vein thrombosis	Cirrhosis—regenerating nodules
Palpable abdominal mass	Area around mass is hyperechoic	Hemangioendothelioma
Elevated serum alpha-fetoprotein levels in 90% of patients	Doppler shows high-velocity, low-resistance flow	Biliary rhabdoma/sarcoma
Fever		Lymphoma
Pain		Metastasis
Infantile Hepatic Vascular Tumors (Infantile Hemangioendotheliomas)		
First 6 months of life	Multiple hypoechoic lesions or solitary mass in liver	Adenoma
Rapid growing benign tumors	Hepatomegaly	Focal nodular hyperplasia
Hepatomegaly	Tumor is heterogeneous or isoechoic with cystic components	Cirrhosis—regenerating nodules
Congestive heart failure		Hepatoblastoma
Cutaneous hemangiomas	Calcification may be present	Biliary rhabdoma/sarcoma
Serum alpha-fetoprotein level rarely elevated	Well circumscribed to poorly marginated	Lymphoma
	Doppler may show arteriovenous shunt	Metastasis

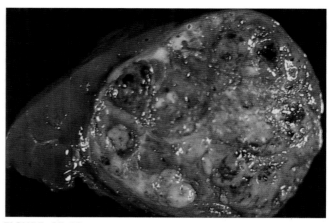

FIGURE 25-12 Hepatoblastoma specimen. Lobular tumor with areas of necrosis.

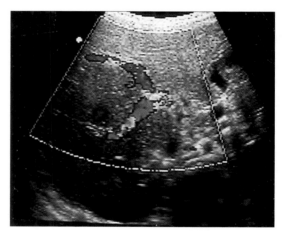

FIGURE 25-13 Hepatoblastoma. The portal veins are displaced by the large mass.

tumor in childhood. It usually affects older children (more than 3 years old) and half will have preexisting liver disease, such as hepatitis or type I glycogen storage disease. This liver tumor is often a multicentric solid mass involving the whole liver, usually without calcification and variable echogenicity on sonography. Color Doppler should be used to evaluate the portal venous and hepatic structures to look for thrombus or tumor invasion, as patients often present with sudden liver failure due to invasion of these vessels.

Benign Liver Tumors. Infantile hepatic vascular tumors (infantile hemangioendotheliomas) are the most common benign liver tumor. They make up the third most common childhood hepatic tumor and account for 12% of all childhood hepatic neoplasms. Mesenchymal hamartoma, adenoma, and focal nodular hyperplasia make up roughly half of all benign liver tumors.

Infantile Hepatic Vascular Tumors (Infantile Hemangioendotheliomas). Perhaps the most perplexing hepatic tumor in infancy is better known as the infantile hemangioendothelioma.

It is not surprising, then, this tumor has recently been divided histologically into two types—hepatic infantile hemangioma (type I) and congenital hepatic vascular malformation (type II). It has been suggested that type I is the hepatic counterpart to the common cutaneous hemangioma, which also has positive immunoreactivity to erythrocyte-type glucose transporter protein 1 (GLUT-1), whereas type II may represent a vascular malformation and does not show GLUT-1 reactivity. Type II tumor histology reports, however, are differing and have been reported as vascular malformations with capillary proliferation and as vascular hepatic lesions that do involute. Likely, these type II tumors represent a heterogeneous type of lesion. Not surprisingly, there is ongoing debate over nomenclature of this pathology that has been previously classified by the clinical appearance of multifocal, focal, or diffuse. It is unclear to which histologic type the diffuse type belongs; however, the uniform appearance and low association with congestive heart failure (CHF) may indicate type I or a combination (Table 25-6).

Regardless, these tumors make up the most common benign vascular liver tumors of early childhood, with a peak diagnosis at 6 months of life, with one third diagnosed in the first month of life. They grow rapidly after birth, causing

TABLE 25-6	Infantile Hepatic Vascular Tumors (Infantile Hemangioendotheliomas) by Type and Histologic Findings
Clinical Findings	**Sonographic Findings**
Type I—Infantile Hepatic Hemangioma	
High association with cutaneous hemangiomas	Multifocal masses
GLUT-1 positive	Small with no central necrosis on pathology, homogeneous in appearance
Proliferation, usually third of fourth month, followed by involution	
Often asymptomatic, but some may have CHF	
Type II—Congenital hepatic vascular malformation (with associated capillary proliferation or vascular hepatic lesions that involute)	
Rarely associated with cutaneous hemangiomas	Large solitary mass
GLUT-1 negative	Large with central hemorrhage, necrosis or fibrosis on pathology, calcifications and mixed heterogeneity
Manifests in perinatal period	
Involute by 12–14 months of age	
Patient is usually symptomatic and may present with CHF	

abdominal distention. Fewer than 5% are diagnosed after the first year.

The clinical presentation for infants with infantile hepatic vascular tumors is hepatomegaly, which may be accompanied by CHF and/or cutaneous hemangioma. CHF and high cardiac output are seen in 50% to 60% of patients, due to increased blood volume and output needed to maintain vascular bed perfusion. Biopsy is not recommended, due to an increased risk of bleeding in these high-flow lesions. The serum alpha-fetoprotein level may be elevated. These benign tumors usually spontaneously regress by 12 to 18 months of age.

Sonographic Findings. The most common sonographic appearance of infantile hepatic vascular tumors is hepatomegaly, with half presenting as multiple hypoechoic lesions (hemangiomatosis) and the other half as a solitary mass. The tumor may be isoechoic or heterogeneous and may contain cystic components from the vascular-stroma structure (Figure 25-14). Speckled areas of calcification may be seen within the mass. Interestingly, infantile hemangiomas do not show calcifications or arteriovenous shunting, whereas congenital vascular malformations may. The tumor may be well circumscribed or poorly marginated. Color Doppler shows high flow in the dilated vascular spaces and may be used to show the arteriovenous shunting that accompanies this lesion. When arteriovenous shunting is severe, the celiac axis, hepatic artery, and veins are dilated and the infraceliac aorta is tapered. Doppler characteristics may overlap with malignancies, showing higher diastolic flow. It is suspected this is likely associated with type II, which may be more aggressive.

Hepatic Hemangiomas. Hepatic hemangiomas may be infantile or juvenile. The juvenile appearance is similar to that of the adult hepatic hemangioma. The hepatic hemangioma is characterized by active endothelial growth. The vessel growth slows down as the tumor matures, but the existing vessels may form "lakes" within the lesion with little blood flow. The sonographic pattern (hyperechoic) is similar to that found in the adult.

Sometimes, infants with common cutaneous hemangiomas (vascular lesions of proliferative endothelium present on the superficial skin) will have a screening ultrasound of the liver, spleen, and brain for concomitant visceral lesions. Risk factors for cutaneous hemangiomas include prematurity, female gender (3:1 to 4:1), and fair skin. The hepatic hemangioma is the most common extracutaneous hemangioma, also with a female prevalence, and is more likely to occur in those patients presenting with five to six cutaneous lesions, with a single one over 5 cm, or with a miliary or disseminated form.

Mesenchymal Hamartoma. This is a rare tumor in the asymptomatic infant under 2 years old. The tumor has multiseptate cystic masses derived from periportal mesenchyma.

Adenoma. This tumor is not commonly seen in the infant unless liver disease is present (i.e., glycogen storage disease). Laboratory values will find that the serum alpha-fetoprotein levels are normal. The sonographic appearance ranges from hyperechoic to hypoechoic and is nonspecific.

GASTROINTESTINAL PATHOLOGY

Although sonography is not commonly used for evaluating adult gastrointestinal conditions, it is routinely used to triage and diagnose common surgical conditions in infants and children. The sonographic evaluation of the gastrointestinal system has been increasing, owing to efforts to reduce ionizing radiation exposure among children. Although considered an inferior imaging modality to computed tomography for gastrointestinal pathology, the increased reliance on ultrasound for appendicitis in pediatric institutions, for example, has resulted in a stable frequency of appendiceal perforations and emergency department revisits, while negative appendectomy rates have slightly decreased.

Common Surgical Conditions

The pediatric patient may appear in the general ultrasound laboratory on an emergent basis for extreme abdominal pain or vomiting with three common surgical conditions: appendicitis, intussusception, and hypertrophic pyloric stenosis (Table 25-7).

Appendicitis. **Appendicitis** is the most common cause of emergent surgical abdominal pain in children. It mostly occurs in patients ages 5 to 15 years old, but may occur as young as 3 months old (although rare under age 2), and has a male (1.7:1) prevalence. Appendicitis occurs when the appendiceal lumen becomes obstructed and subsequently infected. In infants and young children, the progression of acute appendicitis to perforation is more rapid than in older children and adults, sometimes occurring within 6 to 12 hours. Perforation of the appendix is a serious complication of appendicitis,

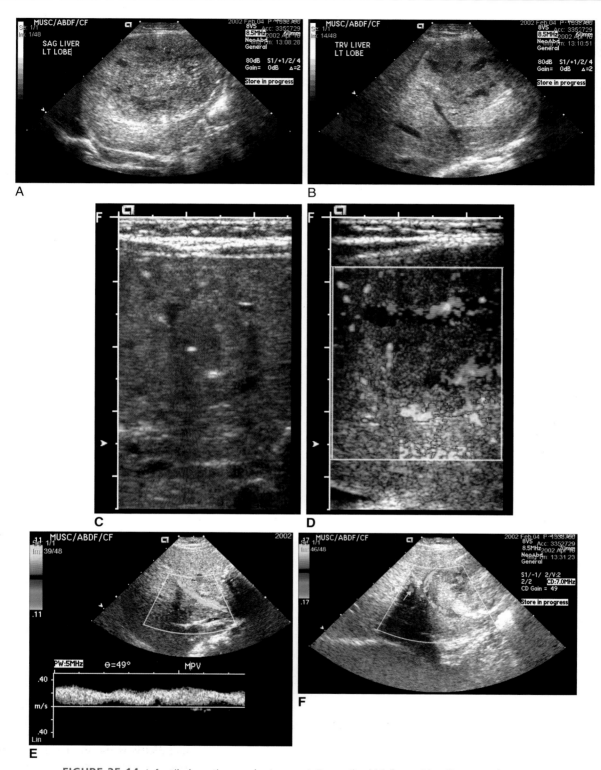

FIGURE 25-14 Infantile hepatic vascular tumor. A 2-month-old infant with a liver vascular tumor (likely infantile hemangioendothelioma type II) shows a well-circumscribed heterogeneous mass with focal areas of calcium in the left lobe of the liver. There is predominant flow around the mass. There were normal waveforms in both the main portal vein and the left hepatic artery. **A,** Sagittal left lobe liver with large heterogeneous mass and right pleural effusion superior to diaphragm. **B,** Transverse left lobe of liver with mass. **C,** Sagittal views of mass showing areas of calcification that appear echogenic on sonography. **D,** Power Doppler shows increased vascularity within the mass (shown), while color Doppler helps to define the vascularity of the mass and the relationships of the portal and hepatic veins to the mass lesion. **E,** Main portal vein flow. **F,** Color flow in portal veins displaced around the mass.

TABLE 25-7	Most Common Gastrointestinal Surgical Conditions	
Clinical Findings	Sonographic Findings	Differential Considerations
Appendicitis		
Right lower quadrant pain	Noncompressible appendix	Mesenteric lymphadenitis
Nausea, vomiting	Diameter >6–7 mm	Gastroenteritis
Increased white blood cell count	Rebound pain	Meckel's diverticulum
Fever		Pelvic mass
		Distal Ileitis
Intussusception		
Colicky abdominal pain	Alternating hypoechoic and hyperechoic rings surrounding an echogenic center ("target sign")	Colic
Vomiting		Intestinal wall thickening
Bloody stools		Inflammatory bowel
Abdominal mass		Colitis
	Free peritoneal fluid	Perforated appendix
		Viral disease
		Lymphoma
		Benign tumors
Hypertrophic Pyloric Stenosis (HPS)		
Male infants	Distended stomach	Pseudoechogenic muscle secondary to beam angulation
Projectile vomiting	Hypertrophied pyloric muscle with a canal >15–16 mm	Antropyloric canal posteriorly oriented
Dehydration and weight loss	Pyloric wall muscle ≥3 mm	Pylorospasm with minimal muscular hypertrophy
		Prostaglandin-induced HPS

along with peritonitis, abscess formation, and sepsis. Classic physical and laboratory findings may be absent or confusing in children, making the diagnosis difficult.

Right lower quadrant pain and vomiting are a common clinical presentation. Pain may originate in the umbilicus area and migrate to **McBurney's point** (Figure 25-15). In addition to appendicitis, diagnostic considerations include mesenteric lymphadenitis, enteritis (inflammation of the small bowel), inflammatory bowel disease, and lymphoma. In girls, the differential broadens to include gynecologic processes, such as ovarian cysts or neoplasms and ovarian torsion.

Examination Technique. Sonography has proven to be very accurate in confirming appendicitis. A survey of the abdomen is first performed using a curved-array transducer, suitable to age and body habitus, to view deeper structures, and in girls the adnexal areas should be examined with the patient having a distended urinary bladder. However, bladder-filling techniques will vary depending on clinical presentation, and it is important to note that females (and those presenting after hours) have significantly increased time to **appendectomy**. Although unusual in the first 12 hours in older children, perforation of the appendix is directly proportional to delayed diagnosis thereafter.

Next, be sure to explain to the patient what you are going to do before beginning the compression portion of the examination. Pain is a limiting factor in effectively performing this technique. Gradual graded compression is slowly applied over the area of the appendix in the right flank and right lower quadrant with a linear array transducer. In infants and young children frequencies of 12 to 17 MHz may be used, whereas with older children 5 to 9 MHz will often suffice. Often more than one probe is necessary. The graded compression technique displaces adjacent bowel loops and gas for better visualization of the appendix. The appendix is usually seen anterior and medial to the psoas muscle and lateral to the iliac vessels. It is best to ask the patient to point to the place of most pain with one finger. It is

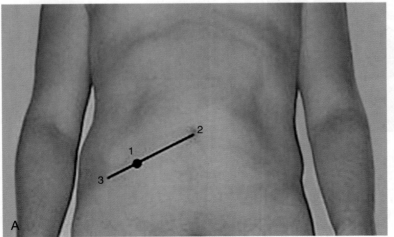
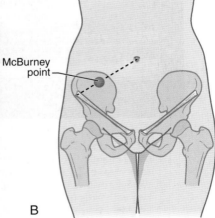

FIGURE 25-15 McBurney's point. Common area of appendiceal attachment to the cecum, one third the distance between the right anterior superior iliac spine and umbilicus.

helpful to follow the ascending colon and cecum inferiorly to the ileocecal junction, where the appendix comes off just postero-medial (inferior) to this valve. The normal appendix appears as a blind-ending, long, tubular structure in the longitudinal plane and as a bull's-eye in the transverse plane. The tip location is variable, but must be seen to rule out focal appendiceal tip appendicitis or appendicolith. A cine clip of the transverse appendix leading to the blind ending is very helpful to the reading radiologist.

The appendix must be visualized for the examination to be deemed diagnostic. Nonvisualization of the appendix (or equivocal examination) may occur for multiple reasons and is not a definite indication of a normal appendix. Appendiceal nonvisualization may result from any of the following: (1) being obscured by overlying bowel; (2) retrocecal position or deep pelvic position of the appendix; (3) overdistention or nondistention of the urinary bladder, which alters the position of the appendix and overlying bowel; or (4) lack of sonographer experience. Also, the child in pain may be moving and the normal appendix moves quite a bit, so changing pressure too fast may move the appendix out of view. Changing the patient's position and emptying or filling the urinary

bladder may facilitate visualization of both the normal and abnormal appendix. A bimanual compression technique may also be used, where the patient lies in a left lateral decubitus position while the sonographer applies pressure with the left hand on the back, while pushing with the transducer in the right scanning hand. Finally, scanning all over is helpful, as the tip may be located as superior as the right kidney.

Sonographic Findings. Peristalsis is not seen in the appendix, allowing differentiation of the normal appendix and adjacent small bowel, which is similar in appearance. The appendix may be tortuous and therefore difficult to visualize in its entirety. The walls are not thickened and maximal mural thickness should measure less than 1.7 mm. The normal appendix compresses easily and the lumen may be empty, or filled with gas or fecal material (Figure 25-16).

Sonographically the acutely inflamed appendix is noncompressible (Figure 25-17). The appendix is measured from outer-to-outer wall, using the anterior-posterior maximum outer diameter (MOD). Measurements are best made in the plane with the most well-defined wall, as acute appendicitis may present with a less defined or ragged wall. MOD $\geq$ 7 mm with compression is consistent with appendicitis in both children

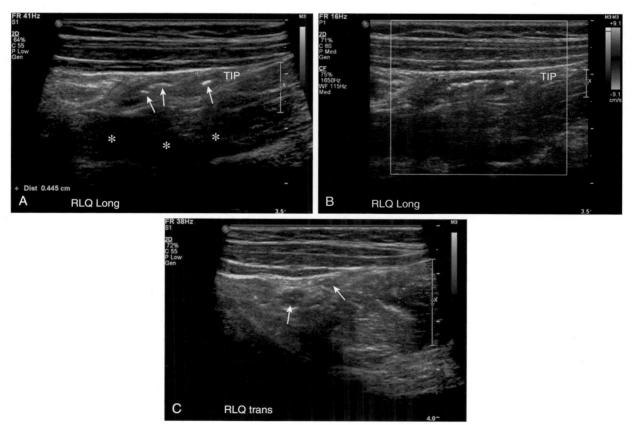

FIGURE 25-16 Normal appendix without secondary signs of appendicitis in 3-year-old with right lower quadrant pain. **A,** Normal appearing distal appendix in the longitudinal plane seen along the iliac vessels (not shown), measuring within normal limits. It is helpful to label the tip, as it can be faint and difficult to see in a static image. *Arrows* point to air in the appendix, and *asterisks* show psoas muscle. **B,** No hyperemia detected with color Doppler. **C,** Transverse view of the same normal appendix; note that two sections of tortuous appendix are visualized *(arrows)*. *(Images courtesy Nationwide Children's Hospital, Columbus, OH.)*

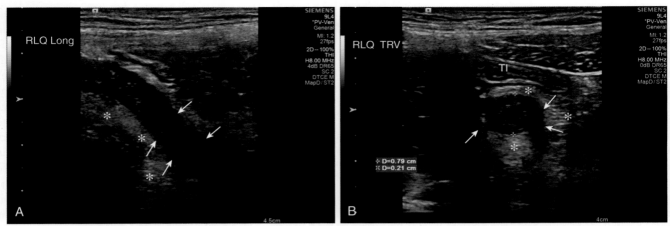

FIGURE 25-17 Appendicitis. Noncompressible appendix, measuring nearly 8 mm in anteroposterior diameter, and wall measuring over 2 mm, indicating appendicitis. Notice the increased periappendiceal fat echogenicity *(asterisks)* and loss of wall delineation *(arrows)*. Terminal ilium *(TI)* is seen superior to appendix in transverse image. **A,** Longitudinal view of inflamed appendix, seen diving posterior. **B,** Transverse or axial view of appendicitis with MOD wall-thickness measurements. *Images courtesy Nationwide Children's Hospital, Columbus, OH.)*

and adults. MOD ≤ 6 mm indicates normal appendix, and MOD between 6 and 7 mm is indeterminate and often established by each institution based on their outcomes. In this case secondary signs of appendicitis may be helpful.

The only statistically significant secondary sign for predicting acute appendicitis is increased echogenic fat. This increased echogenicity may be seen in the surrounding mesentery secondary to inflammation, and subsequently **hypomotility** of bowel peristalsis may be present. Localized pain produced by overlying transducer pressure is an additional clinical finding consistent with appendicitis. Color Doppler is useful to document increased blood flow (hyperemia) of the appendix wall (Figure 25-18). Other findings in appendicitis may include free peritoneal fluid or a loculated fluid collection in the lower abdomen. Mesenteric lymph nodes are another nonspecific secondary finding, and sonographers should report size, number, location, and hyperemia. Confirmation of an appendicolith in a symptomatic patient is virtually diagnostic (Figure 25-19). An **appendicolith** is hyperechoic, produces a classic acoustic shadow, may be single or multiple, and may be intraluminal or surrounded by a periappendiceal phlegmon or abscess. The right kidney may at times be hydronephrotic because of ureteral inflammation.

The perforated appendix may or may not be visualized. If decompressed, an abnormally thick bowel wall may be apparent. A localized, well-defined right lower quadrant phlegmon or abscess with or without an appendicolith may be present (Figure 25-20). Free peritoneal fluid may be the lone abnormal sonographic finding. An abscess far removed from the right lower quadrant is another potential intraabdominal complication of an appendiceal perforation.

Enlarged lymph nodes (Figure 25-21) may be a pitfall in diagnosing appendicitis. The single most common diagnosis mimicking appendicitis is mesenteric lymphadenitis, which may present with prominent lymph nodes (generally defined as three or more lymph nodes, oval in shape, greater than 5 mm short-axis) and symptoms of appendicitis with flulike symptoms previous to the illness. Color Doppler imaging may help the sonographer to determine increased flow in the inflamed appendix from the enlarged node.

Intussusception. **Intussusception** is the most common acute abdominal disorder in early childhood. This condition occurs when the bowel prolapses into a more distal bowel and is propelled in an antegrade fashion. Telescoping of bowel in this manner causes obstruction. The ileum may invaginate into a more distal ileum, causing an ileoileal intussusception, and this often resolves on its own. However, if there is further progression through the ileocecal valve, an ileocolic intussusception results.

Traditionally, intussusception in 90% of cases includes the prolapse of the ileum into the cecum or beyond producing an ileocolic intussusception. Ileocolic intussusception is usually seen in children between the ages of 6 months old and 2 years old. Older children with Henoch-Schonlein purpura are also at risk. A higher incidence has been reported in males (2:1), along with a seasonal prevalence. Frequently, there is a history of an antecedent upper respiratory tract infection. Associated inflammation of lymphoid tissue in the ileocolic region may act as a lead point for the telescoping phenomenon.

Children may present with colicky abdominal pain, vomiting, and bloody (currant jelly) stools. Abdominal distention or a mass may also be palpable in up to 50% of patients with intussusception. In patients with this classic clinical presentation, sonography has established itself as the imaging modality of choice, with sensitivity and specificity of nearly 98% and negative predictive value at nearly 100%. Therapeutic reduction is almost entirely (98% of the time) undergone by fluoroscopic means (often an air enema), although sonographically guided saline enemas may reduce intussusceptions as well. Failure to reduce an intussusception mandates immediate surgical intervention. Likewise,

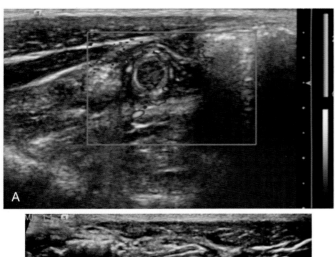

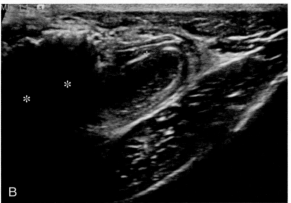

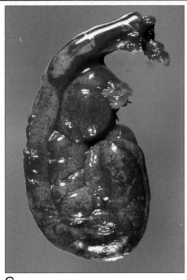

FIGURE 25-18 **A,** Power Doppler demonstrating acute appendicitis in transverse view. **B,** Same acute appendicitis showing the inflamed tip, measuring over 1 cm. Bowel gas (asterisks) is shadowing out the proximal portion of the appendix. **C,** Gross pathology of acute appendicitis demonstrates inflammation extending to the serosa, which appears hyperemic. *(Images A and B courtesy Nationwide Children's Hospital, Columbus, OH.)*

surgical intervention is indicated in patients with a classic clinical presentation of intussusception who have developed fever and peritoneal signs.

Examination Technique. The patient is examined in the supine position. A brief survey of the entire abdomen

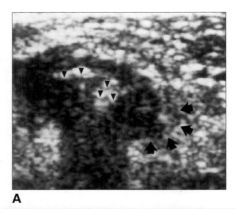

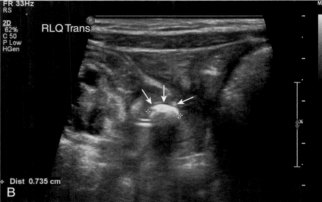

FIGURE 25-19 **Appendicolith(s). A,** Longitudinal image of an inflamed appendix containing multiple echogenic foci (arrowheads) consistent with appendicoliths, which cast acoustic shadows. The blind-ending tip (arrows) confirms that the echogenic foci are within the appendix and are not gas moving through the small bowel. **B,** Transverse image of an inflamed appendix in a different patient. There is a solitary appendicolith (arrows). *(Image B courtesy Nationwide Children's Hospital, Columbus, OH.)*

is performed, dividing the abdomen into four quadrants, followed by an examination focusing on the bowel using a 5- to 12-MHz linear or curved array transducer. The bowel is followed, often starting at the cecum in the right lower quadrant.

Sonographic Findings. The sonographic appearance of intussusception is of alternating hypoechoic and hyperechoic rings surrounding an echogenic center as seen in a short-axis view of the involved area. This is known as the **target** (or **donut**) **sign** (Figure 25-22, *A*). Often the ileoileo intussusception will measure less than 3 cm in the transverse plane, whereas the pathologic ileocolic intussusception will measure greater than 3 cm. In the long-axis view, hypoechoic layers on each side of the echogenic center result in a "pseudokidney" or "sandwich" sign appearance (Figure 25-22, *B*). The sonolucent ring is believed to represent the edematous infolded loop of the intussusceptum, whereas the echogenic central area represents its compressed **mucosa.** Other concentric rings are present resulting from visualization of additional bowel wall layers within the intussusception. Dilated loops of obstructed proximal bowel may also be seen (Figure 25-23). Free peritoneal fluid is not an uncommon

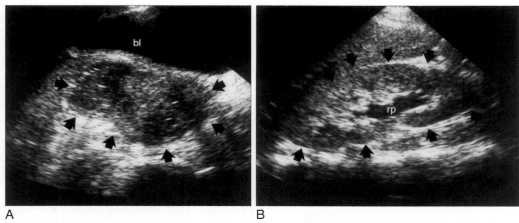

A   B

FIGURE 25-20 A, Midline sagittal image in a boy with an appendiceal abscess *(arrows)* posterior to the urinary bladder *(bl)*. The appendiceal abscess appears heterogeneous in echogenicity and is well demarcated from the surrounding bowel, which was actively peristaltic on real-time examination. **B,** Longitudinal image of the right kidney *(arrows)* in the same patient shows moderate hydronephrosis because of distal ureteral inflammation from the abscess. A fluid-filled right renal pelvis *(rp)* may be a secondary sign of a right lower quadrant or pelvic process.

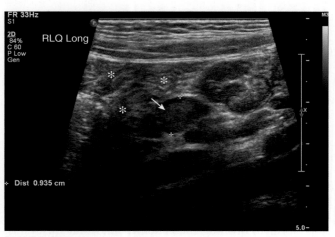

FIGURE 25-21 Patient who was positive for appendicitis has accompanying reactive mesenteric lymph node *(arrow)* seen within the small bowel *(asterisks)*. Short-axis measurement demonstrated. *(Image courtesy Nationwide Children's Hospital, Columbus, OH.)*

finding with uncomplicated intussusception. Color Doppler (Figure 25-24) may help to determine the success of an air reduction enema; if there is good color flow to all areas of the telescoping bowel, the chances are better for a reduction. Poor color Doppler may indicate ischemia to the area of affected bowel and is likely irreducible with air or hydrostatic enema, necessitating surgery.

When an intussusception is documented sonographically an associated mass or cause, though relatively uncommon (5% to 10%), should be sought. A double target sign has been reported as being diagnostic of intussuscepted Meckel's diverticulum. Other causes, such as a small bowel tumor, polyp, or duplication cyst, may likewise be identified.

After reduction an edematous ileocecal valve may be seen on fluoroscopy that may mimic a residual intussusception. Sonography is helpful in distinguishing between persistent

intussusception and an edematous ileocecal valve. The edematous valve appears as a small sonolucent rim with an echogenic center. It is distinguishable from intussusception in that its cross-sectional diameter is smaller than that of an intussusception, and it lacks the concentric rings frequently seen in intussusception.

In addition to intussusception, conditions that can produce a target-like sonographic appearance include primary bowel tumors, such as lymphoma, and thickened bowel wall in post–stem cell transplant or bone marrow transplant patients and in patients with inflammatory bowel disease.

Hypertrophic Pyloric Stenosis. The **pyloric canal** is located between the stomach and duodenum. In some infants, the pyloric muscle can become hypertrophied, resulting in gastric obstruction. Hypertrophy of the circular muscle of the pylorus is an acquired condition that narrows the pyloric canal (Figure 25-25). The pyloric canal itself is not intrinsically stenotic or narrowed, but it functions as if it were as a result of the abnormally thickened surrounding muscle.

Hypertrophic pyloric stenosis (HPS) appears most commonly in male infants (4:1), with 95% of cases occurring between 3 and 12 weeks of age, often peaking at 4 weeks of age. Rarely, it becomes apparent at birth or as late as 5 months of age. The incidence of HPS is approximately 3 in 1000 neonates. Bile-free vomiting in an otherwise healthy infant is the most frequent clinical sign. As the pyloric muscle thickens and elongates, the stomach outlet obstruction increases and vomiting is more constant and projectile. Dehydration and weight loss may ensue. Often acute-onset patients will present very colicky, whereas those who show signs of dehydration and weight loss are often lethargic and too sick to cry and struggle. Peristaltic waves and reverse peristaltic waves crossing the upper abdomen may be observed during or after feeding as the stomach attempts to force its contents through the abnormal canal, often resulting

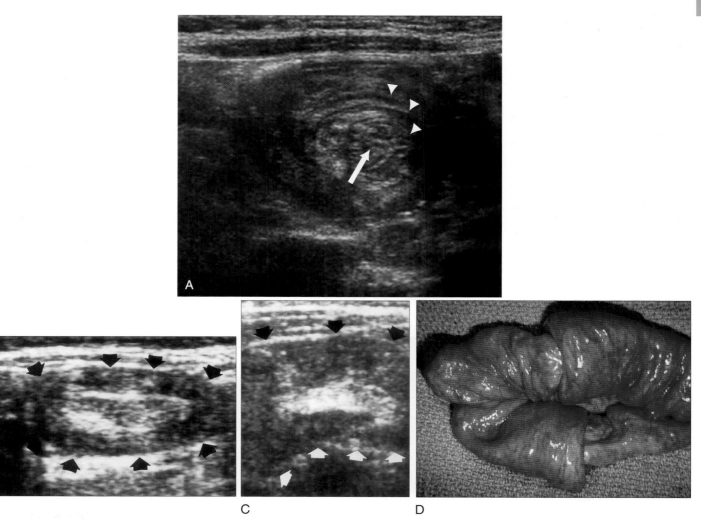

FIGURE 25-22 Intussusception. **A,** "Target" or "donut" sign. Transverse image of an intussusception showing a target sign. There are several circumferential layers of increased and decreased echogenicity *(arrowheads)* because of the telescoping bowel. The lumen *(arrow)* may contain fluid or lymph node. (Image courtesy Nationwide Children's Hospital, Columbus, OH.) **B,** "Pseudokidney" sign. Longitudinal image of the right lower quadrant demonstrates a pseudokidney appearance of an intussusception *(arrows)*. A normal kidney is documented in each renal fossa, so this is not a pelvic kidney. **C,** "Sandwich" sign. Longitudinal image of the right lower quadrant in a different patient with intussusception *(arrows)*. The intussusception has a sandwich appearance. **D,** Gross pathology shows the loops of bowel invaginating one into the other.

in **projectile vomiting.** In these infants, palpation of an olive-shaped mass at the epigastrum is diagnostic and is treated by surgical **pyloromyotomy.** In infants with a suggestive history or an equivocal physical examination, diagnostic imaging is required to provide direct visualization of the pyloric muscle (Figure 25-26).

The neonate with projectile vomiting is frequently sent directly from the physician's office or the hospital emergency department. In pediatric imaging departments and in other ultrasound departments where there is appropriate expertise, sonography is the imaging method of choice to establish the diagnosis of HPS. If HPS is not a primary diagnostic consideration or if the sonogram is not diagnostic, conventional contrast radiography of the upper gastrointestinal tract is necessary to assess for other potential

causes of vomiting. The differential considerations include pylorospasm, gastrointestinal reflux, antral web, hiatal hernia, and duodenal obstruction caused by stenosis or malrotation with bands or volvulus.

Examination Technique. Ideally, the infant will be on nothing-by-mouth (NPO, *nil per os*) status for a couple of hours before scanning, as too much fluid or no fluid in the stomach is undesirable. However, this is rarely the case and it is advised to attempt the examination, warning the parents and medical team that a delay period may be necessary if the stomach is too full. However, in the case of a positive HPS it is often sonographically obvious, regardless of NPO status.

The infant is usually examined first in the supine and then in the right lateral decubitus position, which aids in the visualization of the pylorus. A preliminary survey of the abdomen is

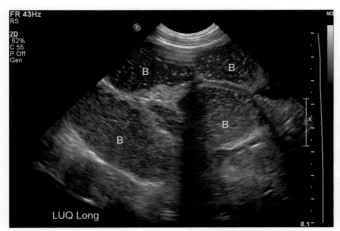

FIGURE 25-23 Dilated fluid-filled bowel loops *(B)* located proximal to an intussusception. Multiple, dilated fluid-filled bowel loops are seen within the left upper quadrant. *(Image courtesy Nationwide Children's Hospital, Columbus, OH.)*

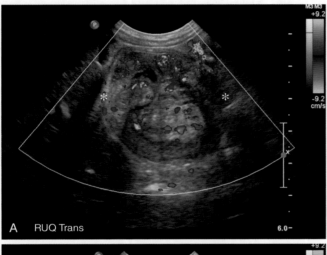

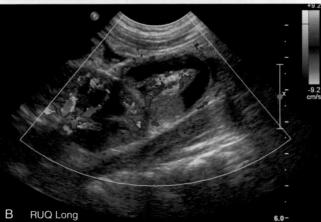

FIGURE 25-24 One-year-old with positive ileocolic intussusception successfully underwent a single air enema for resolution. **A,** Transverse or short-axis view showing good color Doppler flow. Measurement *(asterisks)* was over 3 cm indicating an ileocolic intussusception. **B,** Longitudinal view demonstrating good color Doppler flow. *(Images courtesy Nationwide Children's Hospital, Columbus, OH.)*

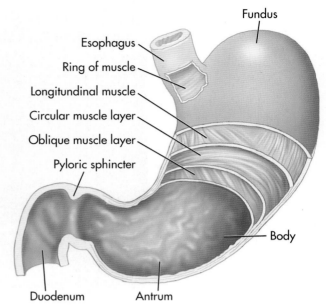

FIGURE 25-25 Diagram of stomach and pyloric canal. The pylorus muscle (sphincter) connects the antrum of the stomach with the duodenum of the small intestine.

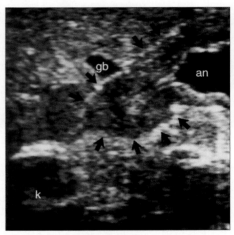

FIGURE 25-26 Transverse image of the right upper quadrant in a 5-week-old boy with hypertrophic pyloric stenosis, using the liver as an acoustic window, shows a longitudinal view of an elongated thickened pyloric muscle *(arrows).* The antrum *(an)* is filled with fluid. The gallbladder *(gb)* is anterior to the pyloric muscle, whereas the right kidney *(k)* is posterior and lateral.

performed in the supine position to exclude adrenal hemorrhage or renal abnormalities, which are increased in the presence of HPS, such as hydronephrosis secondary to ureteropelvic junction obstruction or duplex kidneys. The sonographer should also document the orientation of the superior mesenteric artery and vein to assess for **midgut malrotation**, especially in the case of patients with negative findings of HPS. Real-time imaging is then performed using a high-frequency linear array or small curved array transducer (5 to 12 MHz). Before administering fluid, preliminary imaging of the pylorus is performed to assess the amount of gastric fluid in the antrum of the stomach.

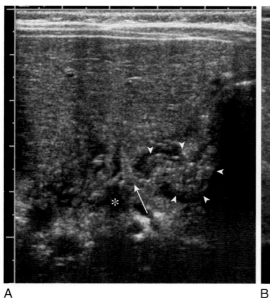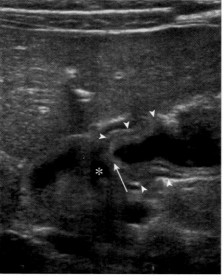

A   B

FIGURE 25-27 Pitfalls of an empty and collapsed antrum. **A,** Long-axis view of empty gastric antrum in a normal pyloric muscle *(arrows).* Antrum is seen anterior and lateral to the muscle *(arrowheads),* while fluid in the duodenum (often triangular in appearance) is seen inferior and medial *(asterisk)* to the muscle. **B,** Long-axis view of properly filled antrum in a normal pylorus. A more clear delineation of the pyloric muscle *(arrow),* gastric antrum *(arrowheads),* and duodenum *(asterisk)* are seen. *(Images courtesy Nationwide Children's Hospital, Columbus, OH.)*

The associated pitfalls of having an improper amount of gastric fluid are as follows: (1) No fluid in the antrum of the stomach. Inadequate gastric fluid will not allow accurate distinction of the normal collapsed antrum from the pylorus (Figure 25-27). (2) Having an overly distended stomach. This can displace the pyloric muscle posteriorly, making sonographic delineation much more difficult or impossible (Figure 25-28). In this instance scanning from a prone approach may do the trick. If not, and the patient is positive for HPS, he or she may vomit the contents out and, rarely, aspiration of gastric contents via a nasogastric tube is required. If the pyloric muscle is normal, the gastric contents will pass through the canal on their own volition, and sending the patient back to wait until this process completes may be necessary.

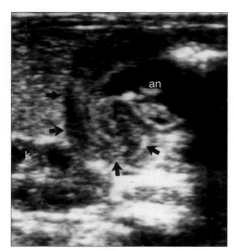

FIGURE 25-28 Transverse view of the right upper quadrant in a 5-week-old boy with hypertrophic pyloric stenosis. The fluid-distended antrum *(an)* has pushed the elongated pyloric muscle *(arrows)* posteriorly, precluding accurate measurement of the length of the pyloric canal. The kidney *(k)* is lateral and slightly posterior to the pyloric muscle.

If there are adequate amounts of fluid in the antrum, the longitudinal images of the pyloric muscle are obtained by placing the transducer transversely across the right upper quadrant, just below the level of the xiphoid process. The transducer is then rotated obliquely until the pyloric muscle is visualized in its long axis. Transverse short-axis images of the pyloric muscle are often obtained from the right coronal plane when the pylorus is abnormal. The gallbladder is initially identified, after which the transducer is angled medially until the hypertrophied pyloric muscle is noted.

If there is not enough residual gastric fluid present, 60 to 120 ml (2 to 4 oz) of glucose water may be administered with a bottle or syringe. Pedialyte (and often breast milk) will have a similar appearance as water; however, formula will appear more echogenic, occluding a good view, and is not advised.

If a positive diagnosis has not been established, the patient is then placed in a right lateral decubitus position and the transducer placed transversely in the right upper quadrant. This allows maximum visualization of the stomach and pyloric canal and is most advantageous for documenting the transit of gastric contents into the duodenum. Sometimes gastrointestinal reflux may be seen as well. This documentation of fluid passing through the canal is important and a cine clip will garner better appreciation.

SONOGRAPHIC MEASUREMENTS AND FINDINGS

Sonographic measurement of pyloric muscle thickness enables the diagnosis of HPS. Pyloric muscle measurements can be made in both the long- and short-axis planes. If the image is oblique, measurements will be overestimated. A muscle thickness greater than or equal to 3 mm and a channel length greater than 15 to 16 mm (often established by institution) on the long-axis view are reliable indicators of HPS. Muscle thickness is the most diagnostic measurement.

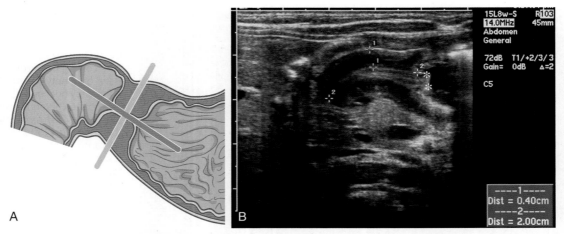

FIGURE 25-29 **A,** Diagram demonstrating long-axis transducer placement in evaluating pylorus. **B,** Positive HPS long-axis "antral nipple" or "cervix" sign, hyperechoic mucosa *(asterisks)* seen bulging into antrum.

If the muscle is thickened and elongated, the mucosa extends into the antrum, and this appearance has been called the "cervix" sign (Figure 25-29). The thickness is measured from the periphery of the hypoechoic muscle to its junction with the echogenic central canal. Pyloric channel length is measured from the proximal to the distal extremes of the echogenic central canal (Figure 25-30).

Transverse axis views will allow measurement of the pylorus overall and muscle wall thickness. A "bagel" or "donut" appearance of a hypertrophied pyloric muscle and echogenic central canal is seen. The pyloric muscle frequently has a nonuniform echo pattern, with the near and far fields appearing more echogenic (Figure 25-31).

In addition to these sonographic findings and measurements, another significant finding is the presence of active antegrade and reverse gastric peristalsis. With positive HPS fluid will often not pass through the canal on fluid-aided real-time sonography. However, occasionally fluid may pass though the crevices of the compressed echogenic mucosa, which appears as the "double-track" sign. This sign may also be seen with pylorospasm, in which the canal is elongated, but the muscle thickness is often within normal limits. In the case of pylorospasm, prolonged observation is necessary, and often will show the pyloric channel opening.

Other Surgical Conditions

In addition to hypertrophic pyloric stenosis, appendicitis, and intussusception, other conditions that may lead to surgical correction may be seen less frequently through the ultrasound department in the neonate. These conditions include midgut malrotation (Figure 25-32), mesenteric or omental cysts (often large in size), duplication cysts of the bowel, duodenal atresia, and meconium peritonitis. Older infants and children may present with Meckel's diverticulum, incarcerated hernia, duplication cysts of the bowel, and hematomas of the bowel resulting from trauma.

Necrotizing Enterocolitis. Necrotizing enterocolitis (NEC) is a very serious condition seen in the premature infant,

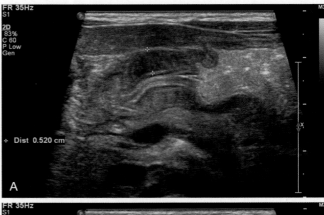
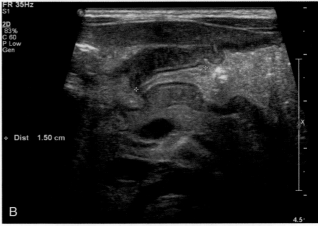

FIGURE 25-30 Positive HPS seen in 26-day-old boy with vomiting. Patient had a positive upper gastrointestinal fluoroscopy study previously (and unnecessarily) at outside hospital. **A,** Long-axis pyloric muscle thickness measurement (anteroposterior) is abnormal at over 5 mm. Pancreas is seen directly posterior to enlarged pylorus. **B,** Pyloric channel length measurement is 15 mm. *(Images courtesy Nationwide Children's Hospital, Columbus, OH.)*

causing high morbidity and mortality. In NEC the bowel undergoes necrosis and must be surgically removed, resulting in **short bowel syndrome.** Once developed, one out of four extremely preterm infants will die from this condition. It is the second leading cause of death in preemies, after

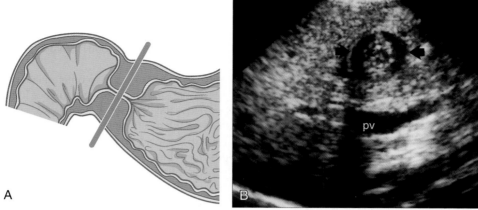

FIGURE 25-31 Positive HPS "bagel" or "donut" sign. **A,** Diagram demonstrating short-axis transducer placement in evaluating pylorus. **B,** Coronal view of the right upper quadrant shows the hypertrophied pyloric muscle in transverse section. The diameter of the muscle *(arrows)* is measured from the outer borders. The muscle thickness *(left arrow to arrowhead)* is measured from the outer border to the mucosal-muscle interface. The portal vein *(pv)* is posterior to the pyloric muscle in this plane.

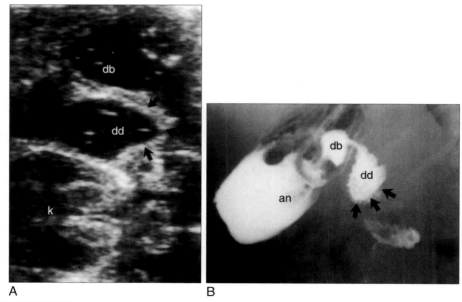

FIGURE 25-32 A, Transverse image of the right upper quadrant using the liver as an acoustic window in a 4-week-old boy with projectile vomiting. There was to-and-fro peristalsis in the fluid-filled duodenal bulb *(db)* and descending duodenum *(dd)*. The descending duodenum tapered abruptly *(arrows)* and could not be traced distally. The right kidney *(k)* is posterior to the descending duodenum. A hypertrophied pyloric muscle was not identified. **B,** Right lateral view from a barium examination in the same patient shows the stomach, antrum *(an)*, duodenal bulb *(db)*, and descending duodenum *(dd)*. The descending duodenum tapers abruptly *(arrows)* and then spirals inferiorly. The barium examination delineates the surgically emergent malrotation, which could not be identified on the sonogram.

respiratory distress. Whereas other causes of mortality in this age-group have declined, NEC mortality has been increasing.

Plain abdominal radiography is the imaging modality of choice, yet sonography can help depict intraabdominal fluid and/or abscess formation before and after surgery in the neonate with abdominal distention or other clinical symptoms. Ultrasound is also helpful in showing bowel wall thickness (Figure 25-33). The most useful sonographic sign, however, is intramural gas, which appears as small punctate hyperechoic foci *within* the intestinal wall, with an associated loss of the normal hypoechoic muscularis halo. Intraluminal gas, on the other hand, will be seen floating within normal intraluminal fluid. Portal venous gas and free intraperitoneal gas may also be detected sonographically.

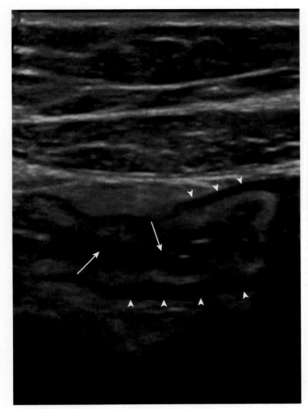

FIGURE 25-33 Slightly thickened bowel in an adolescent, imaged with a high-frequency linear-array transducer. Intraluminal fluid *(arrows)* is seen within the increased hyperechoic mucosal layer, which is surrounded by the muscularis halo *(arrowheads)*. *(Image courtesy Nationwide Children's Hospital, Columbus, OH.)*

 Key Pearls

- Sonography is the imaging modality of choice to evaluate the neonatal and pediatric abdomen, as it provides excellent visualization of the abdominal organs and structures without ionizing radiation.
- Knowledge of a pediatric patient's developmental stage can greatly aid a sonographer in obtaining high-quality diagnostic images.
- Scanning techniques, probe frequencies, and footprints will vary widely across age-groups and continual probe changes and optimization are in order.
- Knowledge of normal organ sizes and reference charts are necessary for the normal pediatric abdominal examination.
- Retroperitoneal and vascular structures should be closely evaluated to rule out malignant processes in the pediatric patient.
- Pancreatitis, trauma, and choledocholithiasis are common reasons for acute abdominal pain.
- Childhood obesity is on the rise and is associated with increased risk of gallstones and nonalcoholic fatty liver disease.
- Acquired and hereditary diseases need to be carefully monitored in children, as there may be increased associated risks of both chronic and malignant processes.

- Most pediatric patients with cystic fibrosis will develop pancreatitis.
- The spleen plays a role in many childhood diseases, as it plays a role in the body's immune response and blood formation.
- Sonography is used to differentiate obstructive from nonobstructive neonatal jaundice in neonates.
- Neonatal hepatitis, biliary atresia, and choledochal cyst are the most common causes of neonatal jaundice.
- Abdominal tumors must be carefully evaluated to determine their organ of origin, blood flow patterns, and morphology and to see if there are any associated lymph nodes or a vessel thrombus.
- Two thirds of all pediatric liver masses are malignant.
- Most malignant pediatric masses are asymptomatic, whereas symptomatic ones tend to be of a gastrointestinal origin.
- The most common surgical conditions diagnosed with sonography are appendicitis, intussusception, and hypertrophic pyloric stenosis.
- Multiple sonographic techniques should be used in evaluating the appendix to overcome an equivocal examination, where the appendix is not visualized.
- Intussusception commonly occurs in children under 2 years old and may cause obstruction of the bowel if in an ileocolic location.
- Hypertrophic pyloric stenosis (HPS) is more commonly seen in males (4:1) and peaks at 1 month of life.
- Too much fluid and too little fluid in the stomach are both pitfalls of HPS imaging.
- Ultrasound may detect other gastrointestinal surgical conditions. Although it may not diagnose them all, ultrasound may be the first imaging procedure in children, so it is good to be aware of these differential diagnoses.

BIBLIOGRAPHY

American Institute of Ultrasound in Medicine: AIUM practice guideline for the performance of an ultrasound examination of the abdomen and/or retroperitoneum, 2012. Available at http://www.aium.org/resources/guidelines/abdominal.pdf.

Amodio J, Fefferman N: Ultrasound of pediatric abdominal and scrotal emergencies, *Appl Radiol* 36(12):22-29, 2007.

Askew N: An overview of infantile hypertrophic pyloric stenosis, *Paediatr Nurs* 22(8):27-30, 2010.

Aziz S, Wild Y, Rosenthal P, Golstein RB: Pseudo gallbladder sign in biliary atresia—an imaging pitfall, *Pediatr Radiol* 41(5):620-626, 2011.

Babcock DS: Sonography of the acute abdomen in the pediatric patient, *J Ultrasound Med* 21:887-899, 2002.

Bachur RG, Dayan PS, Bajaj L, et al: The effect of abdominal pain duration on the accuracy of diagnostic imaging for pediatric appendicitis, *Ann Emerg Med* 60(5):582-590, 2012.

Bachur RG, Levy JA, Callahan MJ, et al: Effect of reduction in the use of computed tomography on clinical outcomes of appendicitis, *JAMA Pediatr* 169(8):755-760, 2015.

Baker ME, Nelson RC, Rosen MP, et al: Expert Panel on Gastrointestinal Imaging: *ACR Appropriateness Criteria®: acute pancreatitis* [online publication], Reston, VA, 2013, American College of Radiology.

Balachandran B, Singhi S, Lal S: Emergency management of acute abdomen in children, *Indian J Pediatr* 80(3):226-234, 2013.

Bhisitkul DM, Listernick R, Shkolnik A, et al: Clinical application of ultrasonography in the diagnosis of intussusception, *J Pediatr* 121:182, 1992.

Butler M, Servaes S, Srinivasan A, et al: US depiction of the appendix: role of abdominal wall thickness and appendiceal location, *Emerg Radiol* 18(6):525-531, 2011.

Centers for Disease Control and Prevention: Child health. Available at http://www.cdc.gov/nchs/fastats/child-health.htm.

Centers for Disease Control and Prevention: Childhood obesity facts. Available at http://www.cdc.gov/healthyschools/obesity/facts.htm.

Chiorean L, et al: Benign liver tumors in pediatric patients—review with emphasis on imaging features, *World J Gastroenterol* 21(28):8541-8561, 2015.

Chung EM, Cube R, Lewis RB, Conran RM: From the archives of the AFIP: pediatric liver masses: radiologic-pathologic correlation part 2. Malignant tumors, *Radiographics* 31(2):483-507, 2011.

Cogley J, O'Connor S, Houshyar R, Dulaimy K: Emergent pediatric US: what every radiologist should know, *Radiographics* 32(3):651-665, 2012.

Coley BD: Pediatric applications of abdominal vascular Doppler imaging: part I, *Pediatr Radiol* 34(10):757-771, 2004.

Cyr J, Johnston DL: Accuracy of physical examination versus ultrasound in the detection of hepatosplenomegaly at diagnosis of pediatric leukemia, *J Hematol Malign* 3(1):24, 2013.

Danon O, et al: Hepatic and splenic involvement in cat-scratch disease: imaging features, *Abdom Imaging* 25(2):182-183, 2000.

Dias SC, Swinson S, Torrão H, et al: Hypertrophic pyloric stenosis: tips and tricks for ultrasound diagnosis, *Insights Imaging* 3(3):247-250, 2012.

Epelman M, et al: Necrotizing enterocolitis: review of state-of-the-art imaging findings with pathologic correlation, *Radiographics* 27(2):285-305, 2007.

Finkelhor D, Turner H, Ormrod R, Hamby S: Trends in childhood violence and abuse exposure: evidence from 2 national surveys, *Arch Pediatr Adolesc Med* 164(3):238-242, 2010.

Fordham LA: Approach to the pediatric patient, *Ultrasound Clin* 4:439-443, 2009.

Goldberg BB, McGahan JP: *Atlas of ultrasound measurements*, ed 2, St Louis, 2006, Mosby.

Goldin AB, Khanna P, Thapa M, et al: Revised ultrasound criteria for appendicitis in children improve diagnostic accuracy, *Pediatr Radiol* 41(8):993-999, 2011.

Haller JO, Slovis TL, Babcock DS, Teele RL: Early history of pediatric ultrasound, *J Ultrasound Med* 23:323-329, 2004.

Heller ME, Veach LM: Evaluation and care of the pediatric patient. In Heller ME, Veach LM, editors: *Clinical medical assisting: a professional, field smart approach to the workplace*, ed 1, New York, 2009, Cengage Learning, pp 426-435.

Herman TE, Siegel MJ: Infantile hepatic hemangioendothelioma, *J Perinatol* 20:447-449, 2000.

Hernanz-Schulman M, Ambrosino MM, Freeman PC, Quinn CB: Common bile duct in children: sonographic dimensions, *Radiology* 195(1):193-195, 1995.

Hilmes MA, Strouse PJ: The pediatric spleen, *Semin Ultrasound CT MRI* 28(1):3-11, 2007.

Humphrey TM, Stringer MD: Biliary atresia: US diagnosis 1, *Radiology* 244(3):845-851, 2007.

Ikeda S, Sera Y, Ohshiro H: Gallbladder contraction in biliary atresia: a pitfall of ultrasound diagnosis, *Pediatr Radiol* 28:451-453, 1998.

Ingram JD, Yerushalmi B, Connell J, et al: Hepatoblastoma in a neonate: a hypervascular presentation mimicking hemangioendothelioma, *Pediatr Radiol* 30:794-797, 2000.

Itagaki A, Uchida M, Ueki K: Double targets sign in ultrasonic diagnosis of intussuscepted Meckel diverticulum, *Pediatr Radiol* 21:148, 1991.

Kendrick A, Phua K, Ooi B, et al: Making the diagnosis of biliary atresia using the triangular cord sign and gallbladder length, *Pediatr Radiol* 30:69-73, 2000.

Kim EH, et al: Clinical features of infantile hepatic hemangioendothelioma, *Korean J Pediatr* 54(6):260-266, 2011.

Kim JS: Acute abdominal pain in children, *Pediatr Gastroenterol Hepatol Nutr* 16(4):219-224, 2013.

Kotagal M, et al: Improving ultrasound quality to reduce computed tomography use in pediatric appendicitis: the Safe and Sound campaign, *Am J Surg* 209(5):896-900, 2015.

Le J, et al: Do clinical outcomes suffer during transition to an ultrasound-first paradigm for the evaluation of acute appendicitis in children? *AJR Am J Roentgenol* 201(6):1348, 2013.

Lee HC, et al: Dilation of the biliary tree in children: sonographic diagnosis and its clinical significance, *J Ultrasound Med* 19:177-182, 2000.

London M, Ladewig P, Ball J, Binler R: Pediatric assessment. In London M, Ladewig P, Ball J, Binler R, editors: *Maternal and child nursing care*, ed 2, London, 2007, Pearson, pp 961-1022.

Loomba, R, Sirlin CB, Schwimmer JB, Lavine JE: Advances in pediatric nonalcoholic fatty liver disease, *Hepatology* 50(4):1282-1293, 2009.

Martin AE, Vollman D, Adler B, Caniano DA: CT scans may not reduce the negative appendectomy rate in children, *J Pediatr Surg* 39(6):886-890, 2004.

Martin-Hirsel A, Cantrell CJ, Hulka F: Antenatal diagnosis of a choledochal cyst and annular pancreas, *J Ultrasound Med* 23:315-318, 2004.

Matz S, Connell M, Sinha M, et al: Clinical outcomes of pediatric patients with acute abdominal pain and incidental findings of free intraperitoneal fluid on diagnostic imaging, *J Ultrasound Med* 32(9):1547-1553, 2013.

Megremis SD, Vlachonikolis JG, Tsilimigaki AM: Spleen length in childhood with US: normal values based on age, sex, and somatometric parameters, *Radiology* 231(1):129-134, 2004.

Milla, SS, Lee EY, Buonomo C, Bramson RT: Ultrasound evaluation of pediatric abdominal masses, *Ultrasound Clin* 2(3):541-559, 2007.

National Institute of Mental Health: What is attention deficit hyperactivity disorder (ADHD, ADD)? Available at http://www.nimh.nih.gov/health/topics/attention-deficit-hyperactivity-disorder-adhd/index.shtml.

National Institute of Mental Health: What is autism spectrum disorder? Available at http://www.nimh.nih.gov/health/topics/autism-spectrum-disorders-asd/index.shtml.

Nielsen JW, et al: Reducing computed tomography scans for appendicitis by introduction of a standardized and validated ultrasonography report template, *J Pediatr Surg* 50(1):144-148, 2015.

Nievelstein RAJ, Robben SJF, Blickman JG: Hepatobiliary and pancreatic imaging in children—techniques and an overview of non-neoplastic disease entities, *Pediatr Radiol* 41:55-75, 2011.

O'Keeffe FN, Stansberry SD, Swischuk LE, et al: Antropyloric muscle thickness at US in infants: what is normal? *Radiology* 178:827, 1991.

Park NH, Park CS, Lee EJ, et al: Ultrasonographic findings identifying the faecal-impacted appendix: differential findings with acute appendicitis, *Br J Radiol* 80(959):872-877, 2007.

Patel RM, Kandefer S, Walsh MC, et al: Causes and timing of death in extremely premature infants from 2000 through 2011, *N Engl J Med* 372(4):331-340, 2015.

Pepper VK, Stanfill AB, Pearl RH: Diagnosis and management of pediatric appendicitis, intussusception, and Meckel diverticulum, *Surg Clin North Am* 92(3):505-526, 2012.

Quillin SP, Siegel MJ, Coffin CM: Acute appendicitis in children: value of sonography in detecting perforation, *Am J Roentgenol* 159:1265, 1992.

Redmon S: Pediatric sonography: funography for kids, *J Diagn Med Sonogr* 23:110-111, 2007.

Restrepo R, Palani R, Cervantes LF, et al: Hemangiomas revisited: the useful, the unusual and the new. Part 1: overview and clinical and imaging characteristics, *Pediatr Radiol* 41(7):895-904, 2011.

Restrepo R, Palani R, Cervantes LF, et al: Hemangiomas revisited: the useful, the unusual and the new. Part 2: endangering hemangiomas and treatment, *Pediatr Radiol* 41(7):905-915, 2011.

Rioux M: Sonographic detection of the normal and abnormal appendix, *Am J Roentgenol* 158:773, 1992.

Saigal G, Therrien JR, Kuo F: Ultrasound in pediatric emergencies, *Appl Radiol* 6-16, Aug 2014. Available at http://appliedradiology.com/articles/ultrasound-in-pediatric-emergencies.

Sato M: Liver tumors in children and young patients: sonographic and color Doppler findings, *Abdom Imaging* 25:596-601, 2000.

Siegel MJ: Pediatric abdominal masses. In Sanders RC, Winter T, editors: *Clinical sonography: a practical guide,* ed 4, Baltimore, MD, 2007, Lippincott Williams & Wilkins, pp 321-340.

Siegel MJ: *Pediatric sonography,* Philadelphia, PA, 2010, Lippincott Williams & Wilkins.

Siegel MJ, Martin KW, Worthington JL: Normal and abnormal pancreas in children: US studies, *Radiology* 165:15-18, 1987.

Sivit CJ: Diagnosis of acute appendicitis in children: spectrum of sonographic findings, *Am J Roentgenol* 161:147, 1993.

Sivit CJ, Newman KD, Boenning DA, et al: Appendicitis: usefulness of US in diagnosis in a pediatric population, *Radiology* 185:549, 1992.

Roos JE, Piffner R, Stallmach T, et al: Infantile hemangioendothelioma, *Radiographics* 23(6):1649-1655, 2003.

Rosenberg HK, et al: Normal splenic sizes in infants and children: sonographic measurements, *AJR Am J Roentgenol* 157:119-121, 1991.

Samuel M: Pediatric appendicitis score, *J Pediatr Surg* 37:877-881, 2002.

Sanchez TRS, Potnick A, Graf JL, et al: Sonographically guided enema for intussusception reduction a safer alternative to fluoroscopy, *J Ultrasound Med* 31(10):1505-1508, 2012.

Sargar KM, Siegel MJ: Sonography of acute appendicitis and its mimics in children, *Indian J Radiol Imaging* 24(2):163, 2014.

Sepulveda A, Buchanan EP: Vascular tumors, *Semin Plast Surg* 28:49-57, 2014.

Spector LJ, Birch J: The epidemiology of hepatoblastoma, *Pediatr Blood Cancer* 59(5):776-779, 2012.

Stranzinger E, Strouse PJ: Ultrasound of the pediatric female pelvis, *Semin Ultrasound CT MRI* 29(2):98-113, 2008.

Stringer MD, Capps SNJ, Pablot SM: Sonographic detection of the lead point in intussusception, *Arch Dis Child* 67:529, 1992.

Swischuk LE, Stansberry SD: Ultrasonographic detection of free peritoneal fluid in uncomplicated intussusception, *Pediatr Radiol* 21:350, 1991.

Trout AT, Sanchez R, Ladino-Torres MF, et al: A critical evaluation of US for the diagnosis of pediatric acute appendicitis in a real-life setting: how can we improve the diagnostic value of sonography? *Pediatr Radiol* 42(7):813-823, 2012.

Trout AT, Sanchez R, Ladino-torres MF: Reevaluating the sonographic criteria for acute appendicitis in children: a review of the literature and a retrospective analysis of 246 cases, *Acad Radiol* 19(11):1382-1394, 2012.

van Rijn RR, Nievelstein RAJ: Paediatric ultrasonography of the liver, hepatobiliary tract and pancreas, *Eur J Radiol* 83(9):1570-1581, 2014.

Varich L: Ultrasound of pediatric liver masses, *Ultrasound Clin* 5(1):137-152, 2010.

Verschelden P, Filiatrault D, Garel L, et al: Intussusception in children: reliability of US in diagnosis—a prospective study, *Radiology* 184:741, 1992.

Vignault F, Filiatrault D, Brandt ML, et al: Acute appendicitis in children: evaluation with US, *Radiology* 176:501, 1990.

Weinberger E, Winters WD: Intussusception in children: the role of sonography, *Radiology* 184:601, 1992.

Wiersma F, Srámek A, Holscher HC: US features of the normal appendix and surrounding area in children, *Radiology* 235(3):1018-1022, 2005.

Wilkinson A: The role of ultrasound in the diagnosis and treatment of intussusception in children, *Ultrasound* 15(2):86-92, 2007.

Zave C: Allergies in children, *Paediatr Child Health* 6(8):555, 2001.

Neonatal and Pediatric Adrenal and Urinary System

Kathryn E. Zale

OBJECTIVES

On completion of this chapter, you should be able to:
- Discuss the sonographic approach to imaging neonatal/pediatric kidneys and adrenal glands
- Distinguish normal anatomy and sonographic findings from abnormal findings
- List and discuss the pathologic conditions covered in this chapter

OUTLINE

KEY TERMS

Adrenal hemorrhage
Angiomyolipomas
Arcuate artery
Autosomal dominant polycystic kidney disease (ADPKD)
Autosomal recessive polycystic kidney disease (ARPKD)
Congenital mesoblastic nephroma
Cortex
Corticomedullary differentiation
Ectasia

Ectopic ureterocele
Hydronephrosis
Medullary pyramids
Multicystic dysplastic kidney (MCDK)
Nephroblastomatosis
Neuroblastoma
Patent urachus
Pelviectasis
Polycystic renal disease
Posterior urethral valves (PUVs)
Potter facies

Prune-belly syndrome
Pulmonary hypoplasia
Pyelonephritis
Renal vein thrombosis
Ureteropelvic junction obstruction
VACTERL
Vesicoureteral reflux (VUR)
Wilms' tumor (nephroblastoma)

Sonography is the diagnostic imaging method of choice when a urinary tract or adrenal abnormality is suspected in the neonate or pediatric patient. There are numerous indications for the renal sonographic examination in the newborn period. One major indication is a renal abnormality detected during prenatal sonography, most commonly congenital hydronephrosis. Some conditions or findings in the newborn associated with renal abnormalities are palpable mass, abdominal distention, anuria, oliguria, hematuria, sepsis or urinary tract infection, myelomeningocele, chromosomal or VACTERL anomalies, abnormal external genitalia, and prune-belly syndrome. Still other indicators include skin tags (usually near the ear and associated with cardiac anomalies)

or a two-vessel umbilical cord. These conditions usually indicate that the renal study in the neonate is for screening the kidneys with no particular renal symptoms present.

In the older infant and child, indications often are for screening of known congenital anomalies and/or for acquired conditions presenting with symptoms, such as flank pain and hematuria.

EXAMINATION PREPARATION

The urinary bladder is considered an important part of the renal sonographic examination, and therefore any child who has bladder control should come to the examination with a full bladder. This preparation and general aspects of the ultrasound examination of the neonate and pediatric patient are described in Chapter 25. Visualization of the bladder includes assessment for distal ureteral dilation (Figure 26-1) or pelvic abnormalities (Figure 26-2). Abnormalities in the urinary tract can often be related to abnormities of the reproductive system, hence the genitourinary system.

A 10-MHz curved array (slightly more curved than an adult footprint) is ideal for scanning neonates and infants, whereas a 7.5-MHz transducer with a similar footprint can provide excellent visualization in a young child (toddler/preschooler) or thin, older (school-age) child. It may be best to use a 9- to 12-MHz linear array in a premature infant or to provide better detail resolution when pathology is suspected. A 3- to 5-MHz curved array is typical for an adolescent.

Scanning is gently initiated over the suprapubic region due to the infant's tendency to urinate spontaneously and a young child's inability to hold the bladder for extended periods of time. If the urinary bladder is not distended at this time, or if voiding occurs before adequate detail can be obtained, this area can be examined after imaging of the kidneys and perirenal areas. Refilling of the urinary bladder is usually relatively rapid if the infant is fed or when parenteral fluids are being administered. A prevoid bladder wall thickness measurement should ideally be obtained with a full bladder.

With the bladder still full, a preliminary view of the kidneys and perirenal areas are scanned via the anterior abdomen or flanks. Longitudinal images of the kidneys are then obtained to document any fluid in the kidney with the bladder full, as well as document the echogenicity comparative to the liver and spleen. In the potty-trained child or older child, the patient is instructed to urinate fully, which may require a short waiting period. The bladder is then reexamined in longitudinal and transverse views, including a postvoid bladder wall thickness. Next, longitudinal and transverse views of the kidneys are documented. Additionally, in both planes, zoomed-up (write zoom) images of the renal superior, mid, and inferior poles are encouraged. In the infant and young child the dedicated renal views are

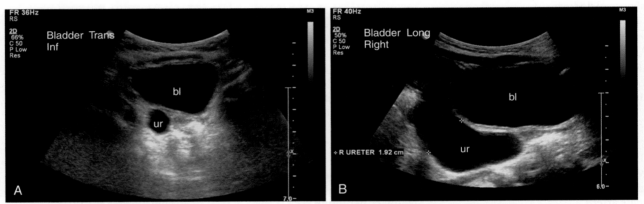

FIGURE 26-1 A, Transverse image of the pelvis in a 28-day-old infant with severe diffuse right hydroureter with primary refluxing megaureter suspected. The urinary bladder *(bl)* is well distended. Dilation of the distal right ureter *(ur)* is seen posterior to the bladder. **B,** Longitudinal view of the same patient shows the distal ureter *(ur)* measuring nearly 2 cm. *(Images courtesy Nationwide Children's Hospital, Columbus, OH.)*

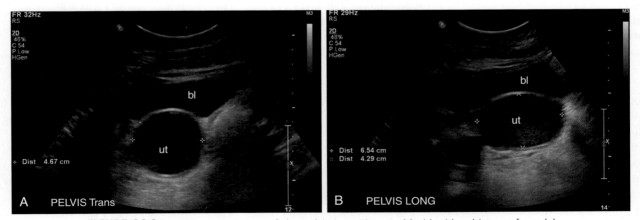

FIGURE 26-2 A, Transverse image of the pelvis in a 12-year-old girl with a history of caudal regression, neurogenic bladder, and left solitary kidney. Hematocolpos/hydrocolpos is detected posterior to the bladder and was confirmed with magnetic resonance imaging, which showed duplicated uteri with fluid in the right uterus. **A,** Transverse image of pelvis shows the urinary bladder *(bl)* and uterus *(ut)* posterior. **B,** Longitudinal view shows bladder *(bl)* and fluid-filled appearance of the uterus *(ut)*. *(Images courtesy Nationwide Children's Hospital, Columbus, OH.)*

often obtained from a prone position, whereas older children and adolescents will be scanned in the decubitus position. Sonographers should keep in mind that renal length may be slightly shorter from a prone position, and position-dependent **pelviectasis** may occur. Renal scanning before and after the infant or child voids can provide useful information. Vesicoureteral reflux, for example, may demonstrate an increase in hydronephrosis as the urinary bladder volume increases. Therefore a prevoid image of the kidney is important in its detection.

NORMAL ANATOMY AND SONOGRAPHIC FINDINGS

Kidneys

The pediatric renal anatomy and sonographic appearance of the kidneys varies widely, depending on the age of the child. This is especially apparent in the young infant. Keep in mind that premature infants are adjusted according to their gestational age in medicine until 2 years of age. Developmentally, in the second trimester the kidney grows from small renunculi that are composed of a central large pyramid with a thin peripheral rim of cortex. As the renunculi fuse progressively, their adjoining cortices form columns of Bertin. The former renunculi are at that point called "lobes." Remnants of these lobes with somewhat incomplete fusion, often termed *fetal* or *renal lobulation,* should not be confused with renal abnormalities or scars when imaging the kidney. Renal lobulation is most prominent at birth and in the neonatal period, often disappearing completely by 6 years of age. The pyramids remain large even after birth in comparison with the thin rim of cortex that surrounds them. The glomerular filtration rate is low right after term birth but increases rapidly thereafter. The cortex continues to grow throughout childhood, whereas the pyramids become smaller. The larger amount of sinus fat is not present in the neonate and pediatric patient, as is often seen in adults.

The normal kidney in the neonate and infant is characterized by a distinct demarcation of the cortex and medullary pyramids or **corticomedullary differentiation,** owed to a larger medullary volume. The **medullary pyramids** are prominent and hypoechoic and should not be mistaken for dilated calyces or cysts. They are typically less prominent by 1 year of age. The surrounding **cortex** is quite thin at birth and echogenicity varies by age. Echogenicity in the full-term neonate is essentially similar to or slightly greater than that of normal liver and splenic parenchyma (Figure 26-3). Premature infants tend to have more echogenic kidneys, owing to underdevelopment of the renal structures. Renal cortical echogenicity normally decreases to less than that of liver parenchyma by 4 to 6 months of age. Increased cortical echogenicity, however, is only seen in the neonatal period (up to 1 month of age). The increased cortical echogenicity may result from glomeruli occupying a larger proportion of cortical volume and the location of 20% of the loops of Henle within the cortex (versus 9% in adults) as opposed to the medulla. Due to a paucity of fat in the renal sinus of the neonate and infant, this area is generally hypoechoic and therefore indistinct.

Children and adolescents have a sonographic renal anatomy similar to adult anatomy. The normal cortex is thick and produces low-level, back-scattered echoes. The medullary pyramids are relatively hypoechoic and arranged around the central, echo-producing renal sinus.

The **arcuate artery** vessels may be seen as intense specular echoes at the corticomedullary junction. Color Doppler is often used to document renal artery and vein in the pediatric renal examination and is best taken in the zoomed-up midtransverse view. This also aids in differentiating a prominent vein from pyelectasis. Pulsed Doppler also aids in detecting cases of renal vein thrombosis, hypertension, or other suspected vascular disease. A dedicated renal duplex examination reports the renal artery resistive index (RI) (along with acceleration time) and the normal RI value varies greatly within the first year: preterm infant, up to 0.9; neonate, 0.6 to 0.8; and by the end of the first

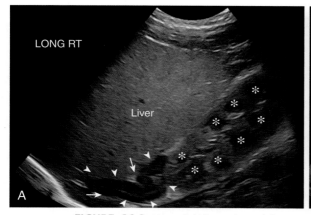 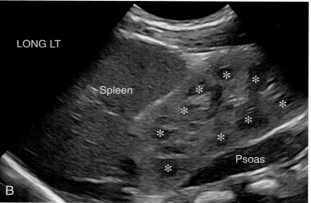

FIGURE 26-3 Normal kidneys in a full-term 1-day-old neonate with congenital heart disease. **A,** Longitudinal supine view of a normal right kidney showing isoechoic cortex echogenicity compared with the liver parenchyma. Normal adrenal gland is also visualized *(arrows)*. The medullary pyramids *(asterisks)* appear as triangular hypoechoic areas. **B,** Longitudinal supine view of a normal left kidney showing hyperechoic cortex echogenicity comparing to the spleen. Adrenal gland is not visualized. The medullary pyramids *(asterisks)* appear as hypoechoic areas. *(Images courtesy Nationwide Children's Hospital, Columbus, OH.)*

year show similar values as adults, 0.5 to 0.7. It is important to keep in mind that cardiac disease, coarctation of the aorta, and patent ductus arteriosus may affect the RI as well.

The normal renal length varies with the age of the neonate or pediatric patient (Figure 26-4). Accurate and consistent measurements are important to document normal growth and to help detect abnormalities. Although the left kidney is somewhat longer, a kidney measurement greater than 1 cm side to side should be monitored closely, and may indicate infection, scarring, or congenital abnormalities, such as hypotrophy or duplicated renal system. A number of renal anomalies may be encountered and include renal agenesis and supernumerary kidney. Anomalies of position, form, and orientation include pelvic kidney, horseshoe kidney (the most common anomaly), crossed ectopy (see Figure 26-6), and renal duplication (see Figures 26-11 and 26-12). See Chapter 15 for further discussion of these anomalies, as the pediatric sonogram may be the first detection of such anomalies, which become increasingly difficult to scan later in life.

Adrenal Glands

The normal adrenal glands are larger and more easily identified in the neonate than in the older infant or young child. In fact, the prominent size of the adrenal gland at birth will normally decrease rapidly within the first 10 days, and then slowly atrophy over the next few weeks. Each gland lies immediately superior to the upper pole of the kidney. The left adrenal gland extends slightly more medial than does the right. Sonographically the gland has an inverted "V" or "Y" shape in the longitudinal plane (Figure 26-5, *A*). In the transverse plane, the portion of the gland delineated has a linear or curvilinear outline (Figure 26-5, *B*). The central adrenal medulla in the neonate is relatively thin, appearing as a distinctly echogenic stripe, surrounded by the more prominent and less echogenic adrenal cortex. When the kidney is absent or ectopic, the ipsilateral adrenal gland remains in the renal fossa, but as a result it may have an altered configuration (Figure 26-6).

Urinary Bladder

The normal urinary bladder is thin walled in the distended state and should measure less than 3 mm (with a mean of 1.5 mm)

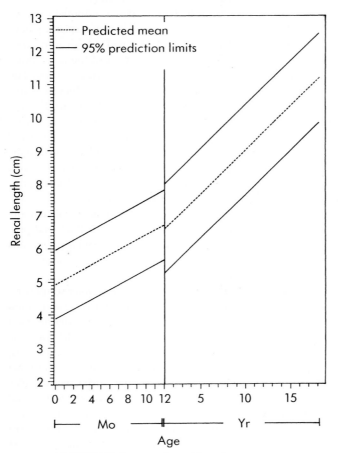

FIGURE 26-4 Normal renal length versus age.

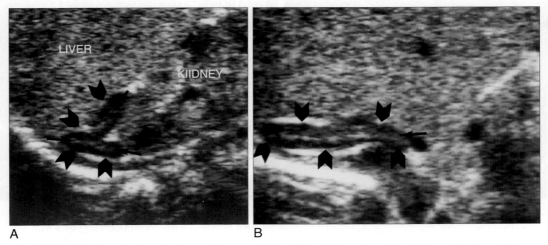

FIGURE 26-5 **A,** Longitudinal view of a normal adrenal gland *(arrowheads)* in a 1-day-old infant with ambiguous genitalia. The adrenal medulla *(arrows)* appears as a central echogenic stripe, surrounded by the less echogenic cortex. The adrenal gland has an inverted-Y configuration. **B,** Transverse view through a portion of a normal adrenal gland *(arrowheads)* demonstrating the curvilinear shape in this plane.

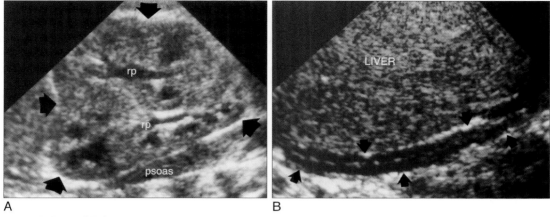

FIGURE 26-6 A, Crossed-fused renal ectopia *(arrows)* in a 1-day-old boy with imperforate anus. Sonogram through the right flank demonstrates the renal pelvis *(rp)* of each kidney. **B,** Longitudinal image through the right flank demonstrates an elongated adrenal gland *(arrows)* resulting from the absence of a kidney in this renal fossa.

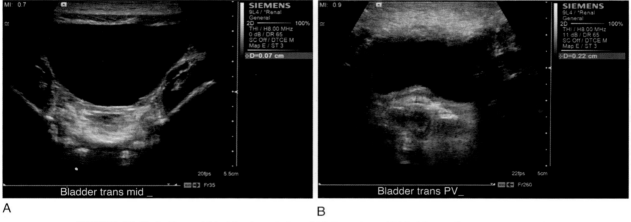

FIGURE 26-7 A, Normal bladder in a 1-day-old infant. Prevoid bladder wall measurement. The urinary bladder is well distended, appearing anechoic with a thin posterior bladder wall. **B,** Sonogram, 2 minutes later after urination, showing postvoid bladder wall measurement still normal at 2.2 mm. Fluid retention in the bladder is normal postvoid in the neonatal period. *(Images courtesy Nationwide Children's Hospital, Columbus, OH.)*

in anterior-posterior dimension. When empty, the wall thickness increases but remains less than 5 mm. Often in pediatrics, the posterior bladder wall is measured, and the posterolateral wall has been suggested to avoid the thickened posterior region of the trigone, which has different characteristics than the detrusor muscle. Likewise, the anterior bladder wall is avoided due to ring-down artifact and the prominent urachal remnant in children. The bladder should normally empty completely or at least 90% of the bladder capacity. Infants are an exception to this, as they often retain urine in the bladder (Figure 26-7). The use of color Doppler may aid in the visualization of the distal ureter as it enters the posterior wall of the bladder.

RENAL, ADRENAL, AND BLADDER PATHOLOGY

The more common congenital anomalies, hereditary renal cystic disease, acquired pathologies, and malignant tumors of the urinary tract and adrenals are presented here. Although discussed separately, it should be understood that congenital or genetic abnormities might contribute to an increased risk of acquired or malignant processes. It should be noted that most of these conditions present as a palpable mass in the neonate. The reasons for both renal and adrenal enlargement, including malignant tumors, are summed up in Tables 26-1 and 26-2.

Congenital Urinary Tract Anomalies

In addition to the many renal anomalies, which may be present in the pediatric patient, hydronephrosis, patent urachus, and multicystic dysplastic kidney disease (MCDK) are other congenital anomalies of the urinary tract found in the neonate and child. Congenital hydronephrosis is a common reason for the pediatric renal sonographic examination, and plays a vital role in the detection and differentiation of the many possible underlying conditions.

TABLE 26-1	Most Common Benign Retroperitoneal Findings	
Clinical Findings	**Sonographic Findings**	**Differential Considerations**
Hydronephrosis		
Flank pain	Pelvocalyceal dilation Ureter is dilated when vesicoureteral reflux or primary megaureter is present	Parapelvic cyst Extrarenal sinus Congenital megacystis Multiple renal cysts Multicystic renal disease Functional dilation Duplicated collecting system
Posterior Urethral Valves		
Decreased urine output	Thickened bladder wall ("keyhole") Hydronephrosis Hydroureter	Megaureter
Multicystic Dysplastic Kidney		
	Unilateral multicystic mass in kidney Contralateral ureteropelvic junction	Hydronephrosis
Polycystic Renal Disease		
Pulmonary hypoplasia Potter's facies	Enlarged kidneys Echogenic kidneys	
Prune-Belly Syndrome		
Absence of abdominal muscle Undescended testes Dilated bladder, ureter, prostatic urethra	Kidney is normal, hydronephrotic, or dysplastic Dysplastic enlarged kidneys Dilated ureters Dilated bladder	Posterior urethral valves
Congenital Mesoblastic Nephroma		
Found in children <1 yr	Hyperechoic or hypoechoic or mixed	Adrenal tumor Neuroblastoma Benign renal tumor Abscess
Adrenal Hemorrhage		
Abdominal mass Jaundice Anemia	Ovoid enlargement of the gland Anechoic to hyperechoic	Adrenal neuroblastoma Adrenal cyst Adrenal neoplasm

TABLE 26-2	Most Common Malignant Retroperitoneal Findings	
Clinical Findings	**Sonographic Findings**	**Differential Considerations**
Neuroblastoma		
Nystagmus Unsteady gait	Mass usually in adrenal gland Echogenic Calcification Look for metastasis to liver	Adrenal hemorrhage Benign renal tumor Abscess
Wilms' Tumor		
Hypertension Palpable abdominal or flank mass Weight loss, fever, anemia, pain	Complex mass in kidney Well-circumscribed mass Isoechoic to echogenic May have calcification Look for tumor extension into renal vein or inferior vena cava	Mesoblastic nephroma Renal cell carcinoma Retroperitoneal sarcoma Adrenal cortical carcinoma Multicystic renal hamartoma

is able to determine the severity of the hydronephrosis, whether the condition is unilateral or bilateral, if the ureters and bladder are dilated, and the status of the renal parenchyma.

Sonographic features found in hydronephrosis include visible renal parenchyma surrounding a central cystic component, small peripheral cysts (dilated calyces) budding off a large central cyst (renal pelvis), and visualization of a dilated ureter. This must be distinguished from the noncommunicating cysts of multicystic dysplastic kidneys. To date, there is no consensus on reporting urinary tract dilation, with roughly two thirds of radiologists using descriptive terminology, one third using the Society for Urology (SFU) grading system, and one third measuring the anteroposterior (AP) diameter of the renal pelvis, leaving a third using two of the above reporting methods. Renal pelvis dilation may be normal up to 10 mm in the AP dimension.

Vesicoureteral Reflux. **Vesicoureteral reflux (VUR)** is a common nonobstructive cause of hydronephrosis and is indicated in up to 33% of prenatally diagnosed hydronephrosis. VUR is the abnormal refluxing of urine from the urinary bladder through the ureters and into the kidney. It has five different grades reflecting severity from I = least severe (reflux limited to ureters only) to V = most severe (severe dilation of ureters and kidney with loss of papillary impressions). It is often treated conservatively because it is nonobstructive. Many cases, often males and an appreciable number of grades IV and V, resolve on their own within the first 2 years. Unilateral or bilateral hydronephrosis may occur and different sides may have different levels of reflux. Although ultrasound can often detect the higher levels of VUR, it may be helpful to detect lower grades by using both prevoid and postvoid renal imaging. Additionally, waiting 7 to 10 days to perform a postnatal ultrasound is recommended, as low

Congenital Hydronephrosis. **Hydronephrosis** describes the dilation of the urinary collecting system and is the most common urinary tract anomaly in children, accounting for 50% of congenital malformations. It is also the most common cause of a palpable mass in the neonate. There are many causes of dilation of the collecting system, the most common being obstruction, reflux, or abnormal muscle development. Sonography is sensitive in detecting small amounts of fluid in the renal pelvis. The sonographer

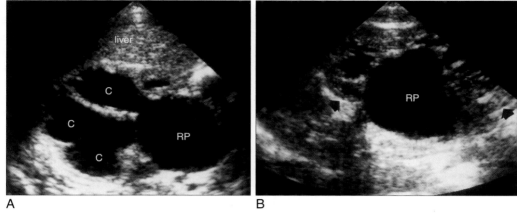

A   B

FIGURE 26-8 A, Ureteropelvic junction obstruction in a 2-week-old girl with an abnormal prenatal ultrasound. Marked dilation of the renal pelvis *(RP)* and calyces *(C)* is present on this transverse view. Parenchymal loss is also noted. The distal ureter was not identified. Radionuclide imaging confirmed the diagnosis. **B,** Ureteropelvic junction obstruction in a 1-day-old infant. Longitudinal image of the kidney *(arrows)* identifies marked dilation of the renal pelvis *(RP)*.

urine output is typical at birth. It is definitively diagnosed by a voiding cystourethrogram.

Sonographic Findings. Sonographic findings for VUR are often nonspecific and may or may not include hydronephrosis, pelvic or ureteral wall thickening (epithelial thickening), intermittent dilation of the collecting system, or displaced ureteral jet in the bladder.

Ureteropelvic Junction Obstruction. **Ureteropelvic junction obstruction** is the most common type of obstruction causing hydronephrosis of the upper urinary tract and occurs in 1 in 2000 children with a male prevalence (3:1), accounting for about 10% of prenatally diagnosed hydronephrosis. It most often results from intrinsic narrowing or extrinsic vascular compression at the level of the ureteropelvic junction. The obstruction produces proximal dilation of the collecting system; however, the ureter is often normal in caliber. There is an increased incidence of abnormalities of the contralateral kidney, such as multicystic dysplastic kidney or vesicoureteral reflux.

Sonographic Findings. Sonographically, there is pelvocalyceal dilation without ureteral dilation (Figure 26-8, *A*). When the obstruction is pronounced, the dilated renal pelvis extends inferiorly and medially (Figure 26-8, *B*). If vesicoureteral reflux or primary megaureter is present, the ureter may be dilated. The best way to demonstrate the dilated ureters at the ureteropelvic junction is with a longitudinal scan plane.

Ureteral Obstruction. The ureter may be obstructed anywhere along its course or at the ureterovesical junction causing hydronephrosis. A secondary process such as abscess, previous surgery (e.g., for appendicitis), lymphoma, and urolithiasis may cause obstruction to the ureter. The presence of a primary megaureter (which may be obstructive or unobstructive), atresia, or an ectopic ureter may be the cause of obstruction as well. With a primary megaureter (see Figure 26-1), sonography shows hydronephrosis and hydroureter with a narrow segment of the distal ureter behind the bladder. The increased peristalsis in the ureter distal to the obstruction may

be seen with sonography as the probe is held over the dilated ureter and the sonographer watches for the peristaltic movement. M-mode may enable a semiquantified assessment of this ureteral peristalsis. A diminished ureteral inflow jet may be seen at the lower margin of the bladder with color Doppler on the side of the obstruction.

Ectopic Ureterocele (and the Duplex Kidney). **Ectopic ureterocele** occurs more commonly in females and more often on the left side. It results from an ectopic bladder insertion and cystic dilation of the distal ureter of the upper moiety of a completely duplicated renal collecting system (Figure 26-9).

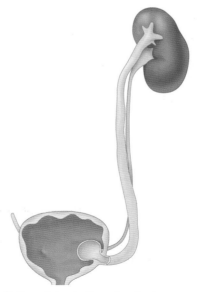

FIGURE 26-9 Complete duplicated collecting system (or duplex kidney) and associated ureterocele diagram. Illustration shows the obstructed ureter, associated with the superior pole, inserting ectopically into an ureterocele resulting in superior hydronephrosis.

These kidneys are commonly referred to as a duplex or "double" kidney.

Sonographic Findings. The ectopic ureterocele, seen as a fluid mass within the urinary bladder, is located inferomedially to the ureteral insertion of the lower pole ureter. Postoperatively, following the incision of the ureterocele, the structure may be seen in a collapsed state. The sonographic delineation of an upper pole fluid mass, in continuity with a dilated ureter and the aforementioned ureterocele, is diagnostic of this entity. Distention and effacement or contraction of the ureterocele may be evident during the real-time study (Figure 26-10).

Bladder Outlet Obstruction. Bilateral hydronephrosis is frequently caused by obstruction at the level of the bladder or bladder outlet. The bladder may be obstructed by a neurogenic bladder, a pelvic mass, or a congenital anomaly, such as posterior urethral valves or prune-belly syndrome. **Posterior urethral valves (PUVs)** are the most common cause of bladder outlet obstruction in the male neonate. A pelvic mass or tumor may be the cause of the bladder obstruction, causing the bladder to be distended with a thickened wall. Vesicoureteral reflux may also be the cause of the dilated renal pelvis. **Prune-belly syndrome** (or abdominal muscle deficiency syndrome), on the other hand, is a rare congenital anomaly of unknown etiology, affecting males in 96% of cases, with severe cases resulting in early infant death from to pulmonary hypoplasia (due to related oligohydramnios in utero). It includes a triad of hypoplasia or deficiency of the abdominal musculature, cryptorchidism, and urinary tract anomalies. This anomaly includes congenital absence or deficiency of the abdominal musculature, large hypotonic dilated tortuous ureters, a large bladder, a patent urachus, bilateral cryptorchidism, and a dilated prostatic urethra. Eighty-five percent of patients with prune-belly syndrome will have associated VUR. Physically, the wrinkled "prunelike" abdomen aids in the clinical diagnosis.

Sonographic Findings. The wall of the urinary bladder appears thickened and trabeculated with PUVs. Midline sagittal imaging with caudal angulation through the bladder may allow visualization of the distended posterior urethra. Alternatively the posterior urethra can be imaged directly from a perineal approach. The resultant hydronephrosis and hydroureter are usually bilateral. Urinary ascites or a perirenal urinoma can result from high-pressure VUR, rupturing a calyceal fornix or tearing the renal parenchyma (Figure 26-11). The

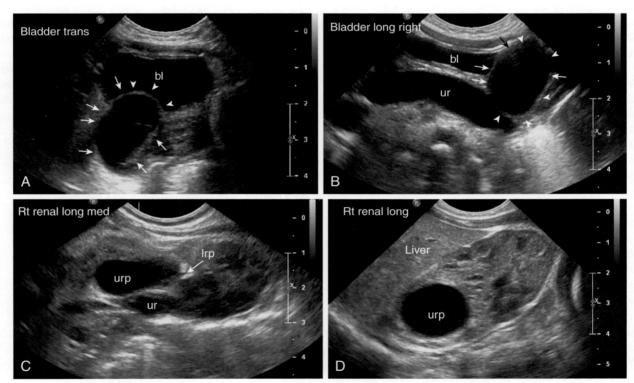

FIGURE 26-10 Duplex kidney with associated ectopic ureterocele in 13-day-old girl with possible right-sided hydronephrosis on prenatal sonogram. A complete duplication of the right kidney with a dilated upper pole and ureter (measuring 1 cm) was seen along the entire course to an inferior ectopic insertion into the bladder terminating in a ureterocele. Bladder wall thickness and left kidney were normal. **A,** Transverse image of the urinary bladder (bl). A large, thin-walled ureterocele (arrows) is seen in the right posterior aspect of the bladder. **B,** Longitudinal view of the bladder in the same patient shows the dilated ureter (ur) and ureterocele (arrows). Low-level echoes seen in the ureter and ureterocele represent debris. **C,** Longitudinal prone view of the medial aspect of the kidney in the same patient demonstrates a duplicated kidney with notable dilation of the upper renal pelvis (urp) and without dilation of the lower renal pelvis (lrp). The ureter from the upper pole segment (ur) is seen posterior to the kidney. **D,** Dilated upper pole (urp), and isoechoic renal parenchyma compared with the liver, as seen from a right supine longitudinal view. (Images courtesy Nationwide Children's Hospital, Columbus, OH.)

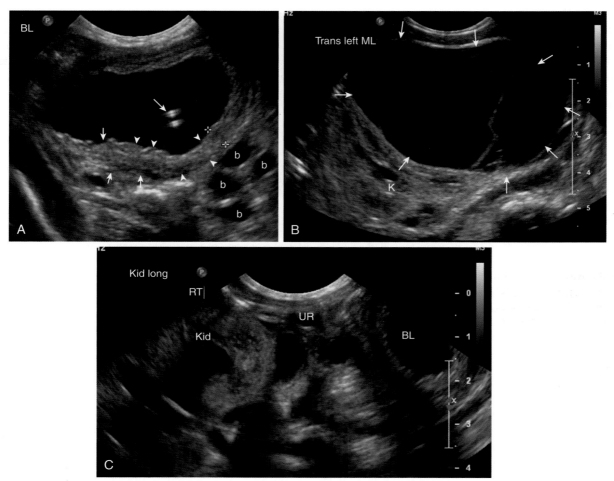

FIGURE 26-11 Posterior urethral valves and urinoma. Posterior urethral valves in an 11-day-old boy. Patient had a bladder catheter placed and a large urinoma drained; however, this follow-up scan showed a distended bladder and the urinoma had reaccumulated. **A,** Transverse view of the urinary bladder shows the thickened bladder wall *(arrows)* and catheter *(arrow)*. Dilated distal ureters were identified in this patient but are not imaged here. Posteriorly, normal fluid-filled bowel *(b)* can be seen peristalsing on real-time imaging. **B,** Longitudinal view of the same patient's left kidney shows a large left perinephric urinoma *(arrows)* measuring 8 cm in its greatest dimension compressing the kidney *(k)* posteriorly. **C,** Right longitudinal image shows the relationship between the kidney *(kid)* with hydronephrosis, dilated ureter *(UR)*, and thickened bladder. *(Images courtesy Nationwide Children's Hospital, Columbus, OH.)*

perirenal urinoma is usually anechoic, but septations may be noted. Other potential causes of perirenal urine extravasation include trauma, ureteropelvic junction obstruction, ureterovesical junction obstruction, and pelvic masses that obstruct the bladder or ureter.

Patent Urachus. The urachus is a long, tubular structure, which connects the dome of the bladder to the umbilicus. Normally it closes during the fourth and fifth months of gestation and is often completely fibrotic at birth, or at least sealed off in the neonatal period. Sometimes, however, the urachus remains patent, either from the bladder end or the umbilical end, and at times from both sides. Sonography plays a role in detecting suspected **patent urachus,** which may present as a cystic mass under the umbilicus at birth or drainage of fluid from the umbilicus. However, often the patent urachus presents with symptoms of infection. This is also called an infected umbilical remnant.

▨ *Sonographic Findings.* High-resolution sonography over the superior bladder will reveal a hypoechoic tract

tracing to the umbilicus. Fluid may be present on either end. In the case where the urachal remnant is patent at the bladder end and closed at the umbilicus, a cyst will form appearing as a hypoechoic mass seen just posterior to the umbilicus. In case of infection, surrounding edema may also be present (Figure 26-12). Color or power Doppler and compression can aid in detecting other signs of infection, such as hyperemia and fluid.

Multicystic Dysplastic Kidney. **Multicystic dysplastic kidney (MCDK)** is the most common cause of renal cystic disease in the neonate, with an incidence of 1 in 4300 live births; when hydronephrosis is excluded, it is the most common cause of an abdominal mass in the newborn. The MCDK is a congenital, usually sporadic, renal dysplasia, which is thought to be secondary to severe, generalized interference with ureteral bud function during the first trimester. The malformation results from ureteral obstruction. High ureteral atresia and pyelocalyceal occlusion are almost always present.

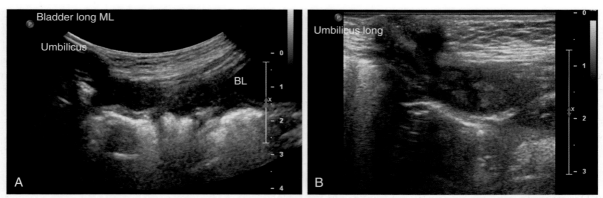

FIGURE 26-12 Infected patent urachus seen in a 4-month-old who presented with purulent drainage from the umbilicus. **A,** Longitudinal image shows a mostly hypoechoic tract extending from the dome of the bladder to the umbilicus. **B,** Longitudinal view over the umbilicus reveals an inhomogeneous mass extending toward the bladder inferiorly. *(Images courtesy Nationwide Children's Hospital, Columbus, OH.)*

In utero the obstruction interferes with ureteral bud division and inhibits the maturation of nephrons in the kidney. Thus the collecting tubules enlarge, becoming cystic and grossly distorting the shape of the kidney. The remaining renal parenchyma becomes virtually nonfunctioning. Nearly half of the cases have contralateral abnormalities (i.e., ureteropelvic junction obstruction and vesicoureteral reflux).

Sonographic Findings. Sonographically the classic appearance of MCDK is of a unilateral mass resembling a "cluster of grapes," which represents multiple discrete noncommunicating cysts, the largest of which are peripheral. There is no identifiable renal pelvis (Figure 26-13). A less common hydronephrotic form of MCDK has been described in which a renal pelvis has been identified. The association with contralateral ureteropelvic junction obstruction has been noted. Bilateral occurrence of MCDK is fatal.

At times, sonographic differentiation of MCDK from severe ureteropelvic junction obstruction may be difficult. In such instances, radionuclide documentation of renal function usually indicates severe hydronephrosis. The use of

ultrasound has led to conservative management of MCDK. These abnormal kidneys most often involute and disappear completely or result in a small dysplastic kidney. If there is evidence of growth, resection is usually undertaken.

Hereditary Renal Cystic Disease

Renal cystic disease is often found as part of the initial workup of renal failure, either through an ultrasound or family history. Prenatal or incidental sonographic findings may also detect these diseases. Hereditary renal cystic diseases, which may present in the neonate or pediatric patient, include autosomal recessive polycystic kidney disease, autosomal dominant polycystic kidney disease, tuberous sclerosis, von Hippel–Lindau disease, and medullary cystic disease/nephronophthisis. These diseases should not be confused with nonhereditary and incidental multiple renal cysts. Just as in the adult, these incidental simple cysts may occur in the child as well, or be associated with a more serious underlying hereditary disease. Furthermore, there may be a high association of cortical renal cysts and the

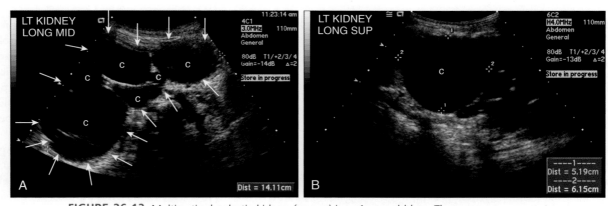

FIGURE 26-13 Multicystic dysplastic kidney *(arrows)* in a 4-year-old boy. There was no apparent left renal pelvis and follow-up imaging a year later showed most of the cysts had involuted. **A,** Longitudinal view of the left flank demonstrates multiple, noncommunicating cysts *(c)* of varying sizes distinguishing it from hydronephrosis. Left MCDK measuring over 14 cm. **B,** Measurement of the largest cyst *(c)* located in the superior pole measuring 6 × 5 cm in longitudinal view. *(Images courtesy Nationwide Children's Hospital, Columbus, OH.)*

development of bilateral Wilms' tumor. Therefore monitoring is important, as well as taking laboratory testing, family history, and associated symptoms or findings into account.

Autosomal Recessive Polycystic Kidney Disease. Polycystic renal disease identified in the neonatal period is most often **autosomal recessive polycystic kidney disease (ARPKD)**, also known as *infantile polycystic disease.* This disease is not common, occurring in 1 in 6000 to 14,000 births, with a female predominance (2:1). As the name suggests it is transmitted by autosomal recessive inheritance. The typical pathologic presentation is diffuse enlargement, sacculations, and cystic diverticula of the medullary portions of the kidneys (Figure 26-14).

ARPKD is associated with biliary **ectasia** and hepatic fibrosis; the severity is proportional to the degree of renal involvement. The most severe form is seen in the neonatal stage, and the least severe form is seen in the infantile to juvenile stage. In the third trimester of pregnancy, the dilated kidneys occupy nearly the entire abdomen and cause the abdomen to protrude. The perinatal form is the most common and is characterized by varying degrees of renal tubular dilation and hepatic fibrosis. The degree of renal cystic disease determines the severity of renal dysplasia, which can lead to renal failure and eventual liver failure. **Pulmonary hypoplasia** with respiratory distress and **Potter facies** may also be associated findings.

In the juvenile form of ARPKD, symptoms can occur later in childhood. The renal tubular ectasia and the resultant renal symptomatology are overshadowed by hepatic fibrosis leading to portal hypertension and gastrointestinal bleeding. In this condition, the dilated renal collecting tubules produce an accentuated medullary echogenicity, and the renal cortex has an essentially normal appearance. Increased liver echogenicity reflects hepatic fibrosis.

Sonographic Findings. The most striking feature is bilateral renal enlargement with diffuse increased echogenicity and loss of definition of the renal sinus, medulla, and cortex. A hypoechogenic outer rim may be present, which represents the cortex compressed by the expanded pyramids. The less severe cases may show hepatosplenomegaly and portal hypertension, with the renal parenchyma normal to echogenic. In utero, oligohydramnios and nonvisualization of the bladder will also be apparent, lending to the development of pulmonary hypoplasia. This diagnosis may be made as early as 16 to 18 weeks of gestation in the presence of severe oligohydramnios and nonvisualization of the bladder.

The macroscopic cystlike appearance throughout both kidneys actually reflects dilated renal tubules that are generally less than 2 mm in diameter. The innumerable acoustic interfaces that present because of this morphologic abnormality result in notable echogenicity, obscuring corticomedullary differentiation. A thin, peripheral, hypoechoic renal rim may be demonstrated, representing either a compressed renal cortex or elongated thin-walled cystic spaces (Figure 26-15). Associated mild

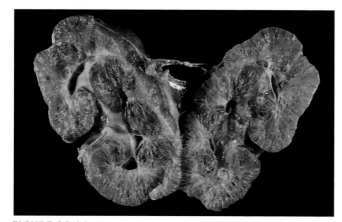

FIGURE 26-14 Gross pathology of autosomal recessive polycystic kidney disease demonstrates bilateral renal enlargement with diffuse cysts replacing the tubules and collecting ducts.

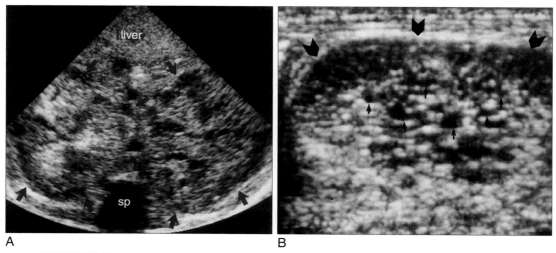

FIGURE 26-15 A, Autosomal recessive polycystic kidney disease (ARPKD) in a 1-day-old boy with abdominal distention. Transverse image of the upper abdomen using the liver as an acoustic window shows the kidneys are enlarged and echogenic with a hypoechoic peripheral rim *(arrows). sp,* Spine. This appearance is typical for ARPKD. **B,** A higher-resolution 7-MHz linear image of the kidney *(arrowheads)* in the same patient reveals multiple small cysts *(arrows).*

hepatic fibrosis and ductal hyperplasia can produce a heterogeneous increase in echogenicity of liver parenchyma.

Autosomal Dominant Polycystic Kidney Disease. More than 90% of patients with **autosomal dominant polycystic kidney disease (ADPKD)** have a gene locus on the short arm of chromosome 16. There is wide variation in the severity of the disease. The adult dominant form of polycystic kidney disease usually appears during middle age. On rare occasions, however, it has been reported in a young infant. Sonography of parents and siblings of patients with ADPKD has proven helpful in identifying this abnormality in afflicted persons who are asymptomatic. More typically the disease becomes manifest during the fourth decade of adulthood, with hypertension, hematuria, and enlarged kidneys.

Sonographic Findings. The sonographic appearance may be similar to slow or late-onset ARPKD. Sonographic findings include bilateral well-defined cysts of various sizes, as the tubular and ductal cells become engorged. Cysts are macroscopic and of varying size and can also form in the liver, spleen, and pancreas. There is an increased incidence of renal cell carcinoma in patients with ADPKD. Cerebral berry aneurysms are also known to occur in 10% to 15% of patients with ADPKD.

Tuberous Sclerosis and von Hippel–Lindau Disease. Just as in the adult patient, renal cysts may appear in the kidney and may be found associated with various multisystemic syndromes such as tuberous sclerosis and von Hippel–Lindau disease. Patients with the autosomal disease of tuberous sclerosis have a 40% incidence of having renal cysts, which may resemble polycystic renal disease. **Angiomyolipomas** may occur and be multiple; their echogenicity is determined by the amount of fatty tissue within the lesion. In patients with von Hippel–Lindau disease, there are multiple cysts. Both tuberous sclerosis and von Hippel–Lindau disease are associated with an increased incidence of renal cell carcinoma.

Medullary Cystic Disease and Nephronophthisis. Medullary cystic disease and nephronophthisis are indistinguishable from, and closely related to, one another. They may be autosomal dominant or recessive and cause renal failure in the child or adolescent. With sonography, the kidneys are small, echogenic, with cysts of variable sizes at the corticomedullary junction and elsewhere in the parenchyma.

Acquired Pathology

Children, like adults, may acquire both acute and chronic pathology of the urinary tract. Often acquired pathology of the kidney and bladder is associated with congenital anomalies, medications, or even prematurity. For example, children with congenital hydronephrosis are at risk for urinary tract infections.

Infection of the Urinary Tract. Urinary tract infection (UTI) is the most common bacterial infection among children. Children under 5 years old with a UTI are often referred for renal sonography to rule out congenital anomalies. Although infection of the urinary system is not as specific to image on sonography as a simple cyst, it is important for the clinician to order a sonogram to rule out the presence of other abnormalities of the kidney that may lead to the infection or renal scarring.

Acute Pyelonephritis. Clinical symptoms of acute **pyelonephritis** include sudden fever, flank pain, and tenderness. The infection usually begins in the bladder and ascends the ureter into the renal pelvis. On sonography, the renal size may be slightly enlarged with an altered renal parenchymal echogenicity secondary to the edema. As the infection spreads into the renal pyramids, there may be increased echogenicity in this triangular area. The renal pelvis and ureter may show some thickening secondary to the inflammation. The infection may be diffuse or localized. Power Doppler may be used in detecting and better defining pyelonephritis, with the area of infection showing an absence or decreased flow (Figure 26-16, *A* and *B*). As the infection begins to wall itself into an abscess formation, a mixed echogenic pattern is demonstrated within the renal parenchyma (Figure 26-16, *C*). Sonography may be useful in following the patient after antibiotic therapy has been given to demonstrate the shrinkage of the lesion.

Chronic Pyelonephritis. This results when repeated episodes of acute pyelonephritis cause the kidney to become scarred and decreased in size. The outline of the kidney may be irregular as the parenchyma becomes scarred. The renal cortex becomes increasingly more echogenic than the liver parenchyma. The renal pyramids become difficult to separate from the renal parenchyma.

Nephrocalcinosis. Nephrocalcinosis is another possible acquired renal pathology. It is the calcification of the renal parenchyma, often in the medulla and rarely in the cortex. Nephrocalcinosis may be encountered in the premature infant, with a wide range reported from 6% to 41%, with the strongest factor associated with very low birth weights. It has many underlying causes, including infants receiving long-term furosemide for lung or heart disease, among other medications, as well as medullary sponge kidney (Cacchi-Ricci disease) or Bartter syndrome.

Renal Vein Thrombosis. **Renal vein thrombosis** is most likely to occur in the dehydrated or septic infant and is more prevalent in infants of diabetic mothers. It may also occur in infants with shock, glomerulonephritis, or nephrotic syndrome. It may also be indicated when malignancy is present, so a full workup is critical. One or both kidneys may be involved. There is renal enlargement, hematuria, proteinuria, and a low platelet count.

Sonographic Findings. Thrombosis occurs initially in the small intrarenal venous branches, and at this stage the enlarged kidney has a nonspecific disordered heterogeneous internal echogenicity corresponding to the extent and severity of the process (Figure 26-17). If the thrombus reaches the renal vein or inferior vena cava, it may be directly visualized within these vascular structures. There may be coexistent adrenal hemorrhage, particularly on the left side where the adrenal vein drains directly into the renal vein. Calcification within the involved veins may eventually result. The use of color and pulsed Doppler helps the sonographer to identify whether the flow is present, reversed, or obstructed.

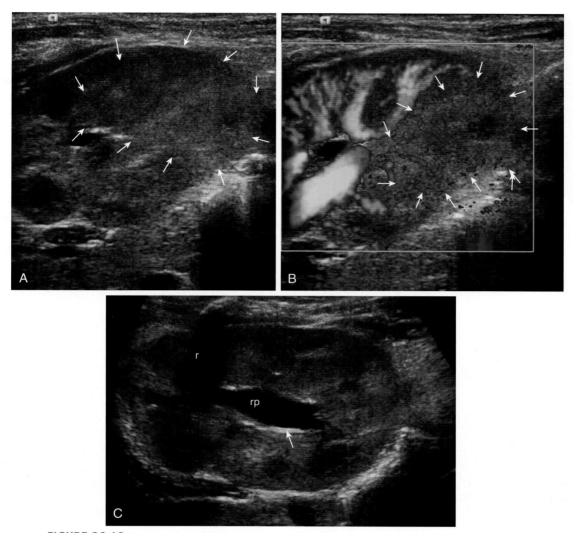

FIGURE 26-16 Focal pyelonephritis seen in a 22-day-old boy with *Escherichia coli* UTI and bacteremia. Right kidney shows focal increased echogenicity in upper pole. There was associated mild pelvic dilation and uroepithelial thickening **A,** Upper pole area of increased echogenicity *(arrows),* suggesting pyelonephritis. Notice a loss of corticomedullary differentiation with gray-scale imaging. **B,** Upper pole view using power Doppler to define area, showing a lack of color filling in the suspected area. **C,** Longitudinal midview showing pelviectasis in the right renal pelvis *(rp)* and associated uroepithelial lining *(arrow)* thickening. Rib shadow *(r)* seen from prone positioning. Pelviectasis was also seen from the supine position, ruling out a prone-position dependent dilation. *(Images courtesy Nationwide Children's Hospital, Columbus, OH.)*

Adrenal Hemorrhage. Difficult delivery, large size, infants of diabetic mothers, stress and hypoxia at delivery, septicemia, and shock all predispose the neonate to the development of an adrenal hemorrhage. The newborn with **adrenal hemorrhage,** however, may have none of these associated factors and still presents with abdominal mass, jaundice, and anemia. Usually the hemorrhage is found secondary to other complications, such as uncontrolled bleeding, jaundice, intestinal obstruction, hypertension, adrenal abscess, or impaired renal function.

Sonographic Findings. Sonographically, adrenal hemorrhage results in ovoid enlargement of the gland or a portion of the gland. The appearance of the hemorrhagic gland can range from anechoic to hyperechoic or may be a mixture of echogenicities, depending on the extent, age, and severity of the process (Figure 26-18). When enlargement is significant, a characteristic blunting of the superior pole of the underlying kidney is produced, along with inferior displacement of the kidney. The initial appearance of adrenal hemorrhage may render it indistinguishable from an adrenal neuroblastoma. Follow-up sonography can differentiate these two entities. Unlike a neoplasm, a hemorrhagic adrenal gland does not enlarge but rather decreases in size. Generally within 4 to 6 weeks, the lesion becomes appreciably smaller and subsequent calcification may be identified on the sonogram or radiographically.

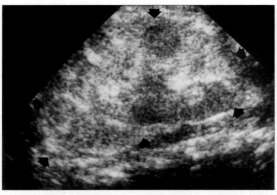

FIGURE 26-17 Renal vein thrombosis in a 3-day-old term newborn with hematuria. Longitudinal sonogram of the left flank demonstrates an enlarged kidney *(arrows)* with patchy areas of increased echogenicity.

Malignant Tumors

Although malignant tumors of the retroperitoneum are far less common than hydronephrosis or multicystic renal dysplasia for palpable mass in the infant or child, they must be considered. When the child presents in the ultrasound department, it is the responsibility of the sonographer to determine the origin of the mass (whether it is part of the liver, kidney, reproductive system, etc.), the internal pattern (cystic, solid, or mixed), and whether the mass has vascular flow. The most common urogenital and adrenal malignant tumors of childhood are presented here.

Nephroblastoma (Wilms' Tumor). Wilms' tumor (nephroblastoma) is the most common intraabdominal malignant renal tumor in young children. The incidence of this tumor peaks between 2 and 5 years of age. This tumor is usually unilateral,

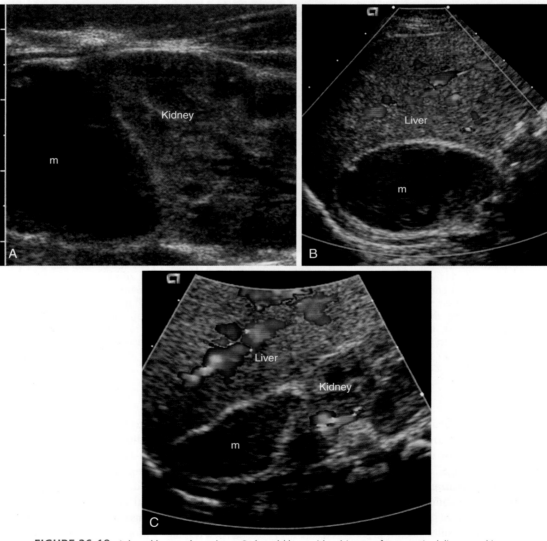

FIGURE 26-18 Adrenal hemorrhage in an 8-day-old boy with a history of traumatic delivery and jaundice. **A,** Longitudinal (zoomed) sonogram demonstrates a suprarenal hypoechoic mass *(m)* just superior to the right kidney. **B,** Longitudinal image of mass *(m)* through the liver without evidence of vascularity. Mass measured 4 × 3.8 × 2.2 cm. A normal adrenal gland was not identified. **C,** Same patient on a follow-up 2 weeks later shows mass *(m)* has decreased in size (2.6 × 3.1 × 1.7 cm) and still without vascularity confirming the diagnosis. *(Images courtesy Nationwide Children's Hospital, Columbus, OH.)*

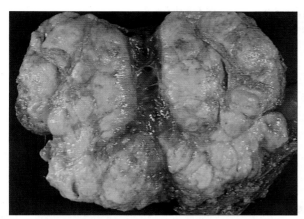

FIGURE 26-19 Gross pathology of a Wilms' tumor demonstrating the multinodular tumor replacing a large portion of the renal parenchyma.

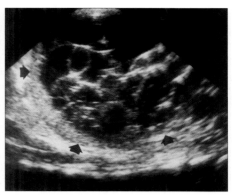

FIGURE 26-20 Wilms' tumor in a 7-month-old with an abdominal mass. Sonogram reveals a large mass with multiple cystic areas occupying the renal fossa (arrows). This represents an unusual presentation of a Wilms' tumor; more frequently a large solid component is present in these masses.

although in a small percentage it may occur bilaterally. Wilms' tumor is bulky and expands within the renal parenchyma, resulting in distortion and displacement of the collecting system and capsule (Figure 26-19). Sonography is used for periodic renal monitoring in those at risk of developing Wilms' tumor, including patients with a previous Wilms' tumor or a family history of the disease. Periodic sonographic monitoring is also performed in patients with either proven or potential **nephroblastomatosis** or with Beckwith-Wiedemann syndrome. In addition to hepatoblastoma and pancreatoblastoma, Beckwith-Wiedemann syndrome also predisposes a child to developing Wilms' tumor. It is important to note that Wilms' tumor may also occur spontaneously. Many pediatric laboratories will sonographically monitor both those predisposed to the tumor and those with a history of Wilms' tumor. In addition, sonography may be used to monitor the size of the tumor while the patient is treated with chemotherapy drugs to shrink the tumor. Therefore the size of the tumor is documented and the appropriate time for surgery is chosen. Early surgical removal and treatment yield a favorable prognosis.

A large differential for Wilms' tumor for children less than 1 year old is neuroblastoma and **congenital mesoblastic nephroma** (also known as *fetal renal hamartoma* or *congenital Wilms' tumor*). Though rare (8 in 1 million births) it is the most common renal tumor of the neonate. This tumor is benign, but is indistinguishable from a Wilms' tumor by any method of imaging. Because the tumor may invade adjacent structures, nephrectomy is indicated.

Sonographic Findings. The sonographic appearance of a Wilms' tumor is variable (Figure 26-20), extending from homogeneous to complex texture. The mass usually has areas of echogenicity and may have calcifications within. The liquefaction may represent necrosis and hemorrhage. The borders are sharply marginated and well defined, but bulky, with a hypoechoic to hyperechoic rim surrounding the mass. The adjacent renal tissue becomes compressed with the growth of the mass. The large solid mass generally is seen to completely distort the renal sinus, pyramids, cortex, and contour of the kidney. The mass may be so large as to protrude into the

hepatic capsule (Figure 26-21). Resultant hydronephrosis may be present.

Sonography is valuable in detecting extension of a Wilms' tumor into the renal vein, inferior vena cava, right atrium, and contralateral kidney. The tumor spreads through direct extension into the renal sinus and peripelvic soft tissues, the lymph nodes in the renal hilum, and the para-aortic areas. Careful evaluation of the renal vein, inferior vena cava, and right atrium of the heart are important to document the possible extension of the tumor. Documentation of tumor extension can have a significant bearing on the surgical approach to the patient. When the tumor extends into the right atrium, cardiopulmonary bypass may be necessary to resect the tumor completely.

Neuroblastoma. **Neuroblastoma** is the most common malignancy in children less than 1 year of age, with an incidence rate twice that of leukemia. It arises in the sympathetic chain ganglia and adrenal medulla and may be detected on prenatal sonography or at birth. This is the second most common abdominal tumor of childhood, occurring between the ages of 2 months and 2 years. About half of these tumors arise in the medulla of the adrenal gland, although tumors have also been found in the neck, mediastinum, retroperitoneum, and pelvis. Clinical findings depend on the location of the tumor. Tumors that arise within the adrenal gland show an abdominal mass, hypertension, diarrhea, and bone pain if metastasis is involved. If the tumor is detected in infants under 1 year old the prognosis is often good, whereas aggressive methods of treatment are often needed in older children. They also carry a worse prognosis than a Wilms' tumor.

Sonographic Findings. Neuroblastoma is usually highly echogenic. Intrinsic calcification may be identified (Figure 26-22). The smaller tumors may appear homogeneous and hyperechoic, whereas the large tumors are more complex in appearance. A cystic form of neuroblastoma has also been described. The adjacent kidney is displaced inferiorly and at times laterally. Doppler evaluation may help to differentiate the tumor from an adrenal hemorrhage because there is increased vascularity within the neoplastic growth.

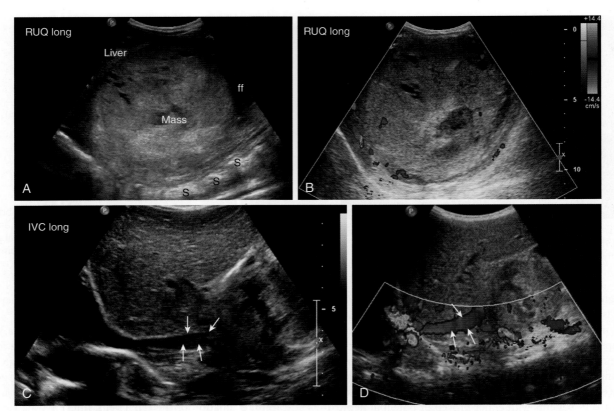

FIGURE 26-21 **Wilms' tumor in a 1-year-old boy presenting with enlarged liver and spleen.** **A,** Longitudinal view of the right renal fossa demonstrates a large (10 × 10 cm) complex mass *(m)* displacing the liver anteriorly. Free fluid *(ff)* is seen inferior to the mass, and the mass can be seen pushing against the spine *(s)*. **B,** Longitudinal evaluation of mass with color Doppler. **C,** Careful evaluation of the inferior vena cava (IVC) showed no extension of the tumor into the IVC and no metastases were seen as well. Proximal IVC *(arrows)* appears to be disrupted by the large tumor. **D,** Color Doppler (shown) in proximal portion of IVC, along with pulsed Doppler, was used for the entire length of the vessel to demonstrate patency. IVC and other midline structures, such as pancreas, were displaced to the left. *(Images courtesy Nationwide Children's Hospital, Columbus, OH.)*

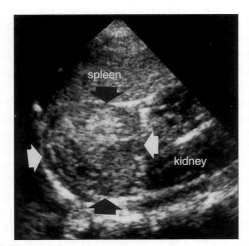

FIGURE 26-22 Adrenal neuroblastoma in a 1-week-old girl with history of a left kidney mass on a fetal sonogram. Longitudinal image through the left flank reveals a large heterogeneous mass *(arrows)* displacing the left kidney inferiorly.

The disease spreads early and widely, so the majority of patients present with metastases. Careful sonographic evaluation of the liver should be made for evidence of metastatic disease. The mass also spreads around the aorta, celiac, and superior mesenteric arteries. This spread of tumor helps to distinguish a neuroblastoma from a Wilms' tumor because this tumor is well encapsulated, although it is somewhat homogeneous and heterogeneous. The neuroblastoma is poorly defined and heterogeneous with irregular hyperechoic areas caused by calcifications. Because intraspinal extension is reported to occur in as many as 15% of patients and because ultrasonography can successfully define the spinal canal in young infants, such examination should be considered in the initial assessment of the infant with suspected neuroblastoma.
Other Malignant Retroperitoneal Tumors. Renal cell carcinoma may infrequently occur in childhood, accounting for 1.8% to 6.3% of all malignant renal tumors in childhood. It appears as an isoechoic to slightly hypoechoic mass within the kidney.

The rhabdomyosarcoma is the fourth most common solid malignancy of childhood, behind central nervous system neoplasms, neuroblastoma, and Wilms' tumor. It often arises from the head and neck, but also the genitourinary system, including the bladder. Average age of presentation for this tumor is 7 years old. It may arise posterior to the bladder causing urethral obstruction. The sonographer should always allow for adequate visualization posterior to the bladder, which in the case of extreme distention may require catheterization.

Adrenal malignant tumors, though rare, include the pheochromocytoma, which is an adrenal neuroendocrine tumor of childhood. Patients present with headache, palpitations, and sweating. Roughly half will present with a palpable abdominal mass, and may also have hypertension. Adrenocortical carcinomas are another malignant adrenal tumor, with most cases occurring before 3 years of age. However, any adrenal tumor or hyperplasia may be indicated in precocious puberty, which is defined as sexual maturation in boys younger than 9 years or girls younger than 8 years.

 Key Pearls

- Neonatal kidneys may appear hyperechoic or isoechoic compared with the liver parenchyma, and this is normal up to 1 month of age. However, they should be less echogenic than liver/spleen parenchyma by 4 to 6 months of age.
- The medullary pyramids are hypoechoic and prominent up to the first year, and should not be mistaken for hydronephrosis or cysts.
- Renal length varies by age, with the left kidney a bit longer. Measurement greater than 1 cm from side to side may indicate a congenital anomaly or possible pathology.
- Accurate and consistent renal measurements are important and allow for the documentation of normal growth and accurate follow-up studies.
- The sonographer should know and recognize renal congenital anomalies, as they are much easier to describe sonographically in the infant or child versus later in the adult.
- It is important to visualize the bladder, often imaged first, and should be properly prepped in those old enough to hold a full urinary bladder.
- Infants are likely to retain urine in the bladder and this is a normal finding.
- Allow for adequate posterior viewing of bladder for identification of dilated ureters, pathology of the uterus, and masses.
- Adrenals may easily be seen in neonates, often prominent at birth and rapidly decrease in size in the first 2 weeks of life.
- It is critical to differentiate communicating cysts (hydronephrosis) from noncommunicating cysts of multicystic dysplastic kidney disease.

- Hydronephrosis is the most common cause of palpable mass in the neonate.
- Ureteropelvic junction obstruction is the most common type of obstruction in hydronephrosis.
- There are many causes of hydronephrosis, including vesicoureteral reflux, ureteropelvic junction obstruction, ectopic ureterocele associated with a duplex kidney, and bladder outlet obstruction (posterior urethral valves and prune-belly syndrome).
- Hereditary renal cystic disease is often found prenatally, incidentally, or as part of a workup for renal failure.
- Multiple simple cysts may be benign or part of a serious hereditary disease; therefore a workup and history are important.
- Multicystic dysplastic kidney disease is the most common renal cystic diagnosis of a neonate.
- Multisystemic diseases, such as tuberous sclerosis and von Hippel–Lindau disease, increase a patient's risk for developing renal cell carcinoma.
- Urinary tract infection is the most common bacterial infection in children, and sonography is used to rule out any underlying congenital anomalies.
- Nephrocalcinosis is often associated with very low birth weight preterm infants.
- Adrenal hemorrhage is often ovoid in shape and will not show any color Doppler flow; follow-up is necessary to confirm this diagnosis.
- Wilms' tumor (nephroblastoma) is the most common intraabdominal malignant tumor in young children, whereas the neuroblastoma is the most common tumor in infants under 1 year of age, although it may present between 2 months and 2 years old.
- Wilms' tumor peaks at 2 to 5 years of age and has a better prognosis than neuroblastoma, which often presents with metastases.
- Careful evaluation of the inferior vena cava and renal veins is important to exclude vascular extension of any abdominal tumor.

BIBLIOGRAPHY

Abdellah A, Selma K, Elamin M, et al: Renal cell carcinoma in children: case report and literature review, *Pan Afr Med J* 20:84, 2015.

American Institute of Ultrasound in Medicine: AIUM practice guideline for the performance of an ultrasound examination in the practice of urology, 2011. Available at http://www.aium.org/resources/guidelines/urology.pdf.

Becker A, Baum M: Obstructive uropathy, *Early Hum Dev* 82(1):15-22, 2006.

Belarmino JM, Kogan BA: Management of neonatal hydronephrosis, *Early Hum Dev* 82(1):9-14, 2006.

Bhansali A, Rajput R, Behra A, et al: Childhood sporadic pheochromocytoma: clinical profile and outcome in 19 patients, *J Pediatr Endocrinol Metab* 19(5):749-756, 2006.

Blane CE, Ritchey M, DiPietro M: Single system ectopic ureters and ureteroceles associated with dysplastic kidney, *Pediatr Radiol* 22:217, 1992.

Chen JJ, Pugach J, Patel M, et al: The renal length nomogram: multivariable approach, *J Urol* 168(5):2149-2152, 2002.

Cohan RH, Ellis JH: Renal masses: imaging evaluation, *Radiol Clin North Am* 53(5):985-1003, 2015.

Coley BD: Pediatric applications of abdominal vascular Doppler: part II, *Pediatr Radiol* 34(10):772-786, 2004.

Creel S, Anderson J, Michael K, Pinkerman B: Evaluation of pediatric renal size by sonography, *J Diagn Med Sonogr* 15(1):1-6, 1999.

Fang SB, Lee H, Sheu J: Prenatal sonographic detection of adrenal hemorrhage confirmed by postnatal surgery, *J Clin Ultrasound* 27:206-209, 1999.

Fenichel G: *Clinical pediatric neurology*, ed 6, Philadelphia, 2009, Saunders.

Fisher JP, Tweddle DA: Neonatal neuroblastoma, *Semin Fetal Neonatal Med* 17(4):207-215, 2012.

Garel L: Renal cystic disease, *Ultrasound Clin* 5(1):15-59, 2010.

Heikkilä J, Taskinen S, Rintala R: Urinomas associated with posterior urethral valves, *J Urol* 180(4):1476-1478, 2008.

Jakubowska A, Grajewska-Ferens M, Brzewski M, Sopyło B: Usefulness of imaging techniques in the diagnostics of precocious puberty in boys, *Pol J Radiol* 76(4):21-27, 2011.

Jequier S, Rousseau O: Sonographic measurements of the normal bladder wall in children, *AJR Am J Roentgenol* 149(3):563-566, 1987.

Kasap B, Soylu A, Türkmen M, Kavukcu S: Relationship of increased renal cortical echogenicity with clinical and laboratory findings in pediatric renal disease, *J Clin Ultrasound* 34(7):339-342, 2006.

Lawande A: Ultrasonography in pediatric renal masses, *Ultrasound Clin* 5(4):433-441, 2010.

Lee HS, Sung IK, Kim SJ, et al: Risk factors associated with nephrocalcinosis in preterm infants, *Am J Perinatol* 31(4):279-286, 2014.

Lee W, Comstock CH, Jurcak-Zaleski S: Prenatal diagnosis of adrenal hemorrhage by ultrasonography, *J Ultrasound Med* 11:369, 1992.

Letourneau K, Harrington C, Reed M, et al: Tuberous sclerosis complex: typical and atypical sonographic findings, *J Diagn Med Sonogr* 21:491-496, 2015.

Leung VY, Chu WC, Yeung CK, et al: Nomograms of total renal volume, urinary bladder volume and bladder wall thickness index in 3,376 children with a normal urinary tract, *Pediatr Radiol* 37(2):181-188, 2007.

Lin CC, Tsai JD, Sheu JC, et al: Segmental multicystic dysplastic kidney in children: clinical presentation, imaging finding, management, and outcome, *J Pediatr Surg* 45(9):1856-1862, 2010.

Luckens JN: Neuroblastoma in the neonate, *Semin Perinatol* 23:263-273, 1999.

Margraf LR: Diagnosis and discussion: autosomal recessive polycystic kidney disease, *Am J Dis Child* 147:77, 1993.

Matos F, Carneiro L, Oeiras L: Retroperitoneal masses in children—beyond neuroblastoma and Wilms tumor, *Eur Congr Radiol* 1970:1-20, 2011.

Mchugh K: Renal and adrenal tumours in children, *Cancer Imaging* 7:41-51, 2007.

Nadler EP, Barksdale EM Jr: Adrenal masses in the newborn, *Semin Pediatr Surg* 9:156-164, 2000.

Orazi C, Fariello G, Malena S: Renal vein thrombosis and adrenal hemorrhage in the newborn: ultrasound evaluation of 4 cases, *J Clin Ultrasound* 21:163, 1993.

Pates JA, Dashe JS: Prenatal diagnosis and management of hydronephrosis, *Early Hum Dev* 82(1):3-8, 2006.

Resontoc LP, Yap HK: Renal vascular thrombosis in the newborn, *Pediatr Nephrol* 31(6):907-915, 2016. doi: 10.1007/s00467-015-3160-0.

Riccabona M: Obstructive diseases of the urinary tract in children: lessons from the last 15 years, *Pediatr Radiol* 40(6):947-955, 2010.

Riccabona M: Urinary tract imaging in infancy, *Pediatr Radiol* 39(Suppl 3):436-445, 2009.

Robert A, Leroy V, Riquet A, et al: Renal involvement in tuberous sclerosis complex with emphasis on cystic lesions, *Radiol Med* 121(5):402-408, 2016.

Rumack CM, Wilson SR, Charboneau JW, Johnson J: *Diagnostic ultrasound,* vol 2, St. Louis, 2010, Elsevier.

Samal SK, Rathod S: Prune belly syndrome: a rare case report, *J Natl Sci Biol Med* 6(1):255-257, 2015.

Scott EM, Thomas A, Mcgarrigle HH, Lachelin GC: Serial adrenal ultrasonography in normal neonates, *J Ultrasound Med* 9(5):279-283, 1990.

Siegel MJ: Pediatric abdominal masses. In Sanders RC, Winter T, editors: *Clinical sonography: a practical guide,* ed 4, Baltimore, MD, 2007, Lippincott Williams & Wilkins, pp 321-340.

Siegel MJ: *Pediatric sonography,* Philadelphia, PA, 2010, Lippincott Williams & Wilkins.

Simanovsky N, Revel-Vilk S, Weintraub M, Hiller N: Association between renal cystic lesions and bilateral Wilms' tumours, *Eur Radiol* 26(6):1665-1669, 2016. doi: 10.1007/s00330-015-3976-9.

Simões e Silva AC, Oliveira EA: Update on the approach of urinary tract infection in childhood, *J Pediatr (Rio J)* 91(6 Suppl 1):S2-S10, 2015. doi: 10.1016/j.jped.2015.05.003.

Sivit CJ: Sonography of pediatric urinary tract emergencies, *Ultrasound Clin* 1(1):67-75, 2006.

Soundappan SV, Lam AH, Cass DT: Traumatic adrenal haemorrhage in children, *Aust N Z J Surg* 76(8):729-731, 2006.

Stark JE, Weinberger E: Ultrasonography of the neonatal genitourinary tract, *Appl Radiol* 22:50, 1993.

Strife JL, et al: Multicystic dysplastic kidney in children: US follow-up, *Radiology* 186:785, 1993.

Sweeney WE, Avner ED: Diagnosis and management of childhood polycystic kidney disease, *Pediatr Nephrol* 26(5):675-692, 2011.

Swenson DW, Darge K, Ziniel SI, Chow JS: Characterizing upper urinary tract dilation on ultrasound: a survey of North American pediatric radiologists' practices, *Pediatr Radiol* 45(5):686-694, 2015.

Teele RL, Share JC: Evaluating an abdominal mass. In Teele RL, Share JC, editors: *Ultrasonography of infants and children,* Philadelphia, 1991, Saunders.

Valdespino RS: The importance of sonography in the evaluation of neonatal adrenal hemorrhage, *J Diagn Med Sonogr* 25(4):221-225, 2009.

Yeung CK, Sreedhar B, Leung YF, Sit KY: Correlation between ultrasonographic bladder measurements and urodynamic findings in children with recurrent urinary tract infection, *BJU Int* 99(3):651-655, 2007.

Zerin JM, Blane CE: Sonographic assessment of renal length in children: a reappraisal, *Pediatr Radiol* 24(2):101-106, 1994.

Neonatal and Infant Head

Kathryn E. Zale

Neurosonography is the primary imaging modality for high-risk and unstable premature infants because it is portable, nonionizing, and noninvasive and can be tolerated by the sickest infants, even immediately after birth. Furthermore, it is safe when adhering to the ALARA (as low as reasonably achievable) principle and is without contraindications, thus allowing for serial imaging of brain maturation and evolution of lesions. In the hands of a skilled sonographer or physician it is a reliable tool for the detection of most hemorrhage cystic and ischemic brain lesions, structural brain anomalies, and calcifications and cerebral infections. Although some conditions are not treatable, neurosonography allows for the assessment of neurologic prognosis, which aids parental counseling, as well as decisions on continuation of neonatal intensive care. Furthermore, it helps to optimize treatment of the infant and provides support to the family both during and after the neonatal period.

TABLE 27-1	Preterm Infants, Gestational Age, and Preterm Weight Categories	
Preterm Definition	**Gestational Age at Birth**	**Birth Weight categories and Median Weight at Gestational Age**
Late preterm (or near-term)	Between 34 and 36 weeks (before 37 weeks)	Most premature births occur in this stage and carry the least amount of mortality and morbidity risks Low birth weight (LBW) defined as weighing less than 2500 g at birth = boys (35 weeks), girls (35.5 weeks)
Moderately preterm	Between 32 and 34 weeks	2000 g at birth = boys (33 weeks), girls (33.5 weeks)
Very preterm	Less than 32 weeks	Very low birth weight (VLBW) defined as less than 1500 g at birth = boys (30.5 weeks), girls (31 weeks)
Extremely preterm	At or before 25 weeks	Extremely low birth weight (ELBW) defined as less than 1000 g at birth = boys (27.5 weeks), girls (28 weeks)

Birth weights are representative of 50th percentile for gestation age. Weight percentile data from Fenton, Tanis R, Kim JH: A systematic review and meta-analysis to revise the Fenton growth chart for preterm infants, *BMC Pediatr* 13(1):59, 2013.

Neurologic impairment is one of the primary concerns about the health of premature infants. (See Table 27-1 for age/weight categories.) Intraventricular and subependymal hemorrhages occur in 40% to 70% of premature neonates under 34 weeks of gestation. Multifocal necrosis of the white matter, referred to as periventricular leukomalacia (PVL), may develop in 12% to 20% of infants weighing less than 2000 g. Additionally, any neonate who suffered a difficult delivery associated with **hypoxia** or **asphyxia** may be examined for PVL. These lesions are associated with increased mortality and an abnormal neurologic outcome.

This chapter aims to provide the reader with an introduction to the neonatal head examination and therefore the focus is on normal cranial anatomy, along with sonographic findings and protocols. Pathology in this chapter includes hydrocephalus, intracranial hemorrhage (ICH), hypoxic-ischemic lesions, congenital malformations, and infection in the neonate.

NORMAL ANATOMY AND SONOGRAPHIC FINDINGS

Knowledge of the normal cranial anatomy is essential to performing the neonatal head examination. The cranial cavity contains the brain and its surrounding meninges and portions of the cranial nerves, arteries, veins, and venous sinuses. The following neonatal head structures and sonographic findings are provided to aid in performing neurosonology.

Fontanels

Fontanels are the spaces between the bones of the skull, which allow for compression at birth and rapid brain growth thereafter. They provide the sonographer with acoustic windows (Figure 27-1) where the transducer is carefully placed to visualize and record brain structures. It is important to note their closure, which heavily hampers or completely impairs sonographic imaging. The anterior fontanel is the largest at birth and provides an optimal sonographic view of the brain until around 9 to 12 months of age, although the median age of closure is 13.8 months, with a range of 9 to 15 months. This fontanel may remain open longer than the normal range in cases of prematurity, hydrocephalus, hypothyroidism, and some bone disorders and chromosomal abnormalities, such as trisomy 13, 18, and 21. If

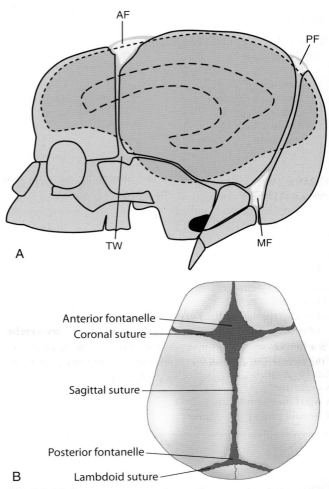

FIGURE 27-1 A, Acoustic windows. The acoustic window often becomes limited at the beginning of the fontanel closure timeframes, which are relative to a term neonate and preterm infants will be adjusted according to their gestational age. *AF,* Anterior fontanel normally closes between 9 and 15 months of age. *PF,* Posterior fontanel closes 8 to 12 weeks after birth, though some may be closed at birth. *TW,* Temporal window, or sphenoidal fontanel, closes around 6 months of age. *MF,* Mastoid fontanel closes between 6 and 18 months after birth. **B,** Top view of the neonatal skull showing the sutures and open anterior and posterior fontanel.

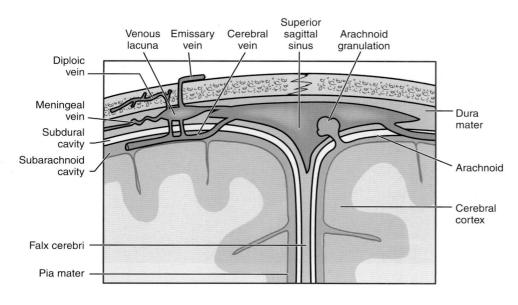

FIGURE 27-2 Coronal diagram showing the three meninges layers and their cavities.

---

hydrocephalus is present, it is felt to be bulging. Compressed or overlapping fontanels, on the other hand, due to oligohydramnios or a difficult delivery, may be difficult to palpate and provide a limited acoustic window to adequately image the structures of the brain.

Meninges

There are three membranes called **meninges** that surround and form a protective covering for the brain: the dura mater, arachnoid, and pia mater membranes. The dura mater, or "soft mother," lies against the delicate brain parenchyma; the arachnoid membrane is in the middle; and the dura mater, or "tough mother," is a double-layered outer membrane that forms the strongest barrier (Figure 27-2). The subarachnoid space is the interface between the vascular channels and the cerebrospinal fluid (CSF), playing an important role in the blood-brain barrier. It connects to the pia matter via the arachnoid trabeculae and to the dura matter via arachnoid granulations. The **falx cerebri** is a fibrous structure separating the two cerebral hemispheres. The **tentorium cerebelli** is an extension of the falx cerebri and separates the cerebrum and cerebellum. Structures above this V-shaped echogenic structure are said to be supratentorial, and structures below it are infratentorial.

Ventricular System

The ventricular system is filled with CSF, which surrounds and protects the brain and spinal cord from physical impact. Putatively, it also acts as a communication route for hormones and transmitters between areas of the central nervous system. The CSF-filled ventricular system includes the ventricles, their connecting foraminae, and subarachnoid space, which are all contiguous with the central spinal column.
Ventricles. The lateral ventricles, located on either side of the brain, are the largest of the CSF-filled cavities located within the cerebral hemispheres and appear anechoic sonographically.

The lateral ventricles are divided into four segments and are generally named after the lobe of the brain into which they project: the frontal horns, central body, temporal horns, and occipital horns. The body is the central section, just posterior to the frontal horn. The **atrium (or trigone) of the lateral ventricle** is the site where the body, occipital, and temporal horns join together (Figure 27-3).

The sonographer should be aware that ventricular size varies with gestational age and that the premature infant will normally have larger-appearing ventricles than the term infant. Dilation of the lateral ventricles often begins in the occipital horns. Minor asymmetry of the lateral ventricles is not uncommon, occurring in 20% to 40% of infants. The left side is often larger than the right. Another more rare variant is coarctation of the ventricle (Figure 27-4), which will appear as a cyst in coronal view at the superior and lateral ventricle(s), often at the level of the intraventricular foramen. In both of these variant cases, care should be taken to make certain the

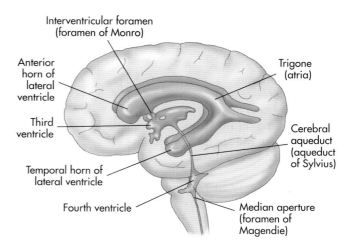

FIGURE 27-3 Sagittal view of the ventricular system. Note that the posterior horns are wider than the anterior ones.

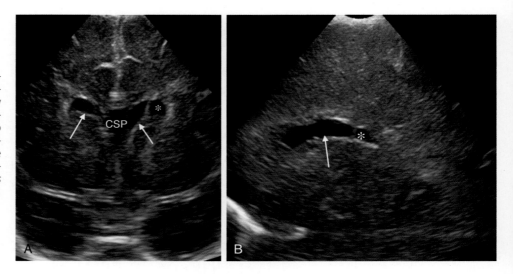

FIGURE 27-4 Coarctation of the lateral ventricles at the level of the intraventricular foramen. **A,** Coronal view shows a cyst *(asterisk)* at the superolateral aspect of the left ventricle. *Arrows* to ventricles; *CSP* is cavum septum pellucidum. **B,** Parasagittal view of the same ventricle demonstrates a large septation-like divide within the cavity. *(Images courtesy Nationwide Children's Hospital, Columbus, OH.)*

cause is not a sequela of **intraventricular hemorrhage (IVH),** either dilation or subependymal cyst, respectively.

The lateral ventricles communicate with the third ventricle through the intraventricular foramen, or foramen of Monroe. The third ventricle is a narrow, irregularly shaped opening, which sits inferior and midline between the lateral ventricles. The roof is formed by the corpus callosum. Often the third ventricle is not visualized beyond 32 weeks of gestation. The cerebral aqueduct, or aqueduct of Sylvius, connects the third and fourth ventricles and is the most narrow passage. It is also the most common site for intraventricular blockage of CSF in the neonate. The medulla oblongata forms the floor of the fourth ventricle. The roof is formed by the cerebellar vermis and posterior medullary vellum. On a coronal view, the fourth ventricle should not be larger than half of the size of the vermis. The lateral angles of the fourth ventricle form the foramen of Luschka. The inferior angle, the foramen of Magendie, is continuous with the central canal of the spinal cord.

Subarachnoid Space and Cisterns. Like the ventricles, the subarachnoid space and cisterns also play a role in the flow of CSF. The narrow subarachnoid space surrounding the brain and spinal cord contains a small amount of CSF. The subarachnoidal cisterns are the spaces at the base of the brain where the arachnoid becomes widely separated from the pia, giving rise to large cavities. The cisterna magna is one of the largest of these subarachnoidal cisterns and is consistently seen with ultrasound, appearing anechoic; it is located in the posterior fossa between the medulla oblongata, cerebellar hemispheres, and occipital bone.

Cerebrospinal Fluid Flow. CSF from the lateral ventricles passes through the foramen of Monroe to the third ventricle. The CSF then passes through the aqueduct of Sylvius to the fourth ventricle. From that point, the CSF may leave through the central foramen of Magendie or the lateral foramen of Luschka into the cisterna magna and the basal subarachnoid cisterns. The anterior flow continues upward through the chiasmatic cisterns, sylvian fissure, and the pericallosal cisterns up over the hemispheres, where it is reabsorbed by the arachnoid granulations in the sagittal sinus. Posteriorly the

CSF flow moves around the cerebelli, through the tentorial incisure, the quadrigeminal cistern, the posterior callosal cistern, and up over the hemispheres. A small amount flows down into the spinal subarachnoid space.

The majority of the CSF results from the production of fluid by the choroid plexuses (Figure 27-5). The ventricular **ependyma,** the intracranial subarachnoid lining, and the spinal subarachnoid lining also produce it. The CSF production does not change appreciably with increased intracranial pressure; however, when the production is significantly increased, there will be a corresponding change in intracranial pressure.

Choroid Plexus. The **choroid plexus** is a mass of specialized cells located in the lateral, third, and fourth ventricles. The main and largest choroid is located in the atrium of the lateral ventricles and is responsible for most of the CSF production. These cells regulate the intraventricular pressure by secretion or absorption of CSF. The choroid is prominent in preterm infants under 25 weeks of gestation and often develops a normal appearance by 30 weeks. The glomus (Figure 27-6) is the largest part of the choroid plexus and tapers posteriorly. It is a major site for bleeding in the term neonate. The choroid

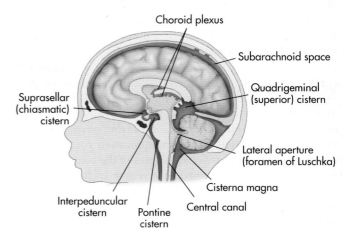

FIGURE 27-5 Sagittal view of choroid plexus and cisterns of the ventricular system.

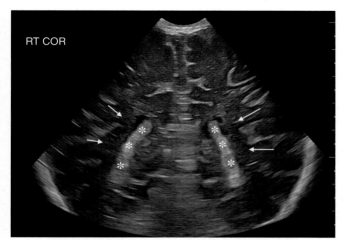

FIGURE 27-6 Normal glomus of the choroid plexus *(asterisks)* in a term 2-week-old, shown on a posterior coronal sonogram. Note that the choroid is more echogenic in relation to the normal surrounding brain parenchyma or periventricular white matter *(arrows)*. *(Image courtesy Nationwide Children's Hospital, Columbus, OH.)*

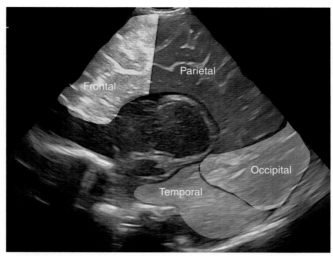

FIGURE 27-7 Lateral parasagittal view at the caudothalamic groove, showing the four lobes of the neonatal cerebrum. *(Image courtesy Nationwide Children's Hospital, Columbus, OH.)*

appears hyperechoic and should be more echogenic than the surrounding brain tissue, where small hemorrhages and areas of infarct within the parenchyma will also appear hyperechoic.

Cavum Septum Pellucidum. The cavum septum pellucidum is a thin triangular space filled with CSF, which lies between the anterior horn of the lateral ventricles and forms the floor of the corpus callosum. Thus the cavum septum pellucidum is anterior to the corpus callosum. The cavum vergae is the posterior extension of the cavum septum pellucidum and is often closed in term neonates. However, it may be seen in preterm infants, as it normally closes around 6 months of gestation. The cavum septum pellucidum is present at birth in 50% to 61% of normal neonates and often closes within 3 to 6 months of life. However, it may persist for life in some individuals.

Cerebrum

Cerebral Hemispheres. There are two cerebral hemispheres connected by the corpus callosum. They extend from the frontal to the occipital bones above the anterior and middle cranial fossae. Posteriorly, they extend above the tentorium cerebelli. They are separated by a longitudinal fissure into which projects the falx cerebri. The **cerebrum** consists of the gray and white matter. The outermost portion of the cerebrum is the cerebral cortex (composed of gray matter). White matter is located at the innermost portion of the cerebrum. The largest and densest bundle of white matter is the corpus callosum.

Lobes of the Brain. The cortex is divided into four lobes: frontal, parietal, occipital, and temporal, which correspond to the cranial bones with the same names (Figure 27-7).

Gyrus and Sulcus. The gyri are convolutions on the surface of the brain caused by infolding of the cortex. The **sulcus** is a groove or depression on the surface of the brain separating the gyri. The sulci further divide the hemispheres into frontal,

parietal, occipital, and temporal lobes. Sulci and gyri development is heavily dependent on the age of an infant. Sulci develop first around 22 weeks of gestation, with most formed by 28 weeks. However, sonographically sulci are not detected until around 26 weeks, and these very premature brains have a smooth appearance. The cingulate sulcus forms fully between weeks 28 and 31. Gyral development occurs after sulci development and even at 32 weeks this may be seen as asymmetric, with the right side more advanced.

Fissures. The interhemispheric fissure is the area in which the falx cerebri sits and separates the two cerebral hemispheres. The sylvian fissure is located along the lateral-most aspect of the brain and is the area where the middle cerebral artery is located (Figure 27-8). The quadrigeminal fissure is located posterior and inferior from the cavum vergae. The vein of Galen is also posterior, so the sonographer must be aware that Doppler should be utilized to make sure it is a fissure and not an enlarged vein of Galen.

Corpus Callosum. The corpus callosum forms broad bands of connecting fibers between the cerebral hemispheres. This structure forms the roof of the lateral ventricles. The corpus callosum sits superior to the cavum septum pellucidum (Figure 27-9). The development of the corpus callosum occurs

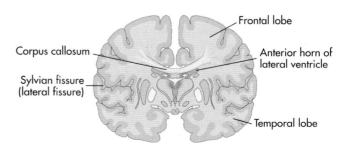

FIGURE 27-8 Coronal view of cerebral lobes, corpus callosum, and sylvian fissure.

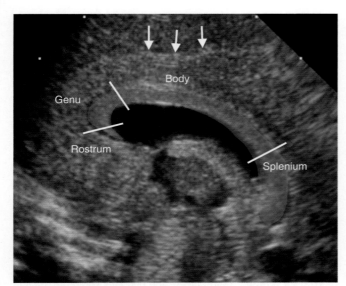

FIGURE 27-9 Sagittal image of the corpus callosum in a very premature infant. Note that it sits superior to the cavum septum pellucidum and cavum vergae. Rostrum, genu, body, and splenium are identified. There is a lack of gyri development in the brain parenchyma. The cingulate sulcus and associated inferior gyri are not well developed in this very premature infant; *arrows* point to the area. *(Image courtesy Nationwide Children's Hospital, Columbus, OH.)*

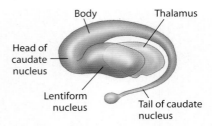

FIGURE 27-10 Lateral view of the basal ganglia with the caudate nucleus.

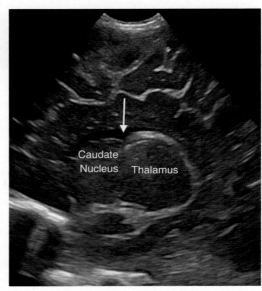

FIGURE 27-11 Normal caudothalamic groove *(arrow),* where the germinal matrix lives; a common site of hemorrhage in the premature infant. *(Image courtesy Nationwide Children's Hospital, Columbus, OH.)*

between the 8th and 18th weeks of gestation, beginning ventrally and extending dorsally. The genu of the corpus callosum develops first, followed by the body and splenium (the posterior element). The rostrum develops last. If a uterine insult occurs, development may be partially arrested or complete agenesis may occur. If partial, the genu will be preserved, whereas the later part(s) will be absent. This is known as agenesis or dysgenesis of the corpus callosum.

Basal Ganglia

The basal ganglia are a collection of gray matter that includes the caudate nucleus, lentiform nucleus, claustrum, and thalamus. The caudate nucleus is the portion of the brain that forms the lateral borders of the frontal horns of the lateral ventricles and lies anterior to the thalamus (Figure 27-10). It is further divided into the head, body, and tail. The head of the caudate nucleus, at the **caudothalamic groove or notch** (Figure 27-11), is a common site for hemorrhage. The caudate nucleus and lentiform nucleus are the largest basal ganglia. They serve as relay stations between the thalamus and the cerebral cortex.

The thalamus consists of two ovoid, egg-shaped brain structures situated on either side of the third ventricle superior to the brainstem. The thalamus borders the third ventricle and connects through the middle of the third ventricle by the massa intermedia, which is composed of gray matter and exists in most neonatal brains. The hypothalamus forms the floor of the third ventricle. The pituitary gland is connected to the hypothalamus by the infundibulum.

The **germinal matrix** includes periventricular tissue and the caudate nucleus. It is located 1 cm above the caudate nucleus in the floor of the lateral ventricle, at the caudothalamic

groove. It sweeps from the frontal horn posteriorly into the temporal horn. It is indicated in 90% of premature brain bleeds and is made up of highly vascular delicate blood vessels, especially in infants under 34 weeks of gestation.

Brainstem

The **brainstem** is the part of the brain connecting the forebrain (cerebral hemispheres, thalamus, and hypothalamus) and the spinal cord. It consists of the midbrain, pons, and medulla oblongata.

Midbrain. The midbrain portion of the brain is narrow and connects the forebrain to the hindbrain. It consists of two halves called the cerebral peduncles, the cerebral aqueduct, the tectum, and tegmentum.

Pons and Medulla Oblongata. The pons and medulla oblongata are part of the brainstem and hindbrain. The pons is found on the anterior surface of the cerebellum below the midbrain and above the medulla oblongata. The medulla oblongata extends from the pons to the foramen magnum where it continues as the spinal cord. This structure contains the fiber tracts between the brain and the spinal cord, and the vital centers that regulate important internal activities of the body (heart rate, respiration, and blood pressure).

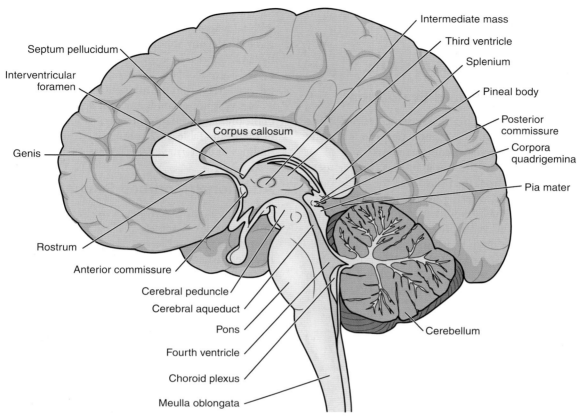

FIGURE 27-12 Sagittal view of midline structures in the brain.

Cerebellum

The **cerebellum,** part of the hindbrain, is composed of two hemispheres that have a cauliflower-like appearance. The cerebellum lies in the posterior cranial fossa under the tentorium cerebelli. The two hemispheres are connected by the vermis. Figure 27-12 summarizes the major midline anatomy.

Cerebrovascular System

The cerebrovascular system consists of the internal cerebral arteries, vertebral arteries, and circle of Willis. When clinically indicated, the circle of Willis and its major branches are evaluated with pulsed-wave and color Doppler ultrasound from a transtemporal approach in determining cerebral blood flow patterns. The cerebrovascular system is discussed in more detail in Chapters 38 and 60.

EXAMINATION PREPARATION

For the premature or sick infant, most neurosonography examinations are performed portably in the neonatal intensive care unit (NICU). Only well, term or older infants may be examined in the ultrasound laboratory, either on the examination table, in a car seat, or on the parent's lap. For inpatients, the sonographer must be aware of the infant's condition before the examination, and therefore should never begin an examination before first contacting the infant's nurse. Two key concerns are keeping premature infants both safe and warm. They can lose a potentially dangerous amount of body heat quickly, so a small amount of warm gel (ideally from an individual packet) should be used, while scanning through the isolette portholes. If a large amount of cold gel is applied to the fontanel, or if the isolette is open for an extended period of time, the infant's temperature may drop, which will often set off the infant's thermal regulation. Likewise, if too much pressure is applied while performing the examination, it may bring an onset of bradycardia or thermal regulation. Additionally, the sonographer should be acutely aware of any lifesaving wires, tubes, and/or monitors (e.g., endotracheal tubes), limit head and neck movement, and practice good infection control techniques to minimize the spread of disease in this vulnerable population.

Neurosonology is performed primarily through the anterior fontanel, or easily felt "soft spot" on top of the head. A curved-array or sector high-frequency transducer of 7 to 10 MHz is best for imaging most preterm infants and neonates, whereas lower frequencies of 5 to 7 MHz may be needed for older infants with closing fontanels or infants with thick hair. A 3- to 5-MHz transducer may also be necessary to visualize deeper structures. More than one transducer may be needed. Often a dedicated neonatal head probe will provide the much-desired small footprint and 110- to 130-degree angle needed to obtain excellent contact and brain visualization. Likewise, specialized settings with low gray-scale contrast and multiple focal zones throughout the depth of the image help to optimize the lateral resolution of brain parenchyma to detect any subtle changes.

NEONATAL HEAD EXAMINATION

Overview of the Standard Evaluation

Sonography of the neonatal brain is initiated through the anterior fontanel in coronal and sagittal views to study the supratentorial and infratentorial compartments (Box 27-1). Although the structures in the infratentorial compartment are located relatively far from the transducer, the alteration of a deep focal placement or lowering the transducer frequency is recommended, particularly in older infants. The posterior cranial bones should always be present in the standard images to ensure the entire brain is being visualized.

The mastoid fontanel is used to better visualize the cerebellum and infratentorial compartment, or posterior fossa, in young infants. Cine clips should be used when possible to show the coronal and sagittal sweeps through the neonatal head. Additional magnified views are also encouraged to provide better resolution of any abnormal or high-risk areas (e.g., the caudothalamic groove in a preterm infant). A color Doppler (and pulsed-wave Doppler when indicated) evaluation of the pericallosal artery from the midsagittal view is also encouraged.

It is very important to note the approximate gestational age of the premature infant when performing a neonatal sonogram of the head. Table 27-2 summarizes the general sonographic findings in the term versus preterm neonate.

Additional/Modified Evaluation

If imaging is restricted due to overlapping bones in the area of the anterior fontanel, or if pathology is suspected in the choroid plexus and lateral ventricles, the posterior fontanel may be used as an alternative window. The posterior fontanel approach may also be useful for any critical neonate on **extracorporeal membrane oxygenation (ECMO),** where the mastoid view is unattainable. The posterior fossa axial images, with the anterior portion of the transducer angled slightly cephalad, will demonstrate the infratentorial structures.

Pathology should always be evaluated in multiple planes, and with color and/or power and spectral Doppler. Additional views of pathology may be obtained from the posterior or mastoid fontanel, the foramen magnum, or thin areas over the temporal and parietal bones. A clot in the occipital horns is best evaluated from the posterior approach, and the foramen magnum is useful to evaluate the proximal end of the spinal canal. Additionally, any open suture, burr hole, or craniotomy defect can also serve as an acoustic window.

BOX 27-1	Supratentorial and Infratentorial Structures

Supratentorial	Infratentorial
Cerebral hemispheres	Cerebellum
Basal ganglia	Brainstem
Lateral and third ventricles	Fourth ventricle
Interhemispheric fissure	Basal cisterns
Subarachnoid space around the hemispheres	

TABLE 27-2	General Term vs. Preterm Normal Sonographic Findings

Term Neonate (after 37 weeks)	Preterm Neonate (before 37 weeks)
Sulci and gyri are well developed.	Sulci and gyri are still developing or may be nearly absent in very preterm infants, also called the "smooth" brain appearance.
Slitlike ventricles or width increasing from 2 mm anteroposterior (AP) at frontal horns to 3–6 mm AP maximum at trigone on coronal study. Height of the bodies of the lateral ventricles are normally less than 7 mm AP at the level of midthalamus on a parasagittal study.	Preterm infants in general will have larger appearing ventricles overall.
Third ventricle not usually seen on coronal study and may only visualize an echogenic formation immediately below the septum pellucidum.	Third ventricle is prominent and easily seen in premature infants less than 32 weeks.
Cavum septum pellucidum (CSP) is seen in 50%–61% of term neonates.	CSP nearly always visualized in preterm infants.
Cavum vergae is not visualized.	Cavum vergae may be present in very preterm infants, seen posterior to CSP.
Choroid plexus between 2–3 mm at the body of the lateral ventricles and 4–5 mm at the atria (or glomus*) between 30–40 weeks.	Choroid plexus is very large in extremely preterm infants (25 weeks or less), should not be mistaken for intraventricular hemorrhages. Appearance similar to term neonate after 30 weeks.
Caudate nuclei show isoechoic or low areas of echogenicity compared with surrounding brain parenchyma.	Caudate nuclei (basal ganglia and thalami†) may have a higher echogenicity than the surrounding brain parenchyma in preterm infants less than 32 weeks.
Periventricular white matter has low echogenicity, with thin echogenic streaks corresponding to small vessels. Should be less echogenic than the choroid.	‡Periventricular area may show a slight increased echogenicity due to anisotropy in preterm infants. Scanning from the posterior fontanel this "blush" or "halo" should disappear.

*Glomus is a common site for bleeding in the full-term neonate.
†Caudothalamic groove is a common site for hemorrhage in preterm infants under 34 weeks.
‡Periventricular area is where most white matter necrosis or PVL occurs in the preterm infant.

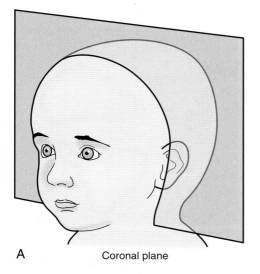

A   Coronal plane

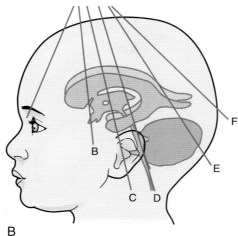

B

FIGURE 27-13 A, The transducer is placed on the anterior fontanel, perpendicular to the neonatal head, with the notch to the right. **B,** The transducer is angled from the anterior to posterior skull as described in the text. *A* through *F* indicate the different coronal scanning planes. *A* is the most anterior, and *F* is the most posterior.

Small linear array, high-frequency transducers (10 to 15 MHz), with or without a standoff pad, may also be used to image near-field pathology. This transducer is used for thrombosis in the superior sagittal sinus, cerebral edema, and subdural hematomas or subdural abscess secondary to meningitis.

Finally, although protocols are provided, additional oblique or axial views may be very helpful and are encouraged for evaluating the neonatal brain. This is true in patients with ventricular shunt tubes, in which oblique angles help to identify the shunt and tip.

Three-Dimensional Neurosonography

Three-dimensional (3D) sonography is showing promise as an emerging method in imaging the neonatal head. This technique can reduce interoperator variability and significantly reduce the time required to perform a neurosonology examination. On average a neonatal head examination will take 10 to 15 minutes, compared with 1 to 2 minutes with the 3D technique. Research now shows this is done without compromising diagnostic quality in comparison to the standard two-dimensional approach. It also allows for later 3D reconstructions and may be useful in better evaluating brain anomalies.

In addition to gray-scale 3D neurosonography, ultrafast Doppler is a new 3D Doppler technique capable of quickly mapping cerebral resistive index (RI) in neonates and infants. It has been called ultrasound angiography. It offers the evaluation of blood flow speed at a subcardiac cycle time scale, which other angiographic modalities are unable to assess. This may be useful for monitoring hypoxic-ischemic injuries in the future, as well as opening up knowledge about cerebrovascular regulation in infants in general.

Coronal Study

To perform the coronal study, the transducer is placed on the anterior fontanel with the scanning plane following the coronal suture (Figure 27-13). When looking at the coronal sections, the vertex of the skull is at the top and the left side of the brain is to the right of the image, and should be annotated as such. The middle of the transducer must be centered in the coronal suture to reduce bone interference and to procure the most extensive image of the brain. It is critical that symmetric images be obtained; this is accomplished by using the skull bones and the middle cerebral arteries at the sylvian fissure as landmarks. The skull bones and the arteries should be the same size bilaterally. In the coronal plane, the transducer is angled from the anterior to the posterior of the skull to completely visualize the lateral and third ventricles, the deep subcortical white matter, and the basal ganglia (Box 27-2).

When the transducer is angled anteriorly, the frontal horns of the lateral ventricles appear as slitlike hypoechoic or cystic formations (Figure 27-14, B, 5). As the transducer is angled posteriorly, the ventricles acquire a comma-like shape and their width increases from the frontal horns to the atria or trigone (Figure 27-14, E, 28). The choroid plexus (Figure 27-14, 15)

BOX 27-2 | Coronal Study

A. Frontal lobes, anterior interhemispheric fissure, and orbits.

B. Frontal horns of the lateral ventricles, head of the caudate nucleus, and fluid-filled cavum septum pellucidum (CSP) between the anterior horns. Corpus callosum is seen anterior to the CSP.

C. Level of the third ventricle. Echogenic choroid plexus seen in the floor of the lateral ventricles, as well as in the middle, in the roof of the third ventricle (may visualize third ventricle in preterm infants as a hypoechoic structure inferior to middle choroid). CSP seen here if present, between the bodies of the lateral ventricles. Brainstem is visualized in the posterior section.

D. Thalami seen anterior to the quadrigeminal cistern (echogenic star shape). Tentorium is also visualized, with echogenic vermis and cerebellum underneath. Cisterna magna is anechoic.

E. Choroid plexus glomi within the trigones of the lateral ventricles and periventricular white matter.

F. Periventricular white matter (periventricular blush), gyri and sulci of occipital lobe, and posterior interhemispheric fissure.

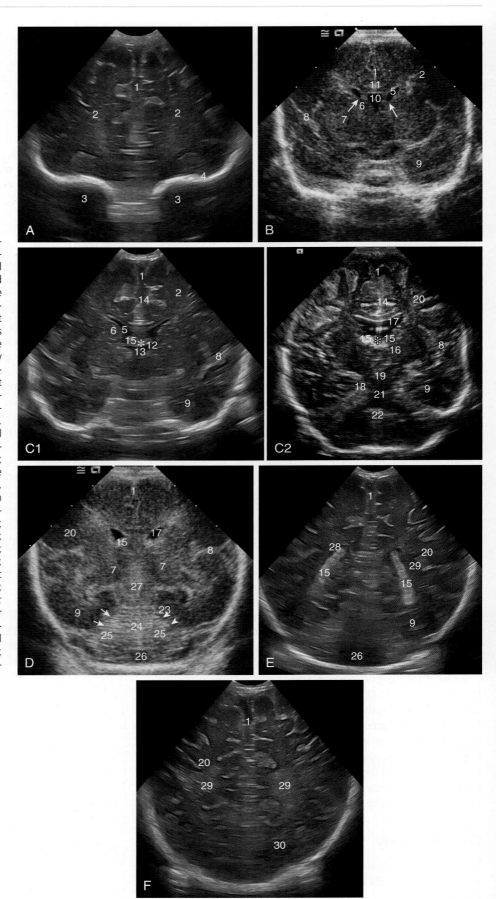

FIGURE 27-14 Normal protocol for coronal images beginning with the transducer angled toward the anterior skull and fanning posteriorly. Images **B** and **D** are from a premature infant, and the remaining are from a term neonate. Notice the increase in gyral development and lack of CSP in term neonate. Images **C-1** and **C-2** show a different appearance of the third ventricle, with **C-1** just slightly more anterior demonstrating the foramen of Monroe, with third ventricle just barely coming into view. Images **A–F** correspond to Table 27-1 and structures correspond to the numbers labeled here. (Bolded numbers correspond to sagittal images as well.) *1,* interhemispheric fissure; *2,* frontal lobe; *3,* orbits; *4,* skull; *5,* frontal horn of lateral ventricle; *6,* caudate nucleus (area of caudothalamic groove, *arrows* on image **B**); *7,* thalamus; *8,* sylvian fissure; *9,* temporal lobe; *10,* CSP; *11,* corpus callosum; *12,* intraventricular foramen; *13,* third ventricle; *14,* cingulate sulcus; *15,* choroid plexus (*asterisk* in the third); *16,* thalamus; *17,* body of lateral ventricle; *18,* hippocampal fissure; *19,* mesencephalic aqueduct; *20,* parietal lobe; *21,* pons; *22,* medulla; *23,* tentorium *(arrows);* *24,* cerebellar vermis; *25,* cerebellar hemispheres; *26,* cisterna magna; *27,* quadrigeminal cistern; *28,* trigone of the lateral ventricle; *29,* periventricular white matter; *30,* occipital lobe. *(Images courtesy Nationwide Children's Hospital, Columbus, OH.)*

is an echogenic structure inside the ventricular cavities surrounding the thalamic nuclei. It lies along the floor of the lateral ventricles, extending from the temporal horn into the atrium and body of the lateral ventricles. It should not appear extending anterior into the frontal horns or posterior into the occipital horns. Increased hyperechoic areas in the floor of the ventricles, anterior to the third ventricle, would indicate hemorrhage at the caudothalamic groove (Figure 27-14, *B, arrows*). At the intraventricular foramen, the choroid plexus enters into the third ventricle (Figure 27-14, *C-1 and C-2, asterisk*). The choroid plexus becomes enlarged at the level of the atria (glomus of the choroid plexus) and can almost entirely fill the ventricular cavity (Figure 27-14, *E, 15*).

The third ventricle is not well visualized in the normal coronal study in the term neonate (Figure 27-14, *C-1, 13*). An off-axis approach and high-frequency transducer may be helpful to identify it. Occasionally, a thin and very echogenic formation can be seen in the midline immediately below the septum pellucidum. This echogenic image corresponds to the choroid plexus extending into the roof of the third ventricle. The septum pellucidum appears as a midline hypoechoic to cystic structure separating the bodies and frontal horns of the lateral ventricles (Figure 27-14, *B, 10*). The cavum septum pellucidum is posterior to the corpus callosum.

Coronal and modified coronal views also visualize the basal ganglia and the white matter. The white matter has low echogenicity, with thin echogenic streaks that correspond to small vessels. In premature infants this area is known as a "watershed zone," which are terminal ends of the vessel bed and may be used to describe the periventricular white matter. This area should be evaluated carefully. The echogenicity should never be greater than that of the choroid plexus; if it is, hemorrhage or infarction should be suspected and follow-up studies are required.

The cerebellar vermis is a very echogenic structure in the midline (Figure 27-14, *D, 24*). The fourth ventricle appears in the midline as a small anechoic space located anteriorly to the vermis and is not always seen in the coronal view. The cerebellar hemispheres (Figure 27-14, *D, 25*) are contiguous with the vermis. The cisterna magna (Figure 27-14, *D, 26*) corresponds to a nonechogenic space between the vermis, the cerebellar hemispheres, and the occipital bone.

Sagittal Study

The sagittal study is made by rotating the coronal plane approximately 90 degrees, positioned over the anterior fontanel, and aligning with the sagittal suture (Figure 27-15). These sections are viewed with the anterior brain to the left and the occipital portion of the brain to the right. Sagittal studies provide the most extensive visualization of the brain.

The straight sagittal view is critical and can rule out many midline anomalies. It should be obtained first and may be used as a guide to stay in axis and determine whether a parasagittal study corresponds to the right or left side. Care must always be taken to properly annotate the images right, left, and midline. Protocol for the sagittal view is often dependent on sonographer or physician preference. One may start midline and scan out to the right, back to center, and then out to the left; or one may start laterally, often the right side, and fan sequentially through to the lateral-most left side if obtaining a cine clip sweep; the latter may be faster. The sagittal study is shown in Figure 27-16, corresponding to Box 27-3.

Midline Sagittal View. The straight sagittal study shows the midline structures in the supratentorial and infratentorial compartments. Supratentorially, the corpus callosum appears as two thin hyperechoic parallel lines separated by a thin hypoechoic space. The cingulate sulcus is found anterior and parallel to the corpus callosum. It may be less defined in the preterm infant (Figure 27-17). The septum pellucidum appears as an anechoic (cystic) structure immediately below the corpus callosum. The third ventricle is normally anechoic and

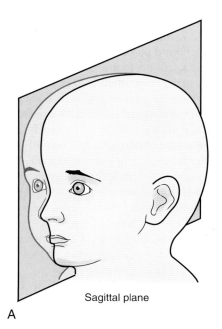

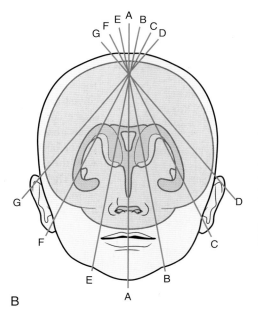

FIGURE 27-15 **A,** The transducer is placed on the anterior fontanel, perpendicular to the skull, and rotated 90 degrees from the coronal plane to the sagittal plane, with the notch to the infant's nose. The transducer uses the midsagittal plane as the primary landmark; slight angulation of the transducer away from the midline will show the parasagittal and midsagittal planes. **B,** Line A indicates the midline sagittal plane and the other lines indicate the lateral sagittal or parasagittal planes.

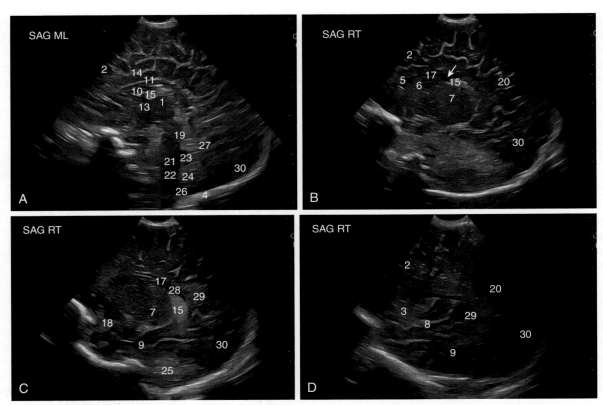

FIGURE 27-16 Normal protocol for sagittal images beginning with the transducer midline parallel to the skull and then angled obliquely to one side, and then the other. Images **A–D** correspond to Box 27-1 and structures correspond to numbers labeled here on a term neonate. (Corresponding **E–G** images are not shown but are the same as the **B–D** images, but for the opposite side; bolded numbers correspond to coronal images as well.) *1,* Massa intermedia; *2,* frontal lobe; *3,* insula; *4,* skull; *5,* frontal horn of lateral ventricle; *6,* caudate nucleus (area of caudothalamic groove, *arrow* on image **B**); *7,* thalamus; *8,* sylvian fissure; *9,* temporal lobe; *10,* CSP; *11,* corpus callosum; *12,* intraventricular foramen; *13,* third ventricle; *14,* cingulate sulcus; *15,* choroid plexus; *16,* thalamus; *17,* body of lateral ventricle; *18,* hippocampal fissure; *19,* mesencephalic aqueduct; *20,* parietal lobe; *21,* pons; *22,* medulla; *23,* fourth ventricle; *24,* cerebellar vermis; *25,* cerebellar hemispheres; *26,* cisterna magna; *27,* quadrigeminal cistern; *28,* trigone of the lateral ventricle; *29,* periventricular white matter; *30,* occipital lobe. *(Images courtesy Nationwide Children's Hospital, Columbus, OH.)*

BOX 27-3 | **Sagittal Study**

A. True sagittal midline
  Gray scale: cavum septum pellucidum, corpus callosum, third ventricle, foramen of Monro, aqueduct of Sylvius, fourth ventricle, cerebellum (tentorium), and cisterna magna.
  Doppler: Pericallosal artery can be evaluated with color and/or spectral Doppler.
B (and E). Parasagittal view of the caudothalamic groove (notch).
C (and F). Parasagittal view of choroid plexus through the body of the lateral ventricle. The periventricular white matter should also be demonstrated.
D (and G). Lateral-most parasagittal angle showing brain parenchyma lateral to the ventricles, should include sylvian fissure and pulsations from the middle cerebral artery *(MCA).*

is located inferiorly to the cavum septum pellucidum (CSP) anteriorly. The echogenic choroid plexus appears to enter the top of the third ventricle through the foramen of Monro.

Infratentorially, in the straight or midline sagittal plane, the vermis of the cerebellum appears as a very echodense formation, separated from the occipital bone by an anechoic space corresponding to the cisterna magna. The other cisterns also are anechoic spaces located above and behind the cerebellar vermis. The fourth ventricle appears as a small "V" with the vertex oriented posteriorly inside the echogenic vermis. The fourth ventricle is limited anteriorly by the brainstem. The brainstem has low echogenicity, with an echodense anterior border demarcated by the basilar artery.

Finally, the pericallosal artery, branch of the anterior cerebral artery, may be seen with color Doppler, shown in Figure 27-18 with spectral Doppler gate placement.

Parasagittal Views. After having studied the midline, the parasagittal views are obtained by angling the transducer to the right or left side of the skull. Three parasagittal studies should

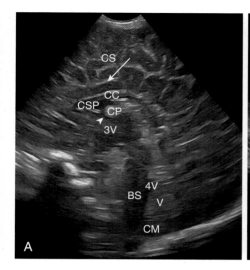
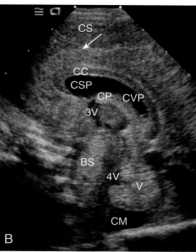

FIGURE 27-17 Normal straight sagittal view of the midline structures in both **A,** a term neonate and **B,** an extremely premature infant. Notice the development of the cingulate sulcus (*CS* with *arrow*) and lack of cavum vergae pellucidum (*CVP*) in the term neonate. Also, the structures are better visualized in the premature infant due to a wider anterior fontanel and more prominent ventricular system. Supratentorial structures: choroid plexus (*CP*), corpus callosum (*CC*), septum pellucidum (*SP*), and third ventricle (*3V, arrowhead* in image **A**). Infratentorial structures: brainstem (*BS*), cerebellar vermis (*V*), cisterna magna (*CM*), and fourth ventricle (*4V*). (*Images courtesy Nationwide Children's Hospital, Columbus, OH.*)

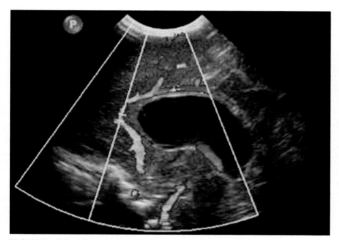

FIGURE 27-18 Color Doppler of the anterior cerebral artery branch (pericallosal artery) in the midline sagittal view seen coursing over the corpus callosum. Spectral Doppler gate placement is also shown. This 12-day-old extremely preterm neonate demonstrates a large cavum septum and cavum vergae pellucidum. (*Image courtesy Nationwide Children's Hospital, Columbus, OH.*)

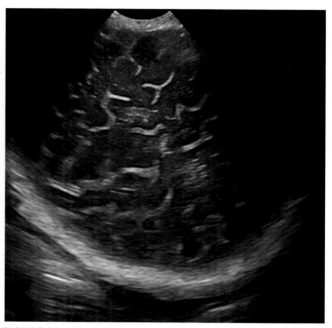

FIGURE 27-19 A common extra parasagittal view, past the sylvian fissure, demonstrating gyri development in the neonatal brain. (*Image courtesy Nationwide Children's Hospital, Columbus, OH.*)

be performed at minimum, and often more are taken at the caudothalamic groove and at the very lateral brain parenchyma, shown in Figure 27-19. The first parasagittal image should be close to the midline to visualize the caudate nuclei in detail, because subependymal hemorrhages begin in the germinal matrix that is located at the caudothalamic groove (see Figure 27-16, *B, arrow*). These views image the frontal horn and body of the lateral ventricles, the thalamus, the head of the caudate nucleus, and the choroid plexus. The frontal horns of the lateral ventricles appear as narrow sonolucent cavities (see Figure 27-16, *B*). The choroid plexus appears as a small (2 to 3 mm height), very echogenic structure lying against the thalamus. The plexus ends at the caudothalamic groove.

The second parasagittal image (see Figure 27-16, *C*) is made slightly lateral to the first image and includes the entire ventricular cavity. Because the ventricular cavity is not entirely parallel to the midline (i.e., the posterior horns are

more lateral or external than the anterior horns), the transducer must be rotated slightly counterclockwise to form an acute angle with the sagittal suture anteriorly. These views show the entire ventricular horns; the choroid plexus, including the glomus; the thalami; the caudate nuclei; and the white matter superior and posterior to the lateral ventricles.

The third parasagittal view images the white matter located lateral (externally) to the lateral ventricles (see Figure 27-16, *D*). This view is useful for studying intraparenchymal hemorrhages, porencephaly, and periventricular leukomalacia. It will also demonstrate the sylvian figure, middle cerebral artery, and insula. The insula (see Figure 27-16, *D, 3*) is considered by some to be the fifth brain lobe and it remains open until 24 to 26 weeks of gestation.

Posterior Fossa Study

The integration of the mastoid view of the posterior fossa (infratentorial compartment) in the routine neonatal head examination increases the detection of congenital anomalies relating to the third and fourth ventricles, as well as the cerebellum. Furthermore, the detection of cerebellar hemorrhages is very limited from the anterior fontanel approach, and this view better visualizes and defines these bleeds.

The transducer is placed just behind the ear after gently bending the auricle forward. If the transducer notch is pointing upward in a vertical position this will correspond to a coronal plane, whereas if the notch is turned to the right in a horizontal position it will correspond to a transverse or axial plane. The side of the head being examined should be clearly annotated, and often one side will clearly visualize both cerebellar hemispheres. However, in the case of difficult visualization of the opposite cerebellar hemisphere, both mastoid fontanels may need to be examined. Figure 27-20 shows the coronal evaluation of the posterior fossa. As with any interrogation, the sonographer should make sure to sweep through the entire viewable area.

Hydrocephalus (Ventriculomegaly). Ventriculomegaly is the most common disorder of the neonatal brain and is marked by the dilation of the ventricular system. Ventricular enlargement may be caused by a variety of conditions leading to the obstruction, overproduction, or decreased absorption of CSF. Often, in regard to the neonatal brain, the terms *ventriculomegaly* and *hydronephrosis* are used interchangeably. Differing definitions of hydrocephalus have emerged, and it may be defined as ventricular enlargement caused by obstruction, or when increased intracranial pressure is present. Nevertheless, hydrocephalus puts neonates at high risk for brain parenchyma loss and subsequent neurodevelopmental impairment.

Neonates may be diagnosed with ventriculomegaly or hydrocephalus in utero, or may present clinically with a bulging anterior fontanel and/or macrocephaly. However, initial ventricular dilation occurs without changes in the head circumference, and hydrocephalus may be silent because the white

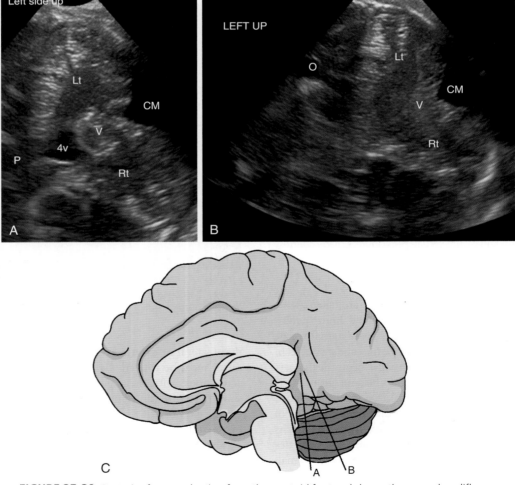

FIGURE 27-20 Posterior fossa evaluation from the mastoid fontanel shows the normal cauliflower-like appearance of the cerebellum. Annotation indicates this coronal image was taken from the left mastoid fontanel. *V,* Vermis; *Rt/Lt,* right and left cerebellar hemispheres; *P,* pons. **A,** View at the level of the fourth ventricle *(4v)* and cisterna magna *(CM)*. **B,** A more posterior view can also show the occipital horns *(O)* of the lateral ventricles. **C,** Diagram of the coronal views (**A** and **B**) from the mastoid fontanel. *(Images A and B courtesy Nationwide Children's Hospital, Columbus, OH.)*

matter of newborn infants is very compliant and easily compressed as the ventricles widen. The head circumference starts to enlarge only after significant compression of the white matter has developed. Therefore screening and sequential neonatal head sonography for infants at risk plays an important role in diagnosing ventricular dilation in the silent phase, as well as determining underlying etiology.

Hydrocephalus may be acquired or congenital. Acquired hydrocephalus may result from CSF obstruction from an intracranial hemorrhage (ICH), also known as posthemorrhagic hydrocephalus (PHH) when severe dilation occurs, or after the loss of deep white matter in PVL. Ex vacuo hydrocephalus describes the dilation of ventricles due to parenchymal loss and can be caused by either ICH or PVL. Congenital hydrocephalus occurs before birth and may be due to structural malformations or congenital brain infections. In general, the earlier that hydrocephalus occurs in utero, the greater the enlargement of the neonatal head.

Hydronephrosis is divided into communicating and noncommunicating forms. The latter is also referred to as obstructive hydronephrosis and is characterized by blockage of the CSF anywhere within the ventricular system itself, causing subsequent enlargement of the ventricular cavities proximal to the obstruction. The most common cause of both acquired and congenital hydrocephalus is **aqueductal stenosis.** The aqueduct of Sylvius, situated in the midbrain, is narrowed or replaced by multiple small channels with blind ends. Occasionally, aqueductal stenosis may be caused by extrinsic lesions posterior to the brainstem, such as congenital aneurysm of the vein of Galen or brain tumors. Congenital brain tumors (which have been defined from birth to 12 months) are quite rare of all pediatric brain tumors, with neuroblastomas making up the largest majority at 26%.

In communicating hydronephrosis, the CSF pathways are open within the ventricular system, but there is either decreased absorption via occluded arachnoid granulations or overproduction of CSF. Hydrocephalus is infrequently caused by overproduction of fluid. Excessive fluid production may occur in infants with papilloma of the choroid plexus, a tumor that actively secretes CSF.

Increased Intracranial Pressure

Of particular concern in the neonate with hydrocephalus is the development of **increased intracranial pressure (ICP),** which is the cause of, or result of, brain injury. Increased ICP restricts cerebral blood flow and is a serious medical condition. Increased ICP, bradycardia, and apnea may follow days or weeks after the onset of ventricular dilation. The drainage of CSF, via a ventricular shunt or reservoir, plays a central role in treatment. Serial sonography aids in this therapeutic decision using both ventricular measurements and spectral Doppler assessment.

Ventricular Measurements

The three most reproducible ventricular biometric measurements are the ventricular index (VI), anterior horn width (AHW), and thalamo-occipital distance (TOD). VI and AHW are taken at the level of the third ventricle in a coronal view, with VI measured at the widest point to the falx and AHW measured at a diagonal at the widest point. The TOD is taken from a parasagittal view and is measured from the outermost part of the occipital horn to the junction of the choroid with the outermost part of the thalamus (Figure 27-21). Some will also measure the midbody height at the level of the thalamus from a parasagittal view or the anterior horn width, which is the anterior-posterior measurement in a coronal view. Measurements beyond the normative 95th percentile represent ventricular dilation. Sonographers should be aware that head position, within 3 hours of a positioning change, could affect measurements.

The VI is the most commonly used metric and shows a considerable increase with maturation (Table 27-3). Although this value may be used as a ratio with hemispheric

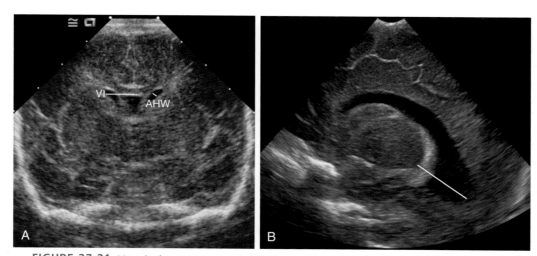

FIGURE 27-21 Ventricular measurements. **A,** Coronal image at the level of the third ventricle shows the ventricular index *(VI)* and anterior horn width *(AHW)*. **B,** Parasagittal view demonstrates the thalamo-occipital distance *(TOD)*. *(Images courtesy Nationwide Children's Hospital, Columbus, OH.)*

TABLE 27-3	Ventricular Index (VI) for Select Gestational Ages	
Gestational Age	Mean VI* (0-6 days)	97.5th Percentile for VI** (0-6 days)
26 weeks	8.5-8.7 mm	10.1-10.3 mm
30 weeks	9.5-9.7 mm	11.2-11.4 mm
34 weeks	10.4-10.6 mm	12.3-12.5 mm
38 weeks	11.3-11.4 mm	13.3-13.5 mm
42 weeks	11.7-11.8 mm	13.8-14.0 mm

*Mean calculation = $0.550280 + (0.359138 * GA) + (-0.002034 * GA^2)$
**97.5 percentile calculation = $0.642056 + (0.424486 * GA) + (-0.002409 * GA^2)$
Data from Brouwer MJ, De Vries LS, Groenendaal F, et al: New reference values for the neonatal cerebral ventricles, *Radiology* 262(1):224-233, 2012.

width (frontal horn ratio), this has been shown to be less useful than absolute VI measurements alone. AHW, regardless of gestational age, over 4 mm may indicate dilation. Preterm infants with a TOD measurement over 19 mm and term infants with a TOD over 21 mm may also indicate ventricular dilation.

These measurements help to define ventricular enlargement in the premature and term neonate, but it is unclear at what degree ventricular dilation is associated with increased ICP, although a VI measurement 4 mm above the 97th percentile for gestational age may be a strong indicator for therapeutic intervention. Additional measurements at the third and fourth ventricle, as well as Doppler assessment, are helpful.

Doppler Measurements

Hemodynamic changes may be recorded by spectral Doppler and used to identify infants with elevated ICP. A tracing from the pericallosal artery is obtained from the anterior fontanel. If a reversal of flow already exists, this is an indication of elevated ICP and fontanel pressure is not recommended. If no reversal is detected, pressure is applied to the anterior fontanel. A reversal of flow in diastole with pressure is also an indication, and no measurement is needed. Often, though, the RI is measured at a state with and without pressure, annotated for clarity. An RI change greater than 0.1 above the baseline is indicated in elevated ICP (Figure 27-22).

Prolonged pressure (greater than 3 to 5 seconds) is not recommended and may cause bradycardia. Also, any change in thermal regulation or desaturation in the neonate during normal compression is a signal to remove pressure immediately, and this should be reported.

Sonographic Findings. The sonographer should look for the blunting of the lateral angles of the lateral ventricles (Figure 27-23). In the setting of aqueductal stenosis there is a widening of the lateral and third ventricles, with a normal-size fourth ventricle. If the hydrocephalus is very large, the posterior fossa is smaller than usual, and the cerebellum is displaced toward the occipital bone with the disappearance of the cisterna magna. However, the cerebellum is not

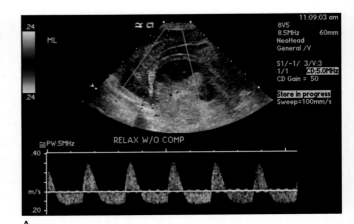

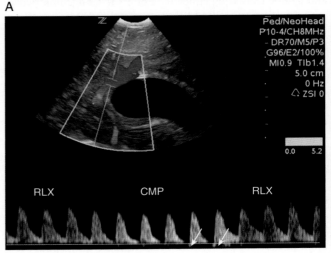

FIGURE 27-22 Spectral Doppler evaluation of the pericallosal artery in the presence of hydrocephalus. **A,** Neonate with bilateral grade IV hemorrhage and a diffusely echogenic and swollen brain demonstrates reversal of diastolic flow without compression. **B,** Premature infant with bilateral periventricular leukomalacia shows an absence (and small bit of reversal shown with *arrows*) of diastolic flow with compression on the anterior fontanel. *(Images courtesy Nationwide Children's Hospital, Columbus, OH.)*

dislodged into the foramen magnum, thus differentiating aqueductal stenosis from the Arnold-Chiari and Dandy-Walker malformations.

Ultrasound is very useful after **ventriculoperitoneal shunt** placements to access tip placement and monitor the drainage of the dilated ventricle. Shunts are often seen as echogenic bright parallel lines in a long-axis view, and echogenic foci in the short-axis view. In a decompressed ventricle they will have a distal shadow.

Extra-Axial Fluid

Increased extra-axial fluid may be detected sonographically. Although often referred to as "benign" extra-axial fluid or benign external hydrocephalus, recent evidence is emerging in linking this finding to autism spectrum disorder (ASD). It is hypothesized that immature arachnoid granulations in infancy may cause CSF to accumulated in

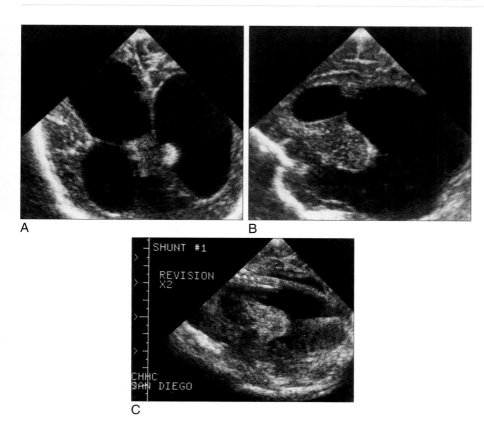

A

B

C

SHUNT #1

REVISION
X2

CHHC
SAN DIEGO

FIGURE 27-23 A 4-month-old infant with hydrocephalus shows gross dilation of the lateral ventricles. **A,** Coronal view. **B,** Sagittal view. **C,** Follow-up study shows shunt tubing in place for drainage of the hydrocephalus.

the subarachnoid space. The arachnoid granulations only form at birth and develop until 18 months. Before birth lymphatic pathways are utilized, this drainage also continues throughout the neonatal period. Twenty percent more extra-axial fluid may be detected in infants with ASD over normal infants at 6 to 9 months, 33% greater fluid at 12 to 15 months, and 22% greater fluid at 18 to 24 months. Infants and toddlers who have the longest persistent extra-axial fluid are at the greatest risk. Sonographically, a transcranial approach has been used to show increased extra-axial spaces in children with ASD.

Sonographic Findings. If cortical vessels are seen passing through the superficial fluid, also known as the cerebral cortical vein sign, it suggests the collection is subarachnoid (Figure 27-24), whereas a subdural collection would show vessels along the periphery. This is not definitive, and

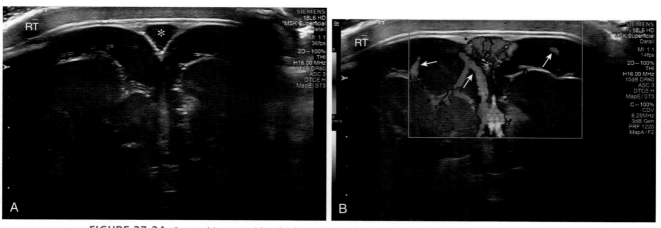

A

B

FIGURE 27-24 Coronal image with a high-resolution linear transducer showing extra-axial fluid in a 12-month-old infant. **A,** Fluid is unable to be differentiated from subarachnoid and subdural fluid collection with gray-scale imaging alone. **B,** Cortical vessels *(arrows)* are seen coursing through the fluid on color Doppler. The superior sagittal sinus is shown here in cross section *(asterisks)* and should also be evaluated for patency and will not fill with color in the presence of thrombus. *(Images courtesy Nationwide Children's Hospital, Columbus, OH.)*

care must be taken to evaluate for debris or compressed vessels posteriorly, which may suggest a subdural bleed, even in the presence of the cortical vein sign.

ACQUIRED BRAIN LESIONS

Sonography is ideal for timing the onset and sequentially following the evolution of brain lesions that may develop in the premature infant.

Intracranial Hemorrhage

The premature neonate is at the greatest risk for intracranial hemorrhage (ICH) and it is a major cause of mortality and morbidity (cerebral palsy) in this population. ICHs, also more specifically termed *germinal matrix–intraventricular hemorrhages (GM-IVHs),* are the most common hemorrhagic lesions in preterm neonates. They are also known as subependymal hemorrhages (SEHs). They affect 40% to 70% of infants less than 34 weeks of gestation, with an increased risk in infants less than 32 weeks of gestational age or less than 1500 g birth weight. ICH is rare beyond the first week of life, with the majority of bleeds occurring within the first 3 days.

GM-IVHs are a developmental disease, as they originate in the subependymal germinal matrix. Although hemorrhage begins there, it can spread throughout the ventricular system and, at worse case, into the parenchyma. The four grades of ICH are described in Box 27-4. Sonography is the most reliable technique to diagnose and follow changes in the ventricular

BOX 27-4	Classification of Intracranial Hemorrhage

Grade I: Germinal matrix (GM)/subependymal hemorrhage only
Grade II: Intraventricular hemorrhage (IVH) without ventricular enlargement
Grade III: IVH with ventricular enlargement
Grade IV: IVH with intraparenchymal hemorrhage (with or without ventricular enlargement)

size and in intraventricular clots. IVHs-SEHs (subependymal hemorrhages) resolve in several days or weeks, depending on the size of the bleed and on the individual patient.

ICH changes in appearance over time, and in the acute stage it will have an echogenicity equal to or greater than the choroid plexus. These GM-IVHs are easily detected with ultrasound as echogenic structures because fluid and clotted blood have higher acoustic impedance than the brain parenchyma and the CSF. As the clot lyses it will become hypoechoic or cystic centrally with the periphery still echogenic. Therefore the degree of echogenicity will depend on the acute-chronic process of the hemorrhage.

Grade I: Germinal Matrix/Subependymal Hemorrhages. Subependymal hemorrhages are caused by capillary bleeding in the germinal matrix. The germinal matrix is the tissue where neurons and glial cells develop before migrating from the subventricular (subependymal) region to the cortex. The germinal matrix is highly cellular, has poor connective supporting tissue, and is richly vascularized with very thin, fragile capillaries, which explains the high frequency of these hemorrhages in tiny infants. By 24 weeks of gestation, most of the neuronal and glial migration has occurred; however, pockets of germinal matrix remain until 40 weeks of gestation in the subependymal area at the head of the caudate nuclei. The most frequent location is at the caudothalamic groove. These lesions are not associated with any morbidity or mortality.

Sonographic Findings. A germinal matrix hemorrhage is usually seen at the caudothalamic notch as a very echogenic lesion pushing up the floor and external wall of the lateral ventricle with partial obliteration of the ventricular cavity. An untrained eye may miss small germinal matrix bleeds (Figure 27-25).

Subependymal cysts. These are most commonly the result of the sequelae of germinal matrix hemorrhage in premature infants. These present as discrete cysts in the lining of the ventricles, and are seen as a smooth-walled spherical cyst in the lateral ventricle at the caudothalamic groove where there was a clot previously.

Grades II and III: Intraventricular Hemorrhage. The germinal matrix or subependymal hemorrhage can extend

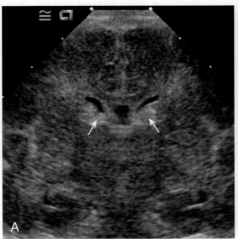
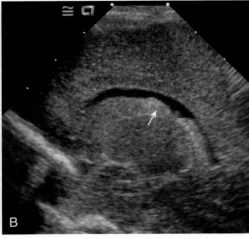

FIGURE 27-25 Grade I: GM/subependymal hemorrhage seen bilaterally in a 1-day-old 28-week preterm infant. **A,** Coronal image showing two small germinal matrix bleeds *(arrows).* **B,** Sagittal image of the left germinal matrix hemorrhage *(arrow).* *(Images courtesy Nationwide Children's Hospital, Columbus, OH.)*

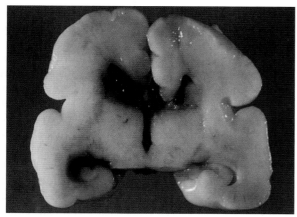

FIGURE 27-26 Intraventricular hemorrhage. Subependymal hemorrhage extending into the ventricles, containing coagulated blood.

by continuous bleeding and perforate the ventricular wall with partial or total flooding of the ventricular system (Figure 27-26), known as a grade II IVH. Depending on the amount of blood, the ventricle can become full and dilated. If dilation occurs, it is said to be a grade III IVH. Subsequently the IVH may obstruct the circulation and absorption of the CSF, causing the ventricles to dilate further with CSF and ultimately resulting in posthemorrhagic hydrocephalus, where intervention is required. This complication occurs in approximately 35% of infants with large hemorrhages. Mild to moderate ventricular dilation usually resolves spontaneously.

IVHs are not a sudden event; they usually expand slowly. Typically, when a small GM-IVH progresses to a large IVH (usually during the first 4 postpartum days), the IVH is asymptomatic. Because approximately 70% of hemorrhages are asymptomatic, it is necessary to have a technique, such as ultrasound, to routinely scan all the infants at risk for these lesions.

However, in some infants the GM-IVH extends very fast; sudden flooding and distention of the ventricles by hemorrhage is associated with the clinical symptoms of shock, seizures, hypoxemia, and a sudden decrease in the hematocrit.

Sonographic Findings. IVHs appear as echogenic structures inside the anechoic ventricular cavities. Blood may fill just a small portion of the ventricle or the entire cavity. Care should be taken for small IVHs because studies from the anterior fontanel may not detect them, as blood tends to "settle out" in the posterior horns. These small IVHs can be diagnosed when the occipital horns are visualized in the axial plane from the mastoid or from the posterior fontanels. Furthermore, even small IVHs may occlude the foramen of Monro or the aqueduct of Sylvius and thereby produce moderate to large dilation of the lateral ventricles by CSF.

When blood fills the entire ventricle it is referred to as a ventricular cast (Figure 27-27). In this case, without

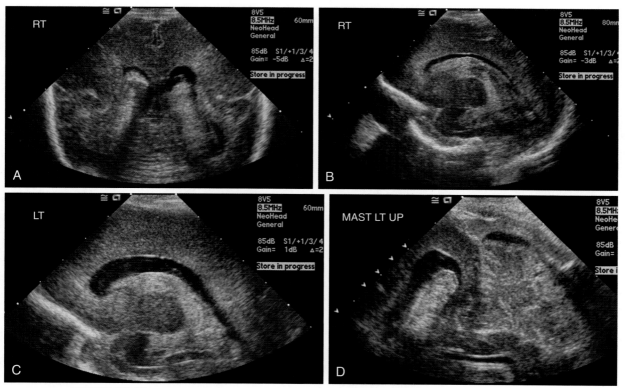

FIGURE 27-27 Grade III: IVH seen in same 1-day-old 28-week preterm infant (Figure 27-25) who had the grade I subependymal bleed bilaterally. Patient had pulmonary hemorrhage on day 2 of life, now grade III IVH seen on follow-up study on day 3 of life. **A,** Coronal view. **B,** Right parasagittal image. **C,** Left parasagittal image. **D,** Mastoid view depicting dilated, blood-filled occipital horns more clearly. (*Images courtesy Nationwide Children's Hospital, Columbus, OH.*)

ventricular dilation the ventricle may become isoechoic with the other structures in the brain, making definition of the borders of the ventricular wall difficult. Large cystic IVH may cause persistent ventricular dilation despite drainage of the CSF by a ventriculoperitoneal shunt.

Grade IV: Intraparenchymal Hemorrhages. Intraparenchymal hemorrhages (IPHs) complicate GM-IVHs in approximately 15% to 25% of infants. IPHs are a severe complication because they indicate that the brain parenchyma has been destroyed. Although IPHs originally were considered an extension of GM-IVHs, evidence suggests this lesion is an infarction of the periventricular and subcortical white matter with destruction of the lateral wall of the ventricle, occurring secondary to GM bleed obstruction of the terminal veins. When the necrotic tissue liquefies, the IVH extends into the necrotic areas.

◤ *Sonographic Findings.* Intraparenchymal hemorrhages appear as very echogenic zones in the white matter adjacent to the lateral ventricles. Echogenic areas in the white matter may correspond to IPHs or to hemorrhagic infarctions or extensive periventricular leukomalacia. In the classic grade IV IPH, there is a clot extending from the white matter into the ventricular cavity (Figure 27-28).

Intraparenchymal clots follow the same evolution as intraventricular clots. A few days after the acute bleeding, the clots become cystic and are reabsorbed completely in 3 or 4 weeks, leaving a cavity communicating with the lateral ventricle (porencephalic cyst).

When GM-IVHs associated with IPH evolve to posthemorrhagic hydrocephalus, the increased intraventricular pressure is transmitted to the porencephalic cyst. Hydrocephalus after hemorrhage associated with porencephaly is an indication for early ventriculoperitoneal shunt placement to minimize the deleterious effects of progressive compression and ischemia of the brain parenchyma.

Intracerebellar Hemorrhages. In premature neonates, there are areas of germinal matrix located around the fourth ventricle in the cerebellar hemispheres. The cerebellar germinal matrix has the same vulnerability to hemorrhage in the telencephalic germinal matrix. Intracerebellar hemorrhages have been reported in approximately 5% to 10% of postmortem studies of neonatal populations. The incidence in live infants is significantly lower.

◤ *Sonographic Findings.* These hemorrhages appear as very echogenic structures inside the less echogenic cerebellar parenchyma (Figure 27-29). Coronal views through the mastoid fontanel may be essential to differentiate intracerebellar hemorrhages from large subarachnoid hemorrhages in the cisterna magna, the supracerebellar cistern, or both. Intracerebellar

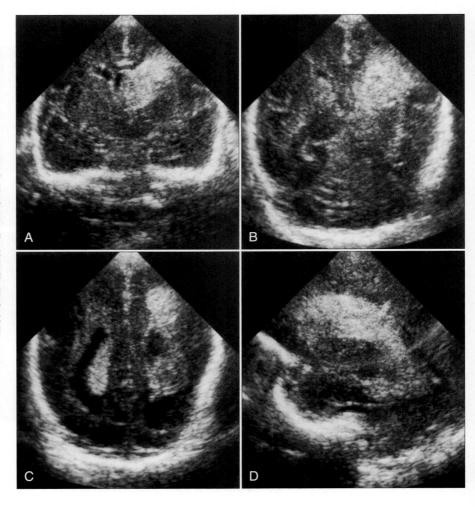

FIGURE 27-28 A 3-day-old premature infant has a grade III bleed on the right and grade IV bleed on the left with extension into the brain parenchyma. **A,** Coronal view at the frontal horns of the lateral ventricles shows hyperechoic hemorrhage extending into brain parenchyma on the left side. **B,** Coronal view just posterior, at the body of the lateral ventricles, shows clot in the right ventricle, as well as a left intraparenchymal bleed. **C,** Coronal view showing dilation of the right and left posterior horn, with bleed anterior to left ventricle and attached to the glomus, distorting its normal shape. **D,** Left parasagittal view showing intraparenchymal bleed.

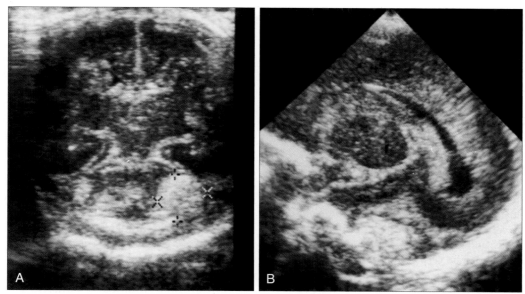

FIGURE 27-29 Multiple coronal and sagittal images in a premature infant born after 27 weeks of gestation with a large cerebellar bleed. In 5 days the bleed had progressed throughout the cerebellar compartment. **A,** Coronal view with largest measurement within a portion of the bleed. **B,** Sagittal view.

hemorrhages become cystic with time, leaving cavitary lesions in the cerebellar hemispheres. These characteristic sequential changes are useful in making a positive diagnosis of intracerebellar hemorrhages.

Epidural Hemorrhages and Subdural Collections. Epidural hemorrhages and subdural fluid collections are better diagnosed by magnetic resonance imaging (MRI) or computed tomography (CT); because these lesions are located peripherally along the surface of the brain, they are often not adequately visualized by ultrasound. However, if superficial fluid is seen, care should be taken to better detail it with color Doppler and proper gray-scale settings, to differentiate it from subarachnoid fluid.

Sonographic Findings. Epidural hemorrhages are seen as echogenic formations located immediately underneath the calvarium. Subdural collections appear as nonechogenic spaces between the echogenic calvarium and the cortex. Also, color Doppler may be helpful to distinguish a subdural hemorrhage from a subarachnoid hemorrhage. Both will produce widening of the interhemispheric fissure, but only a subarachnoid one will cause widening of the sylvian fissures. Additionally, any break in the bone of the calvarium can appear with a step-off or step-down effect, and may be incidentally found imaging the convexities of the brain. In the absence of birth trauma, this may indicate nonaccidental abuse if a subdural bleed is detected.

Extracorporeal Membrane Oxygenation. Neonatal ultrasound is primarily used to monitor hemorrhage in the brain tissue of infants on ECMO. ECMO is used for pulmonary and circulatory support in many neonatal conditions to allow additional time for the lungs to develop. Infants born with diaphragmatic hernia, persistent pulmonary hypertension, meconium aspiration, and congenital heart disease may be recommended for ECMO to give the infant's lungs a

chance to mature. The ECMO cannula is inserted into the right internal jugular vein and carotid artery (the vessels are ligated above their insertion site). Therefore the ECMO pump procedure can cause a notable change in cerebral circulation. After the vessel ligation, there is a 50% abrupt decrease in intracranial blood flow with a return of peak systolic velocities to nearly pre-ECMO levels within 3 to 5 minutes. The end-diastolic velocity is increased, and the Doppler is used to monitor for hypoxic-ischemic encephalopathy.

Hemorrhage and ischemia are common in children on ECMO, both from the effects of ECMO itself and from the conditions leading to the use of ECMO. Preexisting hypoxic-ischemic encephalopathy with an abnormal resistive index has been shown to lead to intracranial hemorrhage in a high percentage of infants. Bleeding may occur in the parenchyma, ventricle, or posterior fossa, but the cerebellum also is a common site. Increased extra-axial fluid is a common finding in children on ECMO.

Hypoxic-Ischemic Injury Lesions

Hypoxic-ischemic injury (HII) is a frequent complication of sick newborn infants. The premature neonate is physiologically delicate at birth and as a result is subject to many stresses that in turn can cause hemorrhage and brain injury. Hypoxia is the lack of adequate oxygen to the brain, whereas ischemia is the lack of adequate blood flow to the brain. These occurrences can result from a variety of insults, including respiratory failure, congenital heart disease, and sepsis.

In the term neonate, HII tends to occur in watershed regions between the vascular territories of the major cerebral vessels, located at the cerebral cortex and subcortical white matter. With severe insults, the basal ganglia and thalami may also be involved. The cortex is usually preserved in the preterm infant as a result of anastomotic communicating vessels from the meningeal circulation that serve to preserve cortical blood flow. The preterm infant suffers injury primarily at their watershed zone located at the periventricular white matter, occurring most commonly near the atria of the lateral ventricles posteriorly and near the foramen of Monro, but can occur anywhere within the corona radiata and even the corpus callosum. White matter ischemia leads to white matter volume loss or PVL (Figure 27-30). These lesions in the brain are usually associated with abnormal neurologic outcome.

Five major types of neonatal hypoxic-ischemic brain injury have been described in the neonatal brain, and MRI is the modality of choice to diagnose them. The initial gray-scale sonographic evaluation for HII is often normal; however, sonography can be very useful in following multifocal white matter necrosis (PVL) and focal ischemic lesion development.

Doppler sonography can be very useful in the earlier detection of neonates with hypoxia/ischemia and may be the only indication that HII has occurred. In an attempt to increase cerebral perfusion, end-diastolic flow rises, leading to a lower RI. The anterior cerebral artery should normally have an RI of 0.70. A low RI (less than 0.6), fluctuating RI, and hyperemia are useful Doppler findings in infants who have suffered HII. Fluctuations in RI likely reflect the loss of cerebrovascular autoregulation.

Periventricular Leukomalacia. Multifocal white matter necrosis, or **periventricular leukomalacia (PVL),** is the most frequent ischemic lesion in the immature brain. This lesion is associated with anomalous myelination of the immature brain and abnormal neurologic development, including cerebral palsy. PVL is probably the most important cause of abnormal neurodevelopmental sequelae in preterm infants.

PVL is found in 20% to 80% of neonatal autopsies. Pathologists describe an acute phase characterized by multiple foci or coagulation necrosis in deep and periventricular white matter, and a chronic phase depicted by cavitation and scarring appearing 1 or more weeks after the cerebral insult. Early in the chronic stage, multiple cavities develop in the necrotic white matter adjacent to the lateral walls of the frontal horns, body, atria, and occipital horns of the lateral ventricles. These lesions are frequently located in the lateral wall of the atria and occipital horns, causing damage to the optic radiations. Eventually the cavities resolve, leaving gliotic scars and diffuse cerebral atrophy. Necrotic lesions with only microscopic cavities may also lead to cerebral atrophy.

◢ ***Sonographic Findings.*** PVL may be detected by sonography only 1 to 2 days after the HII. This "acute" stage of PVL is characterized by highly echogenic areas in the cerebral white matter superior and lateral to the frontal horns, bodies, atria, and occipital horns of the lateral ventricles (Figure 27-31). In preterm infants echogenic areas, or a periventricular blush, are present during the first week after delivery. However, they usually resolve in the following weeks, suggesting the

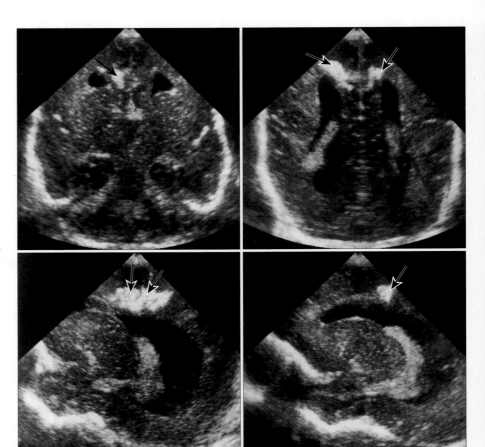

FIGURE 27-30 Periventricular leukomalacia. Chalky white lesions are indicated by *arrows.*

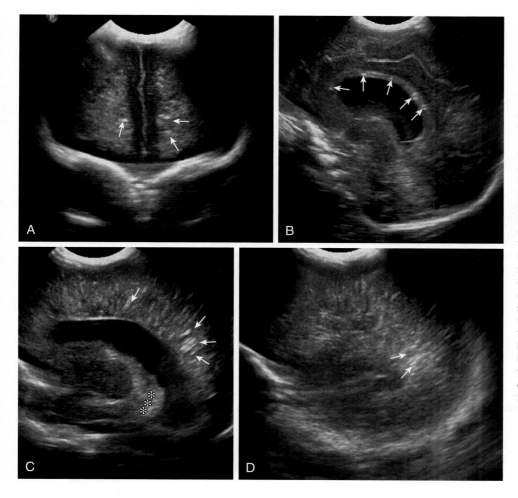

FIGURE 27-31 Acute PVL stage. An 8-day-old extremely premature infant with an acute drop in hematocrit was referred for a head ultrasound to evaluate for intracranial hemorrhage. Bilateral subependymal bleeds were seen, but the major concern was the increased echogenicity of the bilateral periventricular white matter and hyperechoic foci within the corpus callosum. **A,** Coronal view of the anterior periventricular area, *arrows* to increased echogenicity. **B,** Midline sagittal view demonstrating echogenic foci within the corpus callosum *(arrows).* **C,** Left parasagittal view showing increased periventricular white matter *(arrows),* seen more echogenic than the choroid plexus *(asterisks).* **D,** Right parasagittal view showing increased echogenicity of the periventricular white matter *(arrows). (Images courtesy Nationwide Children's Hospital, Columbus, OH.)*

echogenicities may be associated only with congestion and microhemorrhages without necrosis. If necrosis is present in the echogenic areas, cavitary lesions appear 2 or more weeks after the ischemic insult. Therefore careful follow-up studies are required. The chronic stage and definitive diagnosis of PVL with sonography is when echolucencies develop in the echogenic white matter (Figure 27-32).

Keep in mind that cystic lesions in white matter may be microscopic or smaller than the resolution of the ultrasound scanners. Consequently, PVL may exist in the absence of cavitary lesions on ultrasound. Both neuropathologic and MRI studies have shown that a period of 1 to 6 weeks ensues between the acute stage of PVL and the development of cystic lesions. Echogenic areas and cysts decrease in size and eventually disappear 2 to 5 months after the diagnosis of acute necrosis. If the necrosis was extensive, brain atrophy may be the only indication that PVL occurred during the perinatal period. Sonography is also useful to diagnose the chronic atrophic stage of PVL. Brain atrophy is identified by an enlarged subarachnoid space, widened interhemispheric fissure, and persistent ventricular dilation in an infant with a normal or small head circumference.

Focal Brain Necrosis. These necrotic lesions occur within the distribution of large arteries. This complication is present in term and preterm infants, but it is infrequent under

30 weeks of gestational age. Vascular maldevelopment, asphyxia or hypoxia, embolism from the placenta, infectious diseases, thromboembolism secondary to disseminated intravascular coagulation, and polycythemia have been implicated as causal factors in this condition. These insults may occur prenatally or early in postnatal life, leading subsequently to the dissolution of the cerebral tissues and formation of cavitary lesions. The term *porencephaly* is used to describe a single cavity, *multicystic encephalomalacia* for multiple cavities, and *hydranencephaly* for a large single cavity with the entire disappearance of the cerebral hemispheres.

Sonographic Findings. Ultrasound images of these injuries show very echogenic localized lesions within the distribution of the major vessel. The echodense lesions are considered to correspond to cerebral infarctions. After several days, sonolucencies appear within the echogenic areas. Subsequently the infarcted regions are replaced by cavities that may or may not communicate with the ventricle.

Lentriculostriate Vasculopathy. Lentriculostriate vasculopathy (LSV) may be seen in neonates with HII. It is characterized by linear echogenic foci branching within the basal ganglia and thalamus. These lesions have been associated with HII in the neonate. Hemodynamics in the premature brain is indicated in their pathogenesis. LSV has also been associated with congenital anomalies, chromosomal anomalies, prematurity,

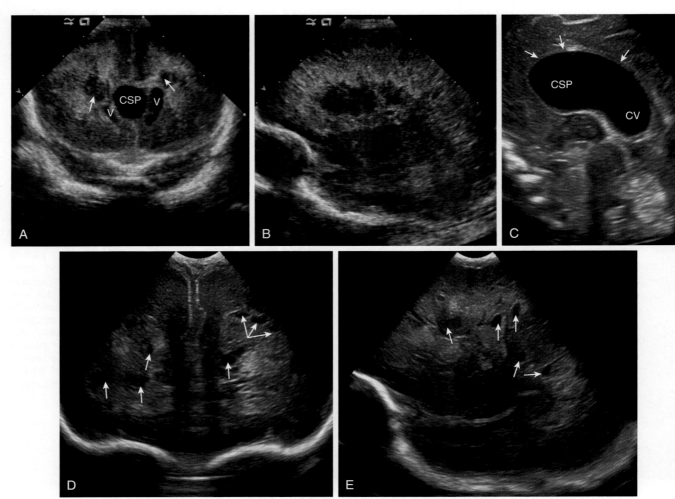

FIGURE 27-32 Chronic PVL stage. Cavitations or cystic formation within the increased periventricular white matter within 2 weeks of hypoxic-ischemic injury (HII) in the same extremely premature infant (Figure 27-31) with bilateral grade I (germinal matrix) bleeds, who also subsequently developed posthemorrhagic hydrocephalus. **A,** At a 4-day follow-up the coronal view of the anterior horns of the lateral ventricles shows increased echogenicity and adjacent hypoechoic areas *(arrows)* are indicative of brain liquefaction. *V,* Ventricle; *CSP,* cavum septum pellucidum. **B,** Right parasagittal view showing same parenchymal pattern lateral to the ventricles. **C,** At a 2-week follow-up there is thinning of the corpus callosum *(arrow). CV,* Cavum vergae. **D,** Coronal view of anterior periventricular white matter confirms an increased number of small cystic spaces *(arrows)* of liquefaction, developing porencephaly. **E,** Right parasagittal view of periventricular white matter with same cysts *(arrows).* (Images courtesy Nationwide Children's Hospital, Columbus, OH.)

perinatal insult, and congenital infection. Isolated findings of LSV have a good prognosis; however, 18.9% to 55% are shown to have neurodevelopmental delay, but this is likely associated with underlying abnormalities and brain insult.

CONGENITAL BRAIN MALFORMATIONS

A number of different malformations may occur in fetal brain development and may be related to neural tube closure, diverticulation, vessel formation, neural tissue migration, or sulcation (sulci development). Congenital brain anomalies are rare and occur in only 3% to 8% of all births, including stillbirths. It is important to keep in mind that brain malformations are often accompanied by characteristic clinical observations, hydrocephalus, and other cerebral malformations. If the anterior fontanel is open, sonography can reliably diagnose these malformations; however, more extensive diagnostics can be achieved through a cranial MRI.

Neural Tube Defects

The more commonly encountered neural tube defects encountered in neonatal head sonography are discussed here. Information on anomalies, such as anencephaly, myelomeningocele, meningocele, and encephalocele, are discussed in more detail in Chapter 60.

Arnold-Chiari Malformation. **Chiari malformations** are some the most common brain anomalies encountered, comprising 50% of all cerebral malformations. There are three types, of which type I and type III are rare. Type I is not usually diagnosed until adulthood, and type III is associated with encephaloceles. The most common is type II, also called Arnold-Chiari malformation, and is of the greatest clinical importance in the setting of the neonatal brain because of its association with myelomeningoceles or myeloceles. In early development of the brain, abnormal neural tube closure may result in a spinal defect, such as a myelomeningocele. About 80% to 90% of infants with myelomeningocele have Chiari malformations.

In Arnold-Chiari malformation the cerebellum and brainstem are pulled toward the spinal cord and secondary hydrocephalus develops. Aqueductal stenosis is present in 40% to 75% of infants with Chiari malformations. Hydrocephalus may also be caused by obstruction at the fourth ventricle or posterior fossa. Myelomeningoceles decompress the ventricles and lead to underdevelopment of the posterior fossa bony structures with a resulting small posterior fossa.

Sonographic Findings. Sagittal studies from the anterior fontanel show a small and dysplastic cerebellum, absence of the cisterna magna, low position of the fourth ventricle, and displacement of the cerebellum through the foramen magnum. The septum pellucidum may be partially or completely absent. With compression of the cerebellum, the cerebellar tonsils and vermis are herniated into the spinal canal through an enlarged foramen magnum, and the cisterna magna is not visualized due to this caudal displacement. The pons and medulla are inferiorly displaced and the fourth ventricle becomes elongated. In addition, enlargement of the massa intermedia may be noted on the coronal and midline sagittal images. Hydrocephalus is present in 90% of cases and to varying degrees, but is often not symmetrically dilated as in the case of posthemorrhagic hydrocephalus. The third ventricle may be slightly dilated and is often dysplastic. Rarely with Arnold-Chiari are the temporal horns dilated. The frontal horns are often small with a batlike configuration, whereas the posterior horns of the ventricles are quite enlarged (Figure 27-33).

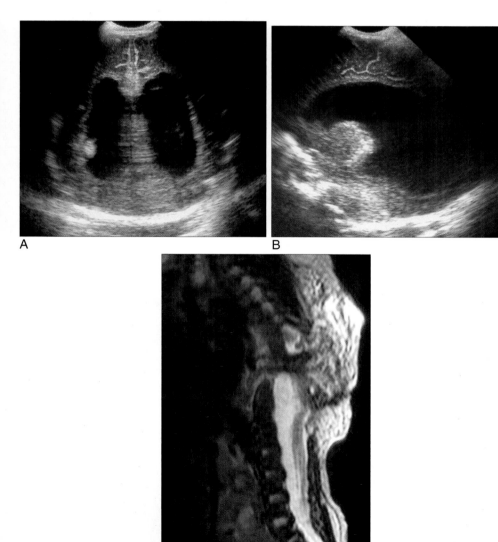

A

B

C

FIGURE 27-33 Infant was delivered by cesarean section at 39 weeks of gestation for thoracic spina bifida. Chiari's malformation, type II, was identified. Enlarged ventricles can be seen in **A,** posterior coronal views and **B,** lateral sagittal view of the head. **C,** Magnetic resonance imaging shows spinal defect.

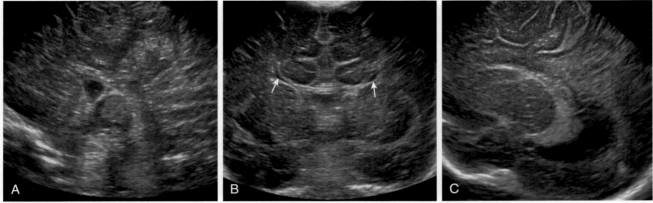

FIGURE 27-34 Agenesis of the corpus callosum in an 11-day-old term infant. **A,** Although randomizing of the cingulate sulcus is not as obvious in this infant, absence of the corpus callosum is easily noted. **B,** Coronal view at the frontal horns shows a winglike or "batman" appearance (*arrows*). **C,** Colpocephaly, or enlargement of the occipital horns, as seen from a coronal view. (*Images courtesy Nationwide Children's Hospital, Columbus, OH.*)

Often ventricular enlargement worsens after the myelomeningocele is repaired, as the CSF cannot enter the spinal defect. Commonly, it necessitates treatment with a ventriculoperitoneal shunt.

Agenesis of the Corpus Callosum. The corpus callosum (or great commissure) is a white matter structure that connects both cerebral hemispheres. The presence of the corpus callosum is important in coordinating information and exchanging sensorial stimuli between the two hemispheres. Development of the corpus callosum occurs between the 8th and 12th weeks of gestation, beginning ventrally and extending dorsally. Depending on the timing of the intrauterine insult, the development of the corpus callosum can be partially arrested or complete agenesis can occur. Absence of the corpus callosum may also be induced by ischemic lesions in the midline or by intrauterine encephalomalacia.

Agenesis of the corpus callosum has been associated with over 80 chromosomal, genetic, and sporadic syndromes, including Arnold-Chiari malformation. Agenesis of the corpus callosum is highly associated with Dandy-Walker malformation, affecting one third of those with it. It is often combined with migrational disorders, such as heterotopias and polymicrogyria. Other defects associated with this defect are porencephaly, hydrocephalus, microgyria, and fusion of the hemispheres. The corpus callosum is absent in severe holoprosencephaly. In neonates with this anomaly, the cerebral hemispheres have ventricles with pointed upper corners (bat-wing appearance).

Sonographic Findings. In neonates with this anomaly, the corpus callosum will be absent. The cingulate sulcus is randomized or spiraled because of the midline defect and the pericallosal artery may have an abnormal course or be absent. The third ventricle may appear to be "high riding," between the ventricles where the CSP normally sits. The CSP is absent when due to developmental destruction and should not be confused for the third ventricle. The cerebral hemispheres have ventricles with pointed upper corners (bat-wing appearance), and colpocephaly is present. Colpocephaly refers to teardrop-like enlarged occipital horns (Figure 27-34). Midline cysts may also be present and may or may not communicate with the lateral ventricles. Partial agenesis of the corpus callosum occurs when the genu, the splenium, and the rostrum are absent.

Dandy-Walker Malformation. Dandy-Walker syndrome is a group of congenital brain anomalies involving the disruption in development of the cerebellar vermis and roof of the fourth ventricle. There are several manifestations of this developmental differentiation just after the neural tube closes, which include both the **Dandy-Walker malformation** and Dandy-Walker variant. Dandy-Walker complex is a newer terminology for Dandy-Walker syndrome and also includes mega cisterna magna and arachnoid cysts of the posterior cranial fossa. Dandy-Walker malformation is the most serious anomaly seen in which a huge fourth ventricle cyst (Figure 27-35) occupies the area where the cerebellum

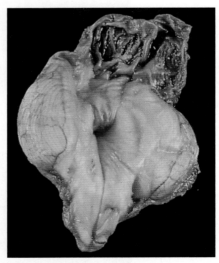

FIGURE 27-35 Dandy-Walker malformation. Hypoplastic vermis and cyst are reflected to expose a dilated fourth ventricle.

usually lies, with secondary dilation of the third and lateral ventricles. The vermis is absent in 25% of the population. The fourth ventricle is enlarged. The posterior fossa is enlarged with the elevation of the tentorium cerebelli, straight sinus, and torcular herophili at the venous sinus confluence. The brainstem may be compressed anteriorly or become hypoplastic. Obstructive hydrocephalus occurs in 70% to 80% of patients and is not often pronounced at birth, but develops within the first 3 months of life.

Dandy-Walker malformation may be associated with other central nervous system (CNS) anomalies, which include hydrocephalus, partial or complete agenesis of the corpus callosum, encephalocele, holoprosencephaly, microcephaly, infundibular hamartomas, or brainstem lipomas.

Sonographic Findings. The typical Dandy-Walker malformation is characterized by absence or hypoplasia of the cerebellar vermis, enlarged fourth ventricle connecting to the development of a large cyst in the posterior fossa (Dandy-Walker cyst), hypoplastic cerebellar hemispheres that are often not connected, displaced laterally by the fourth ventricle, and a small brainstem. A large posterior fossa is present with an elevated tentorium. Ventricular dilation is symmetric. The corpus callosum may be absent as well (Figure 27-36).

In Dandy-Walker variant the posterior fossa is not enlarged and the cerebellar hemispheres are normally developed. Ventricular dilation is rare. The fourth ventricle is only slightly dilated, but communicates with the cyst.

Mega cisterna magna is considered a normal variant with no mass effect that is not associated with the development of hydrocephalus and has a normal cerebellar vermis, fourth ventricle, and cerebellar hemisphere.

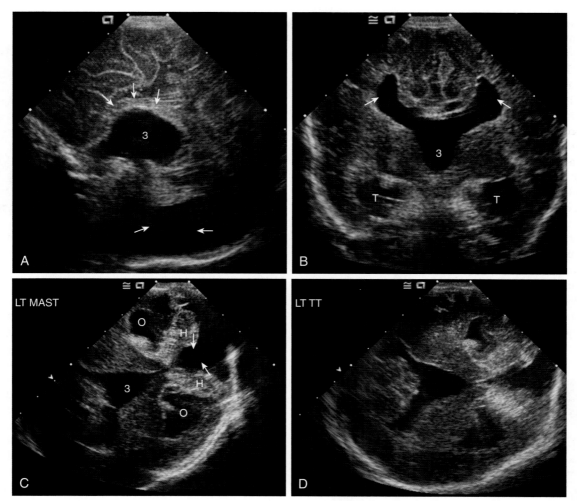

FIGURE 27-36 Dandy-walker malformation and agenesis of the corpus callosum in a term neonate. **A,** Midline sagittal view shows an absence of both the cerebellar vermis and corpus callosum *(arrows)* and a very enlarged third ventricle *(3)* in a higher position. **B,** Coronal view shows grossly enlarged lateral ventricles *(arrows)* with a bat-wing configuration communicating with the third ventricle *(3)*. The temporal horns *(T)* are also seen dilated in this view. **C,** Mastoid view of the cerebellum shows an absent vermis *(arrows)*, the space now occupied with CSF, and hypoplastic cerebellar hemispheres *(H)*. The occipital horns *(O)* are also visualized and are enlarged. **D,** A transtemporal approach demonstrating the anomaly entirely. *(Images courtesy Nationwide Children's Hospital, Columbus, OH.)*

A posterior fossa arachnoid cyst can be differentiated from Dandy-Walker malformation or variant by the lack of communication of the cyst with the fourth ventricle. The arachnoid cyst displaces the normal fourth ventricle, vermis, and cerebellum.

Disorders of Diverticulation and Cleavage

Holoprosencephaly. **Holoprosencephaly** is a complex development abnormality of the brain arising from failure of cleavage of the prosencephalon or forebrain. This failure results early in gestation. It is characterized by a grossly abnormal brain in which there is a common large central ventricle (Figure 27-37). The neuropathologic features include a single cerebrum with a single ventricular cavity, absence of the corpus callosum and frontal horns, and a thin membrane arising from the roof of the third ventricle, which may extend posteriorly forming a supratentorial cyst. In addition, anomalies of the face also accompany this condition.

Holoprosencephaly represents a spectrum of malformations that form a continuum from most severe, with no separation of the telencephalon (alobar), to least severe, with partial separation of the dorsal aspects of the brain (lobar). A third classification of intermediate severity between alobar and lobar is semilobar holoprosencephaly. The mildest form of lobar prosencephaly is septoptic dysplasia, known as De Morsier syndrome, in which there is absence of the septum pellucidum and optic nerve hypoplasia.

Alobar Holoprosencephaly. This is the most severe form of holoprosencephaly. Multiple facial anomalies (i.e., cebocephaly, cyclopia, and ethmocephaly) are present. The brain surrounds a single midline crescent-shaped ventricle with a thin, primitive cerebral cortex surrounding the large ventricle. The thalami and hemispheres are fused; therefore the falx, corpus callosum, and interhemispheric fissure are not present. The fused thalami are seen anterior to the fused hyperechogenic choroid plexus (Figure 27-38). The third ventricle is absent, causing the dilated single ventricle to communicate directly with the aqueduct of Sylvius. A large dorsal cyst may also be present.

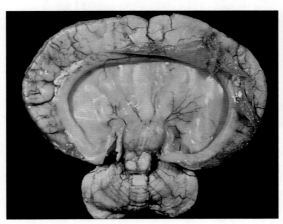

FIGURE 27-37 This posterior coronal view shows the reflected cyst wall communicating with a univentricle.

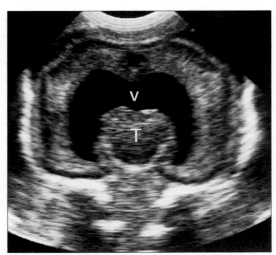

FIGURE 27-38 Alobar holoprosencephaly is identified demonstrating a single ventricle and thalamus. The falx cerebri is absent.

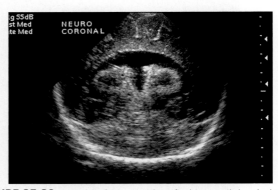

FIGURE 27-39 Variable fusion is identified in semilobar holoprosencephaly shown here with a split thalamus and univentricle.

Semilobar Holoprosencephaly. A single ventricle is evident; however, more brain parenchyma is present. A small portion of the falx and interhemispheric fissure develops in the occipital cortex posteriorly. There may be separate occipital and temporal horns. The splenium and genu of the corpus callosum is often formed and may be seen on midline sagittal images. The thalami are partially separated and the third ventricle is rudimentary (Figure 27-39). Mild facial anomalies (i.e., hypotelorism and cleft lip) may be present.

Lobar Holoprosencephaly. This is the least severe form of holoprosencephaly. There is nearly complete separation of hemispheres with development of a falx and interhemispheric fissure. There may be fusion of the frontal lobes. The septum pellucidum is absent. The anterior horns of the lateral ventricles are fused; however, the occipital horns are separated (Figure 27-40). The third ventricle is present and separates the thalami. The splenium and body of the corpus callosum are present with the absence of the genu and rostrum. Facial anomalies are mild.

Sonographic Findings. When holoprosencephaly is suspected, it is important to obtain coronal studies of the

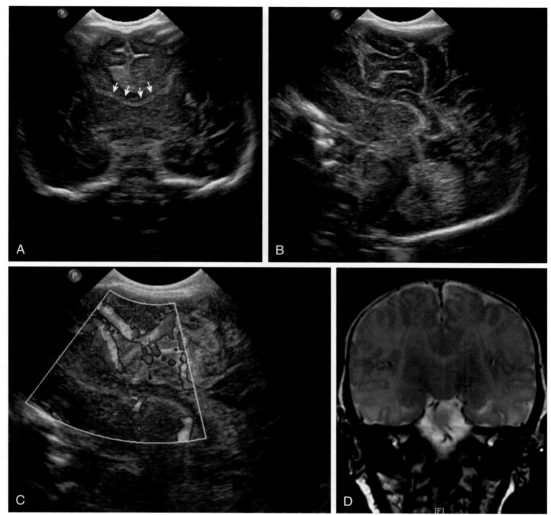

FIGURE 27-40 Lobar holoprosencephaly seen in a 2-day-old with cranial deformity. **A,** Coronal view demonstrates fusion of the anterior lateral ventricles *(arrows)*. The ventricular system is completely decompressed, making visualization of the structures more difficult. **B,** Sagittal midline view does not demonstrate a corpus callosum or cavum septum pellucidum. **C,** Sagittal midline view with color Doppler demonstrates an abnormal pericallosal artery. **D,** Coronal T2-weighted MRI shows same fused anterior horns of the lateral ventricles, and confirmed the patient had lobar holoprosencephaly with partial agenesis of the corpus callosum. *(Images courtesy Nationwide Children's Hospital, Columbus, OH.)*

whole frontal lobes to determine whether one frontal horn or thalamus is present.

Destructive Lesions

Hydranencephaly. Hydranencephaly is an ischemic lesion believed to be the result of bilateral occlusion of the internal carotid arteries during fetal development between the 3rd and 6th months of pregnancy, but it may result from any number of intracranial destructive processes. Brain development is destroyed and replaced by CSF. Because the posterior communicating arteries are preserved, the midbrain and cerebellum are present. The basal ganglia, choroid plexus, and thalamus may also be spared. It has a similar appearance to alobar holoprosencephaly. As in holoprosencephaly,

there is a single ventricular cavity and absence of the corpus callosum. However, the presence of midline structures and two frontal horns or thalami helps differentiate these malformations caused by ischemic lesions from true holoprosencephaly.

Sonographic Findings. There is absence of normal brain tissue with almost complete replacement by CSF (Figure 27-41). Unlike alobar holoprosencephaly, the midline structures, such as the interhemispheric fissure, falx cerebri, and third ventricle, may be preserved. A high-frequency linear transducer may help to visualize the superficial falx. Two thalami and two frontal horns may be identified. The midbrain, basal ganglia, and cerebellum are seen. Macrocephaly may be present. Doppler flow in the carotid arteries is absent.

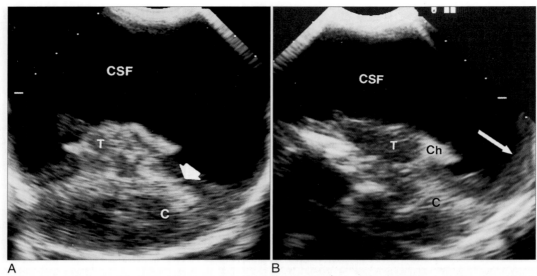

FIGURE 27-41 Hydranencephaly. Coronal **(A)** and sagittal **(B)** midline views. Tentorium cerebelli *(thick arrow)*; thin remnant of cerebral cortex *(thin arrow)*; *T,* thalamus; *C,* cerebellum; *Ch,* choroid plexus.

Porencephalic Cyst. A porencephalic cyst, also known as porencephaly, is a cyst filled with CSF that communicates with the ventricular system or subarachnoid space. These cysts may result from hemorrhage, infarction, delivery trauma, or inflammatory changes in the nervous system. The affected brain parenchyma undergoes necrosis, brain tissue is resorbed, and a cystic lesion remains.

◀ *Sonographic Findings.* A cyst is seen within the brain parenchyma without a mass effect. There may be communication of the cyst with the ventricle or subarachnoid space. A reduction in the size of the affected hemisphere may cause a midline shift and contralateral ventricular enlargement.

Cystic Lesions

Choroid Plexus Cysts. Choroid plexus cysts are common and may be seen in early development, as well as after delivery. The cysts tend to be singular and present as an isolated finding, not associated with other CNS or chromosomal abnormalities. However, when the cysts are greater than 10 mm and multiple, these can be associated with chromosomal abnormalities, particularly trisomy 18.

◀ *Sonographic Findings.* On sonography, the choroid plexus cyst appears as a well-defined anechoic mass within the dorsal choroid plexus. They range in size from 4 to 7 mm and are usually unilateral with the left larger than the right. They should be differentiated from subependymal cysts formed within the ventricular cavity (Figure 27-42).

Galenic Venous Malformation. The galenic venous malformation represents dilation of the vein of Galen within the quadrigeminal cistern caused by a vascular malformation that is fed by large arteries off the anterior or posterior cerebral artery circulation. Infants with this condition usually present with congestive heart failure.

◀ *Sonographic Findings.* This malformation appears as an anechoic, cystic mass between the lateral ventricles. It lies posterior to the foramen of Monro, superior to the third ventricle, and primarily in the midline. The large feeding vessels help to differentiate this lesion from other cystic masses (Figure 27-43). Hydrocephalus may or may not be present and calcification may occur if there is thrombosis in the malformation.

Arachnoid Cysts. Arachnoid cysts are lined by arachnoid tissue and contain CSF and may arise within any of the three meninges. There are three major causes postulated to explain the formation of these cysts: (1) localized entrapment of fluid during embryogenesis, (2) residual subdural hematoma, and (3) fluid extravasation secondary to leptomeningeal tear or ventricular rupture.

The cysts may be located in the infratentorial or supratentorial compartments. Arachnoid cysts in the posterior fossa are associated with a normal vermis and a normal fourth ventricle, which differentiates arachnoid cysts from the Dandy-Walker malformation. In a supratentorial compartment, these cysts usually arise from the suprasellar or quadrigeminal plate cisterns. The most frequent locations are the interhemispheric fissure, the suprasellar region, and the cerebral convexities. These cysts may be symptomatic secondary to cerebral compression or hydrocephalus, or they may be totally asymptomatic.

◀ *Sonographic Findings.* Arachnoid cysts usually appear on sonography as a sonolucent structure arising from the quadrigeminal plate cistern or the suprasellar region (Figure 27-44). Sagittal studies are useful to determine the location and size of these cysts. Sequential studies should be obtained in infants with this complication, as the cysts may have progressive growth and may need to be drained by ventriculoperitoneal shunts. Color Doppler may be used to verify that these are not venous malformations, especially when the cysts occur within the quadrigeminal plate cistern or the suprasellar region.

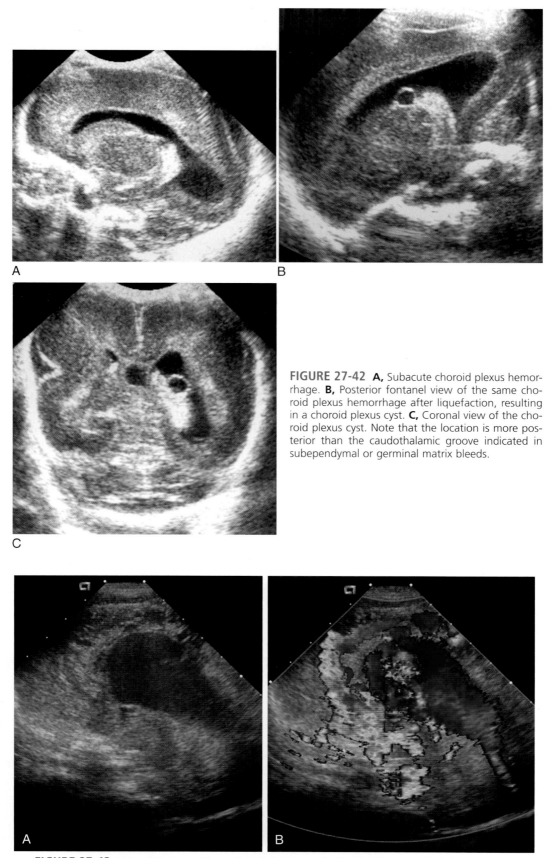

FIGURE 27-42 A, Subacute choroid plexus hemorrhage. **B,** Posterior fontanel view of the same choroid plexus hemorrhage after liquefaction, resulting in a choroid plexus cyst. **C,** Coronal view of the choroid plexus cyst. Note that the location is more posterior than the caudothalamic groove indicated in subependymal or germinal matrix bleeds.

FIGURE 27-43 Vein of Galen malformation. **A,** Large cyst is visualized on a sagittal view. **B,** Color Doppler shows blood flow within the cyst, confirming the diagnosis. *(Images courtesy Nationwide Children's Hospital, Columbus, OH.)*

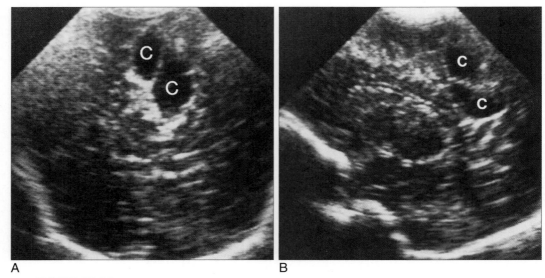

FIGURE 27-44 Midline arachnoid cyst. **A,** Coronal and **B,** sagittal scans show two arachnoid cysts *(C),* one in the interhemispheric fissure, the other just left, both above the lateral ventricle.

BRAIN INFECTIONS

Congenital Infections

Congenital infections of the brain can have serious consequences for the neonate, including death, mental retardation, or developmental delay. The most frequent congenital infections are commonly referred to by the acronym TORCH. This refers to the infections *Toxoplasma gondii,* rubella virus, cytomegalovirus (CMV), and herpes simplex type 2. The "O" stands for *other,* such as syphilis, which may cause acute meningitis. The most common of these infections is CMV, and toxoplasmosis is the second most common.

◼ *Sonographic Findings.* Sonography may detect parenchymal calcifications (Figure 27-45), and/or lenticulostriate vasculopathy (LSV). LSV has been found to be a highly associated with neonatal brain infections. Other complications that may arise include hydrocephalus, abscess, white matter softening or loss (encephalomalacia), and infarctions.

Ventriculitis

Ventriculitis is a common complication of purulent meningitis in newborn infants. Ventriculitis probably is caused by hematogenous spread of the infection to the choroid plexus. The presence of a foreign body in the ventricular cavity, such as a catheter from a ventriculoperitoneal shunt, may provide a nidus for persistent infection of the ventricular cavities.

◼ *Sonographic Findings.* Ventriculitis leads to compartmentalization of the ventricular cavities by inflammatory adhesions extending from wall to wall. The first stage of ventriculitis is seen in ultrasound as thin septations extending from the walls of the lateral ventricles. The septa become thicker and lead to multilocular hydrocephalus and extensive disorganization of the brain anatomy. Sequential studies in patients with meningitis or with ventriculoperitoneal shunts can provide early diagnosis of this severe complication.

FIGURE 27-45 A 1-month-old infant with bright calcifications seen bilaterally secondary to cytomegalovirus. **A,** Coronal image. **B,** Right parasagittal image.

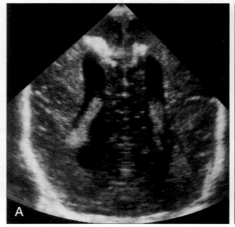
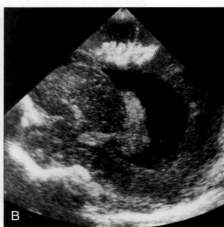

Ependymitis

Ependymitis occurs when the ependymal lining of the ventricles becomes inflamed as a result of irritation from hemorrhage within the ventricle. The ependymal lining will appear thickened and hyperechoic. This is more common and occurs earlier than ventriculitis, which can also develop from intraventricular hemorrhage.

 Key Pearls

- Sonography plays a very important role in the diagnosis and follow-up of intracranial problems in the neonate.
- Care must be taken to keep the infant warm and safe (good disinfectant techniques, minimize movement, etc.).
- It is very important to know the approximate gestational age of the premature infant and the associated sonographic findings.
- Fontanel closure, around 9 months, makes sonographic imaging difficult after this time.
- Sagittal and coronal views are used to image the supratentorial and infratentorial structures. A mastoid view, in most infants under 6 months when the fontanel closes, is very helpful in better depicting the deep infratentorial structures.
- Midline sagittal view is critical to rule out many congenital anomalies.
- Use multiple acoustic windows in the presence of pathology, if possible.
- Ventriculomegaly is very common and ventricular measurements and Doppler of the pericallosal artery can help track enlargement and increased intracranial pressure (ICP).
- Increased ICP is of great clinical concern and is treated with the placement of a ventricular shunt.
- Any superficial fluid should be investigated to determine whether it is subdural or "extra-axial" versus subdural in nature.
- The caudothalamic groove is a common source of subependymal bleeds in infants less than 34 weeks, with increased risk under 32 weeks and under 1500 g.
- In term infants bleeds often occur in the glomus of the choroid plexus
- Intracranial hemorrhages (ICHs) may be classified as grades I through IV depending on the location of the bleed, ventricular dilation, or parenchymal involvement.
- An ICH starts in the germinal matrix or caudothalamic groove and is a progressive disease.
- The periventricular white matter should never appear more hyperechoic than the choroid plexus and is a common place for white matter necrosis (periventricular leukomalacia [PVL]) to occur in the premature infant.
- PVL initially appears hyperechoic, and over the course of weeks cystic areas develop as a result of necrosis.
- Agenesis of the corpus callosum is indicated in many congenital anomalies and the associated cingulate gyri and sulci will have a sunburst appearance.

- Dandy-Walker complex includes an array of anomalies, the most severe of which is the Dandy-Walker malformation, which presents with a large cystic area under the cerebelli tentorium, due to a missing cerebellar vermis. Cerebellar hemispheres may be absent or hypoplastic.
- Chiari malformations involve the hindbrain and type II, called Arnold-Chiari malformation, is nearly always associated with spina bifida.
- Holoprosencephaly is a spectrum of malformations due to abnormal diverticulation in utero. This disorder may be divided into the alobar, semilobar, and lobar types.
- Congenital infections, most commonly the TORCH complex, may present with calcification or lenticulostriate vasculopathy (LSV).
- LSV may also occur in patients who have undergone a hypoxic-ischemic injury.
- Three-dimensional (3D) neurosonography shows promise to decrease neonatal head examination time and improve consistency. 3D ultrafast Doppler is a new method that can provide more hemodynamic information to better understand blood flow within the neonatal brain.

BIBLIOGRAPHY

American Institute of Ultrasound in Medicine: AIUM practice guideline for the performance of neurosonography in neonates and infants, 2009. Available at http://www.aium.org/resources/guidelines/neurosonography.pdf.

Amodio J, Spektor V, Pramanik B, et al: Spontaneous development of bilateral subdural hematomas in an infant with benign infantile hydrocephalus: color Doppler assessment of vessels traversing extra-axial spaces, *Pediatr Radiol* 35(11):1113-1117, 2005.

Bacani M: The neonatal brain. In *Diagnostic medical sonography: abdomen and superficial structures,* ed 3, Philadelphia, PA, 2012, Lippincott Williams & Wilkins, pp 735-747.

Bhat V: Neonatal neurosonography: a pictorial essay, *Indian J Radiol Imaging* 24(4):389-400, 2014.

Bradstreet JJ, Pacini S, Ruggiero M: A new methodology of viewing extra-axial fluid and cortical abnormalities in children with autism via transcranial ultrasonography, *Front Hum Neurosci* 7:934, 2014.

Brouwer MJ, De Vries LS, Groenendaal F, et al: New reference values for the neonatal cerebral ventricles, *Radiology* 262(1):224-233, 2012.

Brouwer MJ, De Vries LS, Pistorius L, et al: Ultrasound measurements of the lateral ventricles in neonates: why, how and when? A systematic review, *Acta Paediatr* 99(9):1298-1306, 2010.

Brown PD, Davies SL, Speake T, Millar ID: Molecular mechanisms of cerebrospinal fluid production, *Neuroscience* 129(4):957-970, 2004.

Chapman T, Mahalingam S, Ishak GE, et al: Diagnostic imaging of posterior fossa anomalies in the fetus and neonate: part 2. Posterior fossa disorders, *Clin Imaging* 39(2):167-175, 2015.

Cinalli G, Spennato P, Nastro A, et al: Hydrocephalus in aqueductal stenosis, *Childs Nerv Syst* 27(10):1621-1642, 2011.

Coley BD, Rusin JA, Boue DR: Importance of hypoxic/ischemic conditions in the development of cerebral lenticulostriate vasculopathy, *Pediatr Radiol* 30(12):846-855, 2000.

Correa FF, Lara C, Bellver J, et al: Potential pitfalls in fetal neurosonography, *Prenat Diagn* 26(1):52-56, 2006.

Daneman A, Epelman M: Neurosonography: in pursuit of an optimized examination, *Pediatr Radiol* 45(Suppl 3):406-412, 2015.

Daneman A, Epelman M, Blaser S, Jarrin JR: Imaging of the brain in full-term neonates: does sonography still play a role? *Pediatr Radiol* 36(7):636-646, 2006.

Deeg KH, Gassner I: Sonographic diagnosis of cerebral malformations in infancy. Part 1: Chiari and Dandy-Walker malformations, *Ultraschall Med* 31(5):446-462, 2010.

Deeg KH, Gassner I: Sonographic diagnosis of brain malformations, part 2: holoprosencephaly—hydranencephaly—agenesis of septum pellucidum—schizencephaly—septo-optical dysplasia, *Ultraschall Med* 31(6):548-560, 2010.

Demené C, Pernot M, Biran V, et al: Ultrafast Doppler reveals the mapping of cerebral vascular resistivity in neonates, *J Cereb Blood Flow Metab* 34(6):1009-1017, 2014.

Duan Y, Sun FQ, Li YQ, et al: Prognosis of psychomotor and mental development in premature infants by early cranial ultrasound, *Ital J Pediatr* 41:30, 2015.

Ecker JL, Shipp TD, Bromley B, et al: The sonographic diagnosis of Dandy-Walker and Dandy-Walker variant: associated findings and outcomes, *Prental Diagn* 20:328-332, 2000.

Engle WA: A recommendation for the definition of "late preterm" (near-term) and the birth weight-gestational age classification system, *Semin Perinatol* 30(1):2-7, 2006.

Evans DH: Doppler ultrasound and the neonatal cerebral circulation: methodology and pitfalls, *Biol Neonate* 62:271, 1992.

Fenton AC, Papathoma E, Evans DH, et al: Neonatal cerebral venous flow velocity measurement using a color flow Doppler system, *J Clin Ultrasound* 19:69, 1991.

Fenton AC, Shortland DB, Papathoma E, et al: Normal range for blood flow velocity in cerebral arteries of newly born term infants, *Early Hum Dev* 22:73, 1990.

Fenton TR, Tanis R, Kim JH: A systematic review and meta-analysis to revise the Fenton growth chart for preterm infants, *BMC Pediatr* 13(1):59, 2013.

Fox LM, Choo P, Rogerson SR, et al: The relationship between ventricular size at 1 month and outcome at 2 years in infants less than 30 weeks' gestation, *Arch Dis Child Fetal Neonatal Ed* 99(3):F209-F214, 2014.

Fox TB: Sonography of the neonatal brain, *J Diagn Med Sonogr* 25(6):331-348, 2009.

Frankel DA, Fessell DP, Wolfson WP: High resolution sonographic determination of the normal dimensions of the intracranial extraaxial compartment in the newborn infant, *J Ultrasound Med* 17(7):411-415, 1998.

Fritz J, Polansky SM, O'Connor SC: Neonatal neurosonography, *Semin Ultrasound CT MRI* 35(4):349-364, 2014.

Govaert P, De Vries LS: *An atlas of neonatal brain sonography,* ed 2, Cornwall, UK, 2010, Mac Keith Press.

Hamrick SE, Miller SP, Leonard C, et al: Trends in severe brain injury and neurodevelopmental outcome in premature newborn infants: the role of cystic periventricular leukomalacia, *J Pediatr* 145(5):593-599, 2004.

Hervey-Jumper SL, Cohen-Gadol AA, Maher CO: Neurosurgical management of congenital malformations of the brain, *Neuroimaging Clin North Am* 21(3):705-717, ix, 2011.

Hong SY, Yang JJ, Li SY, Lee IC: Lenticulostriate vasculopathy in brain ultrasonography is associated with cytomegalovirus infection in newborns, *Pediatr Neonatol* 56(6):1-7, 2015. Available at http://www.ncbi.nlm.nih.gov/pubmed/26073370.

Horbar JD, Leahy KA, Lucey JF: Ultrasound identification of lateral ventricular asymmetry in the human neonate, *J Clin Ultrasound* 11(2):67-69, 1983.

Hwang SW, Su JM, Jea A: Diagnosis and management of brain and spinal cord tumors in the neonate, *Semin Fetal Neonatal Med* 17(4):202-206, 2012.

International Society for Pediatric Neurosurgery: Ultrasound of ventricles in the brains of infants, 2010. Available at http://ispn.guide/book/The%20ISPN%20Guide%20to%20Pediatric%20Neurosurgery/Hydrocephalus%20and%20Other%20Anomalies%20In%20CSF%20Circulation%20In%20Children/Hydrocephalus/2010.

Kliegman RM, et al: *Nelson textbook of pediatrics,* ed 19, Philadelphia, PA, 2011, Saunders Elsevier.

Lowe LH, Bailey Z: State-of-the-art cranial sonography: part 2, pitfalls and variants, *AJR Am J Roentgenol* 196(5):1034-1039, 2011.

Makhoul IR, Eisenstein I, Sujov P, et al: Neonatal lenticulostriate vasculopathy: further characterisation, *Arch Dis Child Fetal Neonatal Ed* 88(5):F410-F414, 2003.

Mandiwanza T, Saidlear C, Caird J, Crimmins D: The open fontanelle: a window to less radiation, *Childs Nerv Syst* 29(7):1177-1181, 2013. doi:10.1007/s00381-013-2073-0.

Mondal P, Mukhopadhyay J, Sural S, et al: A robust method for ventriculomegaly detection from neonatal brain ultrasound images, *J Med Syst* 36(5):2817-2828, 2012.

Monteagudo A: Fetal neurosonography: should it be routine? Should it be detailed? *Ultrasound Obstet Gynecol* 12(1):1-5, 1998.

Orman G, Benson JE, Kweldam CF, et al: Neonatal head ultrasonography today: a powerful imaging tool! *J Neuroimaging* 25(1):31-55, 2015.

Perlman JM: White matter injury in the preterm infant: an important determination of abnormal neuro development outcome, *Early Hum Dev* 53:99-120, 1998.

Rabiner JE, Friedman LM, Khine H, et al: Accuracy of point-of-care ultrasound for diagnosis of skull fractures in children, *Pediatrics* 131(6):e1757-e1764, 2013.

Riccabona M: Neonatal neurosonography, *Eur J Radiol* 83(9):1495-1506, 2014.

Romero JM, Madan N, Betancur I, et al: Time efficiency and diagnostic agreement of 2-D versus 3-D ultrasound acquisition of the neonatal brain, *Ultrasound Med Biol* 40(8):1804-1809, 2014.

Rosenberg HK, et al: Normal splenic sizes in infants and children: sonographic measurements, *AJR Am J Roentgenol* 157:119-121, 1991.

Rumack C, Drose J: Neonatal and infant brain imaging. In *Diagnostic ultrasound,* vol 2, ed 4, St. Louis, 2011, Mosby, pp 1623-1695.

Rumack CM: *Diagnostic ultrasound,* ed 3, St Louis, 2005, Mosby.

Seibert JJ, Avva R, Hronas TN, et al: Use of power Doppler in pediatric neurosonography: a pictorial essay, *Radiographics* 18(4):879-890, 1998.

Shekdar K: Posterior fossa malformations, *Semin Ultrasound CT MRI* 32(3):228-241, 2011.

Shen EY, Weng SM, Kuo YT, et al: Serial sonographic findings of lenticulostriate vasculopathy, *Acta Paediatr Taiwan* 46(2):77-81, 2005.

Shen MD, Nordahl CW, Young GS, et al: Early brain enlargement and elevated extra-axial fluid in infants who develop autism spectrum disorder, *Brain* 136(Pt 9):2825-2835, 2013.

Siegel MJ: Neonatal intracranial problems. In Sanders RC, Winter T, editors: *Clinical sonography: a practical guide,* ed 4, Baltimore, MD, 2007, Lippincott Williams & Wilkins, pp 341-364.

Siegel MJ: *Pediatric sonography,* Philadelphia, PA, 2010, Lippincott Williams & Wilkins.

Taylor GA, Madsen JR: Neonatal hydrocephalus: hemodynamic response to fontanel compression—correlation with intracranial pressure and need for shunt placement, *Radiology* 201(3):685-689, 1996.

van de Bor M, Walther FJ, Sims ME: Acceleration time in cerebral arteries of preterm and term infants, *J Clin Ultrasound* 18:167, 1990.

van Wezel-Meijler G: *Neonatal cranial ultrasonography,* Berlin, 2007, Springer.

van Wezel-Meijler GV, De Vries LS: Cranial ultrasound—optimizing utility in the NICU, *Curr Pediatr Rev* 10(1):16-27, 2014.

Volpe JJ: Brain injury in the premature infant: overview of clinical aspects, neuropathology, and pathogenesis, *Semin Pediatr Neurol* 5:135-151, 1998.

Winter TC, Kennedy AM, Byrne J, Woodward PJ: The cavum septi pellucidi: why is it important? *J Ultrasound Med* 29(3):427-444, 2010.

Whitelaw A: Intraventricular hemorrhage and post-hemorrhagic hydrocephalus: pathogenesis, prevention and future interventions, *Semin Neonatol* 6:135-146, 2001.

Infant and Pediatric Hip

Kathryn E. Zale

Sonographic evaluation of the neonatal hip allows for a dynamic view of the soft tissues and cartilaginous structures, with the added advantages of a low cost and lack of ionizing radiation, contrast media, and sedation. It plays an important role in the diagnosis and management of developmental displacement of the hip (DDH) in the infant. It can also easily detect fluid within the joint space, providing clinicians a quick way to assess for joint effusions or septic arthritis in the child with a painful hip.

Until around 4 to 6 months of age when the femoral head ossifies, sonography is optimal for evaluating DDH in the neonatal/infant hip compared with other imaging modalities. Although magnetic imaging can provide excellent anatomic detail of the hip anatomy in the young infant, it is not dynamic, requires a long scanning period, is expensive, and requires sedation. Computed tomography requires gonadal ionizing radiation and sedation and is also nondynamic, but may be helpful in infants confined to a cast. Radiography, although it was originally used to diagnose DDH in young infants, is

not reliable in detecting the soft cartilaginous structures of the hip that are not yet ossified in this population.

This chapter aims to provide readers with the necessary anatomy, sonographic findings, and techniques to better assess for hip pathology frequently performed in the pediatric setting. Although techniques vary by pathology, this chapter is separated into developmental hip displacement, joint effusions of the hip, and other hip conditions and differential diagnoses. A large majority of attention is given to developmental displacement (dysplasia/dislocation) of the hip.

NORMAL ANATOMY AND SONOGRAPHIC FINDINGS

The anatomy assessed in the pediatric hip consists of the bony pelvic girdle, superior portions of the femur, hip joint (including the acetabulum and acetabular labrum), and supporting ligaments and muscles.

Bones and Cartilage

The sacroiliac joints unite the two pelvic bones, or hipbones, with the sacral part of the vertebral column. The pubic symphysis is where these two hipbones unite with each other anteriorly. The pelvic bones, also referred to as the coxal or innominate bones, consist of the fusion of three separate bones: the ilium, ischium, and pubis. Together they form the **pelvic girdle.** The triradiate cartilage connects these three bones and is made of their three distinct growth plates, or physes, that do not ossify until adulthood, then becoming part of the acetabulum.

The bone of the upper thigh is the femur, which is surrounded by muscles, ligaments, and tendons. The upper part of the femur, the head, articulates with the hipbone to make the hip joint (Figure 28-1).

The three pelvic bones and the shaft (or diaphysis) of the femur are ossified at birth, and sonographically appear hyperechoic, casting an acoustic shadow. The triradiate cartilage is a useful landmark, lying posterior to the femoral head, and appears hypoechoic in the neonate. The greater and less trochanters, as well as the neck and head of the femur, are also cartilaginous and well seen with sonography. The greater

trochanter sits superolateral, whereas the lesser trochanter projects from the posteromedial proximal femoral shaft. The neck of the femur tapers medial, superior, and anterior toward the femoral head.

The head appears as a large hypoechoic circle and may ossify as early as 4 weeks, but typically between 3 and 8 months. Ossification begins centrally, with girls often showing earlier ossification than boys. Sonography can be performed until the femoral head ossifies. Once the femoral head is completely ossified, it is difficult to obtain adequate sonographic images because of beam artifact interference (Figure 28-2).

Hip Joint

The articulation of the rounded head of the femur with the cup-shaped acetabulum of the pelvic bone forms the ball-and-socket **hip joint** (Figure 28-3). The hip joint is not directly palpable because it is surrounded and protected by muscles of the upper thigh. The greater trochanter of the femur forms a palpable knob at the side of the region.

The acetabulum is horseshoe shaped and has a smaller articular surface than the femur's articular surface. The acetabular

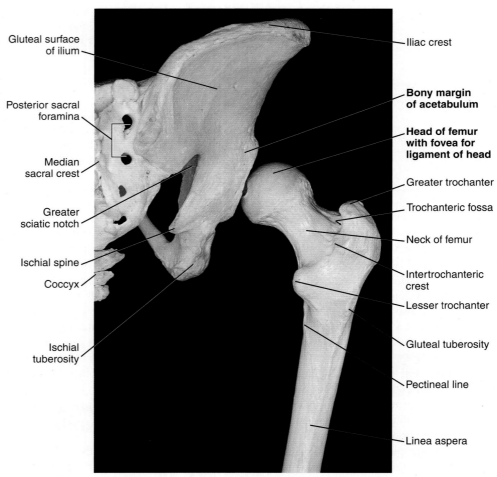

FIGURE 28-1 Hip joint—posterior osteology. Posterior view of the right hip joint. The femur has been partly dislocated so that its posterior surface can be completely visualized.

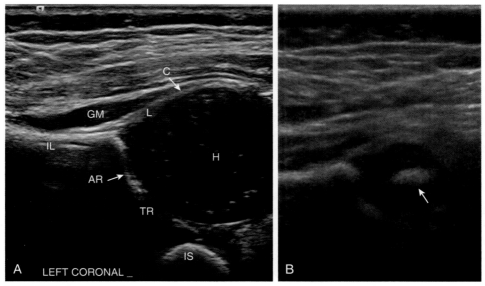

FIGURE 28-2 Normal femoral head development within the hip joint. **A,** This 10-week-old infant has cartilaginous and hypoechoic femoral head with smooth boarders and fine-stippled echoes dispersed throughout. Head of femur *(H),* triradiate cartilage *(TR),* ischium *(IS),* ilium *(IL),* bony acetabular roof *(AR),* labrum *(L),* gluteus medius *(GM),* capsule *(C).* **B,** This 4-month-old infant shows central ossification in the head of the femur *(arrows).* Ossification and structures placed deeper in the body, equates to an overall decrease in image quality. *(Images courtesy Nationwide Children's Hospital, Columbus, OH.)*

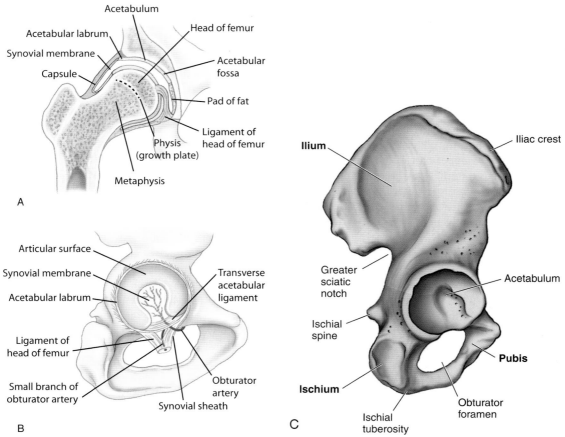

FIGURE 28-3 **A,** Coronal section of the right hip joint. **B,** Posterior view of articular surface of the right hip joint and arterial supply of the head of the femur. **C,** Posterior view of the right hip joint showing the acetabulum and triradiate cartilage.

labrum is a rim of fibrocartilage that surrounds the acetabulum. It also forms an extension of the acetabular roof. The acetabular labrum narrows the acetabulum and increases its depth, functioning to stabilize and support the femoral head articulation within the acetabulum.

The labrum is composed of hyaline cartilage and is hypoechoic, except at its tip, which is echogenic due to its fibrous content. Sonographically, the labrum is best depicted from a coronal view and appears superolateral to the femoral head, adjacent to the ilium. Approximately two thirds of the femoral head should be covered by the labrum.

The acetabular notch is a bony deficiency at the lower part of the acetabulum through which nerves and blood vessels pass, and is covered by a band of fibrous tissue called the transverse ligament. The ligamentum teres of the femur, or rounded ligament, runs from this acetabular notch to the pit or fovea in the head of the femur. In the younger child, this ligament contains the branch of the obturator artery to supply the femoral head. The artery usually disintegrates by 7 years of age.

Supporting Ligaments and Muscles

The hip joint is surrounded by a tough capsule, which attaches to the intertrochanteric line of the femur and is reinforced by outside ligaments and muscles. The psoas tendon crosses the center of the hip joint just inferior to the inguinal ligament. The iliacus muscle sits lateral to the psoas tendon and, along with the psoas muscle, flexes the hip.

The most important hip ligament is the iliofemoral ligament, which passes from the anterior inferior iliac spine to each end of the intertrochanteric line. It is one of the strongest ligaments in the body and is very important for standing and maintaining correct upright balance.

The large gluteus maximus muscle overlies other muscles superior and posterior to the hip joint. The gluteus maximus is a powerful extensor of the hip. The gluteus minimus muscle is the immediate cover for the upper part of the hip joint. The gluteus medius and gluteus minimus pass from the outer surface of the hipbone to the greater trochanter. Together they act as abductors of the hip joint. Their most important function is to prevent adduction and keep the pelvis level during walking.

Movements of the Hip

The movements of the hip are somewhat limited in range because of the tight fit between the femur and acetabulum and because the hipbone is immobile (Figure 28-4). The following are the hip movements and their actions. Note that sonographic evaluation is primarily concerned with the abduction and adduction motions.

Flexion (bending forward) and **extension** (bending backward): The primary flexors of the hip are the psoas major, iliacus, and rectus femoris. Extension is limited to 20 degrees and is brought about by the hamstrings and gluteus maximus.

Adduction (moving sideways inward) and **abduction** (moving sideways outward): An example of hip adduction is crossing your legs when in a seated position, an action performed by the

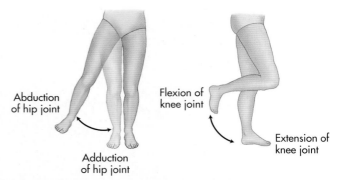

FIGURE 28-4 Anatomic terms used in relation to movement of the hip.

adductor group of muscles. In abduction, the gluteus medius and minimus muscles open the limbs. The more important function of these muscles, however, is to prevent adduction, which is the function they perform during walking.

Medial and lateral rotation: Medial and lateral rotation is related to the angle at which rotation occurs at the head of the femur, which is about 120 degrees angle to the shaft of the femur. When the trochanter moves forward, the femur rotates medially, and when the trochanter moves backward, the femur rotates laterally. Thus the medial rotators are the anterior fibers of gluteus medius and minimus. The lateral rotators are the small muscles at the back of the joint— piriformis, obturator internus, and quadratus femoris, with assistance from the gluteus maximus.

DEVELOPMENTAL DISPLACEMENT OF THE HIP

Developmental dysplasia/dislocation of the hip has been described as far back as Hippocrates. Formerly known as congenital hip dislocation, this misleading term referred to a spectrum of pathology that usually develops after birth. Therefore the term **developmental displacement of the hip (DDH),** or developmental dysplasia of the hip, is now used. DDH encompasses a spectrum of pathologies including subluxated, dysplastic, dislocatable, and dislocated hips.

Development of both sides of the neonatal hip requires the femoral head to be seated normally and congruently within the acetabulum. If the femoral head and acetabulum are not in their normal position, both sides of the hip will develop abnormally. A displacement of the hip is a relatively common abnormality, and when diagnosed in the neonatal period (up to 4 to 6 weeks of age) it is often attributed to normal laxity of the hips. Whereas 90% of mild cases diagnosed with sonography may resolve, in more severe cases DDH can cause impaired function and degenerative joint disease. Diagnosis should be made early and treatment instituted promptly.

In the newborn period, the femoral head may dislocate in a lateral and posterosuperior position relative to the acetabulum (Figure 28-5). When this occurs, the femoral head can usually be reduced without deformity to the joint. However, when the dislocation is not recognized early, the muscles

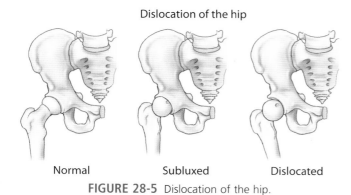

Dislocation of the hip

Normal   Subluxed   Dislocated

FIGURE 28-5 Dislocation of the hip.

tighten and limit movement, which causes the acetabulum to become dysplastic because it lacks the stimulus of the femoral head. In turn, the ligamentous structures stretch and fibrofatty tissue occupies the acetabulum, making it impossible to return the femoral head into the acetabulum. This fibrofatty pulvinar may also develop in subluxation.

Etiology

Incidence of Developmental Displacement of the Hip.
The incidence of hip dislocation is difficult to define as there is no gold standard test, but it is estimated between 1.5 and 20 cases per 1000 live births, and milder forms of displacement, such as subluxation, are more common. When the diagnosis is based on diagnostic sonographic findings it may be as high as 40 to 60 cases per 1000 population. However, epidemiologic and demographic data vary widely, ranging from 0.06 per 1000 live births among Africans, up to 76.1 per 1000 among some Native Americans.

Multiple risk factors may contribute to the condition. Approximately 12% to 16% of all newborns have one or more of these factors and are at a higher risk of developing DDH. The most salient factors include breech presentation in both pregnancy and at delivery, which increases the risk nearly 4 times over the general population. Females are affected 2.5 times more frequently than males, although some population estimates are reported as high as 4 to 6 times. The left hip is affected 64% of the time and occurs unilaterally 64% of the time. It is more common among firstborn children and those with a family history of DDH.

The condition also affects certain races, such as Caucasians and certain North American tribes, more than those of African or Asian decent. Some suspect these differences may be due to swaddling practices. Swaddling has been strongly associated with DDH; DDH has a more prevalent diagnosis in winter months as well. Other risk factors may include maternal hypertension, fetal growth restriction, oligohydramnios, premature rupture of membranes, prolonged gestation, increased birth weight, Potter's syndrome, and neonatal intensive care. Congenital muscular torticollis and congenital foot deformities are also associated factors. Prematurity, however, has not been shown to be a predisposing risk factor for DDH.

Causes of Developmental Displacement of the Hip.
Although the exact etiology of DDH is unknown, the primary root is thought to be increased laxity within the joint capsule, causing a gradual migration of the femoral head away from the acetabulum. Hormonal, mechanical, and genetic factors are thought to play a role.

The hormonal theory suggests that the sex hormones act on the laxity of the connective hip joint tissue. The maternal hormonal effect of estrogen, which increases muscle laxity late in pregnancy (aiding childbirth), is thought to account for increased risk among female neonates, as this effect is reduced by the male sex hormones. Other sex hormones affecting laxity include progesterone and estrogen. Progesterone increases the collagen content in the joint capsule, likely facilitating hip dislocation, whereas estrogen has the opposite effects.

As for the mechanical causes of DDH, swaddling, oligohydramnios, breech presentation, and the primigravid uterus are considered risk factors because each limits the mobility of the hip in its own way. Improper swaddling may keep the hips in an adducted position if swaddled too tight and straight; instead, the legs should be able to bend up and out of the hips. Oligohydramnios limits mobility because there is less than a normal amount of amniotic fluid present for the fetus to move freely within the amniotic sac. In breech presentation, the fetus's hip rests against the maternal sacrum and is usually flexed, which limits movement. This usually affects the left hip. The frank breech presentation of the fetus is the highest risk because the hips are maximally flexed and the knees are extended. The primigravid uterus is smaller than the multigravida uterus and is more confining, limiting mobility.

Genetic factors are currently being investigated in DDH, and findings from family and twin heritability suggest a strong genetic predisposition at onset (although less so with regard to progression or severity). It has been reported that there is a 5% chance that a child will be affected if a sibling has DDH and a 36% chance if one sibling and one parent are affected. There is a 12% chance that an affected individual will have a child with DDH.

Causes of Dislocation of the Hip.
Neonatal hip dislocation is often not present at birth and can be acquired, teratogenic, or developmental. Acquired causes of hip dislocation can be traumatic or nontraumatic (i.e., neuromuscular diseases). Teratogenic dislocations occur in utero and are associated with neuromuscular disorders.

Clinical Examination

A careful physical examination remains the universal screening for DDH and is therefore critical to the diagnosis. DDH detection, however, may vary widely between novice clinicians and experienced pediatric orthopedists. On visual inspection, the dislocated hip shows asymmetric skin folds and shortening of the affected thigh. The knee is lower in position on the affected side when the patient is supine and the knees are flexed, known as the **Galeazzi sign** (Figure 28-6).

Hip instability may resolve after 4 to 6 weeks, due to waning maternal hormones. Therefore neonates with a slightly positive

Early signs (dislocation of right hip)

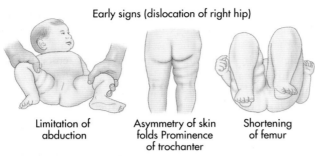

Limitation of abduction

Asymmetry of skin folds Prominence of trochanter

Shortening of femur

FIGURE 28-6 Physical signs of developmental displacement of the hip.

or inconclusive physical examination, and newborns with a risk factor for DDH, should be examined with sonography after this period to reduce false-positive results. Neonates with a grossly positive physical examination result or dislocation, however, are often seen earlier.

Two basic maneuvers are helpful in the diagnosis of DDH. The Barlow maneuver determines whether the hip can be dislocated, and the Ortolani maneuver determines whether the dislocated femoral head can be reduced back into the acetabulum.

Barlow Maneuver. In the **Barlow maneuver** (Figure 28-7) the patient lies in the supine position with the hip flexed 90 degrees and adducted. Downward and outward pressure is then applied. If the hip can be dislocated, the examiner will feel the femoral head move out of the acetabulum with his or her fingers.

Ortolani Maneuver. In the **Ortolani maneuver** (Figure 28-8) the patient lies in the supine position. The examiner's hand is placed around the hip to be examined, with the fingers over the femoral head. The examiner's middle finger lies over the greater trochanter and the thumb is over the lesser trochanter. The hip is flexed 90 degrees and the thigh is abducted. Movement in the normal hip should feel smooth. In cases of DDH, a "clunk" is appreciated as the femoral head returns

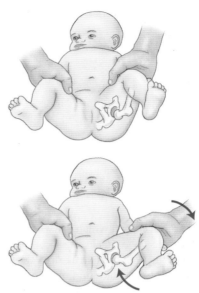

FIGURE 28-8 Ortolani maneuver.

into the acetabulum. A "click" does not imply DDH. Each hip should be examined individually.

Sonographic Examination

Sonography has been found to be more sensitive than physical examination in the detection of DDH. It has been shown to change the diagnosis in over half of cases while changing the management plan in one third of cases presenting to pediatric orthopedist surgeons for suspected DDH. Although universal screening sonography has been recommended, and is currently used in Europe, it is likely cost-prohibitive at this point. Currently, indications for neonatal hip sonography include the presence of certain risk factors for DDH (e.g., female gender with breech presentation, or a family history), an abnormal hip examination, and the need to evaluate the response to treatment. Sonography for DDH is often practical for most infants up to 6 months of age. Exceptions may include older infants if the femoral head is not yet ossified. Typically, after 4 to 6 months of age a radiograph is the preferred modality. If the patient is in a harness, the ordering physician should specify if the ultrasound is to be done in or out of the harness. Infants are often examined in the harness.

Examination Preparation. To achieve a satisfactory examination, the infant should be relaxed and as comfortable as possible. Feeding before or during the examination helps to soothe the infant. Make sure the room is warm and keep blankets close for warmth. Toys and other distractions help to quiet the infant so the examination may be performed. Parental assistance is helpful to keep the infant calm, with the mother or father near the infant's head.

Sonography of the neonatal hip is performed with a high-frequency linear-array transducer (Box 28-1). Sector or curved-array transducers will distort anatomy and are not optimal.

The infant is placed in a supine or decubitus position perpendicular to the table with the feet toward the sonographer.

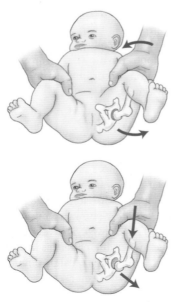

FIGURE 28-7 Barlow maneuver.

In a decubitus view, rolled towels, bolsters, or even specialized cradles may help keep the child on his or her side. It is wise to leave the diaper on through the examination and expose only the side of the hip being examined. Ambidextrous scanning is required for this bilateral examination; the right hip is examined with the transducer in the sonographer's left hand and vice versa. The opposite hand is used for manipulation of the hip being examined. Scanning with the dominant hand first may be helpful. Sonographic imaging is performed from the lateral or posterolateral aspect of the hip.

Sonographic Examination Overview. The sonographic examination for DDH evaluates the degree to which the femoral head is covered by the labrum, as well as the position of the femoral head in the acetabulum at rest and during motion and stress. Throughout the examination, the sonographer is able to assess the position and stability of the femoral head in addition to assessing the development of the acetabulum. The stability of the hip is determined through guided motion and the application of gentle stress. The stress maneuvers are the imaging counterparts of the clinical Barlow (adduction) and Ortolani (abduction) maneuvers.

The sonographic appearance of the femoral head location is described as normal, subluxed, or dislocated. Sonographic description of the acetabulum is assessed visually and described as normal, immature, or dysplastic. Validation of the acetabular morphology by the static sonographic alpha, beta, and femoral head measurements is optimal. Stability testing is reported as normal, lax, subluxable, dislocatable, and reducible or irreducible.

Sonographic Protocol. The basic hip anatomy is imaged in the coronal and transverse views. Views should be properly annotated denoting the view and position of the hips, as appropriate. Figure 28-9 provides images of a normal hip evaluation for DDH.

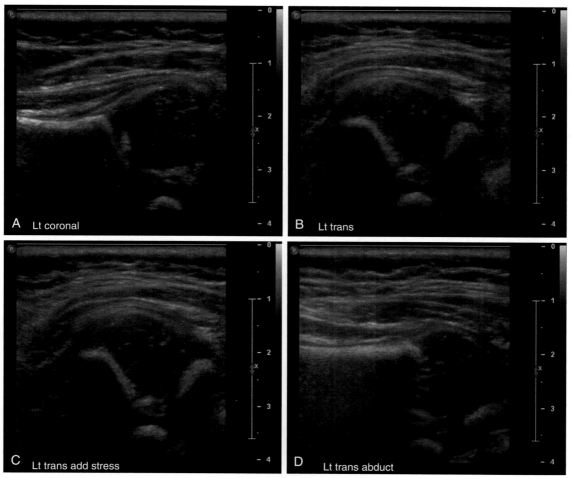

FIGURE 28-9 Normal sonographic study of the left hip of a 10-week-old to rule out DDH. Remember that this is a bilateral examination; in this case the right hip images were nearly identical to the left ones, also normal. **A,** Coronal/flexed view. **B,** Transverse/flexed view. **C,** Transverse view with adduction stress. **D,** Transverse view in abduction position. *(Images courtesy Nationwide Children's Hospital, Columbus, OH.)*

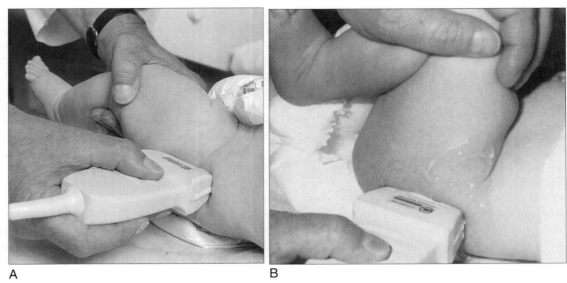

FIGURE 28-10 Coronal view obtained in the neutral and flexed positions. **A,** Coronal/neutral view. The transducer is coronal with respect to the hip. The femur is in physiologic neutral position for the infant (slight hip flexion). **B,** Coronal/flexion view. Transducer is coronal to flexed femur.

Coronal Study. The coronal view is performed with the infant in the supine or lateral decubitus position from the lateral aspect of the hip joint, with the plane of the transducer oriented coronally with respect to the hip joint. The coronal view is crucial for assessing acetabular development. On each side, often two static coronal images are obtained from which measurements are taken. The hip may be evaluated in the neutral or flexed position (Figure 28-10).

In the neutral view, the femur is stabilized with a physiologic amount of flexion, about 15 to 20 degrees, while the flexed view is 90 degrees. For beginners, the head of the femur is a bit more difficult to find in the flexed position, but scanning in a posterior direction along the femoral shaft is helpful. Angulation of the probe in both the flexed and neutral positions should be strictly avoided. It is difficult to make the abnormal hip appear normal; however, one can make the normal hip appear abnormal—this has to do with angling the probe, which results in misalignment, versus moving the entire transducer to align properly with the midacetabular view. Additional dynamic imaging in this plane is optional.

Coronal/Neutral View. This plane must demonstrate a straight iliac line to the inferior tip of the os ilium (ilium bone) at the midportion of the acetabulum. The hypoechoic cartilage of the acetabular roof extends lateral to the acetabular lip. The echogenic tip of the labrum should also be visualized. The femoral head is resting against the bony acetabulum. The acetabular roof should have a concave configuration and cover at least half of the femoral head. According to Graf, the coronal/neutral plane must meet certain checklist criteria to be considered diagnostic (Figure 28-11 and Box 28-2).

Coronal/Flexion View. The coronal/flexion view is also made at the midacetabulum with similar sonographic features to the coronal/neutral view. However, unlike its

FIGURE 28-11 A, Normal coronal/neutral view demonstrating Graf checklist (Box 28-2). *S* demonstrates superior position, *L* the lateral position. *Solid arrow* shows the fibrocartilaginous tip of labrum. *Open arrow* shows the triradiate cartilage. Iliac *(i),* femoral head *(H),* femoral metaphysis *(m),* synovial fold *(SF),* joint capsule *(C),* cartilaginous roof *(CR),* bony acetabular roof *(AR),* bony rim *(Rim).* **B,** Suggested presentation of the coronal/neutral view according to Graf.

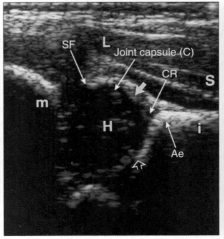

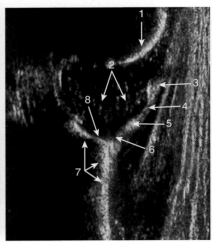

A

B

BOX 28-2	Graf Checklist for Coronal/Neutral View
Checklist 1: Anatomic identification m—Metaphysis or osteochondral boarder H—Femoral head SF—Synovial fold C—Joint capsule CR—Cartilaginous roof Roof—Bony roof Rim—Bony rim (normally concave) Solid arrow—Labrum	**Checklist 2: Usability Check** 1—Lower limb of the os ilium is seen 2—Os ilium contour straight or parallel to the probe 3—Tilting and oblique planes are avoided*

*Graf recommends the use of a specialized cradle and probe guide system to reduce this error.

neutral counterpart, the echogenic femoral metaphysis is not visualized in the coronal/flexed position. Also, the coronal/flexion view provides more of a "ball on a spoon" appearance. The gluteus medius muscle is another landmark of this view and is seen as a hypoechoic structure superolateral to the labrum (Figure 28-12).

Coronal Findings of Hip Displacement. In the coronal view when a hip becomes subluxed, or dislocated, the femoral head gradually migrates laterally and superiorly with progressively decreased coverage of the femoral head. Echogenic soft tissue (fibrofatty pulvinar) may be interposed between the femoral head and the bony acetabulum. In hip dysplasia, the bony acetabular roof is irregular and rounded, and the labrum is defected superiorly and becomes echogenic and thickened. When the hip is frankly dislocated, the labrum may be deformed, which will contribute to irreducibility (Figure 28-13).

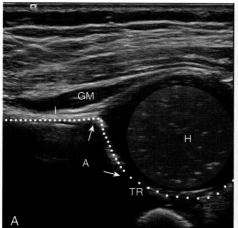
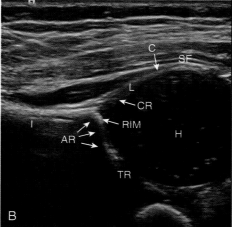

FIGURE 28-12 A, Normal "ball on a spoon" appearance of the coronal/flexion view. The femoral head *(H)* is the ball, the acetabulum *(A)* forms the spoon, and the iliac *(I)* line is the handle. The triradiate cartilage *(TR)* and gluteus medius muscle *(GM)* are also seen. **B,** Corresponding anatomic anatomy with coronal/neutral position (notice metaphysis is missing). Iliac *(i)*, femoral head *(H)*, labrum *(L)*, triradiate cartilage *(TR)*, synovial fold *(SF)*, joint capsule *(C)*, cartilaginous roof *(CR)*, bony acetabular roof *(AR)*, bony rim *(Rim)*. *(Images courtesy Nationwide Children's Hospital, Columbus, OH.)*

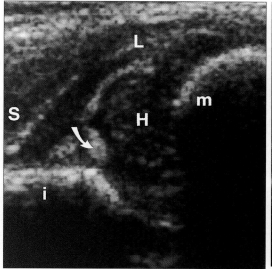
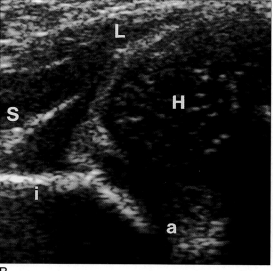

FIGURE 28-13 A, Coronal/neutral view of a dislocated hip shows displacement of the femoral head laterally with deformity of the labrum *(curved arrow)*. **B,** Coronal/flexion view of a dislocated hip has similar findings to Image A, and shows soft tissue echoes in the acetabulum (fibrofatty pulvinar) that may prevent the hip from being reduced without surgical intervention. Femoral head *(H)*, lateral *(L)*, superior *(S)*, iliac line *(i)*, femoral metaphysis *(m)*, acetabulum *(a)*.

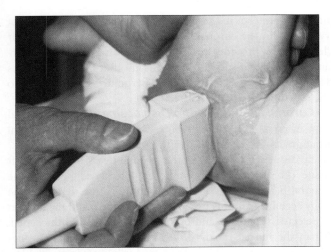

FIGURE 28-14 Transverse/flexion view. The transducer is in the axial plane posterolaterally over the hip joint with the hip flexed.

Transverse Study. In the transverse view, the transducer is rotated 90 degrees and moved posteriorly into a posterolateral position over the hip joint (Figure 28-14). The transverse study is normally performed with the hip flexed 90 degrees, specifically called the transverse/flexion view. One static transverse/flexion view is normally imaged, along with one adduction stress and one abduction image (see Dynamic Harcke Technique, later in this chapter).

The bony shaft of the femur gives off brightly reflected echoes anteriorly, adjacent to the femoral head. The echoes from the bony acetabulum appear posteriorly to the femoral head, and in the normal hip a "U" configuration is produced (Figure 28-15, A).

The relationship of the femoral head to the acetabulum is observed during flexion of the hip from adduction to abduction. In adduction a more "V" appearance is seen, whereas a deep "U" configuration is produced with maximum abduction (Figure 28-15, B). Be careful that the transducer is posterior enough to image the medial bony acetabulum, or the hip may appear falsely displaced. Next, the hip is then stressed with a gentle posterior push in adduction (Barlow maneuver). In the normal hip, the femoral head will remain deeply in the acetabulum in contact with the ischium with stress (Figure 28-15, C).

Transverse Findings of Hip Displacement. In the transverse view if subluxation is present the hip will be normally positioned or mildly displaced at rest and there will be further lateral displacement from the medial acetabulum with stress, but the femoral head will remain in contact with a portion of the ischium. If the femoral head dislocates laterally, the center of the femoral head does not line up with the iliac wing. A line drawn through the iliac wing will pass through the medial aspect of the femoral head. If the femoral head dislocates posteriorly, only an echogenic arc (which represents one side of the head) is seen. With **frank dislocation**, however, the hip will be laterally and posteriorly displaced to the extent that the femoral head has no contact with the acetabulum, and the normal "U" configuration cannot be obtained (Figure 28-16). With abduction (Ortolani maneuver) the dislocated hip may be reduced, or it may return to the acetabulum.

Sonographic Technique/Assessment. Two general sonographic techniques are used in the assessment for DDH: the static (morphologic) Graf technique and the dynamic Harcke technique. A combination of these, as well as their modifications, may be performed across institutions, and the techniques are not mutually exclusive. However, regardless of the Graf method or modification used at an institution, the assessment of hip stability and morphology appears feasible and accurate given a well-organized, high-quality service.

Static Graf and Modified Graf Technique. The standard Graf sonographic image is acquired in the coronal

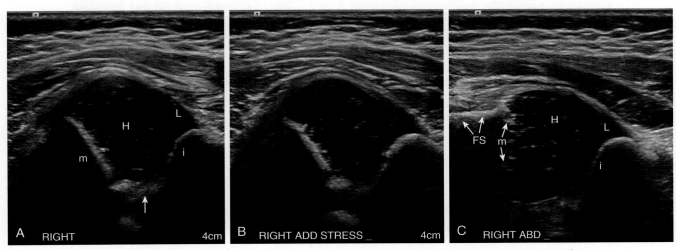

FIGURE 28-15 Normal sonographic appearance of the transverse study. **A,** Transverse image without any added stress—normal "U" shape. **B,** Transverse image with added stress in adduction (ADD)—more of a "V" shape. **C,** Transverse image showing abduction (ABD)—deeper "U" appearance. Head (H), metaphysis (m), labrum (L), ischium (i), femoral shaft (FS). Arrow points to area of triradiate cartilage. (Images courtesy Nationwide Children's Hospital, Columbus, OH.)

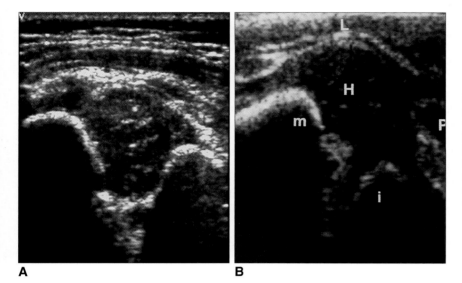

A   **B**

FIGURE 28-16 A, Normal hip sonogram shows echolucent femoral head surrounded by metaphysis (anterior) and ischium (posterior), forming a "U" around the femoral head. **B,** Dislocated hip sonogram shows sonolucent femoral head displaced posterolaterally. The "U" configuration of normal metaphysis and ischium is not seen. *H,* Femoral head; *L,* lateral; *P,* posterior; *i,* ischium; *m,* metaphysis.

plane at the midacetabular level from the lateral aspect of the hip in a neutral position. This image includes the femoral head, acetabulum, labrum, and iliac bone as it meets the triradiate cartilage. Inclusion of these structures ensures a proper image, from which the radiologist or physician can measure the alpha and/or beta Graf angles (Figure 28-17). It is from these angles (Box 28-3) that the neonatal hip is objectively assessed. Software is also available on ultrasound systems making it possible for sonographers to measure these angles.

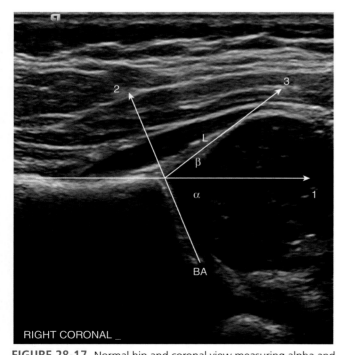

FIGURE 28-17 Normal hip and coronal view measuring alpha and beta angles. Alpha angle (α) is between lines 1 and 2. Beta angle (β) is between lines 1 and 3. *BA,* Edge of the bony acetabulum (deepest point); *L,* labrum. *(Image courtesy Nationwide Children's Hospital, Columbus, OH.)*

BOX 28-3	Graf's Alpha and Beta Angles

Graf used a series of lines and angle measurements to evaluate the morphology of the acetabulum (Figure 28-17):

Line 1: Baseline, drawn along the ilium, extending through the head of the femur

Line 2: Provides the alpha angle, drawn from bony edge of acetabulum at the triradiate cartilage to the lowest point of the ilium.

Line 3: Provides the beta angle, drawn from the ilium along the labrum.

Alpha Angle (α)
- Measures the acetabular depth
- The alpha angle reflects changes in the osseous portion of the acetabulum, which occur gradually
- Normally greater than 60 degrees

Beta Angle (β)
- The beta angle (β) reflects changes in the cartilaginous acetabulum (labrum), which occur more quickly than do changes in the osseous acetabulum
- Normally less than 55 degrees

Modifications to the original Graf technique have allowed for the inclusion of hip shape and stability to be examined. More commonly, the modified Rosendahl method is used and measures the alpha angle only. Meanwhile, Graf encourages the use of the beta angle, as it reflects changes to the cartilaginous acetabulum, which occur more quickly than do changes in the osseous acetabulum, and may be more sensitive than the alpha angle. However, studies have found both techniques to be comparable in their findings. The modified Graf method is taken in the flexed coronal position and also includes the separate dynamic assessment of the hip joint for stability. The usual practice for this modification is having the femur flexed at 90 degrees, allowing for consistency with any possible follow-up examinations when the infant is in a harness.

The four types of neonatal hip displacements are described in Table 28-1, showing the Graf and modified Graf

TABLE 28-1	Classification of Neonatal Hips and Angle Measurements	
Hip Classification Type	**Modified (Rosendahl) Graf Angle Measurements***	**Graf Classification Angle Measurements†**
Type I hip—normal hip at any age	$\alpha \geq 60$ degrees	$\alpha > 60°$, $\beta < 55$ degrees
Type II hip—elastic or physiological hip	50 degrees $\leq \alpha < 60$ degrees	43 degrees $\leq \alpha < 60$ degrees
Type II(a) hip—immature hip	Normal if newborn, or up to 3 months old, may still be due to physiologic laxity Follow-up recommended	
Type II(b) hip	Up to 3 months old, indicates delayed development Follow-up recommended	
Type III hip—dysplastic or unstable hip	43 degrees $\leq \alpha < 50$ degrees, mild dysplasia	$\alpha < 43$ degrees, $\beta > 77$ degrees
Type IV hip—severely dysplastic and/or gross or "frank" dislocation of the hip in either type III or IV	$\alpha < 43$ degrees or immeasurable, with significant dysplasia (with or without changes of the labrum)	$\alpha < 43$ degrees, β is immeasurable

Alpha angle (α), beta angle (β).
*Modified Graf measurements taken from a flexed coronal position.
†Graf measurements taken from a neutral coronal position.

TABLE 28-2	Description of Acetabulum by Graf Type		
Hip Graf Classification Type	**Bony Roof Development**	**Ossific Rim Shape**	**Cartilaginous Rim (Labrum) Appearance**
Type I	Good	Sharp or angular	Extends over femoral head and is narrow
Type II	Deficient or severely deficient	Rounded or rounded/flat	Covers femoral head and may be thinned and compressed
Type III	Poor	Flat	Displaced upward and may be echopoor or more reflective than femoral head, may be thinned or rounded
Type IV	Poor	Flat	Inverted into the acetabulum

(Rosendahl) criteria. Note that there are other subcategories of these classifications, which are not presented here, but may further subdivide dysplasia into mild and severe types. For both of these coronal assessments, type I hips are normal and require no further evaluation. Type II hips must be monitored, and follow-up studies are required. Type III and type IV hips must be treated.

Additional subjective sonographic signs of developmental displacement of the hip are also assessed, which include delayed ossification of the femoral head and acetabular abnormalities (Table 28-2). Fibrofatty pulvinar may also be present.

A recent quality criterion, the osteochondral plate sign (Figure 28-18), may be added for obtaining the standard Graf image in the neutral coronal position. The sign should show a perpendicular angle of the osteochondral boarder, or metaphysis, to the transducer. It may aid in providing better reproducibility of Graf measurements, especially among borderline alpha angle values.

A "normal" sonogram does not absolutely exclude DDH, although the sensitivity and specificity of sonography approach 100%. The accuracy and specificity of this technique increase with age and are highest at 3 months of age and lowest before 4 weeks of age. Furthermore, a learning curve to obtain experience with normal and abnormal hips is important to the reproducibility and accuracy of the

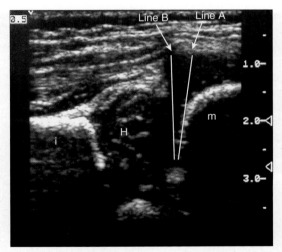

FIGURE 28-18 Osteochondral plate sign shown in a normal hip in the coronal/neutral view. The line (line *A*) is drawn along the osteochondral boarder, or metaphysis *(m)*. For increased reproducibility, this osteochondral boarder line should be angled so it is parallel with the transducer scan lines (line *B*).

sonographic evaluation. Harcke has suggested that at least 100 infant hip examinations should be performed to acquire sufficient experience. Figure 28-19 demonstrates all the different modified Graf hip types, defined by an alpha angle and appearance.

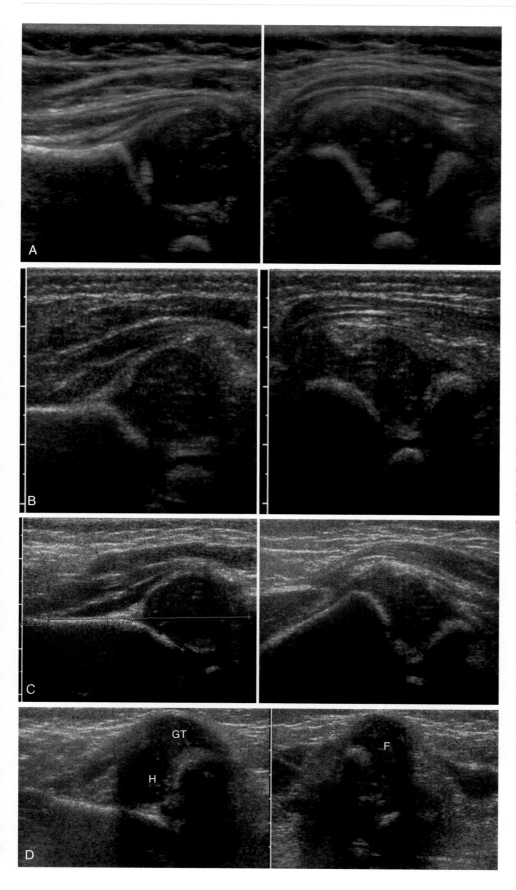

FIGURE 28-19 Graf types I through IV, using the modified Graf with alpha angle and coronal/flexion view. Images on right are coronal/flexed view, and images on the left are a static transverse/flexed view. **A,** Type I—normal. **B,** Type II—immature or delayed development, depending on infant's age. **C,** Type III—dysplasia. Hip click was heard in this patient. **D,** Type IV—frank dislocation and associated severe acetabular dysplasia. *GT,* Greater trochanter; *H,* femoral head. *(Images courtesy Nationwide Children's Hospital, Columbus, OH.)*

Static Femoral Head Coverage Measurement. This is another widely used measurement that can be used in adjunct to the Graf measurements, although not required. Simply, the height of the femoral head is measured and compared with the height of the bony acetabular coverage within the femoral head in a coronal/flexed view (Figure 28-20). Normally, the mean femoral head coverage is between 54% and 56% (in females and males, respectively), with a lower limit of 45%. Fifty percent is considered the limit between normal and potentially abnormal. Subluxation is reached when femoral head coverage reaches lower than 39% and dislocation less than 10%.

Dynamic Harcke Technique. Harcke formulated basic standards for dynamic hip sonography, which are currently used in most clinical situations today. In the flexed position, the hip may be evaluated in the coronal and/or transverse plane. If evaluated in the coronal view, the tip of the labrum must be included in the image. Often, though, the transverse plane is more widely used. It is important to label the appropriate view and stress maneuver used (abduction/adduction).

The thigh of the hip being examined is slightly adducted and abducted while simultaneously exerting a downward force, while imaging is performed with the opposite hand. This is known as the "push-pull" method or "piston maneuver." Images are obtained at rest and at maximum pressure, showing any movement of the femoral head. Cine clips are very useful, too. With added stress in adduction, the femoral head should normally remain resting against the osseous acetabulum. If the hip is unstable, the femoral head will be identified posterior (superior and lateral) to the acetabulum (Figure 28-21). The sonographer will often feel the hip displace out of the joint, and any instability felt in the hip is noted. If the hip does become subluxed or dislocated, the Ortolani maneuver is performed to assess if the hip can be reduced (this is the abduction view). The often accompanying "click" or "clunk" sounds are reported; a "click" sound is not definitive for hip displacement, but a "clunk" diagnoses it.

Hips are classified according to their behavior under stress as normal, unstable, or dislocated. The femoral head should be stable within the acetabulum with stress after 4 weeks of age. Unstable hips are divided into subluxable and dislocatable. A subluxable hip, or an immature hip due to physiologic laxity, is one in which the proximal femur moves (more than 6 mm on the left and 4 mm on the right) within the acetabulum, but it cannot be displaced out of it. A dislocatable hip is one in which the proximal femur can be displaced out of the acetabulum, but it can be reduced. A dislocated hip is one in which the femoral head is displaced out of the acetabulum and cannot be reduced.

Treatment and Sonographic Follow-up

The most important factor influencing the outcome of DDH is the age at which the diagnosis is made and treatment initiated. Treatment should begin before the patient walks, and ideally long beforehand. Delayed diagnosis often requires more complex treatment, and with worse outcomes. The principle of treatment is that a subluxed hip

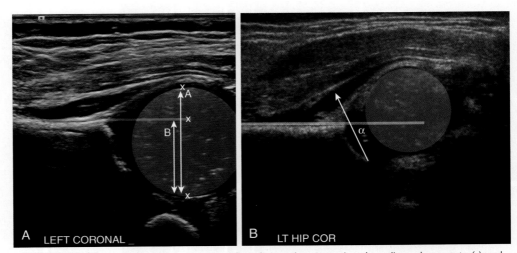

FIGURE 28-20 A, Normal hip in a coronal/flexed view demonstrating the caliper placements *(x)* and line measurements *(double arrows)* for the femoral head coverage technique. Femoral head coverage % = B/A × 100%. **B,** Abnormal hip in a 2-week-old girl with risk factors and abnormal physical examination. Image shows bony roof covering less than 50% of the femoral head. Alpha angle was between 53 and 57 degrees. Acetabular morphology was of concern with labrum slightly more horizontal than normal, while the superior bony rim was a bit more rounded on both sides. Although no hip instability was noted on stress movements, due to acetabular morphology consideration for treatment and a follow-up were strongly suggested. *(Images courtesy Nationwide Children's Hospital, Columbus, OH.)*

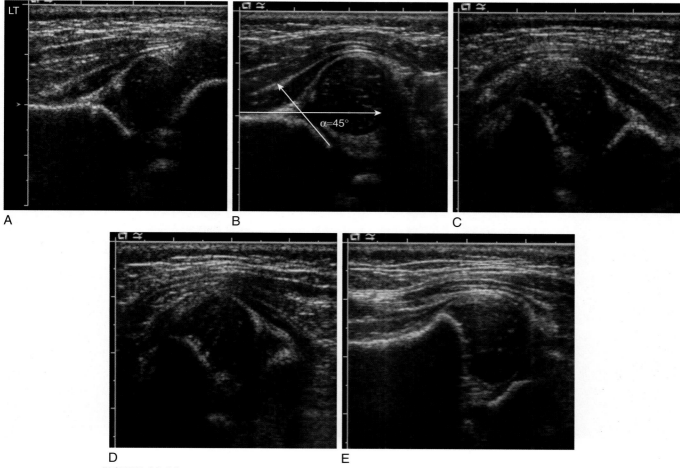

FIGURE 28-21 Dynamic technique of a modified Graf type III hip; sonographer reported a lax unstable hip. **A,** Coronal/neutral position. **B,** Coronal/flexed position with Graf angle measuring at 45 degrees. **C,** Transverse/flexion. **D,** Transverse flexion with stress. Hip appears to move away from the acetabulum, slightly laterally and superiorly. **E,** Transverse in abduction, showing abnormal bony rim morphology. *(Images courtesy Nationwide Children's Hospital, Columbus, OH.)*

in the neutral or rest position will seat itself with continuous flexion and abduction. The initial treatment of uncomplicated DDH is closed reduction. This may be accomplished either by placing two diapers on the neonate or by using a spica cast, brace, or Pavlik harness (Figure 28-22). The hip should be positioned in flexion, with abduction and external rotation.

The position of the femoral head relative to the acetabulum can be determined with follow-up sonography. If the patient has a cast, a "window" must be cut into the cast so the transducer can be placed directly on the skin. Fortunately, the Pavlik harness is more commonly used, allowing for easy access to demonstrate the hip joint's response to treatment (Figure 28-23). Within 6 to 8 weeks of treatment the hip joint often stabilizes.

Causes of failure of closed reduction include inversion of the labrum or capsule and invagination of the iliopsoas muscle, which can be imaged most efficiently by sonography and magnetic resonance imaging. If closed reduction fails or

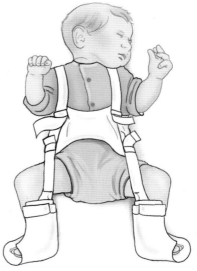

FIGURE 28-22 Pavlik harness may be used in the treatment of hip dysplasia.

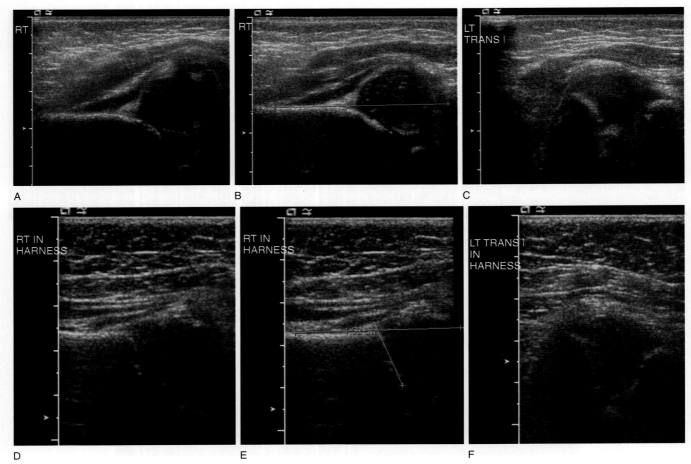

FIGURE 28-23 Pretreatment and posttreatment images of a patient wearing a Pavlik harness for follow-up assessment of DDH. Patient presented with type III hips bilaterally, and both normalized with harness treatment. In the harness, stress maneuvers are not performed. **A,** Pre–right hip coronal/flexion view at 3 weeks of age. **B,** Pre–right hip Graf alpha angle measured 45 degrees, consistent with Graf type III. **C,** Pre–transverse sonogram of left hip, also type III. **D,** Post–right hip coronal/flexion view at 3.5 months of age. **E,** Post–right hip Graf alpha angle measured over 60 degrees on follow-up, consistent with type I—normal hip. **F,** Post–left hip transverse image shows the femoral head seated normally within the acetabulum. *(Images courtesy Nationwide Children's Hospital, Columbus, OH.)*

if the dislocation is teratogenic, the patient usually requires open reduction or surgical means.

JOINT EFFUSIONS OF THE HIP

Joint effusions occur when synovial fluid builds up in the hip capsule—it may be transient or suggest septic arthritis. Transient synovitis is the most common cause of hip pain in children ages 3 to 10 years old. It is more common in males and is thought to be caused by an inflammatory response due to viral infection. Young children often present clinically to the emergency department with localized pain, refusal to bear weight, limping, limited movement of the affected hip, or fever. Before presentation, the child may have had a viral infection 1 to 2 weeks earlier.

Sonography offers a rapid and sensitive technique to detect joint effusions of the hip. If a joint effusion is present, the

synovial fluid needs to be aspirated (arthrocentesis); this is often performed under sonographic guidance. The fluid is then evaluated in the laboratory to determine whether it is transient synovitis versus septic arthritis. Fluid analysis is the definitive diagnosis, although laboratory values may show increased leukocytosis, among others. Transient synovitis can often bring relief with just the removal of the fluid, whereas septic arthritis is a true emergency and is more serious, requiring intravenous antibiotic treatment, orthopedic consultation, and admission. Delayed treatment can result in severe damage to the hip joint and may even necessitate a hip replacement.

Sonographic Technique

A high-frequency linear transducer is used to view the longitudinal anterior femoral neck, where synovial fluid may

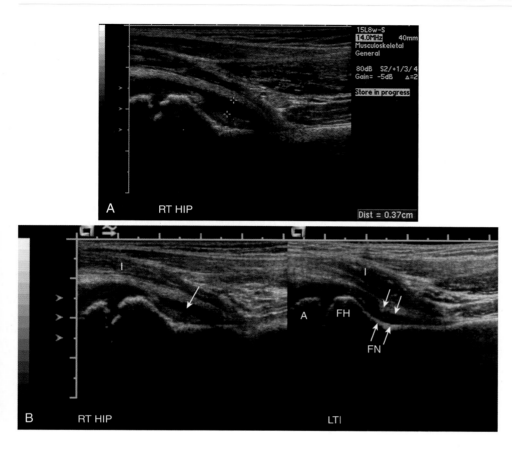

FIGURE 28-24 Sonographic hip evaluation for joint effusion in a young child who presented with hip pain and limping. **A,** Image shows anterior-posterior measurement of nearly 4 mm of fluid found within the symptomatic right hip. **B,** Sonogram shows a side-by-side comparison of the abnormal right hip capsule with an effusion *(left)* and normal left hip capsule *(right)*. *Arrow* points to the fluid and shows an approximate path for fluid aspiration. *Arrowheads* point to the collapsed normal hip capsule of the left hip. Notice the concavity of the normal hip capsule compared with the one distended with fluid. Acetabulum *(A)*, femoral head *(FH)*, and femoral neck *(FN)* are useful landmarks. The iliopsoas muscle *(I)* sits just above the joint capsule. In this case the left iliopsoas appears a bit more distressed and hypertrophied compared with the right, likely attributed to overuse of the asymptomatic limb. *(Images courtesy Nationwide Children's Hospital, Columbus, OH.)*

accumulate in the anterior recess of the joint space. Frequencies will have a wide range, from 5 to 18 MHz, depending on age and body habitus. The patient is placed in a supine position with the legs extended straight in a neutral position. Pain may limit the patient's ability to reach a full neutral position; in this case the use of a small roll under the knee may help the patient relax enough to get a good view. The femoral head and neck are located and the transducer is aligned with the hip capsule and overlying iliopsoas muscle—often at a slight oblique-sagittal plane with the notch end of the footprint more medial. Care should be taken to keep pressure to a minimum so as not to displace the fluid. Two longitudinal images of each hip are taken, along with anterior-posterior measurements of the hip capsule or fluid, as necessary, and power Doppler to detect any soft tissue swelling. Finally, a comparison of the bilateral longitudinal views is taken.

Sonographic Findings. As with any musculoskeletal pathology, it is important to compare the symptomatic side with the asymptomatic side. The normal hip capsule is 2 to 5 mm in thickness and should appear concave and symmetric. Capsular thickness greater than 5 mm or more than 2 mm side-to-side is indicative of a hip effusion. If a hip effusion is detected, fluid within the synovium will be present, and the anterior-posterior diameter is measured. The overlying muscles often appear to bulge toward the transducer as a result of the convex appearance of the

abnormal joint capsule (Figure 28-24). Debris in the synovial fluid and power Doppler detection of hyperemia likely suggest a septic hip, but if these are not present the condition cannot be ruled out, and it may be too early in the course for these findings to show up sonographically.

OTHER HIP CONDITIONS/DIFFERENTIALS

Other conditions of the infant and pediatric hip are often found incidentally on the sonographic evaluation for DDH or painful hip, and may be further evaluated in conjunction with other imaging modalities. So while scanning the hip, although sonographers are focused on a particular disease process, they should also be cognizant of the surrounding areas and differential diagnoses.

There is always potential for neoplasm in the pediatric patient. Rhabdomyosarcoma is the most common malignant soft tissue tumor in children and often occurs in the head, neck, gastrointestinal tract, and extremities. Two thirds of these tumors are found in children under 6 years old. This malignancy, among others, may be detected from associated psoas irritation, and scanning the psoas up into the pelvis is advised. Osteomyelitis and myositis remain as differential diagnoses in the child with a painful hip as well. Deep soft tissue swelling is present, and periosteal fluid or cortical erosion may be seen along the bone. Cellulitis and abscess are additional possibilities.

Finally, in evaluating for DDH, proximal focal femoral deficiency may be identified. Although a rare congenital anomaly, there is a wide range of severity from decreased ossification of the femoral head to complete absence of the hip joint. Half of patients have concomitant limb anomalies. They may have a shortened bowed femur on the affected side, which is a separate abnormality called coxa vera. Radiographs are helpful when available and should be reviewed by the sonographer. Although ultrasound cannot provide an unequivocal diagnosis, the recognition of the normal hip structures may help differentiate it from type IV dysplasia.

Key Pearls

- The infant hip can often be evaluated up to 6 months of age for developmental displacement of the hip (DDH). Thereafter, radiography is used due to bone ossification.
- Sonographic assessment for DDH is often performed after 4 to 6 weeks of age to decrease false-positive results due to physiologic laxity in the neonatal hip joint.
- Risk factors for DDH include breech position, female gender, positive family history, and improper swaddling.
- The Barlow and Ortolani tests are part of the clinical examination and correspond to adduction and abduction, respectively, in the dynamic sonographic techniques.
- Static coronal images and dynamic transverse imaging are standard for the DDH bilateral sonographic evaluation.
- Angulation and misalignment should be avoided, and care should be taken to obtain a precise midacetabular coronal image.
- The coronal view may be evaluated in a neutral or flexed position, corresponding to the Graf or modified Graf technique used.
- There are four types of hip joint classifications, which are based on criteria developed by Graf.
- Sonography is a quick and sensitive way to detect hip joint effusions, and aspiration of fluid is necessary to evaluate for septic arthritis.
- Knowledge of normal anatomy and differential diagnoses can greatly aid in providing patients with the best patient care to get appropriate prompt treatment.

BIBLIOGRAPHY

Abrahams PH, Boon J, Spratt JD: *McMinn's clinical atlas of human anatomy with DVD*, ed 6, St Louis, 2008, Mosby.

Adhikari S, Blaivas M: Utility of bedside sonography to distinguish soft tissue abnormalities from joint effusions in the emergency department, *J Ultrasound Med* 29(4):519-526, 2010.

American College of Radiology: ACR Appropriateness Criteria: developmental dysplasia of the hip—child, 2013. Available at https://acsearch.acr.org/docs/69437/Narrative/.

American College of Radiology: AACR–AIUM–SPR–SRU practice parameter for the performance of the ultrasound examination for detection and assessment of developmental dysplasia of the hip, 2014. Available at http://www.acr.org/~/media/ACR/Documents/PGTS/guidelines/US_Hip_Dysplasia.pdf.

American Institute for Ultrasound in Medicine: AIUM practice guideline for the performance of an ultrasound examination for detection and assessment of developmental dysplasia of the hip. Available at http://www.aium.org/resources/guidelines/hip.pdf.

Arti H, Mehdinasab SA, Arti S: Comparing results of clinical versus ultrasonographic examination in developmental dysplasia of hip, *J Res Med Sci* 18(12):1051-1055, 2013.

Ashby E, Roposch A: Diagnostic yield of sonography in infants with suspected hip dysplasia: diagnostic thinking efficiency and therapeutic efficiency, *AJR Am J Roentgenol* 204(1):177-181, 2015.

Committee on Quality Improvement, Subcommittee on Developmental Dysplasia of the Hip: Clinical practice guideline: early detection of developmental dysplasia of the hip, *Pediatrics* 105(4 Pt 1):896-905, 2000.

Cook MA: Developmental displacement of the neonatal hip. In Haller JO, editor: *Textbook of neonatal ultrasound*, New York, 1998, Parthenon Publishing Group.

Coskun G, et al: Proximal femoral focal deficiency, *Eur J Radiol* 76(3):e99-e101, 2010.

Di Pietro MA: Sonography of the pediatric spine and hip [lecture], 2015. Available at www.sonoworld.com.

Dogruel H, Atalar H, Yavuz OY, Sayli U: Clinical examination versus ultrasonography in detecting developmental dysplasia of the hip, *Int Orthop* 32(3):415-419, 2008.

Falliner A, Schwinzer D, Hahne HJ, et al: Comparing ultrasound measurements of neonatal hips using the methods of Graf and Terjesen, *J Bone Joint Surg Br* 88(1):104-106, 2006.

Filly AL, Robnett-filly B, Filly RA: Syndromes with focal femoral deficiency: strengths and weaknesses of prenatal sonography, *J Ultrasound Med* 23(11):1511-1516, 2004.

Gardiner HM, Dunn PM: Controlled trial of immediate splinting versus ultrasonographic surveillance in congenitally dislocatable hips, *Lancet* 336(8730):1553-1556, 1990.

Gerscovich EO: Infant hip in developmental dysplasia: facts to consider for a successful diagnostic ultrasound examination, *Appl Radiol* 28(3):18-25, 1999.

Graf R: Fundamentals of sonographic diagnosis of infant hip dysplasia, *J Pediatr Orthop* 4:735-740, 1984.

Graf R, Mohajer M, Plattner F: Hip sonography update. Quality-management, catastrophes—tips and tricks, *Med Ultrason* 15(4):299-303, 2013.

Grissom LE, Harcke HT: The pediatric hip. In Rumack C, Wilson S, Charboneau JW, editors: *Diagnostic ultrasound*, ed 3, St Louis, 2005, Mosby.

Gunay C, Atalar H, Dogruel H, et al: Correlation of femoral head coverage and Graf alpha angle in infants being screened for developmental dysplasia of the hip, *Int Orthop* 33(3):761-764, 2009.

Harcke HT: Screening newborns for developmental displacement of the hip: the role of sonography, *Am J Roentgenol* 152:395-397, 1994.

Harcke HT, Grissom LE: Performing dynamic sonography of the infant hip, *Am J Roentgenol* 155:837-844, 1990.

Harcke HT, Grissom LE: Infant hip sonography: current concepts, *Semin Ultrasound CT MRI* 15(4):256-263, 1994.

Henningsen C: *Clinical guide to ultrasonography*, St Louis, 2004, Mosby.

Henningsen C: The infant hip joint. In *Diagnostic medical sonography: abdomen and superficial structures*, ed 3, Philadelphia, PA, 2012, Lippincott Williams & Wilkins, pp 749-748.

Holroyd B, Wedge J: Developmental dysplasia of the hip, *Orthop Trauma* 23(3):162-168, 2009.

Jacobson JA: *Fundamentals of musculoskeletal ultrasound*, ed 2, Philadelphia, PA, 2013, Elsevier Saunders.

Jain N, Sah M, Chakraverty J, et al: Radiological approach to a child with hip pain, *Clin Radiol* 68(11):1167-1178, 2013.

Karnik A: Hip ultrasonography in infants and children, *Indian J Radiol Imaging* 17(4):280, 2007.

Kayser R, Mahlfeld K, Grasshoff H, Merk HR: Proximal focal femoral deficiency—a rare entity in the sonographic differential diagnosis of developmental dysplasia of the hip, *Ultraschall Med* 26(5):379-384, 2005.

Kolb A, Schweiger N, Mailath-Pokorny M, et al: Low incidence of early developmental dysplasia of the hip in universal ultrasonographic screening of newborns: analysis and evaluation of risk factors, *Int Orthop* 40(1):123-127, 2016.

Loder RT, Skopelja EN: The epidemiology and demographics of hip dysplasia, *ISRN Orthop* 2011:238607, 2011.

Mahan ST, Katz JN, Kim YJ: To screen or not to screen? A decision analysis of the utility of screening for developmental dysplasia of the hip, *J Bone Joint Surg Am* 91(7):1705-1719, 2009.

Marks DS, Clegg J, al-Chalabi AN: Routine ultrasound screening for neonatal hip instability. Can it abolish late-presenting congenital dislocation of the hip? *J Bone Joint Surg Br* 76(4):534-538, 1994.

Moraleda L, Albiñana J, Salcedo M, Gonzalez-Moran G: [Dysplasia in the development of the hip], *Rev Esp Cir Ortop Traumatol* 57(1):67-77, 2013.

Neriman D, Basit R, Howlett DC: Imaging of the symptomatic pediatric hip, *Foundation Years* 5(2):84-87, 2009.

Orak MM, Onay T, Gümüştaş SA, et al: Is prematurity a risk factor for developmental dysplasia of the hip? A prospective study, *Bone Joint J* 97-B(5):716-720, 2015.

Ortiz-Neira CL, Paolucci EO, Donnon T: A meta-analysis of common risk factors associated with the diagnosis of developmental dysplasia of the hip in newborns, *Eur J Radiol* 81(3):e344-e351, 2012.

Pillai A, Joseph J, Mcauley A, Bramley D: Diagnostic accuracy of static Graf technique of ultrasound evaluation of infant hips for developmental dysplasia, *Arch Orthop Trauma Surg* 131(1):53-58, 2011.

Rosendahl K, Aslaksen A, Lie RT, Markestad T: Reliability of ultrasound in the early diagnosis of developmental dysplasia of the hip, *Pediatr Radiol* 25(3):219-224, 1995.

Rosendahl K, Toma P: Ultrasound in the diagnosis of developmental dysplasia of the hip in newborns. The European approach. A review of methods, accuracy and clinical validity, *Eur Radiol* 17(8):1960-1967, 2007.

Shipman SA, Helfand M, Moyer VA, Yawn BP: Screening for developmental dysplasia of the hip: a systematic literature review for the US Preventive Services Task Force, *Pediatrics* 117(3):e557-e576, 2006.

Siegel MJ: Developmental dysplasia of the infant hip. In Sanders RC, Winter T, editors: *Clinical sonography: a practical guide,* ed 4, Baltimore, MD, 2007, Lippincott Williams & Wilkins, pp 375-387.

Sewell MD, Rosendahl K, Eastwood DM: Developmental dysplasia of the hip, *BMJ* 339:b44-b54, 2009.

Terjesen T, Holen KJ, Tegnander A: Hip abnormalities detected by ultrasound in clinically normal newborn infants, *J Bone Joint Surg Br* 78(4):636-640, 1996.

Vasilescu D, Cosma D, Vasilescu DE, et al: A new sign in the standard hip ultrasound image of the Graf method, *Med Ultrason* 17(2):206-210, 2015.

Weintroub S, Grill F: Ultrasonography in developmental dysplasia of the hip, *J Bone Joint Surg* 82A:1004-1018, 2000.

Neonatal and Infant Spine

Kathryn E. Zale

The spinal canal and its contents can be demonstrated sonographically with great clarity in the neonatal and early infant period. Thus high-resolution sonography of the spine has emerged as the optimal screening modality for the detection of occult dysraphic conditions, such as a **tethered spinal cord,** with diagnostic sensitivity equal to magnetic resonance imaging (MRI) for certain anomalies. Spinal **dysraphism** includes a wide range of developmental anomalies of the spinal canal and are broadly divided into open and closed types. Neural tube defects are a type of spinal dysraphism involving the absent or incomplete closure of the neural tube. The severity of the defect ranges from mild **spina bifida occulta** to severe **spina bifida aperta.** Open spinal dysraphisms have a skin defect with the neural tissue exposed to the environment, and because spine sonography is contraindicated when the skin is thin or no longer intact, occult or closed conditions are more commonly examined.

Certain lumbosacral stigmata (Box 29-1), or cutaneous back masses and midline deformities, are known to be associated with spinal dysraphism. Clinically, the infant may present with a dimple on the posterior surface of the body along the spinal canal. Although it is not uncommon for the buttocks to contain a shallow dimple near the anus, at times the dimple appears unusually deep or asymmetric. The dimple may also be suspicious if it is more than 2.5 cm above the anus, larger than 5 mm, and most suspicious when associated with other spinal lesions. These findings may suggest the possibility of an underlying maldevelopment of the spinal cord or the adjacent elements, and sonography is used to determine the relationship of these stigmatas to deformities in the spinal canal. If these abnormalities are not recognized early, the patient may have difficulty walking or experience other neurologic problems in infancy or childhood.

Advantages of sonography include the ability to perform the procedure easily, dynamically, and at the bedside without ionizing radiation. The availability of high-frequency transducers now leaves operator inexperience as the main reason for unsuccessful neonatal spinal sonography. The sonographer may observe the spinal cord as it pulsates normally within the spinal canal. The vascular supply to the spinal canal may be evaluated with color Doppler ultrasound. The development of fluid collections, cysts, or fatty tumors (lipomas) may be seen. Malformations of the spinal cord may be imaged and will be presented in this chapter, along with other indications for spine sonography, including the detection of sequelae of spinal cord injury, often from a spinal tap.

EMBRYOGENESIS

The defects of the spinal canal occur in the first 8.5 weeks of life as the fetal nervous system develops. The neural tube and the subsequent spinal cord arise from ectodermal cells. The surface ectoderm separates from the neural tube, with the mesoderm coming to lie between the neural tube and the ectoderm. The mesoderm forms the bony spine, meninges, and muscle. Incomplete separation of the neural tube from the ectoderm may result in cord tethering, **diastematomyelia,** or a dermal sinus. Premature separation of the cutaneous ectoderm from the neural tube can result in abnormal mesenchymal elements, such as lipomas forming between the neural tube and skin. If the neural tube fails to fold and fuse in the midline, defects such as **myelomeningocele** occur. Disorders of the distal cord may lead to fibrolipomas of the **filum terminale.**

NORMAL ANATOMY AND SONOGRAPHIC FINDINGS

The vertebral column extends from the base of the skull to the tip of the coccyx along the posterior surface of the body. The vertebral column is the central bony stabilizer of the body. Within the vertebral cavity lie the spinal cord, the roots of the spinal nerves, and the covering meninges, which provide protection for the vertebral column.

The vertebral column consists of 33 vertebrae: 7 cervical, 12 thoracic, 5 lumbar, 5 sacral (fused to form the sacrum), and 4 coccygeal fused bones (Figure 29-1). The pads of

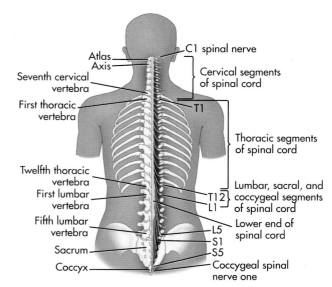

FIGURE 29-1 Spinal cord. Posterior view of the spinal cord showing the origins of the roots of the spinal nerves. On the right, the laminae have been removed to expose the right half of the spinal cord and the nerve roots.

fibrocartilage, called intervertebral disks, are found between each vertebra and allow flexibility in the spine.

Vertebrae

Each vertebra consists of a rounded body anteriorly and a vertebral arch posteriorly (Figure 29-2). These enclose a space called the **vertebral foramen,** through which run the spinal cord and its coverings. The **vertebral arch** consists of a pair of cylindrical pedicles, which form the sides of the arch, and a pair of flattened laminae, which complete the arch posteriorly. The vertebral arch gives rise to seven processes: one spinous, two transverse, and four articular. The two superior articular processes of one vertebral arch articulate with the two inferior articular processes of the arch above, forming two synovial joints.

The pedicles are notched on their upper and lower borders, forming the superior and inferior vertebral notches. On each side, the superior notch of one vertebra and the inferior notch of an adjacent vertebra together form the intervertebral foramen. These foramina transmit the spinal nerves and blood vessels.

In the neonate, problems typically occur in the lower back near the area of the lumbar vertebrae and the sacrum. Characteristics of the lumbar vertebrae include a large and oval body, strong pedicles directed posterior, and thick laminae with a triangular vertebral foramina. Additionally, the transverse processes are short, flat, and project backward.

Although sonography is performed from the back, the anterior vertebral bodies appear echogenic and lie posterior to the hypoechoic spinal canal. The cartilaginous posterior spinous processes appear hypoechoic, allowing for visualization of the canal when scanning directly over them. Laminae

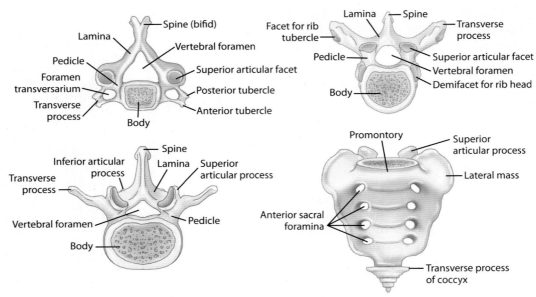

FIGURE 29-2 Basic features of the vertebrae.

are seen when scanning slightly off midline and appear similar to overlapping roof tiles (Figure 29-3).

Sacrum

The sacrum consists of five bones fused together. The upper border articulates with the fifth lumbar vertebra. The narrow inferior border articulates with the coccyx. The coccyx is mostly or completely unossified and is therefore hypoechoic (Figure 29-4). Laterally the sacrum articulates with the two iliac bones to form the sacroiliac joints. The anterior and upper margin of the first sacral vertebra bulges forward as the posterior margin of the pelvic inlet and is known as the sacral promontory.

The vertebral foramina are present and form the sacral canal. The laminae of the fifth sacral vertebra, and sometimes those of the fourth also, fail to meet in the midline and form the sacral hiatus (Figure 29-5). The sacral canal contains the anterior and posterior roots of the sacral and coccygeal spinal nerves, the filum terminale, and fibrofatty material. It also contains the lower part of the subarachnoid space, or dural or thecal sac, down as far as the lower border of the second sacral vertebra (Figure 29-6).

Intervertebral Disks

The intervertebral disks are responsible for one fourth of the length of the vertebral column. They are thickest in the cervical and lumbar regions where the movements of the vertebral column are greatest. Each disk consists of a peripheral part, the annulus fibrosus, and a central part, the nucleus pulposus (Figure 29-7). The annulus fibrosus consists of fibrocartilage. The nucleus pulposus is an ovoid

mass of gelatinous material containing a large amount of water, a small number of collagen fibers, and a few cartilage cells.

Ligaments and Nerves

The anterior and posterior longitudinal ligaments run as continuous bands down the anterior and posterior surfaces of the vertebral column from the skull to the sacrum. Transverse dentate ligaments of the cord are sometimes visible; seen in a transverse view they appear as thin echogenic lines extending laterally from the spinal cord. The small meningeal branches of each spinal nerve innervate the joints between the vertebral bodies.

Spinal Cord

The spinal cord is a cylindrical, grayish white structure that begins above at the foramen magnum, where it is continuous with the medulla oblongata of the brain. In the adult, it terminates below the level of the lower border of the first lumbar vertebra. In the younger child and term neonates, it is relatively longer and should not extend beyond the second lumbar vertebra (Figure 29-8). The conus may end between L2 and L4 in the preterm infant. The cord also has a deep longitudinal fissure in the midline anteriorly, which may be seen on a transverse image.

The spinal cord is hypoechoic with slightly echogenic borders and an echogenic line extending longitudinally along its midline. It is surrounded by cerebrospinal fluid. This central echo complex represents or is close to the cord's central canal (Figure 29-9, A). One should be aware

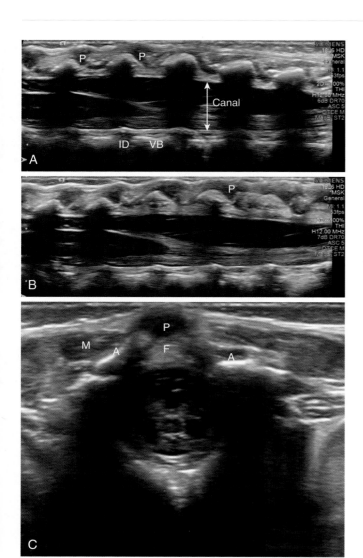

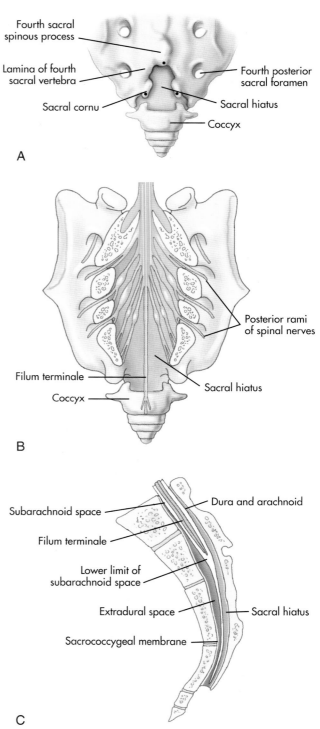

FIGURE 29-3 Longitudinal sonogram of normal thoracic/lumbar spine. A, Approach is slightly off midline. Anterior vertebral bodies *(VB),* intervertebral disks *(ID),* and posterior spinal processes *(P).* **B,** Approach is directly over the hypoechoic posterior spinal processes *(P),* decreasing the amount of shadowing within the central canal. **C,** Transverse view of the lumbar spine. Vertebral arch *(A),* muscle *(M),* and fat *(F)* in the epidural space just anterior to the spinal canal. *(Images courtesy Nationwide Children's Hospital, Columbus, OH.)*

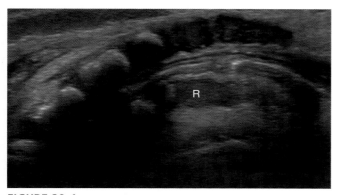

FIGURE 29-4 Longitudinal view over the hypoechoic coccyx. Rectum *(R)* is seen posteriorly. *(Image courtesy Nationwide Children's Hospital, Columbus, OH.)*

FIGURE 29-5 A, The sacral hiatus. The black dots indicate the position of the important bony landmarks. **B,** The dural sheath (thecal sac) around the lower end of the spinal cord and spinal nerves in the sacral canal; the laminae have been removed. **C,** Longitudinal section through the sacrum.

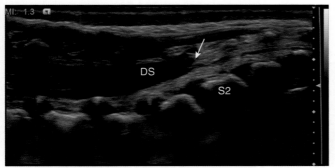

FIGURE 29-6 Sonographic view of the sacrum. The dural sac (*DS*) containing cerebrospinal fluid ends (*arrow*) at the level of the second sacral bone (*S2*). *(Image courtesy Nationwide Children's Hospital, Columbus, OH.)*

that slight prominence or widening of the central canal at the caudal end of the cord (not extending cranially into the thoracic spine) is a common finding in neonates. This normal variant is often referred to as ventriculus terminalis, and typically disappears within the first few months of life (Figure 29-9, *B*).

The size and shape of the spinal cord vary along its length. Its diameter is narrowest in the midthoracic and thoracolumbar junctions. Inferiorly the cord tapers off into the **conus medullaris,** from the apex of which a prolongation of the pia mater, the filum terminale, descends to be attached to the back of the coccyx. The filum terminale appears echogenic and should measure 2 mm or less in thickness. A normal variant to be aware of is the filar cyst. These small cysts in the filum terminale might be remnants of a terminal ventricle or

an arachnoid pseudocyst and have no clinical significance (Figure 29-10).

Roots of the Spinal Nerves

Along the length of the spinal cord are attached 31 pairs of spinal nerves. The spinal nerve roots unite to form a spinal nerve. The lower nerve roots together are called the **cauda equina** (Latin for "horse's tail"). These nerve roots that surround the spinal cord are echogenic. They are especially noticeable at and below the conus forming the cauda equina. Dorsal and ventral nerve roots can have a spider-like configuration at the tip of the conus in the transverse view (Figure 29-11).

Meninges of the Spinal Cord

The spinal cord is surrounded by three meninges: the dura mater, the arachnoid mater, and the pia mater (Figure 29-12).

The dura mater is the most external membrane and is a dense, strong, fibrous sheet that encloses the spinal cord and cauda equina, collectively called the dural/thecal sac or dural sheath. It is continuous through the foramen magnum with the meningeal layer of dura covering the brain. Inferiorly, it ends on the filum terminale at the level of the lower border of the second sacral vertebra.

The arachnoid mater is a delicate impermeable membrane covering the spinal cord, and it lies between the pia mater internally and the dura mater externally. It is separated from the dura by the subdural space, which contains a thin film of tissue fluid. The arachnoid is separated from the pia mater by a wide space, the subarachnoid space, which is filled with cerebrospinal fluid.

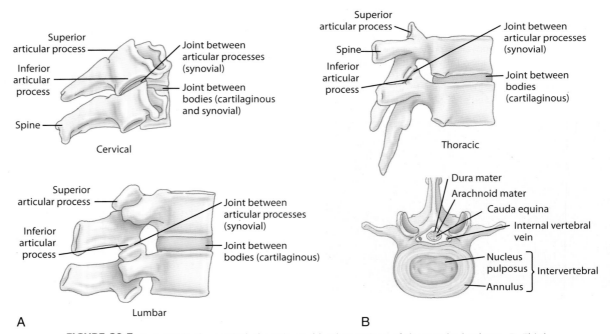

FIGURE 29-7 A, Joints in the cervical, thoracic, and lumbar regions of the vertebral column. **B,** Third lumbar vertebra seen from above showing the relationship between intervertebral disk and cauda equina.

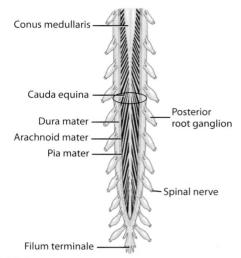

FIGURE 29-8 Lower end of the spinal cord and the cauda equina.

Conus medullaris
Cauda equina
Dura mater
Arachnoid mater
Pia mater
Posterior root ganglion
Spinal nerve
Filum terminale

The pia mater is a vascular membrane that closely covers the spinal cord. It is continuous above the neck through the foramen magnum with the pia covering the brain; below it fuses with the filum terminale (Figure 29-13).

SONOGRAPHIC EVALUATION OF THE NEONATAL AND INFANT SPINE

The incomplete ossification of the posterior spinal elements allows sonography to provide a broad panoramic view of the neonatal spinal canal and its contents (Figure 29-14). Sonography becomes increasingly difficult as the posterior spinous processes ossify and quality decreases at 3 to 4 months of age, and in most infants it is not possible after 6 months of age. The neonatal period is ideal. A posterior approach is used with the patient in a prone or lateral decubitus position. However, movement makes this examination extremely tricky, so it may also be performed with the baby

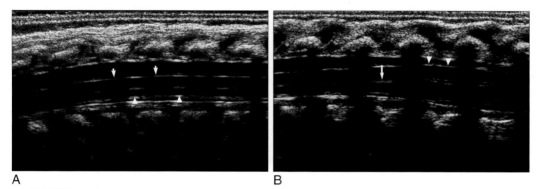

A   B

FIGURE 29-9 **Normal spinal cord. A,** Sagittal view shows the posterior *(arrows)* and the anterior aspects of the thoracic spinal cord *(arrowheads)*. Normal thoracic spinal cord is more anteriorly positioned within the vertebral canal than the more distal spinal cord. **B,** Normal variant of widening of the lumbar spinal cord *(arrowheads)*, caused by the widening of the central canal *(open arrows)*. The central spinal canal is visible as a mid echogenic line *(arrow)*.

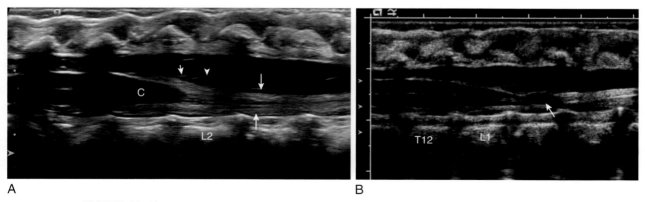

A   B

FIGURE 29-10 **A,** Tip of the conus medullaris *(c)* should taper gradually, not extending past the L2 segment. Individual nerve rootlets are visible *(arrowheads)*, along with the cauda equina *(long arrows)*. **B,** Normal filar cyst variant *(arrow)* appears as a small anechoic fluid collection seen in the nerve roots just below the tip of the conus medullaris, which ends at the mid L2 segment. Line represents the measurement of the filum terminale. *(Images courtesy Nationwide Children's Hospital, Columbus, OH.)*

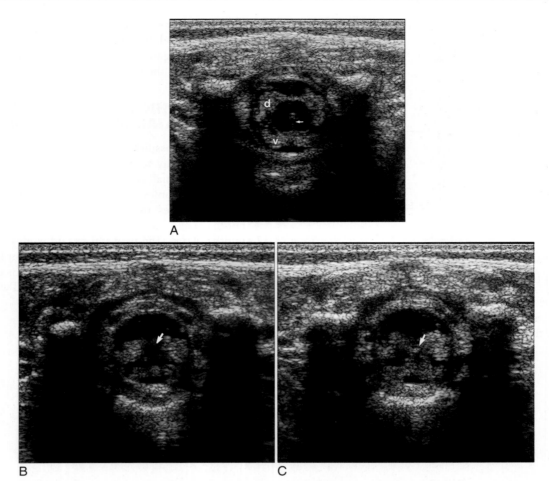

A

B   C

FIGURE 29-11 **A,** On transverse view of the lumbar spinal cord, dorsal *(d)* and ventral *(v)* nerve rootlets, as well as the anterior median fissure, are visible *(arrow)*. **B,** Transverse view near the tip of the conus medullaris demonstrates the relatively hypoechoic substance of the cord *(arrow)* in the center of the more echogenic nerve rootlets. **C,** The beginning of the filum terminale is seen as a central, slightly echogenic focus *(arrow)* in the transverse plane.

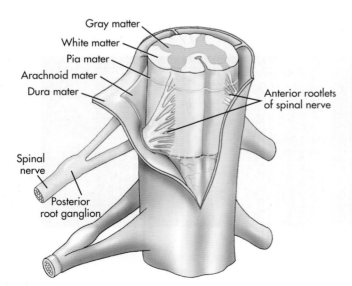

FIGURE 29-12 Section through the thoracic part of the spinal cord showing the anterior and posterior roots of the spinal nerves and meninges.

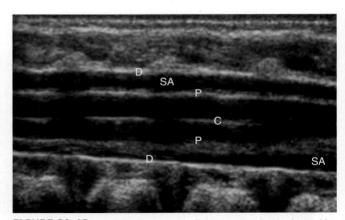

FIGURE 29-13 Normal ultrasound of the neonatal spinal canal by spinal meningeal layers. Thick, fibrous dura mater *(D)* or dural sac enclosing the spinal canal; subarachnoid space *(SA)* filled with cerebrospinal fluid separating the arachnoid mater (dural side) and pia mater (spinal cord side); pia mater *(P)* surrounding the posterior and anterior margins of the spinal cord; central echo complex of the spinal cord *(C)*. *(Image courtesy Nationwide Children's Hospital, Columbus, OH.)*

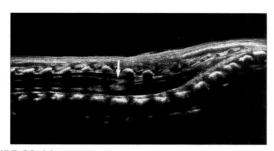

FIGURE 29-14 Lumbosacral spine. Extended field of view image reveals detailed anatomy of the course and contour of the neonatal lumbosacral spine. The tip of the conus medullaris *(arrow)* is clearly visible.

in an upright (against the mother's abdomen) or sitting position when necessary. It is crucial that the spine be flexed or rounded enough to separate the posterior spinal elements. When prone, this is accomplished by having the baby lie over a small pillow or a rolled towel. Slight elevation of the upper part of the body will better distend the caudal aspect of the thecal sac. Care must be taken that flexion is not so extreme as to compromise the infant's breathing. This consideration is amplified if the baby has been sedated. The infant usually falls asleep during the procedure once the warm coupling gel is applied and the transducer is gently rubbed along the spine.

The sonographer should use the highest frequency transducer available to obtain the greatest soft tissue detail. Small neonates will require higher frequencies (15 MHz), whereas chunky babies will require lower frequencies (8 MHz). The linear array transducer works the best to completely scan along the spinal canal. The curved array is used in special situations where the body surface is curved, such as the craniocervical junction or at the margin of a **meningocele**. Sector transducers may be used in older infants with a limited acoustic window.

Scanning is performed in the midline sagittal (longitudinal) and axial (transverse) planes. The longitudinal images are obtained directly over the spine, unless the infant is older and ossification obscures this view, in which case a parasagittal approach is best. Transverse images are taken mainly between the spinous processes. Orientation of the probe is the same as in conventional abdominal imaging.

The spinal canal is usually easily identified, and the depth of the image is adjusted so the vertebral bodies are at the bottom of the image. It is helpful to scan the sacral region first, where the canal is easily identified by the stepwise ascent of the sacral vertebral elements, and then follow the spinal canal in a cranial direction. A standoff pad may be used to examine the soft tissue dorsal to the spine when looking for a sinus tract.

The entire spinal canal is examined. However, because most examinations are performed to exclude an occult tethered spinal cord, determining the vertebral level of the tip of the conus medullaris is most important, and accordingly, the lumbar spinal canal receives the most attention. The

following section describes four particular features important to note.

Important Features Used in the Sonogram Evaluation

Level of the Conus Medullaris. The single most important determination is usually the level of the tip of the tapered conus medullaris. The normal level is in the upper lumbar canal, above the superior endplate of L3, with most cords ending at the mid L2 level.

The lumbar vertebral level may be determined several different ways. This is often achieved by counting cranial from the caudal end of the thecal sac (usually S2), from just beyond the coccyx (starting with S5, the last echogenic structure in the sacrum), or from the lumbosacral junction (L1/S5). Panoramic imaging is especially helpful for these methods (Figure 29-15). A transverse projection across the midline from the lowest palpable rib end is often L2. A similar projection from the palpated apex of the iliac crest is often L5.

One can also sonographically identify the lowest rib over each kidney from the back and follow it medially to its vertebral body (Figure 29-16). That level can be assigned

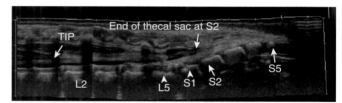

FIGURE 29-15 Counting vertebrae using the panoramic function. Counting may begin with S5, the last ossified bone before the coccyx; the end of the thecal sac at S2; or the lumbosacral junction (L1/S5). This conus medullaris appears to end between L1 and L2. *(Image courtesy Nationwide Children's Hospital, Columbus, OH.)*

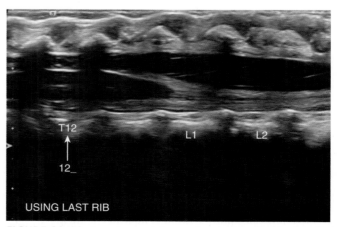

FIGURE 29-16 Counting vertebrae using the last rib. The last rib-bearing vertebral segment is the T12 vertebra, which corresponds to and is followed from the lowest rib over each kidney in the back. This conus medullaris, therefore, ends at the start of the L2. *(Image courtesy Nationwide Children's Hospital, Columbus, OH.)*

as T12, although it could be off by a level if the patient has 11 or 13 pairs of ribs. If the conus tip is midlumbar, its exact level might need to be determined by a correlative radiograph. The conus tip is carefully noted in both longitudinal and transverse sonographic projections, and this position is marked on the skin by a radiopaque marker, such as a nipple "B-B" marker. Most tethered cords, however, are unquestionably low and correlative radiographs are not usually necessary.

Anterior Position of the Spinal Cord. The spinal cord should lay one third to one half way toward the anterior (ventral) vertebrae in the spinal canal. This indicates that the cord's position is gravity dependent and free flowing.

Normal Pulsatile Movement. The spinal cord and roots of the cauda equina are normally observed to move, and may be documented with M-mode or a cine clip. This is observed best when the image persistence or frame averaging is minimized. Dorsoventral oscillations occur at the frequency of the heartbeat, and there is also a superimposed motion, which occurs with respirations. These movements are variably present in neonates but are almost always seen after 1 or 2 months of age.

Clusters of normal nerve roots might be mistaken for an echogenic intracanalicular mass. Nerves, however, will be observed to move and change configuration as one scans along the canal in real-time. In transverse views, nerve roots might appear as an echogenic clump in the middle of the spinal canal or as bilateral clusters, sometimes in an upside-down "V" configuration. Another potential false-positive finding is the bilateral dorsal and ventral roots at the tip of the conus that can superficially mimic a split cord (diastematomyelia). Although they appear similar on the sonographic image, they are readily distinguished during real-time scanning in both projections, above and below the area of concern.

Thickness of the Filum Terminale. Although the filum is normally larger than the cauda equina nerves, it should measure less than 2 mm. Use real-time imaging to be sure and capture just this structure and not a clump of nerve roots.

PATHOLOGY OF THE NEONATAL AND INFANT SPINE

Spinal sonography is performed primarily to evaluate the spinal canal for dysraphic conditions, which are often associated with midline cutaneous abnormalities over the lower back. Midline dimples over the lower back occur in approximately 2% to 4.3% of newborns. Most are low sacral or coccygeal pits without an associated tethered cord. Closed dysraphisms presented in this chapter include tethered spinal cord, along with lipomas, hydromyelia, diastematomyelia, and dermal sinus. Open dysraphisms, myelomeningoceles, and myeloceles are also touched on, along with sequelae of spinal cord injuries, among other indications/conditions. For a more extensive discussion of spinal anomalies, see Chapter 60.

Closed Spinal Dysraphism

Tethered Spinal Cord. The most common request for the sonographic spine study is to search for an occult tethered cord. This may be a primary closed dysraphic condition, known as tight filum terminale syndrome, or it may be associated with other dysraphic conditions. It is suspected in patients with certain associated lumbosacral stigmatas; midline hair patches, fatty lumps, skin tags, pigmented nevi, lumbar dimples, aplasia cutis, and hemangiomas over the back should prompt a search for an occult tethered spinal cord. Hemangiomas seem to have a high association with tethered spinal cord.

The tethered spinal cord is a pathologic fixation of the spinal cord in an abnormal caudal location, so that the cord suffers mechanical stretching, distortion, and ischemia with daily activities, growth, and development. As the child grows, the spinal cord is not able to grow, resulting in terrible consequences if not treated. Children may have pain or lose function of their legs, bowel, or bladder. Onset of symptoms is often seen around 3 years of age.

◤ *Sonographic Findings.* The tethered cord diagnosis corresponds to the four particular features pointed out in the sonographic examination. Positive signs are (1) a low-lying conus medullaris beyond the L2 level, (2) a caudal or posterior position of the spinal cord, (3) absent or dampened pulsations of the spinal cord and nerve roots, and (4) thickened filum terminale (greater than 2 mm) (Figure 29-17).

It is important to note that the normal brisk oscillation of the cord is not as apparent in normal neonates as it is in older infants; therefore looking for dampened or absent oscillations in neonates with tethered cords has limited usefulness (false positives). Most nonoscillating cords in neonates are normal and are not due to tethering. These oscillations usually diminish as the child grows, presumably because the cord is anchored and is being stretched.

Lipoma. A **lipoma** is a benign tumor composed of fat cells. Spinal lipomas are fatty masses that have a connection with the spinal cord. These lipomas may be further divided into four categories of intradural lipomas, lipomyelocele, lipomyelomeningocele, and fibrolipomas of the filum terminale (Figure 29-18). Intradural lipomas are situated in a subpial position in a dorsal cleft of the open spinal cord. The lipomyelocele is analogous to the myelocele, but there is a covering of attached lipoma and intact skin. In patients with lipomyelomeningocele, there is expansion of the subarachnoid space ventral to the placode. Fibrolipomas of the filum terminale are a unique form of lipoma that may represent a variant of normal development.

◤ *Sonographic Findings.* On sonography, fibrolipomas are seen as a thickened, echogenic filum terminale, sometimes with an undulating contour. Lipomas can be isolated to the filum terminale or extend to and infiltrate the spinal cord and conus medullaris to varying degrees. When associated with a tethered cord, it is usually accompanied with a mass of the lower cord or filum terminale

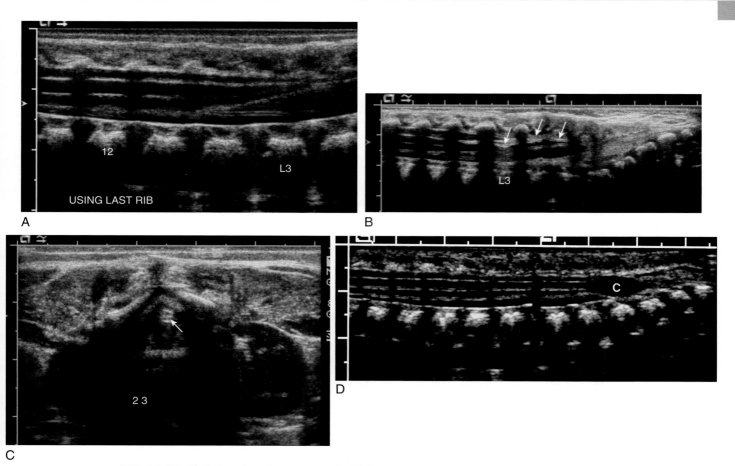

FIGURE 29-17 Tethered cord. A, Two-week-old showing the conus extending below the level of L3. Poor motion of the cauda equina was noted. Cord is located against the posterior portion of the spinal canal. **B,** Another neonate with the conus medullaris extending beyond the L2, with increased filum echogenicity and thickness *(arrows)*. **C,** Transverse view of prominent filum *(arrow)* between the L2 and L3 segments. **D,** Newborn with low-lying tethered cord and filar cyst *(C)*. *(Images A, B, and C courtesy Nationwide Children's Hospital, Columbus, OH.)*

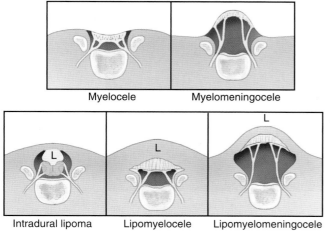

FIGURE 29-18 Diagram of open neural tube defects *(top)* and occult dysraphisms with lipomas *(bottom)*. Each diagram is positioned with the dorsal side up, the position one would use when scanning the spine of an infant (*L,* lipoma).

(Figure 29-19). This anomaly comprises 20% to 50% of the spinal dysplasias. This mass often has lipomatous elements and can be continuous with the subcutaneous tissues and present as a fatty lump on the lower back, constituting a lipomyelocele or lipomyelomeningocele (Figure 29-20). Lipomas are usually echogenic and may present as a small or large mass.

Hydromyelia. **Hydromyelia** is another sonographically observable abnormality of the spinal cord that can be seen in variable degrees. Remember that slight prominence of the central canal at the caudal end of the cord is a common finding in neonates. Focal hydromyelia is often present just cephalad to the site of tethering in dysraphic conditions such as myelomeningocele or lipomyelomeningocele. Hydromyelia might also accompany diastematomyelia (Figure 29-21).

Diastematomyelia. Hydromyelia is a condition in which there is sagittal division of the cord into two hemicords, each containing a central canal, a single dorsal horn, and a single ventral horn. The cord is split at one or more sites by an osseous, cartilaginous, or fibrous septum. The two segments of the cord can be seen most clearly on transverse views (Figure 29-22). They might rejoin caudal to the cleft. The vertebral column is virtually always abnormal on plain radiography in patients with diastematomyelia.

Dermal Sinus (vs. Pilonidal Sinus). The dorsal dermal sinus is a thin tract, lined with epithelium, passing from the skin to the spinal canal. Although they may occur anywhere along the spine, they are most common in the lumbosacral region. Patients are at risk for meningitis due to this open tract directly to the spinal canal. They often present clinically as deep midline pits. A sinus tract will disrupt the echogenic line with possible extension to the dura.

It is important to try to differentiate a true dermal sinus from a pilonidal sinus. A pilonidal sinus is not connected to the spinal canal, nor are they associated with a tethered cord. However, dural penetration may be difficult to ascertain or exclude on sonography, which is why care should be taken

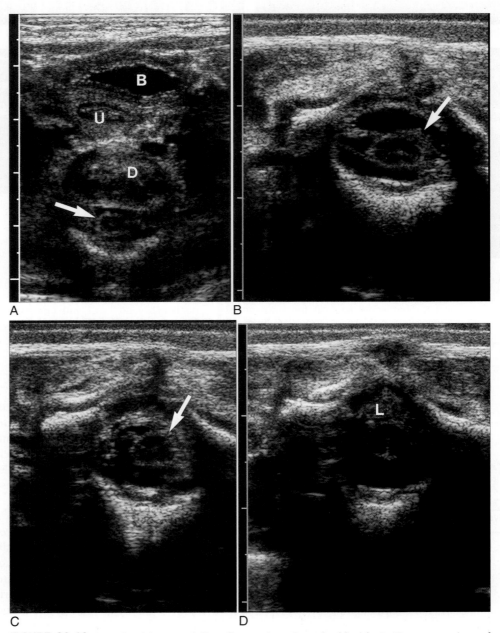

FIGURE 29-19 Intradural juxtamedullary lipoma in a 2-week-old girl. A, Transverse view of the pelvis shows the partially full urinary bladder *(B),* the newborn uterus *(U),* and an intervertebral disk space of the sacrum *(D).* The spinal cord is too low and is visible from an anterior approach *(arrow).* Traditional views of the spine scanning the neonatal back (**B, C,** and **D**) are progressively inferior transverse views revealing the rightward skew of the abnormally low spinal cord *(arrow)* that is also pulled into an abnormally dorsal position by the lipoma *(L).*

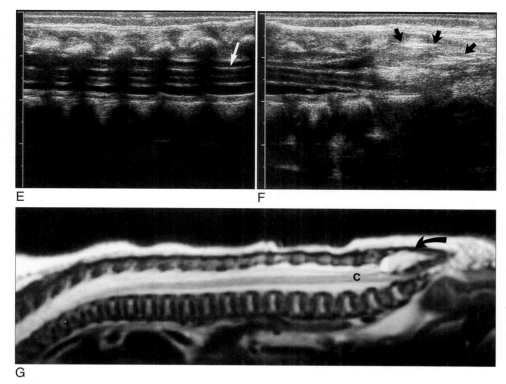

FIGURE 29-19, cont'd E and **F**, Sagittal views of the low cord *(white arrow)* with the clearly visible tethering lipoma *(black arrows)*. **G,** The correlative sagittal T2-weighted MRI, oriented to match the sonogram, reveals the abnormally low cord *(C)* and the lipoma *(curved black arrow)*.

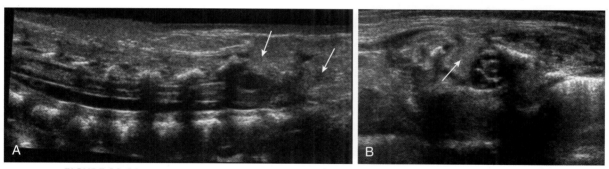

FIGURE 29-20 Lipomyelomeningocele in a 1-day-old infant with an associated back mass (lipoma). **A,** Longitudinal image shows a large lobulated, slightly echogenic mass *(arrows)* tethering the cord inferiorly. **B,** Transverse image shows the mass *(arrow)* against the superiolateral aspect of the spinal canal. *(Images courtesy Nationwide Children's Hospital, Columbus, OH.)*

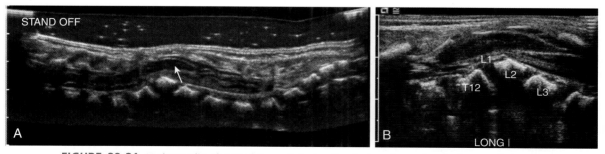

FIGURE 29-21 Hydromyelia observed in an infant with diastematomyelia. **A,** Panoramic image reveals acute kyphosis (flexion) of the spine at the thoracolumbar junction and a dilated central canal *(arrow)*. **B,** Longitudinal image at the level of the thoracolumbar junction. *(Images courtesy Nationwide Children's Hospital, Columbus, OH.)*

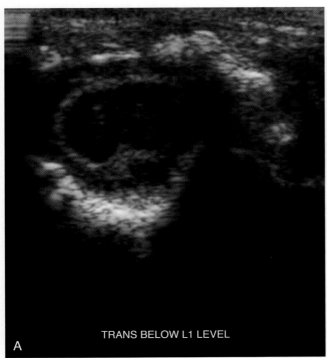

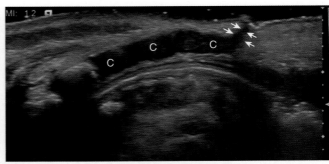

FIGURE 29-23 **Pilonidal sinus.** Newborn with a sacral dimple was referred because the physician was unable to tell if it was open or closed. Tract *(arrows)* seen extending to the very tip of the coccyx *(C)*, demonstrating a pilonidal sinus. There was no evidence for cord tethering. *(Images courtesy Nationwide Children's Hospital, Columbus, OH.)*

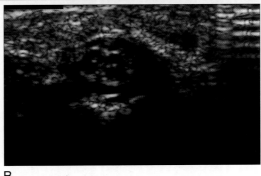

FIGURE 29-22 **Diastematomyelia. A,** Transverse image from same patient in Figure 29-21 helps to better define this pathology. **B,** Transverse scan of the lumbar spinal canal shows left and right hemicords. Each hemicord has an eccentric central canal.

and settings optimized. They frequently occur in the sacral or coccygeal region and may be associated with a sacral dimple. The tract can sometimes be seen and followed (Figure 29-23), especially if it is fluid filled or if it disrupts normal soft tissue planes. Infection is also possible in the pilonidal sinus. The neonatal coccyx is usually of very low echogenicity and should not be mistaken for a cyst or fluid collection in these cases.

Open Spinal Dysraphism

Myelomeningocele and Myelocele. Myelomeningoceles are the most common open spinal defects, occurring 98% of the time, whereas myeloceles are rare, comprising only 2% of open dysraphisms (Figure 29-24). **Myeloschisis** occurs if the defect

is uncovered (Figure 29-25). The primary reason for studying the spinal cord in cases of clinically obvious myelomeningocele or myelocele is to exclude additional cord pathology, such as diastematomyelia, which in conjunction with the myelomeningoceles and myeloceles are called hemimyelomeningocele and hemimyelocele, respectively.

Intraoperative sonography has been successfully used to detect the margin of the skin defect. The anatomy of the cord, adhesion of the cord to the dorsal aspect of the spinal canal cephalad to the defect, and the appearance of the neural placode and nerve roots in the defect can all be seen on a sonogram.

OTHER INDICATIONS AND ASSOCIATIONS

Other indications for spine sonography include following sequelae in spinal cord injury. Injury may occur as a result of birth trauma or a failed lumbar puncture. Although MRI evaluates most birth trauma cases, in the case of a rare cord transection, sonography is useful for a quick and portable examination. Failed spinal taps or lumbar punctures often present with associated epidural hematoma (Figure 29-26). Sonography is used to determine whether the cerebrospinal fluid has leaked and/or reaccumulated, in order to avoid another failed puncture. Additionally, sonographic guidance for lumbar puncture can be beneficial to ensure success.

Sonography of the spine may also be used to assess for cord retethering postoperatively or visualizing the spinal fluid for characteristics of blood products in patients with intracranial hemorrhage.

Finally, although the spectrum of caudal regression syndrome is a dysraphic condition and tethered cord is highly associated in patients with **VACTERL** syndrome, MRI is the imaging modality of choice to depict these more complex conditions associated with anal and urogenital malformations.

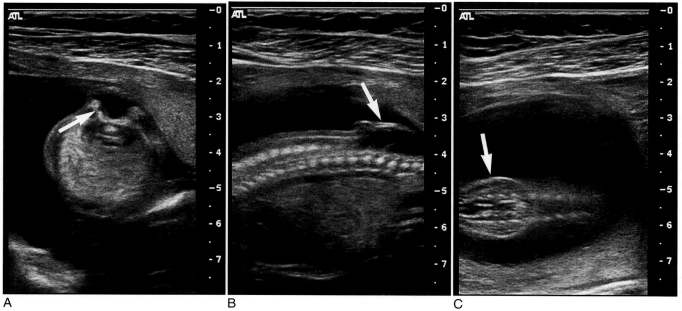

FIGURE 29-24 Lumbosacral myelomeningocele. Transverse **(A)**, sagittal **(B)**, and coronal **(C)** views of an 18-week fetus with a lumbosacral myelomeningocele. The transverse view shows the open nature of the posterior elements of the affected vertebral ring *(arrow)*. The sagittal view shows the protuberance of the covering membrane and neural placode *(arrow)*. The coronal view shows the thin nature of the covering membrane *(arrow)*.

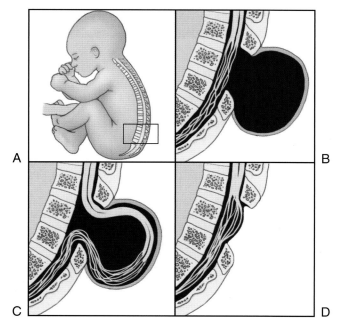

FIGURE 29-25 Spina bifida classifications. Meningoceles **(B)** contain only fluid, whereas myelomeningoceles **(C)** also contain neural elements. The defect is uncovered in myeloschisis **(D)**.

Key Pearls

- Spine sonography is usually diagnostic until 6 months of age and is performed with an 8- to 15-MHz linear-array transducer.
- The most common indication is a midline cutaneous abnormality to look for occult dysraphic conditions, such as tethered cord.
- An extended field of view is optimal and helpful in counting vertebrae.
- A tethered cord may be indicated when a dimple is more than 2.5 cm above the anus, larger than 5 mm, and when associated with other spinal lesions.
- Sonographically, tethering may present with a low-lying conus medullaris, posterior position of the spinal canal, thickened/hyperechoic filum terminale, and normal pulsations and movement within the spinal canal and nerve roots.
- Most defects occur in the lower lumbosacral spine, but they may occur anywhere.
- A dermal sinus should be differentiated from a pilonidal sinus, as the latter is not associated with a tethered cord, but a dermal sinus often is.
- Diastematomyelia is the split of the cord into two complete hemicords.
- Myelomeningocele and myelocele are open dysraphic abnormalities without intact skin, a contraindication to perform a spine sonographic examination.
- Sonography may be indicated for evaluation of spinal cord injury, such as birth trauma or a failed lumbar puncture.

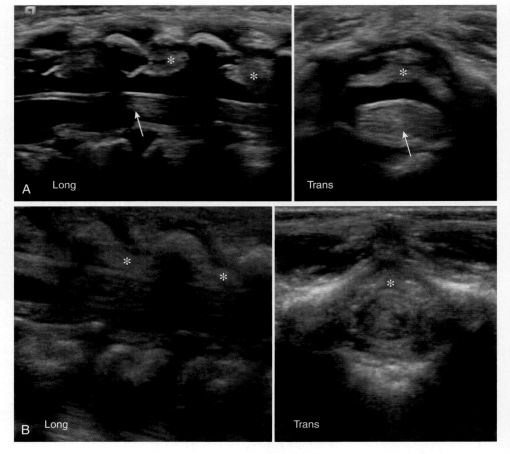

FIGURE 29-26 **A,** Failed or traumatic lumbar puncture attempt in a 2-month-old infant reveals an epidural hematoma *(asterisks);* cauda equina have a tethered cord appearance *(arrows)* (though still in anterior position) from congealed blood. (*Right* is longitudinal view; *left* is transverse view.) **B,** Follow-up 2 days later shows the cerebrospinal fluid (CSF) has leaked out completely, and the hematoma has decreased in size *(asterisks)*. Another lumbar puncture is not indicated until CSF reaccumulates. (*Right* is longitudinal view; *left* is transverse view.) *(Images courtesy Nationwide Children's Hospital, Columbus, OH.)*

BIBLIOGRAPHY

American Institute of Ultrasound in Medicine: AIUM practice guideline for the performance of an ultrasound examination of the neonatal spine, 2011. Available at http://www.aium.org/resources/guidelines/neonatalSpine.pdf.

Baraitser M, Winter RM: *Color atlas of congenital malformation syndromes,* London, 1996, Mosby-Wolfe.

Barnewolt CE: The pediatric spinal canal. In Rumack CM, Wilson SR, Charboneau JW, editors: *Diagnostic ultrasound,* vol 2, ed 3, St Louis, 2005, Elsevier Mosby.

Beek FJA, Bax KMA, Mali WFTM: Sonography of the coccyx in newborns and infants, *J Ultrasound Med* 13:629-634, 1994.

Chern JJ, Kirkma JL, Shannon CN, et al: Use of lumbar ultrasonography to detect occult spinal dysraphism: clinical article, *J Neurosurg Pediatr* 9(3):274-279, 2012.

Dick EA, Patel K, Owens CM: Spinal ultrasound in infants, *Br J Radiol* 75:384-392, 2002.

DiPietro MA: The conus medullaris: normal US findings throughout childhood, *Radiology* 188:149-153, 1993.

DiPietro MA: Sonography of the pediatric spine and hip [lecture], 2015. Available at www.sonoworld.com.

DiPietro MA, Garver KA: Sonography of the neonatal spinal canal. In Haller JO, editor: *Textbook of neonatal ultrasound,* New York, 1998, Parthenon Publishing Group.

Glasier CM, Chadduck WM, Leithiser RE Jr, et al: Screening spinal ultrasound in newborns with neural tube defects, *J Ultrasound Med* 9:339-343, 1990.

Hung PC, Wang HS, Lui TN, Wong AMC: Sonographic findings in a neonate with diastematomyelia and a tethered spinal cord, *J Ultrasound Med* 29(9):1357-1360, 2010.

Irani N, Goud AR, Lowe LH: Isolated filar cyst on lumbar spine sonography in infants: a case-control study, *Pediatr Radiol* 36(12):1283-1288, 2006.

Kriss VM, Desai NS: Occult spinal dysraphism in neonates: assessment of high-risk cutaneous stigmata on sonography, *Am J Roentgenol* 171(4):1687-1692, 1998.

Kriss VM, Kriss TC, Babcock DS: The ventriculus terminalis of the spinal cord in the neonate: a normal variant on sonography, *Am J Radiol* 165:1491-1493, 1995.

McGovern M, et al: Ultrasound investigation of sacral dimples and other stigmata of spinal dysraphism, *Arch Dis Child* 98(10):784-786, 2013.

O'Neill BR, Yu AK, Tyler-Kabara EC: Prevalence of tethered spinal cord in infants with VACTERL: clinical article, *J Neurosurg Pediatr* 6(2):177-182, 2010.

Rypens F, Avni EF, Matos C, et al: Atypical and equivocal sonographic features of the spinal cord in neonates, *Pediatr Radiol* 25:429-432, 1995.

Rufener S, Ibrahim M, Parmar HA: Imaging of congenital spine and spinal cord malformations, *Neuroimag Clin North Am* 21(3):659-676, 2011.

Schenk JP, Herweh C, Günther P, et al: Imaging of congenital anomalies and variations of the caudal spine and back in neonates and small infants, *Eur J Radiol* 58(1):3-14, 2006.

Scottoni F, Iacobelli BD, Zaccara AM, et al: Spinal ultrasound in patients with anorectal malformations: is this the end of an era? *Pediatr Surg Int* 30(8):829-831, 2014.

Siegel MJ: *Pediatric sonography,* Philadelphia, PA, 2010, Lippincott Williams & Wilkins.

Simanovsky N, Stepensky P, Hiller N: The use of ultrasound for the diagnosis of spinal hemorrhage in a newborn, *Pediatr Neurol* 31(4):295-297, 2004.

Unsinn KM, Geley T, Freund MC, et al: US of the spinal cord in newborns: spectrum of normal findings, variants, congenital abnormalities, and acquired diseases, *Radiographics* 20(4):923-938, 2000.

abdominal aortic aneurysm localized dilation of an artery, with an increase in diameter of 1.5 times its normal diameter

abduction to move away from the body

abscess localized collection of pus surrounded by inflamed tissue

absorption process of nutrient molecules passing through wall of intestine into blood or lymph system

accessory spleen results from the failure of fusion of separate splenic masses forming on the dorsal mesogastrium; most commonly found in the splenic hilum or along the splenic vessels of associated ligaments

acholic (stools) describes absence or deficiency of bile secretion or failure of bile to enter the alimentary tract (secondary to obstruction); the stools are claylike and colorless

acini glandular component of the breast lobule; the breast contains hundreds of lobules, each containing several small glands or acini

acini cells cells that perform exocrine function

acoustic emission occurs when an appropriate level of acoustic energy is applied to the tissue, the microbubbles first oscillate and then rupture; the rupture of the microbubbles in random Doppler shifts appearing as a transient mosaic of colors on a color Doppler display

acoustic impedance measure of a material's resistance to the propagation of sound; expressed as the product of acoustic velocity of the medium and the density of the medium

acromioclavicular joint (AC) the joint found in the shoulder that connects the clavicle to the acromion process of the scapula

Addison's disease condition caused by hyposecretion of hormones from the adrenal cortex

adduction to move toward the body

adenoma benign neoplasm characterized by complete fibrous encapsulation

adenomyomatosis small polypoid projections arising from the gallbladder wall

adenopathy multiple, enlarged lymph nodes

adenosis overgrowth of the acini within the terminal ductal lobular unit of the breast

adrenal hemorrhage hemorrhage that occurs when the fetus is stressed during a difficult delivery or a hypoxic insult

adrenocorticotropic hormone (ACTH) hormone secreted by the pituitary gland

afferent arteriole carries blood into the glomerulus of the nephron

aliasing Aliasing in its technical use indicates improper representation of information that has been sampled insufficiently. (Usually occurs in pulsed Doppler imaging in which a high-frequency Doppler shift is interpreted as a lower frequency)

alimentary tract also know as the digestive tract; includes the mouth, pharynx, esophagus, stomach, duodenum, small and large intestine

alkaline phosphatase enzyme of the liver

alpha fetoprotein (AFP) a laboratory test that measures levels of alpha fetoprotein in blood serum; an elevated level could indicate a liver lesion

ALT alanine aminotransferase enzyme of the liver

amplitude strength of the ultrasound wave measured in decibels

ampulla of Vater small opening in the duodenum in which the pancreatic and common bile duct enter to release secretions

amylase enzyme secreted by the pancreas to aid in the digestion of carbohydrates

amyloidosis metabolic disorder marked by amyloid deposits in organs and tissue

anastomosis communication between two blood vessels without any intervening capillary network

anatomic position individual is standing erect, arms are by the sides with the palms facing forward, face and eyes are directed forward, and heels are together, with the feet pointed forward

angiomyolipomas most common benign tumor of the kidney, appear as a hyperechoic mass, composed of blood vessels, muscle cells, and fat cells. Strongly associated with tuberous sclerosis, often bilaterally

angle of incidence angle at which the sound beam strikes the interface

angle of reflection angle at which the beam of the sound is reflected from an interface; the angle of reflection equals the angle of incidence

anisotropy the quality of comprising varying values of a given property when measured in different directions

anterior (ventral) toward the front of the body or in front of another structure

anti-radial plane of imaging on ultrasound that is perpendicular to the radial plane of imaging

aorta largest arterial structure in the body

apnea spontaneous breathing that stops for any reason

apocrine metaplasia form of fibrocystic change in which the epithelial cells of the acini undergo alteration

aponeurosis brandlike flat tendons connecting muscle to the bone

appendicolith a fecalith or calcification located in the appendix

aqueductal stenosis blockage of the duct connecting the third and fourth ventricles, which causes their dilation

arcuate artery small arteries that lie at the bases of the renal pyramids and appear as echogenic structures

areola the pigmented skin surrounding the breast nipple

arrhythmia any irregular heartbeat; also called dysrhythmia

arteries vascular structures that carry blood away from the heart

arteriosclerosis a disease of the arterial vessels marked by thickening, hardening, and loss of elasticity in the arterial walls

arteriovenous fistula communication between an artery and vein

ascites free fluid in the abdominal cavity

asphyxia severe hypoxia, or inadequate oxygenation

AST (aspartase aminotransferase) enzyme of the liver

atherosclerosis condition in which the aortic wall becomes irregular from plaque build-up

atretic describes the congenital absence or closure of a normal body opening or tubular structure

atrium (trigone) of the lateral ventricle junction of the anterior, occipital, and temporal horns of the lateral ventricles

attenuation   reduction in the amplitude and intensity of a sound wave as it propagates through a medium. Attenuation coefficient increases with increasing frequency

atypical hyperplasia   abnormal proliferation of cells with atypical features involving the TDLU

autoimmune hemolytic anemia   anemia caused by antibodies produced by the patient's own immune system

autosomal dominant polycystic renal disease (ADPKD)   hereditary polycystic disease that usually presents in middle age

autosomal recessive polycystic renal disease (ARPKD)   rare, hereditary polycystic disease (infantile polycystic disease)

axial resolution   refers to the minimum distance between two structures positioned along the axis of the beam where both structures can be visualized as separate objects

axilla   the axilla contains lymph nodes that drain the majority of breast tissue

bare area   area superior to the liver that is not covered by peritoneum so that the inferior vena cava may enter the thoracic cavity

Barlow maneuver   the patient lies in the supine position with the hip flexed 90 degrees and adducted; downward and outward pressure is applied; if the hip is dislocated, the examiner will feel the femoral head move out of the acetabulum

BAT   term used to describe blunt abdominal trauma

Beckwith-Wiedemann syndrome   hereditary disorder transmitted as an autosomal recessive trait; clinical manifestations include umbilical hernia (exomphalos), macroglossia, and gigantism. Often accompanied by visceromegaly and dysplasia of the renal medulla; also called exophthalmos-macroglossia-gigantism (EMG) syndrome

biliary atresia   closure or absence of some or all of the major bile ducts

bilirubin   yellow pigment in bile formed by the breakdown of red blood cells; excreted by the liver and stored in the gallbladder

blood urea nitrogen (BUN)   measures amount of nitrogenous waste (along with creatinine); waste products accumulate in the blood when kidneys malfunction

body mechanics   theory and practice of using the correct muscles to complete a task safely, efficiently, and without undue strain on any joints or muscles

body of the pancreas   lies in the mid-epigastrium anterior to the superior mesenteries artery and vein, aorta, and inferior vena cava

Bowman's capsule   part of the filtration process; contains water, salts, glucose, urea, and amino acids

bradycardia   a heart rate of less than 60 bpm

brain stem   part of the brain connecting the forebrain and the spinal cord; consists of the midbrain, pons, and medulla oblongata

branchial cleft cyst   remnant of embryonic development that appears as a cyst in the neck

Budd-Chiari syndrome   thrombosis of the hepatic veins

Bulk modulus   amount of pressure required to compress a small volume of material a small amount

bull's eye (target) lesion   hypoechoic mass with an echogenic central core (abscess, metastases)

BUN   blood urea nitrogen

bursa   a saclike structure containing thick fluid that surrounds areas subject to friction, such as the interface between bone and tendon

bursitis   inflammation of a bursa

calcitonin   a thyroid hormone that is important for maintaining a dense, strong bone matrix and regulating the blood calcium level

calyx   part of the collecting system adjacent to the pyramid that collects urine and is connected to the major calyx

capillaries   minute vessels that connect the arterial and venous systems

cardiac orifice   entrance of the esophagus into the stomach

carpal tunnel   the canal in the wrist bounded by osteofibrous material through which the flexor tendons and the median nerve pass

cartilage interface sign   echogenic line on the anterior surface of the cartilage surrounding the humeral head

cauda equina   bundle of nerve roots from the lumbar, sacral, and coccygeal spinal nerves that descend nearly vertically from the spinal cord until they reach respective openings in the vertebral column

caudal pancreatic artery   branch of the splenic artery that supplies the tail of the pancreas

caudal   toward the feet

caudate lobe   small lobe of the liver situated on the postero-superior surface of the left lobe; the ligamentum venosum is the anterior border

caudothalamic groove or notch   the region at which the caudate nucleus and thalamus join; the most common location of germinal matrix hemorrhage

cavernous transformation of the portal vein   periportal collateral channels in patients with chronic portal vein obstruction

centripetal artery   terminal intratesticular arteries arising from the capsular arteries

cerebellum   area of the brain that lies posterior to the brainstem below the tentorium

cerebrum   largest part of the brain consisting of two equal hemispheres

Chiari malformations   congenital defect in which the cerebellum and brainstem are pulled toward the spinal cord (banana sign seen with sonography); frontal bossing or a *lemon head* can be observed looking at the neonate's head shape

cholangitis   inflammation of the bile ducts

cholecystectomy   removal of the gallbladder

cholecystitis   inflammation of the gallbladder; may be acute or chronic

cholecystokinin   hormone secreted into the blood by the mucosa of the upper small intestine; stimulates contraction of the gallbladder and pancreatic secretion of enzymes

choledochal cyst   cystic growth on the common bile duct that may cause obstruction

choledocholithiasis   stones in the bile duct

cholelithiasis   gallstones in the gallbladder

cholesterosis   variant of adenomyomatosis; cholesterol polyps

choroid plexus   echogenic cluster of cells important in the production of cerebrospinal fluid that lie along the atrium of the lateral ventricles

clapper-in-the-bell sign   hypoechoic hematoma found at the end of a completely retracted muscle fragment

C-loop of the duodenum   forms the lateral border of the head of the pancreas

coagulopathy   a defect in blood-clotting mechanisms

collateral circulation   develops when normal venous channels become obstructed

color flow Doppler velocity in each direction is quantified by allocating a pixel to each area

columns of Bertin bands of cortical tissue that separate the renal pyramids; a prominent column of Bertin may mimic a renal mass on sonography

common bile duct extends from the point where the common hepatic duct meets the cystic duct; drains into the duodenum after it joins with the main pancreatic duct

common hepatic artery arises from the celiac trunk to supply the liver; forms the right superior border of the body and head of the pancreas and gives rise to the gastroduodenal artery

common hepatic duct bile duct drains from the liver to the hepatic duct, which joins the cystic duct to form the common bile duct

common iliac arteries the abdominal aorta bifurcates at the level of the umbilicus into common iliac arteries to supply blood to the lower extremities

compression region of increased particle density

congenital mesoblastic nephroma most common benign renal tumor of the neonate and infant

continuous wave Doppler (CW) one transducer continuously transmits sound while one transducer continuously receives sound; used in high-velocity flow patterns

contrast-enhanced sonography (CES) agent used to reduce or eliminate some of the current limitations of ultrasound imaging and Doppler blood flow detection color flow imaging

conus medullaris the caudal end of the spinal cord, it should taper

converse piezoelectric effect a property of piezoelectric materials whereby an electric stimulus causes the dipolar material to expand and contract, producing a sound wave

Cooper's ligaments connective tissue septa that connect perpendicularly to the breast lobules and extend out to the skin

coronal The coronal plane is a lengthwise plane running from side to side, dividing the body into anterior and posterior portions

cortex (adrenal) outer parenchyma of the adrenal gland that secretes steroid hormones, commonly called corticoids

cortex (kidney) outer parenchyma of an organ; in the kidney, it contains the renal corpuscle and proximal and distal convoluted tubules of the nephron; in the adrenal gland it secretes steroid hormones; in the neonatal kidney it is thin with echogenicity similar to or slightly greater than that of the normal liver parenchyma

corticomedullary differentiation the distinct separation and normal sonographic appearance of the cortex and medulla within the pediatric kidney. When poor, it may be indicative of renal pathology

Courvoisier's gallbladder enlargement of the gallbladder caused by a slow progressive obstruction of the distal common bile duct from an external mass

cranial toward the head

creatinine (Cr) one of the laboratory tests used to measure the ability of the kidney to get rid of waste; waste products accumulate in the blood when the kidneys are malfunctioning

cremasteric artery small artery arising from the inferior epigastric artery (a branch of the external iliac artery), which supplies the peritesticular tissue, including the cremasteric muscle

cremasteric muscle an extension of the internal oblique muscle that descends to the testis with the spermatic cord; contraction of the cremasteric muscle shortens the spermatic cord and elevates the testis

Crohn's disease inflammation of the bowel, accompanied by abscess and bowel wall thickening

cryptorchidism (undescended testes) testicles remain within the abdomen or groin and fail to descend into the scrotal sac

culling process by which the spleen removes abnormal red blood cells as they pass through

curved array probe large footprint that allows good near field and far field visualization with limited intercostal access

Cushing's syndrome condition caused by hypersecretion of hormones from the adrenal cortex

cyanosis bluish discoloration of the skin and mucous membranes caused by lack of oxygen in the blood

cycle a sequence of events occurring at regular intervals; a wavelength cycle is that of a particle density that varies from maximum in the compression zone to a minimum in the reflection zone and back to maximum in the successive compression zone to complete one cycle

cystic duct connects the gallbladder to the common hepatic duct

cystic medial necrosis weakening of the arterial wall

Dandy-Walker malformation abnormal development of the fourth ventricle, often accompanied by hydrocephalus

dartos layer of muscle underneath the scrotal skin

decibel (dB) unit used to quantitatively express the ratio of two amplitudes or intensities

deferential artery arises from the vesicle artery (a branch of the internal iliac artery) and supplies the vas deferens and epididymis

developmental displacement of the hip (DDH) abnormal condition of the hip that results in congenital hip dysplasia; includes dysplastic, subluxated, dislocatable, and dislocated hips

diastematomyelia a congenital fissure of the spinal cord, frequently associated with spina bifida cystica

diffuse hepatocellular disease affects hepatocytes and interferes with liver function

dissecting aneurysm tear in the intima and/or media of the abdominal aorta

distal away from the point of origin or away from the body

diverticulum a pouch-like herniation through the muscular wall of a tubular organ that occurs in the stomach, small intestine, or colon

Doppler angle the angle the reflector path makes with the ultrasound beam; the most accurate velocity is when the beam is parallel to flow

Doppler gate the sample site from which the signal is obtained with PW Doppler

Doppler shift change in frequency of a reflected wave; caused by motion between the reflector and the transducer's beam

dorsal pancreatic artery branch of the splenic artery that supplies the body of the pancreas

dorsiflexion upward movement of the hand or foot

DPT terms used to describe diagnostic peritoneal lavage

dromedary hump normal variant that occurs on the left kidney as a bulge on the lateral border

duct of Santorini small accessory duct found in the head of the pancreas

duct of Wirsung   largest duct that drains the tail, body, and head of the pancreas; it joins the common bile duct to enter the duodenum through the ampulla of Vater

duodenal bulb   first part of the duodenum

dynamic range   ratio of the largest to smallest signals that an instrument or component of an instrument can respond to without distortion

dyspnea   a shortness of breath or the feeling of not getting enough air, which may leave a person gasping

dysraphism   abnormalities associated with incomplete embryologic development of the dorsal aspect of an embryo. Abnormalities of the spine and spinal cord

ectasia   dilation of any tubular vessel

ectopic kidney   located outside of the normal position, most often in the pelvic cavity

ectopic ureterocele   ectopic insertion and cystic dilation of the distal ureter of a duplicated renal collecting system (Duplex kidney); occurs more commonly in females and on the left side

efferent arteriole   blood from this structure supplies the peritubular capillaries, which also supply the convoluted tubules

ejaculatory ducts   connect the seminal vesicle and the vas deferens to the urethra at the verumontanum

endocrine   production of the hormone insulin

enhancement   strengthening of echoes from reflectors that lie behind a weakly attenuating structure

ependyma   the inside lining of the ventricular system, composed of specialized ependymal cells

epicondylitis (lateral and medial)   inflammation of the humerus and surrounding tissues

epididymis   anatomic structure formed by the network of ducts leaving the mediastinum testis that combine into a single, convoluted epidiymal tubule; located on the posterolateral aspect of the testis; the epididymis consists of the head, the body, and the tail; spermatozoa mature and accumulate within the epididymis

epididymal cyst   cyst filled with clear, serous fluid located in the epididymis

epididymitis   inflammation of the epididymis

epigastrium   area between the right and left hypochondrium that contains part of the liver, duodenum, and pancreas

epineurium   the covering of a nerve that consists of connective tissue

ergonomics   the science concerned with fitting a job to a person's anatomical, physiological, and psychological characteristics in a way that enhances human efficiency and well-being

erythrocyte   red blood cell

euthyroid   refers to a normal functioning thyroid gland

exocrine   production and digestion of pancreatic juice

external   outside

extracorporeal membrane oxygenation (ECMO)   intensive treatment for infants with severe respiratory failure who have not responded to maximal conventional ventilator support

extrahepatic   outside the liver

falciform ligament   extends from the umbilicus to the diaphragm in a sagittal plane and contains the ligamentum teres

false pelvis   portion of the pelvic cavity that is above the pelvic brim

falx cerebri   echogenic fibrous structure (portion of the dura mater) that descends through the interhemispheric fissure, separating the cerebral hemispheres

fan   micro movement when the probe is minutely angled, pivoting on a point of interest

far field (Fraunhofer zone)   the field farthest from the transducer during the formation of the sound beam

fasciculi   term describing a small bundle of muscles, nerves, and tendons

FAST exam   FAST (focused assessment with sonography for trauma) is a limited survey of the chest/abdomen/pelvis to evaluate for free fluid or pericardial fluid

fecalith   calculus that may form around fecal material associated with appendicitis

fibroadenoma   most common benign solid tumor of the breast

filum terminale   slender tapering terminal section of the spinal cord, contiguous with the pia mater

fine needle aspiration (FNA)   the use of a fine-gauge needle to obtain cells from a mass

first generation agents   agents containing room air (i.e., Albunex)

focal zone   the region over which the effective width of the sound beam is within some measure of its width at the focal distance

follicular carcinoma   occurs as a solitary malignant mass within the thyroid gland

fontanels   soft space between the bones; the space is usually large enough to accommodate the ultrasound transducer until 9–12 months of age

frame rate   rate at which images are updated on the display; dependent on frequency of the transducer and depth selection

frank dislocation   the hip is laterally and posteriorly displaced to the extent that the femoral head has no contact with the acetabulum and the normal "U" configuration in the transverse view cannot be obtained on ultrasound

frequency   the number of cycles per second that a periodic event or function undergoes per unit of time

fusiform aneurysm   circumferential enlargement of a vessel with tapering at both ends

gain   measure of the strength of the ultrasound signal expressed in decibels

Galeazzi sign   on physical examination, the knee is lower in position on the affected side of the neonate with developmental displacement of the hip (DDH) when the patient is supine and the knees are flexed

gallbladder   storage pouch for bile

gastrin   endocrine hormone released from the stomach that stimulates secretion of gastric acid

gastroduodenal artery   branch of the common hepatic artery to supply to stomach and duodenum

gastrosplenic ligament   ligament between the greater curvature of the stomach and spleen that helps to hold the spleen in place

Gaucher's disease   one of the storage diseases in which fat and proteins are deposited abnormally in the body

germinal matrix   fragile periventricular tissue (includes the caudate nucleus) that easily bleeds in the premature infant

Gerota's fascia   another term for the renal fascia; the kidney is covered by the renal capsule, perirenal fat, Gerota's fascia, and pararenal fat

glomerulus   part of the filtration process in the kidney

glucagon   stimulates the liver to convert glycogen to glucose

goiter   enlargement of the thyroid gland that can be focal or diffuse; multiple nodules may be present

grating lobes   additional beams emitted from an array transducer that are stronger than the side lobes of individual elements

Graves' disease   autoimmune disorder of diffuse toxic goiter characterized by bulging eyes (exophthalmos)

gray scale   B-mode technique that permits the brightness of the B-mode dots to be displayed in various shades of gray to represent different echo amplitudes

gray scale harmonic imaging   allows detection of contrast-enhanced blood flow and organs with grayscale ultrasound; in the harmonic-imaging mode, the echoes from the oscillating microbubbles have a higher signal-to-noise ration than found in conventional ultrasound; regions with microbubbles (e.g., blood vessels and organ parenchyma) are better visualized

greater omentum   known as the "fatty apron" double fold of the peritoneum attached to the duodenum, stomach, and large intestine; helps support the great curve of the stomach

Guyon's canal or tunnel   a fibrous tunnel that contains the ulnar artery and vein, ulnar nerve, and some fatty tissue

gynecomastia   hypertrophy of residual elements that persist behind the nipple in the male

harmonic imaging (HI)   in the HI mode, the ultrasound system is configured to receive only echoes at the second harmonic frequency, which is twice the transmit frequency

Hartmann's pouch   small outpouch of the gallbladder fundus that lies near the cystic duct that may collect gallstones

Hashimoto's thyroiditis   chronic inflammation of the thyroid gland caused by the formation of antibodies against normal thyroid tissue

haustra   normal segmentation of the wall of the colon

head of the pancreas   lies in the C-loop of the duodenum; the gastroduodenal artery is the anterolateral border and the common bile duct is the posterior border

Heimlich maneuver   emergency treatment to clear an upper airway obstruction that is preventing normal breathing

Heister's valve   tiny valves found within the cystic duct

hematocele   blood located between the visceral and parietal layers of the tunica vaginalis

hematopoiesis   blood cell production

hemihypertrophy   excessive development of one side or one half of the body or an organ

hemoglobin   oxygen-binding protein found in red blood cells

hemolytic anemia   anemia resulting from hemolysis of red blood cells

hemoperitoneum   collection of bloody fluid in the abdomen or pelvis secondary to trauma or surgical procedure

hemorrhage   collection of blood

hepatic flexure   ascending colon rises from the right lower quadrant to bend at this point to form the transverse colon

hepatic veins   three large veins that drain the liver and empty into the inferior vena cava at the level of the diaphragm

hepatocellular disease   refers to liver cells or hepatocytes as primary problem

hepatocyte   a parenchymal liver cell that performs all functions ascribed to the liver

hepatofugal   flow away from the liver

hepatopedal   flow toward the liver

hertz (Hz)   unit for frequency, equal to 1 cycle per second

hilus   area of kidney where vessels, ureter, and lymphatics enter and exit

hip joint   formed by the articulation of the head of the femur within the acetabulum of the hip bone

Hodgkin's disease   a malignant disease that involves lymphoid tissue

holoprosencephaly   congenital defect characterized by abnormal single ventricular cavity with some form of thalami fusion; caused by an extra chromosome, the prosencephalon fails to divide into hemispheres during embryonic development

homeostasis   maintenance of normal body physiology

horseshoe kidney   congenital malformation in which both kidneys are joined together by an isthmus, most commonly at the lower poles

hydrocele   fluid formed between the visceral and parietal layers of the tunica vaginalis

hydrocephalus   ventriculomegaly in the neonate; abnormal accumulation of cerebrospinal fluid within the cerebral ventricles, resulting in compression and frequently destruction of brain tissue

hydromyelia   dilation of the central canal of the spinal cord

hydronephrosis   dilation of the renal collecting system

hydrops   massive enlargement of the gallbladder

hypercalcemia   elevated levels of calcium in the blood

hyperglycemia   uncontrolled increase in glucose

hyperlipidemia   congenital condition in which elevated fat levels cause pancreatitis

hyperparathyroidism   disorder associated with elevated serum calcium level, usually caused by a benign parathyroid adenoma

hyperplasia   enlargement

hypertension   high blood pressure, higher than 130/90 mm Hg

hyperthyroidism   oversecretion of thyroid hormones

hypoglycemia   deficiency of glucose

hypomotility   abnormally decreased motility or movement of the bowel can be associated with appendicitis, constipation, and other gastrointestinal conditions. Diarrhea, on the other hand, typically presents with hypermotility of the bowel

hypophosphatasia   low phosphatase level, which can be seen with hyperparathyroidism

hypotension   low blood pressure, lower than 115/75 mm Hg; decreased systolic and diastolic blood pressure below normal; may occur with shock, hemorrhaging, infection, fever, cancer, anemia, neurasthenia, and Addison's disease

hypothyroidism   underactive thyroid hormones

hypoxia   decreased oxygen in the body

incarcerated hernia   imprisonment or confinement of a part of the bowel in which the visceral contents cannot be reduced

increased intracranial pressure (ICP)   increased pressure inside the skull compressing the brain and restricting blood flow; in the neonate it is often caused by hydrocephalus, but may be due to brain edema

induced acoustic emission   after the injection of the tissue-specific UCA Sonazoid, the reflectivity of the contrast-containing tissue increases; when the right level of acoustic energy is applied to tissue, the contrast microbubbles eventually rupture, resulting in random Doppler shifts. These shifts appear as a transient mosaic of colors on the color Doppler display; masses that have destroyed or replaced normal Kupffer cells will be displayed as color-free areas

infarction   an interruption in the blood supply to an area that may lead to necrosis of the area

inferior   below

inferior mesenteric artery   arises from the anterior aortic wall at the level of the third or fourth lumbar vertebra to supply the left transverse colon, descending colon, sigmoid colon, and rectum

inferior mesenteric vein   drains the left third of the colon and upper colon and joins the splenic vein

inferior vena cava   largest venous abdominal vessel that conveys blood from the body below the diaphragm to the right atrium of the heart

infiltrating ductal carcinoma   cancer of the ductal epithelium

infiltrating (invasive) lobular carcinoma   cancer of the lobular epithelium of the breast

inspissated   thickened by absorption, evaporation, or dehydration

insulin   hormone that causes glycogen formation from glucose in the liver and allows cells within insulin receptors to take up glucose to decrease blood sugar

intensity   power per unit area

interface   surface forming the boundary between media having different properties

internal   inside

international normalized ratio (INR)   a method developed to standardize prothrombin time (PT) results among laboratories by accounting for the different thromboplastin reagents used to determine PT

intrahepatic   within the liver

intraperitoneal   within the peritoneal cavity

intravenous (IV) therapy   the practice of giving liquid substances directly into a vein

intraventricular hemorrhage (IVH)   Hemorrhage that has burst through the germinal matrix or subependymal bleed and lies within the ventricular cavity. Depending on severity and location it may or may not cause ventricular enlargement

intussusception   when bowel prolapses into distal bowel (telescoping) and is then propelled in an antegrade fashion causing bowel obstruction

islets of Langerhans   small cells that comprise the endocrine portion of the pancreas for the production of insulin, glucagon, and somatostatin

isolated systolic hypertension   condition that occurs when systolic pressure is above 140 mm Hg but diastolic pressure remains below 90 mm Hg

isthmus   small piece of thyroid tissue that connects the right and left lobes of the gland

jaundice   excessive bilirubin accumulation causes yellow pigmentation of the skin

junctional fold   small septum within the gallbladder, usually arising from the posterior wall

Kasai portoenterostomy   also called a hepatoportoenterostomy, is a surgical procedure often used in the treatment of biliary atresia, anastomosing the jejunum with the porta hepatis region of the liver to the duodenum, allowing bile to flow from the intrahepatic bile ducts to the intestine

kilohertz (kHz)   1000 Hz

Klatskin tumor   cancer at the bifurcation of the hepatic ducts; may cause asymmetric obstruction of the biliary tree

labrum   a piece of fibrocartilage (rubbery tissue) which attaches the rim of a socket to keep the ball joint in place; in the hip, the acetabular labrum has a fibrous echogenic tip and increases the ball (femoral head) depth in the socket

laminar   normal pattern of vessel flow; flow in the center of the vessel is faster than at the edges

lateral   farther from the midline or to the side of the body

lateral resolution   the minimum distance between two objects where they still can be displayed as separate objects

left gastric artery   arises from the celiac axis to supply the stomach and lower third of the esophagus

left hepatic artery   small branch the supplies the caudate and left lobes of the liver

left hypochondrium   left upper quadrant of the abdomen that contains the left lobe of the liver, spleen, and stomach

left lobe of the liver   lies in the epigastrium and left hypochondrium

left portal vein   supplies the left lobe of the liver

left renal artery   arises from the posterolateral wall of the aorta directly into the hilus of the kidney

left renal vein   leaves the renal hilum, travels anterior to the aorta and posterior to the superior mesenteric artery to enter the lateral wall of the inferior vena cava

lesser omentum   suspends the stomach and duodenum from the liver; helps to support the lesser curvature of the stomach

leukocytolysis   destruction of leukocytes

leukopenia   abnormal decrease of white blood corpuscles

lienorenal ligament   ligament between the spleen and kidney which helps support the great curvature of the stomach

ligament   fibrous band of tissue connecting bone or cartilage to bone that aids in stabilizing a joint

ligamentum teres   appears as a bright echogenic foci on transverse images; along with falciform ligament, it divides medial and lateral segments of the left lobe of the liver

ligamentum venosum   separates left lobe from caudate lobe; shown as echogenic line on the transverse and sagittal images

lipase   pancreatic enzyme that breaks down fats; enzyme is elevated in pancreatitis and remains increased longer than amylase

lipoma   common benign tumor composed of fat cells

liver function tests   specific laboratory tests that look at liver function (aspartase or alanine aminotransferase, lactic acid dehydrogenase, alkaline phosphatase, and bilirubin)

longitudinal   The longitudinal plane is parallel to the long axis of the body or part

longus colli muscle   wedge-shaped muscle posterior to the thyroid lobes

loop of Henle   portion of a renal tubule lying between the proximal and distal convoluted portions; reabsorption of fluid, sodium, and chloride occurs in the proximal convoluted tubule and the loop of Henle

lymph   an alkaline fluid found in the lymphatic vessels

lymphoma   malignancy that primarily affects the lymph nodes, spleen, or liver

macro movement   this movement of the probe is used with the sweep and slight motion in which the probe is moved greater than 1 centimeter

main lobar fissure   boundary between the right and left lobes of the liver; seen as hyperechoic line on the sagittal image extending from the portal vein to the neck of the gallbladder

main portal vein   enters the liver at the porta hepatis

major calyces (also known as the infundibulum)   receives urine from the minor calyces to convey to the loop of Henle

mammary layer   middle layer of the breast tissue between the skin and the chest wall that contains the ductal, glandular, and stromal portions of the breast

Marfan syndrome   hereditary disorder of connective tissue, bones, muscles, ligaments, and skeletal structures

McBurney's point site of maximal tenderness in the right lower quadrant; usually with appendicitis; located by drawing a line from the right anterosuperior iliac spine to the umbilicus; at approximately the midpoint of this line lies the root of the appendix

mechanical index (MI) an index that defines the low acoustic output power that can be used to minimize the destruction of microbubbles by energy in the acoustic field; when the microbubbles in microbubble-based ultrasound contrast agents are destroyed, contrast enhancement is lost

Meckel's diverticulum congenital sac or blind pouch found in the lower portion of the ileum

medial nearer to or toward the midline

median plane vertical plane that bisects the body into right and left halves

mediastinum testis central linear structure formed by the convergence of multiple thin septations within the testicle; the septations are invaginations of the tunica albuginea

medulla (aderenal) central tissue of the adrenal gland that secretes epinephrine and norepinephrine

medulla (renal—also known as the pyramid) refers to the inner portion of the renal parenchyma that contains the loop of Henle

medullary carcinoma neoplastic growth that accounts for 10% of thyroid malignancies

medullary pyramids large and hypoechoic in the neonate should not be mistaken for hydronephrosis. Triangular in shape, they consist mainly of tubules, which transport urine from the cortex to the calyces

mega cisterna magna normal variant without associated neurological impairment, in which there is an enlarged cisterna magna without a mass effect

megahertz (MHz) 1,000,000 Hz

meninges three membranes enclosing the brain and spinal cord

meningocele open defect in which the spinal cord, not the nerve roots, just fluid is exposed

mesentery projects from the parietal peritoneum and attaches to the small intestine, anchoring it to the posterior abdominal wall

mesothelium fifth layer of bowel

metastatic disease most common form of neoplasm of the liver; primary sites are colon, breast, and lung

micro movement this movement of the probe is used with the sweep and slight motion in which the probe is moved less than 1 centimeter

midgut malrotation congenital anomaly in which the bowel did not properly rotate during embryogenesis, with sonography may show an inversion of the normal SMA and SMV positioning

minor calyces receives urine from the renal pyramids; forms the border of the renal sinus

mirror image shows structures that exist on one side of a strong reflector as being present on the other side as well

Model for End-Stage Liver Disease (MELD) was initially used to predict death within three months in patients who had a transjugular intrahepatic portosystemic shunt (TIPS) performed. The MELD score is a mathematical calculation based on lab values of bilirubin (measurement of bile pigment), creatinine (kidney function), and International Nationalized Ratio (INR) (blood clotting ability)

molecular imaging agents agents include Optison, Definity, Imagent, Levovist, SonoVue

mononucleosis acute infection caused by the Epstein-Barr virus that most commonly affects teenagers and young adults; symptoms include fever, sore throat, enlarged lymph nodes, abnormal lymphocysts, and hepatosplenomegaly

Morison's pouch right posterior subhepatic space located anterior to the kidney and inferior to the liver where fluid may accumulate

mucosa the most inner layer of the bowel wall, or lining of the gastrointestinal tract, often appearing hyperechoic with sonography (first layer of bowel)

multicystic dysplastic kidney disease (MCDK) multiple cysts replace normal renal tissue throughout the kidney; usually causes renal obstruction; most common cause of renal cystic disease in the neonate; may have contralateral ureteral pelvic junction (UPJ) obstruction

multinodular goiter (MNG) nodular enlargement of the thyroid associated with hyperthyroidism

Murphy's sign positive sign implies exquisite tenderness over the area of the gallbladder upon palpation

muscle a type of tissue consisting of contractile cells or fibers that affects movement of an organ or part of the body

muscularis third layer of bowel

myelin a substance forming the sheath of Schwann cells

myelomeningocele defect in which the spinal cord and nerve roots are exposed, often adhering to the fine membrane that overlies them

myeloschisis cleft spinal cord resulting from failure of the neural tube to close

naked tuberosity sign the deltoid muscle is on the humeral head; seen with a full-thickness tear of the rotator cuff

nasal cannula device for delivering oxygen by way of two small tubes inserted into the nostrils

nasal catheter a piece of tubing longer than a cannula that is inserted through the nostril and into the back of the patient's mouth to provide continual oxygen

near field (Fresnel zone) the field closest to the transducer during the formation of the sound beam

neck of the pancreas small area of the pancreas between the head and the body

neonatal intensive care unit (NICU) Intensive care unit for newborns requiring specialized medical treatment. Includes a very diverse team from doctors and nurses, to social workers and respiratory therapists, etc. There are three levels of accreditation, with level three requiring the highest level of care for the tiniest of infants, often less than 30 weeks gestational age

neoplasm refers to any new growth (benign or malignant)

nephroblastomatosis lesion often found in the cortex or along the columns of Bertin; may replace parenchyma and appear focal, multifocal, or diffuse, appearing hypoechoic

nephron functional unit of the kidney; includes a renal corpuscle and a renal tubule

neuroblastoma malignant, often adrenal, tumor that is seen in pediatric patients; hemorrhagic tumor principally consisting of cells resembling neuroblasts

neuroectodermal tissue early embryonic tissue that will eventually develop into the brain and spinal cord

nodular hyperplasia degenerative nodules within the thyroid

noise Internally generated electronic noise appears if Doppler gain is set too high

non-alcoholic steatohepatitis the most extreme form of NAFLD, causing histologic damage to the liver. Signs of hypertension and cirrhosis may be among the first manifestations

non-Hodgkin's lymphoma   a malignant disease of lymphoid tissue

nonresistive   vessels that have high diastolic component and supply organs that need constant perfusion (i.e., internal carotid artery, hepatic artery, and renal arteries)

non-toxic (simple) goiter or nodule   occurs as a compensatory enlargement of the thyroid gland resulting from thyroid hormone deficiency

nosocomial infections   a hospital-acquired infection

Nyquist limit   The maximum frequency shift that can be measured in PW Doppler without aliasing

obstructive disease   refers to bile excretion blocked within the liver or biliary system

omentum   a double fold of peritoneum attached to the stomach and connecting it with certain of the abdominal viscera

Organ Procurement and Transplantation Network (OPTN)   organ allocation process

Ortolani maneuver   patient lies in the supine position; the examiner's hand is placed around the hip to be examined with the fingers over the femoral head; the hip is flexed 90 degrees and the thigh is abducted

ostomy   surgical procedure in which an opening is made to allow the passage of urine from the bladder or intestinal contents from the bowel to a surgically created opening, or stoma, in the wall of the abdomen

oximetry   noninvasive method of monitoring blood oxygen levels

Paget's disease   surface erosion of the nipple that results from direct invasion of the skin of the nipple from underlying breast cancer

pampiniform plexus   plexus of veins in the spermatic cord that drain into the right and left testicular veins; when a varicocele is present, dilation and tortuosity may develop

pancreatic ascites   occurs when the pancreatic pseudocyst ruptures into the abdomen; free-floating pancreatic enzymes are very dangerous to surrounding structures

pancreatic duct   travels horizontally through the pancreas to join the common bile duct at the ampulla of Vater

pancreatic lipomatosis   the fatty replacement of normal pancreatic tissue

pancreatic pseudocyst   "sterile abscess" collection of pancreatic enzymes that accumulated in the available space in the abdomen, usually near the pancreas

pancreatitis   inflammation of the pancreas

papillary carcinoma   a hormone that is secreted by the parathyroid glands which regulate serum calcium levels

paralytic ileus   dilated fluid-filled bowel loops without peristalsis

parathyroid hormone (PTH)   hormone that is secreted by the parathyroid glands, which regulate serum calcium levels

parathyroid hyperplasia   enlargement of multiple parathyroid glands

partial thromboplastin time (PTT)   laboratory test that can be used to evaluate the effects of heparin, aspirin, and antihistamines on the blood clotting process; PTT detects clotting abnormalities of the intrinsic and common pathways

patent urachus   the urachal remnant (or tube) extending from the superior bladder to the belly button does not properly close (fibrotic by birth), can be open on either ends or both ends; may be a source of infection

patient-focused care (PFC)   national movement to recapture the respect and goodwill of the American public and to ensure that every patient receives the best possible medical care

peau d'orange   descriptive terms for skin thickening of one breast that resembles an orange

pediatric end-stage liver disease (PELD)   for children under 12 years of age

pelvic girdle   formation of the hip bones by the ilium, ischium, and pubis

pelviectasis   (also called pyelectasis) dilation of the renal pelvis only; pelvicaliectasis or pyelocaliectasis would include dilation of the renal pelvis and calyces

pennate   featherlike pattern of muscle growth

perineurium   the surrounding connective tissue of muscle

period   time that it takes for one cycle to occur. Period decreases as frequency increases

peritoneal lavage   invasive procedure that is used to sample the intraperitoneal space for evidence of damage to viscera and blood vessels

peritonitis   inflammation of the peritoneum

periventricular leukomalacia (PVL)   echogenic white matter necrosis (WMN) best seen posterior to the brain or adjacent to the ventricular system

phagocytosis   process by which the red pulp destroys the degenerating red blood cells

Phalen's sign (Phalen's test, Phalen's maneuver, or Phalen's position)   an increase in wrist compression due to hyperflexion of the wrist for 60 seconds; this test is done with the patient holding the forearms upright and pressing the ventral side of the hands together

pheochromocytoma   benign adrenal tumor that secretes hormones that produce hypertension

phrenocolic ligament   ligament between the spleen and the colon

Phrygian cap   gallbladder variant in which part of the funduc is bent back on itself

piezoelectric effect   generation of electric signals as a result of an incident sound beam on a material that has piezoelectric properties

pitting   process by which the spleen removes nuclei from blood cells without destroying the erythrocytes

plantar flexion   pointing of the toes toward the plantar surface of the foot

pneumothorax   a collection of air or gas in the pleural cavity

polycystic renal disease   poorly functioning enlarged kidneys

polycythemia   excess of red blood cells

polycythemia vera   chronic, life-shortening condition of unknown cause involving bone marrow elements; characterized by an increase in red blood cell mass and hemoglobin concentration

polyp   small, well-defined soft tissue projection from the gallbladder wall; a small tumor-like growth that projects from a mucous membrane surface

polysplenia   condition in which there is more than one spleen

porcelain gallbladder   calcification of the gallbladder wall

porta hepatis   central area of the liver where the portal vein, common duct, and hepatic artery enter

portal vein   formed by the union of the superior mesenteric vein and splenic vein near the porta hepatis of the liver

portal venous hypertension   may result from intrinsic liver disease or obstruction of the portal veins, hepatic veins, inferior vena cava, or prolonged congestive heart failure

posterior (dorsal)   toward the back of the body or in back of another structure

posterior urethral valve (PUV)   the presence of a valve in the posterior urethra; occurs only in male fetuses; most common cause of bladder outlet syndrome

potter facies   distinct facial features in infants with severe oligohydramnios in utero, which causes deformation through restraint; shows prominent infraorbital folds, micrognathia, abnormal ear lobulation, and flattened nasal tip

power   rate of energy flow over the entire beam of sound; measured in watts (W) or milliwatts (mW)

prehypertension   blood pressure readings associated with prehypertension are 120 mm Hg to 139 mm Hg systolic pressure, and 80 mm Hg to 89 mm Hg diastolic pressure

primary hyperparathyroidism   oversecretion of parathyroid hormone, usually from a parathyroid adenoma

projectile vomiting   condition found in pyloric stenosis in the neonatal period; after drinking, the infant often experiences violent (across the room) vomiting secondary to obstruction

prone   lying face down

prostate specific antigen (PSA)   laboratory test that measures levels of the protein prostate specific antigen in the body; elevated levels could indicate prostate cancer

prothrombin time (PT)   laboratory test used to detect clotting abnormalities of the extrinsic pathway; measured against a control sample, PT tests the time it takes for a blood sample to coagulate after thromboplastin and calcium are added to it

protocol   standardization of specific anatomical structures that should be imaged in a complete or focused sonographic examination

proximal   closer to the point of origin or closer to the body

prune-belly syndrome   dilation of the fetal abdomen secondary to severe hydronephrosis and fetal ascites; fetus also has oligohydramnios and pulmonary hypoplasia

pseudoaneurysm   pulsatile hematoma that results from leakage of blood into soft tissues abutting the punctured artery with fibrous encapsulation and failure of the vessel wall to heal

pseudodissection   condition seen in a patient with aortic dissection; there is no intimal flap seen, only hypoechoic thrombus near the outer margin of the aorta with echogenic laminated clot

PTLF   Post-transplant lymphoproliferative disorder

pudendal artery   the internal and external pudendal arteries partially supply the scrotal wall and epididymis and occasionally the lower pole of the testis

pulmonary hypoplasia   small, underdeveloped lungs with resultant reduction in lung volume; secondary to prolonged oligohydramnios or as a consequence of a small thoracic cavity

pulse   a way to measure heart rate; recorded as beats per minute (bpm)

pulse duration   time interval required for generating the transmitted pulse; the pulse duration is calculated by multiplying the number of cycles in the pulse times the period

pulse pressure   the difference between the systolic and diastolic blood pressures

pulse repetition frequency (PRF)   the number of times the system is pulsed each second

pulsed wave (PW) Doppler   sound is transmitted and received intermittently with one transducer

pyelonephritis   an infection of the kidneys, often the result of infection spread from the bladder through the ureters

pyloric canal   canal located between the stomach and proximal duodenum; the pyloric sphincter muscle surrounds it

pyloromyotomy   Surgical procedure used in treating hypertrophic pyloric stenosis, in which the pyloric muscle is split longitudinally not to violate the mucosa. Pyloric muscle will appear abnormally large for up to 12 weeks post-op

pyocele   pus located between the visceral and parietal layers of the tunica vaginalis

pyogenic   producing pus

pyogenic abscess   pus-forming collection of fluid

pyramidal lobe   present in small percentage of patients; extends superiorly from the isthmus pyramidal lobe

pyramids   convey urine to the minor calyces

range ambiguity   the misplacement of an interface when the assumption that each echo is derived from the most recent pulse is violated

real-time   ultrasound instrumentation allows the image to be displayed multiple times per second to achieve a "real-time" image of movement

recurrent rami   terminal ends of the centripetal (intratesticular) arteries that curve backward toward the capsule

red pulp   consist of reticular cells and fibers (cords of Billroth); surrounds the splenic sinuses

reducible hernia   capable of being replaced in a normal position, and the visceral contents can be returned to normal intraabdominal location

refractile shadowing (edge artifact)   the bending of the sound beam at the edge of a circular structure, resulting in the absence of posterior echoes

refraction   change in the direction of propagation of a sound wave transmitted across an interface where the speed of sound varies

renal agenesis   interruption in the normal development of the kidney resulting in absence of the kidney; may be unilateral or bilateral

renal autotransplantation   The patient's own kidney is removed from the retroperitoneum and reimplanted into the iliac fossa

renal capsule   first layer adjacent to the kidney that forms a tough, fibrous covering

renal corpuscle   part of the nephron that consists of Bowman's capsule and the glomerulus

renal hilum   area in the midportion of the kidney where the renal vessels and ureter enter and exit

renal pelvis   area in the midportion of the kidney that collects urine before entering the ureter

renal sinus   central area of the kidney that includes the calyces, renal pelvis, renal vessels, fat, nerves, and lymphatics

renal vein thrombosis   obstruction of the renal vein resulting in an enlarged and edematous kidney

resistance   passive force in opposition to another active force; occurs when tissue exerts pressure against the flow

resistive   vessels that have little or reversed flow in diastole and supply organs that do not need a constant blood supply (i.e., external carotid artery and brachial arteries)

resolution   ability of the transducer to distinguish between two structures adjacent to one another

respiration   the process of inhaling and exhaling air

rete testis   network of the channels formed by the convergence of the straight seminiferous tubules in the mediastinum testis; these channels drain into the head of the epididymis

reticuloendothelial certain phagocytic cells found in the liver and spleen comprise the reticuloendothelial system; plays a role in the synthesis of blood proteins and hemopoiesis

retromammary layer deepest of the three layers of the breast

retroperitoneum space behind the peritoneal lining of the abdominal cavity

reverberation Multiple reflections can occur between the transducer and a strong reflector; multiple echoes may be sufficiently strong to be detected by the instrument and to cause confusion on the display (additional echoes that do not represent additional structures). This results in the display of additional reflectors that are not real

right gastric artery supplies the stomach

right hepatic artery supplies the gallbladder via the cystic artery

right hepatic vein supplies the right lobe of the liver; branches into anterior and posterior segments

right hypochondrium right upper quadrant of the abdomen that contains the liver and gallbladder

right renal artery arises from the lateral wall of the aorta, travels posterior to the inferior vena cava to enter the medial segment of the right kidney

right renal vein leaves the medal renal hilum to enter the lateral wall of the inferior vena cava

rock probe is slowly angled back and forth in one place to image the area completely or to follow the anatomical structure

rotate motion used to navigate between the ribs or to change from transverse to longitudinal planes

rugae inner folds of the stomach wall

saccular aneurysm localized dilation of the vessel

sagittal the sagittal plane is a lengthwise plane running from front to back. It divides the body or any of its parts into right and left sides, or two equal halves; this is known as the midsagittal plane

scan window areas in the body that allow the sound beam to penetrate without obstruction

scintigraphy a form of nuclear medicine diagnostic test of photographing the scintillations emitted by radioactive substances injected into the body to determine the outline and function of structures in which the radioactive substance collects or is secreted

scrotum sac containing the testes and epididymis

second generation agents agents containing heavy gases (i.e., Optison)

secondary hyperparathyroidism enlargement of parathyroid glands in patients with renal failure or vitamin D deficiency

secretin released from small bowel as antacid; stimulates secretion of bicarbonate

section thickness The beam width perpendicular to the scan plane results in section-thickness artifacts

sector array probe small face transducer that allows adequate intercostal visualization although the near field is reduced

seminal vesicles reservoirs for sperm located posterior to the bladder

sentinel node represents the first lymph node along the axillary node chain

sepsis the spread of an infection from its initial site of the bloodstream, initiating a systemic response that adversely affects blood flow to vital organs

septa testis multiple septa formed from the tunica albuginea that course toward the mediastinum testis and separate the testicle into lobules

septicemia the presence of pathogenic microorganisms in the blood

seroma accumulation of serous fluid within tissue

serosa fourth layer of bowel

serum amylase pancreatic enzyme that is elevated during pancreatitis

shadowing reduction in echo amplitude from reflectors that lie behind a strongly reflecting or attenuating structure

short bowel syndrome also called short gut syndrome, is a malabsorption disorder often resulting from the surgical removal of the small intestine

sickle cell anemia inherited disorder transmitted as an autosomal recessive trait that causes an abnormality of the globin genes in hemoglobin

sickle cell crisis condition in sickle cell anemia in which the sickled cells interfere with oxygen transport, obstruct capillary blood flow, and cause fever and severe pain in the joints and abdomen

slice thickness thickness of the section in the patient that contributes to echo signals on any one image

slide this motion is used when the probe is physically moved along the area of interest

sludge low-level echoes found along the posterior margin of the gallbladder

spatial pulse length the product of a number of cycles in the pulse and wavelength of the pulse

specific gravity lab tests that measure how much dissolved material is present in the urine

speckle interference pattern incident on a transducer produced by echoes that have undergone multipath scattering. The signal does not exhibit a one-to-one correspondence with the scatters

spectral analysis analysis of the entire frequency spectrum

spectral broadening "fill-in" of the spectral window that is proportional to the severity of the high flow patterns or increased gain

speed error propagation speed error occurs when the assumed value for propagation speed (1.54 mm/μs, leading to the 13 μs/cm round-trip travel-time rule) is incorrect

spermatic cord structure made up of vas deferens, testicular artery, cremasteric artery, and pampiniform plexus that suspends the testis in the scrotum

spherocytosis hereditary condition in which erythrocytes assume a spheroid shape

sphincter of Oddi small muscle that guards the ampulla of Vater

spiculation fingerlike extension of a malignant tumor

spina bifida aperta open (non-skin-covered) neural tube defects, such as myelomeningocele and meningocele

spina bifida occulta closed (skin-covered) neural tube defects, such as spinal lipoma and tethered cord

SPK simultaneous pancreas-kidney transplant

splaying widening

splenic agenesis complete absence of the spleen

splenic artery branch of the celiac axis; arises from the celiac trunk to supply the spleen

splenic flexure the transverse colon travels horizontally across the abdomen and bends at this point to form the descending colon

splenic hilum   site located in the middle of the spleen where the vessels and lymph nodes enter and exit

splenic vein   drains the spleen and travels horizontally across the abdomen, posterior to the pancreas, to join the superior mesenteric vein to form the portal vein; returns blood from the spleen and courses horizontally from the splenic hilum to join the superior mesenteric vein to form the portal vein

splenomegaly   enlargement of the spleen

standard precautions   the basic infection control guidelines used to reduce the risks of infection spread through the following three transmission modes: airborne infections, droplet infection, and contact infection

strangulated hernia   an incarcerated hernia with vascular compromise

strap muscles   group of three muscles (sternothyroid, sternohyoid, and omohyoid) that lie anterior to the thyroid

subacute (de Quervain's) thyroiditis   viral infection of the thyroid that causes inflammation

subcutaneous layer   most superficial of the three layers of the breast

subhepatic   below the liver

submucosa   second layer of bowel

subphrenic   below the spleen

sulcus   groove on the surface of the brain that separates the gyri

superior   above

superior mesenteric artery   arises inferior to the celiac axis to supply the proximal half of the colon and small intestine

superior mesenteric vein   drains the proximal half of the colon and small intestine and travels vertically, slightly anterior to the inferior vena cava, to join the splenic vein to form the portal vein

supine   lying face up

sweep   the probe remains in one area while using a large wrist motion with the probe perpendicular to the skin surface to *sweep* through the area of interest

synovial sheath   membrane surrounding a joint, tendon, or bursa that secretes a viscous fluid called synovia

tachycardia   heart rate more than 100 beats per minute

tadpole sign   seen as narrow bands of acoustic shadowing posterior to the margins of the cyst along the lateral borders of enhancement

tail of Spence   normal extension of breast tissue into the axillary or arm pit region

tail of the pancreas   tapered end of the pancreas that lies in the left hypochondrium near the hilus of the spleen and upper pole of the left kidney

target (donut) sign   characteristic of gastrointestinal wall thickening seen on cross-sectional imaging, consisting of an echogenic center and hypoechoic rim

temporal resolution   the ability of the system to accurately depict motion

tendinitis (tendinopathy, tendinosis, or tenosynovitis)   inflammation of a tendon

tendon   fibrous tissue connecting muscle to bone

tendonitis   inflammation of a tendon

tenosynovitis   inflammation of a tendon sheath

tentorium cerebelli   echogenic V-shaped "tent" structure in the posterior fossa that separates the cerebellum from the cerebrum

terminal ductal lobar units (TDLU)   smallest functional portion of the breast involving the terminal duct and its associated lobule containing at least one acinus

testicle   male gonad that produces hormones that induce masculine features and spermatozoa

testicular artery   artery arising from the aorta just distal to each renal artery; it divides into two major branches supplying the testis medially and laterally

testicular vein   the pampiniform plexus forms each testicular vein; the right testicular vein drains directly into the inferior vena cava, whereas the left testicular vein drains into the left renal vein

tethered spinal cord   fixed spinal cord that is positioned in an abnormal way

thalassemia   group of hereditary anemias occurring in Asian and Mediterranean populations

thoracentesis   surgical puncture of the chest wall for removal of fluids; usually done by using a large-bore needle

thoracic outlet syndrome   a complex symptom caused by conditions in which nerves or vessels are compressed in the neck or axilla

thyroglossal duct cysts   congenital anomalies that present in the midline of the neck anterior to the trachea

thyrotoxicosis   a toxic condition caused by hyperactivity of the thyroid gland

thyroxine   one of the main hormones secreted by the thyroid that increases the use of all food types for energy production and increases the rate of protein synthesis in most tissues

time gain compensation (TGC)   (*also known as depth gain compensation [DGC]*)   ability to compensate for attenuation of the transmitted beam as the sound wave travels through tissues in the body

Tinel's sign (Hoffmann-Tinel sign, Tinel's symptom, or Tinel-Hoffmann sign)   pins-and-needles type tingling felt distally to a percussion site

TIPS   transjugular intrahepatic portosystemic shunt

tissue-specific ultrasound contrast agent   type of contrast agent whose microbubbles are removed from the blood and are taken up by specific tissues in the body; one example is the agent Sonazoid

transducer   in ultrasound, a piezoelectric crystal converts an electrical stimulus into an ultrasound pulse and the returning echo into an electrical signal

transverse   The transverse plane is horizontal to the body

trigger finger   a state in which flexion or extension of a digit is arrested temporarily but is finally completed with a jerk

tunica adventitia   outer layer of the vascular system

tunica albuginea   inner fibrous membrane surrounding the testicle

tunica intima   inner layer of the vascular system

tunica media   middle layer of the vascular system; veins have thinner tunica media than arteries

tunica vaginalis   membrane consisting of a visceral layer (adherent to the testis) and a parietal layer (adherent to the scrotum) lining the inner wall of the scrotum; a potential space between these layers is where hydroceles may develop

ultrasound contrast agents (UCAs)   agents that can be administered intravenously to evaluate blood vessels, blood flow, and solid organs

Ultrasound First   American Institute of Ultrasound in Medicine's (AIUM) endeavor aimed at education and awareness of the effectiveness of ultrasound in improving patient care

umbilical vein catheter   used for vascular access in infants (more commonly premature neonates), which passes through the umbilicus, umbilical vein (which is still patent in neonates), left portal vein, ductus venosus, middle or left hepatic vein, and into the inferior vena cava

uncinate process   small, curved tip of the pancreatic head that lies posterior to the superior mesenteric vein

United Network for Organ Sharing (UNOS)   maintains a centralized computer networking system for all organ procurement organizations and transplant centers while seeking to be fair and effective in selecting transplant candidates

ureteropelvic junction (UPJ) obstruction   most common neonatal obstruction of the urinary tract, causing hydronephrosis; results from intrinsic narrowing or extrinsic vascular compression

ureters   retroperitoneal structures that exit the kidney to carry urine to the urinary bladder

urethra   small, membranous canal that excretes urine from the urinary bladder; tubular structure that extends from the bladder to the end of the penis

urinary bladder   muscular retroperitoneal organ that serves as a reservoir for urine

urinoma   a cyst containing urine

urolithiasis   stone within the urinary system

VACTERL   *v*ertebral abnormalities, *a*nal atresia, *c*ardiac abnormalities, *t*racheo*e*sophageal fistula, and *r*enal and *l*imb abnormalities; VATER excludes cardiac and limb anomalies

VACTERL (VATER)   *v*ertebral abnormalities, *a*nal atresia, cardiac abnormalities, *t*racheo*e*sophageal fistula, and *r*enal and *l*imb abnormalities; VATER excludes cardiac and limb anomalies

valvulae conniventes   normal segmentation of the small bowel

varicocele   dilated veins in the pampiniform plexus

vas deferens   tube that connects the epididymis to the seminal vesicle

vasa vasorum   tiny arteries and veins that supply the walls of blood vessels

vascular ultrasound contrast agents   a type of UCA whose microbubbles are contained in the body's vascular spaces; e.g., Optison, Definity, Imagent, Levovist, and SonoVue

vasovagal   concerning the action of stimuli from the vagus nerve on blood vessels

veins   collapsible vascular structures that carry blood back to the heart

velocity   the rate and direction at which sound propagates through a medium; the average velocity of sound in soft tissues is 1540m/sec

ventriculoperitoneal (VP) shunt   a tube that is placed by a neurosurgeon to relieve intracranial pressure due to increased cerebral spinal fluid (hydrocephalus); it extends from the ventricles in the brain to the lower abdominal (peritoneal) cavity

ventriculoperitoneal (VP) shunt   a tube that is placed by a neurosurgeon to relieve intracranial pressure due to increased cerebral spinal fluid (hydrocephalus); it extends from the ventricles in the brain to the lower abdominal (peritoneal) cavity

vertebral arch   part of the vertebral bones, which make up the vertebral opening or foramen

vertebral foramen   opening in the vertebral bones, through which the spinal cord runs

verumontanum   junction of the ejaculatory ducts with the urethra

vesicoureteral reflux (VUR)   abnormal reflux of urine from the bladder through the ureters, and, at times, back into the renal pelvis and calyces

villi   inner folds of the small intestine

vital signs   medical measurements used to ascertain how the body is functioning

volar   the anterior portion of the body when in the anatomical position

wall echo shadow (WES) sign   sonographic pattern found when the gallbladder is packed with stones

"wandering" spleen   spleen that has migrated from its normal location in the left upper quadrant

wave   propagation of energy that moves back and forth or vibrates at a steady rate

wavelength   length of space over which one cycle occurs. Wavelength decreases as frequency increases

white blood cells   cells that defend the body by destroying invading microorganisms and their toxins

white pulp   consists of lymphatic tissue and lymphatic follicles

Wilms' tumor (nephroblastoma)   most common malignant renal tumor in the neonate and infant; an embryonal tumor arising in the kidneys, which is often unilateral, though may be bilateral

Aehlert B: *Mosby's comprehensive pediatric emergency care,* St. Louis, 2007, Mosby
Figure 2-25, *A*

Becker J, Stucchi A: *Essentials of surgery,* Philadelphia, 2006, Elsevier
Figure 11-8

Chervenak FA and others: Fetal cystic hygroma: cause and natural history, *N Eng J Med* 309:822, 1985
Figure 59-39, *A*

Chikwe J: *Br J Cardio,* 2004, 11(1).
Figure 33-1

Damjanov I, Linder J: *Pathology: a color atlas,* St. Louis, 2000, Mosby
Figures 8-43, *B*; 9-24, *A*; 9-29; 9-33, *A*; 9-44; 9-51, *A*; 9-52, *C*; 9-53, *C*; 9-55; 9-57; 10-19; 10-28; 10-37; 10-51; 10-54; 12-22; 12-23; 12-27; 12-29; 12-31; 12-32, *A*; 12-34, *A*; 12-35; 12-36; 12-40, *B*; 11-21, *A*; 11-21, *C*; 19-16, *C*; 22-8; 22-14; 22-17; 22-18; 22-20; 22-24; 22-26; 22-30; 22-32; 25-12; 25-19, *A*; 25-22; 26-14; 26-19; 27-26; 27-35; 27-37; 44-21; 44-24; 44-29; 44-30; 44-31; 44-34

© Doctor Stock
Figure 10-14

Drake R, et al: Gray's Anatomy for Students, ed 3, Philadelphia, 2015, Churchill Livingstone. (adapted from)
Figure 30-4, 30-5, 30-10 *B*

Elsefteriades JA: Thoracic aortic aneurysm: clinically pertinent controversies and uncertainties: *J Am Coll Cardiol* 55:9, 841–857, 2010
Figure 8-32

England MA: *Color atlas of life before birth,* St. Louis, 1983, Mosby
Figure 49-14

Fliegauf M: When cilia go bad: cilia defects and ciliopathies, *Nature Reviews Molecular Cell Biology* 8, 880-893 (November 2007) Copyright © 2007, Rights Managed by Nature Publishing Group.
Figure 63-11

Goldman L: *Cecil medicine,* ed 23, Philadephia, 2009, Elsevier-Saunders
Figure 26-9

Haaga JR: *CT and MRI of the whole body,* ed 5, St. Louis, 2009, Mosby
Figure 16-3

Hadlock FP, Shah YP, Kanon DJ, Lindsey JV: Fetal crown-rump length: reevaluation of relation to menstrual age (5–18 weeks) with high resolution real time US, *Radiology* 182:501, 1992
Figures 49-26, 49-28

Herlihy B: *The human body in health and illness,* ed 4, St. Louis, 2011, Elsevier
Figure 28-3

Henningsen C: *Clinical guide to ultrasonography,* St. Louis, 2004, Mosby
Figures 15-52; 15-53; 21-29; 27-33; 27-38; 27-39; 25-13; 28-13, *B*; 28-13, *B*; 28-16; 28-18; 55-13; 55-20; 55-25, *A, B*; 55-28; 60-13; 60-32, *A, B*; 60-38, *A, B*; 60-45, *A, B*; 65-4, *A-C*; 65-8, *A, B*; 65-22, *A*

Kasel AM, et al: JACC. Cardiovascular imaging, February 2013, 6(2):249–262.
Figure 30-13*C*

Kisslo J, et al: Basic Doppler echocardiography, New York, 1986, Churchill Livingstone. (redrawn from)
Figure 31-3, 31-4, 31-5, 31-6, 31-10, 31-14, 31-15, 31-16, 31-17, 31-19, 31-21

Kremkau FW: *J Vasc Technol* 15:265–266, 1991. Reprinted with permission by the Society for Vascular Ultrasound (SVU)
Figure 7-27, *C*

Kremkau FW: *Principles and instrumentation.* In Merritt CRB, editor: *Doppler color imaging,* New York, 1992, Churchill Livingstone
Figure 7-31

Kremkau FW: *Principles and pitfalls of real-time color-flow imaging.* In Bernstein EF, editor: *Vascular diagnosis,* ed 4, St. Louis, 1993, Mosby
Figures 7-28, *A-C*; 7-29, *A-E*; 7-33

Kremkau FW: *Semin Roentgenol* 27:6–16, 1992
Figures 7-25; 7-27, *B*

Kremkau FW, Taylor KJW: *J Ultrasound Med* 5:227, 1986
Figure 7-6

Maternal Fetal Medicine Foundation, Washington, D. C.
Figure 49-30 (redrawn)

Mayden KL, et al: Cystic adenomatoid malformation in the fetus: Ultrasound evaluation, *Am J Obstet Gynecol* 148:349, 1984
Figure 61-8

Monin J, et al: Journal of the American College of Cardiology, July 2005, 46(2): 302–309.
Figure 33-2

Moses KP: *Atlas of clinical gross anatomy,* ed 2, Philadelphia, 2013, Elsevier
Figures 11-11, 28-1

Nyberg DA, Mahony BS, Pretorius DH, editors: *Diagnostic ultrasound of fetal anomalies: text and atlas,* St. Louis, 1990, Mosby
Figure 55-23

Oh JK: The Echo Manual, ed 3, 2006. Used with permission of Mayo Foundation for Medical Education and Research. All rights reserved.
Figure 34-22

Patton KT, Thibodeau GA: *Anatomy & physiology,* ed 8, St. Louis, 2013, Elsevier
Figures 8-15, 11-6, 22-28, 30-3*B*, 30-12, 30-13*B*, 34-1

Patton KT, Thibodeau GA: *The human body in health & disease,* ed 6, St. Louis, 2013, Elsevier
Figures 2-28, 4-1, 4-3, 13-4, 13-5

Potter PA, Perry AG, *Fundamentals of nursing,* ed 7, St. Louis, 2009, Mosby
Figures 2-3, *A*; 2-6, *A, B*; 2-9, *B*; 2-12, *A-C*; 2-13; 2-14; 2-18, *B*; 2-20, *A-E*

Roman MJ, Rosen SE, Kramer-Fox R, Deverereux RB: Prognostic significance of the pattern of aortic root dilation in the Marfan syndrome. *J Am Coll Cardiol* 1993; 22: 1470–1476.
Figure 33-33*A*

Rumack C, Wilson S, Charboneau W: *Diagnostic ultrasound,* ed 4, St. Louis, 2011, Mosby
Figures 21-30; 21-41, *A, B*; 21-43, *A, B*; 21-44, *A, B*; 26-4; 28-10 *A, B*; 28-11, *A*; 28-13, *A*; 28-14; 29-14; 29-11, *A-F*; 29-17, *D*; 29-19, *A-G*; 29-24; 43-20; 43-25; 44-9; 44-15; 44-20; 60-21; 64-18, *B*

Sharp JT, Bunnell IL, Holand JF, et al. Hemodynamics during induced cardiac tamponade in man. *Am J Med.* 1960; 25:640.
Figure 34-7

Taylor KJW, Holland S: *Radiology,* 174:297–307, 1990
Figure 7-23, *A-E*

Townsend CM: *Sabiston textbook of surgery,* ed 18, Philadelphia, 2008, Elsevier-Saunders
Figure 8-17, *8-35*

Van Hoorn JH: Pentalogy of Cantrell: two patients and a review to determine prognostic factors for optimal approach. *Eur J Pediatr.* 2008 Jan; 167(1): 29–35.
Figure 36-55*A*, 62-26

Waugh A, Grant A: *Ross and Wilson anatomy and physiology in health and illness,* ed 12, Edinburgh, 2014, Churchill Livingstone
Figure 11-3, *A*

Young AP: *Kinn's the administrative medical assistant: an applied learning approach,* ed 7, Philadelphia, 2011, Saunders
Figures 2-1; 2-2; 2-3, *B*; 2-5, *A*; 2-21; 2-22; 2-24

Zoghbi WA et al: *J Am Soc Echocardiog,* July 2003, 16 (7): 777–802.
Figure 33-18*C*